DIAGNOSTIC PATHOLOGY
LYMPH NODES AND SPLEEN
WITH EXTRANODAL LYMPHOMAS

AMIRSYS®

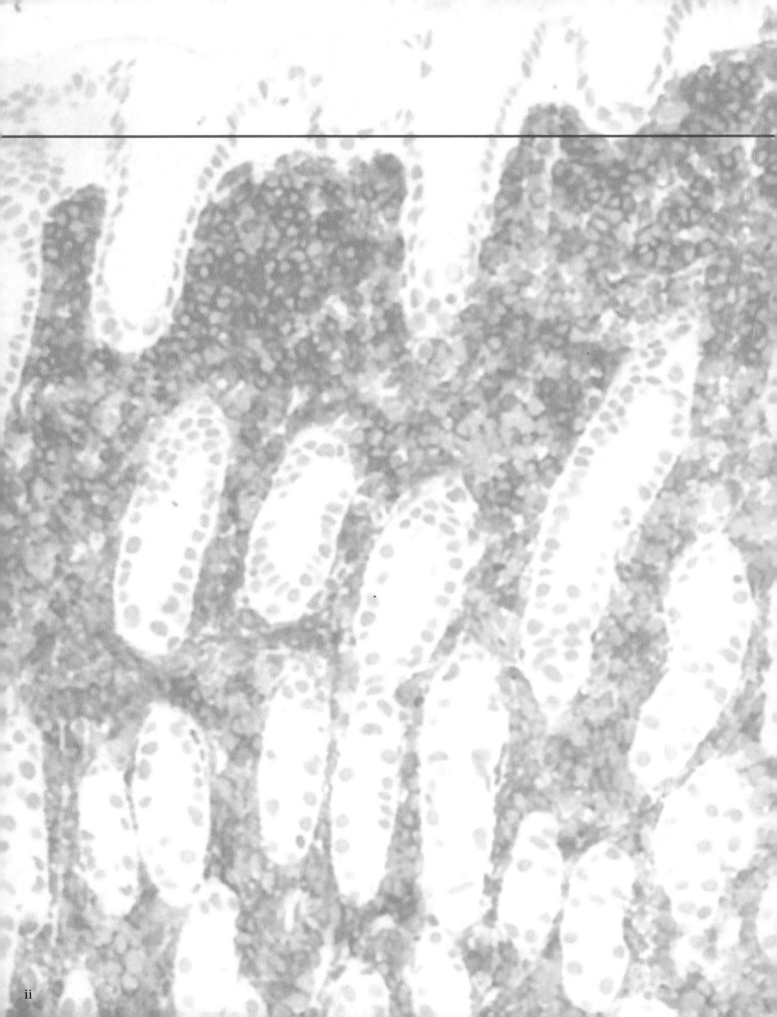
ii

DIAGNOSTIC PATHOLOGY
LYMPH NODES AND SPLEEN
WITH EXTRANODAL LYMPHOMAS

L. Jeffrey Medeiros, MD
Professor and Chair
Department of Hematopathology
The University of Texas M. D. Anderson Cancer Center
Houston, TX

Roberto N. Miranda, MD
Associate Professor
Department of Hematopathology
The University of Texas M. D. Anderson Cancer Center
Houston, TX

Sa A. Wang, MD
Assistant Professor
Department of Hematopathology
The University of Texas M. D. Anderson Cancer Center
Houston, TX

Francisco Vega, MD, PhD
Assistant Professor
Department of Hematopathology
The University of Texas M. D. Anderson Cancer Center
Houston, TX

Tariq Muzzafar, MBBS
Assistant Professor
Department of Hematopathology
The University of Texas M. D. Anderson Cancer Center
Houston, TX

C. Cameron Yin, MD, PhD
Assistant Professor
Department of Hematopathology
The University of Texas M. D. Anderson Cancer Center
Houston, TX

Carlos E. Bueso-Ramos, MD, PhD
Professor
Department of Hematopathology
The University of Texas M. D. Anderson Cancer Center
Houston, TX

Pei Lin, MD
Associate Professor
Department of Hematopathology
The University of Texas M. D. Anderson Cancer Center
Houston, TX

AMIRSYS®
Names you know. Content you trust.®

First Edition

Printed in Canada by Friesens, Altona, Manitoba, Canada

ISBN: 978-1-931884-52-5

Notice and Disclaimer

Library of Congress Cataloging-in-Publication Data

Diagnostic pathology. Lymph nodes and spleen with extranodal lymphomas / [edited by] L. Jeffrey Medeiros, MD, Professor and Chair, Department of Hematopathology, The University of Texas M. D. Anderson Cancer Center, Houston, TX.
    p. ; cm.
  Includes bibliographical references and index.
  ISBN 978-1-931884-52-5
  1. Lymphomas--Diagnosis--Handbooks, manuals, etc. 2. Lymph nodes--Diseases--Diagnosis--Handbooks, manuals, etc. 3. Spleen--Diseases--Pathogenesis--Handbooks, manuals, etc. 4. Lymphomas--Diagnosis--Atlases. 5. Lymph nodes--Diseases--Diagnosis--Atlases. 6. Spleen--Diseases--Pathogenesis--Atlases. I. Medeiros, L. Jeffrey, editor. II. Title: Lymph nodes and spleen with extranodal lymphomas.
  [DNLM: 1. Lymphatic Diseases--diagnosis--Atlases. 2. Lymph Nodes--pathology--Atlases. 3. Lymphoma--diagnosis--Atlases. 4. Spleen--pathology--Atlases. WH 17]
  RC280.L9D53 2011
  616.99'446--dc22
             2010051953

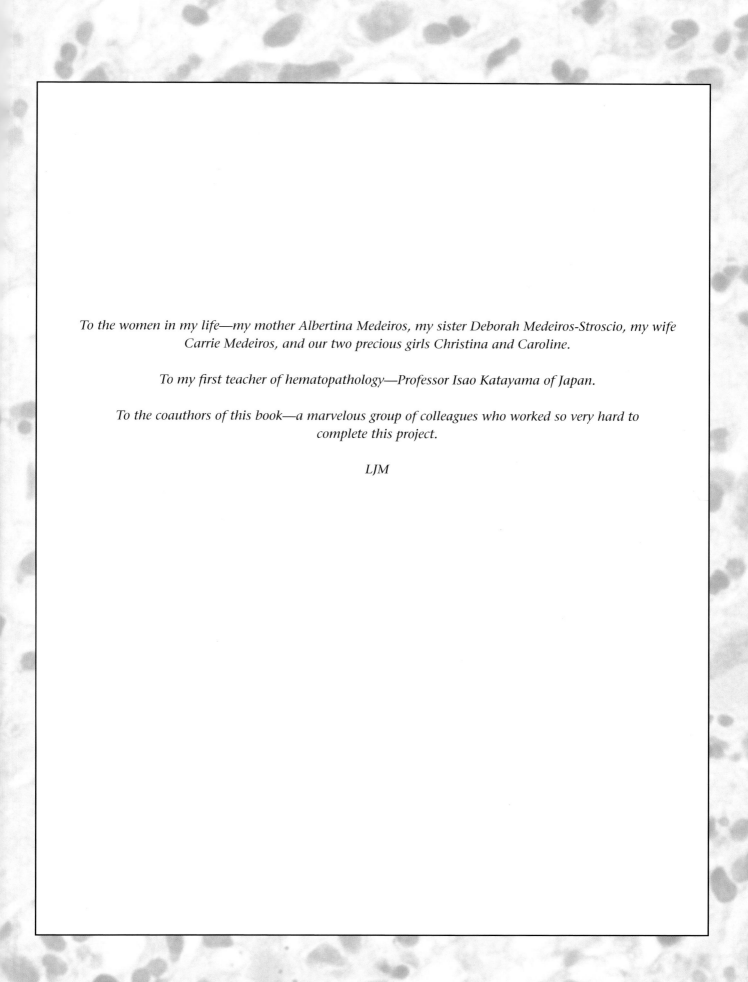

To the women in my life—my mother Albertina Medeiros, my sister Deborah Medeiros-Stroscio, my wife Carrie Medeiros, and our two precious girls Christina and Caroline.

To my first teacher of hematopathology—Professor Isao Katayama of Japan.

To the coauthors of this book—a marvelous group of colleagues who worked so very hard to complete this project.

LJM

CONTRIBUTING AUTHORS

Wesley O. Greaves, MD
Fellow
Department of Hematopathology
The University of Texas M. D. Anderson Cancer Center
Houston, TX

Faisal Alseraye, MD
Fellow
Department of Hematopathology
The University of Texas M. D. Anderson Cancer Center
Houston, TX

Sergej Konoplev, MD, PhD
Assistant Professor
Department of Hematopathology
The University of Texas M. D. Anderson Cancer Center
Houston, TX

Wei Liu, MD, PhD
Fellow
Department of Hematopathology
The University of Texas M. D. Anderson Cancer Center
Houston, TX

Keyur Patel, MD, PhD
Assistant Professor
Department of Hematopathology
The University of Texas M. D. Anderson Cancer Center
Houston, TX

James M. You, MD, PhD
Assistant Professor
Department of Hematopathology
The University of Texas M. D. Anderson Cancer Center
Houston, TX

DIAGNOSTIC PATHOLOGY
LYMPH NODES AND SPLEEN
WITH EXTRANODAL LYMPHOMAS

AMIRSYS®

Amirsys, creators of the highly acclaimed radiology series Diagnostic Imaging, proudly introduces its new Diagnostic Pathology series, designed as easy-to-use reference texts for the busy practicing surgical pathologist. Written by world-renowned experts, the series will consist of 15 titles in all the crucial diagnostic areas of surgical pathology.

The newest book in this series, *Diagnostic Pathology: Lymph Nodes and Spleen with Extranodal Lymphomas*, contains approximately 900 pages of comprehensive, yet concise, descriptions of more than 120 specific diagnoses. Amirsys's pioneering bulleted format distills pertinent information to the essentials. Each chapter has the same organization providing an easy-to-read reference for making rapid, efficient, and accurate diagnoses in a busy surgical pathology practice. A highlighted Key Facts box provides the essential features of each diagnosis. Detailed sections on Terminology, Etiology/Pathogenesis, Clinical Issues, Macroscopic and Microscopic Findings, and the all important Differential Diagnoses follow so you can find the information you need in the exact same place every time.

Most importantly, every diagnosis features numerous high-quality images, including gross pathology, H&E and immunohistochemical stains, correlative radiographic images, and richly colored graphics, all of which are fully annotated to maximize their illustrative potential.

We believe that this lavishly illustrated series, with its up-to-date information and practical focus, will become the core of your reference collection. Enjoy!

Elizabeth H. Hammond, MD
Executive Editor, Pathology
Amirsys, Inc.

Anne G. Osborn, MD
Chairman and Chief Executive Officer
Amirsys Publishing, Inc.

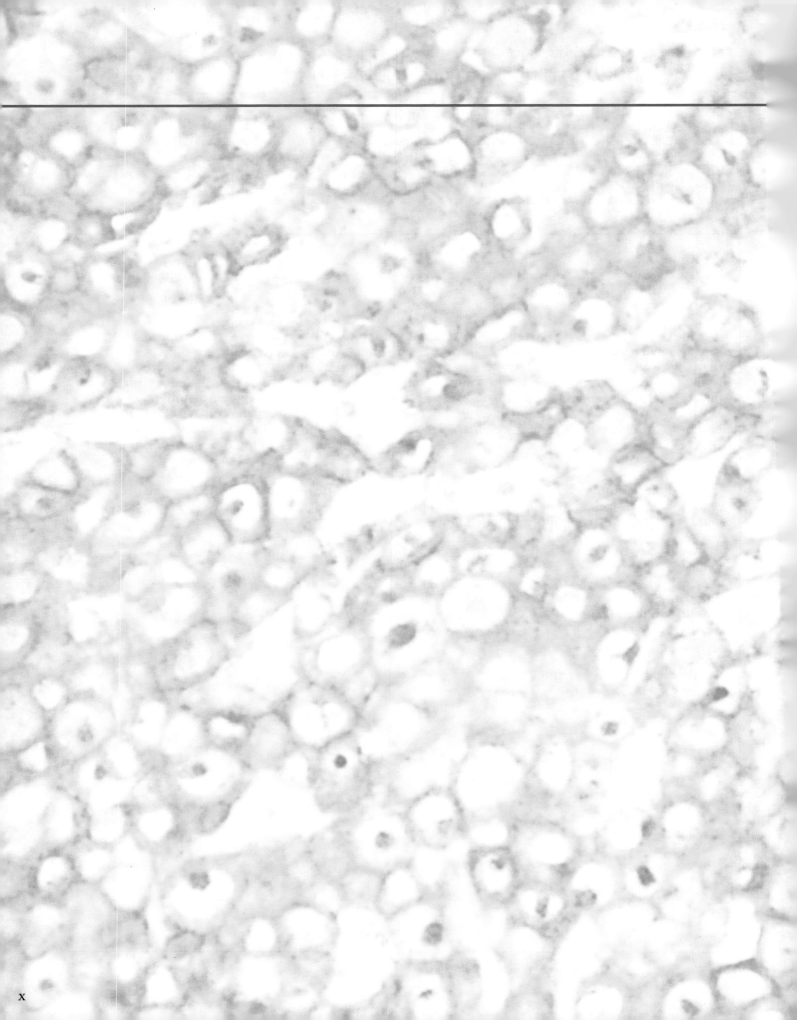

PREFACE

Most likely the reader has heard the lament, often said in jest, "All lymphomas look the same to me." Indeed, lymphomas involving lymph nodes, spleen, and other extranodal sites present many diagnostic difficulties to the practicing pathologist.

Distinguishing benign from malignant lesions can be a challenge in and of itself, requiring histologic and often immunophenotypic analysis, as well as molecular studies in a subset of cases. Once the benign nature of a lesion is established, an etiology needs to be suggested. If the lesion is malignant, both hematopoietic and non-hematopoietic tumors must be identified as such. Even after a lesion is recognized as hematopoietic, the possibilities are vast and include neoplasms of B, T, NK, myeloid, and histiocytic lineage. Complicating matters further is the continuous evolution of the concepts and terminology of the field and the large amounts of data being generated via high throughput technologies. How does one sort and apply this information? What is needed to sign out cases, and what is not?

With these questions in mind, the shared goal of the authors in writing this text was to create a quick, easy-to-use reference. The contents of this volume include benign and malignant lesions of lymph node and spleen as well as extranodal lymphomas. The lymphomas are designated, in large part, using the terminology of the 2008 World Health Organization.

As is the style of the Diagnostic Pathology series, clinical and histologic features, the results of relevant ancillary studies, and a differential diagnosis for each entity are provided in an easy-to-read bulleted format. A Key Facts section captures essential aspects of the entity. References are recent and selected for relevance, rather than encyclopedic coverage. Images have been used generously and illustrate the typical and common variant features of each entity. We also have included standard protocols for the examination and reporting of lymphomas. Finally, the Amirsys eBook Advantage™ license included with each printed copy of this book provides fully searchable text and a complete listing of antibodies.

The authors hope that the reader will find *Diagnostic Pathology: Lymph Nodes and Spleen with Extranodal Lymphomas* to be a useful resource.

L. Jeffrey Medeiros, MD
Professor and Chair
Department of Hematopathology
The University of Texas M. D. Anderson Cancer Center
Houston, TX

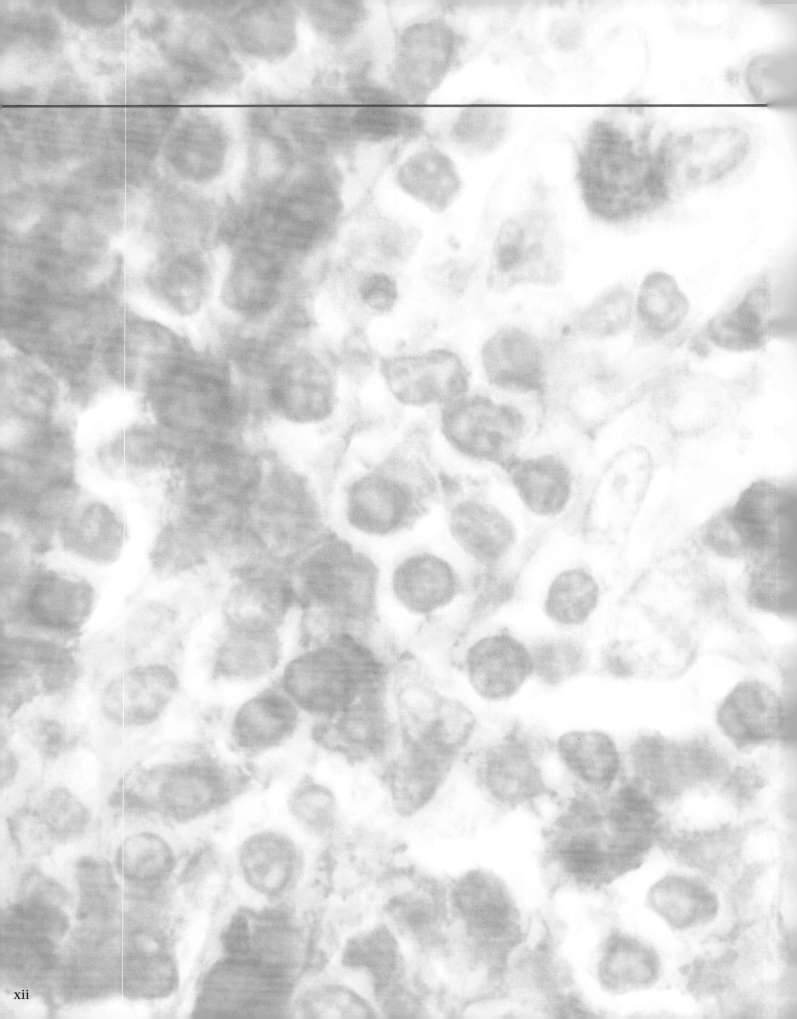

ACKNOWLEDGMENTS

Text Editing

Ashley R. Renlund, MA

Arthur G. Gelsinger, MA

Matthew R. Connelly, MA

Lorna Morring, MS

Alicia M. Moulton

Image Editing

Jeffrey J. Marmorstone

Lisa A. Magar

Medical Text Editing

Carolin J. Teman, MD, MS

Illustrations

Laura C. Sesto, MA

Lane R. Bennion, MS

Richard Coombs, MS

Art Direction and Design

Laura C. Sesto, MA

Assistant Editor

Dave L. Chance, MA

Publishing Lead

Kellie J. Heap

AMIRSYS®

Names you know. Content you trust.®

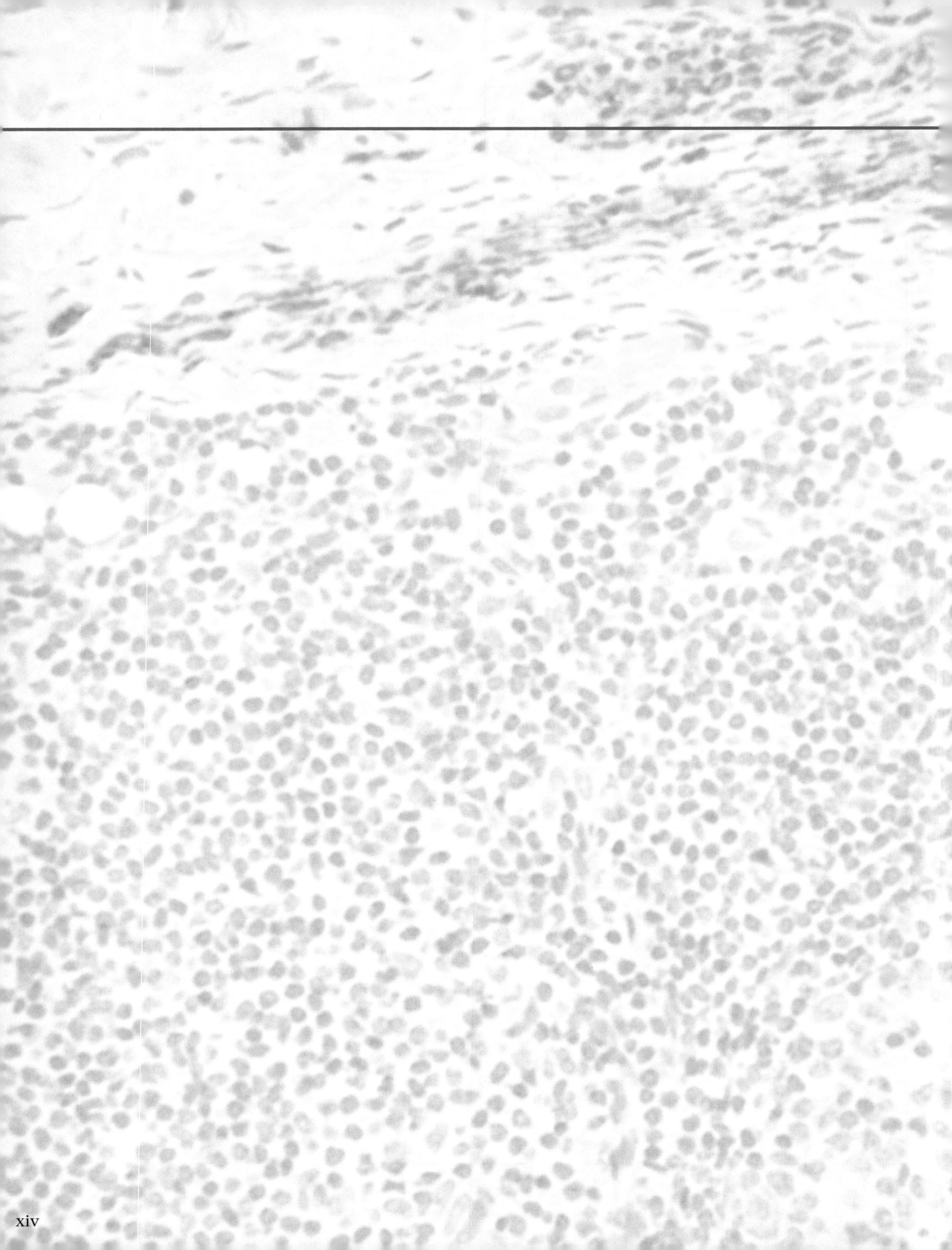

SECTIONS

Reactive Nonspecific Changes

Infectious Causes of Lymphadenitis

Reactive Lymphadenopathies

Hodgkin Lymphomas

Leukemia/Lymphoma of Immature B- or T-cell Lineage

Nodal B-cell Lymphomas

Extranodal B-cell Lymphomas

"Gray Zone" B-cell Lymphomas

Nodal T-cell Lymphomas

Extranodal T-/NK-cell Lymphomas

Immunodeficiency-associated Lymphoproliferations

Non-Hematopoietic Proliferations in Lymph Node

Granulocytic/Histiocytic Tumors

Spleen

Antibody Index

REACTIVE FOLLICULAR HYPERPLASIA

Microscopic and Immunohistochemical Features

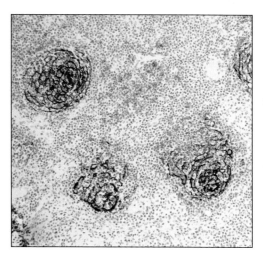

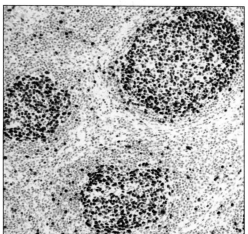

(Left) Immunohistochemical stain for CD23 highlights concentrically arranged follicular dendritic cell networks within hyperplastic follicles. Antibodies specific for CD21 & CD35 (& other markers) also highlight follicular dendritic cells. *(Right)* Immunohistochemical stain for Ki-67 shows high proliferative activity in reactive follicles. Often, reactive follicles are much more proliferative than the neoplastic follicles of follicular lymphoma, especially grades 1-2.

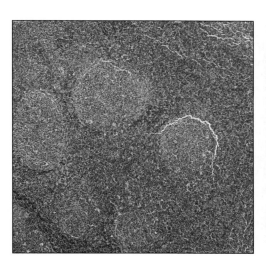

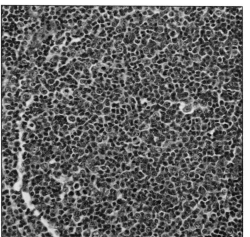

(Left) In this case of low-grade follicular lymphoma, 5 neoplastic follicles are present. Cracking artifact is seen and partially surrounds 2 follicles. The follicles in this field lack well-formed mantle zones, unlike reactive follicles. *(Right)* This case of follicular lymphoma at higher magnification shows a neoplastic follicle composed of a monotonous population of lymphocytes with rare histiocytes.

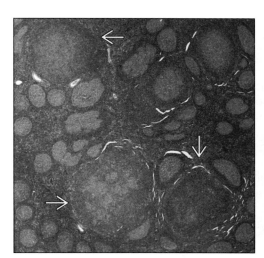

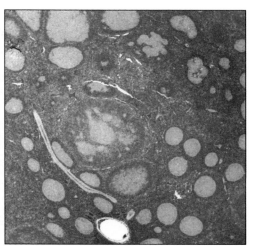

(Left) In this case of progressive transformation of germinal centers (PTGC), there are 3 progressively transformed follicles ➡. These transformed follicles are 3-4 times larger than hyperplastic follicles and are composed of reactive germinal centers infiltrated and disrupted by mantle zone lymphocytes. Many typical hyperplastic follicles are also present in this field. *(Right)* A progressively transformed germinal center is present in the center of this field.

REACTIVE PARACORTICAL HYPERPLASIA

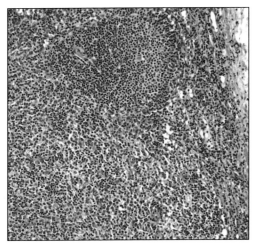

Lymph node with reactive parafollicular hyperplasia demonstrates that the paracortical (interfollicular) area is markedly expanded. A residual follicle is at the top of the field.

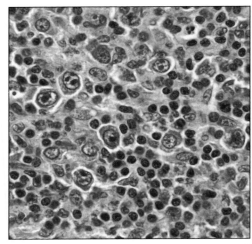

A hyperplastic paracortex with a heterogeneous cell population is shown. Note the large immunoblasts with prominent nucleoli admixed with small lymphocytes and histiocytes.

TERMINOLOGY

Abbreviations
• Reactive paracortical hyperplasia (RPH)

Synonyms
• Diffuse paracortical lymphoid hyperplasia
• Interfollicular hyperplasia, T-zone hyperplasia

Definitions
• RPH is benign reaction, predominantly within paracortical regions of lymph node; manifestation of T-cell immunological response
  ○ Also occurs in extranodal lymphoid tissues
  ○ Often occurs as part of mixed reactive hyperplasia pattern

ETIOLOGY/PATHOGENESIS

Environmental Exposure
• Variety of environmental pollutants and chemicals can cause paracortical hyperplasia
• Therapeutic agents (drugs) are an important cause
  ○ Phenytoin (Dilantin) and other antiseizure medications
• Vaccine administration
  ○ Vaccinia
  ○ Measles (live, attenuated)
  ○ Usually arises 1-3 weeks after vaccination

Infectious Agents
• Viral infection is common cause of RPH
  ○ Epstein-Barr virus (EBV)
  ○ Cytomegalovirus
  ○ Herpes simplex virus (type 1 or 2)
• Necrosis is usually present in viral infection

CLINICAL ISSUES

Presentation
• Patients present with enlarged lymph nodes, either localized or widespread
• Systemic symptoms can be present
  ○ Fever, fatigue, and weight loss
• Laboratory abnormalities may be present
  ○ Leukocytosis, lymphocytosis
• Clues to etiology derived from
  ○ Patient age, duration of symptoms, and site
  ○ Size and consistency of lymph node(s)

Treatment
• Localized lymph node enlargement in absence of other symptoms can be followed
  ○ If no resolution after 3-4 weeks, investigation is needed
• Generalized lymphadenopathy is cause for concern
  ○ Immediate investigation for etiology is usually pursued

Prognosis
• Self-limiting and reversible process with no impact on survival
  ○ Depends, in part, on underlying cause
• Can be associated with other diseases (e.g., autoimmune diseases, malignancy)

IMAGE FINDINGS

Radiographic Findings
• Lymphadenopathy, localized or generalized

MACROSCOPIC FEATURES

General Features
• Lymph nodes mildly to moderately enlarged

REACTIVE PARACORTICAL HYPERPLASIA

Key Facts

Terminology
- Predominantly T-cell response commonly seen in viral and drug-related lymphadenopathies

Clinical Issues
- Patients typically present with enlarged lymph nodes, either localized or widespread
- Systemic symptoms can be present
- Size, location, and consistency of lymph nodes, as well as age and duration, are important factors in identifying etiology

Microscopic Pathology
- Overall lymph node architecture is preserved
- Paracortical areas are markedly expanded by heterogeneous population of cells
  ○ Small lymphocytes, histiocytes, and immunoblasts

- Immunoblasts are large with prominent nucleoli
  ○ Can resemble Hodgkin or Reed-Sternberg cells
  ○ CD30(+), CD45(+), CD15(-)

Ancillary Tests
- Normal T-cell immunophenotype
- No evidence of monoclonal *IgH* or T-cell receptor gene rearrangements

Top Differential Diagnoses
- Dermatopathic lymphadenopathy
- Anaplastic large cell lymphoma
- Myeloid sarcoma
- Marginal zone B-cell lymphoma
- Hodgkin lymphoma
- T-cell/histiocyte-rich large B-cell lymphoma

○ No masses; lymph nodes usually not matted
- Tan-white, soft cut surface
- Focal necrosis may be discernible

MICROSCOPIC PATHOLOGY

Histologic Features
- Overall lymph node architecture is distorted but preserved
- Paracortical areas are markedly expanded by heterogeneous cell population
  ○ Immunoblasts in sea of small lymphocytes (mostly T cells) and histiocytes
  ○ Imparts a mottled or "moth-eaten" pattern at scanning magnification
- Immunoblasts are large with vesicular nuclei and central nucleoli
  ○ Nucleoli are basophilic, often with trapezoidal shape
  ○ Nucleoli often have thin attachments to nuclear membrane ("spider legs")
  ○ Can resemble Hodgkin or Reed-Sternberg (HRS) cells
  ○ Can form sheets in some cases (raising differential diagnosis of large cell lymphoma)
- Eosinophils can be prominent
  ○ Particularly in hypersensitivity causes (e.g., drug reactions)
- High endothelial venules often present
- Other lymph node components can be reactive (so-called mixed pattern)
  ○ Reactive follicles
  ○ Monocytoid B-cell hyperplasia in sinuses
  ○ Nodules of plasmacytoid dendritic cells

Predominant Pattern/Injury Type
- Lymphoid, interfollicular

Predominant Cell/Compartment Type
- Lymphadenopathy

ANCILLARY TESTS

Immunohistochemistry
- Small lymphocytes are usually immunophenotypically normal T cells
  ○ Positive for pan-T-cell antigens (CD3, CD5, CD7, CD43); CD4(+) and CD8(+) subsets
- Immunoblasts can be of either T-cell or B-cell lineage
  ○ CD30(+), CD45(+), CD15(-)
- Evidence of virus in EBV-associated cases
  ○ Positive for EBV-LMP

Flow Cytometry
- Numerous T cells with normal immunophenotype
- Fewer polytypic B cells

In Situ Hybridization
- Evidence of virus in virally induced cases

PCR
- No evidence of monoclonal *IgH* or T-cell receptor gene rearrangements

DIFFERENTIAL DIAGNOSIS

Dermatopathic Lymphadenopathy
- Paracortical distribution
- Marked increase of interdigitating dendritic cells
  ○ S100 protein(+)
- Few or more numerous Langerhans cells
  ○ CD1a(+)

Viral Causes of RPH
- Histologic findings are similar to RPH, not otherwise specified
- Foci of necrosis are common
- Viral inclusions
- Common viruses: EBV, cytomegalovirus, herpes simplex

REACTIVE PARACORTICAL HYPERPLASIA

Drug Reactions
- May manifest as RPH or mixed pattern of RPH and follicular hyperplasia
- Eosinophils often present
- May arise suddenly, raising clinical concern for lymphoma
- Lymphadenopathy often resolves after drug is discontinued

Reaction to Vaccine Administration
- Regional lymph nodes 1-3 weeks after vaccination
- Histologic findings show typical RPH ± follicular hyperplasia

Kikuchi-Fujimoto Lymphadenitis
- Paracortical pattern similar to RPH
- Proliferative phase with many monocytes
- Necrotic and xanthomatous phases
  - No neutrophils

Anaplastic Large Cell Lymphoma
- Replacement of architecture in most cases
- Neoplastic cells often exhibit sinusoidal distribution and cytological atypia
  - Hallmark cells
- Aberrant loss of pan-T-cell antigens
- Usually cytotoxic immunophenotype (e.g., granzyme B, TIA-1) and ALK-1(+/-)
- Monoclonal *TCR* gene rearrangement

Peripheral T-cell Lymphoma, NOS
- Replacement of lymph node architecture
- Cytologically atypical lymphoid cells ± eosinophils or plasma cells
- Aberrant loss of pan-T-cell antigens
- Monoclonal *TCR* gene rearrangement

Myeloid Sarcoma
- Replacement of lymph node architecture
- Eosinophilic myelocytes in subset (~50%)
- Positive for myeloid-associated antigens: lysozyme, myeloperoxidase, CD43, and CD117
  - Subsets of cases express CD34 and TdT (immature) or CD15 (mature)
- Negative for pan-T-cell markers

Nodal Marginal Zone B-cell Lymphoma
- Marginal zone pattern can mimic paracortical distribution
- Neoplastic cells are slightly larger; often monocytoid cytoplasm
- Often associated with prominent, reactive follicles
- Positive for pan-B markers; monotypic Ig(+)
- Monoclonal *Ig* gene rearrangements

Nodular Lymphocyte Predominant Hodgkin Lymphoma
- Numerous small lymphocytes and histiocytes similar to RPH
- Replacement of lymph node architecture by vague nodules
- Large neoplastic LP (L&H or "popcorn") cells

- Small lymphocytes are mixture of B cells and T cells

Classical Hodgkin Lymphoma
- Can have paracortical pattern similar to RPH
- Lymph node architecture usually replaced
- Large neoplastic HRS cells
  - CD15(+), CD30(+), pax-5 (dim+), CD45/LCA(-)

T-cell/Histiocyte-rich Large B-cell Lymphoma
- Replacement of lymph node architecture
- Scattered, large, neoplastic cells in sea of reactive lymphocytes and histiocytes
- Large neoplastic cells of B-cell lineage
- Monoclonal *Ig* gene rearrangements

Diffuse Large B-cell Lymphoma, NOS
- Sheets of large cells that replace lymph node architecture
- Monotypic surface Ig
- Monoclonal *Ig* gene rearrangements

DIAGNOSTIC CHECKLIST

Pathologic Interpretation Pearls
- Overall preservation of architecture
- Paracortical pattern
- "Moth-eaten" appearance at scanning magnification
- Large cells are immunoblasts
- Eosinophils suggest hypersensitivity (e.g., drug reaction)
- Ancillary test results do not support lymphoma

SELECTED REFERENCES
1. Pilichowska ME et al: Histiocytic necrotizing lymphadenitis (Kikuchi-Fujimoto disease): lesional cells exhibit an immature dendritic cell phenotype. Am J Clin Pathol. 131(2):174-82, 2009
2. Medeiros LJ et al: Reactive lymphoid hyperplasia. In: Loachim's Lymph Node Pathology. Philadelphia: Lippincott Williams & Wilkins. 172-80, 2008
3. Kojima M et al: Clinical implication of dermatopathic lymphadenopathy among Japanese: a report of 19 cases. Int J Surg Pathol. 12(2):127-32, 2004
4. Kojima M et al: Autoimmune disease-associated lymphadenopathy with histological appearance of T-zone dysplasia with hyperplastic follicles. A clinicopathological analysis of nine cases. Pathol Res Pract. 197(4):237-44, 2001
5. Ohshima K et al: Clinicopathological study of severe chronic active Epstein-Barr virus infection that developed in association with lymphoproliferative disorder and/or hemophagocytic syndrome. Pathol Int. 48(12):934-43, 1998
6. Abbondazo SL et al: Dilantin-associated lymphadenopathy. Spectrum of histopathologic patterns. Am J Surg Pathol. 19(6):675-86, 1995
7. Dorfman RF et al: Lymphadenopathy simulating the malignant lymphomas. Hum Pathol. 5(5):519-50, 1974
8. Hartsock RJ: Postvaccinial lymphadenitis. Hyperplasia of lymphoid tissue that simulates malignant lymphomas. Cancer. 21(4):632-49, 1968

Microscopic Features and Differential Diagnosis

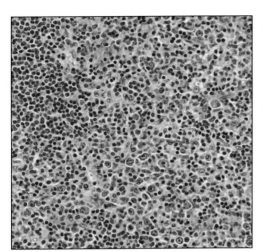

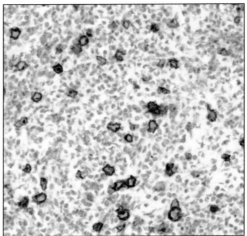

(Left) Lymph node involved by reactive paracortical hyperplasia. The paracortical areas are expanded by a heterogeneous cell population. These histological findings suggest a cell-mediated or T-cell immunologic response but are otherwise nonspecific regarding etiology. (Right) Immunohistochemical stain for CD30 in a lymph node with reactive paracortical hyperplasia. The immunoblasts express CD30 in a membranous and Golgi pattern.

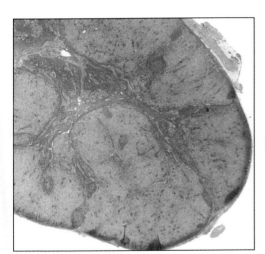

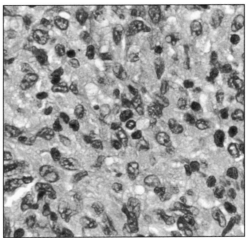

(Left) Lymph node involved by dermatopathic lymphadenopathy. The paracortical areas are markedly expanded by numerous interdigitating dendritic cells. (Right) In dermatopathic lymphadenopathy, the paracortex is expanded by numerous interdigitating dendritic cells with folded nuclei and abundant eosinophilic cytoplasm. Small lymphocytes (T cells) are also present.

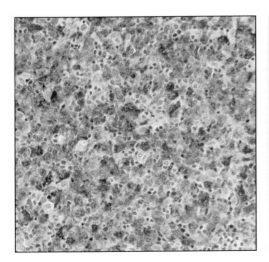

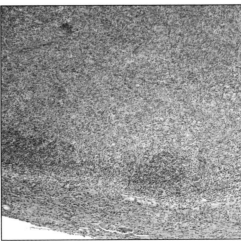

(Left) Immunohistochemical stain for S100 protein highlights numerous interdigitating dendritic cells (and fewer Langerhans cells) in this case of dermatopathic lymphadenopathy. Small lymphocytes are negative. (Right) Lymph node involved by reactive paracortical hyperplasia, here caused by herpes simplex virus (HSV) infection. In this case, HSV was shown by in situ hybridization.

REACTIVE PARACORTICAL HYPERPLASIA

Differential Diagnosis

(Left) Lymph node showing reactive paracortical hyperplasia caused by HSV infection. This field shows a small focus of "punched out" necrosis commonly seen in lymph nodes infected by HSV. Viral inclusions were not seen in this field, but HSV was shown by in situ hybridization. *(Right)* In situ hybridization analysis for herpes simplex virus in a case of reactive paracortical hyperplasia. These positive (brown) nuclei were located in a focus of necrosis.

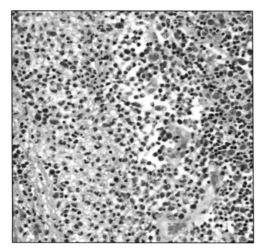
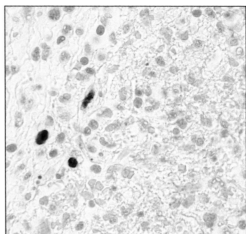

(Left) Lymph node with drug-related reactive paracortical hyperplasia with a minor component of follicular hyperplasia. The architecture of this small lymph node is greatly distorted, and the process extends outside the lymph node borders. *(Right)* Lymph node with drug-related reactive paracortical hyperplasia. Note the heterogeneous cell population including small and large lymphocytes and many eosinophils.

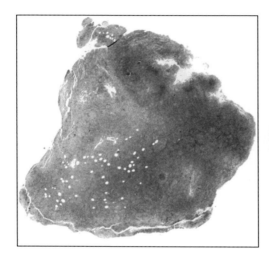
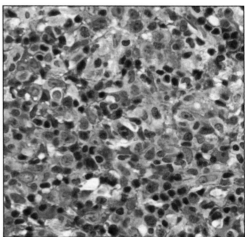

(Left) Immunohistochemical stain for CD3 of a lymph node with drug-related reactive paracortical hyperplasia shows that most of the cells in the paracortical areas are T cells. *(Right)* Immunohistochemical stain for CD20 of a lymph node with drug-related reactive paracortical hyperplasia shows relatively few B cells in the paracortical areas. Most B cells are within reactive lymphoid follicles.

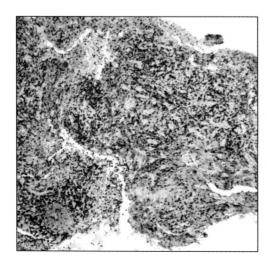
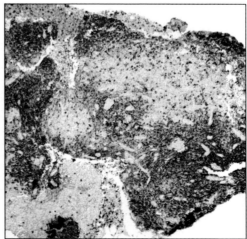

REACTIVE PARACORTICAL HYPERPLASIA

Differential Diagnosis

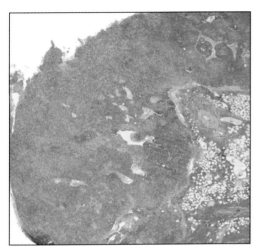
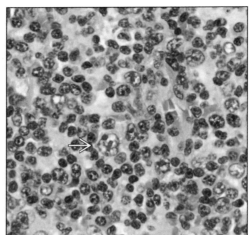

(Left) Low-power view shows a lymph node involved by marked reactive paracortical hyperplasia in a patient with infectious mononucleosis. Note the patent sinuses indicating that the architecture is not completely replaced. *(Right)* Lymph node with reactive paracortical hyperplasia in a patient with infectious mononucleosis. In the paracortex, immunoblasts ➡ are admixed with small lymphocytes.

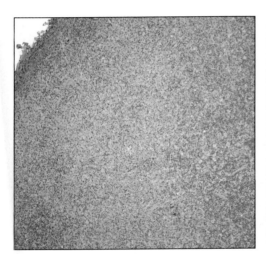
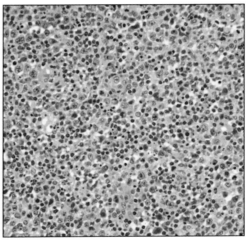

(Left) Lymph node involved by Kikuchi-Fujimoto lymphadenitis during the proliferative phase. The paracortex is expanded by numerous histiocytes. *(Right)* Lymph node involved by Kikuchi-Fujimoto lymphadenitis during the proliferative phase. Note the numerous histiocytes with folded nuclei and abundant cytoplasm in the paracortex. The histiocytes are admixed with small lymphocytes, immunoblasts, apoptotic bodies, and debris.

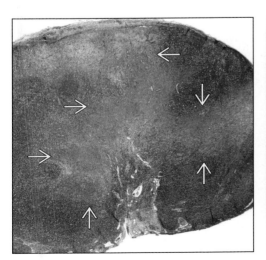
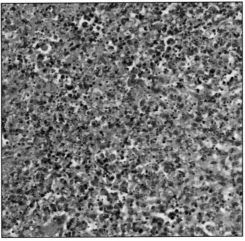

(Left) Lymph node involved by Kikuchi-Fujimoto lymphadenitis during the necrotizing phase. The paracortex is expanded by necrosis ➡ outlined by numerous apoptotic cells and debris. *(Right)* Lymph node involved by Kikuchi-Fujimoto lymphadenitis during the necrotizing phase. The paracortical areas are replaced by numerous necrotic cells, apoptotic bodies, and debris. Note that no neutrophils are present.

REACTIVE PARACORTICAL HYPERPLASIA

Differential Diagnosis

(Left) Lymph node involved by anaplastic large cell lymphoma (ALCL). The architecture is subtotally effaced by the proliferation of large, anaplastic cells. A residual follicle ➡ is also present. *(Right)* Lymph node involved by ALCL. The neoplasm is composed of large cells. Note the so-called hallmark cells ➡ with a horseshoe-shaped nucleus and eosinophilic cytoplasm. There are many in this field.

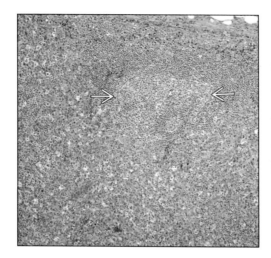
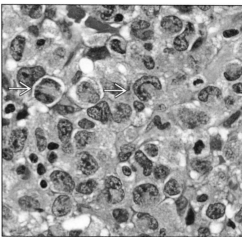

(Left) Immunohistochemical stain for CD30 in a case of anaplastic large cell lymphoma. The neoplastic cells are strongly and uniformly positive for CD30, as is typically observed in ALCL cases. *(Right)* Immunohistochemical stain for ALK-1 in a case of anaplastic large cell lymphoma. The neoplastic cells are strongly positive for ALK-1 in a nuclear and cytoplasmic pattern consistent with t(2;5)(p23;q35).

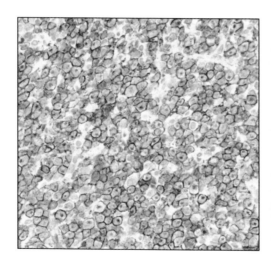
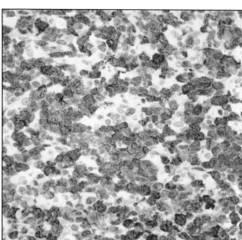

(Left) Lymph node involved by nodular lymphocyte predominant Hodgkin lymphoma (NLPHL). The architecture is replaced by vague nodules. *(Right)* High-power view of a lymph node involved by NLPHL. Scattered large, neoplastic LP cells are admixed with numerous small lymphocytes and histiocytes.

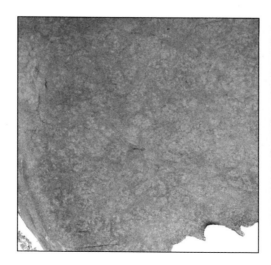
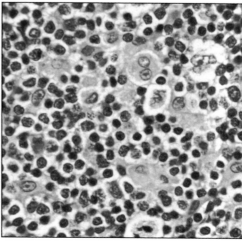

REACTIVE PARACORTICAL HYPERPLASIA

Differential Diagnosis

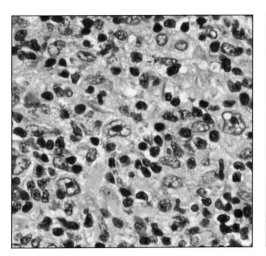
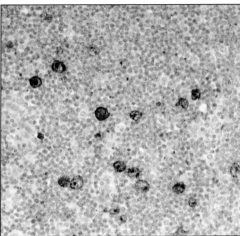

(Left) Lymph node involved by nodular sclerosis Hodgkin lymphoma (NSHL). Scattered HRS cells (mononuclear variants) are seen in a background of small lymphocytes, histiocytes, and eosinophils. (Right) Immunohistochemical stain in NSHL shows that the HRS cells are positive for CD30; they are typically CD15(+) and CD45(-). By contrast, immunoblasts in reactive paracortical hyperplasia are CD30(+), CD15(-), and CD45(+).

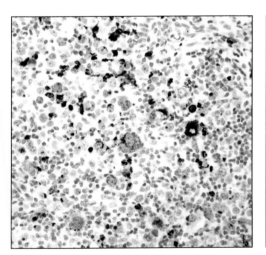
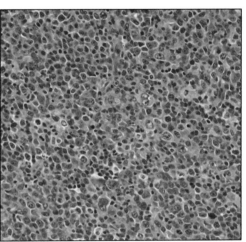

(Left) Immunohistochemical stain for CD15 in a case of NSHL. The HRS cells are positive for CD15. By contrast, immunoblasts in reactive paracortical hyperplasia are CD15(-). (Right) Lymph node involved by diffuse large B-cell lymphoma. The lymph node architecture is replaced by sheets of large neoplastic cells with irregular vesicular nuclei, prominent nucleoli, and a scant to moderate amount of cytoplasm.

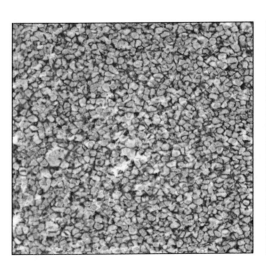
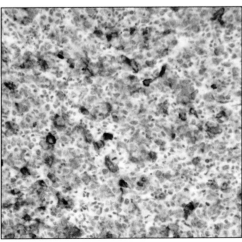

(Left) Immunohistochemical stain for CD20 in a case of diffuse large B-cell lymphoma. The neoplastic cells are strongly and uniformly positive for CD20. (Right) Immunohistochemical stain for CD30 in a case of diffuse large B-cell lymphoma. The neoplastic cells are variably positive for CD30 in a cytoplasmic and membranous pattern.

Infectious Causes of Lymphadenitis

CHRONIC GRANULOMATOUS LYMPHADENITIS

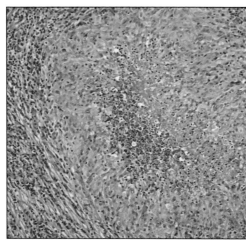

Paraffin section shows necrotizing chronic granulomatous lymphadenitis. The granulomas are composed of central necrosis surrounded by epithelioid histiocytes and inflammatory cells.

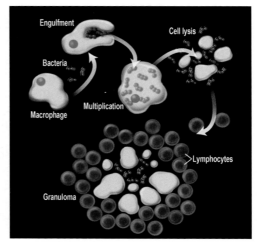

Chronic granulomatous inflammation is formed by a stepwise series of events as listed in this image.

TERMINOLOGY

Abbreviations
- Chronic granulomatous lymphadenitis (CGL)

Synonyms
- Chronic granulomatous inflammation of lymph node

Definitions
- Granulomatous inflammation is a specific type of inflammatory response
  - Characterized by accumulation of modified macrophages (epithelioid cells)
  - Initiated by infectious or noninfectious agents
  - Requires poorly digestible irritants and T-cell mediated immunity directed at irritant
- Chronic granulomatous lymphadenitis is characterized by
  - Accumulation of activated macrophages and inflammatory cells forming granulomas within lymph node
    - Results from deposition of indigestible antigenic material within tissue
  - Often associated with necrosis or acute inflammation

ETIOLOGY/PATHOGENESIS

Infectious Agents
- CGL is usually caused by wide variety of infectious agents including
  - Mycobacteria, bacteria, viruses, fungi, and parasites
    - Chlamydia, spirochetes
- Infectious CGL can be classified into 3 subgroups based on its etiology
  - Infections caused by well-recognized organisms
    - *Mycobacterium tuberculosis* is most common

  - Infections caused by organisms identified by molecular methods but not readily isolated by conventional microbiological methods
  - Infectious etiology is strongly suspected, but causal organisms have not yet been identified
- Advances in molecular diagnostic technology have allowed identification of more organisms
  - Previously, cause of these infections was unknown

Other Causes
- There are a large number of other causes of CGL
  - Foreign bodies or other irritants/antigens
  - Autoimmune diseases/mechanisms
    - e.g., sarcoidosis
    - Granulomas can occur in patients with lymphoma
    - Granulomas also can occur in lymph nodes draining nonhematopoietic neoplasms

Pathogenesis
- CGL is result of complex interplay of events
  - Presence of invading agent (e.g., bacteria) in tissue results in recruitment of monocytes-macrophages from circulation
  - Monocytes-macrophages engulf bacteria
    - Bacteria multiply within macrophages
  - Macrophages process bacteria and present them to activated T-helper cells
  - Release of cytokines and chemokines by activated macrophages and T-helper cells; causes cell lysis
  - Macrophages mature into epithelioid cells or fuse to form multinucleated giant cells
  - Granulomas form when bacteria and debris are surrounded by macrophages and inflammatory cells

CLINICAL ISSUES

Epidemiology
- Age
  - CGL can occur in any age group

CHRONIC GRANULOMATOUS LYMPHADENITIS

Key Facts

Terminology
- Granulomatous inflammation is specific type of inflammatory response
  - Characterized by accumulation of modified macrophages (epithelioid cells)
  - Initiated by infectious or noninfectious agents
  - Requires poorly digestible irritants and T-cell mediated immunity directed at irritant
- Chronic granulomatous lymphadenitis (CGL) is characterized by
  - Accumulation of activated macrophages and inflammatory cells forming granulomas within lymph node
  - Often associated with necrosis or acute inflammation

Etiology/Pathogenesis
- Infections are most common cause of CGL
- Autoimmune diseases (e.g., sarcoidosis)
- Foreign bodies (e.g., talc, suture, lipid)

Clinical Issues
- Cervical lymph nodes most commonly involved

Microscopic Pathology
- CGL may be classified as caseating or noncaseating
  - *M. tuberculosis* is most common cause of caseating granulomas

Ancillary Tests
- PCR allows identification of infectious agents in cases that were previously regarded as unknown etiology

---

- Gender
  - No apparent gender predilection

Site
- Lymph node group involved depends in part on
  - Initiating agent
  - 1st route of entry into body
- Cervical lymph nodes are most common
- Any lymph node or lymph node group can be affected

Presentation
- Lymphadenopathy, localized or general
- May be accompanied by systemic symptoms

Laboratory Tests
- Microbiologic culture and identification by biochemical methods
- Serologic tests are helpful in
  - Identifying infectious agents
  - Determining timing of exposure to organism
- Polymerase chain reaction (PCR) methods detect infectious agents with high sensitivity
  - Infectious agents have been identified in diseases that were previously of unknown etiology

Treatment
- Empiric antibiotics
- Antituberculous therapy
- Surgical manipulation

Prognosis
- Depends on specific etiology and therapy administered
- Benign clinical course with good prognosis

IMAGE FINDINGS

General Features
- Well-defined lymph nodes
  - Increased in number &/or size
- CT scans are 1st-line imaging tool to evaluate lymphadenopathy

- Standard x-rays and CT scans show consolidation
  - With or without central necrosis

MACROSCOPIC FEATURES

General Features
- Cut surface can appear nodular (if macrogranulomas)
- Yellow areas can be seen corresponding to necrotic foci

MICROSCOPIC PATHOLOGY

Histologic Features
- CGL may be classified as immune or foreign body type
- Immune type
  - Caused by insoluble particles (e.g., bacteria) that elicit cell-mediated immune response
  - Can further divide these into caseating and noncaseating granulomas
  - Caseating granulomas
    - Composed of central areas of coagulative necrosis
    - Peripheral concentric layers of epithelioid cells, Langhans giant cells, lymphocytes, and fibroblasts
    - Organisms may be identified by using special stains
    - *M. tuberculosis* is most common cause of caseating granulomas
  - Noncaseating granulomas
    - Composed of collection of epithelioid cells, Langhans giant cells, lymphocytes, and histiocytes
  - Eosinophils can occur in granulomas caused by parasites
  - Acute inflammatory cells common in granulomas caused by fungi
- Foreign body type
  - Caused by inert substances such as talc, suture, lipid
  - Granulomas composed of epithelioid cells, Langhans giant cells, lymphocytes, and histiocytes surround foreign body
    - No caseation occurs usually

CHRONIC GRANULOMATOUS LYMPHADENITIS

- o Can often detect foreign body by using polarized light

Cytologic Features
- Epithelioid histiocytes and inflammatory cells can be identified in fine needle aspiration smears
- In some cases, granulomas can be recognized
- Special stains can be performed on smears

ANCILLARY TESTS

Immunohistochemistry
- Mycobacterial antigens can be detected and typed with monoclonal antibodies conjugated to peroxidase

PCR
- Highly sensitive and has identified infectious agents in diseases that previously had no known etiology

Special Stains
- Acid-fast bacilli can be demonstrated by Ziehl-Neelsen, Kinyoun, or Fite-Faraco stain
- Fungal-like organisms can be highlighted with periodic acid-Schiff (PAS) or Grocott methenamine silver stain
- Gram-positive and Gram-negative organisms can be seen with Gram stain
- Parasites can be highlighted by Giemsa stain

DIFFERENTIAL DIAGNOSIS

Mycobacterium tuberculosis Lymphadenitis
- Decreasing incidence in developed nations
  - o Except resurgence has occurred in HIV(+) patients
- Common in underdeveloped countries and immigrants to developed countries
- Common lymph node groups: Cervical, supraclavicular
- Abnormal chest radiograph common
- Positive tuberculin test
- Histologic findings
  - o Caseating granulomas
  - o Acid-fast bacilli often found within caseating necrosis
  - o Special stains for acid-fast bacilli insensitive
- Cultures for *M. tuberculosis* are reliable but slow
  - o Organism grows slowly over weeks
- PCR is rapid and reliable alternative method for diagnosis

Atypical Mycobacterial Lymphadenitis
- There are a number of nontuberculous or atypical mycobacteria
  - o Most common include
    - *M. marinum, M. fortuitum, M. kansasii*
    - *M. scrofulaceum, M. avium-intracellulare*
- *M. marinum* has been associated with swimming pool use
- *M. kansasii* causes infection of cervical lymph nodes in children
  - o Also displays increased prevalence in patients with hairy cell leukemia

- *M. scrofulaceum* known for causing cervical lymphadenitis in children
  - o a.k.a. scrofula
- *M. avium-intracellulare* is common in HIV(+) patients
  - o Granulomatous inflammation is infrequent
  - o Caseating necrosis is unusual
- Most atypical mycobacterial infections cause granulomatous inflammation
  - o Lesions tend to be more suppurative (than *M. tuberculosis*)
  - o Caseating necrosis may be less or absent (than *M. tuberculosis*)

Fungal Lymphadenitis
- Number of fungi can infect lymph nodes and cause granulomatous lymphadenitis
  - o Common organisms include
    - *Histoplasma capsulatum, Blastomyces dermatitidis, Paracoccidioides brasiliensis*
    - *Coccidioides immitis, Sporothrix schenckii, Cryptococcus neoformans*
    - *Aspergillus, Mucor,* and *Candida* in immunodeficient patients
  - o Histoplasmosis is most common
    - Endemic in central United States
    - Dimorphic fungus with narrow-based budding yeasts at body temperature
  - o Histologic findings
    - Granulomas often associated with acute inflammation
    - Yeast forms are intracellular within histiocytes and multinucleated giant cells
    - GMS stain highlights organisms
    - Caseation often not prominent

Sarcoidosis
- More common in African-Americans than whites or Asians
- Multisystemic disease of unknown etiology
- Hypercalcemia, hypergammaglobulinemia, and elevated angiotensin-converting enzyme common
- Kveim test positive
- Commonly involves lymph nodes and lungs, but any site can be affected
- Histologic findings
  - o Nonnecrotizing/noncaseating granulomas
  - o Typically nonsuppurative

Whipple Disease
- Fever, polyarthritis, diarrhea, weight loss, and lymphadenopathy
- Loose aggregates of histiocytes or sarcoid-like granulomas
  - o Most often involve GI tract and abdominal lymph nodes
- Caused by infection by *Tropheryma whippelii*
  - o Rod-shaped bacilli, PAS(+)
  - o Organism can be identified by electron microscopy or PCR

CHRONIC GRANULOMATOUS LYMPHADENITIS

Subgroups of Chronic Granulomatous Lymphadenitis Based on Etiology

Subgroups	Organisms	Diseases
Group 1	Mycobacteria	Tuberculosis, leprosy
	Chlamydia	Lymphogranuloma venereum
	Spirochetes	Syphilis
	Fungi	Histoplasma lymphadenitis, candidiasis, aspergillosis
	Other bacteria	Brucellosis, actinomycosis
	Parasites	Toxoplasmosis, leishmaniasis
Group 2	*Bartonella henselae, Tropheryma whippelii*	Cat scratch lymphadenopathy, Whipple disease
Group 3	Unknown	Sarcoidosis, Crohn disease

Group 1 = well-recognized organisms; Group 2 = organisms difficult to recognize morphologically but detected by molecular methods.

Nonmycobacterial Infections of Lymph Nodes

- Number of bacterial infections can cause granulomatous lymphadenitis
- Examples of organisms include
  - *Bartonella henselae*, a gram-negative bacillus that causes cat scratch disease
    - Granulomas occur in late phases of infection
    - Often associated with suppuration
  - *Chlamydia* serotypes L1, L2, and L3 cause lymphogranuloma venereum
    - Typically involve inguinal lymph nodes
    - Granulomas occur in late phases of infection
    - Often associated with suppuration
  - *Brucella abortis*, *B. melitensis*, or *B. suis*
    - Related to consumption of unpasteurized milk or cheese
    - Lymph nodes show granulomatous inflammation often associated with suppuration
  - *Francisella tularensis*
    - History of handling rabbits
    - Lymphadenopathy can be prominent
    - Lymph nodes show granulomatous inflammation often associated with suppuration
  - Syphilis
    - Chronic granulomatous inflammation is uncommon but can occur
    - Granulomas are typically noncaseating
    - Spirochetes identifiable by Warthin-Starry silver stain
    - Antitreponemal antibodies detected by serology tests
  - Leprosy
    - Lymph nodes typically show accumulation of large histiocytes ("lepra" cells)
    - No well-formed granulomas
  - *Yersinia pseudotuberculosis* or *Y. enterocolitica*
    - Cause mesenteric lymphadenitis
    - Symptoms can simulate appendicitis
    - Granulomatous inflammation often associated with suppuration

Crohn Disease

- Multisystem involvement, particularly gastrointestinal tract
- Etiology unknown; bacterial infection is suspected
- Transmural inflammation consisting of inflammatory cells with lymphoid aggregates and noncaseating granulomas
  - Peri-intestinal lymph nodes can be involved by granulomas

Foreign Body Granulomas

- Number of foreign bodies can cause chronic granulomatous lymphadenitis
  - Lipid: Causes lipogranulomas
  - Talc: Presents as result of previous surgical procedure
  - Various minerals (e.g., beryllium): Can cause chronic granulomatous inflammation in lungs

DIAGNOSTIC CHECKLIST

Clinically Relevant Pathologic Features

- Chronic granulomatous lymphadenitis has large number of causes
- Microbiologic cultures are essential to work-up of lymph node biopsy
- PCR is a valuable alternative to cultures
  - Very sensitive
  - PCR has identified organisms in diseases that previously were of unknown etiology

SELECTED REFERENCES

1. Ahmed NY et al: A histopathological study of chronic granulomatous lymphadenitis. Saudi Med J. 28(10):1609-11, 2007
2. Darnal HK et al: The profile of lymphadenopathy in adults and children. Med J Malaysia. 60(5):590-8, 2005
3. Moore SW et al: Diagnostic aspects of cervical lymphadenopathy in children in the developing world: a study of 1,877 surgical specimens. Pediatr Surg Int. 19(4):240-4, 2003
4. Kardon DE et al: A clinicopathologic series of 22 cases of tonsillar granulomas. Laryngoscope. 110(3 Pt 1):476-81, 2000
5. Suskind DL et al: Nontuberculous mycobacterial cervical adenitis. Clin Pediatr (Phila). 36(7):403-9, 1997
6. Zumla A et al: Granulomatous infections: etiology and classification. Clin Infect Dis. 23(1):146-58, 1996

CHRONIC GRANULOMATOUS LYMPHADENITIS

Microscopic Features

(Left) Low-power view of a lymph node involved by chronic granulomatous lymphadenitis. Numerous granulomas with abundant central necrosis surrounded by epithelioid histiocytes and inflammatory cells are present. The specific etiology for this case could not be determined. *(Right)* High-power view shows a lymph node involved by chronic granulomatous lymphadenitis. The granuloma in this field is composed of central necrosis surrounded by epithelioid histiocytes and inflammatory cells.

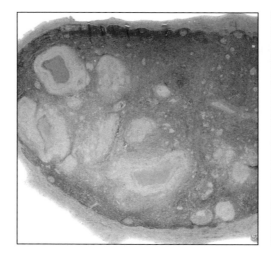
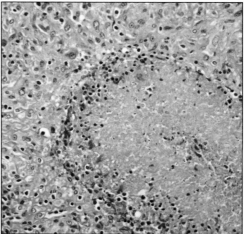

(Left) Paraffin section shows chronic granulomatous lymphadenitis as a result of infection by Coccidioides immitis. This field shows numerous eosinophils, occasional multinucleated giant cells ➡, and reactive follicles. *(Right)* Paraffin section of chronic granulomatous lymphadenitis as a result of infection by Coccidioides immitis. This field illustrates a granuloma with central necrosis. Numerous eosinophils surround the granuloma.

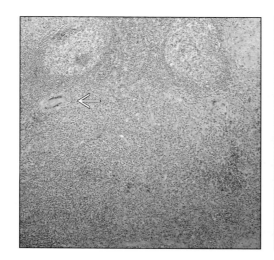
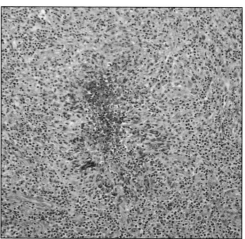

(Left) Paraffin section shows chronic granulomatous lymphadenitis as a result of infection by Coccidioides immitis. The granuloma is composed of numerous epithelioid histiocytes, multinucleated giant cells, and focal central necrosis. *(Right)* Paraffin section of a lymph node involved by chronic granulomatous lymphadenitis as a result of infection by Coccidioides immitis. A cyst form ➡ is present within the cytoplasm of a multinucleated giant cell.

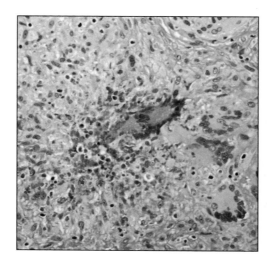
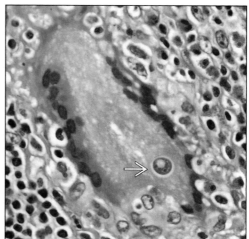

CHRONIC GRANULOMATOUS LYMPHADENITIS

Microscopic Features

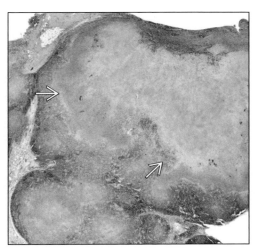 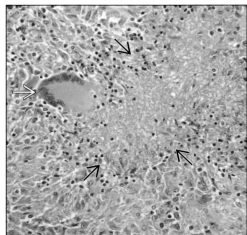

(Left) Chronic granulomatous lymphadenitis as a result of Mycobacterium tuberculosis infection. Note the extensive necrosis ➡, known as caseating necrosis, because its gross appearance resembles cheese. *(Right)* Chronic granulomatous lymphadenitis as a result of Mycobacterium tuberculosis infection. Numerous epithelioid histiocytes, a Langhans-type multinucleated giant cell ➡, and central necrosis ➡ are present.

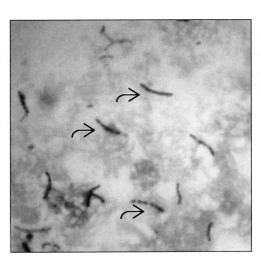 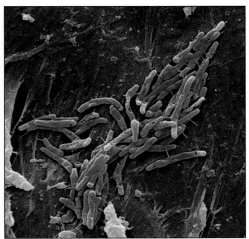

(Left) This photomicrograph reveals Mycobacterium tuberculosis bacteria ➡ using acid-fast Ziehl-Neelsen stain. (Courtesy G. Kubica, CDC Public Health Image Library, #5789.) *(Right)* This scanning electron micrograph shows some of the ultrastructural morphologic details exhibited by rod-shaped Mycobacterium fortuitum bacteria. (Courtesy M. Williams and J. Carr, CDC Public Health Image Library, #11033.)

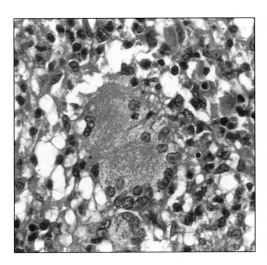 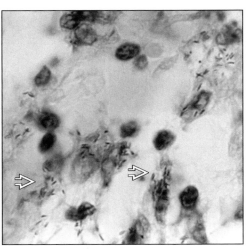

(Left) This field shows a granuloma in the skin in a patient with mycobacterial infection. (Courtesy R. Feldman, CDC Public Health Image Library, #11230.) *(Right)* This light micrograph shows clumps of mycobacteria ➡ highlighted by an acid-fast stain in a patient with a mycobacterial skin infection. (Courtesy R. Feldman, CDC Public Health Image Library, #112327.)

CHRONIC GRANULOMATOUS LYMPHADENITIS

Microscopic Features

(Left) Paraffin section shows chronic granulomatous lymphadenitis as a result of infection by Histoplasma capsulatum. The granuloma ⮞ in this field is composed of epithelioid histiocytes without necrosis and with multinucleated giant cells in the largest granuloma. *(Right)* Gomori methenamine silver stain of a lymph node involved by chronic granulomatous lymphadenitis as a result of infection by Histoplasma capsulatum. The fungal yeast forms are blue-black.

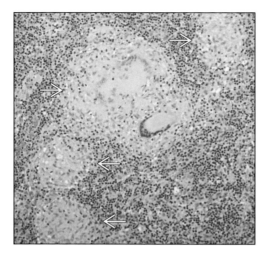
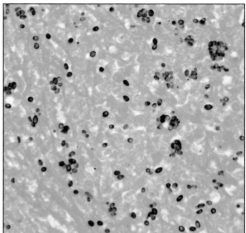

(Left) This micrograph shows chronic granulomatous inflammation associated with histoplasmosis of the lung. *(Courtesy M. Hicklin, CDC Public Health Image Library, #3141.)* *(Right)* Axial contrast-enhanced CT shows bilateral reactive lymphadenopathy ⮞, with the largest node in the right jugulodigastric ⮞, in a child with recent history of cat bite to the tongue.

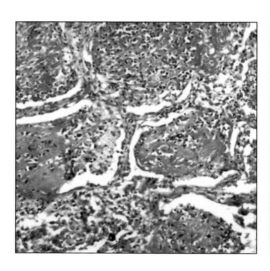
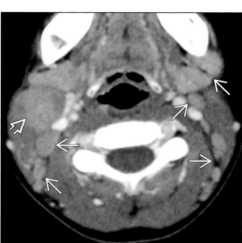

(Left) Paraffin section of a lymph node from a patient with cat scratch lymphadenitis shows granuloma with central acute microabscess, necrosis, and neutrophils. *(Right)* Warthin-Starry stain of a lymph node from a patient with cat scratch lymphadenitis shows clumps of pleomorphic bacilli ⮞ consistent with Bartonella henselae.

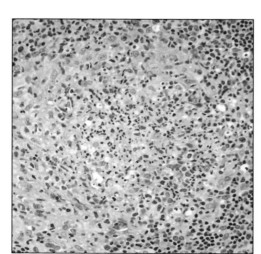
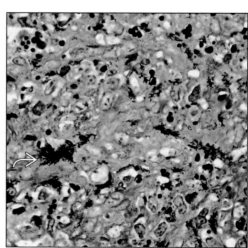

CHRONIC GRANULOMATOUS LYMPHADENITIS

Microscopic Features

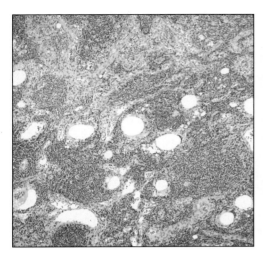
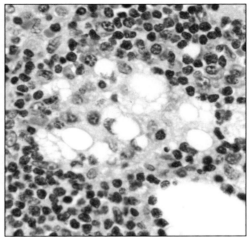

(Left) Paraffin section shows an abdominal lymph node involved by many lipogranulomas. Lipogranulomas are common in abdominal lymph nodes in adult patients. The lipid acts as a foreign body that elicits chronic granulomatous inflammation. (Right) Paraffin section of an abdominal lymph node involved by many lipogranulomas shows that the granuloma is composed of lipid droplets, histiocytes, and lymphocytes.

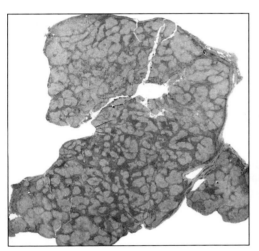
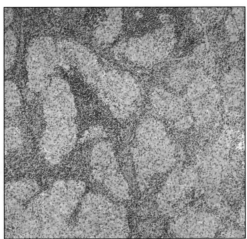

(Left) Paraffin section shows a lymph node involved by sarcoidosis. Note the numerous granulomas that almost completely replace the lymph node parenchyma. (Right) Paraffin section of a lymph node involved by sarcoidosis reveals numerous granulomas that lack evidence of necrosis, a feature useful for distinguishing sarcoidosis from infectious chronic granulomatous inflammation.

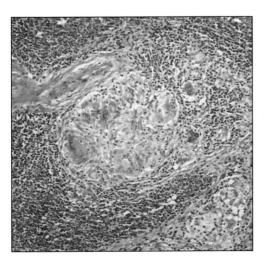
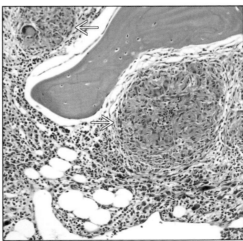

(Left) Paraffin section of spleen shows a sarcoid-like granuloma in a patient with classical Hodgkin lymphoma. There is no evidence of lymphoma in this field. (Right) Paraffin section of bone marrow shows 2 sarcoid-like granulomas ➡ in a patient with plasma cell myeloma.

SUPPURATIVE LYMPHADENITIS

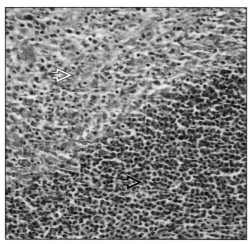

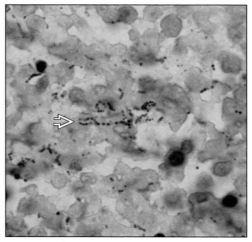

A lymph node obtained from a patient with suppurative lymphadenitis. The lymph node in this field is entirely replaced by granulocytes (pus) ⊇ and surrounded by histiocytes and lymphocytes ⊇.

Gram stain of a smear from a lymph node obtained from a patient with suppurative lymphadenitis. Numerous Gram-positive bacteria are present ⊇.

TERMINOLOGY

Synonyms
- Acute lymphadenitis
- Pyogenic lymphadenitis

Definitions
- Acute lymphadenitis usually caused by bacterial, fungal, or some viral infections

ETIOLOGY/PATHOGENESIS

Infectious Agents
- Common bacteria: *Staphylococcus* and *Streptococcus*
- Nontuberculous mycobacteria
- Variety of fungi
- Can also occur after bacillus Calmette-Guérin (BCG) vaccination

CLINICAL ISSUES

Epidemiology
- Incidence
  - Suppurative lymphadenitis is uncommon in developed countries
    - Due to availability of antibiotic treatment
- Age
  - More common in children
- Gender
  - No gender predilection
- Ethnicity
  - Seen in all ethnic groups

Site
- Regional lymph nodes draining pyogenic inflammation
  - Dental abscess, upper respiratory infection, appendicitis, or infected wound
  - More commonly in superficial nodes, particularly axillary and inguinal nodes

Presentation
- Lymph node(s) variably enlarged
- Soft and tender
- Overlying skin is red and edematous
- Rarely, abscess or sinus formation
- Fever, fatigue

Treatment
- Observation
- Antibiotics
- Surgical drainage

Prognosis
- Self-limiting

MICROSCOPIC PATHOLOGY

Histologic Features
- Preserved lymph node architecture
- Dilated sinuses
  - Weakly eosinophilic proteinaceous fluid
  - Numerous neutrophils and macrophages (sinus catarrh)
- Congested blood vessels
- Neutrophils infiltrate lymph node parenchyma, forming microabscesses
- Bacteria may be free or phagocytosed
- Fungal hyphae or viral inclusions may be present
- Perilymphadenitis
  - Involvement of perinodal fibroadipose tissues by inflammation
- In late stages
  - Acute inflammatory process subsides
  - Macrophages containing ingested cellular debris become predominant

SUPPURATIVE LYMPHADENITIS

Key Facts

Terminology
- Acute lymphadenitis caused by bacterial, fungal, or some viral infections

Etiology/Pathogenesis
- Common bacteria: *Staphylococcus* and *Streptococcus*

Clinical Issues
- Regional lymph nodes draining pyogenic inflammation, e.g., dental abscess, upper respiratory infection, appendicitis, or infected wound

Microscopic Pathology
- Dilated sinuses with weakly eosinophilic proteinaceous fluid and many neutrophils and macrophages
  - So-called sinus catarrh

- Neutrophils infiltrate lymph node parenchyma; form microabscesses
- Bacteria may be free or phagocytosed
- Fungal hyphae; viral inclusions
- Perilymphadenitis due to involvement of perinodal fibroadipose tissue

Ancillary Tests
- Gram stain is useful in identifying presence and nature of bacteria
- Bacteriologic studies, including smears and cultures, are indispensable for identifying etiology

Top Differential Diagnoses
- Cat scratch lymphadenitis
- Lymphogranuloma venereum lymphadenitis
- Classical Hodgkin lymphoma with necrosis

ANCILLARY TESTS

Histochemistry
- Gram stain is useful for identifying presence and nature of bacteria
- Bacteriologic studies, including smears and cultures, are indispensable for identifying etiology
  - Sterile, fresh tissues from area of suppuration
    - Need to be sent immediately to microbiology laboratory
    - Bacterial culture and antibiogram are essential

DIFFERENTIAL DIAGNOSIS

Cat Scratch Lymphadenitis
- Contact with cats
- Unilateral lymphadenopathy
- Matted lymph nodes
- Necrotizing granulomas; central necrosis with neutrophils
- Peripheral palisaded epithelioid cells; ± multinucleated giant cells
- Clumps of pleomorphic bacilli
- *B. henselae*, Gram-negative bacillus
- Capsular and perinodal involvement
- Positive Warthin-Starry silver stain
- Immunoreactive with anti-*B. henselae* antibody

Lymphogranuloma Venereum Lymphadenitis
- Genital and extragenital lesions
- Inguinal, perianal, and pelvic lymph nodes
- Often unilateral
- Stellate abscesses; central necrosis with neutrophils
- Plasma cells and lymphocytes
- Palisaded epithelioid cells; multinucleated giant cells
- Macrophages with vacuoles and intravacuolar *C. trachomatis* bacteria
- Fibrosis, lymphangiectasia, vascular obliteration
- Capsular involvement
- Complement fixation test
- PCR test

Classical Hodgkin Lymphoma with Necrosis
- Necrosis and acute inflammation can be prominent
- Eosinophils or plasma cells often present; can be numerous
- Reed-Sternberg cells, Hodgkin cells, lacunar cells
- CD15(+), CD30(+), CD45(-)

Anaplastic Large Cell Lymphoma, Neutrophil or Eosinophil Rich
- Partial or complete lymph node effacement
- Paracortical or sinusoidal in cases with partial involvement
- Anaplastic large cells with pleomorphic wreath-like nuclei and prominent nucleoli
- CD30(+), ALK-1(+), T-cell markers(+)
- Monoclonal *TCR* gene rearrangements
- t(2;5)(p23;q35)/*NPM-ALK* seen in 80% of cases

Infarcted Malignant Lymphoma
- Ghosts of lymphoma cells are present; usually no inflammatory cells
- Immunohistochemistry is helpful

SELECTED REFERENCES

1. Esparcia A et al: [Fever and suppurative lymphadenitis in a parenteral drug user infected with the human immunodeficiency virus.] Enferm Infecc Microbiol Clin. 19(10):495-6, 2001
2. Naqvi SH et al: Generalized suppurative lymphadenitis with typhoidal salmonellosis. Pediatr Infect Dis J. 7(12):882-3, 1988
3. Toshniwal R et al: Suppurative lymphadenitis with Yersinia enterocolitica. Eur J Clin Microbiol. 4(6):587-8, 1985
4. Hill HR et al: Severe staphylococcal disease associated with allergic manifestations, hyperimmunoglobulinemia E, and defective neutrophil chemotaxis. J Lab Clin Med. 88(5):796-806, 1976
5. Barton LL et al: Childhood cervical lymphadenitis: a reappraisal. J Pediatr. 84(6):846-52, 1974

Microscopic Features

(Left) Low-power view of a lymph node involved by numerous granulomas with abundant central necrosis and granulocytes. This case therefore shows both suppurative ⇨ and necrotizing chronic granulomatous inflammation ⇨. The specific etiology was not determined in this case. (Right) Electron micrograph shows clusters of staphylococcal organisms growing in culture. (Courtesy M. Arduino, CDC Public Health Image Library, #11153.)

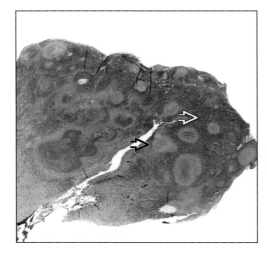
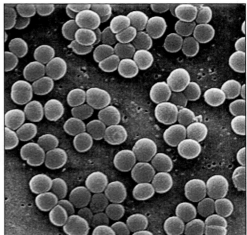

(Left) Paraffin section of a lymph node from a patient with suppurative lymphadenitis due to Actinomyces infection shows numerous neutrophils and "sulfur granules" ⇨. (Right) Paraffin section of a lymph node from a patient with lymphogranuloma venereum lymphadenitis shows stellate microabscesses with central necrosis and neutrophils as well as peripheral palisading epithelioid histiocytes, lymphocytes, and plasma cells.

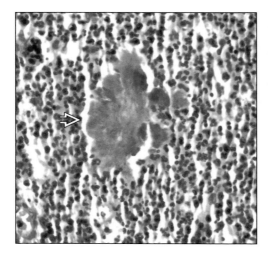
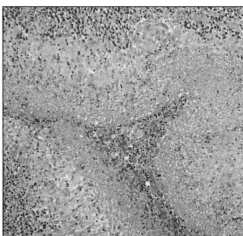

(Left) Paraffin section of a lymph node from a patient with cat scratch lymphadenitis shows microabscess with central necrosis, neutrophils, and lymphocytes. (Right) Warthin-Starry stain of a lymph node from a patient with cat scratch lymphadenitis shows clumps of pleomorphic bacilli ⇨ consistent with Bartonella henselae.

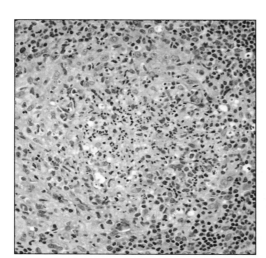
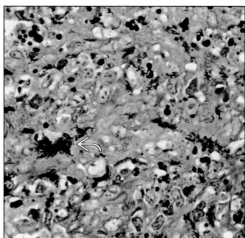

SUPPURATIVE LYMPHADENITIS

Microscopic Features

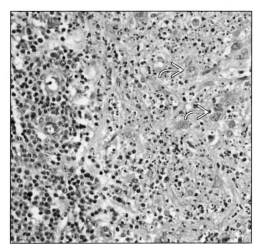
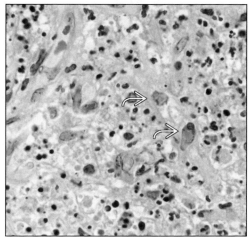

(Left) Paraffin section of a lymph node from a patient with herpes simplex virus lymphadenitis shows necrosis (right of field) within which neutrophils and large cells with ground-glass nuclei ➔ consistent with viral inclusions, are present. *(Right)* High-power magnification of lymph node from a patient with herpes simplex virus lymphadenitis shows a focus of necrosis with inflammatory cells, cell debris, and large cells with intranuclear, Cowdry type A viral inclusions ➔.

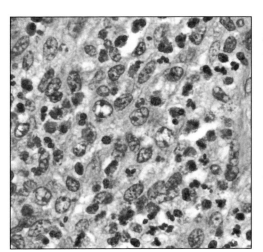
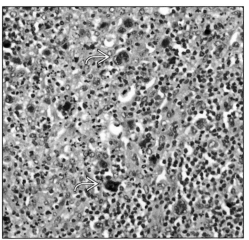

(Left) A case of ALK-1(+) anaplastic large cell lymphoma (ALCL) that is rich in eosinophils. ALCL cases can be rich in neutrophils, eosinophils, or both and may be mistaken for an inflammatory process. *(Right)* Paraffin section of a lymph node from a patient with Hodgkin lymphoma, nodular sclerosis type shows large atypical neoplastic cells with prominent nucleoli ➔ in a mixed population of lymphocytes, plasma cells, histiocytes, and eosinophils.

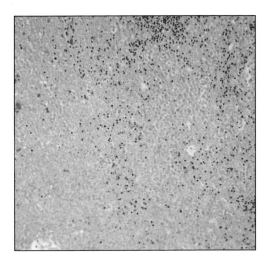
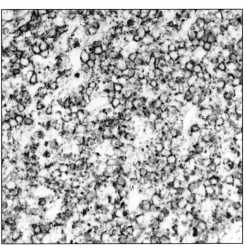

(Left) A lymph node involved by malignant lymphoma that has undergone infarction. The quality of the necrosis in infarct is different from infectious necrosis. Note the many cell ghosts present in this field. *(Right)* A lymph node involved by a malignant lymphoma that has undergone infarction. The anti-CD20 antibody is highlighting the infarcted lymphoma cells in this case. In infectious necrosis, the necrotic cells and material are negative for CD20.

MYCOBACTERIUM TUBERCULOSIS LYMPHADENITIS

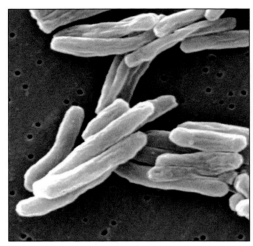

Scanning electron micrograph of M. tuberculosis. The bacterium ranges from 2-4 μm long and 0.2-0.5 μm wide. (Courtesy J. Carr, CDC Public Health Image Library, #9997.)

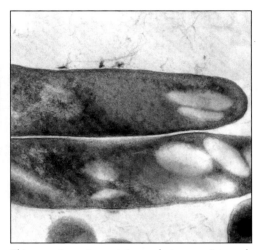

Thin section transmission electron micrograph demonstrates M. tuberculosis bacilli. (CDC Public Health Image Library, #8433.)

TERMINOLOGY

Abbreviations
- Acid-fast bacilli (AFB)
- Tuberculosis (TB)

Definitions
- Lymphadenitis caused by infection with *Mycobacterium tuberculosis*

ETIOLOGY/PATHOGENESIS

Infectious Agents
- *Mycobacterium tuberculosis*

Immunocompetent Patients
- Reactivation of disease at site seeded during primary infection by hematogenous route
- Infection of tonsils, adenoids, and Waldeyer ring
- Abdominal involvement may occur via ingestion of milk or sputum infected with *M. tuberculosis*

Immunocompromised Patients
- Human immunodeficiency virus (HIV) infection most common
- Reactivation of latent infection
- Part of generalized infection, miliary dissemination
  - Greater mycobacterial load than immunocompetent patients

CLINICAL ISSUES

Epidemiology
- Incidence
  - ~ 40% of peripheral lymphadenopathy in developing world
  - Prevalence of TB lymphadenitis in children ≤ 14 years in rural India: 4.4/1,000

  - Lymphadenitis is most common form of extrapulmonary tuberculosis (5-10% of cases)
  - In developed countries, most cases occur in immigrants and travelers to endemic areas
    - Immigrant populations mostly originate from Southeast Asia and Africa
  - In USA, 20% of TB cases are extrapulmonary
    - ~ 30% of these cases present with lymphadenitis
  - *M. tuberculosis* is common in HIV-positive individuals
    - Part of pulmonary or disseminated disease
    - Most extrapulmonary TB cases occur with CD4 counts ≤ 100 cells/μL
- Age
  - Historically, common in children
  - At present, children affected predominantly in developing countries
  - Peak age in developed countries: 20-40 years
- Gender
  - M:F ratio = 1:2
- Ethnicity
  - Asian Pacific Islanders more susceptible

Presentation
- Characteristically, multiple lymph nodes (LNs) involved
- 90% involve superficial LNs in head and neck region
  - Anterior and posterior cervical (most common)
  - Supraclavicular, submandibular, preauricular, submental also involved
- Other LNs: Axillary, inguinal, mesenteric, mediastinal, and intramammary
- Isolated intraabdominal LNs can be involved
  - Periportal, peripancreatic, and mesenteric
- Generalized lymphadenopathy and hepatosplenomegaly in 5%
- Painless progressive swelling in neck
- Parabronchial and paratracheal involvement can lead to airway compromise

MYCOBACTERIUM TUBERCULOSIS LYMPHADENITIS

Key Facts

Clinical Issues
- High index of suspicion essential for diagnosis
- Definitive diagnosis by histology and culture of LN
- Molecular methods enable quicker identification of organism
- FNA is as useful as excisional LN biopsy in HIV(+) patients

Microscopic Pathology
- Granulomas, classically with necrotic center (caseation)
- Concentric layers of epithelioid cells, Langhans giant cells, lymphocytes, and plasma cells
- Fibrosis, hyalinization, calcification present in healing phase
- In LN biopsy specimen, AFB identified morphologically by

- ○ Ziehl-Neelsen, Kinyoun, Fite-Faraco stains
- ○ It is common for stains to be negative in culture (+) cases
- Auramine-rhodamine stain with fluorescent microscopy more sensitive for detection

Top Differential Diagnoses
- *M. avium-intracellulare* lymphadenitis
- Histoplasma lymphadenitis
- Kikuchi-Fujimoto lymphadenitis
- Cat scratch lymphadenitis
- Sarcoidosis lymphadenopathy

Reporting Considerations
- Suspected or confirmed cases of TB should be reported to local public health department
  - ○ Identify contacts for follow-up

- 5% of children develop lymphadenopathy within 6 months of infection
- In adults, TB represents reactivation of previous infection
- Up to 1/3 of patients report previous or family history of TB
- LN on physical examination
  - ○ Firm, rubbery, discrete, and nontender
  - ○ May be swollen and tender due to secondary bacterial infection
- Ulcer &/or sinus tract formation in 10%

Laboratory Tests
- Tuberculin skin test (TST)
  - ○ Positive in 90% of cases with TB lymphadenopathy
  - ○ May be negative in HIV-positive patients with TB
- Interferon-γ release assays
  - ○ Measure in vitro T-cell interferon-γ release in response to 2 unique antigens
    - Sensitivity in active TB: 75-90%
    - Highly specific for *M. tuberculosis*
    - Negative in prior BCG vaccination and in sensitization to nontuberculous mycobacteria
    - Cannot distinguish between latent and active tuberculosis
  - ○ 2 widely studied tests
    - Enzyme-linked immunospot (ELISpot) (T-SPOT.TB; Oxford Immunotec; Oxford, UK)
    - Enzyme-linked immunosorbent assay (ELISA) (QuantiFERON-TB Gold; Cellestis; Chadstone, VIC; Australia)
  - ○ For diagnosis of latent infection
    - Sensitivity of ELISA similar to TST
    - ELISpot more sensitive
- Direct staining
  - ○ Carbolfuchsin stains (Ziehl-Neelsen stain; Kinyoun stain) highlight AFB
    - AFB are bright red against blue or green background, depending on counterstain
    - Must be scanned under oil-immersion

- Time consuming due to limited size of field viewed at 1 time
  - ○ Fluorochrome stain (auramine O, with or without rhodamine)
    - Scanning quicker since slides can be scanned at 25x objective
    - Confirmation may require 40x objective
    - Bacteria bright yellow (auramine) or orange-red (rhodamine) against dark background
- Microbiological culture
  - ○ Loewenstein-Jensen (L) medium
    - Less sensitive
    - Recommended only for chromogenic studies and biochemical tests
  - ○ Middlebrook 7H10 and 7H11 agar medium used for isolation and susceptibility testing
  - ○ Automated Radiometric Detection Systems: BACTEC 460 (BD Diagnostic Systems; Sparks, MD; USA)
  - ○ Automated Nonradiometric Detection Systems
    - MGIT 960 (BD Diagnostic Systems)
    - MB/BacT System (BioMerieux; Durham, NC; USA)
    - BACTEC MYCO/F lytic blood culture bottle (BD Diagnostic Systems)
    - ESP Culture System II (TREK Diagnostic Systems, Inc.; Cleveland, OH; USA)
- Gas-liquid and high-performance liquid chromatography
  - ○ Useful in culture confirmation
- Molecular diagnosis
  - ○ Uses
    - Culture confirmation of isolates
    - Identification of isolates
    - Direct detection
    - DNA fingerprinting
    - Strain-typing
  - ○ Quicker identification than by traditional methods
  - ○ 2 amplification-based methods FDA approved in USA
    - Amplicor *M. tuberculosis* PCR assay (Roche Diagnostics; Indianapolis, IN; USA)

MYCOBACTERIUM TUBERCULOSIS LYMPHADENITIS

- Amplified *M. tuberculosis* Direct Test (Gen-Probe Incorporated; San Diego, CA; USA)
  - Home-brew PCR, including real-time PCR assays, have been developed but need validation by individual laboratories
  - DNA sequencing can make rapid and accurate identification
  - Strain-typing has been used in detection of drug resistance

Treatment
- Surgical approaches
  - Needed in minority of patients
  - Indications: Failure of antimicrobial chemotherapy, pressure effect
  - Excisional biopsy preferred since incisional biopsy may result in sinus tract formation
- Drugs
  - All patients treated with antituberculous agents
  - Treatment may be started prior to culture confirmation
    - Particularly when pathologic features suspicious or in high-risk subject
  - Adults: 6 months of isoniazid, rifampin, pyrazinamide, and ethambutol
  - Children: 2 months of isoniazid, rifampin, and pyrazinamide, plus 2 months of isoniazid and rifampin
  - Mediastinal lymph node involvement treated with same regimen as lung involvement

Prognosis
- Antimicrobial therapy curative; relapse rates of up to 3.5%
- In 30% of patients after beginning therapy
  - Paradoxical increase in LN size
  - New enlarged LNs may develop
  - Mechanism is immune response to mycobacterial killing
  - Must be differentiated from relapse
- HIV-positive patients who begin HAART may develop immune reconstitution inflammatory syndrome with worsening lymphadenopathy
- Residual palpable LNs after completion of therapy may be present in 5–30% of patients
- Retreatment generally considered to be unnecessary if
  - Cultures are negative
  - Compliance with treatment is documented

IMAGE FINDINGS

General Features
- Not definitively diagnostic of TB lymphadenitis

Radiographic Findings
- 80% of children and 20% of adults show evidence of recent or active tuberculosis in lungs

MR Findings
- Discrete, matted, confluent masses; necrosis, soft tissue edema

CT Findings
- Conglomerated masses; hypodense nodes with peripheral enhancement, multilocular appearance

Gallium Scan
- LN "hot" in appearance

MACROSCOPIC FEATURES

General Features
- Cut surface of LNs has distinctive gross features
  - Creamy white patches correspond to caseous, necrotic areas
  - Chalky areas correspond to calcification
  - Periphery may be densely fibrosed
- LNs can be matted
- Extensive areas of necrosis

Sections to Be Submitted
- Solid and caseous areas should be submitted for histopathology and culture
- Caseous areas for direct smears

MICROSCOPIC PATHOLOGY

Histologic Features
- Chronic granulomatous inflammation with caseation necrosis
- LN may be partially or extensively involved
- Granulomas
  - Classically with necrotic center
  - Concentric layers of epithelioid cells
  - Langhans giant cells
    - Have abundant eosinophilic cytoplasm and multiple peripherally arranged nuclei
  - Other multinucleate cells may also be found
  - Lymphocytes and plasma cells
  - Typically, granulocytes absent
  - Fibroblasts present at periphery of granulomas
- Reactive lymphoid follicles often present in uninvolved LN
  - Necrosis can involve follicles
- Fibrosis, hyalinization, calcification present in healing phase
- AFB may be demonstrated by following stains
  - Ziehl-Neelsen
  - Kinyoun
  - Fite-Faraco
  - Auramine-rhodamine with fluorescent microscopy
- Number of bacilli detected is variable
  - Caseous necrosis is best place to search for AFB
  - Often very few; numbers depend upon
    - Phase of disease
    - Past treatment
    - May not be identified in culture-confirmed cases
- Detection of AFB inversely correlated with number of granulomas
  - Rarely in cytoplasm of giant cells

Cytologic Features
- Predominantly necrotic material

MYCOBACTERIUM TUBERCULOSIS LYMPHADENITIS

- Typical caseating epithelioid granulomas & giant cells
- Noncaseating epithelioid cell granulomas ± giant cells
- Nonspecific epithelioid cells

Immunohistochemistry
- Epithelioid histiocytes are CD68(+), lysozyme(+)
- Most lymphocytes are T cells: CD3(+)
- Polytypic plasma cells; few B cells

Flow Cytometry
- Polytypic B cells and T cells with normal immunophenotype

Role of Fine Needle Aspiration (FNA)
- Sensitive, specific, safe, and cost-effective procedure with high yield in assessing peripheral LNs
- 19 or 18 gauge needle should be used
- Smears should be fixed for cytology; air-dried smears for AFB staining
- Specimens should be submitted for culture and PCR testing (if available)
- FNA combined with PCR reportedly as effective as excisional LN biopsy
- Nondiagnostic FNA can be repeated, if needed
- Excisional LN biopsy can be performed in subset with nondiagnostic FNA
- FNA most useful when
  - AFB smear positive
  - LN fluctuant
  - TB present at other body sites
- Identification of granulomas comparable in FNA and excisional biopsy specimens
- Granulomas with necrosis (more specific for TB) more common in biopsy specimens
- Culture positivity rates in FNA comparable to excisional biopsy specimens

DIFFERENTIAL DIAGNOSIS

M. avium-intracellulare Lymphadenitis
- Common in AIDS and other immunocompromised patients
- No single feature definitive
- Sheets of histiocytes
- Ill-defined (nonpalisading), irregular or serpiginous, or sarcoid-like granulomas
- Nonspecific granulomatous response
- Lack of significant caseation
- Neutrophils tend to be in center of necrotic areas
- Abundant AFB, minimal fibrosis, or calcification

Bacillus Calmette-Guérin (BCG) Lymphadenitis
- Attenuated form of *M. tuberculosis* used for immunization
- Lymphadenitis occurs in up to ~ 2% of infants
  - Enlarged LNs appear 2.5 months to 3 years after immunization
- Immunocompetent
  - Enlargement of regional LNs
  - Papular or papulopustular skin lesions
  - Subcutaneous abscess at vaccination site
  - Osteomyelitis, arthritis, and hepatic granulomas ("BCGitis")
  - Multiple epithelioid granulomas and Langhans giant cells
  - Caseous necrosis; minimal neutrophilic infiltration with abscess formation may occur
  - Self-limiting; recover completely, spontaneously, or after excision of suppurative LN
  - Usually do not require antibiotics
  - Bacilli infrequent
- Immunocompromised
  - Large stellate, caseous abscesses without giant cells
  - Numerous bacilli

Histoplasma Lymphadenitis
- May have extensive necrosis
- Neutrophils can be abundant
- Calcification common
- GMS silver staining demonstrates yeast of *H. capsulatum*
  - 2-4 μm with narrow-based buds

Kikuchi-Fujimoto Lymphadenitis
- Necrotic areas
- No neutrophils present
- Sheets of histiocytes and T cells
- No granulomas, giant cells, AFB identified
- No organisms identified by special stains

Cat Scratch Lymphadenitis
- Necrotic areas demonstrate neutrophils
- *Bartonella henselae* bacilli may be identified on Warthin-Starry stain

Sarcoidosis Lymphadenopathy
- Discrete granulomas with fibrosis; minimal necrosis; plasma cells present
- Schaumann and asteroid bodies occasionally identified
- Kveim-Siltzbach test may be positive
- No organisms identified by special stains

SELECTED REFERENCES

1. Lalvani A: Diagnosing tuberculosis infection in the 21st century: new tools to tackle an old enemy. Chest. 131(6):1898-906, 2007
2. Pahwa R et al: Assessment of possible tuberculous lymphadenopathy by PCR compared to non-molecular methods. J Med Microbiol. 54(Pt 9):873-8, 2005
3. Polesky A et al: Peripheral tuberculous lymphadenitis: epidemiology, diagnosis, treatment, and outcome. Medicine (Baltimore). 84(6):350-62, 2005
4. al-Bhlal LA: Pathologic findings for bacille Calmette-Guérin infections in immunocompetent and immunocompromised patients. Am J Clin Pathol. 113(5):703-8, 2000
5. Ellison E et al: Fine needle aspiration diagnosis of mycobacterial lymphadenitis. Sensitivity and predictive value in the United States. Acta Cytol. 43(2):153-7, 1999

MYCOBACTERIUM TUBERCULOSIS LYMPHADENITIS

Microscopic Features

(Left) Lymph node involved by tuberculosis. Numerous well-defined granulomas efface nodal architecture almost entirely. Note central caseation necrosis ➡ at the center of some granulomas. *(Right)* Lymph node involved by tuberculosis. Extensive caseation necrosis almost completely replaces lymph node. A thin rim of chronic inflammatory infiltrate is noted at the periphery.

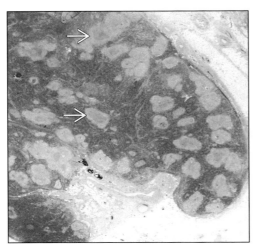
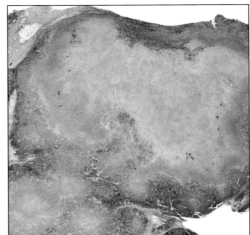

(Left) Lymph node involved by tuberculosis. Caseation necrosis replaces lymph node extensively. Well-defined granulomas ➡ are also present (upper field). *(Right)* Lymph node involved by tuberculosis. Granulomatous inflammation shows extensive caseation necrosis without cellular outlines or nuclear debris (left). Concentric layers of epithelioid cells, Langhans giant cells ➡, lymphocytes, plasma cells, and fibroblasts are also present (right).

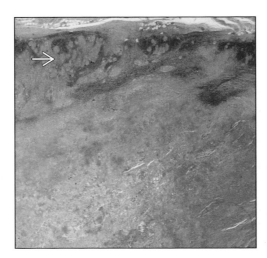
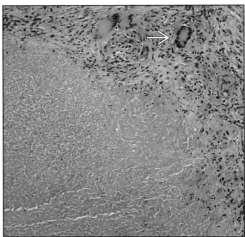

(Left) Lymph node involved by tuberculosis. Confluent epithelioid cell granulomas are present without caseation necrosis. This picture can be confused with sarcoidosis. Note multinucleated Langhans giant cell ➡. *(Right)* Lymph node involved by tuberculosis and extensive granulomatous inflammation with coalescing noncaseating epithelioid cell granulomas. Note dense sclerosis in the center ➡.

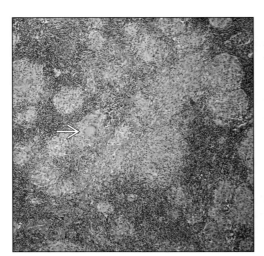
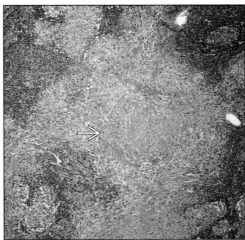

MYCOBACTERIUM TUBERCULOSIS LYMPHADENITIS

Microscopic Features

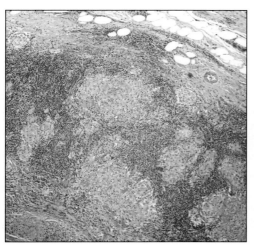
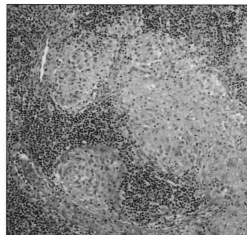

(Left) Lymph node involved by tuberculosis. Numerous granulomas distort nodal architecture. Note epithelioid histiocytes with abundant eosinophilic cytoplasm. *(Right)* Lymph node involved by tuberculosis. Lymph node biopsy specimen shows epithelioid granulomas that are composed of histiocytes with abundant pink cytoplasm.

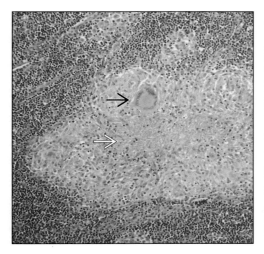
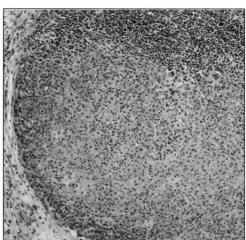

(Left) Lymph node involved by tuberculosis. Lymph node biopsy specimen shows caseating granuloma with epithelioid histiocytes surrounding central necrotic area ➡. Note Langhans giant cell with peripherally arranged nuclei in a "horseshoe" pattern ➡. *(Right)* Lymph node involved by tuberculosis. In this lymph node biopsy specimen, a large granuloma with epithelioid histiocytes and inflammatory cells is present.

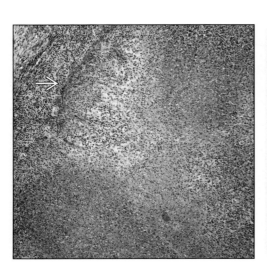
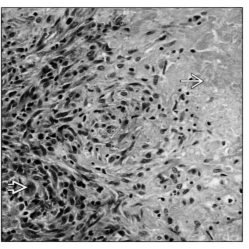

(Left) Lymph node involved by tuberculosis. Lymph node biopsy specimen shows extensive sheets of necrosis. Note chronic inflammatory infiltrate and vascular proliferation ➡. *(Right)* Lymph node involved by tuberculosis. In this lymph node biopsy specimen, extensive necrosis is only partially shown in this field ➡. A prominent histiocytic infiltrate with plasma cells is present at the periphery of the necrosis ➡.

MYCOBACTERIUM TUBERCULOSIS LYMPHADENITIS

Microscopic Features

(Left) Lymph node involved by tuberculosis. Extensive necrosis ➡ is present. Note prominent histiocytic infiltrate ➡. (Right) Lymph node involved by tuberculosis. Caseation necrosis ➡ with a prominent plasmacytic infiltrate ➡ is present in this lymph node biopsy specimen. Note scattered histiocytes in necrotic areas ➡; these have vacuolated cytoplasm giving a bubbly appearance.

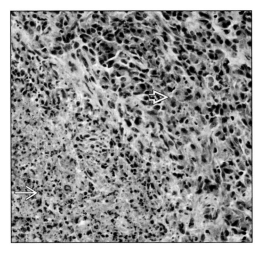 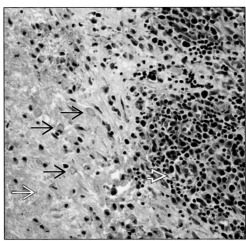

(Left) Lymph node involved by tuberculosis. Granulomatous inflammation with clusters of epithelioid histiocytes are present. Note interspersed fibrillary (fibrinoid) necrosis ➡ and lymphocytes at the periphery. (Right) Lymph node involved by tuberculosis. Fibrillary (fibrinoid) necrosis ➡ is present within an epithelioid cell granuloma. Necrosis is oxyphilic. This special form of necrosis occurs in noncaseating tuberculosis as well as in sarcoidosis.

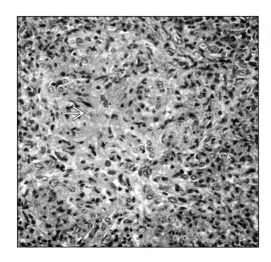 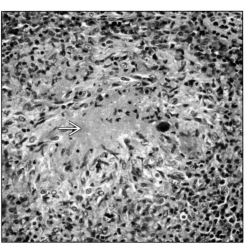

(Left) Lymph node involved by tuberculosis. Giant cells have eosinophilic cytoplasm and multiple peripherally arranged nuclei (Langhans giant cells). (Right) Lymph node involved by tuberculosis. Epithelioid histiocytes surround focal necrotic area ➡. Note Langhans giant cell with peripherally arranged nuclei in a wreath-like pattern ➡.

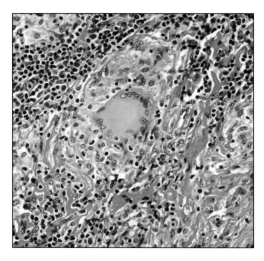 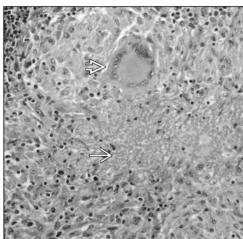

MYCOBACTERIUM TUBERCULOSIS LYMPHADENITIS

Microscopic Features

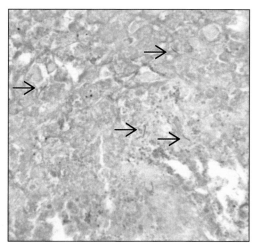
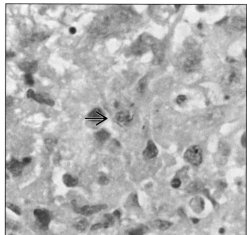

(Left) Lymph node involved by tuberculosis. Ziehl-Neelsen stain demonstrates slender, needle-shaped, slightly curved, bright red bacilli ⇨. (Right) Lymph node involved by tuberculosis. Ziehl-Neelsen stain demonstrates slender, needle-shaped, slightly curved bright red bacilli ⇨.

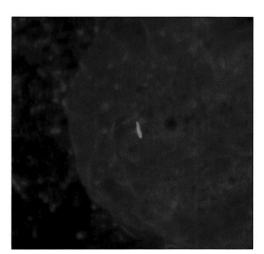
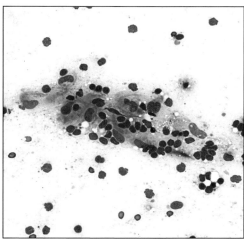

(Left) M. tuberculosis is identified in sputum smear stained with fluorescent auramine with acridine orange counterstain. The bacterium fluoresces yellow under ultraviolet light microscopy. (Courtesy R.W. Smithwick, CDC Public Health Image Library, #2190.) (Right) Fine needle aspirate of lymph node. Noncaseating epithelioid cell granuloma is composed of clusters of epithelioid histiocytes and interspersed lymphocytes.

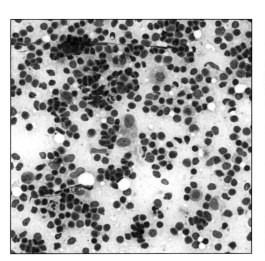
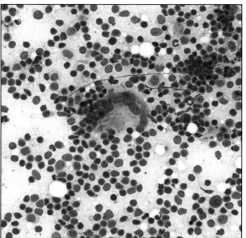

(Left) Fine needle aspirate of lymph node. Epithelioid histiocytes having blue-gray cytoplasm are present in a background of lymphocytes. (Right) Fine needle aspirate of lymph node. Giant cell of Langhans type is present; this cell has abundant cytoplasm and multiple peripherally arranged nuclei.

ATYPICAL MYCOBACTERIAL LYMPHADENITIS

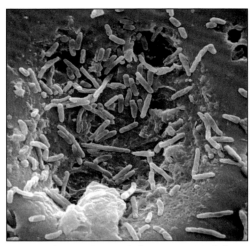

Scanning electron micrograph demonstrates M. chelonae bacteria. (Courtesy J. Carr, CDC Public Health Image Library, #226.)

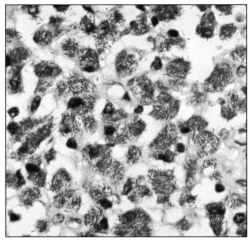

Acid-fast (Ziehl-Neelsen) stain of lymph node in an AIDS patient shows abundant M. avium-intracellulare within histiocytes. (Courtesy E. Ewing, Jr., MD, CDC Public Health Image Library, #965.)

TERMINOLOGY

Abbreviations
- Atypical mycobacteria (AM)

Synonyms
- Nontuberculous mycobacteria (NTM)
- Mycobacteria other than tubercle bacilli (MOT)
- Potentially pathogenic environmental mycobacteria (PPEM)

Definitions
- Lymphadenitis caused by infection by atypical mycobacteria

ETIOLOGY/PATHOGENESIS

Environmental Exposure
- Widely distributed in soil; also present in natural and treated water sources
- No evidence of animal-to-human or human-to-human transmission
- Human infection suspected to be acquired from environmental sources

Infectious Agents
- *M. avium-intracellulare* (MAI) is most common organism implicated in lymphadenitis
- *M. scrofulaceum, M. fortuitum, M. chelonei, M. abscessus, M. kansasii* also occur but are less common
- May cause either asymptomatic infection or symptomatic disease

Pathogenesis
- Nonspecific immunity
  o Epithelial barrier integrity
  o Gastric pH
  o Interleukin (IL)-8, IL-12, chemokine ligand 5 (CCL5)
  o Natural resistance-associated macrophage protein

  o Macrophages initially phagocytose mycobacteria
- Specific immunity
  o Develops over weeks following infection
  o Mediated by CD4(+) T lymphocytes
  o Involves IL-2, interferon (IFN)-γ, tumor necrosis factor (TNF)-γ
  o IFN-γ activates neutrophils and macrophages to kill intracellular mycobacteria
- Host defects predispose to disseminated infection
  o Deficiency of CD4(+) lymphocytes in HIV infection
    ▪ Disseminated AM infection when CD4(+) count < 50/μl
  o Specific mutations resulting in IFN-γ receptor defects and reduced IFN-γ production

CLINICAL ISSUES

Epidemiology
- Incidence
  o Infection rate in North America: 1-12 per 100,000 persons
  o Disease rates: 0.1-2 per 100,000 persons
  o Prevalence of pulmonary AM infection in USA is increasing
  o MAI is most common AM species causing disease
  o Many other species have been implicated
  o Significant percentage of adults have had prior asymptomatic infection with AM as assessed by skin tests
  o Distinguishing infection from disease needs clinical correlation
    ▪ Diagnostic criteria have been defined to guide treatment
    ▪ Infection defined as isolation of viable organisms from uncontaminated specimen in absence of clinical manifestations
    ▪ Disease defined as additional signs or symptoms that suggest pathogenic process

ATYPICAL MYCOBACTERIAL LYMPHADENITIS

Key Facts

Etiology/Pathogenesis
- Peak incidence at 1-5 years
- *M. avium-intracellulare* (in 80% of cases in children)
- *M. scrofulaceum, M. malmoense,* and *M. haemophilum*
- Uncommon in adults with exception of AIDS patients in era of HAART
- Diagnosis requires excluding *M. tuberculosis* infection and
  - Positive culture for AM or
  - Suggestive histologic findings

Microscopic Pathology
- Lymph node architecture partially or totally effaced
- Sheets of large pale histiocytes with abundant foamy cytoplasm
- Acute inflammation can be present
- Rarely, multinucleated giant cells

- Usually no granulomas, necrosis, calcification, fibrosis

Ancillary Tests
- Acid-fast stains: Abundant AFB within histiocytes
- Culture essential for definitive identification
- High-performance liquid chromatography
- Genotypic methods

Top Differential Diagnoses
- *M. tuberculosis* lymphadenitis
- Mycobacterial spindle cell pseudotumor
- Fungal lymphadenitis
- Kikuchi-Fujimoto lymphadenitis

Reporting Considerations
- Not reportable in USA since these are not communicable

- Isolation of a single positive sputum culture does not necessarily represent disease
- No evidence that AM are associated with reactivation of disease
- Prevention of infections not possible at present

Site
- Virtually any body site can be infected by AM

Presentation
- **Pulmonary**
  - Most common clinical manifestation
  - Immunocompetent patients
    - Tuberculosis-like pattern involving upper lobes in men with history of smoking or lung disease
    - Nodular bronchiectasis in slender older nonsmoking women with skeletal deformities; presents with cough
    - Hypersensitivity pneumonitis associated with hot tubs and medicinal baths; presents with dyspnea, cough, and fever
    - *M. kansasii, M. xenopi, M. malmoense,* and MAI implicated in tuberculosis-like pattern
    - MAI implicated in all nodular bronchiectasis and hypersensitivity pneumonitis patterns
    - Isolated pulmonary disease due to MAI occurs typically in immunocompetent adults
  - Immunocompromised (HIV+)
    - AM commonly isolated from respiratory secretions
    - Isolated lung disease uncommon
    - Extrapulmonary or disseminated disease more likely
    - *M. kansasii* can cause lung disease without dissemination
  - Diagnosis of pulmonary MAI based on clinical, microbiological, and radiographic criteria
- **Lymph nodes**
  - Painless swelling of one or more lymph nodes in regional distribution
  - Anterior cervical lymph nodes most commonly affected
    - Submandibular, submaxillary, and preauricular

- Parotid, postauricular, mediastinal lymph nodes can be involved
- Peak incidence at 1-5 years of age
  - MAI isolated in 80% of culture-positive cases in children
  - Other species: *M. scrofulaceum, M. malmoense,* and *M. haemophilum*
  - Recently identified slow-growing mycobacteria have also been implicated
- No systemic symptoms
- Indolent disease
- Unilateral in 95% of cases
- Route of infection hypothesized to be lymphatics draining mouth and oropharynx
- Lymph nodes enlarge and may rapidly soften and rupture
- Chronic, draining fistulae to skin can result
- Spontaneous regression can occur
- Healing usually occurs by fibrosis and calcification
- Uncommon in adults except AIDS patients in era of highly active antiretroviral therapy (HAART)
  - In past, MAI disease in AIDS patients was disseminated process
  - With advent of HAART, lymphadenitis can occur as part of immune reconstitution syndrome
- Diagnosis of AM lymphadenitis requires either positive culture or suggestive histopathology after ruling out *M. tuberculosis* infection
- Most patients have < 10 mm reaction due to cross-reactivity between *M. tuberculosis* and AM proteins
- Induration > 10 mm has been reported in nearly 1/3 of children with AM lymphadenitis
- **Skin and soft tissue**
  - MAI infection
    - Occurs by direct inoculation (trauma, surgery, or injection)
    - Ulceration, abscess with sinus formation, erythematous plaque with crusted base ensue
    - Lesions are indolent
    - Diagnosis requires high index of suspicion

ATYPICAL MYCOBACTERIAL LYMPHADENITIS

- History of exposure to potential source of infection may be helpful
- Combination of excision (or surgical debridement) and chemotherapy required
  - **Buruli ulcer**
    - *M. ulcerans* is causative organism
    - Tropical and subtropical regions: West and Central Africa, Central and South America, and Southeast Asia
    - Infection thought to occur through cut or wound contaminated with water, soil, or vegetation
    - More common in children < 15 years of age
    - Lower limbs involved more than upper limbs
    - Begins as solitary painless subcutaneous nodule or papule
    - Evolves to form ulcer with undermined edges
    - Spontaneous healing in 4–6 months
    - Extensive scar formation
    - Dissemination, including osteomyelitis, can occur, especially in patients < 15 years old
    - Surgical excision with wide margins required
  - **M. marinum infection**
    - Worldwide distribution
    - Infection occurs through injury by fish fins or bites, cutaneous trauma, exposure to contaminated water
    - Infections limited to skin and confined to single extremity
    - Tender, erythematous or bluish papulonodular lesion (0.5–3 cm) enlarges slowly and suppurates
    - Infection may spread to deeper structures, leading to scarring
    - Infection may extend to regional lymph nodes
  - **Rapidly growing atypical mycobacteria (RGM)**
    - Survive in harsh aquatic conditions; piped water systems
    - Resistant to sterilizing agents and disinfectants
    - Immunocompetent: Single lesion after penetrating trauma, surgery; *M. fortuitum* predominant organism
    - Immunocompromised: Multiple/disseminated lesions after penetrating trauma, surgery; *M. chelonae* or *M. abscessus* predominant organisms
    - Identification of RGM at species level essential for deciding treatment regimen
- **Musculoskeletal**
  - Most affected patients are immunocompetent
  - Tendon sheaths, bursae, bones, and joints involved
  - Hand and wrist most common sites
  - Contiguous infection from site of surgical procedure or penetrating trauma
  - Clinically indistinguishable from *M. tuberculosis*-associated infections
  - Rarely, suppuration, necrosis of synovial tissue, osteomyelitis may occur
  - Clinical course protracted
  - *M. marinum* and *M. kansasii* frequently involved
  - *M. chelonae* and *M. haemophilum* only in immunocompromised patients
- **Disseminated**
  - Occurs in immunocompromised patients

- *M. avium* causes > 95% of cases of disseminated disease in AIDS patients
- Most cases occur with CD4(+) count < 50/μL
- Fever, night sweats, weight loss, fatigue, diarrhea, and abdominal pain
- Anemia and elevated alkaline phosphatase
- Diagnosis made by
  - Appreciating signs and symptoms
  - Isolation of MAI from blood, bone marrow, or other normally sterile tissue or body fluids

Laboratory Tests
- **General**
  - Specimen processing
    - Specimens may be collected from any site
    - Contamination by environmental mycobacteria needs to be avoided, especially by tap water
    - Risk of bacterial overgrowth increases with delay between collection and processing
    - Treatment with macrolides and quinolones may decrease AM yield
    - Digestion and decontamination necessary for specimens collected from nonsterile body sites
  - Respiratory specimens
    - Collection of 3 early morning specimens on different days recommended
    - Bronchoscopy and lung biopsy may be needed if sputum cannot be obtained
  - Body fluids, abscesses, and tissues
    - Aseptic collection by needle aspiration or surgical procedures recommended
    - Swabs not recommended for sample collection
- **Smear microscopy**
  - Fluorochrome technique recommended
  - Acid-fast bacilli (AFB) stains (Ziehl-Neelsen, Fite-Faraco, or Kinyoun) are less sensitive
  - Useful in suggesting AM infection
  - Less sensitive and specific than culture
  - RGM are easily decolorized and may not be identified
  - Negative smears do not rule out AM, especially RGM
  - Number of organisms on smears correspond to burden of organisms in clinical material
  - Environmental contamination usually does not result in positive smear
- **Culture**
  - **Liquid (broth) media**
    - Higher yield of AM obtained
    - Results more rapid than those obtained on solid media
    - BACTEC (Becton Dickinson; Sparks, MD; USA)
    - Nonradiometric mycobacteria growth indicator tube (MGIT) (Becton Dickinson)
  - **Solid media**
    - Colony morphology, growth rates, quantitation of organisms possible
    - Identification of > 1 mycobacterial species possible
    - Supplemented for isolating fastidious species of AM
    - Used for susceptibility testing
    - Growth can be slow

- Semiquantitative (0–4) reporting of AM colony counts on solid media recommended
- Used as backup if liquid media cultures contaminated
- Lowenstein-Jensen agar
- Middlebrook 7H10 and 7H11 media
  - **Biphasic media**
    - Septi-Chek System (Becton Dickinson)
    - Provides enhanced recovery of most AM in single system
    - Results take time
  - Culture is cornerstone of diagnosis
  - Fastidious AM require special supplementation for recovery on culture
  - Optimal temperature for most cultures is 28-37°C
  - Optimal recovery of all species may require 2 sets of media at 2 incubation temperatures
  - Most AM grow within 2-3 weeks on subculture
  - *M. ulcerans* and *M. genaven*se isolation requires 8-12 weeks of incubation
- **Phenotypic testing**
  - Growth rate and pigmentation can be used for
    - Preliminary categorization
    - Guiding selection of appropriate media and incubation temperatures
  - Conventional biochemical analysis
    - Slow
    - Does not identify many newly described species
- **High-performance liquid chromatography**
  - Analyzes mycolic acid in bacterial cell walls
  - Advantages
    - Rapid, reliable method for identifying many slowly growing species of AM
    - Direct analysis of primary cultures grown in BACTEC 7H12B medium (Becton Dickinson)
    - Identification of MAI can be performed directly in samples with AFB smear–positive results
  - Disadvantages
    - Recognition of some newer species difficult
- **DNA probes**
  - Acridium ester–labeled DNA probes (AccuProbe; Gen-Probe, Inc., San Diego, CA; USA)
    - Specific for *M. avium, M. intracellulare, M. kansasii, M. gordonae*
    - Technique based on release of target 16S rRNA from organisms
    - Isolates from solid or liquid culture media used
    - Identification achieved within 2 hours
    - 100% specificity; 85-100% sensitivity
    - Limited use at present since probes available for only a few AM species
- **DNA sequence analysis**
  - Analysis of hypervariable sequences of 16S ribosomal DNA
  - Automated commercial system: MicroSeq 500 16S rDNA Bacterial Sequencing Kit (PE Applied Biosystems; Foster City, CA; USA)
  - Limitations
    - Species of recent divergence may contain highly similar 16S rRNA gene sequences
    - No exact species definition based on nucleotide sequence variation established
    - MicroSeq database has only 1 entry per species
    - Hence, isolates reported as "most closely related to" a species depend on sequence difference between the unknown isolate and database

Treatment
- Surgical approaches
  - Uncomplicated AM lymphadenitis
    - Early complete surgical excision recommended to prevent spread and cosmetic damage
    - Curative in 95% of cases of cervical lymphadenopathy in children
    - Incision and drainage not recommended since these can result in sinus tract formation
- Drugs
  - Chemotherapy recommended if
    - Surgery carries high risks in cases of discharging sinus, proximity of facial nerve branches
    - Lymphadenitis recurs after surgery
    - All involved tissue cannot be excised
  - *M. avium-intracellulare*
    - Initial regimen of azithromycin, clarithromycin, and rifabutin, or rifampin and ethambutol
    - Ciprofloxacin or ofloxacin may be added; amikacin in severe illness
  - *M. kansasii*
    - Isoniazid, rifampin, ethambutol
    - Clarithromycin, trimethoprim-sulfamethoxazole, amikacin are alternatives
  - In AIDS, recovery of immune system requires HAART

MACROSCOPIC FEATURES

General Features
- Moderately enlarged lymph nodes

MICROSCOPIC PATHOLOGY

Histologic Features
- Lymph node architecture partially or totally effaced
- Sheets of large pale histiocytes with abundant foamy cytoplasm and small nuclei
  - No pleomorphism or mitotic figures identified
- Rarely, multinucleated giant cells
- Acute inflammation can be present (suppurative)
- Few follicles
- Decreased lymphocytes
- Usually no granulomas, necrosis, calcification, fibrosis
- AFB stains: Abundant acid-fast bacilli within histiocytes
- AIDS patients may show little or no inflammatory reaction to AM infection
- Number of MAI bacilli greater in AIDS patients than in those with medical immunosuppression

Cytologic Features
- Negative imprints of AM in cell cytoplasm in Wright-Giemsa stain
- AFB stains can be performed on smears or touch imprints

ATYPICAL MYCOBACTERIAL LYMPHADENITIS

Runyon Classification of Nontuberculous Mycobacteria

Group	Growth Rate	Pigment Production
Group I (photochromogens)	Grows slowly on culture media (> 7 days)	Colony color changes from buff to bright yellow or orange color after exposure to light
Group II (scotochromogens)	Grows slowly	Demonstrates pigmented colonies when incubated in dark or light
Group III	Grows slowly	Lacks pigment in light or dark
Group IV (rapid growers)	Grows in 3-5 days	Lacks pigment

Nontuberculous Mycobacteria Causing Lymphadenitis

Species	Comments
M. avium complex	Worldwide; most common AM pathogen in USA
M. malmoense	U.K., northern Europe (especially Scandinavia)
M. scrofulaceum	Worldwide; previously common, now rarely isolated in USA
M. abscessus	Rarely isolated
M. chelonae	
M. fortuitum	
M. genavense	Fastidious species
M. haemophilum	Fastidious species
M. kansasii	Rarely isolated
M. szulgai	Rarely isolated

DIFFERENTIAL DIAGNOSIS

M. tuberculosis Lymphadenitis
- Granulomas, classically with central caseating necrosis
- Concentric layers of epithelioid cells, Langhans giant cells
- AFB stains can identify organisms
  - Typically few AFB
  - Most likely to be identified within caseous necrosis
- Auramine-rhodamine stain with fluorescent microscopy helpful to demonstrate AFB

Mycobacterial Spindle Cell Pseudotumor
- Rare entity; predominantly in young men
- History of immunosuppression, especially AIDS
- Spindle cells arranged in fascicles and storiform arrays with eosinophilic to granular cytoplasm
- Clusters of epithelioid histiocytic cells with similar cytoplasmic features
- AFB stain shows numerous bacilli within spindled and epithelioid cells

Fungal Lymphadenitis
- Early acute phase: Neutrophils, histiocytes, eosinophils
- Granulomatous phase
- PAS or GMS stains highlight organisms

Kikuchi-Fujimoto Lymphadenitis
- Necrotic areas with abundant apoptosis
- No neutrophils or granulomas present
- Sheets of crescent-shaped histiocytes
- No organisms identified by special stains

Lymphadenopathy Associated with Joint Prosthesis
- History of prosthesis implant is helpful
- No necrosis identified; AFB stains negative

DIAGNOSTIC CHECKLIST

Clinically Relevant Pathologic Features
- AM disease is defined as isolation of viable organisms plus compatible signs and symptoms
- Diagnosis of AM lymphadenitis requires either
  - Positive culture for AM or
  - Suggestive histologic findings after excluding *M. tuberculosis* infection
- In suspected AM disease, communication between clinician and laboratory is essential
  - Facilitates use of appropriate isolation protocols and laboratory safety

SELECTED REFERENCES

1. Elston D: Nontuberculous mycobacterial skin infections: recognition and management. Am J Clin Dermatol. 10(5):281-5, 2009
2. Piersimoni C et al: Extrapulmonary infections associated with nontuberculous mycobacteria in immunocompetent persons. Emerg Infect Dis. 15(9):1351-8; quiz 1544, 2009
3. Jarzembowski JA et al: Nontuberculous mycobacterial infections. Arch Pathol Lab Med. 132(8):1333-41, 2008
4. Evans MJ et al: Atypical mycobacterial lymphadenitis in childhood--a clinicopathological study of 17 cases. J Clin Pathol. 51(12):925-7, 1998

ATYPICAL MYCOBACTERIAL LYMPHADENITIS

Microscopic Features

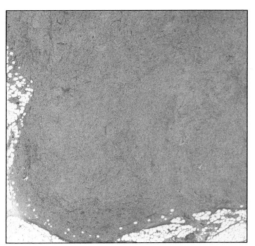
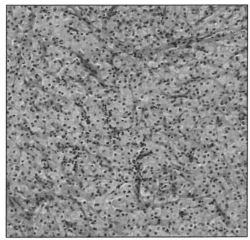

(Left) Lymph node in patient with AIDS demonstrates M. avium-intracellulare infection. The architecture is totally effaced with no intact follicles or lymphocytes appreciated. Sheets of large pale histiocytes with a storiform pattern are present. No granulomas, necrosis, or fibrosis is identified. *(Right)* Lymph node in an AIDS patient with M. avium-intracellulare infection shows numerous histiocytes with abundant foamy cytoplasm; no pleomorphism or mitotic figures are identified.

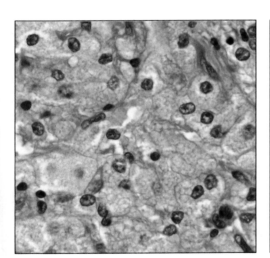
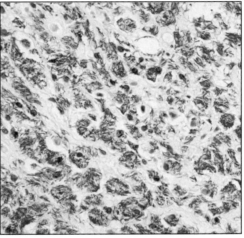

(Left) High-power magnification (oil immersion) of lymph node in an AIDS patient with M. avium-intracellulare (MAI) infection shows small, bland nuclei and the abundant foamy cytoplasm of the histiocytes. *(Right)* Acid-fast stain of lymph node in an AIDS patient with M. avium-intracellulare infection demonstrates abundant acid-fast bacilli within histiocytes. MAI bacilli are typically abundant in infected AIDS patients. The organisms are stained red in this preparation.

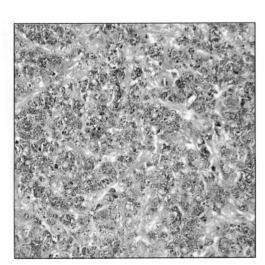
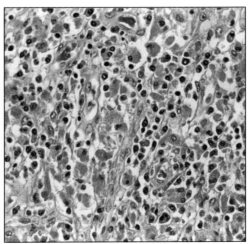

(Left) Gomori methenamine silver stain of lymph node in AIDS patient with M. avium-intracellulare infection demonstrates abundant acid-fast bacilli within histiocytes. Organisms are stained black in this preparation. *(Right)* Lymph node in AIDS patient with M. avium-intracellulare infection demonstrates totally effaced architecture and abundant plump histiocytes. No granuloma formation or necrosis is present. (Courtesy E. Ewing, Jr., MD, CDC Public Health Image Library, #964.)

Infectious Causes of Lymphadenitis

ATYPICAL MYCOBACTERIAL LYMPHADENITIS

Differential Diagnosis

(Left) Lymph node involved by M. tuberculosis reveals granulomatous inflammation and extensive caseating necrosis. Concentric layers of epithelioid cells, Langhans giant cells ➡, lymphocytes, plasma cells, and fibroblasts are also present. **(Right)** Lymph node involved by M. tuberculosis shows granulomatous inflammation. Concentric layers of epithelioid cells, Langhans giant cells ➡, lymphocytes, plasma cells, and fibroblasts are present. Caseation is not shown in this field.

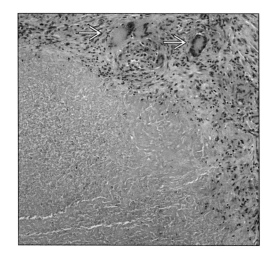
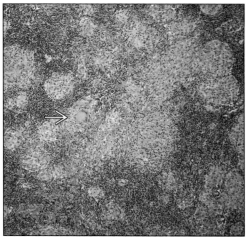

(Left) Mycobacterial spindle cell pseudotumor of lymph node demonstrates spindle-shaped cells with bland nuclei, ill-defined cytoplasmic processes, and eosinophilic, granular cytoplasm. Focal epithelioid histiocytic cells and scattered lymphocytes are also noted. **(Right)** Mycobacterial spindle cell pseudotumor of lymph node demonstrates sheets of epithelioid histiocytic cells with foamy cytoplasm in focal areas. Occasional multinucleated giant cells are noted.

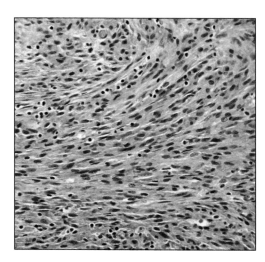
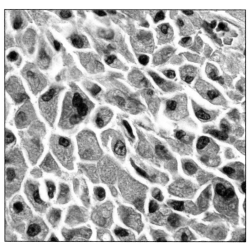

(Left) Acid-fast stain of mycobacterial spindle cell pseudotumor involving lymph node highlights abundant acid-fast bacilli within spindled and epithelioid histiocytes. **(Right)** Granulomatous phase of coccidioidomycosis lymphadenitis demonstrates a dense chronic inflammatory infiltrate composed of lymphocytes and histiocytes in a background of marked vascular proliferation. Note the multinucleated giant cells ➡.

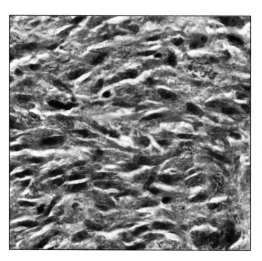
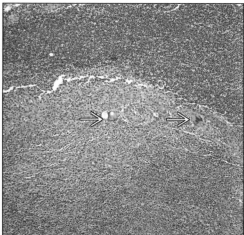

ATYPICAL MYCOBACTERIAL LYMPHADENITIS

Differential Diagnosis

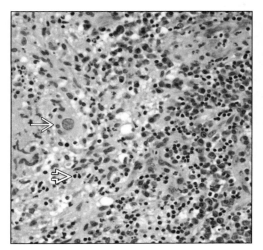

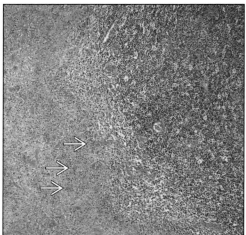

(Left) Granulomatous phase of coccidioidomycosis lymphadenitis demonstrates a mixed lymphoplasmacytic and histiocytic infiltrate. Note spherule containing endospores ➡ and focal neutrophilic reaction ⇒. *(Right)* Lymph node in Kikuchi-Fujimoto lymphadenitis demonstrates effacement with extensive necrosis. Blood vessels within the necrotic area and at the periphery are thrombosed ➡.

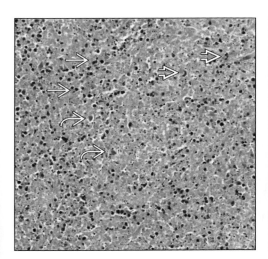

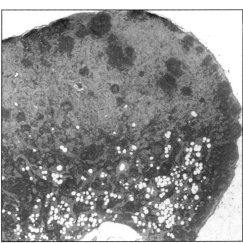

(Left) Lymph node in Kikuchi-Fujimoto lymphadenitis shows necrosis with nuclear fragments ➡. Histiocytes with abundant pale cytoplasm, some with crescentic nuclei, are present ⇒. No neutrophils or eosinophils are seen. Note scattered eosinophilic fibrinoid deposits ➡. *(Right)* Lymphadenopathy in a patient with femur prosthesis with multiple revisions. Markedly distended sinuses filled with sheets of large, foamy histiocytes are present.

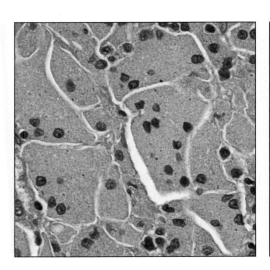

(Left) Lymphadenopathy associated with a joint prosthesis at high-power magnification demonstrates sheets of large histiocytes with bland nuclei and markedly foamy cytoplasm. This is essentially a foreign body reaction to prosthesis debris. *(Right)* Lymphadenopathy associated with a joint prosthesis examined under polarized light demonstrates birefringent small particles within the histiocytes.

MYCOBACTERIAL SPINDLE CELL PSEUDOTUMOR

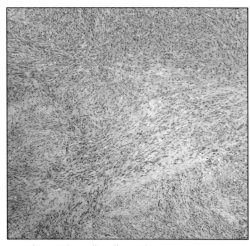

Mycobacterial spindle cell pseudotumor involving lymph node. Fascicles and storiform arrays of spindle cells efface nodal architecture.

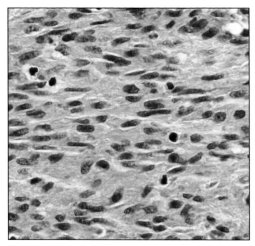

Mycobacterial spindle cell pseudotumor involving lymph node. Fascicles of spindle cells and scattered small lymphocytes are present. Note bland-appearing nuclei and eosinophilic granularity of cytoplasm.

TERMINOLOGY

Definitions
- Tumor-like lesion composed of elongated spindle cells infected by *Mycobacterium avium-intracellulare* (MAI)

ETIOLOGY/PATHOGENESIS

Infectious Agents
- *Mycobacterium avium-intracellulare*
- Cause of distinctive tumor-like appearance is unknown

CLINICAL ISSUES

Epidemiology
- Incidence
  - Rare entity; ~ 20 cases reported in literature
  - Occur in immunocompromised patients
    - Particularly in those with acquired immunodeficiency syndrome (AIDS)
- Age
  - Predominantly affects young individuals
- Gender
  - Predominantly affects males

Site
- Lymph nodes most common
- Other sites: Spleen, skin, bone marrow, lung, and brain

Laboratory Tests
- Traditional media
  - Lowenstein-Jensen media
  - Agar-based Middlebrook medium
  - Growth of organisms is slow
    - Visible colony growth can take up to 6 weeks
- Liquid media (growth takes ~ 2 weeks)
  - BACTEC
  - Mycobacteria growth indicator tubes

Treatment
- Drugs
  - HIV(+): Clarithromycin or azithromycin + ethambutol
  - HIV(-): Clarithromycin or azithromycin plus rifampin or rifabutin and ethambutol

Prognosis
- Anti-MAI drugs are effective, particularly if immunosuppression can be reversed

IMAGE FINDINGS

Radiographic Findings
- Lymphadenopathy

MICROSCOPIC PATHOLOGY

Histologic Features
- Lymph node architecture effaced by elongated spindle cells (histiocytes)
  - Arranged in short fascicles and storiform arrays
- Histiocytes have bland nuclei, eosinophilic to granular cytoplasm
- Admixed small lymphocytes
- No significant mitotic activity
- Acid-fast (Ziehl-Neelsen) stain demonstrates numerous bacilli within cells

Cytologic Features
- In Wright-Giemsa touch imprints
  - Bland histiocytes
  - Negative outlines of MAI bacilli in cytoplasm

Immunohistochemistry
- Both spindled and epithelioid cells express
  - CD68, lysozyme

MYCOBACTERIAL SPINDLE CELL PSEUDOTUMOR

Key Facts

Clinical Issues
- Rare entity; predominantly in young men
- History of immunosuppression and HIV infection

Microscopic Pathology
- Spindle cells arranged in fascicles and storiform arrays with eosinophilic to granular cytoplasm
- Clusters of epithelioid histiocytic cells with similar cytoplasmic features
- Acid-fast stain shows numerous bacilli within spindled and epithelioid cells
- CD68(+), lysozyme(+), vimentin(+)
- CD31(-), CD34(-)

Ancillary Tests
- Culture essential for confirmation

Top Differential Diagnoses
- Kaposi sarcoma
  - Slit-like spaces with erythrocyte extravasation
  - Cytoplasmic eosinophilic globules
  - Presence of mitoses
  - Human herpes virus 8(+)
  - CD31(+), CD34(+)
- Palisaded myofibroblastoma
  - Amianthoid fibers, scattered hemorrhagic foci, pseudocapsule
  - Smooth muscle actin(+), myosin(+), vimentin(+)
- Inflammatory pseudotumor of lymph node
  - Hilum, trabeculae, and capsule of lymph node
  - Abundant lymphocytes, plasma cells, neutrophils
  - Vascular proliferation, flattened endothelial cells

- α-chymotrypsin, vimentin
- S100, desmin(+/-), actin(+/-)
- CD31(-), CD34(-)

DIFFERENTIAL DIAGNOSIS

Kaposi Sarcoma
- Also can occur in HIV(+) patients (skin, lymph nodes)
- Histologic features
  - Prominent fascicular arrangement of spindle cells
  - Slit-like spaces with extravasation of erythrocytes
  - Eosinophilic hyaline globules in cytoplasm
  - Mitoses present and often numerous
- Immunohistochemistry
  - Human herpes virus 8(+)
  - CD31(+), CD34(+)
  - CD68(-), lysozyme(-), S100(-)

Palisaded Myofibroblastoma
- No history of immunosuppression
- Usually solitary, painless mass in inguinal region
- Histologic features
  - Palisading slender, spindle-shaped cells
  - Nuclei tapered with no atypia
  - Stellate deposits of collagen (amianthoid fibers)
  - Pseudocapsule surrounds tumor
  - Focal hemorrhage, rare mitoses
- Immunohistochemistry
  - Smooth muscle actin(+), myosin(+), vimentin(+)
  - Keratin(-), S100(-), FVIIIRAg(-), synaptophysin(-)

Inflammatory Pseudotumor of Lymph Nodes
- No history of immunosuppression
- Patients may have fever, night sweats
- Anemia, hypergammaglobulinemia
- Localized or generalized lymphadenopathy
  - Can persist for weeks to years; often spontaneous remission
  - Often matted lymph nodes adherent to adjacent structures
- Histologic features

- Involves primarily hilum, trabeculae, and capsule of lymph node
  - Histiocytic and fibroblastic spindle-shaped cells
  - Abundant lymphocytes, plasma cells, & neutrophils
  - Vascular proliferation with flattened endothelial cells
  - Infrequent mitoses, no cytologic atypia, no necrosis
  - End stage: Predominantly dense sclerosis
- Immunohistochemistry
  - Vimentin(+), histiocytic markers ([+/-], often focal)
  - FXIIIA(-), CD34(-)

DIAGNOSTIC CHECKLIST

Pathologic Interpretation Pearls
- Eosinophilic and granular cytoplasm of spindle cells is clue for diagnosis

SELECTED REFERENCES

1. Shiomi T et al: Mycobacterial spindle cell pseudotumor of the skin. J Cutan Pathol. 34(4):346-51, 2007
2. Gunia S et al: Mycobacterial spindle cell pseudotumor (MSP) of the nasal septum clinically mimicking Kaposi's sarcoma: case report. Rhinology. 43(1):70-1, 2005
3. Basilio-de-Oliveira C et al: Mycobacterial spindle cell pseudotumor of the appendix vermiformis in a patient with aids. Braz J Infect Dis. 5(2):98-100, 2001
4. Logani S et al: Spindle cell tumors associated with mycobacteria in lymph nodes of HIV-positive patients: 'Kaposi sarcoma with mycobacteria' and 'mycobacterial pseudotumor'. Am J Surg Pathol. 23(6):656-61, 1999
5. Morrison A et al: Mycobacterial spindle cell pseudotumor of the brain: a case report and review of the literature. Am J Surg Pathol. 23(10):1294-9, 1999
6. Wolf DA et al: Mycobacterial pseudotumors of lymph node. A report of two cases diagnosed at the time of intraoperative consultation using touch imprint preparations. Arch Pathol Lab Med. 119(9):811-4, 1995
7. Suster S et al: Mycobacterial spindle-cell pseudotumor of the spleen. Am J Clin Pathol. 101(4):539-42, 1994

LYMPHOGRANULOMA VENEREUM LYMPHADENITIS

Key Facts

Terminology
- Lymphogranuloma venereum (LGV)
- Sexually transmitted disease caused by L1, L2, and L3 serovars of *Chlamydia trachomatis*

Etiology/Pathogenesis
- Obligatory intracellular gram-negative bacterium
- LGV primarily induces lymphoproliferative reaction that extends from primary site to draining LNs

Clinical Issues
- Inoculation site is skin of penis or mucous membranes of vagina, vulva, or rectum
- LNs became enlarged 1-8 weeks after inoculation
- In women, internal lymphadenopathy may lead to chronic pelvic lymphangitis

- *Chlamydia trachomatis* organisms can be isolated and grown in McCoy or HeLa cell lines
- Doxycycline for 3 weeks is preferred therapy

Microscopic Pathology
- Suppurative granuloma with star shape

Ancillary Tests
- PCR can amplify chlamydial DNA from various clinical specimens including urine
- Complement fixation with a titer above 1:256 is considered significant

Top Differential Diagnoses
- Cat scratch disease lymphadenitis
- Tularemia lymphadenitis
- Suppurative lymphadenitis

- Unilateral and less frequently bilateral lymphadenopathy
- Inguinal LNs drain male genitalia whereas deep pelvic or perianal LNs drain cervix
- "Groove" sign occurs when enlarged inguinal and femoral LNs protrude against inguinal ligament
- LN suppurative inflammation may extend to perinodal tissue leading to chronic sinus formation
  ○ In women, internal lymphadenopathy can lead to chronic pelvic lymphangitis
    - Lymphatic obstruction may result in chronic vulvar edema and rectal strictures
- Systemic manifestations occur in 60% of patients
  ○ e.g., fever, myalgia, and headache
- Extragenital involvement may also occur in synovium, heart, lungs, and central nervous system
- Proctitis occurs among homosexual men
  ○ Recent outbreaks among homosexual men in western European countries and North America
  ○ Proctocolitis with fistulae and strictures are common
- Late complications include scarring of inguinal LNs and elephantiasis; infertility, fistulas, and strictures

Laboratory Tests
- *Chlamydia trachomatis* organisms can be isolated and grown in McCoy or HeLa cell lines
  ○ ~ 30% yield from lymph node aspirates
  ○ Low yield from genital ulcers
    - Intracytoplasmic inclusions appear in 2-3 days and can be confirmed with immunofluorescent antibodies
  ○ *Chlamydia* cultures are not usually available outside referral centers

Treatment
- Doxycycline for 3 weeks is preferred therapy
- Therapy cures disease and prevents further tissue damage

Prognosis
- Excellent if treated early; scarring and fistula formation with progressive disease
  ○ Untreated infection can persist and contribute to transmission of infection

MICROSCOPIC PATHOLOGY

Histologic Features
- Early lesion
  ○ Small foci of necrosis and accumulation of neutrophils
- Progressive lesion
  ○ Distinct histiocytes with small or confluent cytoplasmic vacuoles
    - Vacuoles up to 40 μm in diameter
    - Number of vacuoles with microorganisms is variable, and some cases show only rare vacuoles
    - *Chlamydia trachomatis* organisms are 0.2-2 μm in diameter
    - Organisms are larger at periphery of vacuole (reticulate bodies) and smaller in center (elementary bodies)
    - Organisms may be visible with routine hematoxylin and eosin stain
  ○ Lymphocytes and plasma cells surround foci of necrosis
  ○ Clusters of monocytoid B cells may be seen in subcapsular or paratrabecular sinuses
  ○ Coalescence of necrotic foci to render stellate shape
    - Central necrosis admixed with fragmented neutrophils
    - Surrounded by palisading epithelioid histiocytes and few giant cells
- Suppurative lesions may form sinus tracts or become encircled by thick collagen
  ○ Intima of trapped blood vessels may thicken with eventual vascular obliteration
- Late events include collagen fibrosis of LN capsule and perinodal soft tissue

LYMPHOGRANULOMA VENEREUM LYMPHADENITIS

Cytologic Features
- Aspirate from LNs can be examined by immunofluorescence for presence of inclusion bodies
  - Not a sensitive test

ANCILLARY TESTS

Histochemistry
- Giemsa stain highlights light blue bacteria within vacuoles
- Warthin-Starry stain highlights dark, small, round microorganisms within vacuoles
- Brown-Hopp-Gram stain highlights red to violet microorganisms

PCR
- PCR can amplify chlamydial DNA from various clinical specimens including urine
  - Amplification of fragment of 16S ribosomal gene with subsequent sequencing
    - Allows for identification of microorganisms
    - 85% sensitive and 95% specific

Serologic Testing
- Complement fixation, microimmunofluorescence, or counterimmunoelectrophoresis can be used
  - Complement fixation titers above 1:256 are considered significant
  - Serologic tests do not identify serotypes
    - Thus, positive test needs to be correlated with clinical syndrome
- Frei test: Delayed-type skin reaction to inoculation of killed organisms grown in yolk sac
  - Positive test indicates previous exposure to *Chlamydia* antigen
    - Reactivity can persist for years
    - This test is obsolete

Electron Microscopy
- Elementary and reticulate bodies can be identified within vacuoles of macrophages
  - Organisms are 0.2-1.9 μm in diameter and may be admixed with glycogen vacuoles

DIFFERENTIAL DIAGNOSIS

Cat Scratch Disease Lymphadenitis
- Morphologically indistinguishable from LGV lymphadenitis at suppurative stage
- Clinical history of exposure to cat scratch is usually important for diagnosis
  - Serology, immunohistochemistry, and PCR may be necessary to distinguish these infections

Tularemia Lymphadenitis
- Morphologically similar to LGV
- Clinical history, sexual history, sites, circumstances, serologic and PCR testing may be necessary

Suppurative Lymphadenitis
- Infection of LNs by any number of bacteria
- Acute inflammation, necrosis, &/or abscess
- Gram stain and cultures needed to identify etiology

Tuberculous Lymphadenitis
- Necrosis is usually caseous and not stellate-shaped
- Acute inflammation (neutrophils) is usually not present
- Acid-fast stains and culture helpful to establish etiology

DIAGNOSTIC CHECKLIST

Clinically Relevant Pathologic Features
- Sexually transmitted disease

Pathologic Interpretation Pearls
- Stellate suppurative granulomatous inflammation
  - *Chlamydia trachomatis* microorganisms may be found in vacuoles within macrophages

SELECTED REFERENCES

1. Moncada J et al: Evaluation of self-collected glans and rectal swabs from men who have sex with men for detection of Chlamydia trachomatis and Neisseria gonorrhoeae by use of nucleic acid amplification tests. J Clin Microbiol. 47(6):1657-62, 2009
2. Richardson D et al: Lymphogranuloma venereum: an emerging cause of proctitis in men who have sex with men. Int J STD AIDS. 2007 Jan;18(1):11-4; quiz 15. Review. Erratum in: Int J STD AIDS. 18(4):292, 2007
3. Ward H et al: Lymphogranuloma venereum in the United kingdom. Clin Infect Dis. 44(1):26-32, 2007
4. Darville T: Chlamydia trachomatis genital infection in adolescents and young adults. Adv Exp Med Biol. 582:85-100, 2006
5. Cook RL et al: Systematic review: noninvasive testing for Chlamydia trachomatis and Neisseria gonorrhoeae. Ann Intern Med. 142(11):914-25, 2005
6. Morré SA et al: Molecular diagnosis of lymphogranuloma venereum: PCR-based restriction fragment length polymorphism and real-time PCR. J Clin Microbiol. 43(10):5412-3; author reply 5412-3, 2005
7. Kohl KS et al: Developments in the screening for Chlamydia trachomatis: a review. Obstet Gynecol Clin North Am. 30(4):637-58, 2003
8. Hadfield TL et al: Demonstration of Chlamydia trachomatis in inguinal lymphadenitis of lymphogranuloma venereum: a light microscopy, electron microscopy and polymerase chain reaction study. Mod Pathol. 8(9):924-9, 1995
9. Joseph AK et al: Laboratory techniques used in the diagnosis of chancroid, granuloma inguinale, and lymphogranuloma venereum. Dermatol Clin. 12(1):1-8, 1994
10. Martin DH et al: Dermatologic manifestations of sexually transmitted diseases other than HIV. Infect Dis Clin North Am. 8(3):533-82, 1994
11. Brunham RC et al: Mucopurulent cervicitis--the ignored counterpart in women of urethritis in men. N Engl J Med. 311(1):1-6, 1984
12. Thorsteinsson SB: Lymphogranuloma venereum: review of clinical manifestations, epidemiology, diagnosis, and treatment. Scand J Infect Dis Suppl. 32:127-31, 1982

LYMPHOGRANULOMA VENEREUM LYMPHADENITIS

Microscopic Features

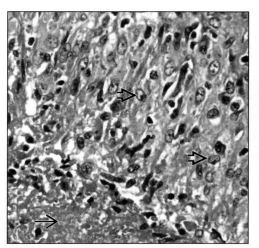

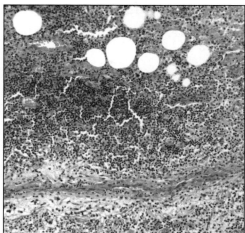

(Left) Edge of a necrotizing granuloma in LGV. Histiocytes arranged in a palisading pattern display vesicular nuclei ⭢ and indistinct pink cytoplasm. Necrosis appears as granular ⭢, amorphous material. **(Right)** Hematoxylin and eosin stain shows LGV with suppuration beyond the lymph node into perinodal adipose tissue as a result of fistula formation and scarring.

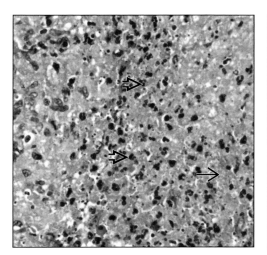

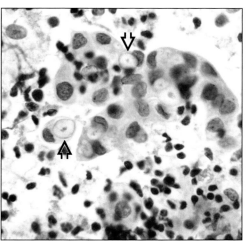

(Left) High magnification at the center of a necrotizing granuloma of LGV shows nuclear fragmentation of neutrophils ⭢ and granular necrosis ⭢. **(Right)** Papanicolaou stain of uterine cervix displays epithelial cells with vacuoles ⭢ suspicious for Chlamydia trachomatis infection. These vacuoles are similar to those seen in histiocytes of LGV; however, serovars D to K infect the cervix. (Courtesy N. Quintanilla, MD.)

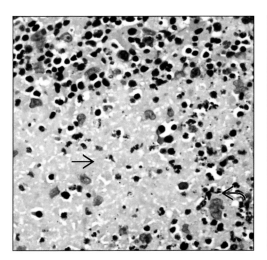

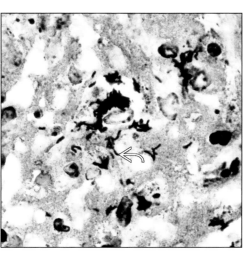

(Left) Necrotizing granuloma of cat scratch disease shows a mixture of granular necrosis ⭢ and karyorrhexis ⭢. **(Right)** Warthin-Starry stain of a lymph node involved by cat scratch disease can be useful in the diagnosis of necrotizing granulomas. This stain can highlight L-shaped bacteria ⭢ individually or in clusters in cat scratch disease but is negative in LGV.

WHIPPLE DISEASE

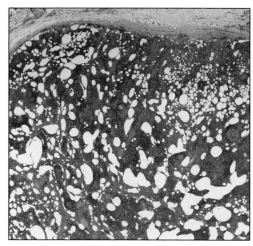

Whipple disease involving mesenteric lymph node. The nodal architecture is obscured by ill-defined lipogranulomas and cystic spaces.

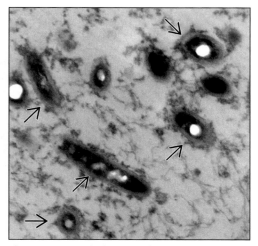

Electron micrograph shows Tropheryma whipplei bacilli (50 to 500 nm) with the characteristic trilaminar cell wall ⇥.

TERMINOLOGY

Synonyms
- Intestinal lipodystrophy

Definitions
- Systemic disease caused by *Tropheryma whipplei* infection

ETIOLOGY/PATHOGENESIS

Infectious Agents
- *T. whipplei*, gram-positive bacilli related to *Actinomycetes*
  - Found primarily in soil and sewage but not in animal hosts
- *T. whipplei* are intracellular organisms
  - Primarily engulfed by and reside within tissue macrophages
  - Can also reside within intestinal epithelial cells and endothelial cells
  - Organism exerts no visible cytotoxic effects upon host cells
- *T. whipplei*: Systemic infection can affect many organs

Host Immune Deficiency Likely Involved in Pathogenesis
- Possibly, immune downregulation is induced by bacterium
- Human host shows remarkable lack of inflammatory response to bacilli
  - Massive accumulation of *T. whipplei* at sites of infection

CLINICAL ISSUES

Epidemiology
- Incidence

- Whipple disease is extremely rare
  - ~ 1,500 cases reported in literature
  - Incidence of ~ 30 cases per year
  - Farmers and persons with occupational exposure to soil or animals have highest incidence
  - Humans remain only known host for disease
  - No evidence exists of person-to-person transmission
    - No outbreaks have been reported
- Age
  - Middle-aged and elderly persons; mean age: 40 years
- Gender
  - M:F = ~ 8-9:1
- Ethnicity
  - North America and Western Europe

Presentation
- Arthralgias, often migratory
  - Large joints more often affected than small joints
  - Rheumatoid factor negative
  - Can precede gastrointestinal symptoms
- Weight loss
- Diarrhea, steatorrhea, abdominal pain
- Central nervous system (CNS) disease
  - Cognitive dysfunction and dementia
  - Oculomasticatory or oculo-facial-skeletal myorhythmia
  - Headache, seizures (focal or generalized)
  - Cerebellar ataxia
  - Psychiatric changes
- Endocarditis
  - Culture negative
- Marked mesenteric and periaortic lymphadenopathy
  - Enlargement of peripheral lymph nodes may occur early

Laboratory Tests
- Cell-free culture of organism has not been achieved
- PCR using primers common to DNA encoding unique bacterial 16S ribosomal RNA is standard test
  - Can test *T. whipplei* in fresh or formalin-fixed tissue

WHIPPLE DISEASE

Key Facts

Etiology/Pathogenesis
- *T. whipplei*, gram-positive bacilli related to *Actinomycetes*
  - Engulfed by tissue macrophages
  - Systemic disease; affects many organ systems
  - Exerts no visible cytotoxic effects upon host cells
- Human host shows remarkable lack of inflammatory response to bacilli

Clinical Issues
- Whipple disease is extremely rare, incidence ~ 30 cases per year
  - Affects predominantly middle-aged white men
  - Farmers and people with occupational exposure to soil or animals have highest incidence

- Laboratory testing: PCR using primers common to DNA encoding unique bacterial 16S ribosomal RNA is standard test
- Treatment: General recommendation is intravenous ceftriaxone x 2 weeks
  - Followed by oral co-trimoxazole or oral trimethoprim-sulfamethoxazole x 1-2 years

Microscopic Pathology
- Histiocytes/macrophages containing undigested bacteria or remnants of bacterial wall
  - DPAS(+), acid-fast(-), specific antibody to *T. whipplei* can be used for immunohistochemistry

Top Differential Diagnoses
- Lysosomal storage disorders, mycobacterial infection, malabsorption syndrome

---

- Test various tissue types: CSF, vitreous fluid, cardiac valves, synovial fluid
- Can be used for treatment monitoring
- Anemia; elevated erythrocyte sedimentation rate (ESR)
- Low serum levels of carotene and albumin
- Other laboratory tests are nonspecific but necessary to exclude other diseases, including
  - Hyperthyroidism
  - Connective tissue disease
  - Inflammatory bowel disease with migratory polyarthropathy
  - Acquired immunodeficiency syndrome (AIDS)

Treatment
- Drugs
  - Antibiotics
    - Intravenous ceftriaxone or penicillin to achieve high CSF levels followed by oral trimethoprim-sulfamethoxazole (TMP-SMX)
    - Followed by oral co-trimoxazole or trimethoprim-sulfamethoxazole (TMP-SMX) x 1-2 years
    - For sulfa allergic patients, alternative maintenance therapy is doxycycline (100 mg PO 2x daily) in combination with hydroxychloroquine
    - For ceftriaxone and penicillin-allergic patients, TMP-SMX plus streptomycin
    - Treatment is based on observations in small patient groups and personal experience
  - Addition of recombinant human interferon-γ might be beneficial

Prognosis
- Whipple disease was uniformly fatal prior to availability of antibiotics
- Most adequately treated patients do well
- Relapses have been reported in as many as 17-35% of patients
- CNS involvement is very difficult to manage
  - Can persist despite antibiotic therapy

IMAGE FINDINGS

Radiographic Findings
- Gastrointestinal findings
  - Upper endoscopy: Bowel dilatation ± prominent mucosal folds of duodenum and jejunum
  - Barium enema: Dilatation of proximal ileum, stomach with thickened nodular folds, and possibly edema of colon
  - Findings are nonspecific; can be found in other diseases such as celiac sprue and lymphoma
- CT scan and MR: Enlarged retroperitoneal and mediastinal lymph nodes
- Neuroimaging (CT scan and MR): Largely nonspecific
  - Atrophy, hydrocephalus, mass lesions with contrast enhancement, ring-enhancing lesions
  - White matter changes suggestive of demyelination

MICROSCOPIC PATHOLOGY

Histologic Features
- Small bowel biopsy
  - Submucosal foamy histiocytes containing mucin and PAS(+) material
    - PAS(+) material is diastase resistant (DPAS)
    - Gram(+), Gomori silver(+), acid-fast(-)
  - Admixed inflammatory infiltrate composed of neutrophils, eosinophils, and lymphocytes can be present
  - Villous shortening can be seen
  - Changes of malakoplakia have been reported
- Lymph node
  - Nodal architecture is obscured by ill-defined lipogranulomas
  - Cystic spaces are often present
  - Giant cells may be seen
  - Necrosis is often absent
  - Associated monoclonal B-cell proliferation or lymphoma has been described
- CNS

WHIPPLE DISEASE

- o Periaqueductal gray matter, hypothalamus, hippocampus, basal ganglia, cerebellum, and cerebral cortex
- o DPAS(+) macrophages surrounded by large reactive astrocytes
- o DPAS(+) cells may extend into white matter and lead to demyelination and neuronal death
- Cardiac valves
  - o Significant fibrosis
  - o Foamy macrophages with mild inflammation
  - o Lack of calcifications
  - o Vegetations

Predominant Pattern/Injury Type

- Histiocytes/macrophages containing undigested bacteria or remnants of bacterial wall

Predominant Cell/Compartment Type

- Large polygonal histiocytes and macrophages with foamy cytoplasm (amphophilic gray-pink color)
  - o Cytoplasm is PAS positive, diastase resistant

ANCILLARY TESTS

Immunohistochemistry

- Antibody specific for *T. whipplei* is available
- Histiocytes: CD68(+), other histiocyte-associated antigens(+)

Electron Microscopy

- Rod-shaped bacilli ranging from 50-500 nm in diameter with trilaminar wall

DIFFERENTIAL DIAGNOSIS

Lysosomal Storage Disorders, PAS(+)

- Fabry disease
  - o Intracellular accumulation of galabiosylceramide (ceramide trihexoside) and digalactosyl ceramide
  - o Involves skin, renal glomeruli, and tubular epithelium, blood vessels, corneal epithelium, myocardium, and ganglion cells
- Gaucher disease
  - o Histiocytes with abundant, finely fibrillar, pale blue-gray cytoplasm that is crinkled or wrinkled paper-like
  - o Confirm diagnosis with absence of glucocerebrosidase in peripheral blood monocytes

Mycobacterium tuberculosis

- Caseating granulomas with Langhans-type giant cells
- PAS(-), acid-fast(+)

Mycobacterium avium-intracellulare

- Granulomas often ill defined, irregular, or serpiginous, with variable plasma cells and neutrophils
- PAS(+), acid-fast(+)

DDx Related to Malabsorption in GI Tract

- Abetalipoproteinemia
  - o Marked fat vacuoles in apical villous cytoplasm
  - o Fat stains highlight lipid vacuoles

- Agammaglobulinemic sprue
  - o No plasma cells in lamina propria
- Disaccharidase (lactase) deficiency
  - o Serum enzyme measurement
- Intestinal lymphangiectasia
  - o Dilated lymphatic channels cause protein-rich fluid in lamina propria and intestinal lumen; causes protein-losing enteropathy

DIAGNOSTIC CHECKLIST

Pathologic Interpretation Pearls

- Systemic disease caused by *Tropheryma whipplei*
- Histiocytes/macrophages contain undigested bacteria or remnants of bacterial wall
  - o DPAS(+), acid-fast(-)
  - o PCR using primers common to DNA encoding unique bacterial 16S ribosomal RNA is standard test
  - o Immunohistochemistry stain using specific antibody to *T. whipplei*
- Lymph node architecture is obscured by ill-defined lipogranulomas
  - o Cases associated with monoclonal B-cell proliferation and lymphoma have been reported
- Differential diagnosis includes
  - o Storage diseases
  - o Mycobacterial infection
  - o GI malabsorption

SELECTED REFERENCES

1. Buckle MJ et al: Neurologically presenting Whipple disease: case report and review of the literature. J Clin Pathol. 61(10):1140-1, 2008
2. Fenollar F et al: Whipple's disease. N Engl J Med. 356(1):55-66, 2007
3. Moreillon P et al: Infective endocarditis. Lancet. 363(9403):139-49, 2004
4. Marth T et al: Whipple's disease. Lancet. 361(9353):239-46, 2003
5. Wang S et al: Systemic Tropheryma whippleii infection associated with monoclonal B-cell proliferation: a Helicobacter pylori-type pathogenesis? Arch Pathol Lab Med. 127(12):1619-22, 2003
6. Gerard A et al: Neurologic presentation of Whipple disease: report of 12 cases and review of the literature. Medicine (Baltimore). 81(6):443-57, 2002
7. Gruner U et al: [Whipple disease and non-Hodgkin lymphoma.] Z Gastroenterol. 39(4):305-9, 2001
8. Walter R et al: Bone marrow involvement in Whipple's disease: rarely reported, but really rare? Br J Haematol. 112(3):677-9, 2001
9. Misbah SA et al: Whipple's disease revisited. J Clin Pathol. 53(10):750-5, 2000
10. Gillen CD et al: Extraintestinal lymphoma in association with Whipple's disease. Gut. 34(11):1627-9, 1993

WHIPPLE DISEASE

Microscopic Features

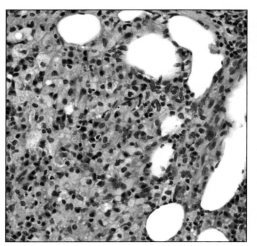

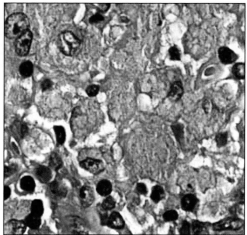

(Left) *Numerous histiocytes with abundant foamy cytoplasm and loosely formed granulomas are admixed with other inflammatory cells.* **(Right)** *The foamy histiocytes contain abundant intracytoplasmic amphophilic material with a bluish hue.*

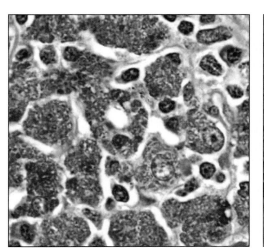

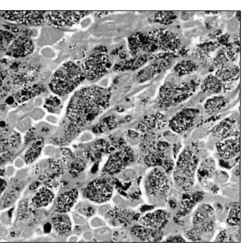

(Left) *The foamy histiocytes contain abundant intracytoplasmic diastase-resistant periodic acid–Schiff (DPAS)–positive material, consistent with undigested Tropheryma whipplei bacilli and remnants.* **(Right)** *Gomori methenamine silver stain shows that the Tropheryma whipplei bacilli cell walls are also positive.*

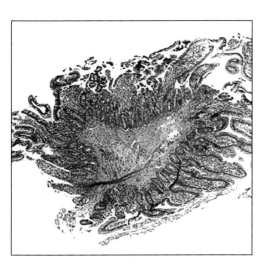

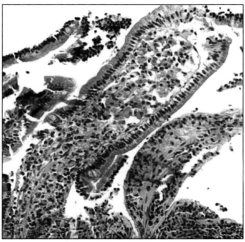

(Left) *Duodenal endoscopic biopsy in patient with Whipple disease shows the villous architecture is well maintained in this specimen.* **(Right)** *High-power magnification of biopsy shows the laminar propria is packed with histiocytes that contain foamy cytoplasm with a bluish hue. This material was PAS(+) and diastase resistant (not shown).*

SYPHILITIC LYMPHADENITIS

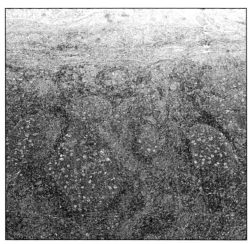

Inguinal lymph node involved by syphilis. There is pericapsular inflammation and fibrosis associated with marked follicular hyperplasia.

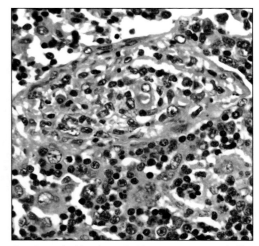

A pericapsular blood vessel with arteritis is surrounded by an inflammatory infiltrate rich in plasma cells. The plasma cells are polytypic.

TERMINOLOGY

Synonyms
- Luetic lymphadenitis, lues

Definitions
- Lymphadenitis in course of syphilis
  - Syphilis: Chronic systemic infection caused by *Treponema pallidum* (*T. pallidum*)
    - Infection usually sexually transmitted, characterized by periods of active disease and latency

ETIOLOGY/PATHOGENESIS

Infectious Agents
- *T. pallidum* is gram-negative spirochete
- At least 4 known subspecies
  - *T. pallidum pallidum*: Causes syphilis
  - *T. pallidum pertenue*: Causes yaws
  - *T. pallidum carateum*: Causes pinta
  - *T. pallidum endemicum*: Causes endemic syphilis or bejel
- *T. pallidum* is slender, spiral organism 5-15 μm long and 0.2 μm thick
  - Cannot be cultured in vitro
  - Human is only known natural host

CLINICAL ISSUES

Presentation
- 3 stages of disease course
  - Primary syphilis
    - Chancre: Usually 1 painless papule that becomes eroded/indurated; lesion heals within 6 weeks
    - Regional (usually inguinal) lymphadenopathy within 1 week of onset

    - Unilateral or bilateral; usually nonsuppurative and painless
    - Lymphadenopathy may persist for months
  - Secondary syphilis
    - Generalized nontender lymphadenopathy
    - Localized or diffuse mucocutaneous lesions (nonpruritic skin rashes)
    - Constitutional symptoms: Sore throat, fever, weight loss, malaise, anorexia
  - Tertiary syphilis
    - In industrialized countries, tertiary disease is nearly eliminated
    - Most common type before antibiotic era
    - Gumma (skin and skeletal system): Granulomatous lesion with central area of necrosis due to endarteritis obliterans
    - Cardiovascular syphilis (usually involving vasa vasorum of ascending aorta)
    - Symptomatic neurosyphilis (tabes dorsalis and paresis)

Laboratory Tests
- 2 types of serologic tests: Nontreponemal and treponemal
  - Nontreponemal antibody tests: Rapid plasma reagin and venereal disease research laboratory tests (screening)
    - Measures IgG and IgM antibodies directed against cardiolipin-lecithin-cholesterol antigen complex
  - Treponemal tests (fluorescent treponemal antibody-absorbed test and several agglutination assays)
    - Measures antibodies to native or recombinant *T. pallidum* antigens

Treatment
- Penicillin G drug of choice for all stages of syphilis
  - For penicillin-allergic patients, doxycycline or tetracycline is recommended

SYPHILITIC LYMPHADENITIS

Key Facts

Terminology
- Syphilis: Chronic systemic infection caused by *T. pallidum* (Gram-negative spirochete)

Clinical Issues
- Course of disease divided into 3 stages: Primary, secondary, and tertiary
- Penicillin G is drug of choice for all stages of syphilis

Microscopic Pathology
- Proliferation of blood vessels with endothelial swelling, phlebitis, and endarteritis
- Follicular hyperplasia
- Spirochetes most frequently found in walls of blood vessels (silver stains)
- Capsular and pericapsular inflammation
- Diffuse plasma cell infiltration; sheets of plasma cells in medulla

Prognosis
- Infection eradicated with antibiotic therapy

MICROSCOPIC PATHOLOGY

Histologic Features
- Capsular and pericapsular inflammation
- Follicular hyperplasia
- Parafollicular expansion with numerous immunoblasts, blood vessels with endothelial swelling, phlebitis, and endarteritis
- Diffuse plasma cell infiltration; sheets of plasma cells in medulla
- Noncaseating epithelioid granulomas
- *T. pallidum* is too thin to be visualized with Gram stain
- Silver stains, Warthin-Starry or Levaditi stains reveal spirochetes
  - More often found in walls of blood vessels

DIFFERENTIAL DIAGNOSIS

Systemic Lupus Lymphadenopathy (SLE)
- In common with lues: SLE shows follicular hyperplasia, increased vascularization, scattered immunoblasts, and plasma cells
  - SLE lacks vasculitis and contains accumulations of basophilic material derived from DNA (hematoxylin bodies)

Rheumatoid Arthritis (RA)
- In common with lues
  - RA shows follicular hyperplasia
  - Vascular proliferation
  - Plasma cell proliferation
  - Capsular infiltration by lymphocytes
- RA usually lacks vasculitis and perivasculitis
- Warthin-Starry stain to detect spirochetes may help

Follicular Lymphoma
- In lues, follicles can be prominent
- Follicles show reactive features (tingible body histiocytes and mitosis)

SELECTED REFERENCES

1. van Crevel R et al: Syphilis presenting as isolated cervical lymphadenopathy: two related cases. J Infect. 58(1):76-8, 2009
2. Moore SW et al: Diagnostic aspects of cervical lymphadenopathy in children in the developing world: a study of 1,877 surgical specimens. Pediatr Surg Int. 19(4):240-4, 2003
3. Singh AE et al: Syphilis: review with emphasis on clinical, epidemiologic, and some biologic features. Clin Microbiol Rev. 12(2):187-209, 1999
4. Choi YJ et al: Syphilitic lymphadenitis: immunofluorescent identification of spirochetes from imprints. Am J Surg Pathol. 3(6):553-5, 1979
5. Dorfman RF et al: Lymphadenopathy simulating the malignant lymphomas. Hum Pathol. 5(5):519-50, 1974

IMAGE GALLERY

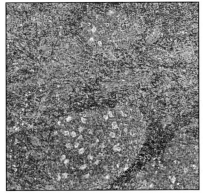 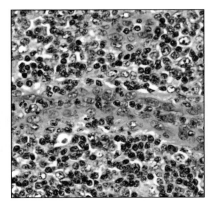 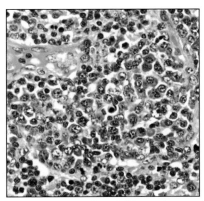

(Left) Follicular hyperplasia and expansion of the paracortex. The paracortex shows numerous vessels, some with endothelial hyperplasia and numerous immunoblasts. *(Center)* The marked hyperplasia of the endothelial cells is shown, which partially obliterates the vascular lumina. *(Right)* Medulla with a prominent infiltrate of plasma cells. They are mature appearing without atypical features.

INFECTIOUS MONONUCLEOSIS

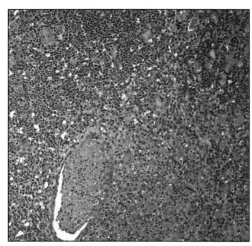

Epstein-Barr virus infection involving tonsil. Marked lymphoid hyperplasia with many tingible body macrophages, with focal karyorrhexis and exudate, are shown.

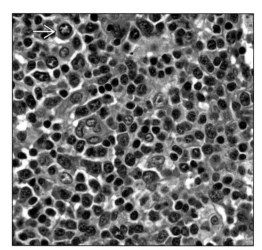

EBV lymphadenitis. Small to large lymphoid cells, eosinophils, and plasma cells are seen. The large cells ➡ are immunoblasts with prominent nucleoli.

TERMINOLOGY

Abbreviations
- Infectious mononucleosis (IM)

Synonyms
- Epstein-Barr virus (EBV) lymphadenitis, Pfeiffer disease, glandular fever

Definitions
- Acute lymphadenitis induced by EBV infection

ETIOLOGY/PATHOGENESIS

Infectious Agents
- Epstein-Barr virus

CLINICAL ISSUES

Epidemiology
- Age
  - Mostly adolescents and young adults in USA
    - Even younger age in developing countries
- Gender
  - No gender preference

Presentation
- Fever
- Pharyngitis
- Lymphadenopathy
- Peripheral blood lymphocytosis of atypical lymphocytes

Laboratory Tests
- Monospot test (a.k.a. heterophile antibody test)
- EBV-specific antibody tests by immunofluorescence
  - Elevated IgM antiviral capsid antigen (VCAs) and absence of antibodies to EBV nuclear antigen (anti-EBNA) indicate acute infection

Treatment
- Options, risks, complications
  - Observation is sufficient in most cases as disease resolves by itself
  - Infection may be complicated by rupture of spleen or hepatitis

Prognosis
- Usually self-limited; EBV rarely fatal, mostly in patients with immunodeficiency
  - EBV can also cause hemophagocytic syndrome or chronic active EBV infection

MICROSCOPIC PATHOLOGY

Histologic Features
- Preserved but distorted lymph node architecture
  - ↑ tingible body macrophages, immunoblasts, and plasma cells; frequent mitoses
  - Immunoblasts may be binucleated resembling Hodgkin cells or Reed-Sternberg cells
  - Predominantly interfollicular process, but follicles are also hyperplastic
- Peripheral blood lymphocytosis with atypical lymphocytes (Downey cells)

Predominant Pattern/Injury Type
- Lymphoid, interfollicular

Predominant Cell/Compartment Type
- Hematopoietic, lymphoid

ANCILLARY TESTS

Immunohistochemistry
- Most lymphocytes are CD3(+), CD8(+) reactive T cells
- Immunoblasts are positive for CD30 and CD45
- EBV-LMP1 is expressed by subset of infected cells

INFECTIOUS MONONUCLEOSIS

Key Facts

Etiology/Pathogenesis
- Epstein-Barr virus infection

Clinical Issues
- Fever
- Pharyngitis
- Lymphadenopathy

Microscopic Pathology
- Follicular and interfollicular hyperplasia
- Range of cells from small mature forms to immunoblasts

Ancillary Tests
- Proliferating lymphocytes in peripheral blood and lymphoid organs are largely CD3(+), CD8(+) T cells
- Immunoblasts are CD30(+) and CD45(+)

- EBV encoded early RNA (EBER) in situ hybridization highlights infected cells

Top Differential Diagnoses
- Classical Hodgkin lymphoma
- Peripheral T-cell lymphoma

Diagnostic Checklist
- Symptom complex
- Preserved overall architecture; marked follicular and interfollicular hyperplasia
- Spectrum of small to large cells with many intermediate forms
- No Reed-Sternberg cells or variants
- Predominantly CD3(+),CD8(+) T cells
- Positive serology or EBER

In Situ Hybridization
- EBV encoded early RNA (EBER) in situ hybridization highlights infected cells

DIFFERENTIAL DIAGNOSIS

Classical Hodgkin Lymphoma
- Mixed cellular background with predominantly small mature forms and occasional HRS cells
  - Unlike spectrum of small to large cells in EBV lymphadenitis
- Immunoblasts are usually weakly positive for CD30 and CD45 and negative for CD15
- Reed-Sternberg cells are usually negative for CD45 and positive for CD30 and CD15

Anaplastic Large Cell Lymphoma (ALCL)
- Large cells usually form sheets and are strongly CD30 positive
- Most ALCL are ALK1(+)

Other Types of Viral-induced Lymphadenitis or Infection
- CMV or early HIV infection may show similar features in lymph nodes
- Serological studies needed to confirm diagnosis

Peripheral T-cell Lymphoma
- Intermixed eosinophils and histiocytes may impart background similar to EBV lymphadenitis
- Neoplastic lymphoid cells are usually cytologically atypical
  - More commonly positive for CD4 than CD8, and usually CD30 negative

DIAGNOSTIC CHECKLIST

Clinically Relevant Pathologic Features
- Symptom complex
- Age distribution

  - Mostly in adolescents but may occur in elderly or immunocompromised individuals

Pathologic Interpretation Pearls
- Marked interfollicular and follicular hyperplasia
- Spectrum of small to large lymphocytes in contrast to predominantly small mature forms and occasional large atypical cells in Hodgkin lymphoma
- May show completely effaced architecture; usually some residual architecture is identified
- Hemophagocytosis may be present
- Lack of true Reed-Sternberg cells with coexpression of CD15 and CD30
  - CD30(+) immunoblasts are also CD45(+)
- Predominantly CD8(+) cytotoxic T cells

SELECTED REFERENCES

1. Hurt C et al: Diagnostic evaluation of mononucleosis-like illnesses. Am J Med. 120(10):911, 2007
2. Imashuku S: Systemic type Epstein-Barr virus-related lymphoproliferative diseases in children and young adults: challenges for pediatric hemato-oncologists and infectious disease specialists. Pediatr Hematol Oncol. 24(8):563-8, 2007
3. Klein E et al: Epstein-Barr virus infection in humans: from harmless to life endangering virus-lymphocyte interactions. Oncogene. 26(9):1297-305, 2007
4. Rezk SA et al: Epstein-Barr virus-associated lymphoproliferative disorders. Hum Pathol. 38(9):1293-304, 2007
5. Auwaerter PG: Recent advances in the understanding of infectious mononucleosis: are prospects improved for treatment or control? Expert Rev Anti Infect Ther. 4(6):1039-49, 2006
6. Kutok JL et al: Spectrum of Epstein-Barr virus-associated diseases. Annu Rev Pathol. 1:375-404, 2006
7. Vetsika EK et al: Infectious mononucleosis and Epstein-Barr virus. Expert Rev Mol Med. 6(23):1-16, 2004

CRYPTOCOCCAL LYMPHADENITIS

Key Facts

Etiology/Pathogenesis
- Infection by *Cryptococcus neoformans*
- Most cases are associated with immunosuppression
  - > 80% of cases associated with AIDS

Microscopic Pathology
- *Cryptococcus neoformans*
  - Single yeasts with narrow-based buds
  - Clear, concentric spaces on H&E due to 3-5 μm thick mucopolysaccharide capsule
  - Fungal organisms highlighted by PAS, GMS, mucicarmine, Fontana-Masson stains
- Tissue reaction
  - Scattered or confluent noncaseous granulomas
  - Cystic spaces composed of gelatinous fluid enclosed by fibrosis

- Often less/minimal reaction in patients with marked immunodeficiency
- Cytologic findings
  - FNA of lymph nodes useful for diagnosis
  - Bronchoalveolar lavage useful for diagnosing lung disease
  - India ink preparation of CSF demonstrates spherical, encapsulated yeast cells, 5-20 μm

Ancillary Tests
- Culture essential for definitive identification
- Fungal antigen in serum and other body fluids can aid in diagnosis

Top Differential Diagnoses
- Tuberculous lymphadenitis
- Histoplasma lymphadenitis

Prognosis
- Generally poor; related to degree of immunosuppression

IMAGE FINDINGS

Radiographic Findings
- Discrete solitary or multiple pulmonary nodules, infiltrates, cavitation, and consolidation in immunocompromised patients
- Other findings: Pleural effusions, hilar lymphadenopathy, endobronchial lesions, and atelectasis

MICROSCOPIC PATHOLOGY

Histologic Features
- *Cryptococcus neoformans*
  - Single yeasts with narrow-based buds
  - Polysaccharide capsule stains red with periodic acid–Schiff (PAS) and mucicarmine stain
  - Gomori methenamine silver (GMS) and Fontana-Masson stain cell wall black
  - Calcofluor can stain fungal chitin
  - Clear, concentric spaces on H&E due to 3-5 μm thick mucopolysaccharide capsule
- Tissue reaction
  - Noncaseating chronic granulomatous inflammation
    - Lymphocytes, epithelioid cells, and multinucleated giant cells
  - Cystic spaces composed of gelatinous fluid released from degenerated yeasts
    - Often surrounded by fibrosis
  - Encapsulated strains elicit liquefactive necrosis
  - Nonencapsulated strains tend to elicit more prominent granulomatous reaction

Cytologic Features
- Fine needle aspiration of lymph nodes or other sites
  - Range of cell types: Lymphocytes, histiocytes

- Can show organisms
- Bronchoalveolar lavage useful for diagnosis of lung disease
- India ink preparation demonstrates spherical, encapsulated yeast cells, 5-20 μm in diameter
  - Can be performed on CSF, sputum, and other liquid specimens

DIFFERENTIAL DIAGNOSIS

Tuberculous Lymphadenitis
- Granulomas, classically with central caseating necrosis
- Concentric layers of epithelioid cells; Langhans giant cells
- Ziehl-Neelsen, Kinyoun, and Fite-Faraco stains
- Auramine-rhodamine stain with fluorescent microscopy to demonstrate acid-fast bacilli

Histoplasma Lymphadenitis
- Yeast forms slightly larger than *C. neoformans*
- Yeast forms not surrounded by thick capsule

Sarcoidosis
- Numerous, back to back, distinct granulomas; no extensive, confluent necrosis
- Scattered multinucleated giant cells of Langhans type

Kikuchi-Fujimoto Lymphadenitis
- Patchy areas of paracortical necrosis without granulocytes
- Abundant nuclear fragmentation (karryorhexis)
- Numerous histiocytes, many with crescentic nuclei (C-shaped histiocytes)

SELECTED REFERENCES
1. Huston SM et al: Cryptococcosis: an emerging respiratory mycosis. Clin Chest Med. 30(2):253-64, vi, 2009
2. Chayakulkeeree M et al: Cryptococcosis. Infect Dis Clin North Am. 20(3):507-44, v-vi, 2006

CRYPTOCOCCAL LYMPHADENITIS

Microscopic Features

(Left) Plate culture of C. neoformans grown at 37°C demonstrates mucoid appearance. Some strains are poorly encapsulated and lack the mucoid appearance. *(Courtesy W. Kaplan, CDC Public Health Image Library, #3204.)* *(Right)* Hematoxylin and eosin stain of lymph node obtained at time of autopsy demonstrates spherical fungal yeast forms consistent with C. neoformans ➡. This image also shows marked autolytic changes in the tissue.

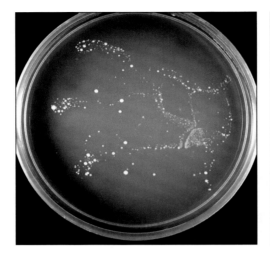
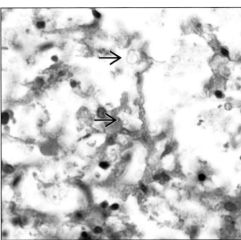

(Left) Mucicarmine stain of lymph node obtained at autopsy highlights many fungal yeast forms consistent with C. neoformans. The mucicarmine stain highlights polysaccharides (red) that are part of the thick capsule of this organism ➡. *(Right)* Mucicarmine stain of heart tissue obtained at autopsy highlights fungal yeast forms (red) within myocardium.

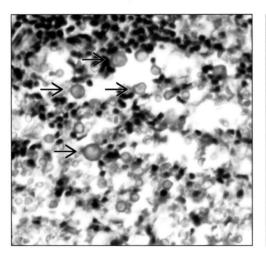
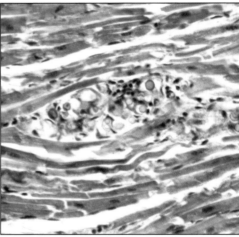

(Left) Bone marrow biopsy specimen demonstrates histiocytic infiltrate with scattered clear concentric fungal yeast forms with a thick mucopolysaccharide capsule consistent with C. neoformans ➡. *(Right)* Mucicarmine stain of bone marrow biopsy specimen highlights fungal yeast forms (red) ➡ consistent with C. neoformans.

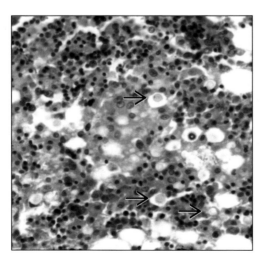
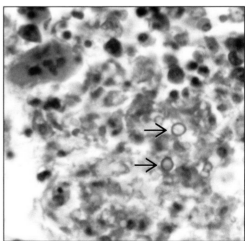

CRYPTOCOCCAL LYMPHADENITIS

Imaging and Microscopic Features

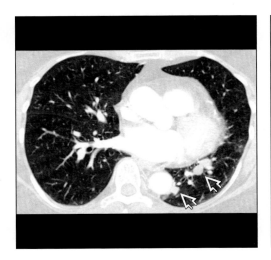
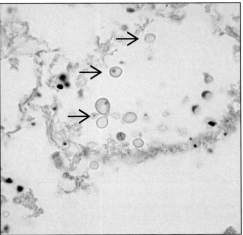

(Left) CT scan of the lungs shows multiple nodules ⇨ within the left lung as a result of infection by C. neoformans (cryptococcal pneumonia). *(Right)* Gomori methenamine silver (GMS) stain of lung alveolar parenchyma highlights fungal yeast forms consistent with C. neoformans. This GMS stains cell walls black ⇨.

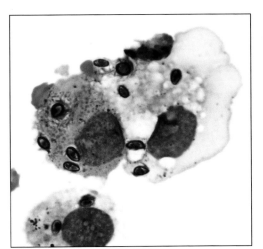
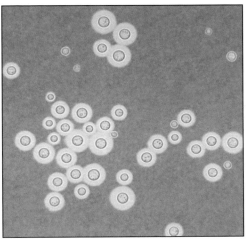

(Left) Wright-Giemsa stain of cytospin of bronchoalveolar lavage specimen demonstrates numerous fungal yeast forms consistent with C. neoformans located within histiocyte cytoplasm. *(Right)* C. neoformans using a light India ink staining preparation demonstrates the thick capsule surrounding these organisms. (Courtesy L. Haley, Public Health Image Library, CDC, ID #3771.)

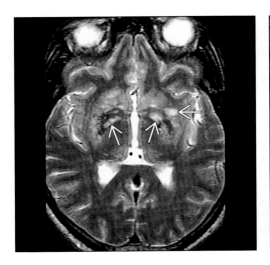
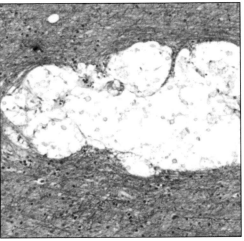

(Left) Axial T2-weighted MR of the brain in an HIV-positive patient with a cryptococcal infection shows multiple areas of abnormal high signal ⇨ that proved to be cryptococcal gelatinous pseudocysts. *(Right)* Luxol fast blue stain of brain demonstrates cryptococcal gelatinous pseudocyst within white matter. Note numerous fungal yeast forms consistent with C. neoformans within gelatinous material in the background.

TOXOPLASMA LYMPHADENITIS

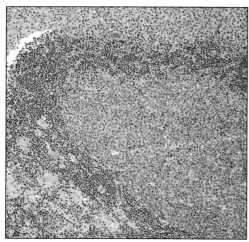

Toxoplasma lymphadenitis. Note enlarged follicles with reactive germinal centers, clusters of epithelioid cells encroaching on lymphoid follicles, and monocytoid cells.

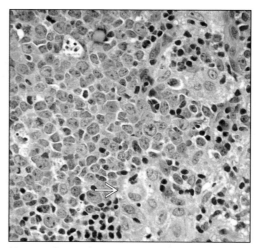

Hematoxylin and eosin stain shows a reactive germinal center with many centroblasts, tingible-body macrophages, and epithelioid cells encroaching into the germinal center from the right ➡.

TERMINOLOGY

Synonyms
- Toxoplasmic lymphadenitis
- Glandular toxoplasmosis
- Piringer-Kuchinka lymphadenopathy

Definitions
- Inflammation of lymph node caused by infection by *Toxoplasma gondii*

ETIOLOGY/PATHOGENESIS

Toxoplasma gondii Infection
- *T. gondii is* protozoan that can invade many cell types
- Cat is definitive host for sexual stage of reproduction
  - Trophozoites reproduce in intestinal epithelium
  - Oocysts are generated that are eliminated in feces
- Humans and animals are intermediate hosts
  - Ingest oocysts from contaminated soil
  - Humans can ingest oocysts from undercooked meat
- In humans and animals, oocysts are digested by digestive enzymes
  - Trophozoites are released into intestine
    - Organisms are carried by macrophages
    - Spread via lymphatics and blood vessels to internal organs
  - Within macrophages, trophozoites can multiply and become crescent-shaped tachyzoites
- In immunocompetent patients, tachyzoites usually become segregated into cysts synthesized by host
  - Within cysts, organisms are slow-growing bradyzoites
  - Infection typically resolves
- In immunodeficient patients, tachyzoites widely disseminate, causing acute infection

CLINICAL ISSUES

Epidemiology
- Incidence
  - Toxoplasmosis is common parasitic disease worldwide
    - More prevalent in warm and humid climates
  - In USA, toxoplasmosis is most common parasitic infection
    - 50% of USA citizens have serum antibodies to *T. gondii*: Evidence of chronic infection
  - *T. gondii* can be spread transplacentally from mother to fetus
    - 1 in every 1,000 live births in USA
    - ~ 3,000 births are affected annually
    - Potential damage to fetus is greatest with infection in 1st trimester
  - Rarely, *T. gondii* infection can be transmitted via transplanted organ
  - Active infection may result from reactivation of earlier infection
    - Common in patients with cancers and diabetes mellitus
- Age
  - Children and young adults most often affected
- Gender
  - No sex preference

Site
- Lymph nodes are commonly affected
  - Posterior cervical lymph nodes are characteristic site
    - Often unilateral
  - Any group of lymph nodes can be involved
    - Other cervical, supraclavicular, occipital, parotid, intramammary regions
  - Generalized lymphadenopathy or hepatosplenomegaly can occur but is unusual

TOXOPLASMA LYMPHADENITIS

Key Facts

Etiology/Pathogenesis
- *Toxoplasma gondii is* parasitic protozoan
- Cat is definitive host for sexual stage of reproduction
- Oocysts containing trophozoites are generated that are eliminated in feces
- Humans and animals are intermediate hosts
- Humans ingest oocysts from contaminated soil or undercooked meat

Clinical Issues
- Self-limited clinical course in most patients
- Children and young adults (65%) most often affected
- Unilateral lymphadenopathy, commonly posterior cervical

Microscopic Pathology
- Diagnostic triad
  - Florid reactive follicular hyperplasia
  - Monocytoid B-cell hyperplasia in sinuses
  - Epithelioid histiocytes in paracortical areas that encroach into germinal centers
- No multinucleated giant cells; no necrosis

Ancillary Tests
- Sabin-Feldman dye test
- IgM screening antibody test positive in 1st 3 months
- Positive *Toxoplasma*-specific antibodies are detected by enzyme immunoassays
- Anti-*Toxoplasma* immunohistochemistry detects presence of parasites
- *Toxoplasma* genomes can be detected by PCR

Presentation
- Asymptomatic infection is common in immunocompetent individuals
- Mild illness also can occur manifested by malaise, fever, myalgia
- Physical examination of lymph nodes
  - Tender or nontender
  - Firm but not rock hard
  - 0.5-3.0 cm

Laboratory Tests
- Sabin-Feldman dye test
  - Highly sensitive and specific
  - *T. gondii* organisms do not stain with alkaline methylene blue if they have been exposed to serum anti-*T. gondii* antibodies
  - Positive result: Change from negative to positive or rapidly increasing titers
- Antibodies to *T. gondii* can be detected by enzyme immunoassays or indirect immunofluorescence
  - IgM or IgG antibodies against cell wall antigens
  - IgM antibodies present within few days after infection
    - Titers of 1:80 or higher indicate recent infection
  - IgG antibody titers of 1:1,000 occur at 6-8 weeks after infection
    - Can persist for years
- Latex agglutination test and ELISA assays available
- PCR can be used to amplify *T. gondii* DNA
  - Commonly used on amniotic fluid

Treatment
- Pyrimethamine/sulfadiazine

Prognosis
- In immunocompetent patients, infection is self-limiting
- In immunodeficient patients, great risk of acute dissemination
  - Encephalitis, chorioretinitis, pneumonia, and cardiac involvement
  - Death as result of above conditions

MICROSCOPIC PATHOLOGY

Histologic Features
- Lymph node
  - Architecture: Preserved
  - Capsule/pericapsule: Minimal involvement
  - Sinuses: Distended by monocytoid B cells
    - Large cells with sharp, visible cell borders, clear cytoplasm, and small darkly stained nuclei
  - Follicles: Florid reactive follicular hyperplasia
    - Numerous tingible body macrophages
    - Germinal centers can have ragged, indistinct margins
  - Numerous epithelioid histiocytes in interfollicular and paracortical regions
    - Encroach upon and invade into germinal centers
    - Form collections of less than 25 epithelioid cells (microgranulomas)
  - Plasma cells and immunoblasts in medullary cords
  - Toxoplasma cysts and bradyzoites are rare (1% of cases)
    - Can identify by routine histologic examination in ~ 1% of cases
  - Necrosis is absent
  - Well-formed (sarcoid-like) granulomas do not occur
  - No multinucleated giant cells; no fibrosis

Cytologic Features
- Diagnosis can be established by fine needle aspiration of lymph node
  - Diff-Quik smears show polymorphous cell population
    - Small and large lymphocytes
    - Clusters of epithelioid histiocytes (microgranulomas)
    - Plasma cells
  - Rarely, parasitic cysts can be detected

TOXOPLASMA LYMPHADENITIS

ANCILLARY TESTS

Immunohistochemistry
- Anti-*T. gondii* antibodies can be used to detect presence of parasites in tissues

PCR
- Toxoplasma genomes are detected by conventional and nested polymerase chain reaction
  - Often not detected in lymph nodes with changes of *Toxoplasma* lymphadenitis
- Does not distinguish active from latent infection

Electron Microscopy
- Transmission
  - *T. gondii* has distinctive features
    - Paired organelles, dense bodies
    - Conoid nuclei at rounded posterior end
    - Double-layered pellicles

DIFFERENTIAL DIAGNOSIS

Human Immunodeficiency Virus (HIV) Lymphadenitis
- Early stage of HIV infection can be associated with changes that can mimic toxoplasmosis
- Explosive follicular hyperplasia
- Sinusoidal and paracortical monocytoid B-cell proliferation
- Epithelioid histiocytes can be present or absent
- Positive immunohistochemical staining for HIV p24

Leishmaniasis Lymphadenitis
- Histologic findings can closely mimic toxoplasmosis
- Multinucleated giant cells are usually present
- Leishman-Donovan bodies may be seen in cytoplasm of histiocytes

Dermatopathic Lymphadenopathy
- Paracortical distribution
  - Numerous histiocytes, many with twisted nuclei
    - S100 protein(+), CD1a([+], subset)
  - Melanin pigment

Sarcoidosis
- Well-formed granulomas unlike toxoplasmosis
- Multinucleated giant cells often present
- Usually monocytoid B-cell hyperplasia is absent or minimal

Systemic Lupus Erythematosus (SLE) Lymphadenopathy
- Areas of paracortical necrosis; ± hematoxylin bodies
- Clinical history and serologic findings of SLE

Infectious Mononucleosis
- Paracortical and polymorphous lymphoid proliferation
- Numerous immunoblasts and foci of necrosis
- No epithelioid histiocytes encroaching on germinal centers

Non-Hodgkin Lymphoma (NHL)
- Clusters of epithelioid histiocytes can be present in many NHL types
  - Lymphoepithelioid variant of peripheral T-cell lymphoma (so-called Lennert lymphoma)
- Lymph node architecture is altered
- Monocytoid B-cell hyperplasia absent or minimal

Nodular Lymphocyte Predominant Hodgkin Lymphoma
- Epithelioid histiocytes can be numerous
- Large, vague nodules that are closely packed and lack mantle zones
  - Follicular dendritic cell networks in nodules
- LP cells (a.k.a. "popcorn" or L&H cells) are present
  - CD20(+), pax-5([+], strong), CD45/LCA(+)

Classical Hodgkin Lymphoma
- Epithelioid histiocytes can be numerous
- Most common in mixed cellularity type
- Reed-Sternberg and Hodgkin cells present
  - CD15(+), CD30(+), CD45/LCA(-)

DIAGNOSTIC CHECKLIST

Clinically Relevant Pathologic Features
- Persistent unilateral lymphadenopathy
  - Posterior cervical lymph nodes commonly affected

Pathologic Interpretation Pearls
- Diagnostic triad is characteristic of *Toxoplasma* lymphadenitis and correlates with serologic data
  - Marked reactive follicular hyperplasia
  - Monocytoid B-cell hyperplasia in sinuses
  - Epithelioid histiocytes in paracortex that encroach upon and invade germinal centers

SELECTED REFERENCES

1. Boothroyd JC: Toxoplasma gondii: 25 years and 25 major advances for the field. Int J Parasitol. 39(8):935-46, 2009
2. Shin DW et al: Seroprevalence of Toxoplasma gondii infection and characteristics of seropositive patients in general hospitals in Daejeon, Korea. Korean J Parasitol. 47(2):125-30, 2009
3. Eapen M et al: Evidence based criteria for the histopathological diagnosis of toxoplasmic lymphadenopathy. J Clin Pathol. 58(11):1143-6, 2005
4. Viguer JM et al: Fine needle aspiration of toxoplasmic (Piringer-Kuchinka) lymphadenitis: a cytohistologic correlation study. Acta Cytol. 49(2):139-43, 2005
5. Held TK et al: Diagnosis of toxoplasmosis in bone marrow transplant recipients: comparison of PCR-based results and immunohistochemistry. Bone Marrow Transplant. 25(12):1257-62, 2000
6. Tenter AM et al: Toxoplasma gondii: from animals to humans. Int J Parasitol. 30(12-13):1217-58, 2000
7. Saxen E et al: Glandular toxoplasmosis: a report of 23 histologically diagnosed cases. Acta Pathol Microbiol Scand. 44:319, 1958

TOXOPLASMA LYMPHADENITIS

Diagrammatic and Microscopic Features

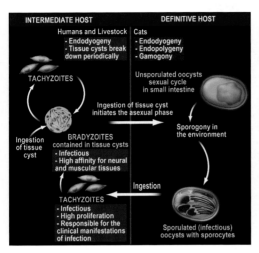

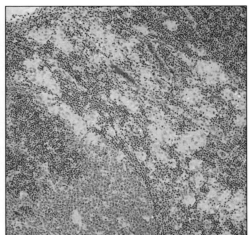

(Left) Life cycle of T. gondii. The infectious stages are tachyzoites, bradyzoites contained in tissue cysts, and sporozoites contained in sporulated oocysts. *(Right)* Toxoplasma lymphadenitis. Numerous clusters of epithelioid cells are seen in interfollicular areas of the lymph node. Epithelioid histiocytes encroach on follicles.

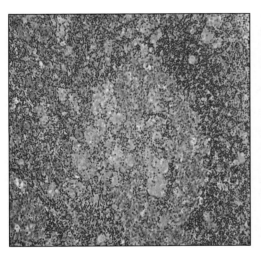

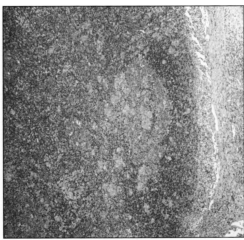

(Left) Microgranulomas can be seen within a follicle center in this case of Toxoplasma lymphadenitis. *(Right)* This case of Toxoplasma lymphadenitis shows the diagnostic triad of reactive follicular hyperplasia, clusters of epithelioid histiocytes in the paracortical area encroaching upon follicles, and monocytoid B-cell hyperplasia expanding the subcapsular sinus.

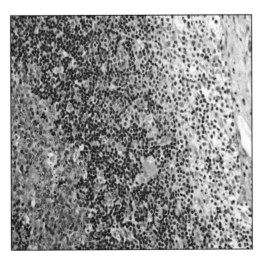

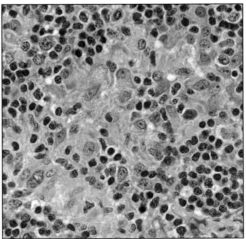

(Left) High-power magnification of a case of Toxoplasma lymphadenitis shows a reactive follicle, epithelioid histiocytes, and monocytoid B cells expanding the sinus. *(Right)* Hematoxylin and eosin stain shows epithelioid cells without formation of granulomas in this case of Toxoplasma lymphadenitis.

TOXOPLASMA LYMPHADENITIS

Microscopic Features and Differential Diagnosis

(Left) In this field from a case of Toxoplasma lymphadenitis, numerous monocytoid B cells are present. These cells are monomorphic with abundant pale cytoplasm and round, dark, centrally located nuclei. *(Right)* This field in a case of Toxoplasma lymphadenitis shows monocytoid B cells (lower left) and scattered epithelioid histiocytes (lower right).

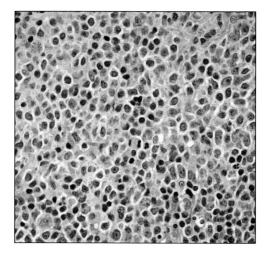 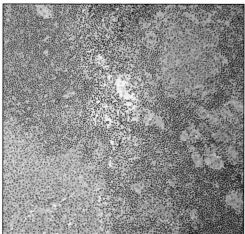

(Left) Microgranulomas are present in this field of a case of Toxoplasma lymphadenitis. Note that there are no multinucleated giant cells, and caseation is absent. *(Right)* Monocytoid cells are between 2 large, reactive follicles in this field of a case of Toxoplasma lymphadenitis.

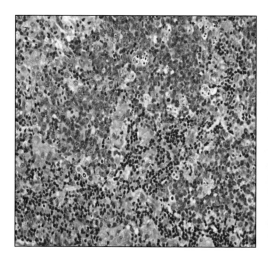 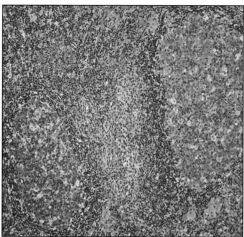

(Left) Anti-Toxoplasma gondii immunohistochemistry detects the presence of a Toxoplasma pseudocyst containing bradyzoites in the brain of this immunosuppressed patient with encephalitis. *(Right)* Clusters of epithelioid histiocytes are present in this case of peripheral T-cell lymphoma, lymphoepithelioid variant (so-called Lennert lymphoma). Note the architectural replacement and lack of reactive follicles in this case.

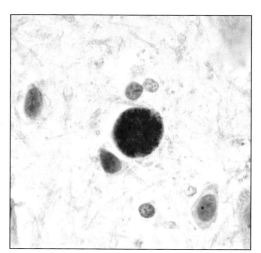 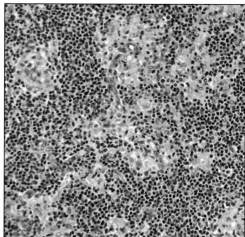

Differential Diagnosis

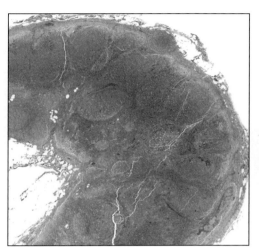
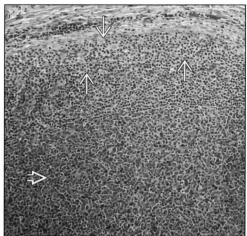

(Left) A lymph node biopsy specimen from an HIV(+) patient. This lymph node shows florid follicular hyperplasia and monocytoid B-cell hyperplasia and therefore has features in common with Toxoplasma lymphadenitis. *(Right)* Lymph node biopsy specimen from an HIV(+) patient. This field shows monocytoid B-cell hyperplasia in the subcapsular sinus ➡ and a reactive germinal center ⮞ surrounded by a poorly formed mantle zone.

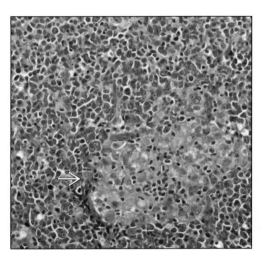
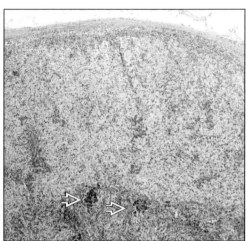

(Left) Paraffin section of lymph node biopsy specimen from an HIV(+) patient. Clusters of epithelioid histiocytes ➡ are present within the germinal center. Cases of HIV lymphadenitis can exhibit the diagnostic triad of histologic features that typically occur in Toxoplasma lymphadenitis. *(Right)* A case of dermatopathic lymphadenopathy shows marked expansion of the paracortex by histiocytes. Melanin pigment is also present in this field ⮞.

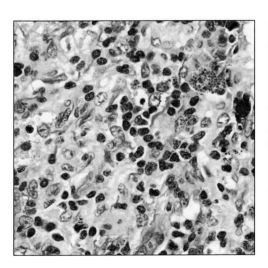
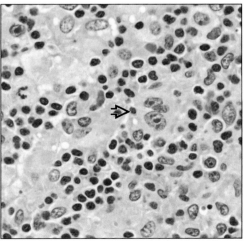

(Left) A case of dermatopathic lymphadenopathy shows many cells with twisted nuclei and abundant cytoplasm consistent with interdigitating dendritic cells and Langerhans cells. Pigment is also present in this field (upper right). *(Right)* Classical Hodgkin lymphoma involving lymph node. A Reed-Sternberg cell ⮞ is present in this field associated with numerous epithelioid histiocytes and small lymphocytes.

COCCIDIOIDES LYMPHADENITIS

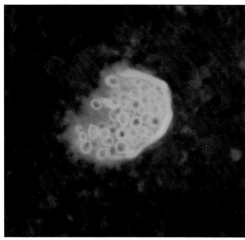

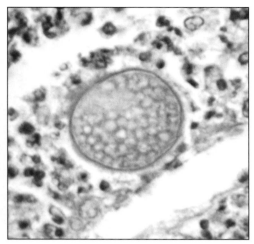

Spherule of C. immitis with endospores is demonstrated by Calcofluor white stain. (Courtesy B.J. Harrington, MD.)

Mature spherule with endospores of C. immitis in lung is demonstrated by PAS stain. Note the dense neutrophilic infiltrate. (Courtesy L. Georg, MD, CDC Public Health Image Library, #480.)

TERMINOLOGY

Definitions
- Inflammation of lymph nodes due to *Coccidioides immitis* or *Coccidioides posadasii*

ETIOLOGY/PATHOGENESIS

Infectious Agents
- 2 species recognized
  - *C. immitis*, predominant in California, USA
  - *C. posadasii*, predominant in other regions

Epidemiology
- Endemic in semi-arid to arid areas of
  - Southwest USA
  - Parts of South America
- Organism
  - Grows in warm, sandy soil
  - Prevalent in areas having hot summers, mild winters, and < 20 inches of rainfall annually
  - Does not grow at altitudes above 3,700 feet
  - Occasional epidemics in past 30 years
  - Outbreaks can follow dust storms, earthquakes, and droughts
- High-risk factors include
  - Occupational soil exposure
    - Agricultural workers
    - Military personnel
    - Archaeologists
  - Immunocompromised status as a result of
    - Organ transplant
    - Immunosuppressive agents
    - Acquired immune deficiency syndrome (AIDS)
    - Malignant diseases
  - Pregnancy
- High risk of dissemination in
  - Filipinos
  - African-Americans
  - Subjects with blood group B
- Incidence rising rapidly in USA due to
  - People settling in endemic areas
  - Growing immunocompromised population
  - New construction in uninhabited regions resulting in arthrospore dissemination
  - Increased awareness of disease entity
- Cases seen in nonendemic areas due to increased travel
  - Travel history should be sought
  - High level of suspicion necessary
- Incidence expected to rise in future

Pathogenesis
- *Coccidioides* spp. are dimorphic
- Mycelial phase
  - Grows in soil
  - Branching, septate hyphae
  - Can remain viable in dry desert soil for years
  - Multiplies after rainfall, forming arthroconidia
- Arthroconidia
  - Separated by empty, thin-walled cells (disjunctors)
  - Dispersed into air and inhaled
  - Transform into multinucleated spherules within lung
- Spherule phase
  - Spherules increase in size
  - Form thick outer wall
  - Divide to form numerous uninucleated endospores
  - Break open and release endospores, which form new spherules
  - Cycle continues
- Spherules disseminate hematogenously to meninges, bones, skin, and soft tissue
- Cell-mediated immunity crucial to limiting infection
- Primary pulmonary infections asymptomatic in 60% of patients
- Usual course of infection is healing without sequelae

COCCIDIOIDES LYMPHADENITIS

Key Facts

Etiology/Pathogenesis
- 2 species: *C. immitis* prevalent in California, USA; *C. posadasii* in other regions

Clinical Issues
- May be seen in nonendemic areas
- Travel history should be sought
- 60% of infections are asymptomatic

Microscopic Pathology
- Early acute phase: Neutrophils, histiocytes, eosinophils
- Granulomatous phase
- Round spherules (10-100 μm) in progressive developmental stages
- Internal and external endospores (2-5 μm)

Ancillary Tests
- Calcofluor white fluorescense sensitive
- GMS and PAS stains highlight spherules
- Recognition of endospores within spherules diagnostic
- Culture yield variable and depends on site and phase of disease

Top Differential Diagnoses
- Tuberculous lymphadenitis
- Histoplasma lymphadenitis
- Sarcoidosis
- Kikuchi-Fujimoto lymphadenitis

Reporting Considerations
- Classified as agents of potential bioterrorism in USA
- Isolates should be reported to CDC within 7 days

- Localized lesion (coccidioidoma) may persist

Reporting Considerations
- *C. immitis* and *C. posadasii* classified as select agents of potential bioterrorism in USA
- Laboratories must report findings to Centers for Disease Control (CDC) within 7 calendar days

Safety Considerations
- Laboratory workers potentially at risk of accidental exposure
- Biosafety level 2 practices and facilities recommended
- Manipulation of clinical material conducted in class II biological safety cabinets

CLINICAL ISSUES

Presentation
- General comments
  - Signs and symptoms
    - Wide spectrum
    - Similar to community-acquired pneumonia
  - 60% of patients are asymptomatic
  - Most common infections self-limited and misdiagnosed
  - Disseminated disease in < 5% of symptomatic patients
- Acute pneumonia
  - Presents 1-3 weeks after inhalation of arthroconidia
  - Profound fatigue
  - Lobar infiltrates and lymphadenopathy in patient who has traveled to endemic area are suggestive
  - Pleural effusion in 5-10% cases
  - Erythema multiforme, erythema nodosum, toxic erythema (immune mediated)
- Diffuse pneumonia
  - Due to
    - Inhalation of large number of arthrospores
    - Hematogenous spread
    - Immunocompromised status
  - Severe illness, high fever, dyspnea, hypoxemia

- Can progress to acute respiratory distress syndrome
- Chronic progressive pneumonia
  - Persistent illness lasting > 3 months in small percentage of patients
  - Persistent coughing, sputum production, hemoptysis
  - Weight loss
  - Serologic testing positive
- Pulmonary nodules and cavities
  - Can be initial presentation of primary infection
  - Can occur in immunocompetent hosts after infiltrate resolves
  - 1-2 cm nodule or cavity
  - Cavity may wax and wane
  - Usually do not cause symptoms
  - Cough, chest pain, and hemoptysis may occur
  - Rupture of cavity near pleural surface may lead to hydropneumothorax
- Extrapulmonary noncentral nervous system disease
  - Occurs in < 5% of immunocompetent patients and in high-risk groups
  - Skin, lymph nodes, bones, and joints involved
  - Diagnosed several months after onset of pulmonary symptoms
  - Surgical excision may be necessary
- Central nervous system disease
  - Granulomatous meningitis or coccidioidoma
  - Headache, mental status changes, neurologic deficits
  - Serologic studies essential for diagnosis

Laboratory Tests
- Peripheral blood
  - Elevated erythrocyte sedimentation rate
  - Eosinophilia
- Pleural fluid
  - Usually exudative
  - May show eosinophilia
- Cerebrospinal fluid (CSF)
  - Increased white blood cells, predominantly lymphocytes
  - Increased protein, decreased glucose
- Light microscopy

COCCIDIOIDES LYMPHADENITIS

- o Round spherules (10–100 μm) in progressive developmental stages
- o Internal and external endospores (2–5 μm)
- o Recognition of endospores within spherules considered diagnostic
- o Few spherules without internal structures considered presumptive evidence
- o May be seen in giant cells, microabscesses, and in acute presentations
- o Less likely to be found in caseous, calcified, or liquefactive foci
- o Rarely seen in CSF in meningitis
- o Immature spherules in contact may simulate *Blastomyces*
- o Endospores without spherules (especially in CSF) may simulate *Histoplasma, Cryptococcus, Candida*
- o Mycelia may be identified in
  - Boundaries of old cavitary lung lesions
  - Skin lesions
  - Ventricular fluid in CNS infection
- o Mycelia without spherules not diagnostic
- o Culture isolates show slender, hyaline, and septate hyphae
- o Arthroconidia
  - Unicellular, barrel-shaped (3–4 x 3–6 μm)
  - Arise from side branches
  - Alternate with thin-walled, empty disjunctor cells
  - Released at maturity
- o **Calcofluor white (CFW) fluorescence**
  - Binds chitin and cellulose in fungal cell wall
  - Sensitive but may stain plant material
  - Rapid results
  - May be used on tissue, body fluids, respiratory secretions
- o **KOH wet mount**
  - Not as sensitive as CFW
- o **Grocott methenamine silver**
  - Most sensitive histopathologic stain
  - However, may obscure endospores within spherules
- o **Periodic acid-Schiff (PAS) reaction**
  - Stain fungi red
  - Delineate fungal morphology
  - More sensitive than H&E
- o **Lactophenol cotton blue**
  - Used on tease-mounts prepared from culture isolates
- Culture
  - o Colonies detected in 2-16 days
    - Initially, white to cream, glistening, glabrous, and tenacious
    - After 4–5 days, develop discrete concentric rings with filamentous areas containing the following
    - Arthroconidia (barrel shaped with intercalated ghost cells)
    - Tan, yellow, pale to gray-brown colonies also reported
    - Appear woody with aging
  - o Organism recovered in variety of specimens
  - o Yield depends on
    - Site
    - Clinical presentation at time of sampling

- o Respiratory tract has highest yield, and blood has lowest yield
- o CNS usually negative since density of organisms is low
- o Specimens with potentially mixed flora should be inoculated onto selective media additionally
- o Culture media include
  - Brain–heart infusion (BHI) agar
  - Potato dextrose agar (PDA) or potato flakes agar (PFA)
  - Sabouraud dextrose agar (SDA) (selective and nonselective)
  - Blood agar
  - Chocolate agar
  - Buffered charcoal-yeast extract (selective and nonselective)
  - Bordet-Gengou and Regan-Lowe (selective and nonselective)
- Molecular studies
  - o AccuProbe nucleic acid hybridization assay (Gen-Probe; San Diego, CA; USA) used for confirmation of isolates
  - o Identification to species level (*C. immitis* and *C. posadasii*) reported
  - o Uses chemiluminescent-labeled, single-stranded DNA probe complementary to rRNA of fungus
  - o Not commercially available for use in surgical tissue
- Serology
  - o Humoral immunity
    - Not protective
    - Indicates disease burden
    - Used for diagnosis and prognosis
    - Includes early (IgM) and late (IgG) antibodies
  - o Serological studies not 100% sensitive
  - o Responses diminished or absent in immunocompromised patients
  - o Positive results may be helpful in diagnosis
  - o Negative results cannot rule out disease, especially early in course
  - o Enzyme immunoassays (EIA)
    - Can detect IgM and IgG
    - Most sensitive method
    - Positive results, especially for IgM, may be less specific
    - Cross reactivity to *H. capsulatum* and *P. braziliensis* can give false-positive results
    - Require confirmation by immunodiffusion or complement-fixation if clinically incompatible with diagnosis
    - Qualitative; not quantitative
  - o Immunodiffusion (IMDF)
    - Can detect IgM and IgG
    - Requires incubation periods of up to 4 days to rule out negative results
    - Can be modified to quantify titers
    - Useful when CF test cannot be used in sera having anticomplement activity
  - o Complement-fixation (CF)
    - Less sensitive than EIA and IMDF tests
    - Essential for diagnosis of meningeal disease
  - o Ideally must be performed at reference laboratories with high-volume testing

COCCIDIOIDES LYMPHADENITIS

○ IgM
- Detected by week 1 in 50%; by week 3 in 90%
- Tube precipitin method commonly used
- EIA and latex agglutination highly sensitive but less specific

○ IgG
- Detected by CF 8-28 weeks after disease onset
- Less sensitive
- Indicates intensity of immune response
- May not be reliable in immunocompromised patients
- May remain positive for years
- Quantitative titer
- Serial testing used to assess treatment response in immunocompetent patient
- Titer of 1:2 or 1:4 is associated with favorable outcome
- Titer of 1:16 or greater is associated with disseminated disease
- Sequential specimens from patient must be tested in parallel by same laboratory

- Cell-mediated immunity
  ○ Skin testing for cell-mediated cellular response using fungus-specific antigen
  ○ Not available in USA at present

Treatment
- Azoles in
  ○ Chronic pulmonary disease
  ○ Chronic disseminated disease
  ○ Central nervous system disease
- Amphotericin B in
  ○ Acute progressive or persistent pneumonia

IMAGE FINDINGS

Acute Pneumonia
- Lobar, segmental, or subsegmental infiltrates
- Hilar or paratracheal adenopathy in 25% of cases

Diffuse Pneumonia
- Bilateral, diffuse, small, fluffy nodules

Chronic Progressive Pneumonia
- Dense unifocal or multifocal consolidation
- Cavitation

Pulmonary Nodules and Cavities
- Present as coin lesions raising concern for tumor
- Rupture can lead to pneumothorax, pleural effusion

CNS
- Meningeal enhancement
- Cerebral infarction, hydrocephalus

MICROSCOPIC PATHOLOGY

Histologic Features
- 2 phases of inflammation in immunocompetent patients
  ○ Early acute phase

- Neutrophils, histiocytes, occasionally eosinophils surrounding organisms
  ○ Granulomatous phase
  - Spherules with endospores identified
  - Scattered or confluent granulomas
  - Caseating necrosis may be present
  - Lymphocytes, plasma cells, epithelioid histiocytes, numerous multinucleated giant cells
- Organisms stain black with GMS stain; red with PAS stain

Cytologic Features
- Organisms can be identified in fine needle aspiration smears
- Cellular infiltrate similar to that observed in tissue sections

DIFFERENTIAL DIAGNOSIS

Tuberculous Lymphadenitis
- Granulomas, classically with central caseating necrosis
- Concentric layers of epithelioid histiocytes; Langhans giant cells
- Acid-fast bacilli demonstrated by
  ○ Ziehl-Neelsen, Kinyoun, and Fite-Faraco stains
  ○ Auramine-rhodamine stain with fluorescent microscopy

Histoplasma Lymphadenitis
- Yeast forms are round or oval; diameter of 2-4 μm
  ○ Have narrow-based buds

Sarcoidosis
- Numerous, back to back, well-defined granulomas; no extensive, confluent necrosis
- Scattered multinucleated giant cells of Langhans type

Kikuchi-Fujimoto Lymphadenitis
- Patchy areas of paracortical necrosis without granulocytes
- Abundant nuclear fragmentation (karryorhexis)
- Numerous histiocytes, many with crescentic nuclei (C-shaped histiocytes)

DIAGNOSTIC CHECKLIST

Pathologic Interpretation Pearls
- Immature spherules in contact may simulate *Blastomyces*
- Endospores without spherules (especially in CSF) may simulate *Histoplasma, Cryptococcus, Candida*

SELECTED REFERENCES

1. Saubolle MA et al: Epidemiologic, clinical, and diagnostic aspects of coccidioidomycosis. J Clin Microbiol. 45(1):26-30, 2007
2. Saubolle MA: Laboratory aspects in the diagnosis of coccidioidomycosis. Ann N Y Acad Sci. 1111:301-14, 2007
3. Sutton DA: Diagnosis of coccidioidomycosis by culture: safety considerations, traditional methods, and susceptibility testing. Ann N Y Acad Sci. 1111:315-25, 2007

COCCIDIOIDES LYMPHADENITIS

Ancillary Techniques

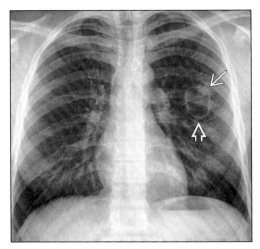
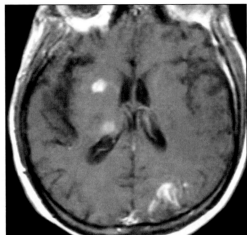

(Left) Pulmonary cavity ➡ is present in a patient 7 months after primary infection with Coccidioides species. Note the mural nodularity ➡. *(Right)* Axial T1WI C+ MR shows enhancing lesions in the right basal ganglia and thalamus and in the left occipital lobe due to infection with Coccidioides spp.

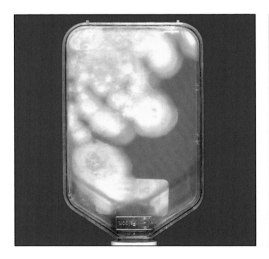
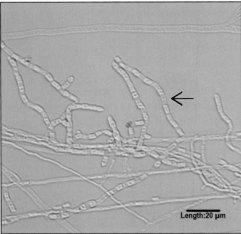

(Left) Sabouraud dextrose agar demonstrates cob web-like floccose, gray-white- to buff-colored colonies of C. immitis. (Courtesy L. Haley, MD, CDC Public Health Image Library, #4187.) *(Right)* Lactophenol cotton blue tease-mount of C. immitis demonstrates chains of arthroconidia separated by empty disjunctor cells ➡. (Courtesy D. Sutton, MD.)

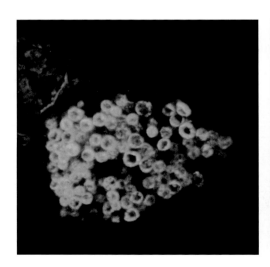
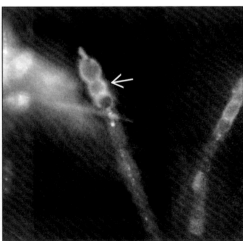

(Left) Spherule with endospores of C. immitis in lung is demonstrated by calcofluor white stain. Endospores, and not the spherule wall, are stained. (Courtesy CDC Public Health Image Library, #488.) *(Right)* C. immitis hyphae from ventriculoperitoneal catheter tip stained with calcofluor white stain demonstrates barrel-shaped arthroconidia ➡ and empty disjunctor cells. (Courtesy L. Davis, MD.)

COCCIDIOIDES LYMPHADENITIS

Microscopic Features

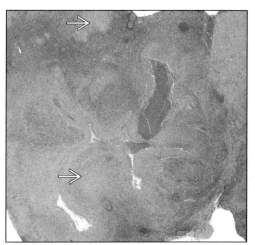

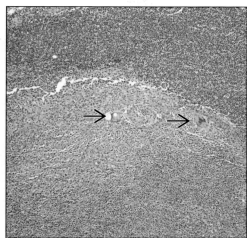

(Left) Granulomatous phase of coccidioidomycosis lymphadenitis demonstrates effaced architecture with capsular thickening at low power. Note the nodular areas with caseating necrosis at the center ➡. *(Right)* Granulomatous phase of coccidioidomycosis lymphadenitis demonstrates a dense chronic inflammatory infiltrate composed of lymphocytes and histiocytes in a background of marked vascular proliferation. Note the multinucleated giant cells ➡.

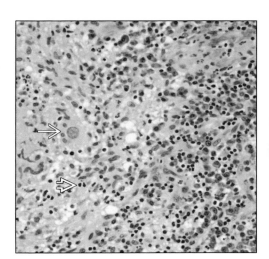

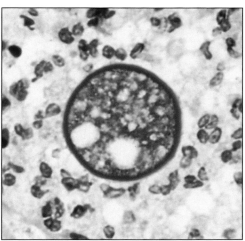

(Left) Granulomatous phase of coccidioidomycosis lymphadenitis demonstrates a mixed lymphoplasmacytic and histiocytic infiltrate. Note the spherule containing endospores ➡ and focal neutrophilic reaction ➡. *(Right)* A thick-walled spherule of C. immitis containing endospores is demonstrated by PAS stain. Note the surrounding neutrophilic reaction.

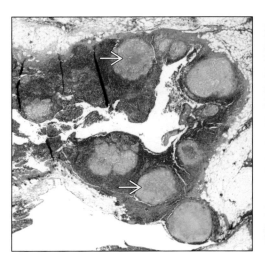

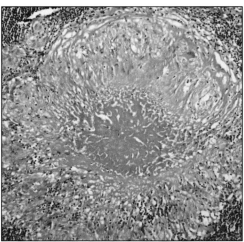

(Left) Granulomatous phase of coccidioidomycosis lymphadenitis demonstrates numerous well-defined granulomas with central caseating necrosis ➡ surrounded by pale pink histiocytic cells. *(Right)* Granulomatous phase of coccidioidomycosis lymphadenitis demonstrates caseating necrosis surrounded by layers of pale epithelioid histiocytic cells.

COCCIDIOIDES LYMPHADENITIS

Microscopic Features

(Left) Granulomatous phase of coccidioidomycosis lymphadenitis demonstrates extensive caseating necrosis ➡ with a chronic inflammatory reaction and fibrosis ➡. *(Right)* Spherule of C. immitis is demonstrated by GMS stain. Note the endospore abutting the spherule wall ➡. A few spherules with no endospores identified is considered presumptive evidence of infection. (Courtesy A. Husain, MD.)

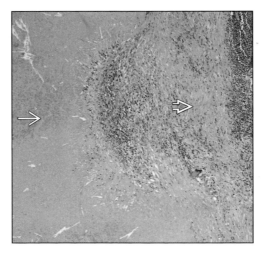
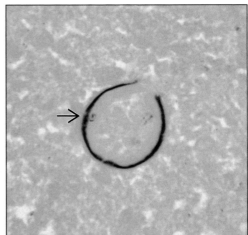

(Left) Spherule of C. immitis containing endospores is demonstrated by GMS stain. Identification of endospores within spherules is considered diagnostic. (Courtesy A. Husain, MD.) *(Right)* Immature spherule of C. immitis containing endospores is demonstrated by PAS in pus specimen harvested from a skin lesion in a case of cutaneous coccidioidomycosis. (Courtesy G. Carroll, MD, CDC Public Health Image Library, #11031.)

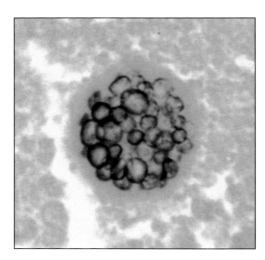
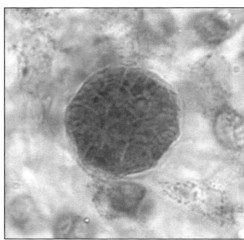

(Left) Spherule of C. immitis is demonstrated by PAS stain. Note rupture of the wall releasing the endospores. (Courtesy A. Husain, MD.) *(Right)* Spherule of C. immitis is demonstrated by PAS stain. Note the well-defined endospores. (Courtesy CDC Public Health Image Library, #487.)

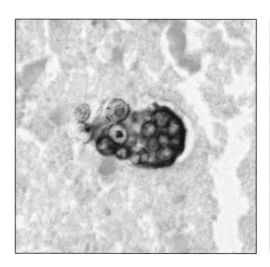
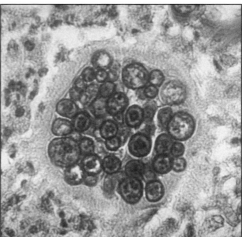

COCCIDIOIDES LYMPHADENITIS

Microscopic Features

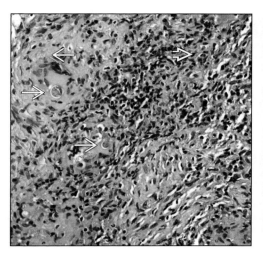

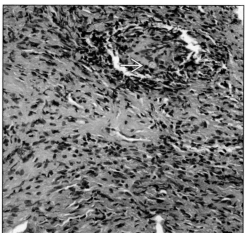

(Left) Granulomatous phase of coccidioidomycosis lymphadenitis involving lymph node demonstrates endospores containing spherules within giant cells ➡. Scattered eosinophils are admixed with an exuberant histiocytic infiltrate ➡. This HIV(+) patient presented with generalized lymphadenopathy and systemic symptoms. *(Right)* Granulomatous phase of coccidioidomycosis lymphadenitis demonstrates spherule of C. immitis containing endospores within a granuloma ➡.

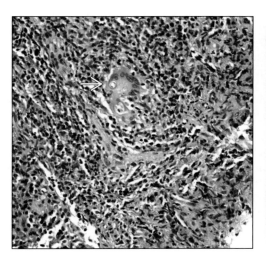

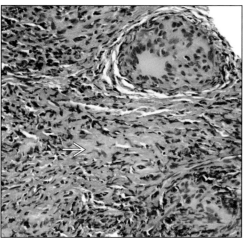

(Left) Granulomatous phase of coccidioidomycosis lymphadenitis demonstrates a single spherule of C. immitis containing endospores within a giant cell ➡. *(Right)* Numerous multinucleated giant cells are seen in this case of granulomatous phase of coccidioidomycosis lymphadenitis. Note the surrounding fibrosis ➡.

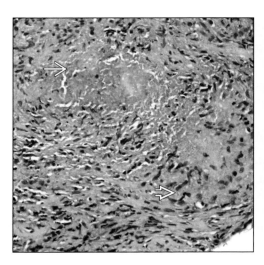

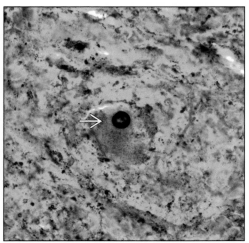

(Left) Granulomatous phase of coccidioidomycosis lymphadenitis demonstrates necrosis ➡ surrounded by epithelioid histiocytes ➡. *(Right)* Grocott methenamine silver stain highlights spherule of C. immitis with endospores ➡ in this case of coccidioidomycosis lymphadenitis (1,000x oil immersion).

HERPES SIMPLEX LYMPHADENITIS

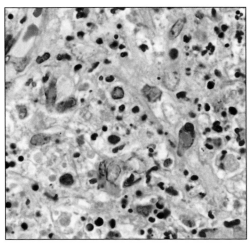

Cells with eosinophilic intranuclear inclusions (Cowdry type A) in a background of necrosis. These findings are typical of herpes simplex infection.

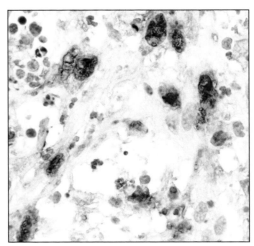

HSV1/2 shows many cells with nuclei that are strongly positive for herpes virus types 1 and 2. The cells infected in this field are spindled and appear to be endothelial.

TERMINOLOGY

Abbreviations
- Herpes simplex virus (HSV)

Synonyms
- HSV lymphadenitis, herpetic lymphadenitis

Definitions
- Lymph node infection by herpes simplex virus (type 1 or 2)

CLINICAL ISSUES

Presentation
- Lymphadenopathy, localized
  - Most common; often involves inguinal or femoral regions 4-7 days after exposure
  - Generalized lymphadenopathy or disseminated viral infection can occur, often in immunocompromised patients
- Skin lesions most common and occur as bilateral clusters of vesicles or papules
  - Lesions can be painful with burning or itching
  - Skin lesions commonly recur
- HSV lymphadenitis or skin lesions can occur in patients with malignant neoplasms

Treatment
- Drugs
  - Antiviral agents commonly used include acyclovir, valacyclovir, and famciclovir
    - Drugs ameliorate symptoms or decrease outbreaks but are not curative

Prognosis
- Infection usually resolves in immunocompetent patients; herpes infection can reactivate with recurrent lesions

MICROSCOPIC PATHOLOGY

Histologic Features
- Interfollicular/paracortical regions usually focally involved, imparting "punched out" appearance
  - Necrotic areas show "ghost cells," debris, neutrophils, and infected cells
- Lymphocytes, epithelial, and endothelial cells can be infected
  - HSV-infected cells show multinucleation, ground-glass nuclei, and intranuclear inclusions
  - Inclusions are eosinophilic and intranuclear
  - Inclusions are known as Cowdry type A
- Surrounding necrotic areas show spectrum of inflammatory cells including immunoblasts
- Follicular hyperplasia can be present
- HSV infection can be associated with lymphomas
  - Can occur simultaneously with lymphoma in same or different anatomic sites
  - Chronic lymphocytic leukemia/small lymphocytic lymphoma (CLL/SLL) is most common

Predominant Pattern/Injury Type
- Lymphoid, interfollicular

Predominant Cell/Compartment Type
- Lymphocyte

ANCILLARY TESTS

Immunohistochemistry
- Predominance of T cells in interfollicular regions and necrotic areas; increased CD8(+) T cells
- No evidence of monotypic Ig

Flow Cytometry
- Flow cytometry shows mixture of T cells and polytypic B cells; no evidence of monoclonality

HERPES SIMPLEX LYMPHADENITIS

Key Facts

Terminology
- Lymph node infection by HSV (type 1 or 2)

Clinical Issues
- Localized lymphadenopathy is most common, often involves inguinal or femoral regions
  - 4-7 days after exposure
  - Often associated with constitutional symptoms
- Generalized lymphadenopathy or disseminated herpes virus infection also can occur
  - Most common in immunocompromised patients

Microscopic Pathology
- Interfollicular/paracortical regions usually focally involved
  - Imparts a low-power "punched out" appearance

- HSV-infected cells show multinucleation, ground-glass nuclei, and inclusions
  - Inclusions are eosinophilic and intranuclear
- Surrounding necrotic areas show spectrum of inflammatory cells
  - Lymphocytes, immunoblasts, eosinophils, and macrophages
- Flow cytometry shows mixture of T cells and polytypic B cells
- Immunohistochemistry: T cells > B cells
- No evidence of monoclonal gene rearrangements

Top Differential Diagnoses
- Cat scratch lymphadenitis
- Kikuchi-Fujimoto disease
- Classical Hodgkin lymphoma
- Diffuse large B-cell lymphoma

PCR
- Gene rearrangement studies show no evidence of monoclonal *Ig* or *TCR* gene rearrangements

DIFFERENTIAL DIAGNOSIS

Cat Scratch Lymphadenitis
- Foci of necrosis in paracortical regions but form stellate microabscesses
  - Caused by bacterium *B. henselae*
- Later stages can exhibit granulomas

Mycobacterial Tuberculosis Lymphadenitis
- Caseating necrosis surrounded by granulomatous inflammation
  - Acid-fast stain helpful to detect bacilli
  - Bacilli most often detected in caseating necrosis

Kikuchi-Fujimoto Disease
- Paracortical distribution
- Early phase shows many histiocytes
- Later phases show necrosis
  - No neutrophils
- Unknown etiology; unknown virus suspected

Classical Hodgkin Lymphoma (CHL)
- Immunoblasts in HSV may be confused with Hodgkin and Reed-Sternberg (HRS) cells
  - HRS cells are CD15(+), CD30(+), CD45(-)
- Many eosinophils often in HL; unusual in HSV

Diffuse Large B-cell Lymphoma (DLBCL)
- Sheets of immunoblasts in HSV may be confused with DLBCL
  - Large cells are CD20(+); may express monotypic Ig
- DLBCL has monoclonal *Ig* gene rearrangements

DIAGNOSTIC CHECKLIST

Pathologic Interpretation Pearls
- Presence of paracortical necrosis should alert search for evidence of HSV infection
  - Inguinal lymph nodes are suspicious site
  - Necrosis
  - Multinucleation, ground-glass nuclei, and intranuclear inclusions

SELECTED REFERENCES
1. Arduino PG et al: Herpes Simplex Virus Type 1 infection: overview on relevant clinico-pathological features. J Oral Pathol Med. 37(2):107-21, 2008
2. Cernik C et al: The treatment of herpes simplex infections: an evidence-based review. Arch Intern Med. 168(11):1137-44, 2008
3. Gattenlohner S et al: Concomitant Herpes simplex and Epstein-Barr virus lymphadenitis with simultaneous lymph node metastases of an occult squamous cell carcinoma in a patient with chronic lymphocytic leukemia. Leuk Lymphoma. 49(12):2390-2, 2008
4. Koelle DM et al: Herpes simplex: insights on pathogenesis and possible vaccines. Annu Rev Med. 59:381-95, 2008
5. Gupta R et al: Genital herpes. Lancet. 370(9605):2127-37, 2007
6. Pilichowska ME et al: Concurrent herpes simplex viral lymphadenitis and mantle cell lymphoma: a case report and review of the literature. Arch Pathol Lab Med. 130(4):536-9, 2006
7. Joseph L et al: Localized herpes simplex lymphadenitis mimicking large-cell (Richter's) transformation of chronic lymphocytic leukemia/small lymphocytic lymphoma. Am J Hematol. 68(4):287-91, 2001
8. Howat AJ et al: Generalized lymphadenopathy due to herpes simplex virus type I. Histopathology. 19(6):563-4, 1991
9. Tamaru J et al: Herpes simplex lymphadenitis. Report of two cases with review of the literature. Am J Surg Pathol. 14(6):571-7, 1990

HERPES SIMPLEX LYMPHADENITIS

Microscopic Features

(Left) Inguinal lymph node is seen with capsular thickening and marked expansion of the paracortical/interfollicular areas by a spectrum of lymphoid cells, including many immunoblasts. *(Right)* Lymph node at the junction of the expanded paracortex/interfollicular region and residual, uninvolved lymphoid tissue ➡. Numerous large centroblasts and immunoblasts are present.

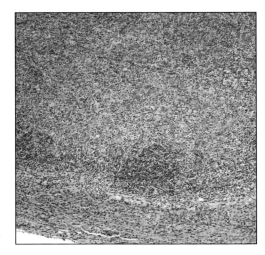
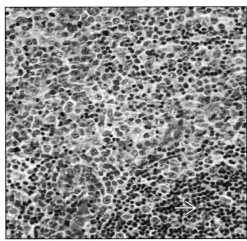

(Left) Lymph node with a focus of necrosis and acute inflammation in the subcapsular region. Viral inclusions, although not easily seen in a routine histologic section, were shown by in situ hybridization for HSV. *(Right)* In situ hybridization shows a lymph node in which evidence of an HSV infection was identified. In this field, 4 virally infected cells ➡ are seen in an area of subcapsular necrosis.

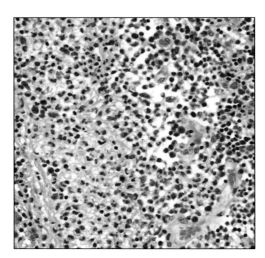
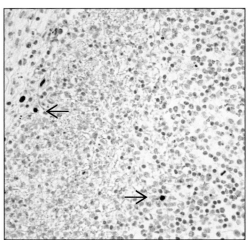

(Left) Lymph node involved by CLL/SLL (left) and HSV infection (right). The HSV-infected area shows extensive necrosis. *(Right)* Lymph node with CLL/SLL and HSV infection. This is a high-power magnification of area of an HSV infection. There are many spindled cells with intranuclear inclusions and one with a multinucleation, consistent with viral infection.

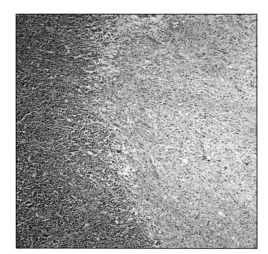
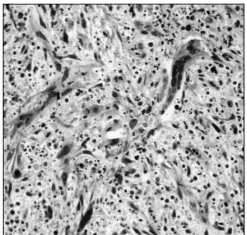

HERPES SIMPLEX LYMPHADENITIS

Microscopic and Immunohistochemical Features

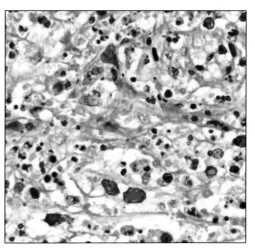

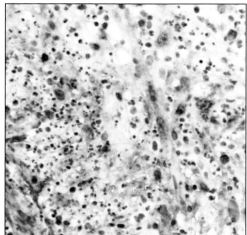

(Left) Lymph node with CLL/SLL and HSV infection. In this field of HSV infection, there are many cells with large nuclei and prominent intranuclear (Cowdry type A) inclusions. The virally infected cells are present in a background of necrotic cell ghosts, nuclear debris, and inflammatory cells. (Right) HSV1/2 immunohistochemical stain of lymph node with CLL/SLL and HSV infection. This high-power field of HSV infection shows nuclei strongly positive for HSV.

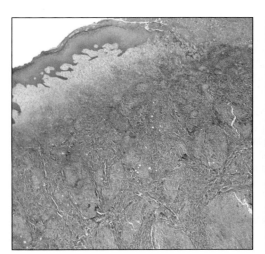

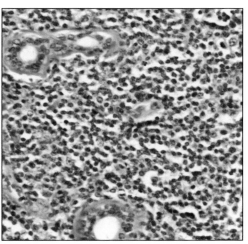

(Left) Hematoxylin and eosin stain shows skin involved by CLL/SLL in the dermis and HSV infection causing an epidermal ulcer (upper right). (Right) Skin with CLL/SLL and HSV infection. This field shows numerous small CLL/SLL cells that replace the dermis. There is no evidence of HSV shown in this field.

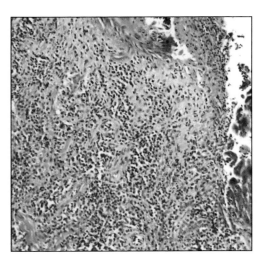

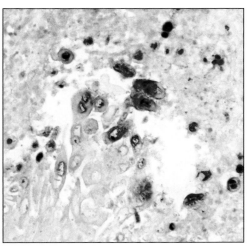

(Left) CLL/SLL involving the dermis. In addition, an epidermal ulcer is shown, the result of an HSV infection. Many epidermal cells in this field (lower right) show ground-glass nuclei, consistent with HSV infection. (Right) In situ hybridization shows epidermal cells with many nuclei positive for HSV DNA.

CYTOMEGALOVIRUS LYMPHADENITIS

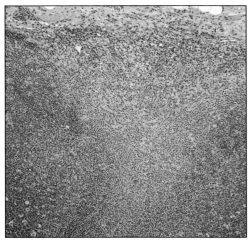

CMV lymphadenitis. This field shows that the sinus is expanded by monocytoid B cells between 2 large, reactive follicles (left and right).

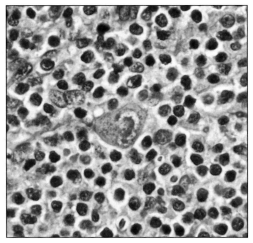

The high-power view of CMV lymphadenitis shows a large cell infected by CMV, which has a prominent intranuclear inclusion surrounded by a halo and multiple, small cytoplasmic inclusions.

TERMINOLOGY

Abbreviations
- Cytomegalovirus (CMV)

Definitions
- Lymphadenitis caused by CMV infection

ETIOLOGY/PATHOGENESIS

CMV
- Member of β-herpes virus family
  - Double-stranded DNA virus with 162 hexagonal protein capsomeres surrounded by lipid membrane
- Lytic virus that causes cytopathic effect in vitro and in vivo
- Productive (lytic) infection leads to synthesis of immediate-early, early, and late viral proteins
- Viral DNA has been detected in monocytes, dendritic cells, megakaryocytes, and myeloid progenitor cells in bone marrow
- Virus infects T cells but not B cells
- Monocytes and endothelial cells are also commonly infected by CMV
- Can be transmitted by a number of means
  - Person-to person via saliva, respiratory secretions, or sexual fluids
  - Blood transfusions
  - Transplacental passage
- Immunology
  - Body produces neutralizing antibodies upon primary infection
  - Cell-mediated immunity is most important factor in controlling CMV infection

CMV Infection in Immunocompetent Host
- Mostly primary infection

CMV Infection in Immunocompromised Patients
- Reactivation of CMV, either iatrogenic or secondary to underlying medical conditions
  - Solid organ or bone marrow transplantation
  - Acquired immunodeficiency syndrome (AIDS)

CMV Infection in Pregnancy
- Maternal primary CMV infection
- In utero transmission of CMV, either due to primary CMV infection or reactivation
  - Can be lethal with damage to central nervous system (CNS)

CLINICAL ISSUES

Epidemiology
- Incidence
  - Infection with CMV is common as determined by presence of serum antibodies
    - In developed countries, 60-80% of population is infected by adulthood
    - In developing countries, most children are infected by 3 years of age
    - > 90% of homosexual men are infected by CMV
  - Age, geography, cultural and socioeconomic status, and child rearing practices affect prevalence
- Age
  - Congenital
    - 1% of newborns are infected by CMV
  - Perinatal infection due to
    - Maternal cervicovaginal secretions during delivery
    - Breast feeding
  - Daycare toddlers
    - Horizontal transmission of virus to both children and adult daycare center workers
  - Adolescence
    - Sexual transmission

CYTOMEGALOVIRUS LYMPHADENITIS

Key Facts

Terminology
- Lymphadenitis caused by cytomegalovirus (CMV) infection

Etiology/Pathogenesis
- Member of β-herpes viruses
- Causes cytopathic changes
- Lytic infection: Immediate-early, early, and late viral proteins
- Immunocompetent hosts: Often primary infection
- Immunocompromised patients: Reactivation

Clinical Issues
- Diagnosis of CMV infection
  ○ Serology
  ○ Shell vial culture
  ○ CMV antigenemia assay
  ○ Molecular amplification
- Treatment: Ganciclovir
- Prognosis
  ○ In immunocompetent patients: Self-limited
  ○ CMV pneumonia in immunocompromised patients has high mortality rate

Microscopic Pathology
- Follicular hyperplasia can be florid
- Paracortical, interfollicular, and subcapsular areas
  ○ Immunoblasts, monocytoid B cells
  ○ Focal necrosis can be seen
  ○ CMV infected cells

Top Differential Diagnoses
- Infectious mononucleosis
- Other types of viral lymphadenitis

  ○ Immunocompromised patients, all ages
  ○ Blood or tissue exposure, all ages
- Gender
  ○ No sex preference
- Ethnicity
  ○ No preferences

Presentation
- Immunocompetent patients
  ○ Asymptomatic or flu-like syndrome
  ○ Symptoms similar to infectious mononucleosis-type syndrome, but milder
    ▪ Fever of unknown origin
    ▪ Lymphadenopathy, often cervical
    ▪ Pharyngitis
    ▪ Hepatosplenomegaly
    ▪ Blood: Lymphocytosis with atypical lymphocytes
  ○ CMV reactivation is common in critically ill immunocompetent patients
    ▪ Can be associated with prolonged hospitalization
- Immunocompromised patients
  ○ Organ transplant recipients and patients with immunodeficiency syndromes
  ○ Interstitial pneumonitis
    ▪ Respiratory symptoms, fever, and dyspnea
    ▪ Can be life-threatening
  ○ Gastrointestinal infection
    ▪ Esophagus: Dysphagia
    ▪ Upper gastrointestinal tract: Ulcer
    ▪ Colon: Bloody diarrhea, fever, and abdominal pain
  ○ CMV retinitis
    ▪ Frequent in HIV patients with a CD4 count < 50 cells/μL
    ▪ Decreased/impaired visual acuity, floaters, and loss of visual fields on 1 side
    ▪ Can progress to bilateral involvement if untreated
  ○ Neurologic manifestations
    ▪ CMV encephalitis
    ▪ Guillain-Barré syndrome
    ▪ Other peripheral neuropathies
  ○ CMV hepatitis

    ▪ Often subclinical
    ▪ Unexplained fever
    ▪ Abnormal liver function tests
    ▪ Portal vein thrombosis (rare)
  ○ Pericarditis and myocarditis
  ○ Myeloradiculopathy
  ○ Disseminated CMV infection is criterion for AIDS
- Congenital infection
  ○ At birth
    ▪ Small size for gestational age
    ▪ Hepatosplenomegaly
    ▪ Petechiae and purpura of the skin, jaundice
    ▪ Neurologic involvement: Microcephaly, seizures, and feeding difficulties
  ○ Sequelae in children
    ▪ Sensorineural hearing loss
    ▪ Chorioretinitis
    ▪ Microcephaly, seizures, or paresis/paralysis
    ▪ Mental retardation

Laboratory Tests
- Serology
  ○ Recent and acute CMV infection
    ▪ Detection of CMV-specific IgM antibodies
    ▪ At least 4x increase in CMV-specific IgG titers in specimens obtained at least 2-4 weeks apart
  ○ To determine past exposure to CMV infection
    ▪ If positive for past infection, monitor those at risk for CMV reactivation syndromes
    ▪ If negative for past infection, monitor for new infection if transplanted with CMV seropositive organ
- Early antigen detection (shell vial cultures)
  ○ Methods
    ▪ Centrifugation of clinical samples (e.g., urine, blood) to increase absorption of virus
    ▪ Infected cell monolayers incubated with monoclonal antibodies specific for CMV
  ○ Results typically available within 2-3 days
    ▪ Accelerates time to diagnosis
- CMV antigenemia assays
  ○ Methods

CYTOMEGALOVIRUS LYMPHADENITIS

- Using monoclonal antibodies specific to pp65 lower matrix protein of CMV to detect CMV-infected leukocytes in peripheral blood
- Results are reported as number of cells with staining per total number of cells counted
  - o Advantage
    - Results generally available within 24 hours
    - Antigenemia appears to correlate with viremia
- Molecular methods for detecting CMV
  - o Hybrid Capture System CMV DNA test
    - Signal amplification method using RNA probe that targets CMV
  - o COBAS Amplicor test
    - PCR assay that amplifies 365 base pair region of CMV polymerase gene
  - o Nucleic acid sequence-based amplification (NASBA)
    - Detects both immediate-early gene *UL123 (IE1)* and late gene expression (*pp67*)
  - o Utility
    - Sensitive and specific for organ transplant patients
    - Not sensitive in detecting acute CMV infection
- Other laboratory findings
  - o Heterophile antibody is negative
  - o Hematologic findings: Absolute lymphocytosis and atypical lymphocytes
    - CD4:CD8 ratio reversed
    - Increased large granular lymphocytes, NK cells
- Viral cultures
  - o CMV grows slowly in cell culture
    - Not a rapid confirmatory test
  - o Positive result does not confirm active CMV disease
  - o Limited sensitivity

Treatment

- Drugs
  - o Antiviral agents have value
    - Ganciclovir
    - Foscarnet (Foscavir)
    - Valganciclovir
    - Cidofovir (Vistide)
- Therapy for bone marrow or solid organ transplant patients
  - o Prophylaxis
    - Patients who have positive CMV serology
    - CMV-positive donor with CMV-negative recipient
  - o Preemptive therapy
    - Patients who have evidence of ongoing viral replication
- In HIV(+) or AIDS patients
  - o Greatly reduced frequency of CMV infection as result of highly active antiretroviral therapy
- CMV hyperimmune globulin-prophylactic therapy of CMV disease

Prognosis

- Immunocompetent patients
  - o Infection usually self-limited
- Immunocompromised patients
  - o CMV pneumonia
    - High mortality rate, especially in bone marrow transplant patients

- Mortality: 30-60% with ganciclovir vs. 85% without ganciclovir
  - o CMV hepatitis
  - o CNS: Infection can leave neurological deficits
  - o Prognosis determined by underlying disease
- Congenital infection
  - o Can cause impairment of hearing or cognitive or motor functions

IMAGE FINDINGS

Radiographic Findings

- CMV interstitial pneumonia
  - o Changes on chest radiograph or CT scan

MICROSCOPIC PATHOLOGY

Histologic Features

- Lymph nodes show mixed reactive pattern
  - o Follicular hyperplasia
    - Often florid with prominent "starry sky" pattern
    - May not be prominent in immunocompromised or older patients
  - o Paracortical and interfollicular hyperplasia
    - Diffuse pattern ± mottled appearance
    - Mixed cell population: Lymphocytes of varying size, histiocytes, and immunoblasts
    - Immunoblasts can form sheets
    - Increased vascularity
    - Clusters of plasmacytoid monocytes (type 2 dendritic cells)
    - Foci of necrosis can be present
  - o Monocytoid B-cell hyperplasia
    - Located within and distends sinuses
    - Associated with neutrophils

Cytologic Features

- Virus infects lymphocytes, monocytes, and endothelial cells
  - o Infected cells can be cytologically normal or show characteristic changes
  - o Endothelial cells in sinuses are likely place for viral inclusions
    - Often surrounded by acute inflammatory cells
- Large cells with nuclear inclusions
  - o Usually single, 15 μm
  - o Brightly eosinophilic, surrounded by clear space
  - o "Owl's eye" appearance
- CMV-infected cells also have cytoplasmic inclusions
  - o 2-4 μm, eosinophilic, multiple
- Immunohistochemistry or in situ hybridization required to detect all infected cells
  - o Subset of infected cells are cytologically normal

Histopathology of CMV Infection Involving Other Anatomic Sites

- Gastrointestinal tract
  - o CMV infects endothelial cells, fibroblasts, and smooth muscle cells
  - o In colon: Usually affects ileocecal area

- May cause vasculitis, luminal thrombosis, and associated severe necrotizing disease
- Liver
  - In immunocompetent patients
    - Predominantly sinusoidal infiltrate of atypical lymphocytes
    - Minimal necrosis
    - Variable mitotic figures and small epithelioid granulomas can be seen
  - In immunocompromised patients
    - Microabscesses are often present
    - Other findings similar to immunocompetent patients
- Placenta
  - Chronic villitis with lymphocytes and plasma cells
  - Rare cells with CMV inclusions (nuclear or cytoplasmic)
- Lung
  - CMV usually infects both endothelial and epithelial cells
  - Lymphocytic infiltrate, edema, and pneumocyte hyperplasia
  - Hemorrhagic necrosis may be present
- Retina
  - Coagulative necrosis with secondary choroidal inflammation
  - Retinal cells can have prominent CMV inclusions (nuclear and cytoplasmic)
- Brain
  - Infects neurons and glial cells
  - Cells with CMV inclusions common
- Kidney
  - Virus infects glomerular cells, tubular epithelial cells, and peritubular capillary endothelial cells
  - Cells with CMV inclusions usually detected; inflammatory infiltrate
- Skin
  - Endothelial cells and fibroblasts are infected
  - Epidermal cells are usually not involved
- Adrenal gland
  - Many cells with viral inclusions can be detected
    - Commonly associated with necrosis
    - Usually examined at autopsy
  - CMV infection in early stages may stimulate cortisol production

ANCILLARY TESTS

Immunohistochemistry
- Sensitive method for detecting cells infected by CMV
  - More sensitive for detecting nuclear than cytoplasmic virus
- More cells infected by virus revealed by IHC than morphological assessment of viral inclusions
- Infected lymphocytes are T cells, either CD4(+) or CD8(+)
  - B cells are usually negative for CMV
- CMV-infected endothelial cells can be negative for factor VIII-related antigen
- Cells with CMV inclusions can be CD15(+) and CD45(-)

In Situ Hybridization
- This method is interchangeable with IHC for CMV detection
- Flow cytometry immunophenotyping
  - No evidence of a monotypic B-cell or aberrant T-cell population
- Molecular testing
  - No evidence of a monoclonal B-cell or T-cell population
  - Detection of CMV virus

DIFFERENTIAL DIAGNOSIS

Infectious Mononucleosis (IM)
- Infection by Epstein-Barr virus (EBV)
- CMV lymphadenitis can closely resemble IM clinically
- CMV lymphadenitis also can resemble IM histologically
  - Diffuse paracortical/interfollicular proliferation
    - Spectrum of cells, including immunoblasts
    - Immunoblasts can form sheets
  - Follicular hyperplasia can be marked
    - Ragged or mottled borders and "starry sky" pattern
    - Increased mitotic activity
  - Capsular/extranodal infiltration
  - Early CMV infections have prominent monocytoid B-cell reaction
- IM can be distinguished from CMV lymphadenitis by
  - Heterophil antibody in serum is often positive
  - Serology for EBV IgM is often positive in acute infection
  - In situ hybridization for EBV encoded RNA (EBER) is positive in lymph nodes
  - No cells with viral inclusions in lymph nodes
  - IHC or in situ hybridization negative for CMV

Other Viral or Viral-like Lymphadenitis
- Postvaccinal lymphoid hyperplasia: Smallpox, measles
  - Diffuse or nodular paracortical hyperplasia
    - Proliferation of immunoblasts
    - Other cells: Eosinophils, plasma cells
  - Follicular hyperplasia is usually not prominent
  - In measles, polykaryocytes (Warthin-Finkeldey) cells may be present
- Herpes simplex virus (HSV)
  - Changes can be similar to infectious mononucleosis
  - "Punched out" necrosis can be present
    - Usually in paracortex
  - HSV infects lymphocytes or endothelial cells in lymph node
  - Cells with intranuclear inclusions may be seen in or near necrotic areas
    - Mononucleated or multinucleated cells
    - Ground-glass intranuclear inclusions with peripheral margination of chromatin (Cowdry type A)
    - No cytoplasmic inclusions (unlike CMV)
    - Reactive for anti-HSV antibody

HIV Lymphadenopathy
- In early stages

CYTOMEGALOVIRUS LYMPHADENITIS

- o Florid reactive hyperplasia with follicle lysis
- o Foci of hemorrhage
- o Monocytoid B-cell hyperplasia in sinuses
- In later stages
  - o Interfollicular area shows vascular proliferation and increased plasma cells and histiocytes
  - o Progressive depletion of lymphocytes
  - o Presence of opportunistic infections
  - o Presence of neoplasms (e.g., lymphomas, Kaposi sarcoma)
- HIV lymphadenopathy can coexist with CMV infection

Kikuchi-Fujimoto Disease

- Paracortical, well-circumscribed necrotic lesions
  - o Karyorrhexis/apoptosis; fibrin deposits
  - o No neutrophils in necrotic zones
- Surrounding necrotic regions, following changes often present
  - o "Starry sky" pattern in viable lymphoid tissue
  - o Plasmacytoid monocytes are often prominent
  - o Follicular hyperplasia can be present

Drug-induced Lymphadenopathy

- Very common with anti-seizure medications
  - o Phenytoin (Dilantin) and carbamazepine (Tegretol)
- Often a time relationship between drug administration and lymphadenopathy
- Diffuse paracortical hyperplasia with increased immunoblasts
  - o Eosinophils are helpful clue
  - o Immunoblasts can form sheets
- No evidence of CMV by morphology (i.e., no inclusions) or IHC/in situ hybridization

Non-Hodgkin Lymphoma (NHL)

- Sheets of immunoblasts in CMV lymphadenitis may suggest large cell lymphoma
- Clues to diagnosis of NHL
  - o Large cells usually do not resemble benign immunoblasts
  - o No CMV viral inclusions
  - o Cells in background are usually not polymorphous in NHL
  - o Immunophenotypic or molecular evidence of monoclonality

Classical Hodgkin Lymphoma (CHL)

- Large CMV-infected cells may be misinterpreted as Reed-Sternberg or Hodgkin cells
  - o CMV cells can be CD15(+) and CD45(-) similar to HL
- Clues to diagnosis of CHL
  - o Reed-Sternberg and Hodgkin cells are usually numerous (unlike CMV inclusions)
  - o Greater mixture of population of cells (eosinophils and plasma cells)
  - o No CMV viral inclusions
  - o Reed-Sternberg and Hodgkin cells are CD30(+) and pax-5(+) (unlike CMV cells)

DIAGNOSTIC CHECKLIST

Clinically Relevant Pathologic Features

- Asymptomatic or acute self-limited illness in immunocompetent patients
  - o Usually primary infection
- Can cause severe illness in immunocompromised patients
  - o Often reactivation of latent viral infection

Pathologic Interpretation Pearls

- Mixed pattern of hyperplasia
  - o Follicular hyperplasia can be florid
  - o Paracortical and interfollicular diffuse infiltrate
    - Polymorphous cell population with increased immunoblasts
  - o Distension of sinuses by monocytoid B cells
  - o Focal necrosis
- CMV-infected cells can be recognized by
  - o Prominent, single intranuclear inclusion
  - o Multiple small cytoplasmic inclusions
- IHC is more sensitive than visual inspection for detecting CMV
- IHC and in situ hybridization are equivalent methods for detecting CMV

SELECTED REFERENCES

1. Trevisan M et al: Human cytomegalovirus productively infects adrenocortical cells and induces an early cortisol response. J Cell Physiol. Epub ahead of print, 2009
2. Valenzuela M et al: Strategies for prevention of cytomegalovirus infection in renal transplant patients. Transplant Proc. 41(6):2673-5, 2009
3. Fernández-Ruiz M et al: Cytomegalovirus myopericarditis and hepatitis in an immunocompetent adult: successful treatment with oral valganciclovir. Intern Med. 47(22):1963-6, 2008
4. Sun HY et al: Prevention of posttransplant cytomegalovirus disease and related outcomes with valganciclovir: a systematic review. Am J Transplant. 8(10):2111-8, 2008
5. Torres-Madriz G et al: Immunocompromised hosts: perspectives in the treatment and prophylaxis of cytomegalovirus disease in solid-organ transplant recipients. Clin Infect Dis. 47(5):702-11, 2008
6. Staras SA et al: Seroprevalence of cytomegalovirus infection in the United States, 1988-1994. Clin Infect Dis. 43(9):1143-51, 2006
7. Griffiths P: Cytomegalovirus infection of the central nervous system. Herpes. 11 Suppl 2:95A-104A, 2004
8. Barry SM et al: Cytopathology or immunopathology? The puzzle of cytomegalovirus pneumonitis revisited. Bone Marrow Transplant. 26(6):591-7, 2000
9. Eddleston M et al: Severe cytomegalovirus infection in immunocompetent patients. Clin Infect Dis. 24(1):52-6, 1997
10. Mutimer D: CMV infection of transplant recipients. J Hepatol. 25(2):259-69, 1996
11. Zaia JA et al: Cytomegalovirus infection in the bone marrow transplant recipient. Infect Dis Clin North Am. 9(4):879-900, 1995
12. Rushin JM et al: Cytomegalovirus-infected cells express Leu-M1 antigen. A potential source of diagnostic error. Am J Pathol. 136(5):989-95, 1990

CYTOMEGALOVIRUS LYMPHADENITIS

Microscopic Features

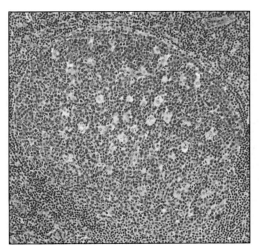

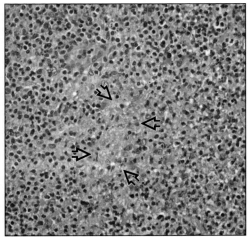

(Left) CMV lymphadenitis. A markedly reactive lymphoid follicle is seen. The follicle shows polarization with dark (upper) and light (lower) zones and a prominent "starry sky" pattern. *(Right)* CMV lymphadenitis. Note foci of necrosis. Necrosis can be present, especially in cases of severe infection ⊵.

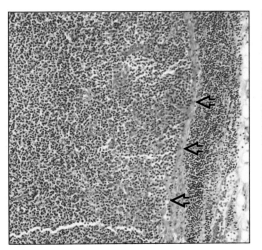

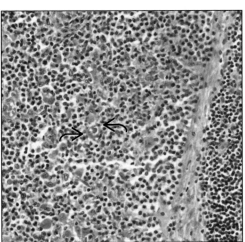

(Left) CMV lymphadenitis. A focus of subcapsular necrosis ⊵ is seen. Cells with viral inclusions are often present in areas with necrosis or inflammation. *(Right)* At high power, a large cell with a CMV intranuclear inclusion ⊅ is present in this focus of subcapsular necrosis.

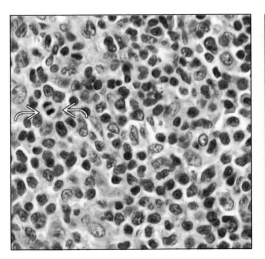

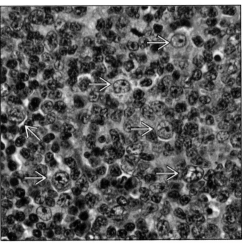

(Left) CMV lymphadenitis. Paracortical hyperplasia is seen with a polymorphous population of cells. A mitotic figure is present in the upper left region of this field ⊅. *(Right)* The paracortical and interfollicular areas contain many immunoblasts ⊅.

CYTOMEGALOVIRUS LYMPHADENITIS

Microscopic Features

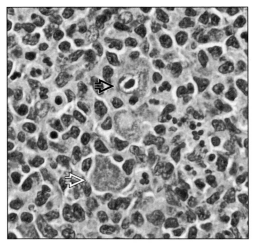 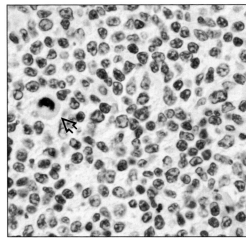

(Left) This field shows 2 large CMV-infected cells within a sinus, associated with monocytoid B cells and granulocytes. The upper cell ⮕ shows a prominent intranuclear inclusion and multiple cytoplasmic inclusions of CMV. The lower cell ⮕ shows cytoplasmic viral inclusions. *(Right)* An immunohistochemical stain using an anti-CMV antibody highlights nuclear viral inclusion ⮕. Cytoplasmic inclusions are often negative.

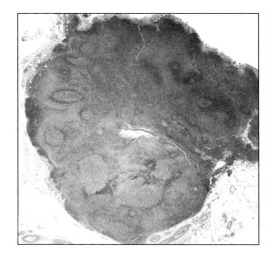 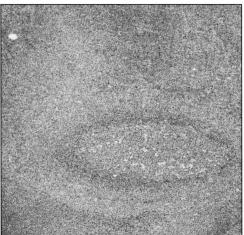

(Left) A low-power view of CMV lymphadenitis demonstrates follicular hyperplasia, monocytoid B cell hyperplasia in sinuses, and paracortical hyperplasia. *(Right)* CMV lymphadenitis. High magnification shows a central reactive follicle surrounded by monocytoid B-cell hyperplasia distending the sinuses.

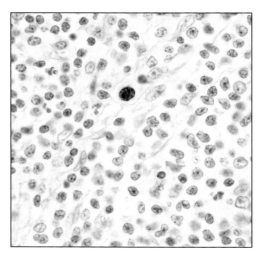 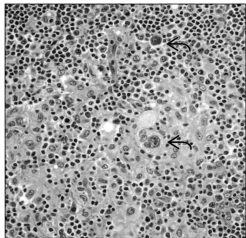

(Left) A case of CMV lymphadenitis in which typical CMV inclusions were very rare. However, an immunohistochemical stain using an anti-CMV antibody highlighted cells with positive nuclei. This case illustrates the point that IHC or in situ hybridization for CMV is more sensitive than morphologic examination and that IHC highlights cells that cytologically are not diagnostic of CMV infection. *(Right)* Tumor cells ⮕ in classical Hodgkin lymphoma can resemble CMV inclusions.

CYTOMEGALOVIRUS LYMPHADENITIS

Microscopic Features

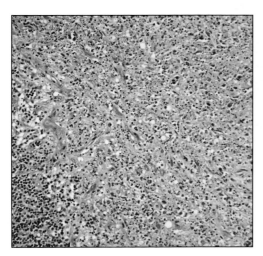
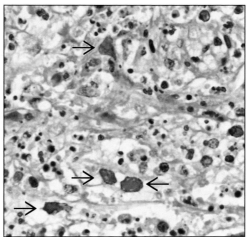

(Left) Herpes simplex viral (HSV) lymphadenitis. An area of "punched out" necrosis. Residual lymphoid tissue is at lower left. *(Right)* HSV lymphadenitis. Many cells with Cowdry type A intranuclear inclusions ⇨ are present in this field.

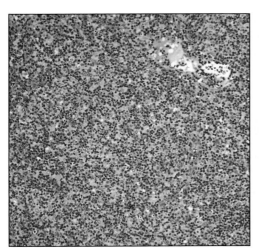
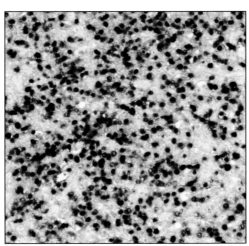

(Left) Infectious mononucleosis caused by infection by EBV. Marked interfollicular expansion by a mixed cell population, including activated lymphocytes, immunoblasts, histiocytes, and scattered eosinophils, is seen. *(Right)* In situ hybridization for Epstein-Barr virus encoded RNA (EBER) shows numerous infected cells.

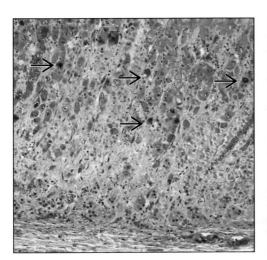
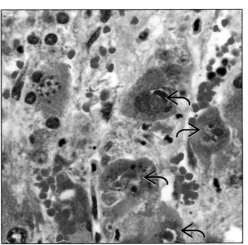

(Left) Disseminated CMV infection in the adrenal gland of a child with congenital immunodeficiency. This specimen was obtained at autopsy. This field shows necrosis and many large cells ⇨ that contain viral inclusions. *(Right)* CMV infection of the adrenal gland. Numerous prominent intranuclear inclusions and cytoplasmic inclusions ⇨ within adrenal cortical cells are present in this field.

HUMAN IMMUNODEFICIENCY VIRUS LYMPHADENITIS

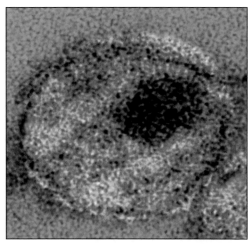

Thin section transmission electron micrograph of HIV. The viral core is the dark area in the center. (Courtesy A. Harrison, P. Feorino, CDC Public Health Image Library, #10860).

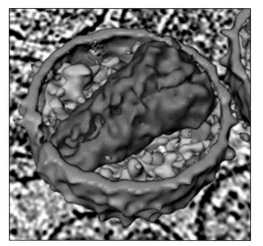

This 3D rendering of HIV demonstrates the viral membrane (blue), the density between the membrane and core (yellow), and the capsid (red). (Courtesy J. Briggs, PhD.)

TERMINOLOGY

Abbreviations
- Human immunodeficiency virus (HIV)

Synonyms
- Acquired immune deficiency syndrome (AIDS) lymphadenitis
- HIV lymphadenopathy

Definitions
- Lymphadenitis caused by HIV infection

ETIOLOGY/PATHOGENESIS

Infectious Agents
- HIV-1 underwent single cross-species transmission from chimpanzees to humans 100 years ago
  - Virus diversified in humans into many genetic subtypes: A-D
- Most sexually transmitted HIV infections are initiated by a single variant
  - Initial target cells are CD4(+) T cells
- HIV, a retrovirus belonging to the lentivirus family has
  - 9 genes
  - 2 copies of single-stranded RNA in core
  - Reverse transcriptase generates double-stranded DNA copy that integrates into host genome
    - Covalently forms a provirus
  - Provirus can remain latent or be highly expressed, forming progeny viruses
- Icosahedral structure with 72 external spikes composed of envelope proteins gp120 and gp41
  - Crucial for cell attachment and entry
- HIV has tropism for CD4(+) T cells, monocytes, and follicular dendritic cells
  - gp120 binds with CD4 receptor and subsequently with chemokines CR5 and CXCR4

  - Leads to fusion of viral and cellular membranes and internalization of viral complex
- 4 nucleocapsid proteins: p24, p17, p9, and p7

Pathogenesis of HIV Lymphadenopathy
- High HIV antigen density, marked inflammation, and adhesion molecule expression by lymphocytes
  - Leads to lymphocyte sequestration
- Exposure to increased cytokine levels results in lymphocyte death
- Prolonged inflammation leads to fibrosis resulting in
  - Disrupted maturation of T cells
  - Decreased naive circulating CD4(+) T cells
- Follicular dendritic cells in germinal centers entrap HIV

CLINICAL ISSUES

Epidemiology
- Incidence
  - 2.7 million new HIV infections per year in 2007 globally
  - Prevalence is stable at 0.8%
  - 33.2 million people have HIV infection or AIDS
  - 2 million deaths per year related to AIDS
- Age
  - Patients 15-24 years old represent 45% of new HIV infections globally
  - Estimated 370,000 children < 14 years old were infected in 2007
  - 2 million children with HIV
- Gender
  - No sex preference; stable globally
- Ethnicity
  - Sub-Saharan Africa accounts for 67% of total people and 90% of children living with HIV
    - Predominantly heterosexual transmission in general population
    - Accounts for 75% of AIDS-related deaths

HUMAN IMMUNODEFICIENCY VIRUS LYMPHADENITIS

Key Facts

Terminology
- Human immunodeficiency virus (HIV)
- Lymphadenitis caused by HIV infection

Clinical Issues
- History of high-risk exposure should be sought

Microscopic Pathology
- Histologic findings can be divided into stages
- Florid follicular hyperplasia
  - Irregularly shaped follicles, attenuation of mantle zones, follicle lysis, hemorrhage
- Mixed pattern
  - Transitional stage
- Follicular involution
  - Small, hypocellular, hyalinized follicles
  - Expanded paracortical regions

- Moderate lymphocyte depletion, plasmacytosis, vascular proliferation
- Lymphocyte depletion
  - Predominantly medullary cords and sinusoids
  - Marked lymphocyte depletion with absence of follicles and paracortical areas
  - Predominance of histiocytes and plasma cells; subcapsular and sinusoidal fibrosis
- Histologic changes partially reversed by HAART

Top Differential Diagnoses
- Other causes of acute lymphadenitis
  - Infectious mononucleosis (EBV+)
- Castleman disease, hyaline-vascular variant
- AIDS-related lymphomas
  - Non-Hodgkin lymphoma
  - Hodgkin lymphoma

- Asia overall has shown a trend toward a decrease in new HIV infections and an increase in AIDS-related deaths
  - National trends vary considerably
  - Recreational drug use, commercial sex work, and male-male sex are major factors in transmission
- Eastern Europe and Central Asia have shown a rising trend in number of people living with HIV infection
  - Number of new infections has been slowing
  - Recreational drug use and commercial sex work are major factors in transmission
- Western and Central Europe show stable trends
  - Heterosexual transmission is major mode of transmission
- Caribbean basin, South and North America show stable trends
  - Male-male sex is major mode of transmission, followed by heterosexual transmission
  - Number of persons living with HIV infection has increased as result of therapy

Presentation
- Acute (primary) phase of HIV infection
  - Can present as flu-like or mononucleosis type of syndrome with nonspecific symptoms
    - Findings: Fever, lymphadenopathy, skin rash, myalgia, arthralgia, headache, diarrhea, oral ulcers
    - Clinical diagnosis of acute HIV infection can be challenging
  - Usually lasts several weeks
  - Opportunistic infections can occur during transient CD4 lymphopenia
    - Most common: Oral and esophageal candidiasis
- Chronic phase of HIV infection is characterized by dysregulated or suppressed immunity
  - HIV infection can generally be latent for a number of years
  - Eventually patients develop symptoms and abnormalities related to low CD4(+) count
    - Polyclonal hypergammaglobulinemia
    - Altered levels of cytokines (e.g., IL-6, TNF-α) and activation markers (e.g., CD38 on T cells)

- Opportunistic infections: *Mycobacterium tuberculosis*, *Pneumocystis jiroveci* (formerly known as *P. carinii*)
    - Neoplasms: Lymphomas, Kaposi sarcoma
- ~ 50% of HIV(+) patients with lymphadenopathy are asymptomatic
  - Usually, lymph node biopsy shows follicular hyperplasia

Laboratory Tests
- Acute (primary) phase of HIV infection
  - Leukopenia, thrombocytopenia, elevated serum transaminase level
  - Viremia at high titers; CD4(+) T cells and monocytes infected
  - 3rd generation enzyme immunoassays used in clinical practice and in blood banks in USA do not detect HIV antibodies until 3-7 weeks after infection
- Chronic phase of HIV infection
  - Drop in CD4(+) counts to < 200/mm³
  - Findings related to specific opportunistic infections
- Diagnosis of acute infection is established by demonstrating
  - High viral load
  - p24 antigen in patient with typical clinical features and negative or indeterminate HIV serologic test
- Serologic testing
  - Based on detection of IgG against HIV antigens in serum
    - p24, a nucleocapsid protein
    - gp120 and gp41, envelope proteins
  - Centers for Disease Control (CDC) criteria for positive serology include
    - Antibodies to gp120 plus antibodies to either gp41 or p24
  - Antibodies to gp41 and p24 antigens are 1st detectable serologic markers following HIV infection
    - IgG antibodies appear 6-12 weeks following infection in most patients (by 6 months in 95%)
    - Antibodies persist for life
  - Results are reported as positive, negative, or indeterminate

HUMAN IMMUNODEFICIENCY VIRUS LYMPHADENITIS

- o Criteria for a positive test: Repeatedly positive enzyme immunoassay test followed by a positive Western blot analysis
  - ▪ Positive test should be confirmed by repeat testing or corroborating laboratory data
- o Accuracy of HIV serologic testing is high
  - ▪ 99.3% sensitivity and 99.7% specificity according to CDC survey
- o Rapid tests can be done at point of care and read by provider
  - ▪ High diagnostic accuracy comparable to standard serological tests and much cheaper
  - ▪ Results can be available in minutes

Treatment

- • Drugs
  - o Highly active antiretroviral therapy (HAART)
    - ▪ Increases disease-free survival by suppressing viral replication and improving immunologic function
  - o Indications for HAART
    - ▪ History of AIDS-defining illness, CD4 count < 350 cells/mm³, pregnant women, and HIV-associated nephropathy
  - o Syndrome resembling primary HIV infection occurs in patients 2-4 weeks after HAART is discontinued
    - ▪ Fever, lymphadenopathy, and rash; plasma viremia rises and CD4(+) counts fall

Prognosis

- • HIV infection can be indolent for years but will eventually become lethal without HAART
- • Lymph nodes in HIV(+) patients show histologic progression without therapy, from follicular hyperplasia to lymphocyte depletion
- • Lymph node biopsy findings in HIV(+) patients correlate, in part, with outcome
  - o Patients with follicular hyperplasia or mixed pattern have
    - ▪ Longer survival
    - ▪ Lower incidence of opportunistic infections
  - o Patients with lymphocyte depletion have very poor prognosis
- • HIV(+) patients have increased risk of non-Hodgkin and Hodgkin lymphoma
  - o HAART has reduced risk of non-Hodgkin lymphoma but not Hodgkin lymphoma

MACROSCOPIC FEATURES

General Features

- • Enlarged lymph nodes in follicular hyperplasia
- • Small, shrunken lymph nodes in lymphocyte depletion
  - o Often not biopsied but detected at autopsy

MICROSCOPIC PATHOLOGY

Histologic Features

- • Florid (explosive) follicular hyperplasia
  - o Markedly hyperplastic lymphoid follicles in cortex and medulla

- ▪ Follicles with irregular shapes (e.g., serpiginous)
- ▪ Attenuated mantle zones
- ▪ Follicle lysis, often associated with hemorrhage
- ▪ Hyperplastic germinal centers: Mitoses, apoptosis, tingible body macrophages ("starry sky")
- o Interfollicular areas show foci of hemorrhage
- o Sinuses can be expanded by monocytoid B cells
- o Multinucleated giant cells (Warthin-Finkeldey type)
  - ▪ Derived from follicular dendritic cells
- o Follicular involution may be focally present
- o Immunohistochemistry: Expression of viral antigens in germinal centers
- o Flow cytometry
  - ▪ No evidence of monoclonal B-cell population
- o Immunohistochemistry
  - ▪ Expression of viral antigens in germinal centers
  - ▪ Decreased CD4(+) T cells; increased CD8(+) and cytotoxic T cells in interfollicular areas
- • Mixed pattern
  - o Considered to be transitional phase
  - o Mixture of follicular hyperplasia and areas of follicular destruction
  - o Increased plasma cells and vascularity
- • Follicular involution
  - o Atrophic burnt-out follicles
  - o Small, depleted, and frequently hyalinized follicles
    - ▪ Intrafollicular blood vessels can be prominent (so-called "lollipop" lesions)
  - o Interfollicular areas show
    - ▪ Lymphocyte depletion
    - ▪ Increased histiocytes and plasma cells
    - ▪ Increased vascularity
- • Lymphocyte depletion
  - o Normal architecture effaced
    - ▪ Follicles and paracortical regions absent or poorly defined
    - ▪ Lymph nodes composed mainly of medullary cords and sinusoids
  - o Marked lymphocyte depletion with predominance of histiocytes and plasma cells
  - o Subcapsular and sinusoidal fibrosis
  - o Opportunistic infections common at this stage
- • Effect of HAART on lymph node histology
  - o Changes substantially reversed but usually do not entirely disappear
  - o Restoration of architecture with recovery of follicular structures
  - o CD4(+) T cells increase; CD8(+) and cytotoxic T cells decrease in interfollicular areas
  - o Increased naive (CD45RA[+]) and memory (CD45RO[+]) T cells
  - o Viral load and p24 expression in follicular dendritic cells decrease but persist
  - o If HAART discontinued, follicular hyperplasia recurs in 1-2 months
- • HIV-polymorphic lymphoproliferative disorders (PLD)
  - o Analogous, morphologically and genetically, to those arising after organ transplantation
  - o Continuous morphologic spectrum of increasing numbers of atypical cells to monomorphic DLBCL
  - o Most patients show localized nodal or extranodal presentation

HUMAN IMMUNODEFICIENCY VIRUS LYMPHADENITIS

- ▪ Extranodal sites: Lungs, parotid, and skin
- o Pathologic findings
  - ▪ Diffuse pattern
  - ▪ Polymorphous cell population
  - ▪ Foci of coagulative necrosis
  - ▪ Immunophenotype: B cells predominant
  - ▪ Monoclonal B cells in ~ 75% of cases (usually small population)
- o Viral data
  - ▪ Monoclonal EBV infection in ~ 40%
  - ▪ Human herpes virus 8 infection in ~ 20%
- o No *MYC*, *BCL6*, *RAS*, or *P53* gene abnormalities
- o Risk for transformation to overt B-cell lymphoma poorly characterized

Cytologic Features
- Fine needle aspiration of lymph node is useful to exclude
  - o Opportunistic infections
  - o Neoplasms

DIFFERENTIAL DIAGNOSIS

General Considerations
- Differential diagnosis is broad and includes benign and malignant diseases
- Varies according to stage of disease

Florid (Explosive) Follicular Hyperplasia
- Infectious mononucleosis (Epstein-Barr virus positive)
- Cytomegalovirus lymphadenitis
- Toxoplasma lymphadenitis
- Serologic studies required for specific diagnosis

Follicular Involution
- Castleman disease, hyaline-vascular variant
  - o Occurs in immunocompetent subjects
  - o Usually involves a single lymph node or group of lymph nodes (unicentric)
    - ▪ Thoracic region common
  - o No systemic signs and symptoms
  - o Lymphoid follicles have distinctive morphologic findings
    - ▪ "Lollipop" lesions and "onion skin" changes
  - o Vascular proliferation in interfollicular areas

Lymphocyte Depletion
- Late-stage lymphadenitis with fibrosis
  - o Diverse etiology
  - o History and serology essential for diagnosis

HIV-Polymorphic Lymphoproliferative Disorders (PLD)
- AIDS-related non-Hodgkin lymphomas
  - o Usually monomorphous
  - o Often stage III or IV disease
  - o Large monoclonal B-cell population
  - o Common abnormalities of *MYC*, *BCL6*, and *P53* genes
- AIDS-related classical Hodgkin lymphoma
  - o HRS cells present
    - ▪ CD15(+), CD30(+), EBV(+), CD45(-)

DIAGNOSTIC CHECKLIST

Pathologic Interpretation Pearls
- Changes in florid follicular hyperplasia that raise possibility of HIV infection
  - o Florid reactive follicles with attenuated mantle zones
  - o Foci of hemorrhage
  - o Follicle lysis, especially if associated with hemorrhage

SELECTED REFERENCES

1. Kilmarx PH: Global epidemiology of HIV. Curr Opin HIV AIDS. 4(4):240-6, 2009
2. Davenport MP et al: Understanding the mechanisms and limitations of immune control of HIV. Immunol Rev. 216:164-75, 2007
3. de Paiva GR et al: Discovery of human immunodeficiency virus infection by immunohistochemistry on lymph node biopsies from patients with unexplained follicular hyperplasia. Am J Surg Pathol. 31(10):1534-8, 2007
4. Branson BM et al: Revised recommendations for HIV testing of adults, adolescents, and pregnant women in health-care settings. MMWR Recomm Rep. 55(RR-14):1-17; quiz CE1-4, 2006
5. Alòs L et al: Immunoarchitecture of lymphoid tissue in HIV-infection during antiretroviral therapy correlates with viral persistence. Mod Pathol. 18(1):127-36, 2005
6. Nador RG et al: Human immunodeficiency virus (HIV)-associated polymorphic lymphoproliferative disorders. Am J Surg Pathol. 27(3):293-302, 2003
7. Orenstein JM et al: Rapid activation of lymph nodes and mononuclear cell HIV expression upon interrupting highly active antiretroviral therapy in patients after prolonged viral suppression. AIDS. 14(12):1709-15, 2000
8. Quijano G et al: Histopathologic findings in the lymphoid and reticuloendothelial system in pediatric HIV infection: a postmortem study. Pediatr Pathol Lab Med. 17(6):845-56, 1997
9. Wenig BM et al: Lymphoid changes of the nasopharyngeal and palatine tonsils that are indicative of human immunodeficiency virus infection. A clinicopathologic study of 12 cases. Am J Surg Pathol. 20(5):572-87, 1996
10. Burke AP et al: Systemic lymphadenopathic histology in human immunodeficiency virus-1-seropositive drug addicts without apparent acquired immunodeficiency syndrome. Hum Pathol. 25(3):248-56, 1994
11. Baroni CD et al: Lymph nodes in HIV-positive drug abusers with persistent generalized lymphadenopathy: histology, immunohistochemistry, and pathogenetic correlations. Prog AIDS Pathol. 2:33-50, 1990
12. Wood GS: The immunohistology of lymph nodes in HIV infection: a review. Prog AIDS Pathol. 2:25-32, 1990
13. Chadburn A et al: Progressive lymph node histology and its prognostic value in patients with acquired immunodeficiency syndrome and AIDS-related complex. Hum Pathol. 20(6):579-87, 1989

Microscopic Features

(Left) Inguinal lymph node demonstrates florid follicular hyperplasia in an HIV(+) patient. This low-power magnification shows numerous nodules composed of prominent germinal centers, many of which are surrounded by thin and attenuated mantle zones. In addition, some follicles in this field completely lack mantle zones. (Right) Lymph node shows florid follicular hyperplasia in an HIV(+) patient. This follicle lacks a surrounding mantle zone.

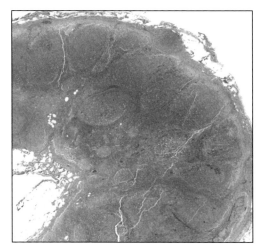 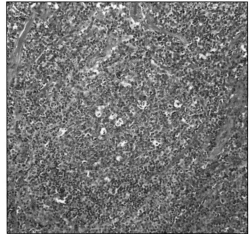

(Left) Inguinal lymph node demonstrates florid follicular hyperplasia in an HIV(+) patient. The germinal center in this field is not surrounded by a mantle zone and is composed of many centroblasts with fewer tingible body macrophages. (Right) Inguinal lymph node demonstrates follicular hyperplasia and monocytoid B-cell hyperplasia in an HIV(+) patient. This field shows monocytoid B cells in the subcapsular sinus ➡ and a germinal center ➡.

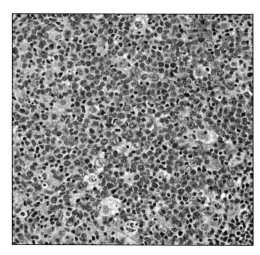 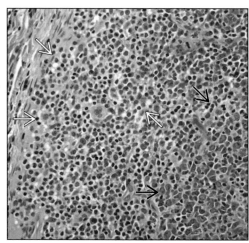

(Left) Inguinal lymph node demonstrates florid follicular and monocytoid B-cell hyperplasia in an HIV(+) patient. The anti-CD20 antibody highlights B cells within prominent follicles and monocytoid B cells in the subcapsular sinus. (Right) Inguinal lymph node demonstrates florid follicular hyperplasia in an HIV(+) patient. The B cells within the follicles are negative for Bcl-2, supporting reactive follicular hyperplasia.

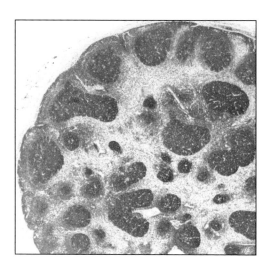 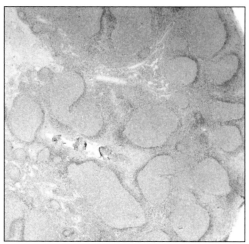

HUMAN IMMUNODEFICIENCY VIRUS LYMPHADENITIS

Microscopic Features

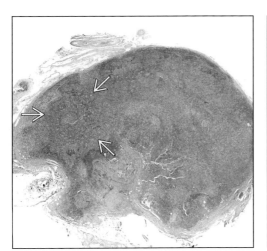

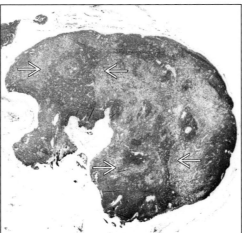

(Left) Lymph node in an HIV(+) patient reveals a mixed pattern of follicular hyperplasia and partial involution. There are numerous expanded and partially disrupted follicles with 1 extremely large follicle ➡ present. (Right) Lymph node in an HIV(+) patient shows a mixed pattern of follicular hyperplasia and partial involution. The follicles ➡ contain many B cells that are highlighted by the anti-CD20 antibody.

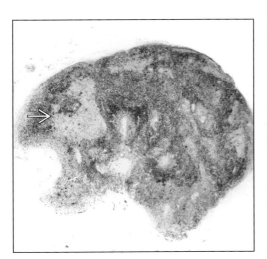

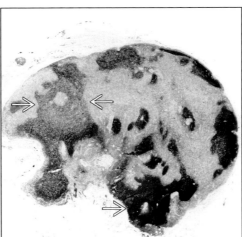

(Left) Lymph node in an HIV(+) patient reveals a mixed pattern of follicular hyperplasia and partial involution. The anti-CD3 antibody highlights T cells between the follicles. A large follicle ➡ is devoid of T cells. (Right) Lymph node in an HIV(+) patient shows a mixed pattern of follicular hyperplasia and partial involution. The anti-CD21 antibody highlights expanded and distorted networks of follicular dendritic cells ➡.

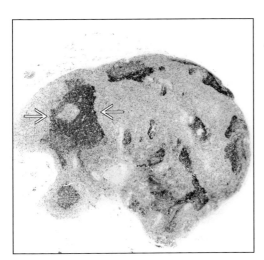

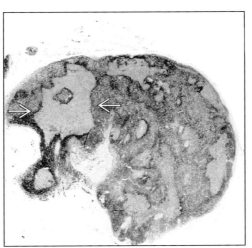

(Left) Lymph node in an HIV(+) patient assessed for Ki-67 shows a high proliferation rate in follicles ➡. (Right) Lymph node in an HIV(+) patient shows a mixed pattern of follicular hyperplasia and partial involution. Germinal center B cells within follicles are negative for Bcl-2, supporting reactive follicular hyperplasia. A very large follicle is noted ➡.

HUMAN IMMUNODEFICIENCY VIRUS LYMPHADENITIS

Microscopic Features

(Left) Lymph node demonstrates follicle lysis in an HIV(+) patient. A follicle is partially disrupted by infiltration of numerous small lymphocytes and increased vascularity. Also note the absence of a mantle zone. *(Right)* Lymph node shows HIV lymphadenitis assessed with anti-CD10 antibody. This field illustrates follicle lysis as the CD10(+) germinal center cells are infiltrated and disrupted by CD10(-) mantle zone small lymphocytes.

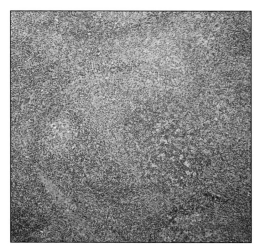 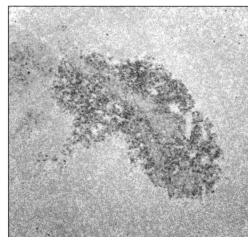

(Left) Lymph node from an HIV(+) patient demonstrates evidence of follicular hyperplasia and follicle lysis. The anti-CD20 antibody highlights B cells within distorted and partially confluent follicles. *(Right)* Lymph node studied with anti-CD21 antibody in an HIV(+) patient. The pattern of CD21 expression highlights irregular networks of follicular dendritic cells. This is an early stage of follicular involution.

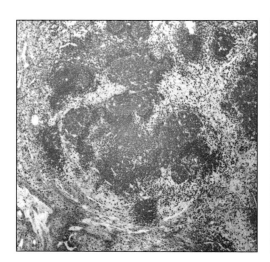 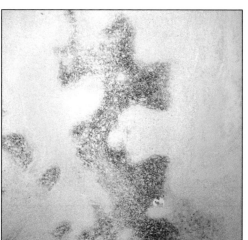

(Left) Lymph node from an HIV(+) patient demonstrates follicular involution. In this field, an atrophic, "burned-out," hyalinized follicle is present. *(Right)* Lymph node from an HIV(+) patient demonstrates follicular involution. In this field there is marked vascular proliferation with a polymorphous infiltrate in the paracortex that includes numerous plasma cells and scattered immunoblasts.

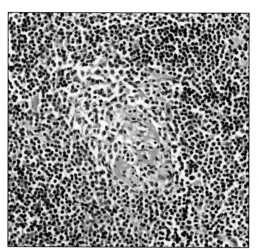 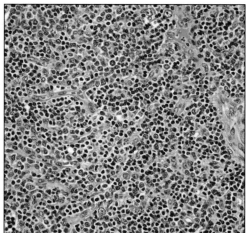

Microscopic Features and Differential Diagnosis

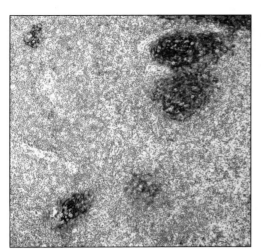

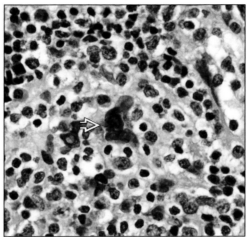

(Left) Lymph node from an HIV(+) patient demonstrates partial involution as shown by the presence of small, atrophic, and lymphocyte-depleted follicles. The anti-CD21 antibody highlights follicular dendritic cells within these follicles. *(Right)* Lymph node from an HIV(+) patient showing a multinucleated giant (Warthin-Finkeldey) cell ➡.

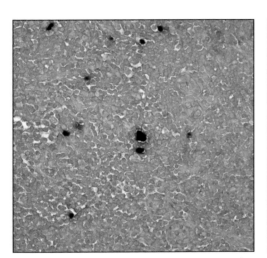

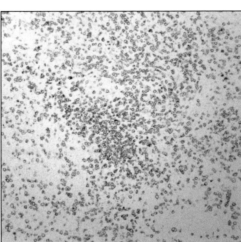

(Left) Lymph node from an HIV(+) patient assessed by in situ hybridization studies for Epstein-Barr virus small encoded RNA (EBER) shows scattered large and small cells positive for EBER. *(Right)* Lymph node from an HIV(+) patient shows evidence of partial involution. Immunohistochemical studies highlighted numerous CD30(+) immunoblasts present throughout the lymph node. These immunoblasts were negative for CD15 (not shown).

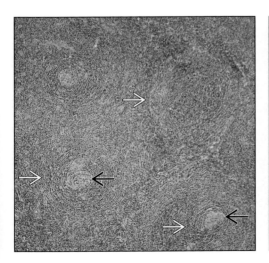

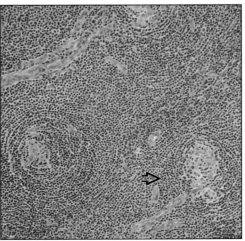

(Left) Lymph node involved by Castleman disease, hyaline-vascular variant, demonstrates numerous follicles with prominent mantle zones composed of small lymphocytes in a concentric ("onion skin") pattern ➡. Germinal centers in these follicles are atrophic and lymphocyte-depleted ➡. *(Right)* Lymph node involved by Castleman disease, hyaline-vascular variant, shows a germinal center penetrated by a sclerotic blood vessel ("lollipop" lesion) ➡.

HUMAN IMMUNODEFICIENCY VIRUS LYMPHADENITIS

Differential Diagnosis

(Left) Touch imprint of lymph node in AIDS patient demonstrates Burkitt lymphoma. Intermediate-sized lymphoid cells with basophilic cytoplasm & prominent vacuoles are shown. *(Right)* Lymph node of an AIDS patient demonstrates Burkitt lymphoma. The tumor is composed of sheets of monotonous, intermediate-sized cells with round nuclei, multiple nucleoli, & basophilic cytoplasm. Numerous mitotic figures & apoptotic bodies are present, imparting a "starry sky" pattern.

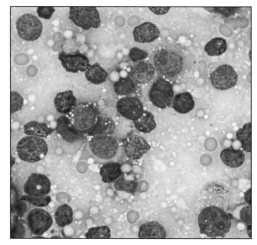 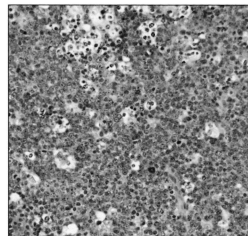

(Left) Lymph node in an AIDS patient demonstrates Burkitt lymphoma. Immunohistochemical studies for Ki-67 demonstrate a proliferation index of almost 100%. This extremely high proliferation rate is characteristic of Burkitt lymphoma. *(Right)* Lymph node in an AIDS patient involved by Burkitt lymphoma assessed by in situ hybridization for EBER shows that almost all of the tumor cells are positive for EBER.

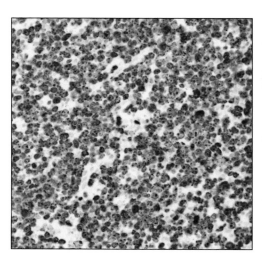 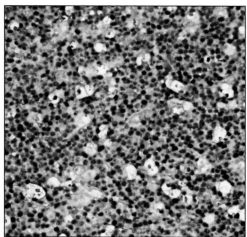

(Left) Biopsy of a "groin mass" in an AIDS patient demonstrates soft tissue infiltrated by diffuse large B-cell lymphoma. This neoplasm is composed of diffuse sheets of pleomorphic large cells with variably dispersed chromatin, multiple nucleoli, and abundant basophilic cytoplasm. A "starry sky" pattern can be appreciated. *(Right)* Biopsy of "groin mass" in an AIDS patient shows diffuse large B-cell lymphoma. The neoplastic cells express CD20.

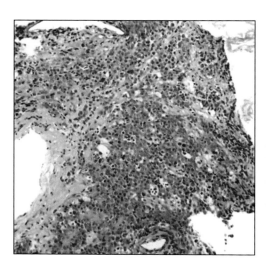 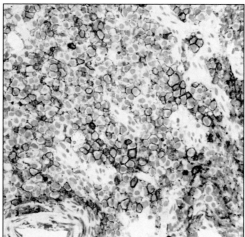

INFLAMMATORY PSEUDOTUMOR

Key Facts

Terminology
- Inflammatory reaction with multifactorial pathogenesis
  - Infectious etiologies account for subset of cases

Clinical Issues
- Young adults with fever and constitutional symptoms
- Localized or involving several lymph node groups
- Excellent prognosis

Microscopic Pathology
- Initially centered on hilum, trabeculae, and capsule of lymph nodes
- Fascicles and whorls of spindle cells
- Vascular proliferation
- Polymorphic inflammatory infiltrate
  - Plasma cells often numerous

- Pronounced follicular hyperplasia occurs in syphilitic lymphadenitis

Ancillary Tests
- Spindle cells positive for markers of fibroblastic reticulum cells &/or histiocytes
- Lack of chromosomal translocations involving *ALK* or lack of ALK1 protein expression
- No evidence of monoclonality

Top Differential Diagnoses
- Inflammatory myofibroblastic tumor
- Kaposi sarcoma
- Mycobacterial spindle cell pseudotumor
- Follicular dendritic cell sarcoma
- Hemorrhagic spindle cell tumor with amianthoid fibers (palisaded myofibroblastoma)

ANCILLARY TESTS

Immunohistochemistry
- Spindle cells can have immunophenotype of fibroblastic reticulum cells (FRC) or histiocytes
- FRC are often
  - Positive for actin, desmin, and vimentin
  - Negative for CD34, S100, CD1a, and ALK1, and largely negative for CD68
- Histiocytes are positive for CD11c, CD68, and CD163
- Plasma cells are polytypic

Cytogenetics
- No specific or consistent abnormalities
- No chromosomal translocations involving *ALK* at 2p23

PCR
- No evidence of monoclonal *Ig* or *TCR* rearrangements

DIFFERENTIAL DIAGNOSIS

Inflammatory Myofibroblastic Tumor
- Children and adolescents
- Abdomen and pelvis are common sites
- Multiple recurrences (up to 80%)
- Myofibroblastic spindle cells associated with inflammatory cells
- Cytoplasmic ALK1(+) ~ 60%, particularly pediatric cases
- Clonal, neoplastic
- Chromosomal translocations involving *ALK* gene at 2p23 and ALK1(+)
  - Pattern of *ALK* expression correlates with partners
- Metastatic potential is confined to ALK1(-) cases
  - Metastatic spread (< 5%)

Kaposi Sarcoma
- Spindle cells forming slits containing red blood cells
- Hyaline bodies (PAS positive)
- Spindle cells are HHV8(+); virtually 100%
- Spindle cells are CD31(+), CD34(+),and factor VIII(+)

Mycobacterial Spindle Cell Pseudotumor
- Most common in HIV(+) patients (AIDS)
- Infection by *Mycobacterium avium intracellulare*
  - Highlighted by acid-fast stain
- Spindled cells are histiocytes (CD68[+])

Follicular Dendritic Cell Sarcoma
- Spindle cell sarcoma with frequent nuclear pseudoinclusions associated with small lymphocytes
- Tumor cells are positive for 1 or more markers associated with follicular dendritic cells
  - CD21, CD23, CD35, clusterin, fascin, EGFR

Hemorrhagic Spindle Cell Tumor with Amianthoid Fibers (Palisaded Myofibroblastoma)
- Inguinal lymph nodes
- Bland-looking spindle cells with indistinct cell borders and nuclear palisading
- Rosette-like collagen ("amianthoid fibers")
- Positive for vimentin and actin (myofibroblasts)

SELECTED REFERENCES

1. Facchetti F et al: Nodal inflammatory pseudotumor caused by luetic infection. Am J Surg Pathol. 33(3):447-53, 2009
2. Coffin CM et al: Inflammatory myofibroblastic tumor: comparison of clinicopathologic, histologic, and immunohistochemical features including ALK expression in atypical and aggressive cases. Am J Surg Pathol. 31(4):509-20, 2007
3. Trevenzoli M et al: Inflammatory pseudotumor of lymph nodes. Ann Med Interne (Paris). 154(8):557-9, 2003
4. Moran CA et al: Inflammatory pseudotumor of lymph nodes: a study of 25 cases with emphasis on morphological heterogeneity. Hum Pathol. 28(3):332-8, 1997
5. Perrone T et al: Inflammatory pseudotumor of lymph nodes. A distinctive pattern of nodal reaction. Am J Surg Pathol. 12(5):351-61, 1988

INFLAMMATORY PSEUDOTUMOR

Microscopic Features

(Left) IPT involving lymph node. Note the dense sclerosis (stage III) and the effacement of the lymph node parenchyma. *(Right)* IPT characterized by marked pericapsular involvement ⇨. Note the presence of open subcapsular sinuses ⇾ and noninvolved lymph node parenchyma ↗.

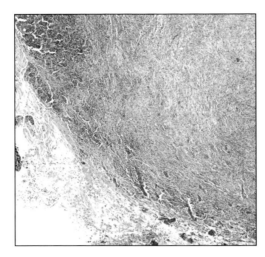 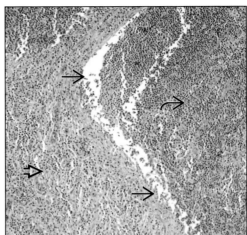

(Left) IPT involving lymph node with predominant sclerosis extending into the perinodal adipose tissue. *(Right)* IPT characterized by proliferation of spindle cells, histiocytes, and small vessels in a polymorphic inflammatory background.

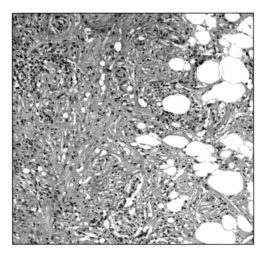 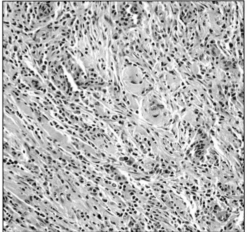

(Left) Vasculitis of small vessels can be frequently seen in IPT involving lymph node, often best observed in perinodal adipose tissue. *(Right)* Most cases of IPT of lymph node show variable degrees of follicular hyperplasia in the noninvolved lymphoid parenchyma. Prominent follicular hyperplasia is common in IPT as a result of syphilis infection.

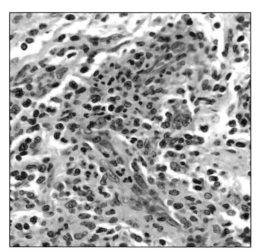 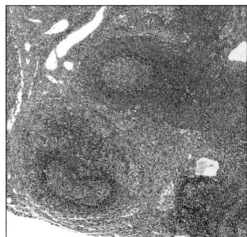

INFLAMMATORY PSEUDOTUMOR

Differential Diagnosis

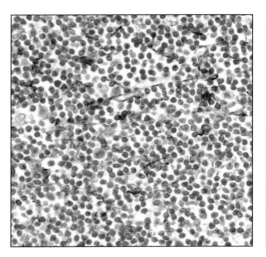 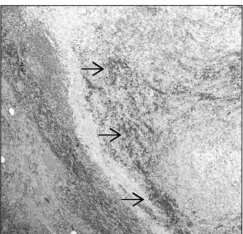

(Left) Fibroblastic reticulum cells (FRC) are part of the proliferating cells in IPT. They maintain the nodal architecture, support the reticulin fibers, have features of myofibroblasts, and are positive for vimentin, desmin (shown), keratins (8/18), and transglutaminase. (Right) Hemorrhagic spindle cell tumor involving inguinal lymph node and showing areas of recent hemorrhage ➡. Note that the tumor is well circumscribed and separated from the lymph node parenchyma by a fibrous pseudocapsule.

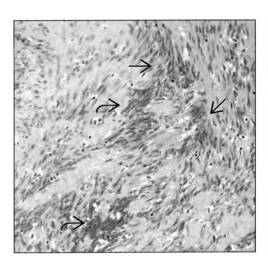 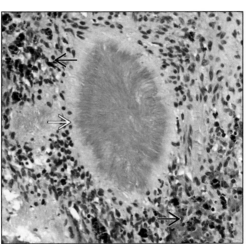

(Left) Hemorrhagic spindle cell tumor involving inguinal lymph node. Note bland spindle cells with indistinct borders, a focal palisading pattern ➡, and areas of recent hemorrhage ➡. (Right) Hemorrhagic spindle cell tumor involving lymph node shows characteristic giant rosette-like collections of collagen "amianthoid fiber" ➡. Note the hemosiderin-laden macrophages ➡ consistent with presence of old hemorrhage.

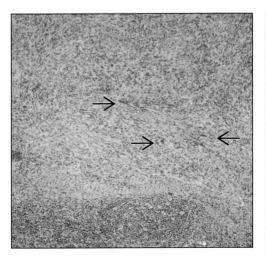 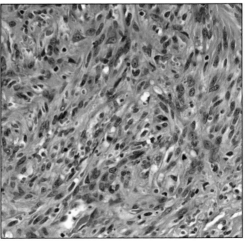

(Left) Metastatic Kaposi sarcoma in lymph node characterized by proliferation of spindle cells displacing normal lymph node architecture. Note the extravasated erythrocytes ➡ within the neoplasm. (Right) Metastatic Kaposi sarcoma in lymph node shows spindle cells separated by slits containing red blood cells.

INFLAMMATORY PSEUDOTUMOR

Differential Diagnosis

(Left) Metastatic Kaposi sarcoma in lymph node shows spindle cells and cytoplasmic and extracellular hyaline globules ➡. The globules are the end result of ingestion and degradation of erythrocytes.
(Right) Kaposi sarcoma positive for HHV8. In addition, in this case the tumor cells were also focally positive for vascular markers including CD34, CD31, and factor VIII (not shown).

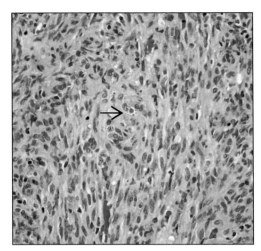
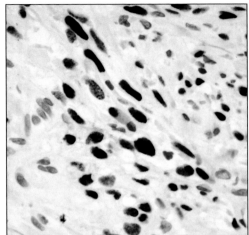

(Left) Inflammatory myofibroblastic tumor involving the mesentery of a child is characterized by elongated spindle cells and focal inflammation. (Courtesy M. Lim, MD.) *(Right)* Inflammatory myofibroblastic tumor shows cells that strongly express ALK1. (Courtesy M. Lim, MD.)

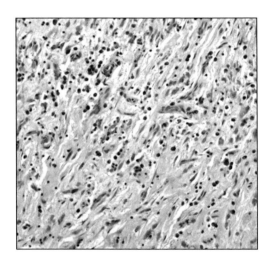
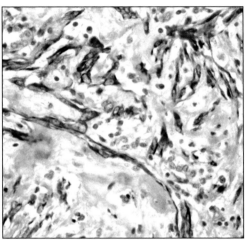

(Left) Follicular dendritic cell (FDC) sarcoma shows proliferation of spindle cells with indistinct cell borders. Note that FDC sarcomas typically contain an infiltrate of small lymphocytes.
(Right) Follicular dendritic cell sarcoma composed of numerous epithelioid tumor cells. The neoplastic cells are large with indistinct borders, vesicular nuclear chromatin, and prominent nucleoli. Note the presence of small lymphocytes admixed with the neoplastic cells.

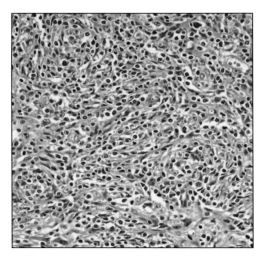
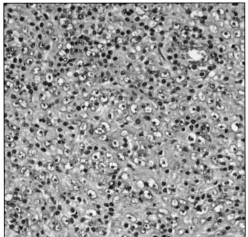

INFLAMMATORY PSEUDOTUMOR

Differential Diagnosis

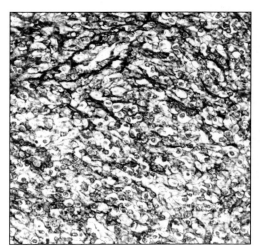

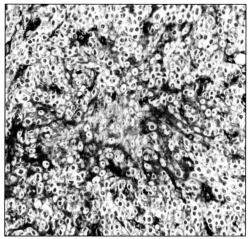

(Left) Follicular dendritic cell sarcoma positive for CD21. Other markers that are often positive in FDC sarcomas include CD23, CD35, clusterin, fascin, and epidermal growth factor receptor (EGFR). *(Right)* In this case of follicular dendritic cell sarcoma, a subset of the tumor cells is positive for fascin.

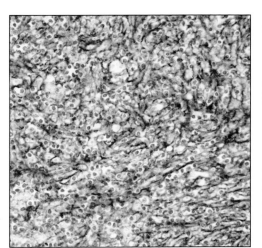

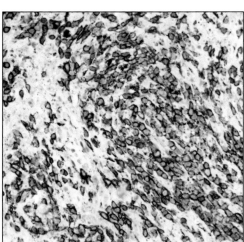

(Left) Follicular dendritic cell sarcoma positive for epidermal growth factor receptor (EGFR). Some studies suggest that EGFR may be the most sensitive marker for these neoplasms. *(Right)* A small subset of cases of follicular dendritic cell sarcoma is positive for CD20.

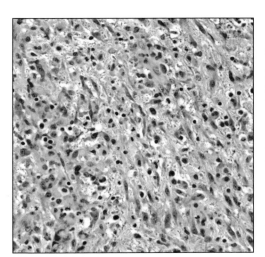

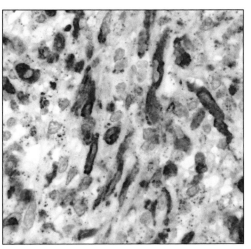

(Left) The differential diagnosis of IPT also includes lymphomas with spindle cell component. Here, we show a case of ALCL with a spindle cell component & a myxoid background. Immunohistochemical studies showed that the neoplastic cells were positive for ALK1, CD30 (bright), CD43, & granzyme B. *(Right)* Anaplastic large cell lymphoma (ALCL) with a spindle cell component. The neoplastic cells are granzyme B(+), a cytotoxic protein often expressed by ALCL.

PROGRESSIVE TRANSFORMATION OF GERMINAL CENTERS

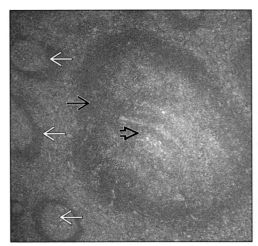

Progressive transformation of germinal centers (PTGC). The PTGC follicle ⇒ is 4-5x larger than normal reactive follicles ➡. Note the expanded mantle zone ⇨ of the PTGC follicle.

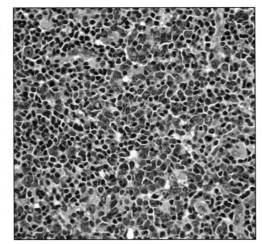

Center of a PTGC follicle at high-power magnification. Centroblasts and centrocytes are intermixed with small mature lymphocytes from the mantle zone. However, LP cells are not present.

TERMINOLOGY

Abbreviations
- Progressive transformation of germinal centers (PTGC)

Synonyms
- Progressively transformed germinal centers
- Progressively transformed follicular centers

Definitions
- Reactive hyperplasia of follicles characterized by
  o Large follicles with hyperplastic germinal centers
  o Disruption of germinal centers due to infiltration by mantle zone B cells
  o Affected follicles typically are at different stages of dissolution

ETIOLOGY/PATHOGENESIS

Unknown
- Viral cause suspected

CLINICAL ISSUES

Presentation
- PTGC can occur at any age but is common in young adults
  o Median age: 28 years
  o ~ 20% of cases occur in children
- Men are more often affected than women
- PTGC usually involves peripheral lymph nodes
  o Cervical lymph nodes are most commonly involved (50% of cases)
  o Axillary and inguinal lymph nodes less common
- PTGC can be the predominant change in lymph nodes prompting biopsy
- Patients with PTGC can present with or without symptoms

o Most frequent presentation is asymptomatic and localized lymphadenopathy
o Generalized lymphadenopathy can occur in subset of patients
  ▪ Adolescents who present with viral-like illness
  ▪ Patients with autoimmune diseases
o PTGC can be incidental finding in patients with lymphoma
  ▪ PTGC can be detected at initial diagnosis or after therapy
  ▪ Interval between PTGC and lymphoma can be > 10 years
  ▪ PTGC also rarely can precede diagnosis of lymphoma
- PTGC usually spontaneously resolves but can recur
  o Same or different lymph nodes
  o Recurrence occurs more often in children than adults
- PTGC is not associated with human immunodeficiency virus infection

Treatment
- Observation

Prognosis
- Excellent

IMAGE FINDINGS

Radiographic Findings
- Lymphadenopathy in subset of patients

MICROSCOPIC PATHOLOGY

Histologic Features
- Follicles with PTGC are usually large
  o 4-5x the size of normal reactive secondary follicles
- PTGC is usually focal; involves only a few follicles in lymph node

PROGRESSIVE TRANSFORMATION OF GERMINAL CENTERS

Key Facts

Terminology
- Progressive transformation of germinal centers (PTGC)

Clinical Issues
- Young adults most commonly affected
- Asymptomatic localized lymphadenopathy in most patients
  - Cervical lymph nodes in ~ 50%
- Generalized lymphadenopathy occurs in subset of patients
- Can be incidental finding in patients with lymphoma
  - NLPHL most common
- PTGC usually resolves spontaneously
  - Can recur
- PTGC not associated with HIV

Microscopic Pathology
- Scattered large follicles in otherwise reactive lymph node with follicular hyperplasia
- Mantle zone cells migrate into and disrupt hyperplastic germinal centers
- Each affected follicle at different stage of PTGC (asynchronous)

Top Differential Diagnoses
- Nodular lymphocyte-predominant Hodgkin lymphoma (NLPHL)
- Lymphocyte-rich classical Hodgkin lymphoma, nodular variant
- Follicular lymphoma, floral variant
- HIV-associated lymphadenopathy

- Process of PTGC appears to proceed in stages
  - Initially germinal centers become hyperplastic
    - "Starry sky" pattern can occur but unusual
  - 2-3 germinal centers per follicle fuse together
  - Mantle zone B cells infiltrate and disrupt germinal centers
  - Eventually germinal centers disappear
    - Centroblasts and follicular dendritic cells are scattered among small mantle zone B cells
- Follicles involved by PTGC appear to be at different stages (i.e., asynchronous)
- PTGC is almost always accompanied by follicular hyperplasia
  - Interfollicular hyperplasia often present
- PTGC follicles can show Castleman-like changes; uncommon
- Clusters of epithelioid cells can surround PTGC follicles
  - More common in pediatric cases
- PTGC can coexist with Hodgkin or non-Hodgkin lymphoma
  - Nodular lymphocyte predominant Hodgkin lymphoma (NLPHL) most common
    - No data to support PTGC as precursor of NLPHL
  - Other lymphoma types uncommonly associated with PTGC
    - Classical Hodgkin lymphoma (nodular sclerosis or mixed cellularity)
    - Plasma cell myeloma
  - PTGC may involve same lymph node involved by lymphoma or different lymph node
- In generalized cases of PTGC, histologic findings are more florid
  - Rarely associated with lymphoma

Cytologic Features
- Mixed population of small and large lymphocytes
  - Small round lymphocytes are mantle zone B cells and reactive T cells
  - Germinal center centrocytes and centroblasts
- No LP cells; no Hodgkin or Reed-Sternberg (HRS) cells
- No plasma cells, neutrophils, or eosinophils

ANCILLARY TESTS

Immunohistochemistry
- Preserved B-cell and T-cell compartments of lymph node
  - Prominent follicular pattern
- In PTGC follicles
  - Germinal centers
    - B-cell antigens(+), T-cell antigens(-)
    - CD10(+), Bcl-6(+), Bcl-2(-)
    - Disruption of follicular dendritic cells that are CD21(+), CD23(+)
  - Mantle zones
    - B-cell antigens(+), T-cell antigens(-)
    - IgD(+), Bcl-2(+)
    - CD10(-), Bcl-6(-)
- T cells are relatively few in PTGC follicles

Flow Cytometry
- No evidence of monoclonal B-cell population

Cytogenetics
- Little data available
  - 1 case reported showed t(3;22)(q27;q11)
    - Possibly involved BCL6 gene at 3q27

Molecular Genetics
- No evidence of monoclonal gene rearrangements

DIFFERENTIAL DIAGNOSIS

Nodular Lymphocyte-Predominant Hodgkin Lymphoma (NLPHL)
- Neoplastic nodules are more numerous and replace lymph node architecture
- Neoplastic nodules more irregular than those of PTGC
- Lymphocyte predominant (LP) cells are present
  - Previously known as L&H or "popcorn" cells
  - Large with multilobated contours, clear nucleoplasm, and inconspicuous nucleoli
  - CD20(+), CD45/LCA(+), CD15(-), CD30(-/+)

PROGRESSIVE TRANSFORMATION OF GERMINAL CENTERS

Immunohistochemistry

Antibody	Reactivity	Staining Pattern	Comment
CD20	Positive	Cell membrane	Germinal center (GC) B cells and mantle zone B cells that infiltrate GC
IgD	Positive	Cell membrane	Mantle zone B cells
Bcl-2	Positive	Cytoplasmic	Mantle zone B cells, negative in germinal center B cells
Bcl-6	Positive	Nuclear	Germinal center B cells, negative in mantle zone B cells
CD3	Positive	Cell membrane	Minor component in PTGC, small mature T cells, may also express CD57
CD57	Positive	Cell membrane	More uniformly distributed, and may rarely form rosettes around GC B cells

- ○ Bcl-6(+), Bcl-2(-)
- ○ CD3(+) CD57(+) T cells form rosettes around LP cells

Lymphocyte-rich Classical Hodgkin Lymphoma, Nodular Variant
- Neoplastic nodules are more numerous and replace lymph node architecture
- Residual germinal centers are common within neoplastic nodules
  - ○ Often eccentrically located and small
- HRS cells are present
  - ○ Large cells; usually 1-2 prominent nucleoli
  - ○ CD15(+/-), CD30(+), CD45/LCA(-)
  - ○ CD20(-/+; weak), Bcl-2(+/-)

Follicular Lymphoma, Floral Variant
- Neoplastic follicles are numerous; back to back
- Composition of follicles is relatively homogeneous
  - ○ Mixture of centrocytes and centroblasts
- No LP cells identified
- Monotypic Ig(+), CD10(+), Bcl-6(+), and Bcl-2(+)

HIV-associated Lymphadenopathy
- Follicle lysis is common in HIV(+) lymphadenopathy
  - ○ Most common in early stages of infection
- Follicle lysis superficially resembles PTGC but
  - ○ Follicles are usually not enlarged (unlike PTGC)
  - ○ Hemorrhage is common in affected follicles
  - ○ Follicles are infiltrated by T cells

DIAGNOSTIC CHECKLIST

Clinically Relevant Pathologic Features
- Young patients; male > female
- Most patients are asymptomatic
  - ○ Single enlarged lymph node
- Generalized lymphadenopathy with florid PTGC can occur
  - ○ Adolescents
  - ○ Patients with autoimmune diseases
- Small number of cases are associated with lymphoma
  - ○ Nodular lymphocyte predominant Hodgkin lymphoma is most common
  - ○ PTGC may precede, coexist with, or follow diagnosis of lymphoma

Pathologic Interpretation Pearls
- Lymph node architecture is preserved

- Large and well-defined follicles that have expanded mantle zones and disrupted germinal centers
- Usually involve small number of follicles in background of follicular hyperplasia
- No LP or HRS cells
- No evidence of monoclonal B-cell population

SELECTED REFERENCES
1. Bouron-Dal Soglio D et al: A B-cell lymphoma-associated chromosomal translocation in a progressive transformation of germinal center. Hum Pathol. 39(2):292-7, 2008
2. Kojima M et al: Follicular lymphoid hyperplasia of the oral cavity representing progressive transformation of germinal center. APMIS. 113(3):221-4, 2005
3. Kojima M et al: Progressive transformation of germinal center presenting with histological features of hyaline-vascular type of Castleman's disease. APMIS. 113(4):288-95, 2005
4. Lin P et al: The activation profile of tumour-associated reactive T-cells differs in the nodular and diffuse patterns of lymphocyte predominant Hodgkin's disease. Histopathology. 44(6):561-9, 2004
5. Chang CC et al: Follicular hyperplasia, follicular lysis, and progressive transformation of germinal centers. A sequential spectrum of morphologic evolution in lymphoid hyperplasia. Am J Clin Pathol. 120(3):322-6, 2003
6. Kojima M et al: Progressive transformation of germinal centers: a clinicopathological study of 42 Japanese patients. Int J Surg Pathol. 11(2):101-7, 2003
7. Hicks J et al: Progressive transformation of germinal centers: review of histopathologic and clinical features. Int J Pediatr Otorhinolaryngol. 65(3):195-202, 2002
8. Nguyen PL et al: Progressive transformation of germinal centers and nodular lymphocyte predominance Hodgkin's disease: a comparative immunohistochemical study. Am J Surg Pathol. 23(1):27-33, 1999
9. Ferry JA et al: Florid progressive transformation of germinal centers. A syndrome affecting young men, without early progression to nodular lymphocyte predominance Hodgkin's disease. Am J Surg Pathol. 16(3):252-8, 1992
10. Osborne BM et al: Progressive transformation of germinal centers: comparison of 23 pediatric patients to the adult population. Mod Pathol. 5(2):135-40, 1992
11. Hansmann ML et al: Progressive transformation of germinal centers with and without association to Hodgkin's disease. Am J Clin Pathol. 93(2):219-26, 1990

Microscopic Features

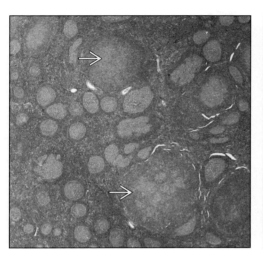 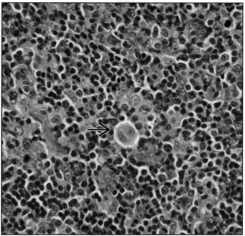

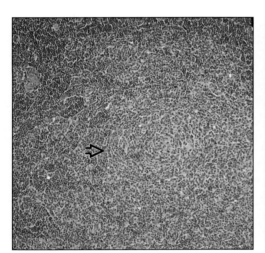 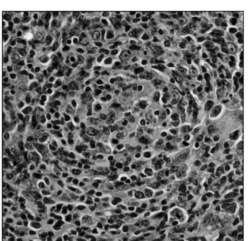

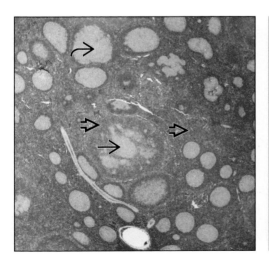 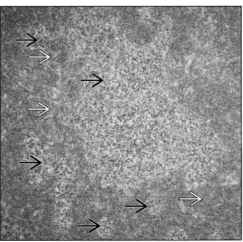

(Left) Paraffin section of a lymph node shows PTGC with follicles at various stages of the process. Two of the largest follicles involved by PTGC ➡ are substantially larger than the reactive follicles also present. The PTGC follicles have a variegated appearance with dark and light areas. The normal polarization of the germinal centers is lost. (Right) In PTGC, binucleated follicular dendritic cells ➡ can be present and may resemble HRS cells.

(Left) In this case of PTGC, some follicles show involution of their germinal centers, imparting a hyaline vascular Castleman disease-like appearance ➡. (Right) PTGC with Castleman-like changes. High-power magnification is characterized by some degree of lymphocyte depletion in the germinal center.

(Left) Lymph node involved by PTGC. A central, large follicle ➡ shows infiltration by Bcl-2(+) mantle zone B cells ➡. The germinal center B cells in the large PTGC follicle, other smaller PTGC follicles, and reactive follicles are negative for Bcl-2 ➡. (Right) Lymph node with a central, large PTGC follicle. In this field, germinal center cells (Bcl-6[+]) ➡ are being infiltrated and disrupted by mantle zone cells that are Bcl-6(-) ➡.

PROGRESSIVE TRANSFORMATION OF GERMINAL CENTERS

Differential Diagnosis

(Left) Lower power view of a lymph node involved by nodular lymphocyte predominant Hodgkin lymphoma (NLPHL). The neoplasm has a nodular pattern ⇥. The nodules are large with a "moth-eaten" appearance. Reactive follicles are not seen in this field.
(Right) Paraffin section of case of NLPHL. The neoplastic LP cells ⇥ are surrounded by small, reactive lymphocytes ⇥ and histiocytes ⇥.

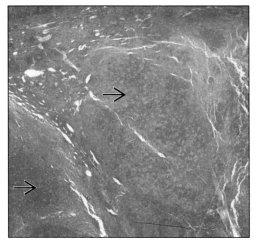
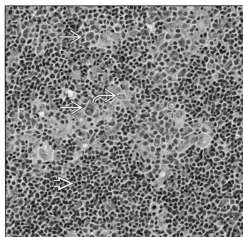

(Left) Anti-CD20 of a case of NLPHL highlights the LP cells as well as numerous reactive small lymphocytes ⇥ in the background. Note that the reactive lymphocytes are predominantly B cells rather than T cells in this case.
(Right) In this case of NLPHL, CD3(+) T cells represent the minority of small reactive lymphocytes and form rosettes around LP cells ⇥.

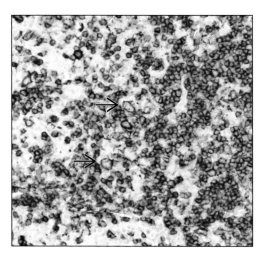
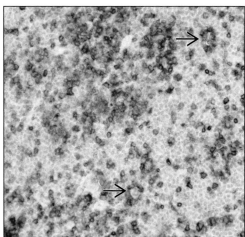

(Left) Lymph node involved by reactive follicular hyperplasia. Four reactive follicles are shown. In contrast to PTGC follicles, reactive follicles are much smaller, the germinal centers show polarity, and mantle zones are thinner.
(Right) An immunostain for Bcl-2 performed on lymph node involved by reactive follicular hyperplasia. Bcl-2 highlights the mantle zone B cells and the interfollicular T cells. Germinal T cells are positive whereas germinal center B cells are negative for Bcl-2.

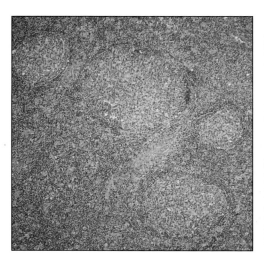
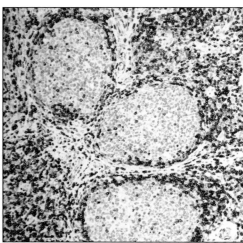

Differential Diagnosis

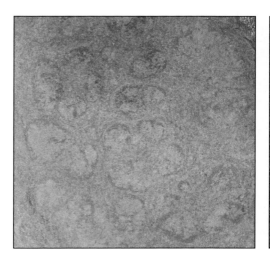
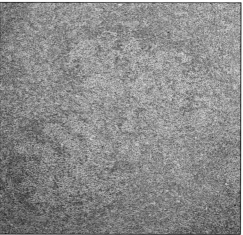

(Left) Paraffin section of a lymph node involved by the floral variant of follicular lymphoma. The neoplastic follicles are arranged back-to-back. *(Right)* Paraffin section of a lymph node involved by the floral variant of follicular lymphoma. The neoplastic cells are monotonous, composed predominantly of centrocytes with occasional centroblasts. The mantle zones are thin.

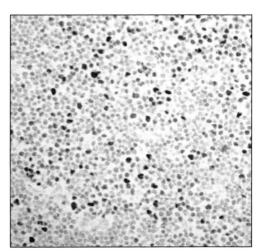
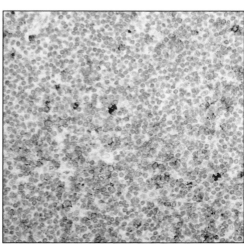

(Left) Bcl-6 immunostain highlights numerous neoplastic cells in a case of floral variant of follicular lymphoma, confirming the germinal center origin of this neoplasm. *(Right)* CD10 immunostain highlights numerous neoplastic cells in a case of floral variant of follicular lymphoma, confirming the germinal center origin of this neoplasm.

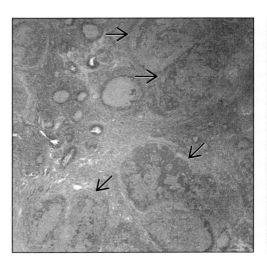
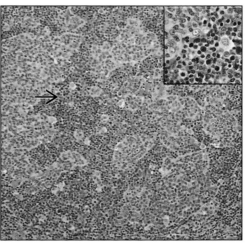

(Left) Lymph node showing well-developed follicle lysis. Note that several follicles ➔ at variable levels of lysis are involved. The follicles are not as large as is seen in PTGC. *(Right)* High-power view of follicle lysis. Note that the lymphoid cells between the broken-apart germinal center cells are of variable size and mixed with hemorrhage. The border between the germinal center cells and other lymphoid cells ➔ is shown in the inset.

KIKUCHI-FUJIMOTO DISEASE

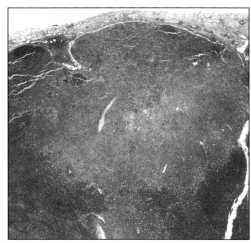

Cervical lymph node involved by Kikuchi-Fujimoto disease. The paracortex shows a circumscribed, wedge-shaped area of necrosis that extends to the capsule.

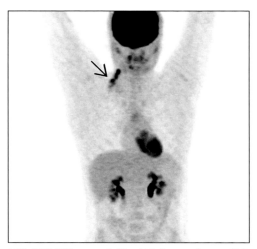

MIP FDG-PET scan of Kikuchi-Fujimoto disease. This image reveals an area of FDG uptake in the right cervical region that was interpreted as suspicious for lymphoma ⇒.

TERMINOLOGY

Abbreviations
- Kikuchi-Fujimoto disease (KFD)

Synonyms
- Necrotizing lymphadenitis without granulocytic infiltration
- Histiocytic necrotizing lymphadenitis
- Kikuchi-Fujimoto lymphadenopathy

Definitions
- Self-limited, benign form of lymphadenopathy characterized by
  - Proliferation of histiocytes and plasmacytoid monocytes
  - Apoptosis with abundant karyorrhectic debris
  - Systemic symptoms and low-grade fever in subset of patients

ETIOLOGY/PATHOGENESIS

Unknown
- Viral, infectious, or autoimmune cause has been suggested
- Exuberant T-cell-mediated response to variety of stimuli in genetically susceptible people
- Cytokine-mediated mechanisms
  - ↑ interleukin-6, interferon-α, FAS ligand
- Viruses suggested to be involved in KFD include
  - Epstein-Barr virus (EBV) and human herpes virus 6 (HHV6)
  - Identified in small subset of cases; unlikely to be cause

CLINICAL ISSUES

Epidemiology
- Age
  - Usually < 30 years (range: 2-75 years)
- Gender
  - Women are affected more often
    - Female to male ratio is 4:1
- Ethnicity
  - KFD has been described in a variety of ethnic backgrounds
    - Asian descent most common

Site
- Lymphadenopathy
  - Cervical lymph nodes most often involved

Presentation
- Fever typically lasts for 1 week
  - Can persist for up to 1 month
- Upper respiratory symptoms
- Most common initial manifestations are
  - Tender and painful lymphadenopathy
  - Lymphadenopathy with fever
- Uncommon manifestations
  - Weight loss, night sweats, nausea, vomiting
  - Generalized lymphadenopathy
  - Joint pain
  - Extranodal involvement by KFD
  - Splenomegaly, hepatomegaly

Laboratory Tests
- Rule out other causes of necrotizing lymphadenopathy
- No specific tests are available for detecting KFD
- Anemia
- Elevated lactate dehydrogenase levels
- Granulocytopenia and atypical lymphocytosis in peripheral blood (50%)
- Elevated erythrocyte sedimentation rates
- Polyclonal hypergammaglobulinemia

KIKUCHI-FUJIMOTO DISEASE

Key Facts

Clinical Issues
- Self-limited clinical course in most patients
- Might represent phenotype of diverse disease entities
- Prognosis is different according to underlying cause
- Young patients
- Acute tender cervical lymphadenopathy
- Low-grade fever; systemic symptoms
- Systemic survey and follow-up is recommended to rule out systemic lupus erythematosus

Microscopic Pathology
- Multiple, pale circumscribed foci are found in paracortical area of lymph node
- Lack of extension of process into perinodal tissue
- 3 phases: Proliferative, necrotizing, xanthomatous
- Lesions are composed of mononuclear cells with round to irregular nuclei
- Abundant karyorrhectic debris
- Plasmacytoid dendritic cells are present
- Paracortical areas of coagulative necrosis are seen
- Large numbers of histiocytes, including crescentic histiocytes and activated lymphoid cells
- Absence of neutrophils

Ancillary Tests
- Predominance of CD3(+), CD8(+) T cells
- Histiocytes express myeloperoxidase, lysozyme and CD68
- ↑ plasmacytoid dendritic cells expressing CD68, CD123, CD303
- No evidence of monoclonal *Ig* or *TCR* rearrangements

- Negative serologic studies for
  - EBV, Cytomegalovirus, influenza, adenovirus
  - Toxoplasmosis, *Mycoplasma*, Q fever
- Usually negative autoimmune laboratory studies
  - Antinuclear antibodies, rheumatoid factor, anti-double-strand DNA antibodies
  - Rare patients with KFD are subsequently diagnosed to have systemic lupus erythematosus

Natural History
- Diagnosis is usually established by lymph node biopsy
  - Excisional biopsy is often required because KFD can be patchy
    - Assessment of lymph node architecture is very helpful in establishing diagnosis
- Spontaneous resolution occurs, usually within 1-4 months
- Small (~ 3%) subset of patients develop relapse

Treatment
- No specific therapy required
- Anti-inflammatory agents

Prognosis
- Excellent

IMAGE FINDINGS

CT Findings
- Computed tomography (CT) is preferred modality
- Cervical lymph nodes in KFD tend to be located in posterior triangle
- Lymph nodes appear as clusters
  - < 4 cm in greatest dimension
  - Nonenhancing necrosis
- Any lymph node group can be involved in KFD

MACROSCOPIC FEATURES

General Features
- Size: 0.5-4.0 cm

MICROSCOPIC PATHOLOGY

Histologic Features
- Lymph node
  - Architecture: Partial or extensive involvement
    - Often patchy in early stages
  - KFD begins in paracortex and near capsule
    - Degree of apoptosis/necrosis varies from one case to another
    - No granulocytes identified in necrotic areas
    - Plasma cells usually absent or rare
    - Process does not extend into perinodal tissues
    - Immunoblasts are numerous in viable paracortex contiguous with necrosis
    - No hematoxylin bodies identified
  - Sinuses are patent or compressed
    - Can be filled by histiocytes or monocytoid B cells
  - Hyperplastic lymphoid follicles in uninvolved areas
  - ± thrombosed blood vessels
  - 3 histologic subtypes of KFD have been described
    - Lymphohistiocytic/proliferative; thought to be early stage
    - Necrotic
    - Phagocytic/foamy cell; thought to be late stage
  - > 1 stage of KFD can be present within lymph node
  - Lymphohistiocytic/proliferative type
    - Proliferation of histiocytes (including C-shaped forms)
    - Increased plasmacytoid dendritic cells
    - Small lymphocytes and immunoblasts are present
    - Relatively little apoptosis or necrotic debris
  - Necrotic type
    - Abundant apoptosis within distinct foci of necrosis associated with eosinophilic debris
    - Histiocytes and plasmacytoid dendritic cells undergo apoptosis
    - Fibrin thrombi may be present in blood vessels
  - Phagocytic/foamy cell type
    - Numerous histiocytes containing phagocytosed debris (foamy cytoplasm)

3

■ Histiocytes often form rim surrounding necrotic areas

Cytologic Features
- Diagnosis can be suggested in touch imprints of lymph node
  - Highlights cytologic characteristics of plasmacytoid dendritic cells (pDC)
  - Touch imprint often better than fine needle aspiration (FNA) smears
- Frequency of CD123(+) pDC is high in KFD
  - Valuable indicator for diagnosis of KFD
  - Useful for distinguishing KFD from reactive lymphadenopathy and neoplasms

Skin
- Most frequently located on face or upper body
- KFD in skin can grossly present as
  - Erythematous papules
  - Indurated lesions or plaques
  - Ulcers
- Histologic findings in skin include
  - Dermal lymphohistiocytic infiltrate; most common
  - Epidermal changes
    ■ Necrotic keratinocytes
    ■ Nonneutrophilic karyorrhectic debris
    ■ Basal vacuolar change
  - Edema of papillary dermis

ANCILLARY TESTS

Immunohistochemistry
- Histiocytes are CD4(+), CD68(+), lysozyme(+), myeloperoxidase(+, dim)
- Plasmacytoid dendritic cells are
  - CD68(+), CD123(+), CD303(+)
  - Myeloperoxidase(-), fascin(-)
- T cells are predominantly CD8(+)
- Immunoblasts are CD30(+) and of CD8(+) T-cell lineage
- B cells are rare or absent in areas of necrosis

Flow Cytometry
- Predominance of CD8(+) T cells without aberrancies
- Rare polytypic B cells
- Insufficient to establish diagnosis of KFD
  - Helpful to exclude non-Hodgkin lymphoma

PCR
- No evidence of monoclonal *IgH* gene rearrangements
- No evidence of monoclonal *TCR* rearrangements
- No known chromosomal translocations or gene mutations

Electron Microscopy
- KFD has high frequency of cytoplasmic inclusions in histiocytes and immunoblasts, including
  - Intracytoplasmic rodlets
  - Tubulo-reticular structures
    ■ Interferon-α is related to presence of tubulo-reticular structures
    ■ Interferon-α has been identified in many histiocytes of KFD

DIFFERENTIAL DIAGNOSIS

Systemic Lupus Erythematosus (SLE) Lymphadenitis
- Pattern of lymph node involvement can be similar to KFD
  - Prominent foci of necrosis and histiocytic infiltrates
  - Degenerated nuclear debris (hematoxylin bodies)
  - Azzopardi phenomenon can be present
    ■ Encrustation of blood vessel walls by degenerated nuclear material
  - Plasma cells can be numerous
  - Uninvolved areas of lymph node can show prominent reactive follicular hyperplasia
- Serologic studies for anti-nuclear antibodies and anti-double-strand DNA antibodies support SLE
- SLE patients often have other systemic manifestations of disease

Herpes Simplex-associated Lymphadenitis
- "Punched-out" lesions in paracortex of lymph node can mimic KFD
  - Necrotic debris and histiocytic infiltrate often prominent
- Features of herpes lymphadenitis that distinguish it from KFD
  - Viral inclusions; both Cowdry type A and multinucleated cells
  - Abundant neutrophils
  - Skin and mucous membranes have ulcerative lesions near sites of lymphadenopathy

Necrotizing Granulomatous Lesions
- Tuberculosis, atypical mycobacteria, and fungi
  - Usually not restricted to paracortical regions of lymph node
  - Epithelioid cells, giant cells, and granuloma formation
  - Neutrophils and plasma cells are usually numerous
  - Identification of etiologic agents by special stains
- No infiltrate of C-shaped histiocytes and plasmacytoid dendritic cells

Cat Scratch Disease
- Paracortical areas of necrosis show some resemblance to KFD but
  - Stellate-shaped necrosis with abundant neutrophils in earlier stages
  - Granulomatous inflammation in later stages
  - Caused by *Bartonella henselae*
    ■ Can detect in Warthin-Starry stain in some cases

Kawasaki Disease
- Mostly occurs in children younger than 5 years old
- Geographic necrosis; fibrinoid thrombosis
- Neutrophilic infiltration is usually present
- No infiltrate of C-shaped histiocytes and plasmacytoid dendritic cells

Diffuse Large B-cell Lymphoma (DLBCL)
- Early proliferative phase of KFD can mimic DLBCL

KIKUCHI-FUJIMOTO DISEASE

o Sheets of histiocytes and plasmacytoid dendritic cells can be mistaken for sheets of large B cells
o Histiocytes are CD68(+), CD123(+), and B-cell antigens(-)
• Rare cases of DLBCL can show abundant apoptosis and mimic proliferative phase of KFD
o Expression of B-cell antigens (e.g., CD20) supports diagnosis of DLBCL
o Monoclonal *IgH* rearrangements

Peripheral T-cell Lymphoma (PTCL)

• Proliferative/early necrotic phases of KFD can mimic PTCL
o T-immunoblasts and CD8(+) predominance can be mistaken for neoplastic T cells
• Features against diagnosis of PTCL
o No proliferation of C-shaped histiocytes and plasmacytoid dendritic cells
o Most cases of PTCL are CD4(+)
o Histiocytes in PTCL are MPO(-)
o No evidence of aberrant T-cell immunophenotype in KFD
o No evidence of monoclonal T-cell receptor gene rearrangements in KFD

Classical Hodgkin Lymphoma (HL)

• Paracortical areas of necrosis can occur in classical HL possibly mimicking KFD
• Features against diagnosis of KFD
o No infiltrate of C-shaped histiocytes and plasmacytoid dendritic cells
o Neutrophils, eosinophils, &/or plasma cells often numerous
o Hodgkin and Reed-Sternberg cells
  ▪ Often located around necrotic foci
  ▪ CD15(+), CD30(+), pax-5(+, dim), CD45/LCA(-)

Acute Myeloid Leukemia (AML)/Myeloid Sarcoma

• Sheets of neoplastic cells, especially monocytes, can mimic early phase of KFD
• Features against diagnosis of KFD
o Neoplastic cells have immature nuclear chromatin
o Immunophenotype is myeloid or monocytic
  ▪ CD13(+), CD33(+), CD34(+), CD117(+), HLA-DR(+), CD123(-)
  ▪ CD68 is not helpful in this differential diagnosis
• Most patients with AML are older and have systemic manifestations of disease
o Peripheral blood involvement
o Bone marrow involvement
o History of AML

DIAGNOSTIC CHECKLIST

Clinically Relevant Pathologic Features

• Young patients
• Acute tender cervical lymphadenopathy
• Low-grade fever (±)

Pathologic Interpretation Pearls

• 3 general, often overlapping types or phases of disease
o Lymphohistiocytic/proliferative
  ▪ Striking infiltrate of histiocytes and plasmacytoid dendritic cells with minimal apoptosis
  ▪ Type of KFD most often misdiagnosed as non-Hodgkin lymphoma
o Necrotic
  ▪ Paracortical areas of necrosis
  ▪ Abundant apoptosis with eosinophilic debris
  ▪ Lack of neutrophils
  ▪ Abundance of CD3(+), CD8(+) T cells
o Phagocytic/foamy cell type
  ▪ Numerous lipid-laden or foamy histiocytes surround areas of necrosis
• Systemic lupus erythematosus can closely mimic KFD
o Recommend serologic testing for every patient in whom diagnosis of KFD is considered

SELECTED REFERENCES

1. Hutchinson CB et al: Kikuchi-Fujimoto disease. Arch Pathol Lab Med. 134(2):289-93, 2010
2. Khanna D et al: Necrotizing lymphadenitis in systemic lupus erythematosus: is it Kikuchi-Fujimoto disease? J Clin Rheumatol. 16(3):123-4, 2010
3. Pilichowska ME et al: Histiocytic necrotizing lymphadenitis (Kikuchi-Fujimoto disease): lesional cells exhibit an immature dendritic cell phenotype. Am J Clin Pathol. 131(2):174-82, 2009
4. Song JY et al: Clinical outcome and predictive factors of recurrence among patients with Kikuchi's disease. Int J Infect Dis. 13(3):322-6, 2009
5. Atwater AR et al: Kikuchi's disease: case report and systematic review of cutaneous and histopathologic presentations. J Am Acad Dermatol. 59(1):130-6, 2008
6. Jun-Fen F et al: Kikuchi-Fujimoto disease manifesting as recurrent thrombocytopenia and Mobitz type II atrioventricular block in a 7-year-old girl: a case report and analysis of 138 Chinese childhood Kikuchi-Fujimoto cases with 10 years of follow-up in 97 patients. Acta Paediatr. 96(12):1844-7, 2007
7. Bosch X et al: Enigmatic Kikuchi-Fujimoto disease: a comprehensive review. Am J Clin Pathol. 122(1):141-52, 2004
8. Onciu M et al: Kikuchi-Fujimoto lymphadenitis. Adv Anat Pathol. 10(4):204-11, 2003
9. Menasce LP et al: Histiocytic necrotizing lymphadenitis (Kikuchi-Fujimoto disease): continuing diagnostic difficulties. Histopathology. 33(3):248-54, 1998
10. Medeiros LJ et al: Lupus lymphadenitis: report of a case with immunohistologic studies on frozen sections. Hum Pathol. 20(3):295-9, 1989
11. Dorfman RF et al: Kikuchi's histiocytic necrotizing lymphadenitis: an analysis of 108 cases with emphasis on differential diagnosis. Semin Diagn Pathol. 5(4):329-45, 1988

KIKUCHI-FUJIMOTO DISEASE

Microscopic and Immunohistochemical Features

(Left) Kikuchi-Fujimoto disease involving lymph node. This image shows the lymphohistiocytic or proliferative phase of disease with numerous histiocytes and plasmacytoid dendritic cells and relatively less apoptosis and karyorrhectic debris. *(Right)* A high-power view of Kikuchi-Fujimoto disease, lymphohistiocytic/proliferative phase, shows numerous histiocentic including crescentic or C-shaped histiocytes ⇒ and scattered apoptotic cells. No neutrophils are present.

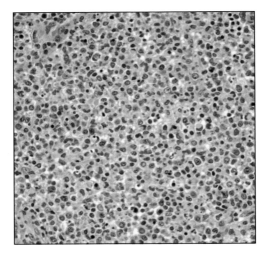
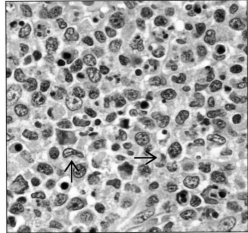

(Left) Kikuchi-Fujimoto disease involving lymph node, lymphohistiocytic/proliferative phase. Numerous histiocytes and plasmacytoid dendritic cells (also known as plasmacytoid monocytes) are CD68(+). *(Right)* Kikuchi-Fujimoto disease involving lymph node, lymphohistiocytic/proliferative phase. Many of the histiocytes and mononuclear cells are positive for myeloperoxidase (MPO).

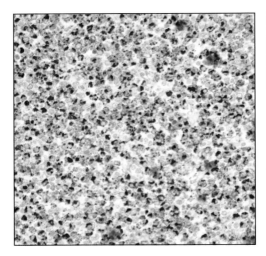
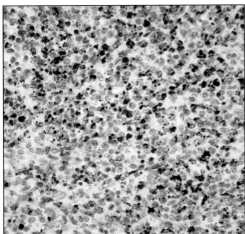

(Left) Kikuchi-Fujimoto disease involving lymph node, lymphohistiocytic/proliferative phase. Scattered CD30(+) immunoblasts are present. *(Right)* Kikuchi-Fujimoto disease involving lymph node, lymphohistiocytic/proliferative phase. Many small T cells are present that are CD3(+).

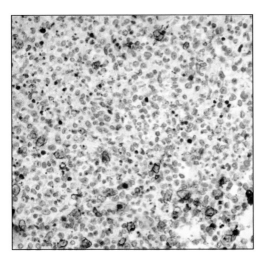
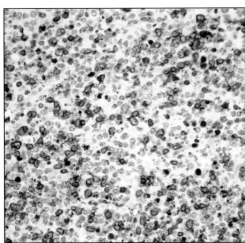

KIKUCHI-FUJIMOTO DISEASE

Microscopic and Immunohistochemical Features

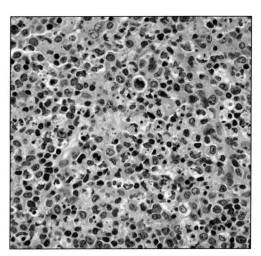
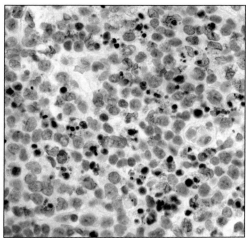

(Left) Kikuchi-Fujimoto disease, proliferative phase, involving lymph node. A number of apoptotic cells are present, suggesting that the lesions are beginning to evolve into necrotic phase. *(Right)* Kikuchi-Fujimoto disease involving a lymph node. Numerous CD68(+) plasmacytoid dendritic cells are present. These are also positive for CD123 (not shown) and CD303 (not shown).

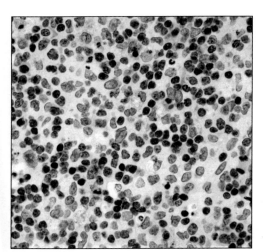
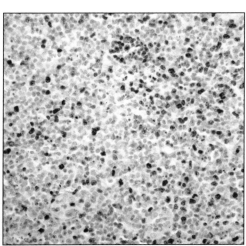

(Left) Kikuchi-Fujimoto disease involving lymph node. Histiocytes and plasmacytoid monocytes are mostly CD15(-). Note the absence of CD15(+) granulocytes. The absence of CD15 is evidence against the diagnosis of classical Hodgkin lymphoma. *(Right)* Kikuchi-Fujimoto disease involving lymph node. Note the relatively high proliferative fraction as shown by the number of Ki-67(+) cells in this field.

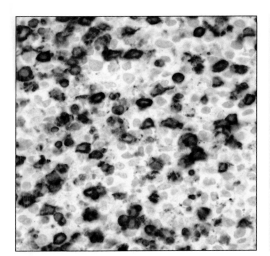
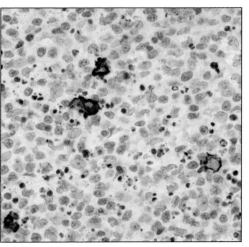

(Left) Kikuchi-Fujimoto disease involving lymph node. Approximately 60% of the cells in this field are CD3(+) T cells. The presence of T cells and necrosis should not be misinterpreted as peripheral T-cell lymphoma. *(Right)* Kikuchi-Fujimoto disease involving lymph node. CD20 is negative in most of the cells in this case. Lack of expression of CD20, CD79a, or pax-5 within the large cell population is evidence against the diagnosis of B-cell non-Hodgkin lymphoma.

KIKUCHI-FUJIMOTO DISEASE

Microscopic and Immunohistochemical Features

(Left) Kikuchi-Fujimoto disease involving lymph node with some features of both the proliferative and necrotic phases. Note numerous plasmacytoid monocytes/dendritic cells and many apoptotic cells. *(Right)* Kikuchi-Fujimoto disease involving lymph node with some features of both the proliferative and necrotic phases. Histiocytes and plasmacytoid dendritic cells are seen in association with apoptotic cells.

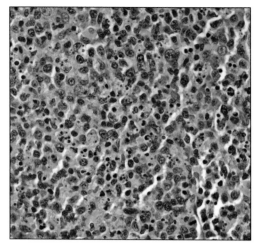
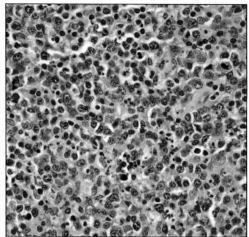

(Left) Cervical lymph node involved by Kikuchi-Fujimoto disease, necrotic phase. This field shows an area of necrosis with abundant eosinophilic debris. Viable lymphocytes and histiocytes are present in the lower right of the field. *(Right)* Cervical lymph node involved by Kikuchi-Fujimoto disease, necrotic phase. Necrosis with extensive fibrinoid deposits and apoptotic cells are seen. Note the absence of neutrophils or plasma cells in this field.

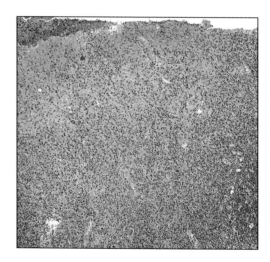
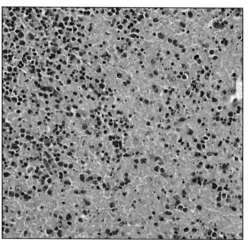

(Left) Cervical lymph node involved by Kikuchi-Fujimoto disease, necrotic phase. The histiocytes in this field in are CD68(+). *(Right)* Cervical lymph node involved by Kikuchi-Fujimoto disease, necrotic phase. Many T cells in this field are CD3(+).

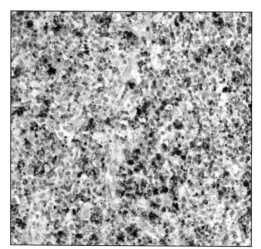
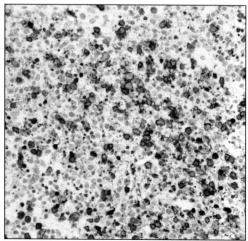

3

KIKUCHI-FUJIMOTO DISEASE

Microscopic and Immunohistochemical Features

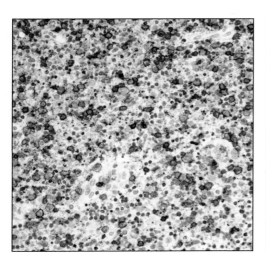

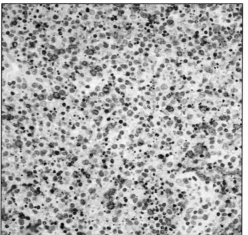

(Left) Cervical lymph node involved by Kikuchi-Fujimoto disease, necrotic phase. Most of the T cells in areas of necrosis are T-cytotoxic/suppressor cells that are CD4(-) and CD8(+). This field shows numerous CD8(+) T cells. *(Right)* Cervical lymph node involved by Kikuchi-Fujimoto disease, necrotic phase. This anti-CD4 antibody highlights relatively few CD4(+) T cells (bright) as well as a subset of histiocytes (dim). Apoptotic cells also stain nonspecifically.

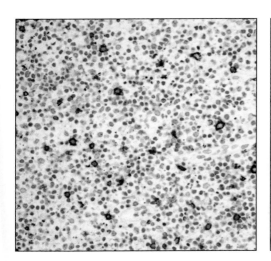

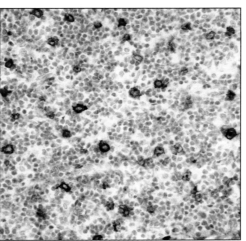

(Left) Cervical lymph node involved by Kikuchi-Fujimoto disease, necrotic phase. Few CD20(+) B cells are present in the necrotic areas. *(Right)* Cervical lymph node involved by Kikuchi-Fujimoto disease, necrotic phase. Scattered CD30(+) immunoblasts are identified within and near the necrotic area. These immunoblasts are of T-cell lineage (not shown).

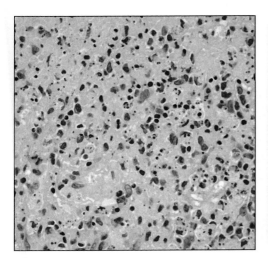

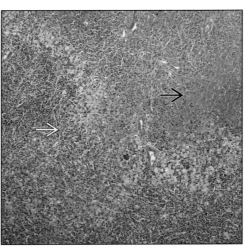

(Left) Hematoxylin and eosin stain shows a lymph node involved by Kikuchi-Fujimoto disease, fully developed necrotic phase. This field shows abundant eosinophilic and karyorrhectic debris. No neutrophils or eosinophils are present. *(Right)* Kikuchi-Fujimoto disease involving lymph node shows evidence of the necrotic and phagocytic/xanthomatous phases. Necrosis ⇨ is surrounded by numerous foamy histiocytes ⇶.

KIKUCHI-FUJIMOTO DISEASE

Microscopic Features and Differential Diagnosis

(Left) Kikuchi-Fujimoto disease involving lymph node shows evidence of the necrotic and phagocytic/xanthomatous phases. Foamy histiocytes predominate ➡. Necrosis is present at upper left ⊡. *(Right)* Kikuchi-Fujimoto disease involving lymph node shows evidence of the necrotic ⊡ and phagocytic/xanthomatous phases. This is high-power magnification of foamy histiocytic proliferation adjacent to the necrotic area.

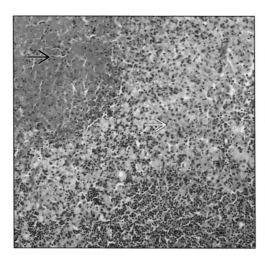 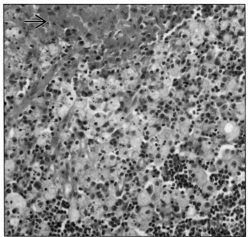

(Left) CT scan of Kikuchi-Fujimoto disease shows enlarged homogeneously enhancing lymph nodes in the mediastinum on the right side ➡, which was considered suspicious for lymphoma. The largest lymph node is about 2 x 1 cm. *(Right)* Kikuchi-Fujimoto disease involving lymph node. This image shows the lack of extension of KFD into perinodal tissues. Regions peripheral to the necrotic areas in KFD may show thrombosed blood vessels, but these are not always present.

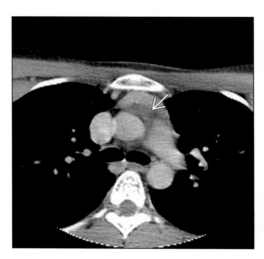 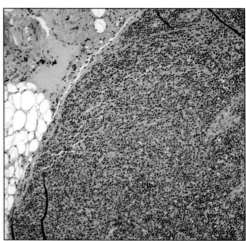

(Left) Lupus lymphadenitis. In this field, a zone of necrosis is present at the upper left ⊡. The necrosis is surrounded by lipid-laden histiocytes ➡. In the remainder of the lymph node, the paracortical areas are expanded by lymphocytes and immunoblasts. *(Right)* Lupus lymphadenitis. Within the necrosis, nuclear debris (dust-like) and basophilic hematoxylin bodies can be seen. Hematoxylin bodies do not occur in KFD and are helpful in differential diagnosis.

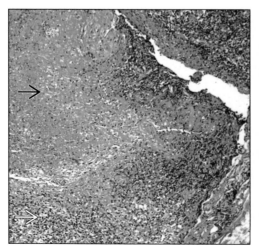 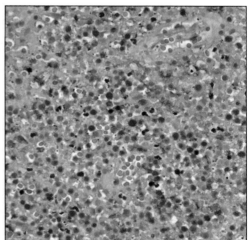

KIKUCHI-FUJIMOTO DISEASE

Differential Diagnosis

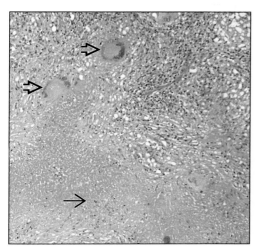

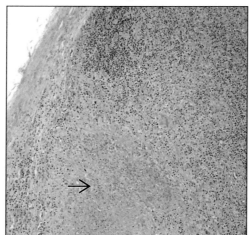

(Left) Mycobacterium tuberculosis involving lymph node. Note caseating necrosis ➡ and multinucleated giant cells ▷. *(Right)* Classical Hodgkin lymphoma involving lymph node. Note the expanded paracortex with necrosis ➡, histiocytes, lymphocytes, eosinophils, and plasma cells. Scattered large HRS cells are present but are difficult to appreciate at this magnification.

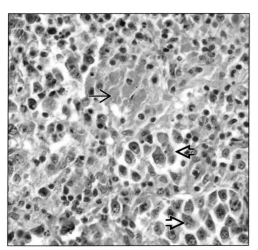

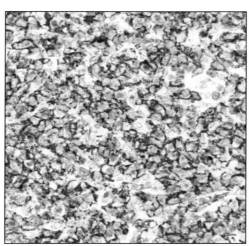

(Left) Diffuse large B-cell lymphoma involving lymph node with many viable cells ▷, apoptotic cells, and fibrinoid necrosis ➡. This degree of necrosis can mimic, in part, the proliferative phase of Kikuchi-Fujimoto disease, but immunohistochemical analysis readily resolves this differential diagnosis. *(Right)* Diffuse large B-cell lymphoma involving lymph node. All of the large cells are CD20(+) and CD68(-) (not shown) supporting the diagnosis.

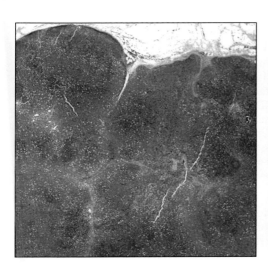

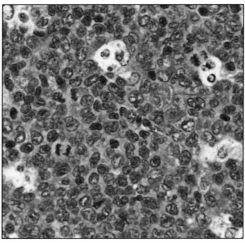

(Left) Myeloid (granulocytic) sarcoma involving lymph node. The paracortical regions are replaced by a diffuse proliferation of immature cells with a "starry sky" pattern. *(Right)* Myeloid (granulocytic) sarcoma involving lymph node. The immature cells have myelomonocytic cytologic features and numerous mitoses are present. There are also scattered eosinophilic metamyelocytes.

ROSAI-DORFMAN DISEASE

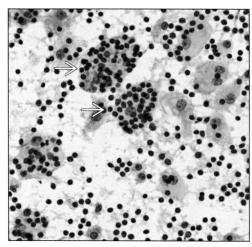

Touch imprint of lymph node involved by Rosai-Dorfman disease. Numerous histiocytes with emperipolesis and small lymphocytes are present. The histiocytes show emperipolesis, particularly prominent in some cells ➡️.

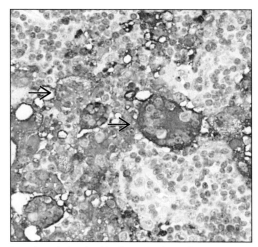

Lymph node involved by Rosai-Dorfman disease (RDD). S100 stain highlights the cytoplasm of RDD histiocytes. S100 negatively outlines intracytoplasmic lymphocytes ➡️ in cells with emperipolesis.

TERMINOLOGY

Abbreviations
- Rosai-Dorfman disease (RDD)

Synonyms
- Sinus histiocytosis with massive lymphadenopathy (SHML)
- Histiocytose lipidique ganglionnaire pseudotumorale de Destombes

Definitions
- Benign proliferation of histiocytes with characteristic cytologic features
  - Histiocytes show emperipolesis (engulfment of lymphocytes)
  - Histiocytes express S100

ETIOLOGY/PATHOGENESIS

Unknown
- RDD has been reported in identical twins or families suggesting genetic predisposition
- Associated with autoimmune lymphoproliferative syndrome

CLINICAL ISSUES

Epidemiology
- Incidence
  - Rare; worldwide geographic distribution
- Age
  - Wide range
    - Newborn to ~ 75 years; more common in children
- Gender
  - M:F = 3:2 (1.5)
- Ethnicity
  - All races affected

Site
- Lymph nodes
- Extranodal sites in ~ 40% of patients
  - Head and neck region common
    - Upper respiratory tract, skin
  - Other common sites
    - Skin, soft tissues, gastrointestinal tract
    - Bones, breast, dura
    - Almost any site can be involved

Presentation
- Lymphadenopathy, often without any symptoms
  - Usually localized
  - Cervical lymph nodes most often involved
  - Often bilateral with massive enlargement
- B symptoms are uncommon but can occur
  - Fever, night sweats can precede lymphadenopathy
- Laboratory abnormalities in subset of patients
  - Polyclonal hypergammaglobulinemia common
  - Blood lymphocytes with low CD4 to CD8 ratio
  - Hemolytic anemia

Treatment
- In most patients, RDD regresses spontaneously
  - No specific therapy needed
  - RDD often persists for months before regression
  - Rarely RDD can persist for years before regression
- Rare subset of patients have aggressive RDD and require therapy
  - Therapies: Steroids, radiation therapy, chemotherapy
  - Surgical excision for patients with obstruction/compression-type symptoms

Prognosis
- Excellent for most affected patients
- Rare cases can be clinically aggressive
  - No effective therapy for these rare aggressive cases
  - Fatalities can occur as a result of
    - Accompanying immune dysregulation
    - Mass effect in vital organs

ROSAI-DORFMAN DISEASE

Key Facts

Terminology
- Rosai-Dorfman disease (RDD) and sinus histiocytosis with massive lymphadenopathy are equivalent terms

Etiology/Pathogenesis
- Unknown; histologic features are suggestive of virus

Clinical Issues
- Spontaneous regression occurs in most patients
- No specific therapy required

Macroscopic Features
- Large, often massive lymph nodes
- Often matted with capsular fibrosis

Microscopic Pathology
- Lymph nodes show dilated sinuses
- Associated small lymphocytes and plasma cells

- RDD histiocytes characterized by
  - Abundant eosinophilic cytoplasm
  - Central vesicular nucleus
  - Small but distinct, central nucleolus
  - Emperipolesis
- In extranodal sites
  - Emperipolesis often focal or absent

Ancillary Tests
- Immunohistochemistry
  - S100(+), CD1a(-)

Top Differential Diagnoses
- Langerhans cell histiocytosis
- Chronic granulomatous inflammation
- Metastatic neoplasms to lymph node sinuses
- Anaplastic large cell lymphoma

IMAGE FINDINGS

Radiographic Findings
- Lymphadenopathy

MACROSCOPIC FEATURES

General Features
- Enlarged lymph nodes: Often massive
  - Often matted with capsular fibrosis

MICROSCOPIC PATHOLOGY

Histologic Features
- Lymph nodes
  - Overall lymph node architecture is intact but distorted
  - Marked dilatation of sinuses
    - Filled with RDD histiocytes
    - Associated with small lymphocytes and plasma cells
    - Granulocytes not present, unless superimposed necrosis or infection
  - RDD histiocytes show emperipolesis
    - Engulf cells that become located in histiocyte cytoplasm
    - Small lymphocytes, plasma cells, or erythrocytes
    - Cells surrounded by intracytoplasmic vacuole
    - Engulfed cells are usually viable
  - Often marked plasmacytosis between sinuses
  - Reactive follicles often present
  - Mitotic figures are uncommon
  - Rarely affected lymph nodes can undergo infarct
- Extranodal sites
  - RDD histiocytes can be sparse in areas
    - Emperipolesis can be absent
  - Small lymphocytes and plasma cells often numerous
  - Fibrosis can be prominent
- RDD can be associated with Hodgkin or non-Hodgkin lymphomas

  - Most common types
    - Nodular lymphocyte predominant Hodgkin lymphoma
    - Follicular lymphoma
  - RDD is often a small focus in this setting
  - Incidental finding without impact on prognosis

Cytologic Features
- RDD histiocytes are characterized by
  - Large size with abundant eosinophilic cytoplasm
    - Well-defined cell borders
  - Central, often round nucleus
    - Distinct central nucleolus
  - ± emperipolesis

Predominant Pattern/Injury Type
- Sinusoidal

Predominant Cell/Compartment Type
- Histiocyte

ANCILLARY TESTS

Immunohistochemistry
- RDD histiocytes are
  - S100(+), CD1a(-), langerin(-)
  - Histiocyte markers: CD4(+/-), CD14(+), CD68(+), CD163(+)
  - Adhesion molecules: CD11b(+), CD11c(+), CD18(+), CD31(+)
  - B-cell antigens(-), T-cell antigens(-)
- Intracytoplasmic lymphocytes include both B and T cells
- Plasma cells are polytypic

Flow Cytometry
- Polytypic B cells
- T cells with normal immunophenotype

Cytogenetics
- Rare cases reported in literature; noncontributory

ROSAI-DORFMAN DISEASE

In Situ Hybridization
- Epstein-Barr virus(-)
- Human herpes virus: HHV6(-), HHV8(-)

Molecular Genetics
- X-linked polymorphic human androgen receptor assay (HUMARA)
  - RDD histiocytes are polyclonal
- No evidence of monoclonal *Ig* or *TCR* rearrangements

DIFFERENTIAL DIAGNOSIS

Langerhans Cell Histiocytosis (LCH)
- LCH can be confined to lymph node sinusoids similar to RDD
- Eosinophils and necrosis are common
- LCH cells have twisted nuclei with nuclear grooves
  - Less cytoplasm than RDD histiocytes
  - No emperipolesis
- Birbeck granules present as shown by electron microscopy
- Immunohistochemistry
  - S100(+), CD1a(+), langerin/CD207(+)
- HUMARA assay
  - LCH cells are monoclonal unlike RDD histiocytes

Chronic Granulomatous Inflammation
- Usually not confined to lymph node sinuses
- Associated necrosis and acute and chronic inflammation
- Epithelioid histiocytes and multinucleated cells
  - Histiocytes do not resemble RDD histiocytes
  - S100([-/+] focal)

Metastatic Melanoma or Carcinoma
- Metastases to lymph node often involve sinuses
- Cytologic atypia present; mitoses common
- Immunohistochemistry of melanoma
  - S100(+), HMB-45(+), Mart-1(+)
- Immunohistochemistry of carcinoma
  - Keratins(+), S100(-)
- Clinical history of primary tumor

Anaplastic Large Cell Lymphoma
- Can selectively involve and expand lymph node sinuses
- Neoplastic cells are large with horseshoe-shaped nuclei (hallmark cells)
- Immunohistochemistry
  - CD30(+), T-cell antigens(+), ALK1(+/-), S100(-)
- Monoclonal T-cell receptor gene rearrangements(+)
- t(2;5)(p23;q35) in up to 75% of ALK(+) cases

Histiocytic Sarcoma
- Typically replaces lymph node architecture, not sinusoidal
- Cytologic atypia and mitotic figures
- Neoplastic histiocytes lack cytologic features of RDD histiocytes
- Phagocytosis by neoplastic histiocytes can occur
  - Usually not prominent and not true emperipolesis

Classical Hodgkin Lymphoma
- Can rarely be localized to lymph node sinuses
- Hodgkin and Reed-Sternberg cells are present
- ± associated granulocytes and plasma cells
- Immunohistochemistry
  - CD15(+/-), CD30(+), CD45/LCA(-), S100(-)

Toxoplasma Lymphadenitis
- Caused by infection by *Toxoplasma gondii*
- Diagnostic histologic triad includes
  - Sinusoidal expansion by monocytoid B cells
  - Follicular hyperplasia
  - Epithelioid histiocytes encroaching upon reactive germinal centers
- No RDD histiocytes; no emperipolesis

Sinus Histiocytosis
- Nonspecific reaction pattern in lymph node sinuses
- Histiocytes do not cytologically resemble RDD histiocytes
  - Smaller, less cytoplasm; no emperipolesis
- Immunohistochemistry
  - S100([-/+] focal): Different pattern than RDD

DIAGNOSTIC CHECKLIST

Clinically Relevant Pathologic Features
- Usually asymptomatic lymphadenopathy in young patient

Pathologic Interpretation Pearls
- Lymph nodes
  - Sinusoidal distribution
  - Large histiocytes with abundant cytoplasm
    - Central vesicular nuclei and small, distinct nucleoli
    - Emperipolesis present in lymph nodes
    - S100(+), CD1a(-)
  - Associated small lymphocytes and plasma cells
- Extranodal sites
  - Emperipolesis can be absent or very focal

SELECTED REFERENCES

1. La Barge DV 3rd et al: Sinus histiocytosis with massive lymphadenopathy (Rosai-Dorfman disease): imaging manifestations in the head and neck. AJR Am J Roentgenol. 191(6):W299-306, 2008
2. Hsiao CH et al: Clinicopathologic characteristics of Rosai-Dorfman disease in a medical center in northern taiwan. J Formos Med Assoc. 105(9):701-7, 2006
3. Lussier C et al: Cytology of Rosai-Dorfman disease. Diagn Cytopathol. 24(4):298-300, 2001
4. Lu D et al: Sinus histiocytosis with massive lymphadenopathy and malignant lymphoma involving the same lymph node: a report of four cases and review of the literature. Mod Pathol. 13(4):414-9, 2000
5. Foucar E et al: Sinus histiocytosis with massive lymphadenopathy (Rosai-Dorfman disease): review of the entity. Semin Diagn Pathol. 7(1):19-73, 1990
6. Komp DM: The treatment of sinus histiocytosis with massive lymphadenopathy (Rosai-Dorfman disease). Semin Diagn Pathol. 7(1):83-6, 1990

ROSAI-DORFMAN DISEASE

Microscopic Features

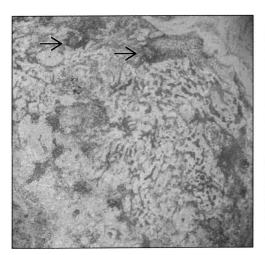

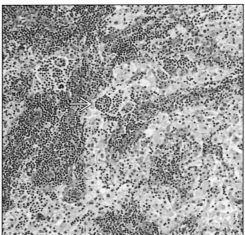

(Left) Lymph node involved by RDD. The overall architecture of the lymph node is intact, and the sinuses are markedly dilated with numerous histiocytes. Histiocytes have abundant pale cytoplasm accounting for the pale appearance of the expanded sinuses. Note reactive follicles ⇨ between the sinuses. (Right) Lymph node involved by RDD. This field shows dilated sinuses and prominent emperipolesis that can be seen at this power ➡.

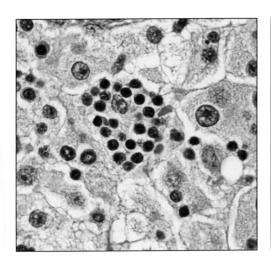

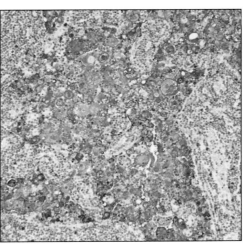

(Left) Lymph node involved by Rosai-Dorfman disease (RDD). The RDD histiocytes have abundant eosinophilic cytoplasm that can be granular or vacuolated in some cases. RDD histiocytes have centrally located and vesicular nuclei and most also have a distinct nucleolus. Emperipolesis is shown in the center of the field. (Right) Paraffin section of lymph node involved by RDD. S100 highlights the abundant cytoplasm of RDD histiocytes within the sinuses.

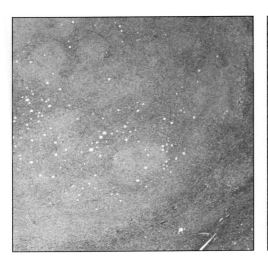

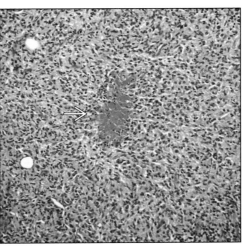

(Left) Axillary adipose tissue involved by Rosai-Dorfman disease (RDD). In extranodal sites, RDD does not exhibit a sinusoidal pattern, and the process is infiltrative. (Right) Axillary adipose tissue involved by Rosai-Dorfman disease (RDD). In this case, small foci of necrosis ➡ were present. Necrosis is unusual in RDD and superimposed infection cannot be excluded in this case.

ROSAI-DORFMAN DISEASE

Microscopic Features

(Left) Axillary adipose tissue involved by Rosai-Dorfman disease (RDD). Small lymphocytes, plasma cells, and fibroblasts are present. It can be difficult to identify RDD histiocytes or emperipolesis in extranodal lesions. *(Right)* Axillary adipose tissue involved by RDD. This field shows abundant pale histiocytes, small lymphocytes, and plasma cells. This combination is a clue to the diagnosis of RDD.

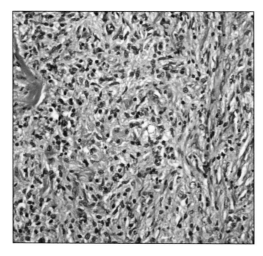 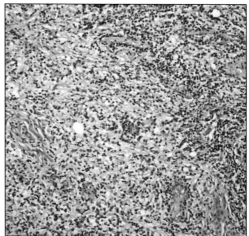

(Left) Axillary adipose tissue involved by Rosai-Dorfman disease (RDD). This high-power magnification illustrates an RDD histiocyte with emperipolesis ➡. Very few RDD histiocytes showed emperipolesis in this case. The diagnosis was confirmed by immunohistochemical stain for S100 protein. *(Right)* Mediastinal soft tissue involved by Rosai-Dorfman disease (RDD). Relatively few small lymphocytes and plasma cells were present in this case.

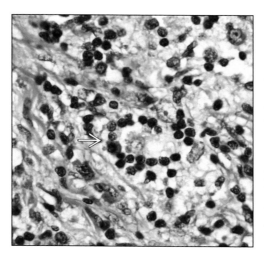 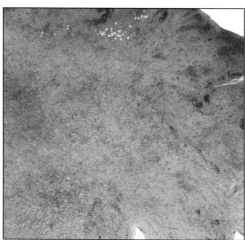

(Left) Mediastinal soft tissue involved by Rosai-Dorfman disease (RDD). In areas where aggregates of small lymphocytes were identified, RDD histiocytes were found. Emperipolesis was minimal in this case. *(Right)* Mediastinal soft tissue involved by Rosai-Dorfman disease (RDD). The RDD histiocytes in this field do not show emperipolesis. The diagnosis was confirmed by S100 stain.

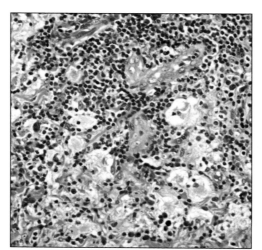 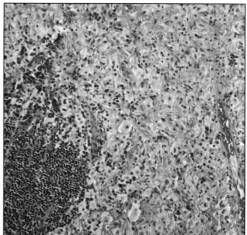

ROSAI-DORFMAN DISEASE

Microscopic Features and Differential Diagnosis

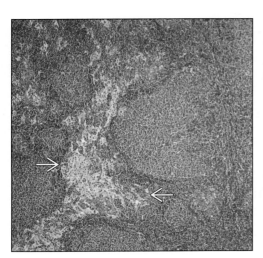

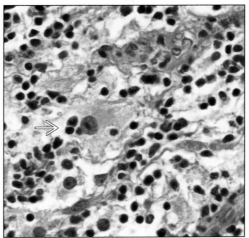

(Left) Paraffin section of a lymph node involved by low-grade follicular lymphoma and focal RDD. A number of neoplastic follicles in this field partially surround a focus of RDD within a sinus ➡. The discovery of RDD was an incidental finding that had no impact on therapeutic decisions. *(Right)* Lymph node involved by low-grade follicular lymphoma and focal RDD. This is a high-power view of the RDD focus. Emperipolesis is present but not prominent ➡.

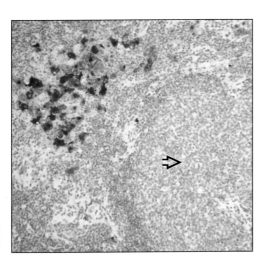

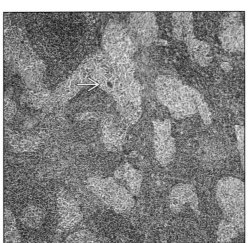

(Left) Lymph node involved by low-grade follicular lymphoma and focal Rosai-Dorfman disease. S100 immunohistochemical stain highlights RDD histiocytes within the sinus. A neoplastic follicle is also present in the right ➡ of this field. *(Right)* Lymph node involved by Langerhans cell histiocytosis (LCH). The process is located within and expands lymph node sinuses. A multinucleated giant cell can be seen at this low power ➡.

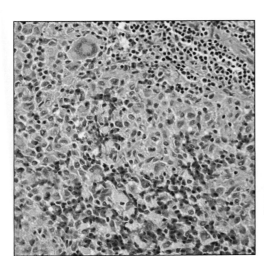

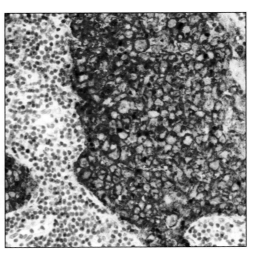

(Left) Lymph node involved by LCH. High-power magnification shows sinus expanded by Langerhans cells with folded nuclei and abundant cytoplasm. These cells are associated with numerous eosinophils and scattered multinucleated giant cells. Eosinophils and multinucleated giant cells are not a feature of RDD. *(Right)* Lymph node involved by LCH. CD1a highlights the numerous CD1a(+) Langerhans cells within sinuses, supporting the diagnosis.

KIMURA DISEASE

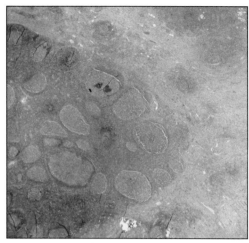

Lymph node and perinodal soft tissue involved by Kimura disease. This field reveals hyperplastic lymphoid follicles, marked eosinophilia, and fibrosis.

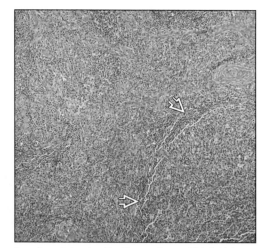

Lymph node involved by Kimura disease. This field shows marked replacement of the interfollicular regions by lymphocytes and eosinophils. A reactive follicle is present ➡.

TERMINOLOGY

Abbreviations
• Kimura disease (KD)

Synonyms
• Kimura lymphadenopathy
• Eosinophilic lymphogranuloma
• Eosinophilic lymphoid follicular hyperplasia

Definitions
• Rare chronic inflammatory disorder of unknown etiology
  ○ Commonly occurs in head & neck region and involves subcutaneous tissues and lymph nodes
• Unrelated to angiolymphoid hyperplasia with eosinophilia (ALHE)
  ○ Historically, these entities were once considered to be the same

ETIOLOGY/PATHOGENESIS

Infectious Agents
• History and histologic findings suggest infectious etiology
  ○ No definite pathogen has been identified

Other Proposed Causes
• Allergy
• Autoimmunity

CLINICAL ISSUES

Epidemiology
• Age
  ○ Mainly occurs in young adults
    ▪ Peak age of onset in 3rd decade
• Gender
  ○ Predominantly males

• Ethnicity
  ○ Asians are most commonly afflicted
  ○ Named after T. Kimura from Japan who reported a case in 1948

Site
• Usually in head & neck region
• Involves deep subcutaneous tissues
  ○ Regional lymph nodes
• Often involves major salivary glands
  ○ Parotid
  ○ Submandibular

Presentation
• Nontender masses in head & neck
  ○ Most often in periauricular region
• Rarely patients have generalized lymphadenopathy
• Systemic symptoms are uncommon
• Nephrotic syndrome may occur in up to 60% of patients

Laboratory Tests
• Peripheral blood eosinophilia almost invariable
• Elevated serum IgE level
• Elevated erythrocyte sedimentation rate (ESR)
• Imbalance between Th1 and Th2 cytokines with
  ○ Increased TNF-α, IL-4, IL-5, IL-13, etc.

Natural History
• Insidious onset
• Slow-growing mass
  ○ Interval from onset of swelling to presentation may be several years
  ○ Often persists unchanged for years

Treatment
• Adjuvant therapy
  ○ Radiation therapy usually yields best outcome
  ○ Patients treated with surgical excision &/or steroid therapy have high rate of recurrence

KIMURA DISEASE

Key Facts

Terminology
- Chronic inflammatory disease that affects subcutaneous tissue and regional lymph nodes

Etiology/Pathogenesis
- Unknown; infectious cause suspected

Clinical Issues
- Mainly in young Asian males
- Head & neck region
  - Nontender subcutaneous masses
  - Regional lymphadenopathy
- Peripheral blood eosinophilia and elevated serum IgE
- Benign clinical course; recurrence common

Microscopic Pathology
- Skin
  - Typically located in deep subcutaneous tissue
  - Reactive follicles with prominent germinal centers
  - Eosinophilia and vascular hyperplasia
- Lymph nodes
  - Hyperplastic follicles
  - Eosinophilia with eosinophilic microabscesses
  - Stromal and perivascular sclerosis

Ancillary Tests
- Immunohistochemistry and molecular studies
  - IgE deposits in germinal centers
  - Polytypic B cells and normal T cells

Top Differential Diagnoses
- Angiolymphoid hyperplasia with eosinophilia
- Langerhans cell histiocytosis
- Dermatopathic lymphadenopathy
- Parasitic infection

- Advantages of surgical excision: Short treatment duration and provides tissue for histopathologic diagnosis

Prognosis
- Indolent clinical course
- Recurrence after excision is common

IMAGE FINDINGS

General Features
- Ultrasound, CT, or MR scans are useful for determining extent of disease
- Combination of ultrasonography and MR has been shown to have high diagnostic value
  - Hypoechoic center and hyperechoic margin with enriched blood vessels on ultrasonography and Doppler
  - Hypointensity replaces normal hyperintense subcutaneous fat on MR
  - Lymph nodes are enlarged with well-defined outline
- CT scan shows nonspecific findings

MICROSCOPIC PATHOLOGY

Histologic Features
- Lymphoid infiltrate in deep subcutis
  - Formation of follicles with germinal centers
  - Accompanied by many eosinophils, plasma cells, and mast cells
    - Eosinophilic microabscesses can be present
  - Vascular hyperplasia
- Lymph nodes show preserved but distorted overall architecture with
  - Hyperplastic follicles with well-formed germinal centers and mantle zones
  - Deposition of IgE in germinal centers forms hyaline proteinaceous material
  - Eosinophilia

- Eosinophilic microabscesses and eosinophilic follicle lysis
- Involvement of perinodal soft tissues
  - Necrosis (±); usually not extensive
  - Vascular proliferation in interfollicular regions
    - Endothelial cells lack cuboidal/polygonal shape with cytoplasmic vacuoles
    - i.e., endothelial cells lack "hobnail" or "tombstone" appearance (seen in ALHE)
  - Stromal and perivascular sclerosis

Cytologic Features
- Fine needle aspiration (FNA) yields polymorphous cell population with many eosinophils
  - Difficult to establish diagnosis of KD based on FNA findings alone

ANCILLARY TESTS

Immunohistochemistry
- IgE deposits in the germinal centers can be shown by immunohistochemistry or immunofluorescence
- Polytypic B cells and normal T cells

Molecular Genetics
- No evidence of monoclonal gene rearrangements
- No known translocations or oncogene abnormalities
- No evidence of infectious organism identified

DIFFERENTIAL DIAGNOSIS

Angiolymphoid Hyperplasia with Eosinophilia (ALHE)
- ALHE has number of other names
  - Epithelioid hemangioma is probably best name
    - Lesion is thought to be benign vascular neoplasm
  - Other names
    - Histiocytoid hemangioma
    - Pseudo- or atypical pyogenic granuloma
    - Inflammatory angiomatous nodule

- Intravenous atypical vascular proliferation
- Occurs more often in
  - Caucasians
  - Young to middle-aged adults
- Presents as multiple papules or nodules
  - Usually occurs in head and neck region
  - Common around ear
- Peripheral blood eosinophilia occurs in ~ 15% of ALHE patients
- Histologic findings of ALHE differ from Kimura disease as follows
  - Located in superficial dermis
  - Lesion has low-power lobular pattern of capillary or medium-sized blood vessels
  - Hypertrophic cuboidal/polygonal endothelial cells
    - Protrude into or occlude vascular lumina
    - Described as "hobnail" or "tombstone" appearance
  - Lesion can be located within large blood vessel
  - No lymph node involvement
- Local recurrence can occur in ~ 33% of patients

Langerhans Cell Histiocytosis
- Young children, adolescents, and young adults
- Can involve lymph nodes or extranodal sites
  - However, deep subcutis is unlikely site of involvement (in contrast with KD)
- Lymph nodes
  - Often sinusoidal; can be both sinusoidal and paracortical
- Skin
  - Superficial dermis
- Characteristic Langerhans cells cytologic features
  - Convoluted nuclei with linear grooves and thin nuclear membranes
- Inflammatory background: Eosinophils, neutrophils, lymphocytes, and histiocytes
- Necrosis and eosinophilic microabscesses common
- Immunohistochemistry: CD1a(+), S100(+), langerin(+)
- Birbeck granules shown by electron microscopy

Dermatopathic Lymphadenopathy
- Most patients (but not all) have skin disease
- Affects lymph nodes without extranodal disease
  - Axillary or inguinal lymphadenopathy most common
- Paracortical expansion by
  - Increased interdigitating dendritic cells and Langerhans cells
  - Scattered plasma cells and eosinophils
  - Deposits of hemosiderin, melanin, and lipids

Parasitic Infection
- Histologic findings can overlap with KD
  - Reactive follicles
  - Eosinophilia
  - Granulomatous inflammation
- Identification of parasitic remnants helpful for diagnosis

Drug Reactions
- History of medications very helpful
- Onset immediately after beginning drug therapy or can occur later

- Associated fever &/or skin rash common
- Generalized or localized lymphadenopathy
  - Paracortical expansion by polymorphous cellular infiltrate
  - Eosinophilia can be prominent
  - Hodgkin-like and Reed-Sternberg-like cells can be present
- Regression after cessation of medication

Castleman Disease, Hyaline Vascular Type
- Most often involves peripheral lymph nodes or mediastinum
- Does not usually involve deep subcutis (unlike KD)
- Large follicles with lymphocyte depletion of germinal centers
  - Small atretic germinal centers
  - Penetrating sclerotic arterioles (hyaline-vascular or "lollipop" lesions)
  - Hyaline deposits in germinal centers
  - Concentric layering of mantle zone lymphocytes ("onion skin")
- Interfollicular vascular and stromal proliferation
- Lacks eosinophilia

Florid Reactive Follicular Hyperplasia, Unspecified
- Large follicles with reactive germinal centers
  - Frequent mitoses, apoptotic bodies, and tingible-body macrophages
- Prominent eosinophilia and vascular proliferation are not present

Angioimmunoblastic T-cell Lymphoma
- Middle-aged to elderly patients
- Patients typically present with systemic symptoms and have aggressive clinical course
  - Generalized lymphadenopathy: Almost all patients
  - Hepatosplenomegaly common
  - Laboratory abnormalities are common
    - Polyclonal hypergammaglobulinemia
    - Autoimmune phenomena
- Lymph nodes, bone marrow, spleen, liver, and skin are frequently involved
- Histologic findings
  - Paracortical or complete effacement of lymph node architecture
  - Polymorphous cellular proliferation with spectrum of lymphocytes, histiocytes, eosinophils, and plasma cells
  - Arborizing high endothelial venules
  - Follicular dendritic cells (CD21[+]) surrounding blood vessels
- Thought to be neoplasm of follicular T-helper cell origin
  - T-cell antigens(+)
  - CD10(+), Bcl-6(+)
  - CXCL13(+), PD-1(+)
- EBV(+) in B cells common
- Monoclonal T-cell receptor gene rearrangements

Hodgkin Disease, Mixed Cellularity Type
- Typically involves lymph nodes

KIMURA DISEASE

Differential Diagnosis between Kimura Disease and Angiolymphoid Hyperplasia with Eosinophilia

Features	Kimura Disease	Angiolymphoid Hyperplasia with Eosinophilia
Race	Asians	Caucasians
Age	Young	Young to middle-aged
Gender	Predominantly male	Predominantly female
Presentation	Subcutaneous mass	Papules or nodules
Location	Deep, head and neck	Superficial, head and neck
Number	Single or multiple	Usually multiple
Overlying skin	Usually normal	Usually erythematous
Regional lymphadenopathy	Common	Uncommon
Blood eosinophilia	Common	Uncommon (~ 15%)
Serum IgE	Usually elevated	Usually normal
Lymphoid infiltrate	Hyperplastic follicles	More diffuse, occasionally forms follicles
Eosinophils	Abundant	Variable, sparse to abundant
Eosinophilic abscesses	Often present	Rare
Vascular proliferation	Some degree, usually thin-walled	Florid, thick-walled
Low-power pattern	None apparent	Lobular
Endothelium	Flat to low cuboidal	Hypertrophic, epithelioid or histiocytoid
Sclerosis	Significant at all stages	Not a prominent feature
Behavior	Insidious onset; indolent; persistent	Benign
Recurrence	Common after surgical excision	~ 33%

- Extranodal involvement is rare without adjacent nodal disease
- Hodgkin and Reed-Sternberg cells
  - CD15(+), CD30(+), pax-5(+ dim), CD45/LCA(-)
- Mixed population of small lymphocytes, plasma cells, eosinophils, and histiocytes

DIAGNOSTIC CHECKLIST

Clinically Relevant Pathologic Features
- Peripheral blood eosinophilia and elevated serum IgE level
- Organ distribution
  - Subcutaneous tissue and regional lymph nodes
  - Head & neck region
  - Peripheral blood eosinophilia and elevated serum IgE level

Pathologic Interpretation Pearls
- Reactive follicular hyperplasia
- IgE deposits in germinal centers
- Eosinophilia

SELECTED REFERENCES

1. Cham E et al: Epithelioid hemangioma (angiolymphoid hyperplasia with eosinophilia) arising on the extremities. J Cutan Pathol. Epub ahead of print, 2009
2. Gopinathan A et al: Kimura's disease: imaging patterns on computed tomography. Clin Radiol. 64(10):994-9, 2009
3. Abuel-Haija M et al: Kimura disease. Arch Pathol Lab Med. 131(4):650-1, 2007
4. Chitapanarux I et al: Radiotherapy in Kimura's disease: a report of eight cases. J Med Assoc Thai. 90(5):1001-5, 2007
5. Iwai H et al: Kimura disease: diagnosis and prognostic factors. Otolaryngol Head Neck Surg. 137(2):306-11, 2007
6. Meningaud JP et al: Kimura's disease of the parotid region: report of 2 cases and review of the literature. J Oral Maxillofac Surg. 65(1):134-40, 2007
7. Ohta N et al: Serum concentrations of eosinophil cationic protein and eosinophils of patients with Kimura's disease. Allergol Int. 56(1):45-9, 2007
8. Takeishi M et al: Kimura disease: diagnostic imaging findings and surgical treatment. J Craniofac Surg. 18(5):1062-7, 2007
9. Chong WS et al: Kimura's disease and angiolymphoid hyperplasia with eosinophilia: two disease entities in the same patient: case report and review of the literature. Int J Dermatol. 45(2):139-45, 2006
10. Wang TF et al: Kimura's disease with generalized lymphadenopathy demonstrated by positron emission tomography scan. Intern Med. 45(12):775-8, 2006
11. Chen H et al: Kimura disease: a clinicopathologic study of 21 cases. Am J Surg Pathol. 28(4):505-13, 2004
12. Seregard S: Angiolymphoid hyperplasia with eosinophilia should not be confused with Kimura's disease. Acta Ophthalmol Scand. 79(1):91-3, 2001
13. Kini U et al: Cytodiagnosis of Kimura's disease. Indian J Pathol Microbiol. 41(4):473-7, 1998
14. Chun SI et al: Kimura's disease and angiolymphoid hyperplasia with eosinophilia: clinical and histopathologic differences. J Am Acad Dermatol. 27(6 Pt 1):954-8, 1992
15. Chan JK et al: Epithelioid haemangioma (angiolymphoid hyperplasia with eosinophilia) and Kimura's disease in Chinese. Histopathology. 15(6):557-74, 1989
16. Hui PK et al: Lymphadenopathy of Kimura's disease. Am J Surg Pathol. 13(3):177-86, 1989

3

KIMURA DISEASE

Microscopic Features

(Left) Upper lip lesion involved by Kimura disease shows a moderately dense lymphoid infiltrate based in the deep dermis. Note the many hyperplastic lymphoid follicles that can be seen in this field. Eosinophilia is also present but not easy to appreciate at this magnification. *(Right)* Upper lip lesion involved by Kimura disease shows lymphocytes and eosinophils surrounding skeletal muscle. Eosinophils are not easily appreciated at this magnification.

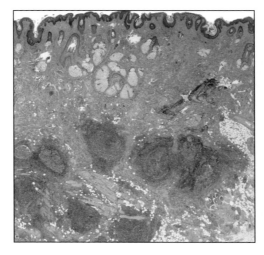
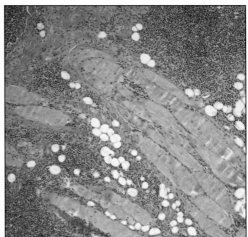

(Left) High-power magnification of upper lip lesion involved by Kimura disease. This field shows marked eosinophilia, vascular proliferation, and lymphocytes including a reactive germinal center ➡ surrounded and partially infiltrated by small lymphocytes and eosinophils. *(Right)* Biopsy of subcutaneous tissue shows findings of Kimura disease. The lesion is located in the deep dermis and extends into deeper adipose tissue. Many hyperplastic follicles can be seen at this magnification.

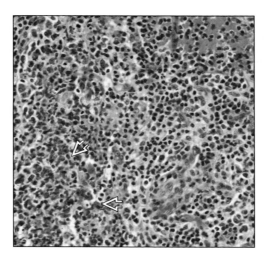
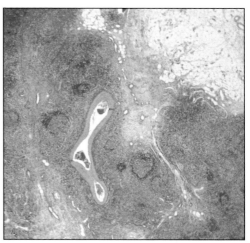

(Left) Biopsy of lesion in subcutaneous tissue shows findings of Kimura disease. This field shows numerous eosinophils forming a microabscess ➡ and a reactive lymphoid follicle with a germinal center at the bottom of the field ➡. *(Right)* Biopsy of subcutaneous tissue shows findings of Kimura disease. In this field, a large reactive lymphoid follicle (bottom left of filed) is surrounded by numerous eosinophils (upper right).

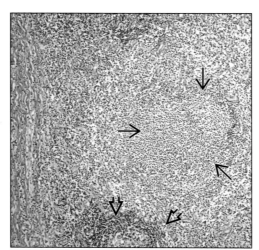
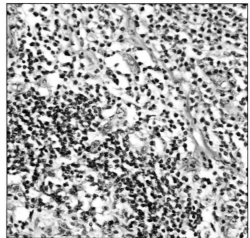

KIMURA DISEASE

Imaging and Microscopic Features

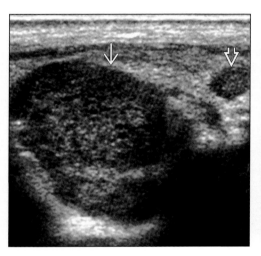
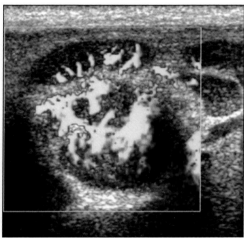

(Left) Transverse grayscale US shows a well-defined, solid, hypoechoic homogeneous mass ➡ in the superficial parotid in a patient with Kimura disease. There is no necrosis. Note another smaller adjacent nodule ➡. After grayscale imaging, Doppler should always be performed to evaluate vascularity. *(Right)* Power Doppler shows marked vascularity within the mass. In an Asian male, consider nodal Kimura disease in an intraparotid node. Diagnosis was confirmed at biopsy.

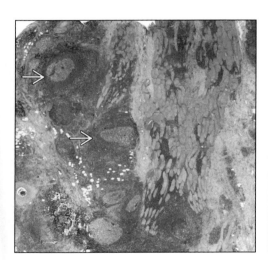
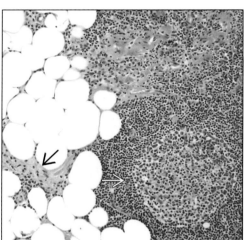

(Left) Biopsy specimen from the submaxillary region of 45-year-old man shows Kimura disease involving primarily skeletal muscle. Large reactive follicles ➡ can be seen. Eosinophils cannot be appreciated at this magnification. *(Right)* Biopsy specimen from the submaxillary region shows Kimura disease involving adipose tissue. A reactive germinal center is present ➡. Eosinophils in adipose tissue are barely appreciable at this magnification ➡.

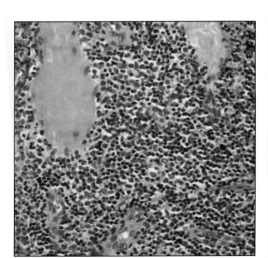
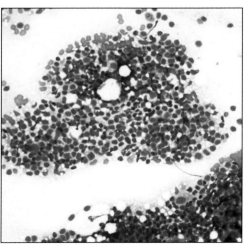

(Left) Biopsy specimen from the submaxillary region of a 45-year-old man with Kimura disease. Many lymphocytes and eosinophils infiltrate skeletal muscle. *(Right)* Touch imprint of lymph node involved by Kimura disease. The nodular arrangement of cells suggests a nodular or follicular pattern. The cell population is polymorphous with eosinophils.

KIMURA DISEASE

Microscopic Features and Differential Diagnosis

(Left) Lymph node involved by Kimura disease shows hyperplastic lymphoid follicles and marked eosinophilia. *(Right)* Lymph node involved by Kimura disease shows a hyperplastic lymphoid follicle (right) and marked eosinophilia (left). Eosinophils infiltrate the follicle (follicle lysis) in this field.

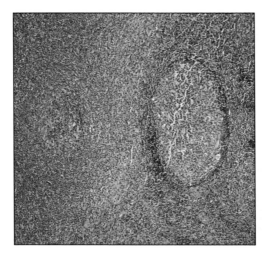 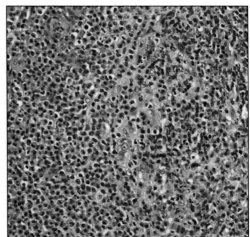

(Left) Lymph node involved by Kimura disease. In this case, numerous histiocytes and eosinophils replaced lymph node parenchyma. Reactive follicular hyperplasia was not a prominent feature in this case. *(Right)* Lymph node involved by Kimura disease. This image shows an eosinophilic microabscess (upper portion of field). Histiocytes are also present (bottom of field).

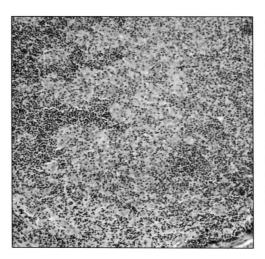 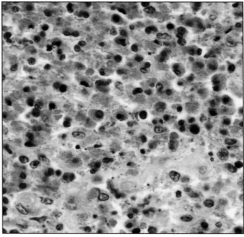

(Left) A case of angiolymphoid hyperplasia with eosinophilia (epithelioid hemangioma) from the lip region of a 28-year-old man. This field shows soft tissue involved by a large reactive lymphoid follicle ➡ and increased blood vessels and eosinophils (top of field). *(Right)* Angiolymphoid hyperplasia with eosinophilia (epithelioid hemangioma) from the lip region. Vascular proliferation, small lymphocytes, and eosinophils are present. (Courtesy B. L. Kemp, MD.)

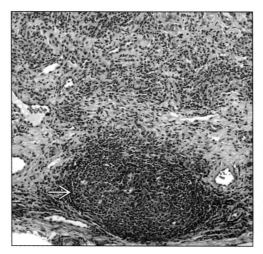 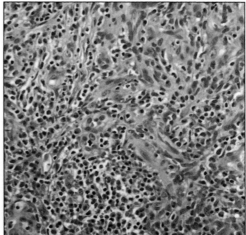

KIMURA DISEASE

Differential Diagnosis

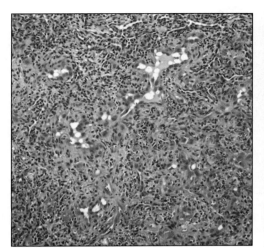

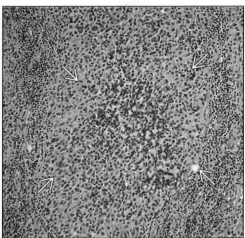

(Left) Angiolymphoid hyperplasia with eosinophilia (epithelioid hemangioma) from the lip. Blood vessels with prominent, cuboidal endothelial cells are characteristic of this lesion. *(Right)* Lymph node involved by Langerhans cell histiocytosis (LCH). The numerous eosinophils are similar to Kimura disease; however, Langerhans cells tend to involve sinuses (outlined by ➡) and have distinctive cytologic and immunophenotypic features.

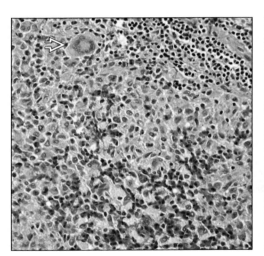

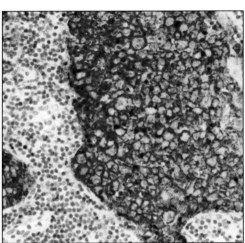

(Left) Lymph node involved by Langerhans cell histiocytosis (LCH). This field shows the distinctive Langerhans cells and a multinucleated giant cell ➡. *(Right)* Lymph node involved by Langerhans cell histiocytosis (LCH). The Langerhans cells are strongly positive for CD1a as well as S100 protein (not shown) and langerin (not shown).

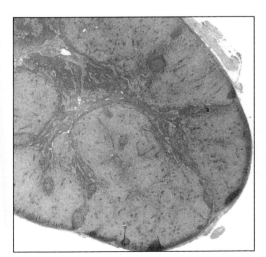

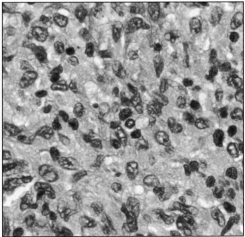

(Left) Lymph node involved by dermatopathic lymphadenopathy shows marked expansion of paracortical regions by interdigitating dendritic cells and Langerhans cells. *(Right)* High magnification of dermatopathic lymphadenopathy (DL) shows numerous interdigitating dendritic cells and fewer Langerhans cells with folded nuclei, grooves, and abundant pale cytoplasm.

UNICENTRIC HYALINE VASCULAR VARIANT CASTLEMAN DISEASE

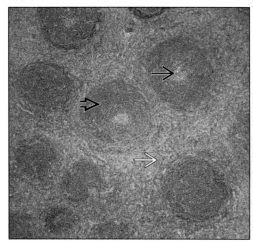

Castleman disease, hyaline-vascular variant (HV-CD). Regressed germinal centers ⇒ are surrounded by expanded mantle zones ⇒. There is also marked interfollicular blood vessel proliferation ⇒.

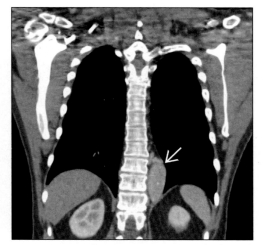

Positive CT scan shows a 4.5 cm mass in the low left paraspinal region ⇒. The site of disease in this patient is unusual but is otherwise consistent with unifocal HV-CD.

TERMINOLOGY

Abbreviations
- Castleman disease, hyaline-vascular variant (HV-CD)

Synonyms
- Angiofollicular lymph node hyperplasia
- Giant lymph node hyperplasia
- Angiomatous lymphoid hamartoma

Definitions
- Typically unicentric and reactive lymphoproliferation of unknown etiology involving lymph nodes

ETIOLOGY/PATHOGENESIS

Unknown
- Possible factors in pathogenesis
  - Dysregulation of vascular endothelial growth factor
  - Follicular dendritic cell (FDC) dysplasia may be precursor

CLINICAL ISSUES

Epidemiology
- Incidence
  - Rare
- Age
  - Young adults; median age: 4th decade
- Gender
  - No preference

Presentation
- Patients present with localized mass
  - Mass often detected incidentally
- Rarely symptoms related to compression of adjacent tissues by enlarged lymph nodes
- Lymphadenopathy, localized
  - Mediastinal or thoracic lymph nodes most commonly involved
  - Other sites: Cervical and retroperitoneal lymph nodes
  - Extranodal sites of involvement are rare
- Patients may develop secondary amyloidosis

Treatment
- Surgical approaches
  - Surgery to remove enlarged lymph nodes
- Adjuvant therapy
  - Usually not necessary
  - Radiation therapy has been used to alleviate compression symptoms

Prognosis
- Excellent
- Surgical removal is usually curative; relapse can occur uncommonly
- Malignant neoplasms can arise in association with HV-CD
  - Follicular dendritic cell sarcomas are most common
  - Vascular neoplasms
  - Secondary neoplasms in HV-CD are often low grade but metastases are reported

IMAGE FINDINGS

Radiographic Findings
- Enlarged lymph node or group of lymph nodes, but any site can be involved
  - Mediastinal or thoracic lymph nodes most common

MICROSCOPIC PATHOLOGY

Histologic Features
- Numerous follicles in cortex and medulla of lymph node
- Obliteration of subcapsular sinuses

UNICENTRIC HYALINE VASCULAR VARIANT CASTLEMAN DISEASE

Key Facts

Clinical Issues
- Young adults
- Lymphadenopathy, localized
- Excision is usually curative

Microscopic Pathology
- Large follicles with regressed (involuted) germinal centers
- 2 or more germinal centers per follicle ("twinning")
- Concentric rings of mantle zone lymphocytes ("onion skin")
- Hyaline-vascular ("lollipop") follicles
- Increased vascular proliferation in interfollicular zones
- Plasma cells and immunoblasts are not abundant

Ancillary Tests
- Polytypic B cells and normal T cells
- Increased FDCs in germinal centers: CD21(+), CD23(+), CD35(+), &/or EGFR(+)
- No evidence of monoclonal *Ig* or *TCR* gene rearrangements
- No consistent cytogenetic or molecular abnormalities known

Top Differential Diagnoses
- Castleman disease, plasma cell variant
- Thymoma
- Angioimmunoblastic T-cell lymphoma
- HIV lymphadenitis
- Castleman-like changes associated with various lymphomas

- 2 or more germinal centers in a follicle ("twinning")
- Follicles typically large with regressed (or involuted) germinal centers
  - Germinal centers are composed mostly of FDC with few lymphocytes
  - FDCs often hyperplastic and can show dysplasia
- Many follicles show so-called "lollipop" features characterized by
  - Concentric rings of the mantle zone lymphocytes ("onion skin" appearance)
  - Sclerotic blood vessels radially traversing into germinal center
- Interfollicular or stromal component is also important
  - Increased number of high endothelial venules with hyalinized walls
  - Stromal component can predominate with only few hyaline-vascular follicles
- Clusters of plasmacytoid dendritic cells (plasmacytoid monocytes) can be prominent
- Plasma cells and immunoblasts are not abundant in HV-CD
  - Much more common in plasma cell variant of CD

ANCILLARY TESTS

Immunohistochemistry
- Human herpes virus-8 (HHV8) is absent
- Polytypic B cells and T cells
- Increased FDCs in involuted germinal centers often positive for CD21, CD23, CD35, or EGFR
  - Dysplastic FDCs often stain variably for FDC markers
- Plasma cells are polytypic

Flow Cytometry
- Polytypic B cells and T cells with normal immunophenotype

Cytogenetics
- Rare cases reported with chromosomal translocations or other clonal abnormalities

- No consistent cytogenetic findings
- Del(12q13-15) resulted in intragenic *HMGIC* gene rearrangement reported in 1 case

PCR
- No evidence of monoclonal immunoglobulin (*Ig*) or T-cell receptor (*TCR*) gene rearrangements

DIFFERENTIAL DIAGNOSIS

Castleman Disease, Plasma Cell Variant (PC-CD), HHV8(-)
- PC-CD represents 10-20% of localized (unicentric) CD cases
- Any lymph node group can be affected
  - Mediastinal involvement less common than HV-CD
- Preserved overall lymph node architecture
- Sheets of plasma cells in interfollicular areas
  - No cytologic atypia
- Variable follicular hyperplasia with focal, less well-developed hyaline-vascular lesions
- Lymph node sinuses not obliterated

Castleman Disease, Plasma Cell Variant, HHV8(+)
- Most patients present with multicentric disease
- High association with HIV infection
- Constitutional symptoms and laboratory abnormalities common
- Histologic resistance to HHV8(-) PC-CD but
  - Often greater vascularity
  - Often shows greater overall cell depletion
- HHV8(+) defines this variant of CD
  - Plasmablasts present in mantle zones and paracortical regions
- Associated with increased risk of HHV8(+) plasmablastic lymphoma

Castleman Disease, Plasma Cell Variant, Associated with POEMS Syndrome
- Resembles PC-CD in other patients

UNICENTRIC HYALINE VASCULAR VARIANT CASTLEMAN DISEASE

- Association with HHV8 unclear in literature
  - Some studies report antibodies to HHV8 antigens in serum of POEMS patients

Thymoma
- Epithelial neoplasm
- Cytokeratin immunohistochemical stain highlights epithelial cell network
- Lymphocytes in thymoma are of immature T-cell lineage (TdT[+])
- Unlike HV-CD, thymomas lack
  - Hyaline-vascular follicles ("lollipop" lesions)
  - Stromal proliferation
  - FDC dysplasia

Angioimmunoblastic T-cell Lymphoma (AITL)
- Hyperplastic follicles are present in only subset of cases (~ 10%)
  - Follicles are "burnt-out" and can resemble involuted germinal centers of HV-CD
- Unlike HV-CD, AITL is characterized by
  - Paracortical distribution
  - Proliferation of high endothelial venules
  - Neoplastic cells are cytologically atypical and often have clear cytoplasm
  - Often numerous reactive eosinophils are present
  - Markers of FDC show pattern of proliferation quite different from HV-CD

HIV Lymphadenitis
- Prominent reactive follicular hyperplasia in early stages of infection
- Involuted follicles and vascular proliferation in interfollicular zones can occur in later stages
  - When present, hyaline-vascular lesions tend to be focal and not well developed
- HIV serological testing needed to confirm diagnosis

Castleman Disease-like Changes
- Some features of HV-CD can be observed in association with various lymphoma types
  - Most common: Hodgkin lymphoma, follicular lymphoma
- May be associated with interleukin-6 dysregulation
- Usually manifested as focal hyaline-vascular lesions and plasmacytosis
- No apparent clinical significance

Kaposi Sarcoma (KS)
- Rarely associated with HV-CD unlike multicentric CD in HIV(+) patients
- Proliferating neoplastic endothelial cells of KS show cytological atypia
- Routinely positive for HHV8 using anti-LNA-1

Follicular Lymphoma
- Numerous follicles that replace lymph node architecture
- Hyaline-vascular lesions uncommon
  - When present, focal and not well developed
- Immunophenotyping shows monoclonal B-cell population
  - CD10(+) &/or Bcl-6(+)

- Monoclonal Ig gene rearrangements and t(14;18) (q32;q21)/*IgH-BCL2* in 80-90%

Mantle Cell Lymphoma, Mantle Zone Variant
- Follicles can be prominent with concentric rings of lymphocytes
- Usually no hyaline-vascular lesions or stromal vascular proliferation
- Immunophenotyping shows monoclonal B-cell population
  - CD5(+), Cyclin-D1(+)
- Monoclonal Ig gene rearrangements and t(11;14) (q13;q32)/*CCND1-IgH* in 90-95%

DIAGNOSTIC CHECKLIST

Clinically Relevant Pathologic Features
- Organ distribution

Pathologic Interpretation Pearls
- Both follicular and interfollicular (stromal) changes
- Follicular component
  - Large follicles with small, regressed germinal centers
  - Onion skin-like mantle zones
  - Hyaline-vascular lesions
  - Dysplastic FDCs can be present in germinal centers
- Vascular proliferation in interfollicular regions

SELECTED REFERENCES

1. Cronin DM et al: Castleman disease: an update on classification and the spectrum of associated lesions. Adv Anat Pathol. 16(4):236-46, 2009
2. Cokelaere K et al: Hyaline vascular Castleman's disease with HMGIC rearrangement in follicular dendritic cells: molecular evidence of mesenchymal tumorigenesis. Am J Surg Pathol. 26(5):662-9, 2002
3. Lin O et al: Angiomyoid and follicular dendritic cell proliferative lesions in Castleman's disease of hyaline-vascular type: a study of 10 cases. Am J Surg Pathol. 21(11):1295-306, 1997
4. Oksenhendler E et al: Multicentric Castleman's disease in HIV infection: a clinical and pathological study of 20 patients. AIDS. 10(1):61-7, 1996
5. Zarate-Osorno A et al: Hodgkin's disease with coexistent Castleman-like histologic features. A report of three cases. Arch Pathol Lab Med. 118(3):270-4, 1994
6. Danon AD et al: Morpho-immunophenotypic diversity of Castleman's disease, hyaline-vascular type: with emphasis on a stroma-rich variant and a new pathogenetic hypothesis. Virchows Arch A Pathol Anat Histopathol. 423(5):369-82, 1993
7. Krishnan J et al: Reactive lymphadenopathies and atypical lymphoproliferative disorders. Am J Clin Pathol. 99(4):385-96, 1993
8. Keller AR et al: Hyaline-vascular and plasma-cell types of giant lymph node hyperplasia of the mediastinum and other locations. Cancer. 29(3):670-83, 1972
9. Castleman B et al: Localized mediastinal lymphnode hyperplasia resembling thymoma. Cancer. 9(4):822-30, 1956

UNICENTRIC HYALINE VASCULAR VARIANT CASTLEMAN DISEASE

Microscopic Features

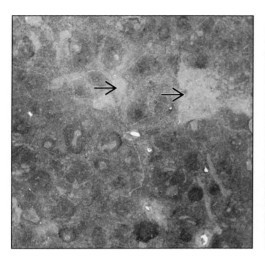

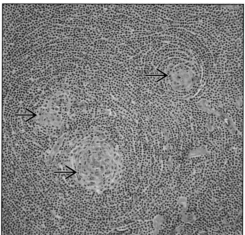

(Left) Castleman disease, hyaline-vascular variant (HV-CD). Markedly increased follicles are present throughout the lymph node parenchyma. The follicles are located in the cortex as well as the medulla. Areas of fibrosis ➨ are also noted. (Right) Castleman disease, hyaline-vascular variant. Three involuted germinal centers ➨ are surrounded by concentric layers of small lymphocytes. The presence of multiple germinal centers within a follicle is known as "twinning."

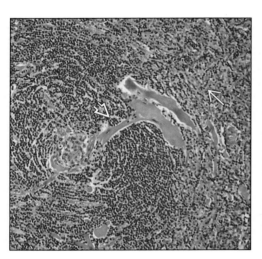

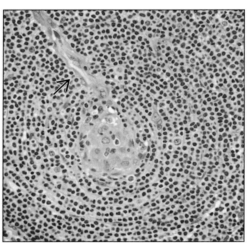

(Left) A hyaline-vascular or "lollipop" lesion in HV-CD. A hyalinized blood vessel ➨ exiting radially from an involuted follicle is surrounded by an expanded mantle zone. Also note the increased blood vessels ➨ in the interfollicular area. (Right) A hyaline-vascular lesion in a different case of HV-CD. Note the lymphocyte-depleted germinal center surrounded by layers of mantle zone lymphocytes and a sclerotic blood vessel radially exiting the germinal center ➨.

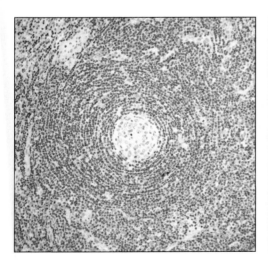

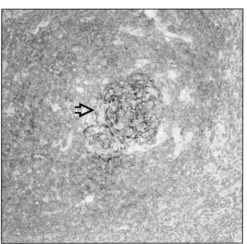

(Left) Castleman disease, hyaline-vascular variant. The lymphocytes in the expanded mantle zone are positive for Bcl-2, whereas the cells within the small regressed germinal center cells are negative. (Right) Castleman disease, hyaline-vascular variant. Immunohistochemistry for CD21 highlights many follicular dendritic cells in small germinal center ➨.

Variant Microscopic Features

(Left) Castleman disease, hyaline-vascular variant. Increased follicular dendritic cells and lymphocyte depletion are shown in a regressed germinal center surrounded by concentric layers of mantle zone small lymphocytes. (Right) Castleman disease, hyaline-vascular variant. Clusters of plasmacytoid dendritic cells ⮕ (plasmacytoid monocytes) are prominent in the interfollicular areas in this case.

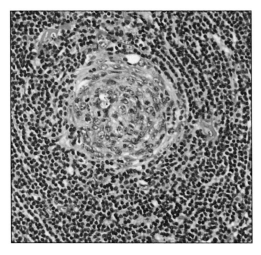
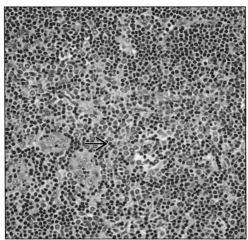

(Left) Marked vascular and spindle cell proliferation in Castleman disease, hyaline-vascular variant may resemble Kaposi sarcoma, but the endothelial cells show no cytological atypia, and mitotic figures are rare. (Right) In this case of HV-CD, the stromal proliferation ⮕ is prominent (stroma rich), and the follicle is atretic ⮕.

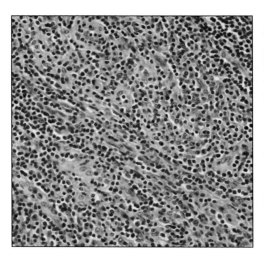
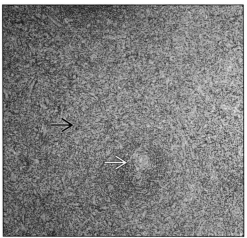

(Left) Higher power view of Castleman disease, hyaline-vascular variant. Note prominent stromal changes. (Right) CD21 immunostain in a case of HV-CD illustrates abundant follicular dendritic cell proliferation in the interfollicular regions. This case of HV-CD had marked interfollicular changes also known as being stroma rich.

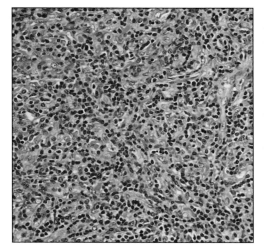
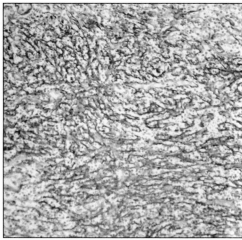

UNICENTRIC HYALINE VASCULAR VARIANT CASTLEMAN DISEASE

Differential Diagnosis

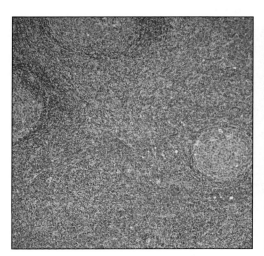

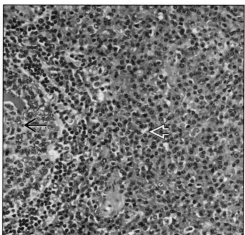

(Left) Plasma cell variant of CD (PC-CD). The follicles are not as atretic as seen in HV-CD and are often hyperplastic. The interfollicular areas are expanded by plasma cells. *(Right)* High-power view of plasma cell variant of CD (PC-CD). The germinal centers ➡ do not show prominent FDC proliferation. The most striking feature is the presence of sheets of mature plasma cells ➡ in the interfollicular regions.

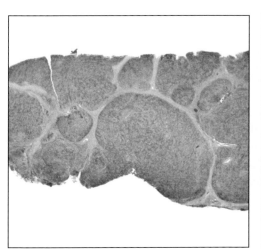

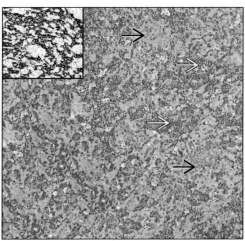

(Left) Thymoma. A mass in the mediastinum poses a differential diagnosis of thymoma versus HV-CD. The presence of broad fibrous bands forming nodules in this case is more common in thymoma. *(Right)* Thymoma. The proliferating cells are epithelial ➡ with plump nuclei and moderate cytoplasm. The cells form large clusters with interspersed mature and immature lymphoid cells ➡. The neoplastic cells are positive for cytokeratin (inset).

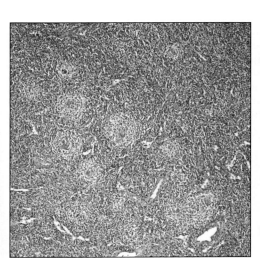

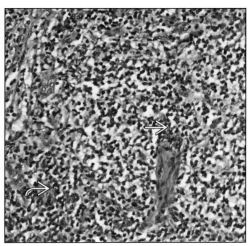

(Left) Follicular lymphoma. The follicles are numerous and sclerotic. Vascular proliferation in the interfollicular areas is also noted. These features resemble those of HV-CD at low power. *(Right)* Follicular lymphoma. The neoplastic follicles are composed of mostly centrocytes ➡ in this case. The vessel ➡ traversing the follicle is not hyalinized. Vascular proliferation is prominent in this case but stromal proliferation is uncommon in follicular lymphoma.

UNICENTRIC PLASMA CELL VARIANT CASTLEMAN DISEASE

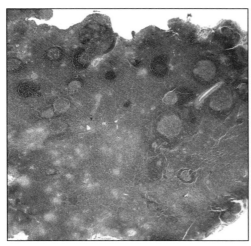

Lymph node involved by unicentric Castleman disease, plasma cell variant (CD-PV). Multiple follicles are present and the interfollicular zones are expanded by plasma cells.

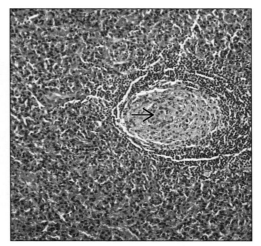

Lymph node involved by unicentric CD-PV. This field shows interfollicular plasma cells and a follicle with a small germinal center with involution (regressive changes) ➔.

TERMINOLOGY

Abbreviations
- Castleman disease, plasma cell variant (CD-PV)

Synonyms
- Unicentric Castleman disease, plasma cell variant
- Angiofollicular lymph node hyperplasia
- Giant lymph node hyperplasia
- Angiomatous lymphoid hamartoma
- Benign giant lymphoma

Definitions
- Histologically distinctive reaction pattern in lymph node characterized by
  - Marked interfollicular plasmacytosis
  - Regressive (hyaline-vascular) changes in small subset of follicles in subset of cases

ETIOLOGY/PATHOGENESIS

Unknown
- Data supporting role for dysregulation of interleukin-6 (IL-6) in pathogenesis
  - Lymphocytes in CD-PV express IL-6
  - B cells express IL-6 receptor (CD126)
    - Autocrine or paracrine mechanisms may be involved
  - In mice, forced expression of IL-6 in bone marrow cells causes syndrome that resembles, in part, CD-PV
- Immune dysregulation also may be involved
- As defined in this chapter, there is no evidence of human herpes virus 8 (HHV8) infection

CLINICAL ISSUES

Epidemiology
- Incidence

  - Accounts for 10-20% of localized or unicentric cases of CD
- Age
  - Broad range; median in 3rd-4th decade
- Gender
  - No preference

Site
- Peripheral lymph nodes most common
- Mediastinal involvement less common (than hyaline vascular variant of CD)

Presentation
- Most patients present with lymphadenopathy without systemic symptoms
- 10-20% of patients reported in literature had systemic symptoms
  - Fever, night sweats, weight loss, malaise
  - However, it seems likely that many of these patients were HHV8(+)
    - Therefore better classified as HHV8-associated &/or multicentric CD
- Small subset of patients reported were associated with POEMS syndrome
  - POEMS = peripheral neuropathy, organomegaly, endocrinopathy, monoclonal M protein, skin lesions
  - These patients also likely to be HHV8(+)
    - Probably better classified as HHV8-associated &/or multicentric CD

Laboratory Tests
- Many patients lack laboratory abnormalities
- Subset of patients (~ 10-20%) can have cytopenias
  - Anemia and thrombocytopenia
- Serum IL-6 levels can be increased

Treatment
- Surgical approaches
  - Usually curative by excision

UNICENTRIC PLASMA CELL VARIANT CASTLEMAN DISEASE

Key Facts

Terminology
- Histologically distinctive reaction pattern in lymph node characterized by
  - Marked interfollicular plasmacytosis
  - Regressive (hyaline-vascular) changes in small subset of follicles
- Defined in this chapter as HHV8(-) and not associated with either multicentric CD or POEMS syndrome

Clinical Issues
- ~ 10-20% of localized/unicentric cases of CD
- Broad age range; median 3rd-4th decade
- Peripheral lymph nodes are most commonly affected
- ~ 10-20% of patients have systemic symptoms &/or laboratory abnormalities
  - Subset of cases reported with these abnormalities may be unrecognized multicentric CD
- Usually cured by surgical excision

Microscopic Pathology
- Preserved lymph node architecture
- Marked plasmacytosis in interfollicular areas
  - No cytologic atypia
- Germinal centers are hyperplastic and usually subset are atretic with changes resembling CD-HV

Ancillary Tests
- No evidence of HHV8 infection
- No evidence of monoclonality

Top Differential Diagnoses
- HHV8(+) multicentric CD
- Autoimmune diseases
- Marginal zone B-cell lymphoma

Prognosis
- Good
- Small subset of patients may evolve to multicentric CD
  - Possibly were cases of multicentric CD at time of initial biopsy

IMAGE FINDINGS

Radiographic Findings
- Lymphadenopathy
  - Often multiple lymph nodes in an anatomic group are large
- PET scan shows increased FDG uptake

MACROSCOPIC FEATURES

Size
- Usually lymphadenopathy is of modest size

MICROSCOPIC PATHOLOGY

Histologic Features
- Less well defined than HV-CD
- Preserved overall lymph node architecture
- Marked plasmacytosis in interfollicular areas
  - Some plasma cells can be binucleated
- Vascularity in interfollicular areas can be prominent
- Sinuses usually patent
- Widely spaced lymphoid follicles
- Lymphoid follicles contain hyperplastic germinal centers, but small subset of germinal centers often show regressive changes
  - Resemble follicles seen in CD-HV
  - Others have used term "mixed or transitional" type because of these follicles
  - Atretic follicles are usually present and part of spectrum of CD-PV
- Mantle zones are usually well defined and can be expanded
  - Plasmablasts are absent or rare in mantle zones

Cytologic Features
- Plasma cells are cytologically normal without atypia
- Lymphocytes show range in cytologic appearance
- Difficult to establish specific diagnosis of CD-PV by fine needle aspiration

ANCILLARY TESTS

Immunohistochemistry
- Interfollicular plasma cells express polytypic immunoglobulin light chains
- Follicles composed of polytypic B cells and T cells
  - Germinal centers are Bcl-2(-)
  - Atretic follicles show increased follicular dendritic cells
    - CD21(+), CD23(+), CD35(+)
- Rare cases are reported with monoclonal plasma cells
  - These cases most likely HHV8(+) &/or multicentric CD

Flow Cytometry
- Polytypic B cells and normal T cells
- Specific diagnosis cannot be suggested based on immunophenotype

Cytogenetics
- Very few cases studied
- No specific abnormalities reported

Molecular Studies
- Most cases lack monoclonal *Ig* gene rearrangements
  - Small subset of cases carry *IGH* gene rearrangements
  - Monoclonal cases may be HHV8(+) &/or multicentric CD in retrospect
- No specific chromosomal translocations

Associated Lymphoid Neoplasms
- Small subset of CD-PV can be associated with lymphoma
  - Classical Hodgkin lymphoma is most common

- ■ Mixed cellularity type
- ■ CD changes can obscure large HRS cells
- o Non-Hodgkin lymphomas also occur
  - ■ Diffuse large B-cell lymphoma
  - ■ Mantle cell lymphoma
  - ■ Peripheral T-cell lymphoma

DIFFERENTIAL DIAGNOSIS

HHV8(+) Multicentric CD
- Clinically aggressive disease commonly associated with HIV infection and rarely POEMS syndrome
- Affected lymph nodes usually show blurred boundaries between germinal centers and mantle zones
  - o Plasmablasts in mantle zones are HHV8(+)
    - ■ Can be identified using antibody specific for latency associated nuclear antigen (LANA-1)
- Plasmablasts can be present in clusters and are monotypic Igλ(+), known as "microlymphoma"

Autoimmune Diseases
- Rheumatoid arthritis may be best example
- Lymph nodes show florid interfollicular plasmacytosis and follicular hyperplasia
- Serological studies such as testing for anti-CCP antibody helpful to confirm diagnosis
- No evidence of monoclonality

Marginal Zone B-cell Lymphoma with Marked Plasmacytic Differentiation
- Follicular hyperplasia and sheets of plasma cells can be prominent in some cases
- Nodal architecture is usually altered or replaced by lymphoma
  - o Neoplastic B cells often with monocytoid features
  - o Monotypic Ig expression or monoclonal *Ig* gene rearrangements

Plasmacytoma
- Plasma cells form sheets that replace lymph node architecture
  - o Plasma cells are cytologically atypical
  - o Residual follicles are usually small and overtaken by neoplastic cell proliferation
  - o Neoplasm may extend into perinodal adipose tissue
- Plasma cells are monotypic and monoclonal

Classical Hodgkin Lymphoma (HL)
- Marked plasmacytosis can occur in some cases of classical HL
- HRS cells in classical HL
  - o CD15(+), CD30(+), pax-5(dimly [+]), CD45/LCA(-)

Angioimmunoblastic T-cell Lymphoma
- Rare cases have marked plasmacytosis and hyaline-vascular type changes in germinal centers
- Lymph node architecture is replaced
  - o Polymorphous cell population including cells with pale/clear cytoplasm

- T-cells express CD10, Bcl-6, CXCL13, or PD-1 in many cases
- Monoclonal *TCR* rearrangements

DIAGNOSTIC CHECKLIST

Clinically Relevant Pathologic Features
- Patients with unicentric/localized CD-PV as defined in this chapter
  - o Have variable clinical presentation associated with lymphadenopathy
  - o Are HHV8(-) and usually lack systemic symptoms or laboratory abnormalities
- Small subset of patients reported in literature have symptoms or laboratory abnormalities
  - o Part of multicentric CD that initially presented with unicentric lymphadenopathy?
  - o Associated with unappreciated HHV8 &/or HIV infection?
  - o Associated with POEMS syndrome?
- Once other conditions are excluded, unicentric CD-PV may not be disease but simply a nonspecific reaction pattern in lymph nodes
  - o More research is needed to clarify relationship between CD-HV, CD-PV, and multicentric CD

Pathologic Interpretation Pearls
- Preserved lymph node architecture
- Marked interfollicular polytypic plasmacytosis
- Histologic features are not specific and can be observed in other conditions
- Must exclude HHV8(+) multicentric CD

SELECTED REFERENCES

1. Cronin DM et al: Castleman disease: an update on classification and the spectrum of associated lesions. Adv Anat Pathol. 16(4):236-46, 2009
2. Choi JH et al: Unicentric castleman disease is not clearly distinguished from multicentric type: a case report. Clin Lymphoma Myeloma. 8(4):256-9, 2008
3. Vasudev Rao T et al: Follicular dendritic cell hyperplasia in plasma cell variant of Castleman's disease with interfollicular Hodgkin's disease. Pathol Res Pract. 203(6):479-84, 2007
4. Dispenzieri A et al: Treatment of Castleman's disease. Curr Treat Options Oncol. 6(3):255-66, 2005
5. Brousset P et al: Colocalization of the viral interleukin-6 with latent nuclear antigen-1 of human herpesvirus-8 in endothelial spindle cells of Kaposi's sarcoma and lymphoid cells of multicentric Castleman's disease. Hum Pathol. 32(1):95-100, 2001
6. Zarate-Osorno A et al: Hodgkin's disease with coexistent Castleman-like histologic features. A report of three cases. Arch Pathol Lab Med. 118(3):270-4, 1994
7. Mandler RN et al: Castleman's disease in POEMS syndrome with elevated interleukin-6. Cancer. 69(11):2697-703, 1992
8. Leger-Ravet MB et al: Interleukin-6 gene expression in Castleman's disease. Blood. 78(11):2923-30, 1991
9. Schlosnagle DC et al: Plasmacytoma arising in giant lymph node hyperplasia. Am J Clin Pathol. 78(4):541-4, 1982

UNICENTRIC PLASMA CELL VARIANT CASTLEMAN DISEASE

Microscopic Features

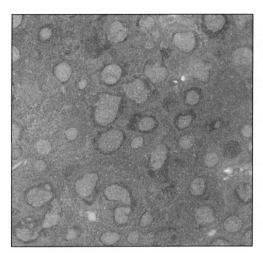 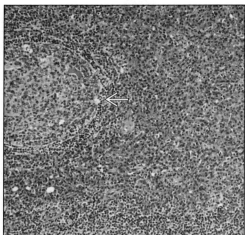

(Left) Lymph node involved by unicentric CD-PV. Lymph node architecture is relatively preserved. Numerous follicles are surrounded by marked interfollicular plasmacytosis. A few patent sinuses are present. At low power, CD-PV in lymph node has some resemblance to spleen, a clue to the diagnosis. (Right) A lymph node involved by CD-PV. The plasma cells convey a purple-pink appearance. A small follicle is also present ➡.

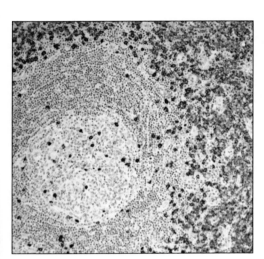 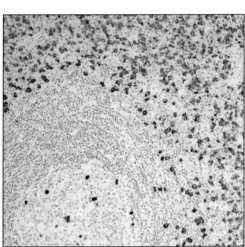

(Left) Lymph node involved by unicentric CD-PV. Many plasma cells in the interfollicular region and a few cells within the central follicle express cytoplasmic Igκ light chain. (Right) Lymph node involved by unicentric CD-PV. Plasma cells in the interfollicular region and a few cells within the central follicle express cytoplasmic Igλ light chain. κ outnumbered λ in this case but the ratio supports polytypic plasma cells.

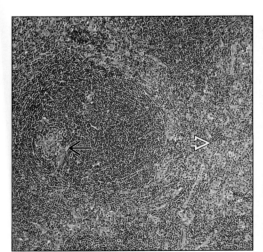 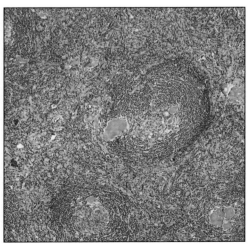

(Left) Lymph node involved by CD-PV shows germinal center with involution ➡, surrounded by prominent mantle zone lymphocytes. Interfollicular areas are expanded by plasma cells and lymphoid cells with prominent vasculature ➡. Cases such as this have been designated as "mixed" or "transitional" type in the literature but are part of the spectrum of CD-PV. (Right) A case of CD-hyaline-vascular variant is shown for comparison.

UNICENTRIC PLASMA CELL VARIANT CASTLEMAN DISEASE

Microscopic Features and Differential Diagnosis

(Left) Lymph node involved by unicentric CD-PV. The lymph node architecture is generally preserved and sinuses are patent. Interfollicular areas are expanded by plasma cells. Residual follicles with small or atretic germinal centers are present in this field ⇾. *(Right)* Lymph node involved by unicentric CD-PV. A follicle with small germinal center ⇾ and interfollicular plasmacytosis ⇾ are present.

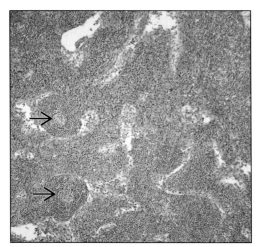
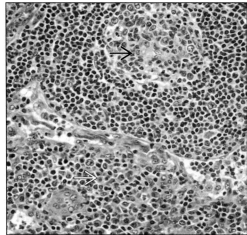

(Left) Lymph node involved by unicentric CD-PV. The plasma cells are cytologically bland without atypia. Rare plasma cells can be binucleated in CD-PV but were not found in this case. Vascular proliferation can also be appreciated in this field. *(Right)* Lymph node involved by unicentric PC-CD. Vasculature in the interfollicular areas ⇾ is prominent. A follicle with a small germinal center is also shown ⇾.

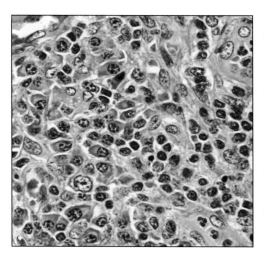
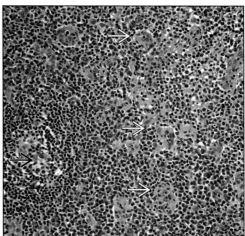

(Left) Lymph node involved by multicentric CD, plasma cell variant, HHV8(+), in an HIV-infected patient with AIDS. This field shows a follicle with hyaline-vascular changes: Prominent, fibrotic blood vessels and lymphocyte depletion. *(Right)* Lymph node involved by multicentric CD-PV, HHV8(+), in an HIV-infected patient. Note the large immunoblasts/plasmablasts ⇾ in this field and the blurring between germinal center and mantle zone.

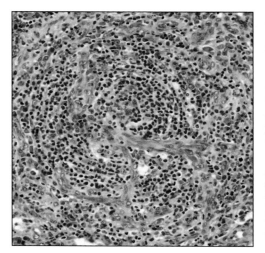
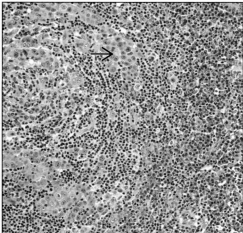

UNICENTRIC PLASMA CELL VARIANT CASTLEMAN DISEASE

Differential Diagnosis

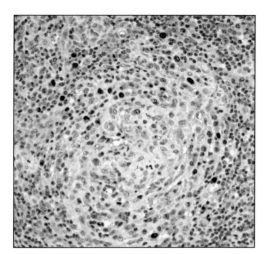 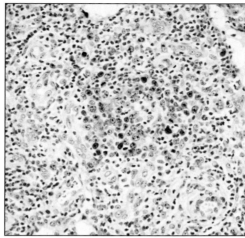

(Left) Lymph node from an HIV(+) patient with multicentric CD-PV. LANA1 antibody highlights plasmablasts in the mantle zone of a regressed lymphoid follicle. (Right) Lymph node involved by multicentric CD, PV, HHV8(+), in an HIV-infected patient with AIDS. LANA1 antibody highlights a cluster of plasmablasts consistent with a so-called microlymphoma. These plasmablasts usually express Igλ light chain.

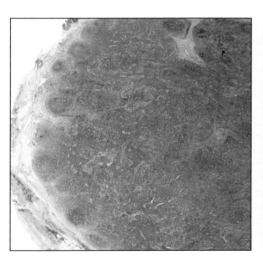 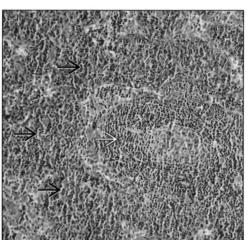

(Left) Lymph node in a patient with active rheumatoid arthritis and lymphadenopathy. Numerous mature plasma cells are present in the interfollicular areas resembling unicentric CD-PV, HHV8(-). (Right) Lymph node in a patient with active rheumatoid arthritis and lymphadenopathy. Numerous cytologically bland or mature plasma cells are present in interfollicular areas. ⊟ A follicle with a small germinal center is also present ➡.

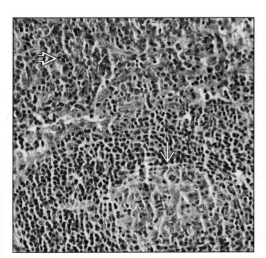 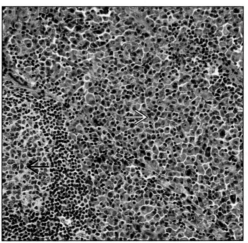

(Left) Lymph node in a patient with active rheumatoid arthritis and lymphadenopathy. This high-power view shows plasmacytosis ➡ and reactive follicle with atretic, regressed germinal center ➡. (Right) Lymph node involved by plasmacytoma. A residual germinal center ⊟ is present, surrounded by a small rim of mantle/marginal zone cells. The interfollicular area contains sheets of neoplastic plasma cells ➡.

MULTICENTRIC CASTLEMAN DISEASE

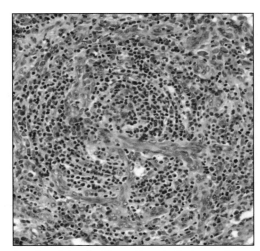

Lymph node involved by multicentric Castleman disease, HHV8(+) in an HIV(+) patient. Scattered hyaline-vascular follicles are present.

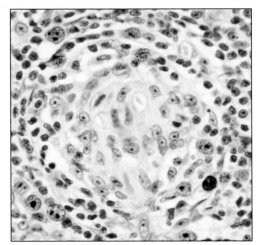

Lymph node involved by multicentric Castleman disease in an HIV(+) patient. Antibody specific for latency-associated nuclear antigen (LANA-1) of HHV8 shows positive immunoblasts within the mantle zone.

TERMINOLOGY

Abbreviations
- Multicentric Castleman disease (MCD)

Synonyms
- Angiofollicular lymph node hyperplasia
- Angiomatous lymphoid hamartoma
- Giant lymph node hyperplasia

Definitions
- Systemic lymphoproliferative disease that occurs in patients with immunodeficiency or immune dysregulation
  - Usually associated with human herpesvirus type 8 (HHV8) infection

ETIOLOGY/PATHOGENESIS

Infectious Agents
- HHV8
  - a.k.a. Kaposi sarcoma herpesvirus (KSHV)
  - γ-herpesvirus with estimated seroprevalence of 25% in USA
  - Virus load in peripheral blood mononuclear cells correlates with disease severity
  - HHV8 encodes for homolog of human interleukin-6 (IL-6)
  - Viral IL-6 stimulates human IL-6 induced cellular pathways
  - Human IL-6 is B-cell growth factor that regulates differentiation of B lymphocytes to plasma cells
    - Regulates T-cell function and induces C-reactive protein (CRP) production by hepatocytes
    - Endogenous pyrogen
  - B cells derived form MCD overexpress IL-6 receptor CD126
    - Cells within lymph nodes express high levels of IL-6

- This suggests paracrine and autocrine mechanisms involved in pathophysiology of MCD
- Immunodeficiency or immune dysregulation/ dysfunction
  - HIV infection
    - Most HIV(+) patients with MCD are HHV8(+)
  - Wiskott-Aldrich syndrome
  - Autoimmune diseases or phenomena
    - Associated with autoantibody-induced paraneoplastic pemphigus
    - Associated with myasthenia gravis
  - POEMS syndrome
    - **P**eripheral neuropathy, **o**rganomegaly, **e**ndocrinopathy, monoclonal **M** protein, **s**kin lesions
    - Serologic evidence of HHV8(+) in many patients
    - Poorly understood syndrome associated with immune dysregulation

CLINICAL ISSUES

Epidemiology
- Incidence
  - MCD occurs most often in HIV(+) patients with AIDS
    - Therefore, incidence correlates with that of AIDS
- Age
  - Broad age range
- Gender
  - More often in males (correlates with AIDS)

Presentation
- Lymphadenopathy is constant finding; any lymph node group can be involved
  - Peripheral, abdominal, or mediastinal lymphadenopathy
- B-type symptoms in over 95% of patients
  - Fever, night sweats, weight loss
- Splenomegaly in ~ 75%, hepatomegaly in ~ 50%

MULTICENTRIC CASTLEMAN DISEASE

Key Facts

Terminology
- Systemic lymphoproliferative disease occurs in patients with immunodeficiency or immune dysregulation and is usually associated with human herpesvirus type 8 (HHV8) infection

Etiology/Pathogenesis
- HHV8 (KSHV) infection important
  - Virus has pleiotropic effects, including encoding homolog of IL-6
- Immunodeficiency (e.g., HIV) plays important role
- POEMS syndrome is commonly associated with MCD

Clinical Issues
- Lymphadenopathy constant; any lymph node group
- B symptoms in over 95% of patients
- Splenomegaly in ~ 75%; hepatomegaly ~ 50%

- Patients with MCD have increased frequency of other neoplasms
  - Plasmablastic lymphoma, Kaposi sarcoma, primary effusion lymphoma

Microscopic Pathology
- Sheets of plasma cells in interfollicular zones
- Extensive vascular proliferation
- Blurring of boundary between mantle zone and interfollicular area
- HHV8(+) cells are usually localized in mantle zones of follicles
  - Plasmablasts or immunoblasts

Ancillary Tests
- LANA1 antibody recognizes HHV8(+) cells
- Monoclonal *Ig* gene rearrangements

- Edema, body cavity effusions, and skin rash in subset of patients
- Central nervous system abnormalities in small patient subset
- Higher risk for coexistent chronic infections
  - Epstein-Barr virus, hepatitis C, CMV

Laboratory Tests
- Abnormal serum findings
  - Elevated serum IL-6 levels during symptomatic episodes
  - Elevated erythrocyte sedimentation rate
  - Elevated lactate dehydrogenase (LDH) levels
  - Hypergammaglobulinemia
- Hematologic
  - Cytopenias
    - Anemia &/or thrombocytopenia

Treatment
- Chemotherapy and steroids have been used for patients with MCD
  - Not very effective for MCD patients who are HIV(+) or have POEMS syndrome

Prognosis
- Poor in patients with POEMS syndrome or HIV infection
  - Patients usually die within a few months of diagnosis

Frequently Associated Neoplasms
- Plasmablastic lymphoma (PBL)
  - HHV8(+) patients; often also EBV(+)
  - PBL usually involves lymph nodes and spleen; leukemia rare
  - Can affect HIV(-) patients in HHV8 endemic regions (Africa and Mediterranean countries)
- Kaposi sarcoma
  - More common in HIV(+) patients
- Primary effusion lymphoma (PEL)
  - Occurs in HHV8(+) patients
  - Usually coinfected with EBV

- Glomeruloid hemangioma
  - Distinctive skin tumor highly suggestive of POEMS syndrome
- Increased frequency of classical Hodgkin lymphoma (HL), diffuse large B-cell lymphoma, mantle cell lymphoma, and peripheral T-cell lymphoma
  - Mixed cellularity is most common type of classical HL

IMAGE FINDINGS

Radiographic Findings
- Lymphadenopathy and hepatosplenomegaly
- CT scan: Lesions enhance with IV contrast
- PET scan: ~ 50-60% of lesions have increased FDG uptake
- Radiographic findings are not specific
  - Biopsy required for diagnosis

MICROSCOPIC PATHOLOGY

Histologic Features
- Lymph nodes
  - Most MCD cases have features that fit best as plasma cell variant
  - Hyaline-vascular follicles are also usually present
    - Others in past have designated these cases as mixed or transitional type of CD
    - These changes are part of spectrum of plasma cell (PC) variant
- Sheets of polytypic plasma cells in interfollicular regions
- Extensive vascular proliferation
- Some features of HHV8(+) MCD differ from HHV8(-) plasma cell variant
  - Greater degree of lymphocyte depletion
    - Particularly in HIV(+) patients
  - Blurred border between mantle zones and surrounding interfollicular areas

RHEUMATOID ARTHRITIS-RELATED LYMPHADENOPATHY

Microscopic Features

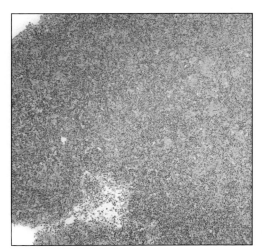

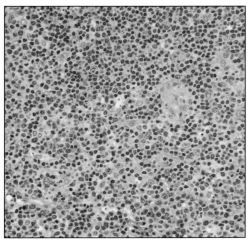

(Left) Diffuse lymphoplasmacytic infiltrate involving lymph node in a rheumatoid arthritis (RA) patient on immunosuppressive therapy. No lymphoid follicles can be appreciated in this field. *(Right)* Diffuse lymphoplasmacytic infiltrate involving lymph node in RA patient on immunosuppressive therapy. At this magnification, the heterogeneity of the cell population can be appreciated.

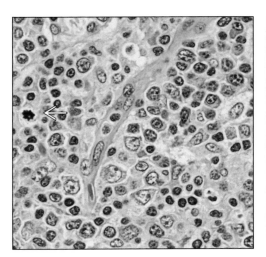

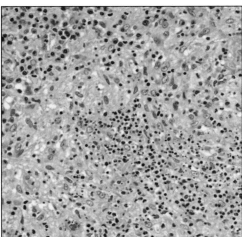

(Left) Diffuse lymphoplasmacytic infiltrate involving lymph node in RA patient on immunosuppressive therapy. This image shows various cell types, including plasma cells, small lymphocytes, and immunoblasts. A mitotic figure is also present ➡. *(Right)* Diffuse lymphoplasmacytic infiltrate involving lymph node in a RA patient on immunosuppressive therapy. A focus of necrosis with neutrophils is shown. Necrotic foci can occur in RA lymph nodes.

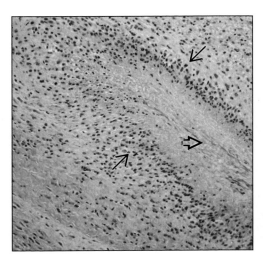

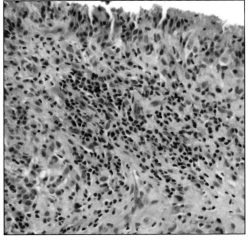

(Left) Patient with rheumatoid arthritis who underwent joint replacement. Synovial tissue from the joint shows a rheumatoid nodule. Note the central area of necrobiosis ⊅ surrounded by palisading histiocytes ➡. *(Right)* Patient with rheumatoid arthritis who underwent joint replacement. Synovial tissue from the joint shows a chronic inflammatory infiltrate composed of lymphocytes and plasma cells. Synovial lining is at the top of the field.

RHEUMATOID ARTHRITIS-RELATED LYMPHADENOPATHY

Microscopic Features

(Left) Lymphoplasmacytic infiltrate involving the lung in a patient with rheumatoid arthritis. The alveolar parenchyma is irregularly replaced by small lymphocytes in nodular aggregates (dark blue color) and plasma cells (purple color). *(Right)* Lymphoplasmacytic infiltrate involving the lung in a patient with rheumatoid arthritis. High magnification shows a mixture of small lymphocytes and plasma cells.

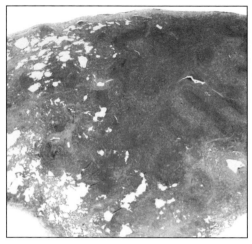
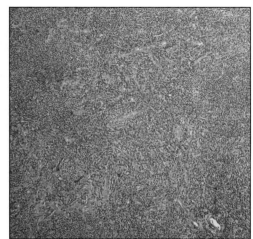

(Left) Lymphoplasmacytic infiltrate involving the lung in a patient with rheumatoid arthritis. Anti-CD20 antibody highlights collections of B cells consistent with primordial lymphoid follicles. *(Right)* Lymphoplasmacytic infiltrate involving the lung in a patient with rheumatoid arthritis. Anti-CD3 antibody highlights small T cells. B cells within lymphoid follicles ➡ are CD3(-).

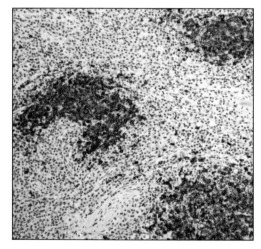
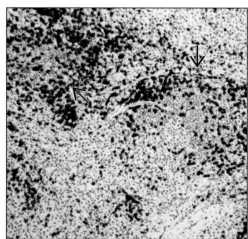

(Left) Lymphoplasmacytic infiltrate involving the lung in a patient with rheumatoid arthritis. Many plasma cells between follicles express cytoplasmic κ light chain. Follicles are negative. *(Right)* Lymphoplasmacytic infiltrate involving the lung in a patient with rheumatoid arthritis. Many plasma cells between follicles express cytoplasmic λ light chain. Follicles are negative.

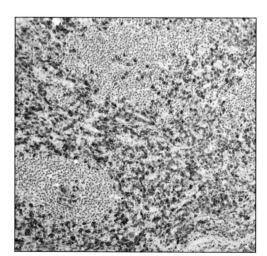
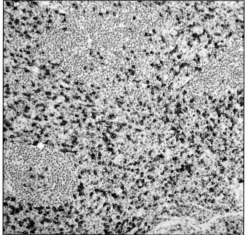

RHEUMATOID ARTHRITIS-RELATED LYMPHADENOPATHY

Differential Diagnosis

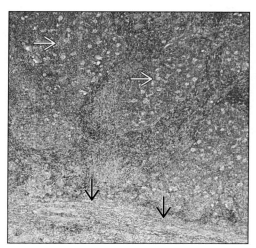

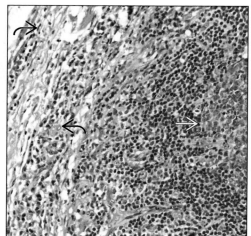

(Left) Syphilitic lymphadenopathy. This image shows marked follicular hyperplasia ➡ and capsular thickening by inflammation and fibrosis �””. *(Right)* Syphilitic lymphadenopathy. This field shows the edge of a hyperplastic follicle ➡ and lymph node capsule ➚ thickened by inflammation and fibrosis.

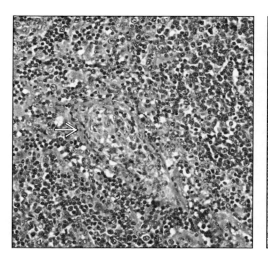

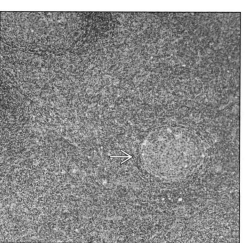

(Left) Syphilitic lymphadenopathy. A blood vessel ➡ is surrounded and infiltrated by inflammatory cells, evidence of vasculitis. Small lymphocytes and plasma cells are also numerous in this field. *(Right)* Unicentric Castleman disease, plasma cell variant, HHV8(-), involving lymph node. A small, lymphocyte-depleted follicle ➡ is surrounded by sheets of mature plasma cells.

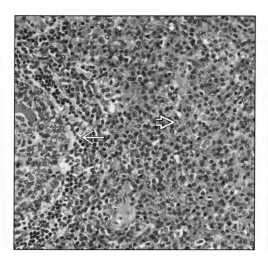

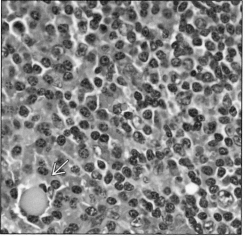

(Left) Unicentric Castleman disease, plasma cell variant, HHV8(-), involving lymph node. A lymphoid follicle ➡ and sheets of mature plasma cells ➡ are shown. *(Right)* Unicentric Castleman disease, plasma cell variant, HHV8(-), involving lymph node. This high magnification shows numerous plasma cells without atypia. A plasma cell filled with immunoglobulin, known as a Russell body, is shown ➡.

SARCOID LYMPHADENOPATHY

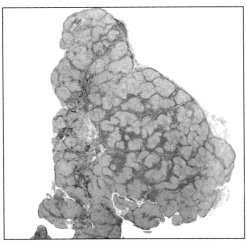

The lymph node parenchyma is substantially effaced by multiple granulomas.

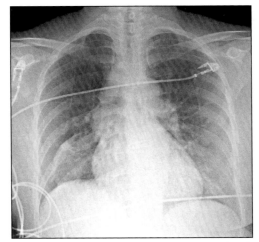

Chest radiograph shows bilateral enlarged hilar lymph nodes. Fine linear and reticular opacities are present in the perihilar lung parenchyma.

TERMINOLOGY

Definitions
- Multisystemic granulomatous disease of unknown etiology
- Diagnosis of exclusion

ETIOLOGY/PATHOGENESIS

Exact Etiology and Pathogenesis Unknown
- Occupational and environmental exposure
  - Inorganic particles, insecticides, and moldy environments
- Probable role of genetics as shown by assessment of major histocompatibility complex
  - Positive association with HLA-A1, -B8, and -DR3
  - Negative association with HLA-B12 and -DR4
- Possible role of infectious agents
  - *Mycobacterium tuberculosis*
  - *Propionibacterium acnes*
- T-cell abnormalities
  - Increased CD4(+) T cells and CD4(+) and CD25(+) regulatory T- cells
  - Decreased CD1d-restricted natural killer cells
  - Oligoclonal TCR-αβ T-cell repertoire
- Cytokines: Increased interferon-γ and interleukin-2

CLINICAL ISSUES

Epidemiology
- Incidence
  - 10-20 per 100,000 population
- Age
  - All ages; peak 20-39 years
- Gender
  - Female preponderance
- Ethnicity

- Lifetime risk in USA is 2.4% in African-Americans and 0.85% in Caucasians
- More likely to be chronic and fatal in African-Americans

Presentation
- Constitutional symptoms are common
  - Fatigue, malaise, fever, night sweats, and weight loss
- Symptoms related to organ involvement
  - Lungs: Dyspnea and cough
  - Heart: Loss of ventricular function and sudden death
  - Eyes: Keratoconjunctivitis, uveitis, retinal vasculitis
  - Skin: Maculopapular eruptions, nodules, plaque-like lesions
  - Erythema nodosum
    - Painful, red, subcutaneous lesions on anterior surface of legs
    - Associated with sarcoidosis but not specific
  - Musculoskeletal: Arthritis
  - Kidneys and electrolytes: Abnormal calcium metabolism
    - Extrarenal production of calcitriol by activated macrophages
  - Nervous system: Central and peripheral nervous system can be affected
    - Hypothalamic hypopituitarism
    - Diabetes insipidus
    - Lymphocytic meningitis
  - Other organs: Symptoms directly related to organ involvement
    - Endocrine system, reproductive system, gastrointestinal tract
- Lofgren syndrome: Occurs in subset of patients
  - Erythema nodosum, hilar lymphadenopathy, migratory polyarthralgias, and fever
- In approximately 50% of cases, patients are asymptomatic when 1st diagnosed
  - Incidental detection by radiographic studies
  - Most children are asymptomatic

SARCOID LYMPHADENOPATHY

Microscopic Features and Differential Diagnosis

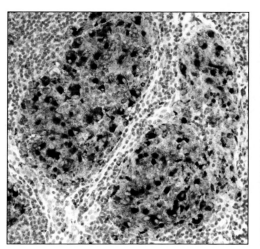

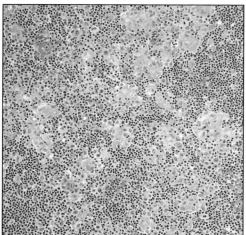

(Left) In sarcoidosis, the epithelioid histiocytes are strongly CD68 positive. *(Right)* A case of classical Hodgkin lymphoma with numerous epithelioid granulomas. At this low-power magnification, the histologic appearance, in part, resembles sarcoidosis.

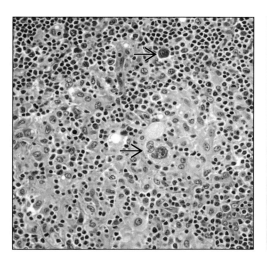

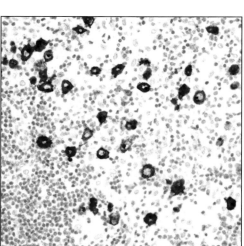

(Left) Classical Hodgkin lymphoma. At high-power magnification, large atypical cells with cherry-red nucleoli can be seen, consistent with HRS cells ➡. Many eosinophils are also present. *(Right)* Classical Hodgkin lymphoma. The HRS cells are positive for CD30. Small lymphocytes and histiocytes are negative.

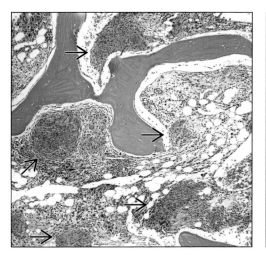

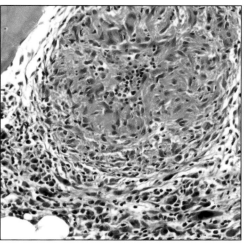

(Left) A case of plasma cell myeloma associated with sarcoid-like granulomas ➡ in the bone marrow is illustrated. Atypical plasma cells involve the bone marrow between the granulomas. *(Right)* Plasma cell myeloma. The granuloma in this field contains histiocytes, Langhans giant cells, and small lymphocytes that closely resemble sarcoidosis granuloma. Atypical plasma cells are also present (bottom of field).

DERMATOPATHIC LYMPHADENOPATHY

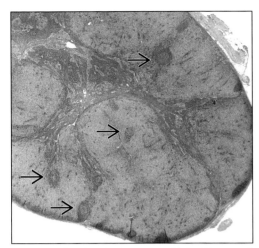

Dermatopathic lymphadenopathy (DLA). The overall architecture is maintained, but the paracortical zones are markedly expanded. Lymphoid follicles are compressed and atrophic ➡.

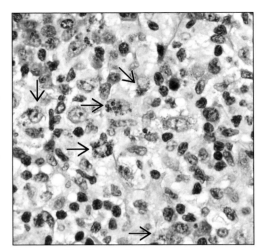

Dermatopathic lymphadenopathy. The expanded paracortical zones are composed of macrophages containing melanin pigment ➡, Langerhans cells, interdigitating dendritic cells, and reactive T cells.

TERMINOLOGY

Abbreviations
- Dermatopathic lymphadenopathy (DLA)

Synonyms
- Dermatopathic lymphadenitis
- Lipomelanosis reticularis of Pautrier

Definitions
- Reactive lymphadenopathy characterized by paracortical hyperplasia composed of
  o Interdigitating dendritic cells (IDCs), Langerhans cells (LCs), and macrophages containing melanin

ETIOLOGY/PATHOGENESIS

Disease Associations
- Usually associated with chronic skin disease
  o Benign or malignant

T-cell Response to Skin Antigen Processing
- Skin antigens processed and presented by LCs and IDCs
- LCs are specialized dendritic cells that reside in skin
  o Upon activation, LCs migrate to lymph node
- IDCs are specialized dendritic cells that reside in lymph node paracortex
  o IDCs may be derived from LC
- Both LCs and IDCs are derived from bone marrow precursor cells

CLINICAL ISSUES

Epidemiology
- Age
  o All ages, but often middle-aged to elderly patients
- Gender
  o Males affected more frequently

- Ethnicity
  o No preference

Presentation
- Lymphadenopathy; usually superficial
  o Most often axillary or inguinal lymph nodes
  o Generalized lymphadenopathy is less common
- May occur in association with any chronic inflammatory skin disorder
  o Usually generalized dermatitis, especially exfoliative and eczematoid dermatitis
    ▪ Toxic shock syndrome, pemphigus, psoriasis, neurodermatitis, eczema, atrophia senilis
  o Skin conditions may precede lymphadenopathy by months to years
  o Mild to moderate dermatopathic changes also can occur in patients without skin disease
    ▪ ~ 10% of patients do not have skin disease
- DLA often associated with mycosis fungoides (MF) or Sézary syndrome (SS)
  o ~ 75% of patients with MF/SS present with lymphadenopathy
    ▪ DLA, involvement by MF/SS, or both

Laboratory Tests
- Increased erythrocyte sedimentation rate
- Hypereosinophilia
- Autoimmune antibodies can be detected in some patients, related to skin conditions

Treatment
- No current guidelines exist on appropriate management of patients with DLA
  o Benign DLA requires no specific therapy
  o If DLA is associated with lymphoma, appropriate diagnosis and staging of lymphoma is needed
    ▪ Therapy is directed at lymphoma

DERMATOPATHIC LYMPHADENOPATHY

Key Facts

Terminology
- Paracortical hyperplasia characterized by
  - Interdigitating dendritic cells (IDCs), Langerhans cells (LCs), and macrophages
  - Melanin pigment (variable)
- Usually associated with skin disorders
  - Exfoliative or eczematoid dermatitis

Etiology/Pathogenesis
- T-cell response to skin antigens processed and presented by IDCs and LCs

Clinical Issues
- Prognosis is related to underlying skin disease or other associated systemic diseases
  - Specific therapy is not required for DLA

Ancillary Tests
- Immunohistochemistry
  - IDCs and LCs are S100(+)
  - Only LCs are CD1a(+) and langerin/CD207(+)
  - Macrophages are CD68(+); T-cells are CD3(+)
- Electron microscopy
  - Birbeck granules only in LCs
- Flow cytometry immunophenotyping and gene rearrangement analysis
  - Useful to exclude T-cell clone and early involvement by MF/SS

Top Differential Diagnoses
- Langerhans cell histiocytosis
- Classical Hodgkin lymphoma
- Mycosis fungoides/Sézary syndrome

Prognosis
- In benign DLA, related to underlying skin or systemic disease

MACROSCOPIC FEATURES

General Features
- Lymph node is enlarged
- Cut surface is bulging, pale yellow
- In some extreme cases, black peripheral lines can be observed due to clumps of melanin pigment

MICROSCOPIC PATHOLOGY

Histologic Features
- Continuum exists between early changes & fully developed DLA
  - Early stage/mild
    - Accumulation of IDCs, LCs, and macrophages in paracortical zones
    - Subset of macrophages contain melanin pigment
    - Follicular hyperplasia
    - Lymph node architecture generally preserved
  - Middle stage/moderate
    - Continuous expansion of paracortical zones by IDCs, LCs, and macrophages
    - Lymphoid follicles are compressed, become atrophic
  - Later stage/severe
    - Nodular or confluent expansion of paracortical zones with further accumulation of IDCs, LCs, and macrophages
    - Relative depletion of small lymphocytes
    - Atrophic/compressed follicles
    - Plasmacytosis in medullary cords can be prominent
    - Plasma cells, eosinophils, and immunoblasts can be prominent
- Vascular proliferation is often mild

- Difficult to distinguish DLA from DLA with early involvement by MF/SS using histologic criteria
  - Lymph node involvement by MF/SS can be subtle
  - Small, cerebriform lymphocytes can be seen in DLA associated with either MF/SS or benign skin diseases

Cytologic Features
- Clusters of IDCs and LCs are present in paracortex
  - IDCs and LCs are morphologically indistinguishable by light microscopy
    - Elongated convoluted nuclei with lineage grooves ("twisted towel" appearance)
    - Pale or eosinophilic cytoplasm and pseudonucleoli
- Macrophages with variable pigment
  - Mostly melanin but hemosiderin also can be present
  - Histiocytes can have cytoplasmic lipid droplets
- Absent or rare tingible body macrophages

ANCILLARY TESTS

Immunohistochemistry
- IDCs, LCs, and subset of macrophages are S100(+)
- Only LCs are CD1a(+) and langerin/CD207(+)
- IDCs and LCs are CD4([+] weak), CD68([+] variable), and IDCs can express fascin
- LCs can show variable lysozyme(+)
- IDCs and LCs are CD21(-), CD35(-), CD123(-), CD163(-), and TCL1(+)
- Macrophages are CD68(+)
- Small lymphocytes express T-cell antigens
- Immunoblasts are CD30(+)
- If involvement by MF/SS is suspected, assessment for CD3, CD4, CD7, and CD8 can be helpful
  - T-cell markers will highlight MF/SS cells and may show aberrant immunophenotype

Molecular Genetics
- Assessment for T-cell receptor (*TCR*) gene rearrangements can be helpful if MF/SS suspected
  - No monoclonal *TCR* rearrangements excludes MF/SS

DERMATOPATHIC LYMPHADENOPATHY

o *TCR* gene rearrangement analysis more sensitive than morphology to detect MF/SS
o No evidence of monoclonal *Ig* rearrangements

Electron Microscopy
- Birbeck granules are present in cytoplasm of LCs but not IDCs
- Both LCs and IDCs have irregular nuclear contours and finger-like cytoplasmic projections

Cytochemistry
- Fontana silver: Melanin
- Prussian blue: Hemosiderin
- Oil red O: Lipid

DIFFERENTIAL DIAGNOSIS

Langerhans Cell Histiocytosis (LCH)
- Early involvement by LCH tends to be sinusoidal
- Partial or total effacement of lymph node with more extensive involvement by LCH
- LCs often associated with eosinophils &/or necrosis
- LCs are CD1a(+), langerin/CD207(+), and S100(+)
- Electron microscopy shows Birbeck granules
- Patients with LCH can have visceral involvement (unlike patients with DLA)

Classical Hodgkin Lymphoma
- The interfollicular pattern is especially problematic
- HRS cells are always present
- The HRS cells are typically CD15(+/-), CD30(+), pax-5 (+ dim), CD20(-/+), CD45/LCA(-)

Mycosis Fungoides/Sézary Syndrome
- Early lymph node involvement is especially problematic
- Small, cerebriform lymphocytes may not be appreciable
- Flow cytometry immunophenotyping is often more sensitive
  o Altered expression of CD2, CD3, CD4, CD5, or CD7
  o Decreased or absent CD26 expression
  o *TCR* Vβ clonality analysis is helpful
    ▪ Presence of clone supports MF/SS
- *TCR* gene rearrangement analysis is helpful to identify minimal/early MF/SS
  o Identification of monoclonal *TCR* gene rearrangement
    ▪ Supports involvement by MF/SS
    ▪ Correlates with poorer prognosis

Monocytic Leukemia/Sarcoma
- Paracortical expansion by leukemic cells with preservation of follicles
- Blasts/immature monocytes are of medium to large size with delicate nuclear membranes and distinct cytoplasmic borders
- CD34(+/-), CD43(+), CD68(+), CD117(+), lysozyme(+), MPO usually (-)
- Patients usually have bone marrow and systemic disease (unlike DLA)

Metastatic Malignant Melanoma
- In florid cases of DLA, melanin pigment and S100(+) may suggest possibility of melanoma
- DLA lacks nuclear atypia and mitotic rate of metastatic melanoma

Lymph Nodes with Other Pigments
- Drainage from tattoo; black pigment
- Hemosiderosis following blood transfusions
- Drainage after local trauma or surgery; hemosiderin
- Anthracotic pigment
- In most cases, IDCs and LCs are not markedly increased
- Dermatitis is not present

DIAGNOSTIC CHECKLIST

Clinically Relevant Pathologic Features
- Often associated with skin disorders
  o Especially generalized and exfoliative dermatitis

Pathologic Interpretation Pearls
- Grossly enlarged lymph nodes; sometimes pigmented
- Paracortical hyperplasia with
  o IDCs, LCs, and macrophages containing melanin pigment and lipid vacuoles
- Histologic features of DLA do not exclude early involvement by MF/SS
- Ancillary testing for clonality assessment can be helpful
  o Flow cytometry immunophenotyping
  o *TCR* gene rearrangement analysis

SELECTED REFERENCES

1. Edelweiss M et al: Lymph node involvement by Langerhans cell histiocytosis: a clinicopathologic and immunohistochemical study of 20 cases. Hum Pathol. 38(10):1463-9, 2007
2. Winter LK et al: Dermatopathic lymphadenitis of the head and neck. J Cutan Pathol. 34(2):195-7, 2007
3. Assaf C et al: Early TCR-beta and TCR-gamma PCR detection of T-cell clonality indicates minimal tumor disease in lymph nodes of cutaneous T-cell lymphoma: diagnostic and prognostic implications. Blood. 105(2):503-10, 2005
4. Iyer VK et al: Fine needle aspiration cytology of dermatopathic lymphadenitis. Acta Cytol. 42(6):1347-51, 1998
5. Kern DE et al: Analysis of T-cell receptor gene rearrangement in lymph nodes of patients with mycosis fungoides. Prognostic implications. Arch Dermatol. 134(2):158-64, 1998
6. Gould E et al: Dermatopathic lymphadenitis. The spectrum and significance of its morphologic features. Arch Pathol Lab Med. 112(11):1145-50, 1988

DERMATOPATHIC LYMPHADENOPATHY

Microscopic Features

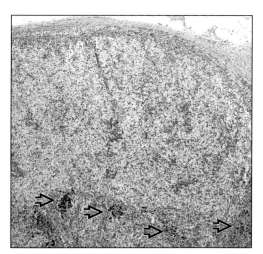

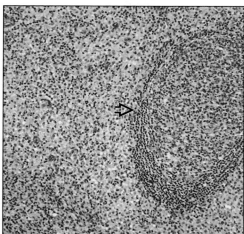

(Left) In some cases of dermatopathic lymphadenopathy, macrophages containing melanin pigment are prominent and form clusters ⇗ that can be visible grossly. *(Right)* Hyperplastic follicles ⇗ are often seen in cases of dermatopathic lymphadenopathy in which there is mild/early or a moderate degree of involvement.

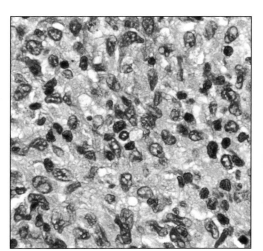

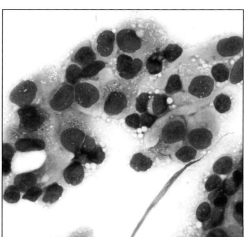

(Left) Dermatopathic lymphadenopathy. Both Langerhans cells (LCs) and interdigitating dendritic cells (IDCs) have elongated nuclei, some with nuclear grooves and vesicular chromatin. LCs and IDCs are morphologically indistinguishable by light microscopy. *(Right)* Touch imprint of a case of DLA. Numerous Langerhans cells, interdigitating dendritic cells, macrophages, and small lymphocytes are present in this field. A subset of macrophages contain cytoplasmic lipids.

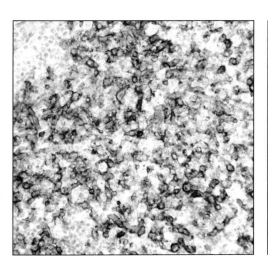

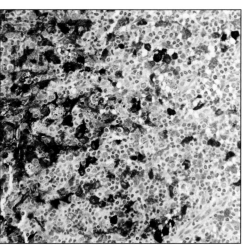

(Left) CD1a immunostain highlights numerous Langerhans cells in a case of advanced DLA. Interdigitating dendritic cells and macrophages are negative for CD1a. *(Right)* S100 immunostain highlights Langerhans cells, interdigitating dendritic cells, and a subset of macrophages. This is a case with a moderate degree of DLA.

DERMATOPATHIC LYMPHADENOPATHY

Microscopic Features and Differential Diagnosis

(Left) CD68 immunostain brightly highlights macrophages in DLA. Langerhans cells and interdigitating dendritic cells are weakly positive or negative for CD68. *(Right)* Langerhans cell histiocytosis (LCH). In contrast to DLA, Langerhans cells in LCH have abundant acidophilic cytoplasm and often are accompanied by numerous eosinophils or necrosis (not shown).

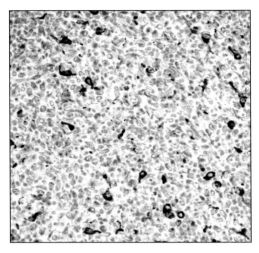
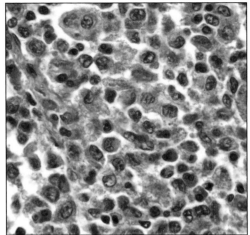

(Left) Skin biopsy of mycosis fungoides (MF) shows parakeratosis and an epidermal infiltrate of atypical cerebriform lymphocytes. The presence of collections of atypical lymphoid cells in the epidermis (Pautrier microabscesses) is a highly characteristic feature of MF ⊳. *(Right)* CD3 immunostain highlights numerous intra-epidermal and dermal T cells in a case of mycosis fungoides.

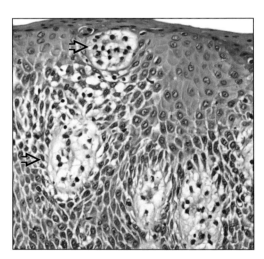
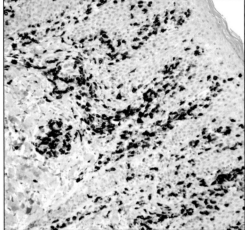

(Left) Lymph node biopsy specimen obtained from a patient with mycosis fungoides shows changes histologically consistent with dermatopathic lymphadenopathy. *(Right)* In addition to the changes of dermatopathic lymphadenopathy in this lymph node, small clusters of atypical, cerebriform lymphocytes are also present, suggestive of mycosis fungoides cells ➚.

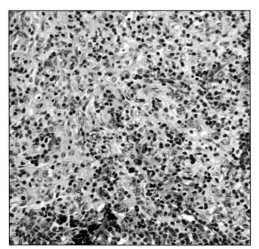
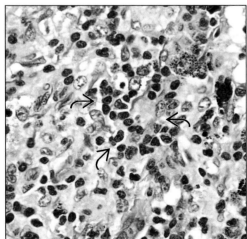

DERMATOPATHIC LYMPHADENOPATHY

Flow Cytometry of Lymph Node Involvement by MF

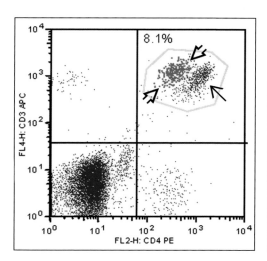

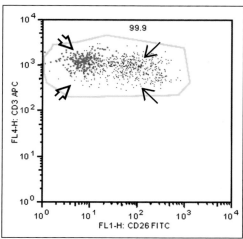

(Left) Flow cytometry immunophenotyping of lymph node fine needle aspiration (FNA) specimen with early involvement by mycosis fungoides. CD4:CD8 ratio is increased. A subset of CD4(+) T cells show dimmer expression of CD4 ⧐ (red), in contrast with normal CD4(+) T cells ⧐ (blue). *(Right)* FNA of lymph node involved by MF. Dim CD4(+) T cells show complete loss of CD26 ⧐ (red) expression, while the normal CD4 T cells show normal expression of CD26 ⧐ (blue).

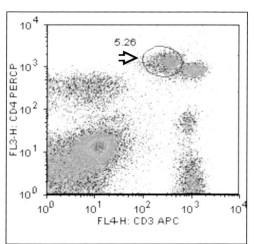

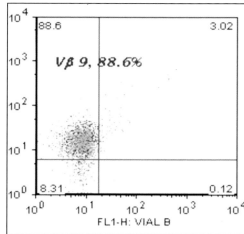

(Left) Flow cytometry immunophenotyping of a lymph node FNA specimen with early involvement by mycosis fungoides reveals an aberrant T-cell population that is CD3 (dim +) and CD4 (bright +) ⧐. *(Right)* Lymph node FNA specimen involved by mycosis fungoides. Flow cytometric Vβ analysis: CD4 (dim) and CD3 (bright +) T cells are preferentially expressing Vβ 9 (in 88.6% cells), indicative of T-cell clonality.

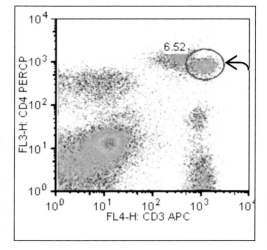

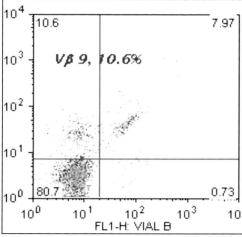

(Left) Lymph node FNA specimen involved by mycosis fungoides. Flow cytometry immunophenotyping of the same case shows that normal T cells with a normal expression of CD3 and CD4 ⧐ are also present. *(Right)* Lymph node FNA specimen involved by mycosis fungoides. Flow cytometry Vβ analysis shows that the normal T cells are polyclonal.

HEMOPHAGOCYTIC LYMPHOHISTIOCYTOSIS

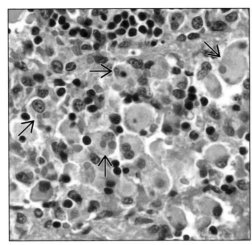

Hemophagocytic lymphohistiocytosis (HLH). The lymph node sinus is expanded by numerous mature histiocytes/ macrophages, some exhibiting phagocytosis of mostly erythrocytes in this field ⇥.

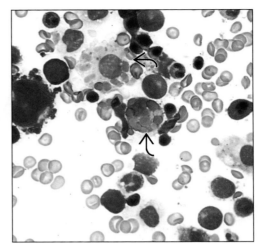

HLH in bone marrow aspirate smear (Wright-Giemsa stain). Histiocytes ⇥ show erythrophagocytosis. This patient presented with fever and pancytopenia prompting bone marrow examination.

TERMINOLOGY

Abbreviations
- Hemophagocytic lymphohistiocytosis (HLH)

Synonyms
- Hemophagocytic syndrome
- Erythrophagocytic lymphohistiocytosis
- Viral-associated hemophagocytic syndrome

Definitions
- Cytokine dysfunction, either due to inherited or secondary causes
  - Results in overwhelming activation of normal T lymphocytes and macrophages
    - Leads to systemic symptoms and organ damage

ETIOLOGY/PATHOGENESIS

Inherited vs. Secondary/Acquired Defects
- **Inherited genetic defects**
  - Result in depressed natural killer (NK) and cytotoxic T-cell activity
  - Perforin (*PRF1*) mutation
    - Localized at 10q21-22
    - Results in decrease or absence of perforin in NK or CD8(+) T cells
  - Griscelli syndrome-*MUNC13-4* defect
    - Lack of protein rab27a which controls secretion of lytic granules in NK and cytotoxic T cells
  - Chediak-Higashi syndrome-*LYST* gene defect
    - Cytotoxic T-lymphocyte-associated antigen 4 (CTLA-4) is involved
    - Failure to move CTLA-4 from secretory lysozymes to cell membrane
  - Syntaxin gene mutations
    - NK cells fail to degranulate when encountering susceptible targets
  - X-linked lymphoproliferative disease (XLP)
    - *SH2D1A* gene mutation
    - Defect in T-cell signal transduction
    - T-cell lytic defect against EBV infected B-lymphocytes
    - Trigger vigorous cytotoxic cellular responses
    - a.k.a. Duncan syndrome
  - Defect in apoptosis-caspase 3
    - Accumulation of T cells
- **Acquired/secondary defects**
  - It is not clear how NK and T-cell function is impaired
  - Many infectious agents are reported to be associated with HLH
  - Viruses
    - Epstein-Barr virus is most common, cytomegalovirus, parvovirus B19, herpes simplex
    - Herpes varicella-zoster, measles, human herpes virus 8, human immunodeficiency virus (HIV)
    - Adenovirus, respiratory syncytial virus, parainfluenza virus, enteroviruses
  - Bacteria
    - *Pseudomonas aeruginosa*, staphylococci, streptococci
    - *Escherichia coli* and *Brucella abortus*
    - Mycobacteria: *Mycobacterium tuberculosis*
  - Parasites: *Leishmania donovani*; *Plasmodium* species
  - Fungal infections
    - *Histoplasma capsulatum*, *Penicillium marneffei*; aspergillosis
    - Cryptococcal meningitis, histoplasmosis, and disseminated *Trichosporon beigelii*
  - Autoimmune disorders have been reported associated with HLH
    - Systemic lupus erythematosus, rheumatoid arthritis
    - Still disease, polyarteritis nodosa
    - Mixed connective tissue disease, systemic sclerosis, Sjögren syndrome
  - Malignancies associated with HLH

HEMOPHAGOCYTIC LYMPHOHISTIOCYTOSIS

Key Facts

Terminology

- Cytokine dysfunction, resulting in activation of T lymphocytes and macrophages
  - Leads to systemic symptoms and organ damage

Etiology/Pathogenesis

- Inherited genetic or acquired defect
  - Leads to depressed NK- &/or cytotoxic T-cell activity

Microscopic Pathology

- In lymph nodes
  - Sinuses are infiltrated by bland histiocytes showing phagocytic activity
  - Underlying etiology may coexist in same lymph node

Top Differential Diagnoses

- Rosai-Dorfman disease
- Histiocytic sarcoma
- Langerhans cell histiocytosis

Diagnostic Checklist

- Clinical and laboratory criteria (5 out of 8 criteria)
  - Fever
  - Splenomegaly
  - Cytopenias
  - Hypertriglyceridemia &/or hypofibrinogenemia
  - Serum ferritin > 500 μg/L
  - Hemophagocytosis
  - Low or absent NK-cell activity
  - Soluble CD25 (sIL-2 receptor) > 2,400 U/mL
- HLH diagnosed by molecular testing

- ▪ T- and NK-cell lymphomas
- ▪ Acute myeloid leukemias and myelodysplastic syndromes
- ▪ Acute lymphoblastic leukemia/lymphoma (B or T cell)
- ▪ B-cell lymphomas
- ▪ Carcinomas
- Other diseases associated with HLH
  - ▪ Post-transplantation
  - ▪ Pulmonary sarcoidosis

Common Etiologies of Inherited & Secondary/Acquired HLH

- Inappropriate immune reaction caused by
  - Proliferation &/or activation of T cells either due to genetic defects or secondary causes
  - Production of large quantities of cytokines including
    - ▪ Interferon-γ, TNF-α, and granulocyte-macrophage colony-stimulating factor
    - ▪ Interleukin-1 (IL-1) and interleukin-6 (IL-6)
    - ▪ Associated with macrophage activation
    - ▪ Inadequate apoptosis of immunogenic cells
  - Lead to tissue damage and injury

CLINICAL ISSUES

Epidemiology

- Incidence
  - 1.2 children per million per year
    - ▪ 1 case per every 50,000 births
  - Incidence in adults is unknown
- Age
  - Familial form frequently affects infants
    - ▪ Birth to age 18 months most common (70-80%)
    - ▪ Rare familial cases can affect adolescents and adults
  - Acquired form can occur at any age
- Gender
  - M = F
- Ethnicity
  - No predilection for any race

Presentation

- Fever
  - 7 or more days of fever as high as 38.5°C (101.3°F)
- Easy bruisability and pallor related to cytopenia(s) or coagulopathy
- Splenomegaly
  - Spleen palpable > 3 cm below costal margin
- Central nervous system symptoms
  - Seizures, ataxia, hemiplegia, mental status changes, irritability
- Skin rash
  - Scaly and waxy lesions; rashes on scalp and behind ear
- Lymphadenopathy
- Hepatomegaly, jaundice
- Pleural effusion
- Ascites

Laboratory Tests

- Cytopenia(s), often pancytopenia
  - Hemoglobin < 9.0 g/dL
  - Platelets < 100,000/μL
  - Absolute neutrophil count < 1,000/μL
- Hypofibrinogenemia
  - Fibrinogen < 1.5 g/L, or > 3 standard deviations (SD) below normal value for age
- Hypertriglyceridemia
  - Fasting triglycerides ≥ 2.0 mmol/L, or > 3 SD above normal value for age
- Increased serum ferritin
  - > 500 μg/L
  - Glycosylated ferritin < 20% of total ferritin
  - Levels parallel to course of disease
    - ▪ Can use to monitor disease activity
  - 80% specific for diagnosis of HLH
- Abnormal liver function
  - Hyperbilirubinemia
  - Hypoalbuminemia
  - Increased aspartate aminotransferase (AST) and alanine aminotransferase (ALT) levels
- Serum lactate dehydrogenase (LDH) increased

HEMOPHAGOCYTIC LYMPHOHISTIOCYTOSIS

- Defect in NK-cell activity; adequate NK-cell number
  - Decreased cytotoxic activity
    - Using peripheral blood mononuclear cells as effector cells and fluorescein isothiocyanate-labeled K562 cells as target cells
    - Measure by flow cytometry
  - Can differentiate between the HLH subtypes
- Increased concentrations of circulating soluble interleukin receptor (sIL-2R)
- Molecular diagnosis
  - Gene mutation analysis

Treatment

- HLH-2004 protocol recommended by Histiocytosis Association of America
  - 8-week period with dexamethasone, etoposide, and cyclosporine
    - Resolved nonfamilial HLH does not require continuation of therapeutic regimen
    - Children with persistent nonfamilial disease or familial disease continue therapy with cyclosporine, plus etoposide and dexamethasone pulses, until stem cell transplant
  - Intrathecal methotrexate is used for persistently abnormal CSF or progressive neurologic symptoms
- Stem cell transplantation for patients with
  - Familial HLH
  - Children and adults with persistent nonfamilial disease

Prognosis

- With HLH-2004 protocol
  - 3-year probability of survival was 51% for verified familial cases
  - 55% for entire group of HLH patients
- Stem cell transplant
  - Matched transplant: Long-term disease-free rate about 70%

Special Form of HLH-Macrophage Activation Syndrome

- Occurs in children and adults with autoimmune diseases, especially
  - Systemic onset juvenile rheumatoid arthritis
  - Adult-onset Still disease
  - Lupus erythematosus
- Clinical and laboratory features
  - Share many characteristics with HLH
    - Defective NK-cell function and low perforin expression
    - Clinical signs and symptoms similar to HLH
    - Hemophagocytosis is present in bone marrow, spleen, lymph node
    - High ferritin levels
  - Features that differ from HLH
    - Less severe cytopenias
    - More severe cardiac impairment
    - More pronounced coagulopathy
    - Very high C-reactive protein level
- Therapy
  - Cyclosporine and steroids
  - If does not work, use HLH-2004 protocol

IMAGE FINDINGS

General Features

- No specific imaging patterns are diagnostic of HLH
- CT or ultrasonography findings
  - Ascites, pleural effusion
  - Gallbladder wall thickening
  - Lymphadenopathy
- MR for CNS involvement

MICROSCOPIC PATHOLOGY

Histologic Features

- Proliferation of small mature histiocytes
  - Histiocytes show phagocytic activities
  - Tissue infiltrate and cellular injury
  - Increased lymphocytes; mostly T cells

Cytologic Features

- Histiocytes are mature and cytologically benign
  - Have vesicular nuclei and abundant cytoplasm
- Histiocytes engulf
  - Erythrocytes (nucleated and anucleated)
  - Platelets
  - Occasionally lymphocytes and neutrophils

Lymph Nodes

- Overall architecture is maintained
  - Foci of hemorrhage are common
  - Focal necrosis may be present
- Sinuses are infiltrated by bland histiocytes containing erythrocytes and occasionally lymphocytes and neutrophils
  - Mainly erythrophagocytosis (anucleated red blood cells)
- Evidence of hemophagocytosis may be less pronounced in lymph node, compared to bone marrow or spleen
- Underlying etiology of HLH may be present in lymph node
  - Lymphoma
    - Mainly of T-cell or NK-cell lymphomas
    - Rarely associated with B-cell lymphoma
  - Infections
    - HLH associated with EBV or CMV; lymph node may show changes of infectious mononucleosis
    - HLH in HIV; changes of HIV lymphadenopathy may occur
    - HLH of bacteria infection, may show changes of bacteria lymphadenitis
    - Fungal infection may show changes of fungal lymphadenitis
    - Mycobacterial infection may show changes of granulomatous lymphadenitis
- Immunohistochemistry
  - Histiocytes are CD68(+), S100(+/-), and CD1a(-)
  - Lymphocytes have normal immunophenotype

Bone Marrow

- Increased histiocytes
  - Many are phagocytes, better appreciated on aspirate smears or touch imprints

HEMOPHAGOCYTIC LYMPHOHISTIOCYTOSIS

■ Engulfing anucleated red cells, nucleated red cells, platelets, neutrophils
  ○ In some cases, histiocytes can exhibit slightly immature morphology and increased Ki-67 activity
- Increased mature-appearing T cells
- Hematopoietic cells, especially erythrocytes, can show dysplastic features associated with acute bone marrow injury
  ○ Should not be interpreted as myelodysplasia

Spleen
- Splenomegaly
- Expanded red pulp, filled with mature histiocytes
  ○ Many are phagocytes
- Focal necrosis can be present
- White pulp is usually spared
- Underlying etiology of HLH can be present in spleen
- Extramedullary hematopoiesis can be present

Liver
- Portal lymphohistiocytic infiltrates
- Hyperplasia of Kupffer cells with hemophagocytosis
- Hepatocyte injury

Skin Involvement
- Occurs in ~ 10-60% of patients
- Erythematous macules and plaques
- Increased T cells and histiocytes
- Often nondiagnostic and only rarely shows hemophagocytosis
- Rule out subcutaneous panniculitis-like T-cell lymphoma, which is often associated with HLH

Brain
- Meningeal lymphohistiocytic infiltration
- Focal subarachnoid hemorrhage

DIFFERENTIAL DIAGNOSIS

Rosai-Dorfman Disease (Sinus Histiocytosis with Massive Lymphadenopathy)
- Lymph nodes or extranodal sites
- Patients can present with
  ○ Fever, leukocytosis, anemia
  ○ Elevated sedimentation rate, polyclonal hypergammaglobulinemia
- Histiocytes are S100(+), CD68(+), CD1a(-)
- Lymph nodes
  ○ Marked dilation of sinuses filled with large histiocytes
  ○ Histiocytes have round, vesicular nuclei, prominent central nucleoli, and abundant cytoplasm
  ○ Histiocytes contain intact lymphocytes (emperipolesis, lymphocytophagocytosis)
  ○ Plasmacytosis usually present; often Russell bodies seen
- Extranodal sites
  ○ Emperipolesis often focal or absent
  ○ Fibrosis commonly superimposed on process

Histiocytic Sarcoma Involving Lymph Node
- Systemic symptoms are common, can be confused with HLH
- In lymph node, can diffusely replace architecture or involve sinuses
- Histiocytes are cytologically malignant
  ○ Large and pleomorphic
  ○ Often have abundant and eosinophilic cytoplasm
  ○ Vesicular chromatin, increased N/C ratio
  ○ Mitotic figures are often present
  ○ Can show hemophagocytosis
  ○ Proliferation rate (Ki-67) is increased
- Immunohistochemistry
  ○ CD68(+), CD4(+), S100(+/-)
  ○ CD1a(-), B-cell and T-cell antigens(-)

Langerhans Cell Histiocytosis
- Langerhans cells have abundant, pale eosinophilic cytoplasm
- Irregular and elongated nuclei with prominent nuclear grooves and folds
- Increased eosinophils in background; necrosis common
- Early lesions are often sinusoidal; but extensive disease replaces lymph node
- Langerhans cells do not exhibit phagocytosis
- Immunohistochemistry
  ○ CD1a(+), S100(+), CD68(+/-)
  ○ CD4(-), B-cell and T-cell antigens(-)

Sinus Histiocytosis in Lymph Node
- Very common nonspecific histologic finding
- No clinical significance
- Often no systemic symptoms
- Associated with various etiologies (benign or malignant)
- Histologic findings
  ○ Dilated and prominent sinuses; contain increased macrophages
  ○ Often absence of phagocytes
  ○ Histiocytes and macrophages are CD68(+); can be S100([+] focal)

Lymph Nodes and Other Organs Post Blood Transfusion
- Can show erythrophagocytosis
  ○ Common in lymph nodes and bone marrow
- Patients often exhibit lack of other criteria for HLH

Histiocytosis in Lymph Nodes Draining Prosthesis
- Increased benign histiocytes filling sinuses and parenchyma
- Histiocyte cytoplasm may exhibit granular quality attributable to foreign material
- Polarized light may show polarizable foreign material

Mycobacterial Infections
- Most common in immunocompromised patients
- *Mycobacterium avium intracellulare, M. tuberculosis* (MTB), or *M. leprae*

Diagnostic Criteria for Hemophagocytic Lymphohistiocytosis (HLH)

Description

Familial disease or known genetic defect*

Clinical and laboratory criteria (5 out of 8 criteria)

1. Fever: Peak temperature > 38.5°C for 7 or more days

2. Splenomegaly: Spleen palpated > 3 cm below left costal margin

3. Cytopenia involving 2 or more cell lines

    Hemoglobin < 9.0 g/dL

    Platelets < 100,000/μL

    Absolute neutrophil count < 1,000/μL

4. Hypertriglyceridemia &/or hypofibrinogenemia

    Fasting triglycerides ≥ 2.0 mmol/L, or > 3 standard deviations (SD) above normal value for age

    Fibrinogen < 1.5 g/L, or > 3 SD below normal value for age

5. Serum ferritin > 500 μg/L

6. Hemophagocytosis in bone marrow, CSF, spleen, or lymph nodes**

7. Low or absent natural killer-cell activity

8. Soluble CD25 (sIL-2 receptor) > 2,400 U/mL

Supportive evidence: Cerebral symptoms with moderate pleocytosis, elevated transaminases, bilirubin, LDH

*Patients with molecular diagnosis of HLH do not need to fulfill all other diagnostic criteria. **Inability to demonstrate hemophagocytosis on initial specimen should not prevent prompt institution of therapy, provided other clinical criteria are fulfilled.*

- o Granulomas often are ill-defined, irregular, or serpiginous
- o Langhans-type giant cells are often present
- o Necrosis is common in MTB; often caseating
- o Variable plasma cells and neutrophils
- o Acid-fast stain reveals organisms

DIAGNOSTIC CHECKLIST

Pathologic Interpretation Pearls

- HLH is clinicopathological diagnosis
  - o 5 of 8 diagnostic criteria for HLH need to be met
- Diagnosis also can be established by molecular testing
- Pathologists must be vigilant about diagnosis
  - o Presence of phagocytes is not specific for diagnosis of HLH
  - o Inability to demonstrate hemophagocytosis in initial specimen does not exclude diagnosis of HLH
    - But, other clinical criteria must be fulfilled
- Histiocytes are usually cytologically bland
- Lymphocytes are often increased, mainly small T cells
- In bone marrow, hematopoietic cells can exhibit dysplastic features
  - o This should not be interpreted as myelodysplasia
  - o Myelodysplastic syndromes associated with HLH have been reported

SELECTED REFERENCES

1. Chung HJ et al: Establishment of a reference interval for natural killer cell activity through flow cytometry and its clinical application in the diagnosis of hemophagocytic lymphohistiocytosis. Int J Lab Hematol. Epub ahead of print, 2009
2. Doyle T et al: Haemophagocytic syndrome and HIV. Curr Opin Infect Dis. 22(1):1-6, 2009
3. Gupta AA et al: Experience with hemophagocytic lymphohistiocytosis/macrophage activation syndrome at a single institution. J Pediatr Hematol Oncol. 31(2):81-4, 2009
4. Suzuki N et al: Characteristics of hemophagocytic lymphohistiocytosis in neonates: a nationwide survey in Japan. J Pediatr. 155(2):235-8, 2009
5. Wang Z et al: Early diagnostic value of low percentage of glycosylated ferritin in secondary hemophagocytic lymphohistiocytosis. Int J Hematol. Epub ahead of print, 2009
6. Wood SM et al: Different NK cell activating receptors preferentially recruit Rab27a or Munc13-4 to perforin-containing granules for cytotoxicity. Blood. Epub ahead of print, 2009
7. Bhattacharyya M et al: Hemophagoctic lymphohistiocytosis--recent concept. J Assoc Physicians India. 56:453-7, 2008
8. Filipovich AH: Hemophagocytic lymphohistiocytosis and other hemophagocytic disorders. Immunol Allergy Clin North Am. 28(2):293-313, viii, 2008
9. Henter JI et al: HLH-2004: Diagnostic and therapeutic guidelines for hemophagocytic lymphohistiocytosis. Pediatr Blood Cancer. 48(2):124-31, 2007
10. Janka GE: Hemophagocytic syndromes. Blood Rev. 21(5):245-53, 2007
11. Rouphael NG et al: Infections associated with haemophagocytic syndrome. Lancet Infect Dis. 7(12):814-22, 2007
12. Wang S et al: Hemophagocytosis exacerbated by G-CSF/GM-CSF treatment in a patient with myelodysplasia. Am J Hematol. 77(4):391-6, 2004
13. Grom AA: Macrophage activation syndrome and reactive hemophagocytic lymphohistiocytosis: the same entities? Curr Opin Rheumatol. 15(5):587-90, 2003

HEMOPHAGOCYTIC LYMPHOHISTIOCYTOSIS

Microscopic Features

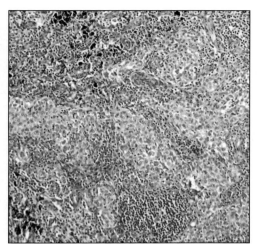
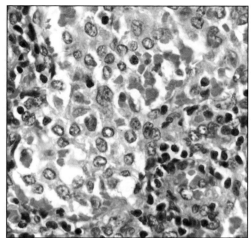

(Left) Lymph node biopsy specimen involved by HLH. This field shows markedly increased histiocytes expanding the lymph node sinuses. Pigmented histiocytes are also present in this field. *(Right)* HLH in lymph node biopsy specimen. The histiocytes within sinuses are cytologically mature with abundant cytoplasm and vesicular nuclei. Phagocytosis of erythrocytes can be seen in this field, but in some cases phagocytosis can be difficult to appreciate.

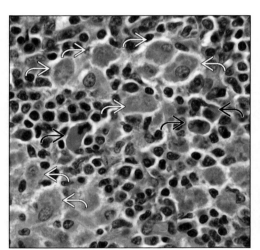
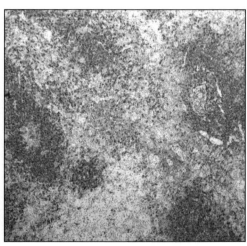

(Left) HLH in lymph node biopsy specimen. In this case, hemophagocytosis (mainly erythrophagocytosis) is very prominent ➡. Increased plasma cells containing Russell bodies are also present ➡ in the field. *(Right)* HLH involving lymph node biopsy specimen. Immunohistochemical stain for CD20 shows maintained lymph node architecture with B cells confined to the follicles. The sinuses are expanded by histiocytes, which are CD20(-).

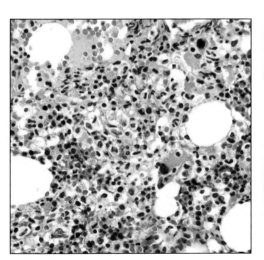
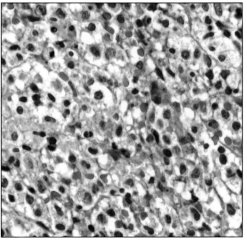

(Left) HLH involving bone marrow biopsy specimen. This field shows increased histiocytes and small lymphocytes (T cells). The histiocytes show phagocytosis of erythrocytes. *(Right)* HLH involving bone marrow biopsy specimen. In this field, histiocytes are present in sheets, raising the possibility of a histiocytic neoplasm. However, the histiocytes are cytologically benign, with cellular features distinct from monocytic leukemia or histiocytic neoplasm.

HEMOPHAGOCYTIC LYMPHOHISTIOCYTOSIS

Microscopic Features and Differential Diagnosis

(Left) HLH involving bone marrow biopsy specimen. Immunohistochemical stain for CD68 highlights histiocytes (and other myeloid cells) in the bone marrow. (Right) HLH involving bone marrow biopsy specimen. In situ hybridization for Epstein-Barr virus-encoded RNA (EBER) shows positive cells ⤢, suggesting that this case of HLH is triggered by EBV infection.

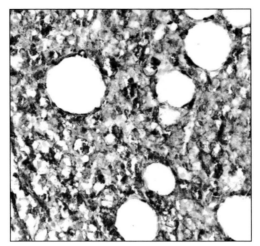
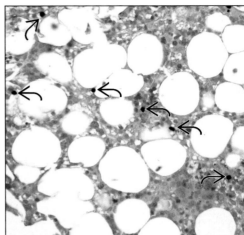

(Left) HLH bone marrow aspirate smear. The presence of histiocytes engulfing nucleated erythrocytes ⇨ is more specific for macrophage activation than histiocytes engulfing only anucleated erythrocytes. (Right) HLH involving bone marrow aspirate smear (Wright-Giemsa stain). Dyserythropoiesis ⤢ can be seen in the bone marrow of HLH patients, and this finding should not be misinterpreted as myelodysplasia. Hemophagocytosis is not present in this field.

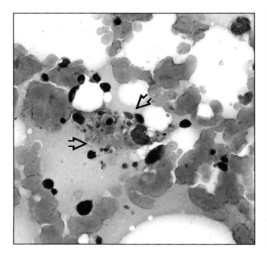
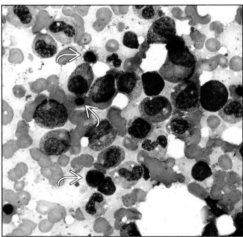

(Left) Lymph node involved by Rosai-Dorfman disease. Numerous histiocytes expand lymph node sinuses. (Right) Lymph node involved by Rosai-Dorfman disease. The histiocytes are large with abundant cytoplasm, central nuclei, and distinct nucleoli. Emperipolesis ⇨ is present within sinuses, and numerous small lymphocytes and plasma cells are present between sinuses.

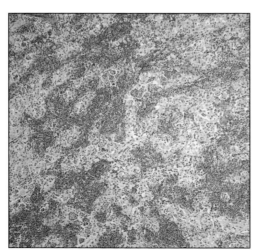
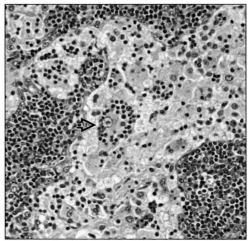

HEMOPHAGOCYTIC LYMPHOHISTIOCYTOSIS

Differential Diagnosis

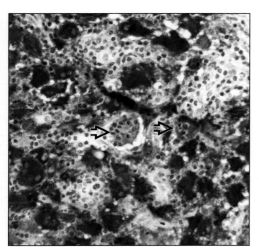
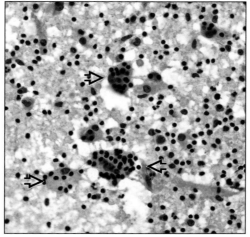

(Left) Lymph node involved by Rosai-Dorfman disease. The histiocytes are strongly positive for S100. This immunostain also negatively outlines emperipolesis ⊵ in histiocytes. *(Right)* Lymph node involved by Rosai-Dorfman disease. Emperipolesis ⊵ is often better visualized in a touch imprint preparation as shown here.

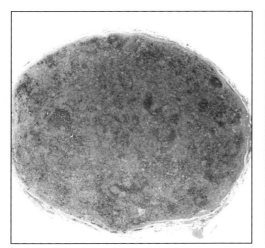
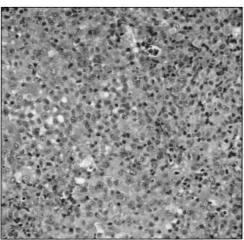

(Left) Langerhans cell histiocytosis (LCH) involving lymph node. Most of the lymph node architecture is replaced by LCH, but residual lymphoid follicles can be seen at this magnification. *(Right)* Langerhans cell histiocytosis (LCH) involving lymph node. The Langerhans cells have abundant eosinophilic cytoplasm. Recent hemorrhage and hemosiderin are present in this field.

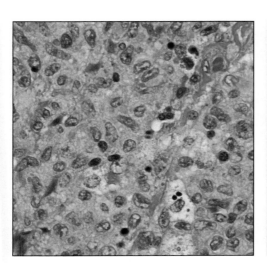
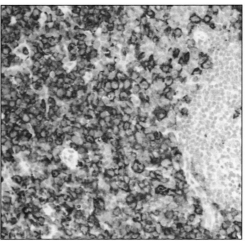

(Left) Langerhans cell histiocytosis (LCH) involving lymph node. The Langerhans cells have nuclei with folded or twisted nuclear membranes ("twisted towel" appearance) and abundant eosinophilic cytoplasm. Eosinophils are common in LCH and can be seen in this field. Mitotic figures can be present but are usually infrequent in LCH. *(Right)* Langerhans cell histiocytosis (LCH) involving lymph node. The Langerhans cells strongly express CD1a (shown), S100, and langerin/CD207.

HEMOPHAGOCYTIC LYMPHOHISTIOCYTOSIS

Differential Diagnosis

(Left) *Histiocytic sarcoma involving lymph node. The lymph node architecture is replaced by neoplasm. The neoplasm has a pale, eosinophilic appearance at low-power magnification because the neoplastic cells have abundant cytoplasm.* *(Right)* *Histiocytic sarcoma involving lymph node. The neoplastic histiocytes have highly atypical nuclei and abundant eosinophilic cytoplasm.*

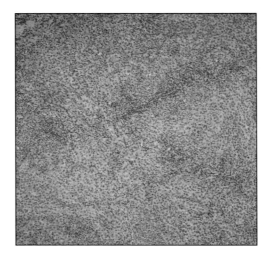 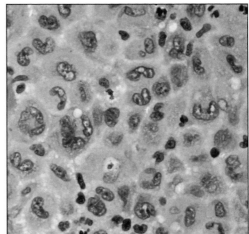

(Left) *Histiocytic sarcoma involving lymph node. This touch imprint preparation shows large and atypical histiocytes with small lymphocytes and neutrophils in the background.* *(Right)* *Histiocytic sarcoma involving lymph node. The neoplastic cells strongly express CD68, indicating that the cytoplasm of the cells contain numerous lysosomes, consistent with histiocytic lineage.*

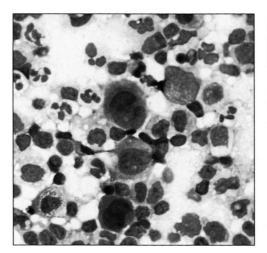 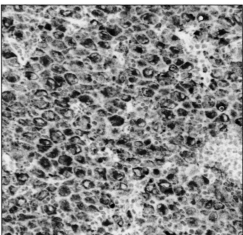

(Left) *Histiocytic sarcoma involving lymph node. The neoplastic cells strongly express CD4.* *(Right)* *Histiocytic sarcoma involving lymph node. S100 is variably and weakly expressed by the neoplastic histiocytes in this case, as is common in histiocytic sarcoma, and unlike Langerhans cell histiocytosis.*

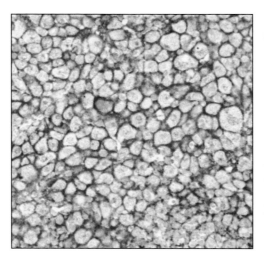 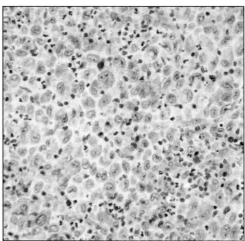

HEMOPHAGOCYTIC LYMPHOHISTIOCYTOSIS

Differential Diagnosis

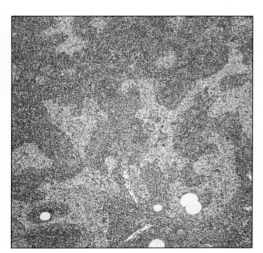
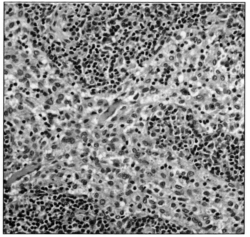

(Left) Sinus histiocytosis of lymph node. This lymph node was part of an axillary lymph node dissection in a patient with breast carcinoma. The sinuses are expanded and lymph node architecture is preserved in this field. (Right) Sinus histiocytosis of lymph node. This lymph node was part of an axillary lymph node dissection in a patient with breast carcinoma. The sinuses are expanded by benign histiocytes. There is no evidence of hemophagocytosis.

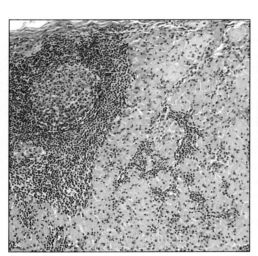
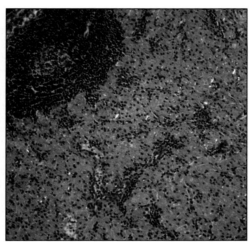

(Left) Lymph node draining an area of a prosthesis. Histiocytes are markedly increased within lymph node parenchyma and sinuses. There is no evidence of hemophagocytosis. (Right) Lymph node draining an area of a prosthesis. The histiocytes contain foreign material that can be appreciated by using polarized light.

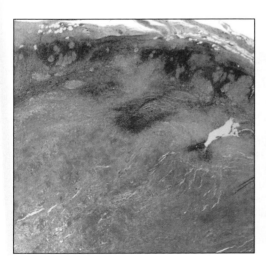
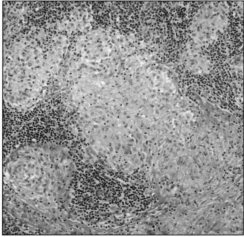

(Left) Mycobacterium tuberculosis involving lymph node. This field shows marked caseating necrosis with granulomas present at the periphery, underlying the capsule. (Right) Mycobacterium tuberculosis involving lymph node. Granulomas present at the periphery of necrosis are shown. The histiocytes do not show evidence of hemophagocytosis.

LANGERHANS CELL HISTIOCYTOSIS

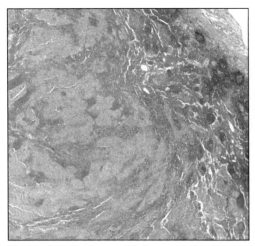

The lymph node shows partial effacement of architecture by Langerhans cell histiocytosis (LCH). Note that LCH preferentially involves and distends lymph node sinuses.

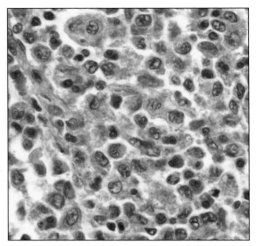

Lymph node involved by Langerhans cell histiocytosis. Langerhans cells have irregular nuclear contours, nuclear grooves, and abundant pale cytoplasm. Eosinophils are also present.

TERMINOLOGY

Abbreviations
- Langerhans cell histiocytosis (LCH)

Synonyms
- Langerhans cell granulomatosis
- Histiocytosis X
- Eosinophilic granuloma
- Letterer-Siwe disease
- Hand-Schüller-Christian disease
- Diffuse reticuloendotheliosis

Definitions
- Proliferation of Langerhans cells characterized by distinctive cytologic features and
  - Expression of CD1a, S100 protein, and langerin (CD207)
  - Birbeck granules shown by ultrastructural examination
  - Monoclonality (in most types of LCH)

ETIOLOGY/PATHOGENESIS

Normal Langerhans Cells
- Bone marrow-derived dendritic cells
- Important antigen-presenting cells, particularly in skin

Etiology of LCH Unknown
- Connection with human herpesvirus 6 (HHV6) has been suggested but is not proven
- LCH has been shown to be monoclonal by X-linked androgen receptor gene assay (*HUMARA*)
  - Some cases of adult pulmonary LCH are not monoclonal
    - Related to cigarette smoking in many cases
  - No cytogenetic abnormalities have been found
- LCH may be related to immunological dysfunction
  - Aberrant chemokine receptor expression

- GM-CSF, interferon-γ, interleukin (IL)-1, and IL-10 are increased in LCH lesions
- LCH and extent of disease are associated with specific HLA types
  - HLA-DRB1*03
  - Cw7 and DR4

LCH Associated with Other Hematopoietic Tumors ("Incidental LCH")
- Pathogenesis is unclear
  - Does it represent true neoplasm?
    - Collision tumor, i.e., not clonally related to other tumor?
    - Stem cell neoplasm clonally related to other tumor?
  - Is LCH in this context an unusual form of host response?
    - Elicited by some antigenic stimulus or substance produced by neoplastic cells?
    - Some studies have shown that incidental LCH is polyclonal

CLINICAL ISSUES

Epidemiology
- Incidence
  - 4.0-5.4 per million/year
- Age
  - All age groups, ranging from neonates to adults
  - Peak in childhood
  - Patients with single system involvement are usually older than those with multisystem involvement
    - Letterer-Siwe disease occurs predominantly in children younger than 2 years of age
    - Hand-Schüller-Christian syndrome: Peak of onset in children aged 2-10 years
    - Localized eosinophilic granuloma: Most frequently in patients 5-15 years of age

LANGERHANS CELL HISTIOCYTOSIS

Microscopic Features

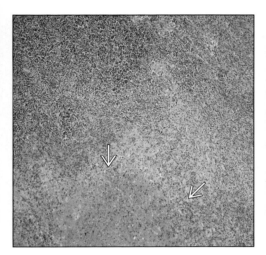

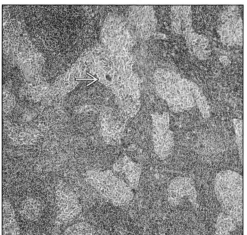

(Left) Partial replacement of lymph node by Langerhans cell histiocytosis with large areas of necrosis ➡️. *(Right)* Lymph node shows extensive sinusoidal involvement by Langerhans cell histiocytosis. A multinucleated giant Langerhans cell is seen in this field ➡️.

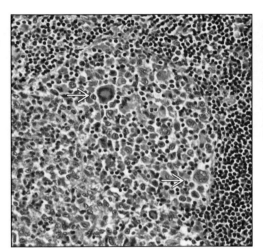

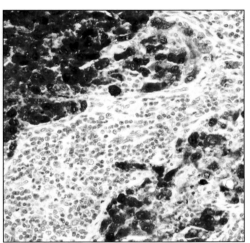

(Left) Lymph node shows involvement and expansion of sinus by Langerhans cell histiocytosis. In addition to Langerhans cells and eosinophils, scattered multinucleated giant cells are present ➡️. *(Right)* Lymph node shows involvement of sinuses by Langerhans cell histiocytosis. The Langerhans cells are strongly positive for S100 protein.

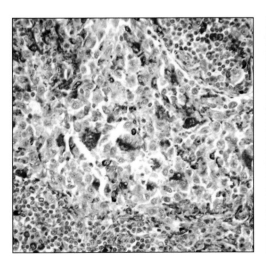

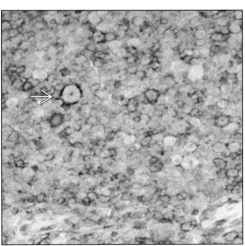

(Left) Lymph node shows involvement of sinus by Langerhans cell histiocytosis. The Langerhans cells are weakly positive for CD68. Scattered macrophages in this field are strongly CD68(+). *(Right)* Lymph node involved by Langerhans cell histiocytosis. The Langerhans cells are weakly and variably positive for CD4. Multinucleated giant cell ➡️ is more brightly CD4(+).

LANGERHANS CELL HISTIOCYTOSIS

Microscopic and Radiographic Features

(Left) Low-power view of a lymph node involved by LCH shows sinusoidal and paracortical infiltrate of Langerhans cells, with preservation of some lymphoid follicles. This patient was a young adult man who presented with systemic symptoms and widespread disease. *(Right)* Lymph node involved by LCH shows sinusoidal and paracortical infiltrate of Langerhans cells. Multinucleated giant macrophages ➡ are also present in this field.

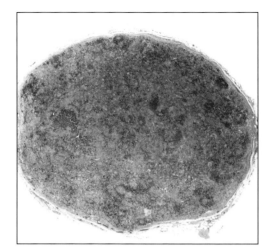
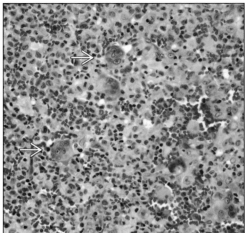

(Left) Lymph node involved by Langerhans cell histiocytosis shows paracortical infiltrate of Langerhans cells. The Langerhans cells are strongly CD1a(+). *(Right)* Radiograph of the distal femur in a child shows a well-defined lytic femoral lesion as a result of Langerhans cell histiocytosis (LCH). Notice the sclerotic margin ➡, typically indicating healing phase of LCH.

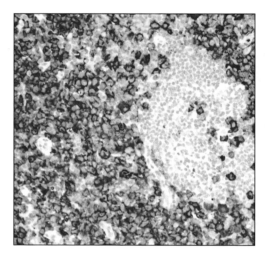
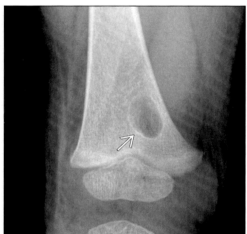

(Left) Langerhans cell histiocytosis involving bone shows a Langerhans cell infiltrate, destruction of the bone trabeculae with focal necrosis ➡, fibrosis, and reactive changes. *(Right)* Langerhans cell histiocytosis (LCH) involving bone shows numerous Langerhans cells, eosinophils, and a giant cell. Note the mitotic figure ➡ present in this field. LCH lesions often have rare to occasional mitotic figures.

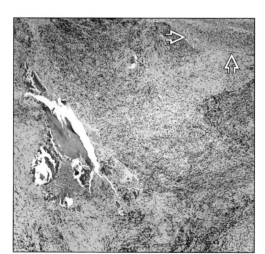
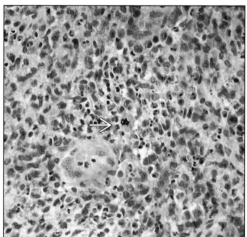

LANGERHANS CELL HISTIOCYTOSIS

Imaging and Microscopic Features

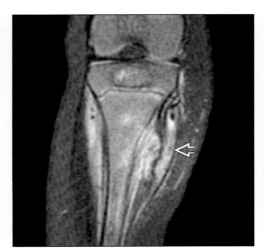

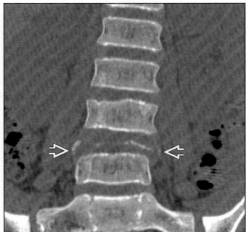

(Left) MR of Langerhans cell histiocytosis involving the proximal tibia shows extensive periosteal reaction and "onion skin" appearance ⮕ along the metadiaphysis. *(Right)* Coronal reconstructed bone CT of a 12-year-old boy with Langerhans cell histiocytosis (LCH) shows a dramatic but typical example of LCH of the spine with compression of the 4th lumbar vertebral body ⮕.

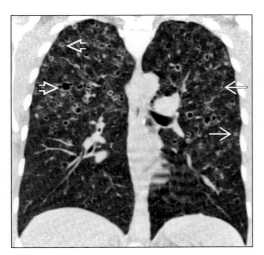

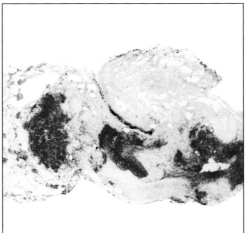

(Left) Coronal reformatted CT image of a patient with pulmonary Langerhans cell histiocytosis (LCH) shows the characteristic predominance of irregular nodules ⮕ and variably shaped cysts ⮕ in the upper and mid-lung zones, with relative sparing of the lung bases. *(Right)* Paraffin section of Langerhans cell histiocytosis (LCH) involving the lung shows patchy involvement by LCH. The Langerhans cells are strongly CD1a(+).

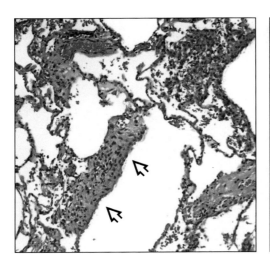

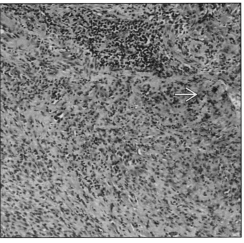

(Left) Lung involved by Langerhans cell histiocytosis (LCH). This field shows an area of alveolar lung parenchyma with a minute LCH lesion ⮕. *(Right)* Langerhans cell histiocytosis (LCH) involving the lung. This field shows an area of alveolar lung parenchyma with a large LCH lesion. In this field, there are many Langerhans cells and eosinophils and fibrosis. Macrophages with hemosiderin pigment are also present ⮕.

LANGERHANS CELL HISTIOCYTOSIS

Microscopic and Radiographic Features

(Left) Skin with extensive involvement of dermis by Langerhans cell histiocytosis. This patient presented with skin lesions without evidence of lymphadenopathy or bone lesions. *(Right)* Skin involved by Langerhans cell histiocytosis shows the characteristic cytologic features of Langerhans cells including irregular nuclear contours, nuclear grooves, and abundant cytoplasm.

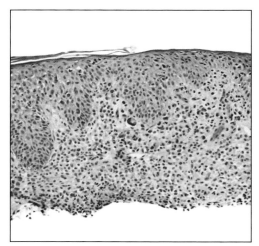 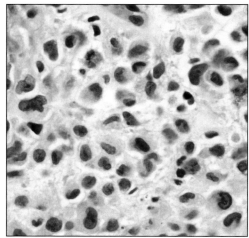

(Left) Thyroid gland with extensive involvement ⟹ by Langerhans cell histiocytosis (LCH). LCH can rarely present in endocrine organs. *(Right)* Thyroid gland involved by Langerhans cell histiocytosis shows strong expression of CD1a by Langerhans cells, supporting the diagnosis.

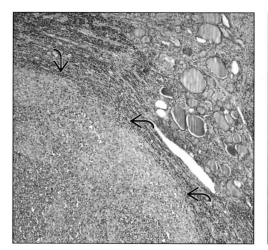 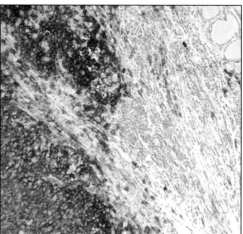

(Left) Lateral radiograph of a child with disseminated Langerhans cell histiocytosis shows multiple well-defined lytic lesions ⟹ involving the calvarium. This finding is common in children with Hand-Schüller-Christian syndrome. *(Right)* Sagittal T1WI MR shows thickening of the pituitary infundibulum ⟹ and absence of the normal posterior pituitary ⟹, which would normally appear as a bright spot, as a result of Langerhans cell histiocytosis. This can occur in children with Hand-Schüller-Christian syndrome.

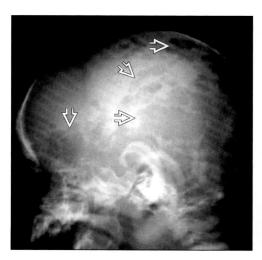 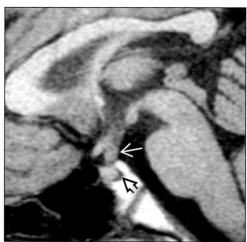

LANGERHANS CELL HISTIOCYTOSIS

"Incidental" Langerhans Cell Histiocytosis

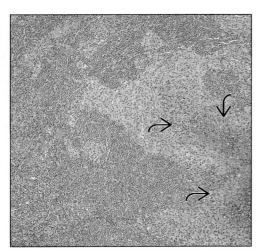

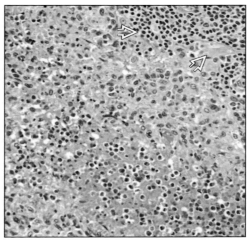

(Left) A case of Langerhans cell histiocytosis associated with mantle cell lymphoma shows proliferation of Langerhans cells. Necrosis is present ⊅. *(Right)* A case of Langerhans cell histiocytosis associated with mantle cell lymphoma shows proliferation of Langerhans cells. Intermediate-power view of Langerhans cells shows eosinophilic abscess as well as monotonous, small mantle cell lymphoma cells in the upper right corner ⧩.

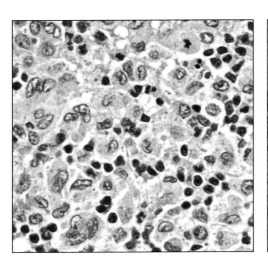

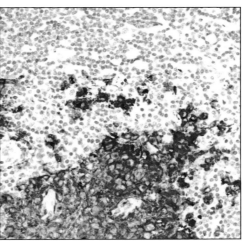

(Left) A case of Langerhans cell histiocytosis associated with mantle cell lymphoma shows that the Langerhans cells have abundant cytoplasm and deep nuclear grooves. Eosinophils are also present. *(Right)* A case of Langerhans cell histiocytosis (LCH) associated with mantle cell lymphoma shows Langerhans cells that are strongly CD1a(+), supporting the diagnosis of LCH.

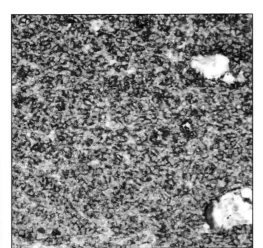

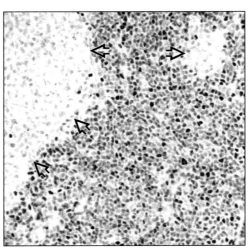

(Left) A case of Langerhans cell histiocytosis (LCH) associated with mantle cell lymphoma shows that the anti-CD20 antibody highlights the mantle cell lymphoma cells. *(Right)* A case of Langerhans cell histiocytosis associated with mantle cell lymphoma shows that the anti-Cyclin-D1 antibody highlights the mantle cell lymphoma cells. Langerhans cells are Cyclin-D1 negative ⧩.

LANGERHANS CELL HISTIOCYTOSIS

"Incidental" Langerhans Cell Histiocytosis

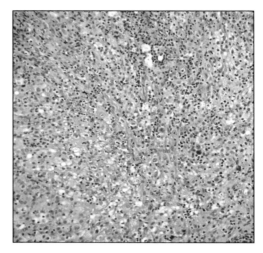
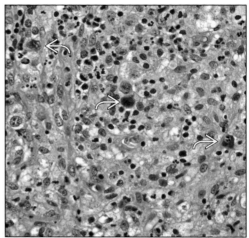

(Left) A case of classical Hodgkin lymphoma associated with Langerhans cell histiocytosis shows proliferation of Langerhans cells with numerous eosinophils. Necrosis is present. (Right) A case of classical Hodgkin lymphoma associated with Langerhans cell histiocytosis shows HRS cells ⮑. Many Langerhans cells and eosinophils are present in the background.

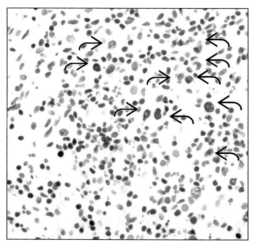
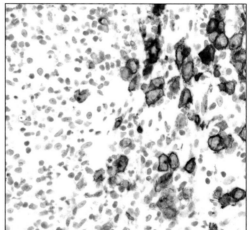

(Left) A case of classical Hodgkin lymphoma associated with Langerhans cell histiocytosis shows HRS cells that are weakly positive for pax-5 ➔. (Right) A case of classical Hodgkin lymphoma associated with Langerhans cell histiocytosis shows HRS cells that are CD30(+) in a membrane and peri-Golgi pattern.

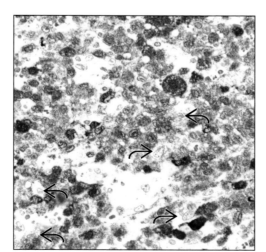
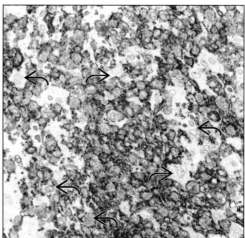

(Left) A case of classical Hodgkin lymphoma associated with Langerhans cell histiocytosis shows that the Langerhans cells are S100(+). Of note, the HRS cells ➔ are negative for S100. (Right) A case of classical Hodgkin lymphoma associated with Langerhans cell histiocytosis shows that the Langerhans cells are CD1a(+). Of note, the HRS cells ➔ are CD1a(-).

LANGERHANS CELL HISTIOCYTOSIS

Differential Diagnosis

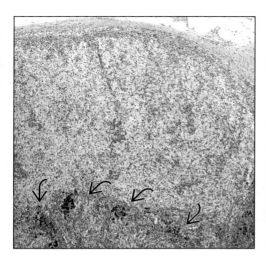

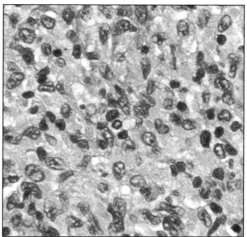

(Left) A case of dermatopathic lymphadenopathy shows marked expansion of paracortical areas with proliferation of Langerhans cells, interdigitating dendritic cells, and macrophages containing melanin pigment ➔. *(Right)* Dermatopathic lymphadenopathy. Langerhans cells and interdigitating dendritic cells have elongated nuclei, some with nuclear grooves, and a small amount cytoplasm. Eosinophils are either absent or not a prominent feature.

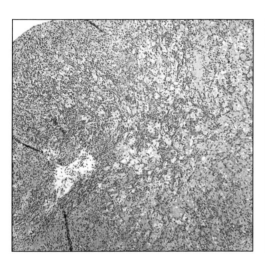

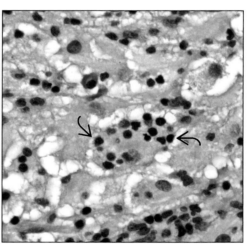

(Left) A case of Rosai-Dorfman disease involving lymph node shows dilated sinuses filled with large histiocytes. *(Right)* Rosai-Dorfman disease involving lymph node. Histiocytes contain intact lymphocytes (emperipolesis, lymphocytophagocytosis) ➔ and lipid.

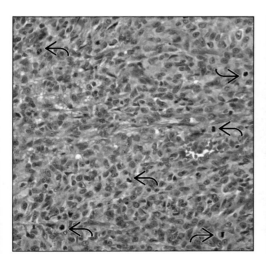

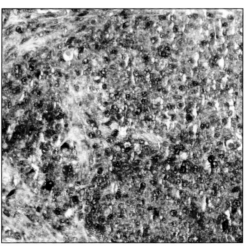

(Left) A case of Langerhans cell sarcoma shows that the Langerhans cells are overtly malignant, with nuclear hyperchromasia, numerous mitotic figures ➔, and a high nucleus:cytoplasm ratio. *(Right)* A case of Langerhans cell sarcoma shows that the Langerhans cells express 1 or more antigens in common with LCH. This image illustrates S100(+) sarcomatous cells.

LYMPHADENOPATHY ASSOCIATED WITH JOINT PROSTHESES

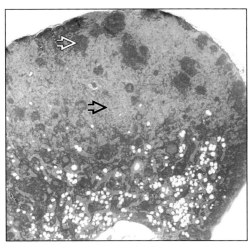

Enlarged lymph node associated with joint prosthesis. There is marked interfollicular expansion by histiocytes ⊳ and hyperplastic lymphoid follicles ⊳.

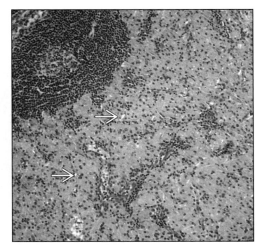

Lymph node of pelvic region examined under polarized light shows needle-shaped birefringent crystals ⊳ within histiocytes.

TERMINOLOGY

Definitions
- Lymphadenopathy caused by abraded metal debris and cementing substances drained from sites of joint prostheses

ETIOLOGY/PATHOGENESIS

Environmental Exposure
- Lymphadenopathy associated with use of metal prostheses to replace large joints
  - Hip and knee replacements are most frequent sites
- Abraded metallic debris can be found in regional or distant lymph nodes
  - Rarely found in bone marrow, liver, and spleen
- Various materials used in construction of hip and knee replacements may be found in lymph nodes
  - Materials include stainless steel, cobalt, chromium, titanium, zirconium, nickel, barium, and ceramic
    - Most modern joint prostheses are made of stainless steel or cobalt-chrome alloy
  - Cementing materials include mainly polyethylene, which is birefringent
    - Polyethylene or ceramic are mostly used to fashion articulating surface
- Titanium dioxide appears as black dusty pigment within histiocytes
- Wear debris is released in periarticular tissues
  - When wear is excessive, local foreign body giant cell reaction occurs in joint
  - Tissue macrophages clear debris by draining particulate material to regional lymph nodes

CLINICAL ISSUES

Presentation
- Pelvic lymph nodes are enlarged in patients who undergo hip prostheses
  - Incidentally found in patients undergoing genital or urinary tract staging surgery
    - May raise concern of malignancy
- Distant sites to prosthesis may also show histiocytic reaction
- Wear debris that is released into periarticular tissue elicits histiocytic reaction
  - Inflammatory reaction contributes to further wear of prosthesis and occasionally leads to fracture

Treatment
- Lymph node removal confirms diagnosis of lymphadenopathy associated with prostheses
  - Excludes other causes of lymphadenopathy
  - No other therapy required

Prognosis
- Lymphadenopathy associated with prosthesis is benign; no impact on survival

MACROSCOPIC FEATURES

General Features
- Lymph nodes are usually 1-2 cm in diameter
- Cut surface of lymph nodes appears dark brown or black

MICROSCOPIC PATHOLOGY

Histologic Features
- Sinuses are markedly distended and occupied by polygonal histiocytes with abundant granular or foamy cytoplasm

LYMPHADENOPATHY ASSOCIATED WITH JOINT PROSTHESES

Key Facts

Terminology
- Lymphadenopathy caused by abraded metal debris and cementing substances drained from sites of joint prostheses

Etiology/Pathogenesis
- Hip and knee replacements are most frequent sites
- Cementing materials include mainly polyethylene, which is birefringent

Clinical Issues
- Pelvic lymph nodes are enlarged in patients who undergo hip replacement

Macroscopic Features
- Cut surfaces of enlarged lymph nodes appear dark brown or black

Microscopic Pathology
- Sinuses are markedly distended by histiocytes
- Histiocytes are polygonal with abundant granular or foamy cytoplasm
  - Black pigment can be present
- Polyethylene is transparent on routine stains; upon polarized light examination appears as birefringent
  - 0.5-50 μm slender needles or flakes
- Usually no acute inflammation or necrosis

Top Differential Diagnoses
- Nonspecific sinus histiocytosis
- Infectious etiologies of histiocytosis
- Storage diseases
- Rosai-Dorfman disease
- Metastatic carcinoma to lymph nodes

- Occasionally granulomatous reaction &/or necrosis is also present
- On routinely stained H&E sections, metals appear as black nonrefringent 0.5-2 μm particles
  - Rarely these particles can be up to 100 μm
- Polyethylene is transparent on routine stains; upon polarized light examination it is birefringent
  - Polarized light examination shows birefringent 0.5-50 μm slender needles or flakes
- Histiocytes are PAS positive

ANCILLARY TESTS

Immunohistochemistry
- Histiocytes are: Lysozyme(+), α-1-antitrypsin(+), α-1-antichymotrypsin(+), and cathepsin-D(+)
- Cytokeratin(-), CD1a(-) and S100 protein(-)

Electron Microscopy
- Histiocytes demonstrate abundant lysosomes
- Energy dispersive x-ray elemental analysis (EDXEA) shows characteristic peaks for cobalt-chromium and titanium

DIFFERENTIAL DIAGNOSIS

Sinus Histiocytosis
- Nonspecific histiocytic reaction in sinuses of lymph node
- Expansion of sinuses due to histiocytes, which usually lack abundant foamy cytoplasm

Fungal Lymphadenitis
- *Aspergillus*, *Candida*, and *Histoplasma* species most common
- More common in immunosuppressed patients
- Histiocytosis can be present in any lymph node compartment
  - Lack pigment; no polarizable material
- Often associated with necrosis, acute inflammation, and foreign-body giant cells

- Stains for fungi (GMS, PAS) should be performed
- Cultures are valuable to identify specific organism

Mycobacterial Infections
- Mycobacteria associated with histiocytosis include *M. tuberculosis*, *M. avium*, and *M. leprae*
- Histiocytosis present in paracortical areas and sinuses
  - Lack pigment; no polarizable material
- Epithelioid histiocytes, giant cells, granulomas, and necrosis are common
- Stains for acid-fast bacilli should be performed
- Cultures are valuable to identify specific organism

Storage Diseases
- A number of storage diseases can cause histiocytosis in lymph nodes
- Histiocytes can involve any lymph node compartment

Metastatic Carcinoma in Lymph Nodes
- Metastatic carcinoma in lymph nodes can morphologically mimic histiocytosis
- Lobular carcinoma of breast may mimic sinusoidal hyperplasia
  - Neoplastic cells can have abundant foamy cytoplasm and bland-appearing nuclei
- Other primary sites of cancer in which cells can be histiocyte-like or foamy
  - Prostate, bladder, uterine cervix

Silicone Lymphadenopathy
- Lymphadenopathy secondary to breast prosthesis shows sinus histiocytosis with fine or coarse vacuolization
- Usually involves axillary lymph nodes

Rosai-Dorfman Disease
- This histiocytic disorder typically begins in sinuses but can extend into other areas
- Histiocytes are large with abundant cytoplasm and single central nucleus
- Emperipolesis is usually present; can be obvious or more subtle
- Histiocytes are strongly S100 protein(+)

Differential Diagnosis of Lymphadenopathy Associated with Joint Prostheses

	Associated with Joint Prostheses	Mycobacterial or Fungal Infection	Storage Diseases	Rosai-Dorfman Disease	Whipple Disease
Clinical Features					
	Adults with history of joint prostheses	Immunosuppression or history of exposure	Children with systemic disease; adults with organomegaly	Young patients with massive lymphadenopathy	Fever, diarrhea, weight loss, malabsorption
Site					
	Near surgical site; sometimes distant sites	Peripheral lymphadenopathy	Generalized lymphadenopathy	Cervical lymph nodes, less commonly any nodal region	Abdominal mesenteric lymphadenopathy
Histopathologic Features					
	Interfollicular expansion with distended sinuses	Interfollicular or random expansion; granulomas and necrosis	Interfollicular sinusoidal or diffuse nodal expansion	Confluent expansion of sinuses with plasmacytosis	Interfollicular and random expansion
Cytologic Features					
	Large histiocytes with granular or foamy cytoplasm, and fine dark pigment	Foamy histiocytes in Mycobacterium infection; yeasts in fungal infection	Foamy histiocytes; "wrinkled paper" in Gaucher disease	Large histiocytes with emperipolesis, large nucleus with prominent nucleoli	Intermediate size histiocytes with foamy cytoplasm
Special Studies					
	Needle-shaped crystals upon polarized light; cobalt-chromium or titanium with x-ray elemental analysis	Acid-fast stains for *Mycobacterium*; GMS, PAS, or mucicarmine stains for fungal organisms	PAS(+) or electron microscopy to detect storage organelles	S100(+), CD68(+), CD1a(-) immunohistochemistry	PAS(+) and ultrastructural analysis for intracellular bacterial structures

Whipple Disease

- Caused by bacterium *Tropheryma whipplei*
- Patients commonly present with fever, diarrhea, and substantial weight loss
- Lymph nodes in mesentery and abdomen most often affected
- Histiocytes with foamy cytoplasm involving sinuses and other lymph node compartments
  - Histiocytes contain abundant PAS(+), diastase-resistant material
- Cystic spaces, granulomatous inflammation, and epithelioid histiocytes are common
- Presence of organisms can be shown by
  - Immunohistochemistry: Monoclonal antibody specific for *T. whipplei* is available
  - Electron microscopy: Rod-shaped bacillary body with trilaminar plasma membrane
  - PCR analysis is very sensitive

DIAGNOSTIC CHECKLIST

Clinically Relevant Pathologic Features

- History of joint prosthesis

Pathologic Interpretation Pearls

- Sinus histiocytosis due to large polygonal histiocytes with dark particles and birefringent needle-shaped material

- Systemic dissemination of debris may indicate loose or worn prosthesis due to local inflammatory tissue reaction

SELECTED REFERENCES

1. Clark CR: A potential concern in total joint arthroplasty: systemic dissemination of wear debris. J Bone Joint Surg Am. 82(4):455-6, 2000
2. Baslé MF et al: Migration of metal and polyethylene particles from articular prostheses may generate lymphadenopathy with histiocytosis. J Biomed Mater Res. 30(2):157-63, 1996
3. Hicks DG et al: Granular histiocytosis of pelvic lymph nodes following total hip arthroplasty. The presence of wear debris, cytokine production, and immunologically activated macrophages. J Bone Joint Surg Am. 78(4):482-96, 1996
4. Albores-Saavedra J et al: Sinus histiocytosis of pelvic lymph nodes after hip replacement. A histiocytic proliferation induced by cobalt-chromium and titanium. Am J Surg Pathol. 18(1):83-90, 1994
5. Case CP et al: Widespread dissemination of metal debris from implants. J Bone Joint Surg Br. 76(5):701-12, 1994
6. Santavirta S et al: Aggressive granulomatous lesions in cementless total hip arthroplasty. J Bone Joint Surg Br. 72(6):980-4, 1990
7. Gray MH et al: Changes seen in lymph nodes draining the sites of large joint prostheses. Am J Surg Pathol. 13(12):1050-6, 1989

LYMPHADENOPATHY ASSOCIATED WITH JOINT PROSTHESES

Microscopic Features

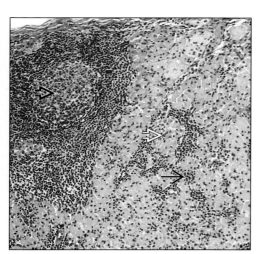

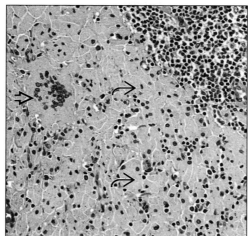

(Left) Joint prosthesis-associated lymphadenopathy. Hyperplastic lymphoid follicle with prominent germinal center ⇗ is surrounded by sheets of histiocytes ⇒ with abundant cytoplasm, which are admixed with scattered reactive lymphocytes and plasma cells ⇒. *(Right)* A case of joint prosthesis-associated lymphadenopathy is shown with interfollicular sheets of histiocytes ⇒ and an occasional multinucleated giant cell ⇗.

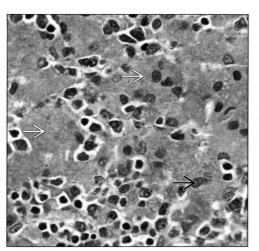

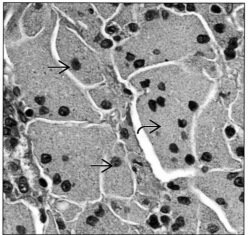

(Left) A case of joint prosthesis-associated lymphadenopathy shows histiocytes with abundant cytoplasm ⇒ and central to eccentric vesicular nuclei ⇒. *(Right)* Joint prosthesis-associated lymphadenopathy. This field reveals many histiocytes with ample pink, granular cytoplasm. Some histiocytes show a single nucleus ⇒, while others show multinucleation ⇗.

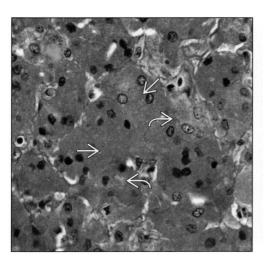

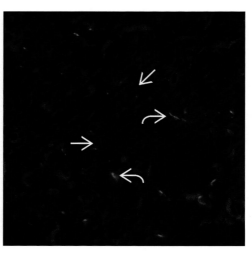

(Left) This H&E stained section shows rare black particles contained within the cytoplasm of histiocytes ⇒. Nonstaining areas ⇗ are present, which are birefringent upon use of polarized light. *(Right)* Birefringent particles ⇗ were transparent with light microscopy whereas pigmented areas on H&E are nonbirefringent ⇒ using polarized light.

LYMPHADENOPATHY SECONDARY TO DRUG-INDUCED HYPERSENSITIVITY SYNDROME

Microscopic Features and Differential Diagnosis

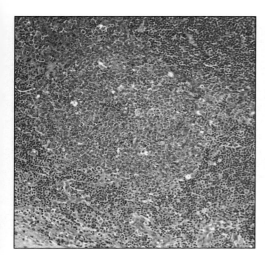
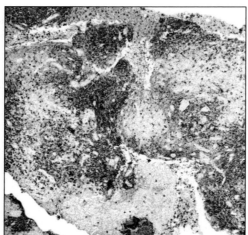

(Left) Lymph node in a patient with drug-induced hypersensitivity syndrome (phenytoin) demonstrates reactive follicles with sharply demarcated, polarized germinal centers and mantle zones. Prominent apoptosis with tingible body macrophages is present. *(Right)* Immunohistochemical study performed on lymph node specimen shows DIHS (phenytoin). The anti-CD20 antibody highlights B cells in follicles.

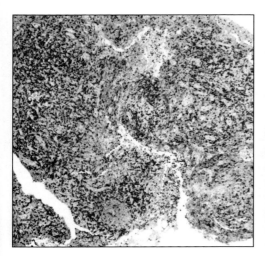
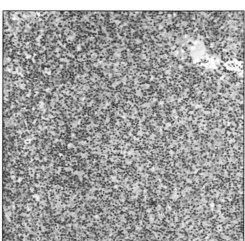

(Left) Immunohistochemical study performed on lymph node specimen shows DIHS (phenytoin). The anti-CD3 antibody highlights many T cells in interfollicular/paracortical regions. *(Right)* Lymph node biopsy specimen involved by infectious mononucleosis secondary to Epstein-Barr virus (EBV) shows paracortical expansion by a polymorphous cell population, including small and larger lymphocytes, immunoblasts, histiocytes, and plasma cells.

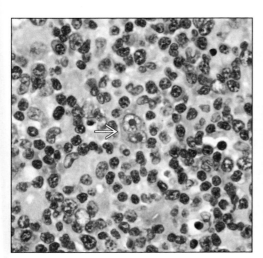
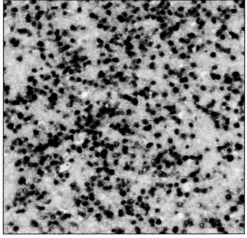

(Left) Lymph node biopsy specimen involved by infectious mononucleosis shows large Reed-Sternberg-like cells ➡. *(Right)* In situ hybridization for Epstein-Barr virus-encoded small RNA (EBER) performed on lymph node biopsy specimen involved by infectious mononucleosis shows many small and large EBER(+) cells.

3

LYMPHADENOPATHY SECONDARY TO DRUG-INDUCED HYPERSENSITIVITY SYNDROME

Differential Diagnosis

(Left) Lymph node biopsy involved by angioimmunoblastic T-cell lymphoma (AITL) demonstrates effaced architecture by a diffuse and polymorphous cellular infiltrate. Exuberant vascular proliferation with arborizing branching can be seen. (Right) Lymph node involved by AITL demonstrates atypical small to intermediate-sized lymphoid cells with many lymphoid cells having clear cytoplasm ➡. Scattered eosinophils ➡ and vascular proliferation can be appreciated in this field.

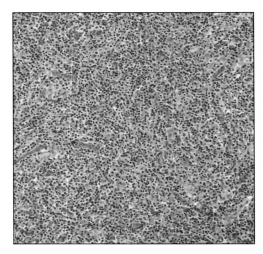
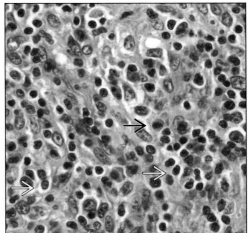

(Left) Immunohistochemical study of lymph node involved by AITL demonstrates that the atypical lymphoid cells are CD3(+), indicating T-cell lineage. (Right) Lymph node biopsy specimen involved by Hodgkin lymphoma, mixed cellularity type. The architecture is effaced in this field.

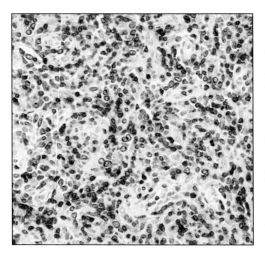
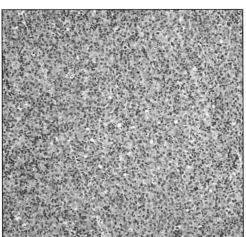

(Left) Paraffin section of lymph node involved by Hodgkin lymphoma, mixed cellularity type. This field shows a large Hodgkin (mononuclear) cell variant ➡ in a background of numerous histiocytes and scattered small lymphocytes and eosinophils. (Right) Immunohistochemical study for CD30 performed on lymph node involved by Hodgkin lymphoma, mixed cellularity type. The HRS cells express CD30 with membranous and Golgi pattern of staining ➡.

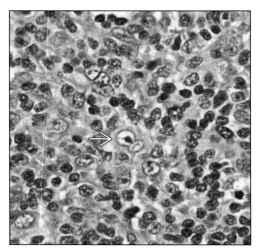
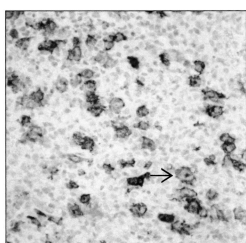

LYMPHADENOPATHY SECONDARY TO DRUG-INDUCED HYPERSENSITIVITY SYNDROME

Differential Diagnosis

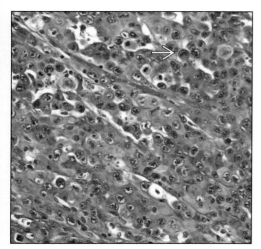

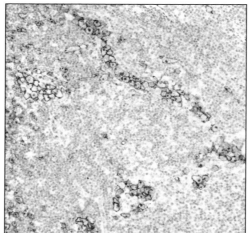

(Left) Lymph node involved by ALK(+) anaplastic large cell lymphoma (ALCL) demonstrates architectural effacement by sheets of large pleomorphic cells with vesicular nuclei, prominent nucleoli, and abundant basophilic cytoplasm. Numerous cells with horseshoe-shaped nuclei, consistent with hallmark cells ➡, are identified. **(Right)** Lymph node biopsy specimen involved by ALK(+) ALCL shows large pleomorphic lymphoid cells expressing CD30 infiltrating lymph node sinuses.

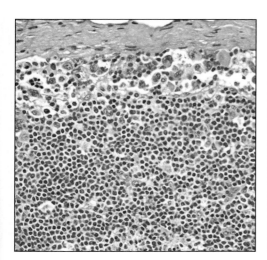

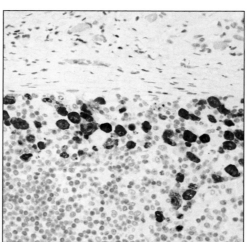

(Left) Lymph node biopsy specimen involved by ALK(+) ALCL demonstrates large pleomorphic lymphoid cells infiltrating subcapsular sinus. **(Right)** Lymph node biopsy specimen involved by ALK(+) ALCL demonstrates large pleomorphic lymphoid cells expressing ALK in a subcapsular sinus. The ALK is expressed in a nuclear and cytoplasmic pattern consistent with t(2;5) (p23;q35).

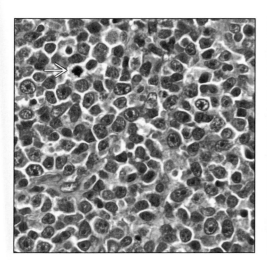

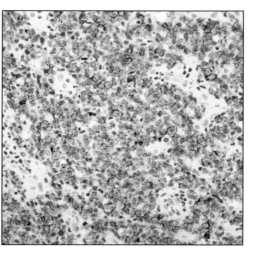

(Left) Lymph node biopsy specimen involved by diffuse large B-cell lymphoma (DLBCL), immunoblastic variant. This field demonstrates large cells, each with relatively abundant eosinophilic cytoplasm, a central nucleus, and a single, prominent central nucleolus. Mitotic figures are easily identified ➡. **(Right)** Immunohistochemical study of lymph node involved by DLBCL shows that the neoplastic cells are uniformly CD20(+), supporting B-cell lineage.

Hodgkin Lymphomas

Hodgkin Lymphoma Specimen Examination

NODULAR LYMPHOCYTE PREDOMINANT HODGKIN LYMPHOMA

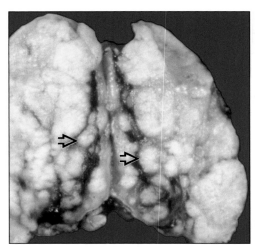

Nodular lymphocyte predominant Hodgkin lymphoma (NLPHL) in a lymph node. There are multiple nodules of variable size ⊟ throughout the lymph node parenchyma.

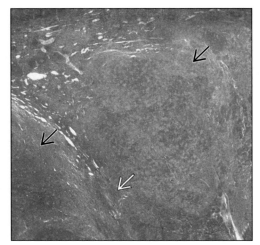

NLPHL involving lymph node. The nodal architecture is effaced by multiple expansile nodules ⊡ with compressed interfollicular zones ➡. The nodules have a "moth-eaten" appearance.

TERMINOLOGY

Abbreviations
- Nodular lymphocyte predominant Hodgkin lymphoma (NLPHL)

Synonyms
- Nodular lymphocyte predominant Hodgkin disease (REAL, 1994)
- Lymphocytic-predominant Hodgkin disease (Rye, 1966)
- Lymphocytic &/or histiocytic predominance Hodgkin disease (Lukes and Butler, 1966)
- Paragranuloma (Jackson and Parker, 1944)

Definitions
- Nodular proliferation of scattered large neoplastic B cells associated with numerous inflammatory cells
  - Neoplastic cells are designated as lymphocyte-predominant (LP) cells
    - a.k.a. "popcorn" cells because of their hyperlobated nuclei with vesicular chromatin
    - Formerly called L&H (lymphocytic &/or histiocytic) cells
  - Neoplastic cells are usually confined within follicular dendritic cell meshworks
  - Background infiltrate of nonneoplastic small lymphocytes and histiocytes
    - Inflammatory cells greatly outnumber neoplastic LP cells
- Diffuse form of NLPHL
  - Term derived from Lukes and Butler classification, but its existence has been challenged
  - Most cases in this category have been reclassified as
    - T-cell/histiocyte-rich large B-cell lymphoma (THRLBCL)
    - NLPHL with diffuse THRLBCL-like areas
    - Classical Hodgkin lymphoma (CHL)

  - Rare cases of diffuse NLPHL probably exist, i.e., "moth-eaten" B-cell-rich pattern of NLPHL

ETIOLOGY/PATHOGENESIS

Postulated Normal Counterpart
- Germinal center B lymphocyte at centroblast stage of differentiation

Associated Lesions
- NLPHL is associated with progressive transformation of germinal centers (PTGC)
  - PTGC and NLPHL can involve same lymph node biopsy specimen
  - In past, PTGC often identified in staging laparotomy specimens of NLPHL patients
  - However, prospective studies of patients with PTGC show no increased risk of NLPHL

CLINICAL ISSUES

Epidemiology
- Incidence
  - 5-6% of all Hodgkin lymphomas
- Age
  - Median: 35 years
  - All age groups are affected
- Gender
  - Male predominance
  - Male to female ratio > 2:1

Site
- Lymph nodes
- Most commonly affected groups include cervical, axillary, or inguinal lymph nodes
  - Paraaortic and iliac lymph nodes less often involved
- Liver &/or spleen involved in ~ 10% of cases
- Mediastinum involved in ~ 7%
- Bone marrow rarely involved (~ 2%)

NODULAR LYMPHOCYTE PREDOMINANT HODGKIN LYMPHOMA

Key Facts

Clinical Issues
- Peak incidence in 4th decade, affects all age groups
- Patients often present with stage I or II nodal disease
- Cervical, axillary, or inguinal lymph nodes
- Slow progression and frequent relapses
- Excellent prognosis
- ~ 3-5% of patients develop large B-cell lymphoma

Microscopic Pathology
- Nodular or nodular and diffuse patterns
- LP cells scattered in background of small lymphocytes and histiocytes
  - LP cells have vesicular chromatin, inconspicuous nucleolus, and thin nuclear membrane
- Mixture of different cell types gives "moth-eaten" pattern on low-power view
- No necrosis or thick fibrous bands

- Uninvolved lymph node shows reactive follicular hyperplasia &/or PTGC

Ancillary Tests
- Immunophenotype of LP cells
  - CD20(+), CD22(+), CD45/LCA(+), CD79a(+)
  - Bcl-6(+), pax-5(+), OCT2(+), BOB1(+)
  - CD15(-), CD30(-), EBV(-), Bcl-2(-)
- Single-cell PCR
  - LP cells carry monoclonal *IgH* gene rearrangements

Top Differential Diagnoses
- Lymphocyte-rich classical Hodgkin lymphoma
- T-cell/histiocyte-rich large B-cell lymphoma
- Progressive transformation of germinal centers
- Follicular lymphoma
- Nodular sclerosis Hodgkin lymphoma

- Bone marrow involvement is usually evidence of transformation to large B-cell lymphoma

Presentation
- Peripheral lymphadenopathy
  - Stage I or II in ~ 80% of patients
- B symptoms are uncommon (~ 10%)

Laboratory Tests
- Normal complete blood count; no leukemic phase
- Serum lactate dehydrogenase (LDH) or β-2-microglobulin levels are rarely elevated

Natural History
- NLPHL is clinically indolent disease with frequent relapses
- Relapse-free survival curves show "staircase"
  - No plateau suggestive of cure
  - Early and late (> 10 years) relapses occur
  - Risk of relapse is independent of stage of disease or therapy
  - Relapse can be localized or generalized (~ 20%) disease
- ~ 3-5% of NLPHL transform to large B-cell lymphoma (LBCL)
  - Large B-cell lymphoma typically follows NLPHL but can coexist with or precede NLPHL
    - Subset of transformed cases resembles diffuse large B-cell lymphoma (DLBCL)
    - Clinically indolent when compared with de novo diffuse large B-cell lymphoma
  - 2nd subset resembles THRLBCL
- ~ 15% of patients die of disease with prolonged follow-up
  - Deaths related to therapy-refractory disease or 2nd malignancies
  - 2nd malignancies represent ~ 4% of all deaths
    - Acute leukemia (2%), non-Hodgkin lymphoma (1%), solid organ tumors (1%)

Treatment
- Options, risks, complications

- "Watch and wait" has been advocated for pediatric patients with localized disease
- Drugs
  - Combination chemotherapy employed most often
  - Recommended regime: Doxorubicin, bleomycin, vinblastine, dacarbazine (ABVD)
  - Rituximab (anti-CD20) monoclonal antibody is often used
    - As part of ABVD regimen, upfront (R-ABVD)
    - At time of refractory disease
- Radiation
  - Localized disease may be treated with involved field radiation alone
    - This option is avoided in pediatric and adolescent patients to avoid injuring growth plates of bones

Prognosis
- Good prognosis with > 80% 10-year survival
  - Better survival for patients with low- vs. high-stage disease
  - Patients with NLPHL have better survival than patients with classical Hodgkin lymphoma
- Transformation to diffuse large B-cell lymphoma or THRLBCL is often associated with poorer prognosis
  - Bone marrow involvement is associated with aggressive clinical behavior
  - Prognosis may not be impacted if large B-cell lymphoma is localized and treated appropriately

IMAGE FINDINGS

Radiographic Findings
- Peripheral lymphadenopathy
- NLPHL lesions are not FDG-PET avid

MICROSCOPIC PATHOLOGY

Histologic Features
- Complete or partial effacement of lymph node architecture

NODULAR LYMPHOCYTE PREDOMINANT HODGKIN LYMPHOMA

- Nodular or nodular and diffuse patterns
- Expansile nodules composed mostly of small lymphocytes and fewer histiocytes
  - Reactive lymphoid follicles usually absent within nodules
  - Absent or rare centrocytes or centroblasts within nodules
- Nodules larger than normal lymphoid follicles
- LP cells are large and scattered amongst abundant small lymphocytes and histiocytes
  - Represent ~ 1% of all cells
  - LP cells have variety of appearances
    - Multilobated "popcorn" cells with vesicular chromatin and multiple small nucleoli
    - Multinucleated or mummified cells
    - LP cells also can be round without multilobation
- Various architectural patterns have been described
  - Classical nodular pattern is most common
  - Serpiginous nodular pattern
    - Confluent irregular nodules
  - Nodular with extranodular LP cells
    - Pattern more commonly seen in patients with recurrence
  - Nodular pattern with T-cell-rich background
  - THRLBCL-like
    - Always associated with at least 1 typical nodule of NLPHL
    - Diffuse areas indistinguishable from primary THRLBCL
    - Most background lymphocytes are T cells and histiocytes
    - Absence of underlying follicular dendritic cell meshworks
    - Associated with B symptoms and higher clinical stage
  - Diffuse, B cell-rich with "moth-eaten" appearance
    - Uncommon pattern (< 5% of cases)
    - Most background lymphocytes are B cells
    - Underlying follicular dendritic cell meshworks positive
- Histiocytes may be epithelioid &/or form small granulomas
- Features common in classical Hodgkin lymphoma are usually absent in NLPHL
  - Eosinophils, neutrophils, and plasma cells are unusual
  - Classical Hodgkin and Reed-Sternberg (HRS) cells are absent or rare
  - Necrosis is rare; no fibrous bands around nodules
- Residual/uninvolved lymph node in biopsy specimens of NLPHL
  - Reactive follicular hyperplasia is usually present
  - PTGC commonly present
- Recurrent/relapsed NLPHL
  - Depletion of small lymphocytes with increased histiocytes
  - Fibrosis in up to 40% of cases with recurrence
  - Diffuse areas present; often increased in size

Cytologic Features
- Diagnosis of NLPHL difficult to establish in fine needle aspirate specimens
  - Nodular architecture difficult to appreciate in smears
  - Small lymphocytes, histiocytes, and large LP cells present
  - No granulocytes or plasma cells

Transformation of NLPHL to Large Cell Lymphoma
- Large cell lymphoma may coexist with or follow NLPHL
  - Large cells may form sheets, as in de novo diffuse large B-cell lymphoma, or be scattered, as in THRLBCL
- No consensus on pathologic criteria to distinguish between
  - NLPHL with diffuse THRLBCL-like areas vs. transformation to THRLBCL
- Transformation of NLPHL to THRLBCL can be diagnosed when
  - Diffuse areas of THRLBCL are identified, and
  - Patients have high-stage disease, including bone marrow involvement, &/or other clinical evidence of transformation, such as
    - High serum lactate dehydrogenase or β-2-microglobulin levels
    - Lytic bone lesions
  - Bone marrow involvement in patients with NLPHL is usually evidence of transformation
  - Extensive liver involvement is usually associated with transformation
- Transformation of NLPHL to diffuse large B-cell lymphoma
  - Sheets of large neoplastic cells outside nodules of NLPHL

ANCILLARY TESTS

Immunohistochemistry
- LP cells
  - CD20(+), CD22(+), CD79a(+), CD75(+)
  - pax-5(+), OCT2(+), BOB1(+), PU.1(+)
  - CD40(+), CD80(+), CD86(+)
  - Bcl-6(+), AID(+), SWAP-70(+)
  - CD45/LCA(+), Ki-67 (proliferation) high
  - EMA and MUM1(+) in ~ 50% of cases
  - IgD(+) in ~ 25% of cases
    - IgD correlates with younger patient age
  - Pan-T-cell antigens(-), Bcl-2(-)
  - CD15(-) and CD30(-)
    - CD30(+) LP cells reported in ~ 10% of NLPHL cases
    - CD30(+) reactive immunoblasts are common in NLPHL
    - CD15(+) LP cells very rare; often at time of relapse
  - Epstein-Barr virus (EBV)-LMP1(-)
    - Rare (< 1%) cases of NLPHL with EBV(+) LP cells reported in developed countries
- Background inflammatory infiltrate
  - Small lymphocytes are mixture of B and T cells
  - B cells
    - CD19(+), CD20(+), CD22(+), pax-5(+)
    - IgM(+), IgD(+)

- ▪ CD10(-), Bcl-6(-)
  - o T cells
    - ▪ CD2(+), CD3(+), CD5(+), CD7(+)
    - ▪ Form "rosettes" around LP cells
  - o Minor population of CD3(+) cells is of follicular T-helper cell lineage
    - ▪ CD3(+), CD4(+), CD57(+)
    - ▪ CD10(+), Bcl-6(+) < PD-1(+)
    - ▪ Form "rosettes" around LP cells in ~ 50% of cases
  - o Follicular dendritic cell meshworks are present in nodular areas
    - ▪ CD21(+), CD23(+), &/or CD35(+)
  - o Histiocytes
    - ▪ CD68(+)
- Recurrent/relapsed NLPHL
  - o Depletion of background small B cells
  - o Decreased or absent follicular dendritic cells
  - o Increased numbers of background T cells and histiocytes
  - o LP cells may express CD30 or rarely CD15

Flow Cytometry
- Polytypic B cells
- Mature T cells
  - o CD4(+), CD8(+) T cells in ~ 50% of cases
- Large neoplastic cells are lost or overlooked in routine flow cytometric analysis

Cytogenetics
- Usually complex structural karyotypic aberrations
- Chromosome 3q27 (*BCL6* locus) involved in up to 60% of cases

In Situ Hybridization
- EBER(-) in LP cells
  - o < 1% of NLPHL cases are EBER(+) in Western countries
  - o EBV may be more common in LP cells of NLPHL in developing countries

PCR
- Monoclonal *IgH* or light chain gene rearrangements when using single-cell PCR analysis
- Rearrangements often not detectable using standard PCR or Southern blot methods and whole biopsy specimens

Array CGH
- 30-60% of cases may show gains or losses of chromosomes
  - o Gains: Chromosomes 1, 2q, 3, 4q, 5q, 6, 8q, 11q, 12q, and X
  - o Loss: Chromosome 17

Molecular Genetics
- Frequent somatic mutations of *IgH* variable region
  - o Evidence of ongoing mutations
- *BCL6* gene rearrangements in ~ 50% of cases
  - o *IgH* is most common partner
  - o Other partners: Chromosome loci 2q23; 5q31, 6q22, 9q22, and 17p21

DIFFERENTIAL DIAGNOSIS

Lymphocyte-rich Classical Hodgkin Lymphoma, Nodular Variant
- Form of classical Hodgkin lymphoma with prominent nodular pattern that can closely mimic NLPHL
- Nodules composed of prominent mantle zones with atrophic or absent germinal centers
- HRS cells in mantle zones of enlarged lymphoid follicles
- Immunophenotype
  - o HRS cells are CD15(+), CD30(+), EBV-LMP1(+/-), CD45/LCA(-)

T-cell/Histiocyte-rich Large B-cell (THRLBCL) Lymphoma
- Affects elderly patients; rare in children and adolescents
- B symptoms, high stage, and elevated serum LDH levels
- Usually not associated with reactive follicular hyperplasia or PTGC
- Diffuse growth pattern
- Large neoplastic cells represent < 10% of all cells in specimen

Nodular Sclerosis Hodgkin Lymphoma
- Uncommonly, cases of NLPHL are associated with fibrosis
  - o Inguinal region is common site of fibrosis
  - o Fibrosis is more often present at time of relapse
- Fibrosis in NLPHL is not birefringent/polarizable
  - o Fibrous bands surrounding nodules are not present
- Immunophenotype
  - o HRS cells are CD15(+), CD30(+), EBV-LMP1(+/-), CD45/LCA(-)

Follicular Lymphoma
- Usually stage IV disease on presentation
- Neoplastic follicles typically smaller than those seen in NLPHL
  - o Neoplastic follicles commonly found in perinodal soft tissue
- Abundant neoplastic small and large centrocytes and large centroblasts
- Immunophenotype
  - o CD10(+), Bcl-6(+), Bcl-2(+)
  - o Flow cytometry immunophenotype shows monotypic B-lymphocytes, CD10(+)

Progressive Transformation of Germinal Centers
- Rare patients can present with florid syndrome with generalized lymphadenopathy
- Lymph node architecture is preserved
- Markedly enlarged lymphoid follicles (often 3-4x larger than typical reactive follicle)
- Lymphoid follicles extensively colonized by mantle zone lymphocytes
  - o Can infiltrate and obliterate germinal centers

NODULAR LYMPHOCYTE PREDOMINANT HODGKIN LYMPHOMA

Immunohistochemistry

Antibody	Reactivity	Staining Pattern	Comment
CD45	Positive	Cell membrane	Almost always positive
Pan-B-cell Marker			
CD20	Positive	Cell membrane	Almost always positive
Transcription Factors			
pax-5	Positive	Nuclear	Stronger than reactivity in HRS cells of CHL
OCT2	Positive	Nuclear	Stronger than reactivity in HRS cells of CHL
BOB1	Positive	Nuclear	Stronger than reactivity in HRS cells of CHL
CHL Markers			
CD30	Negative	Nuclear & cytoplasmic	May rarely be positive; reactive immunoblasts are positive in interfollicular areas
CD15	Negative	Cytoplasmic	May rarely be positive in subset of cases
Germinal Center B-cell-associated Antigen			
Bcl-6	Positive	Nuclear	
Other Useful Markers			
EMA	Positive	Cell membrane	Positive in 50% of cases
EBER	Negative	Nuclear	Usually negative but may be positive in patients from underdeveloped countries
EBV-LMP	Negative	Cytoplasmic	Usually negative but may be positive in patients from underdeveloped countries

- Enlarged follicles with underlying follicular dendritic cell meshwork
- LP cells are absent
- CD4(+), CD8(+) T cells are increased (similar to NLPHL)

Reactive Lymphoid Hyperplasia
- Lymph node architecture is preserved
- Well-defined germinal centers with polarization and distinct mantle zones
- Small and large centrocytes and centroblasts without atypia
- Tingible body macrophages usually abundant and prominent

DIAGNOSTIC CHECKLIST

Clinically Relevant Pathologic Features
- Clinically indolent disease that responds to therapy but frequently relapses
- Survival curves show early and late relapses without plateau
  - Suggests that no patients with NLPHL are "cured"

Pathologic Interpretation Pearls
- Expansile nodules with LP cells in small lymphocytic background
  - Pattern can be purely nodular or nodular and diffuse
  - Nodules are larger than lymphoid follicles of reactive conditions or follicular lymphoma
    - Most cells within nodules are reactive T and B cells
    - Histiocytes and follicular dendritic cell meshworks in nodules

- LP cells represent < 1% of cells within nodules
- LP cells are B cells with germinal center-like immunophenotype

SELECTED REFERENCES

1. Biasoli I et al: Nodular, lymphocyte-predominant Hodgkin lymphoma: a long-term study and analysis of transformation to diffuse large B-cell lymphoma in a cohort of 164 patients from the Adult Lymphoma Study Group. Cancer. 116(3):631-9, 2010
2. Churchill HR et al: Programmed death 1 expression in variant immunoarchitectural patterns of nodular lymphocyte predominant Hodgkin lymphoma: comparison with CD57 and lymphomas in the differential diagnosis. Hum Pathol. Epub ahead of print, 2010
3. Lee AI et al: Nodular lymphocyte predominant Hodgkin lymphoma. Oncologist. 14(7):739-51, 2009
4. Mourad WA et al: Morphologic, immunphenotypic and clinical discriminators between T-cell/histiocyte-rich large B-cell lymphoma and lymphocyte-predominant Hodgkin lymphoma. Hematol Oncol Stem Cell Ther. 1(1):22-7, 2008
5. Yang DT et al: Nodular lymphocyte predominant Hodgkin lymphoma at atypical locations may be associated with increased numbers of large cells and a diffuse histologic component. Am J Hematol. 83(3):218-21, 2008
6. Stamatoullas A et al: Conventional cytogenetics of nodular lymphocyte-predominant Hodgkin's lymphoma. Leukemia. 21(9):2064-7, 2007
7. Khoury JD et al: Bone marrow involvement in patients with nodular lymphocyte predominant Hodgkin lymphoma. Am J Surg Pathol. 28(4):489-95, 2004
8. Boudová L et al: Nodular lymphocyte-predominant Hodgkin lymphoma with nodules resembling T-cell/histiocyte-rich B-cell lymphoma: differential diagnosis between nodular lymphocyte-predominant Hodgkin lymphoma and T-cell/histiocyte-rich B-cell lymphoma. Blood. 102(10):3753-8, 2003

NODULAR LYMPHOCYTE PREDOMINANT HODGKIN LYMPHOMA

Microscopic Features

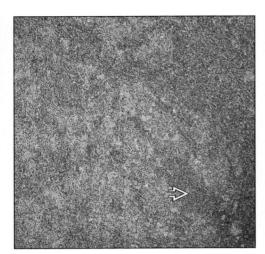

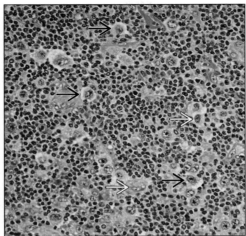

(Left) Nodular lymphocyte predominant Hodgkin lymphoma (NLPHL). The large nodule has a "moth-eaten" pattern at low power due to the presence of larger cells in a background of small lymphocytes ⇨. *(Right)* NLPHL involving lymph node. At high power, the large neoplastic lymphocyte predominant (LP) cells ⇨ are scattered among numerous small lymphocytes and a few histiocytes ⇨.

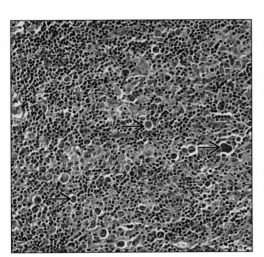

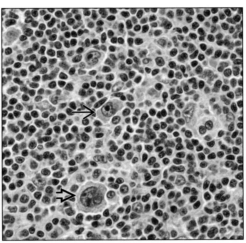

(Left) Nodular lymphocyte predominant Hodgkin lymphoma (NLPHL). The cytology of the LP cells spans a spectrum. Some are mummified or have irregular nuclear contours, as in this case ⇨. *(Right)* NLPHL involving lymph node. H&E shows various morphologic appearances of LP cells, including "popcorn" cells ⇨ and 1 with a prominent nucleolus ⇨, similar to the HRS cells of classical Hodgkin lymphoma.

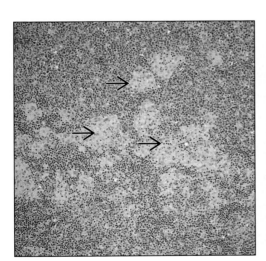

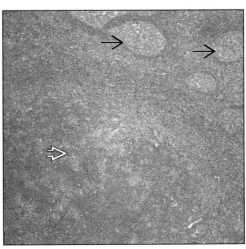

(Left) Nodular lymphocyte predominant Hodgkin lymphoma. Small clusters of histiocytes can be seen forming noncaseating granulomata ⇨. *(Right)* Hyperplastic lymphoid follicles ⇨ as well as an expansile lymphoid follicle showing progressive transformation of germinal centers (PTGC) ⇨ may be identified at the periphery of NLPHL. No atypical or LP cells were found in the follicle with PTGC.

Immunohistochemical Features

(Left) Nodular lymphocyte predominant Hodgkin lymphoma (NLPHL). The large LP cells ➡ as well as many of the small background lymphocytes are CD20(+). The small background lymphocytes are predominantly B cells in NLPHL. *(Right)* NLPHL involving lymph node. The LP cells are strongly positive for pax-5 ➡. In contrast, the HRS cells of classical Hodgkin lymphoma are dimly pax-5(+). Note also that LP cells can be multilobated.

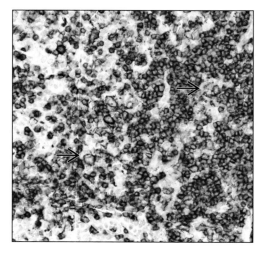
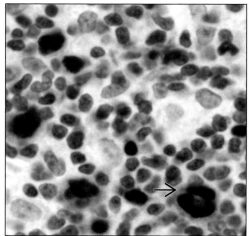

(Left) Nodular lymphocyte predominant Hodgkin lymphoma (NLPHL). Low-power magnification shows that the neoplastic nodules ➡ contain scattered small CD3(+) T cells ➡. Most cells in the infiltrate are negative ➡, suggesting that they are B lymphocytes. *(Right)* NLPHL involving lymph node. Small CD3(+) cells surround some LP cells, forming so-called "rosettes" ➡.

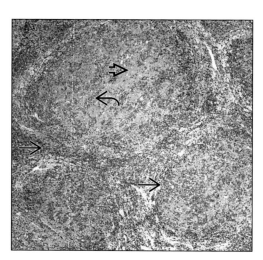
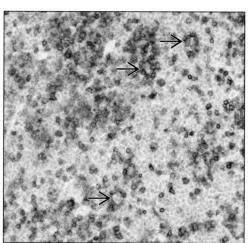

(Left) Nodular lymphocyte predominant Hodgkin lymphoma (NLPHL). Small CD57(+) T cells ➡ surround one LP cell ➡, forming a "rosette." CD3 is more sensitive than CD57 in identifying rosettes in NLPHL. *(Right)* NLPHL involving lymph node. The LP cells of NLPHL are negative for CD30 ➡. Interfollicular immunoblasts of intermediate size ➡ are commonly CD30(+) in NLPHL and in reactive follicular hyperplasia.

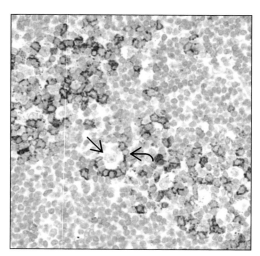
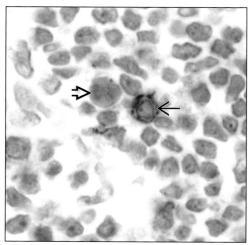

NODULAR LYMPHOCYTE PREDOMINANT HODGKIN LYMPHOMA

Immunohistochemical and Microscopic Features

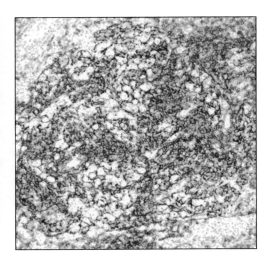

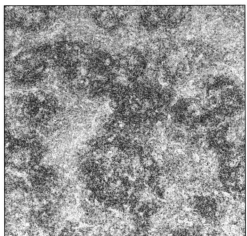

(Left) Nodular lymphocyte predominant Hodgkin lymphoma (NLPHL) shows a classical nodular pattern. CD21 highlights a follicular dendritic cell meshwork underlying an enlarged nodule. This is the most common pattern identified in NLPHL. *(Right)* NLPHL, nodular serpiginous pattern, involving lymph node. pax-5 highlights confluent nodules of B-lymphocytes, which convey a "serpiginous" pattern.

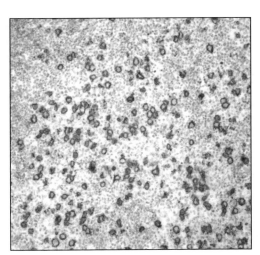

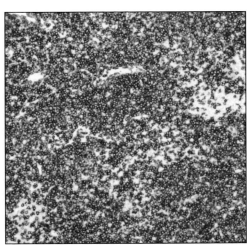

(Left) Nodular lymphocyte predominant Hodgkin lymphoma (NLPHL), nodular T-cell-rich pattern. CD20 immunohistochemistry highlights lymphocyte predominant (LP) cells in a nodule of NLPHL. The majority of small lymphocytes in the background are CD20(-). *(Right)* NLPHL, T-cell-rich pattern, involving lymph node. CD3 immunohistochemistry highlights numerous positive cells. This pattern is uncommon.

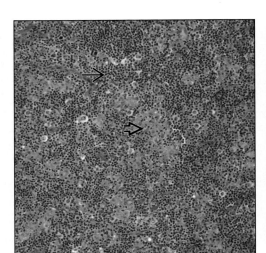

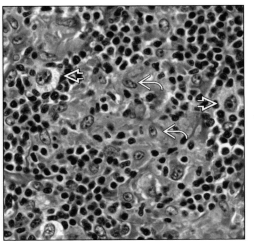

(Left) Nodular lymphocyte predominant Hodgkin lymphoma (NLPHL), histiocyte-rich pattern. Many cells in the background are histiocytes ⇗, which are admixed with small lymphocytes ⇘. *(Right)* NLPHL, histiocyte-rich pattern, involving lymph node. The histiocytes ⇗ may form loose clusters, and only rare (~ 1%) LP cells ⇗ are present.

NODULAR LYMPHOCYTE PREDOMINANT HODGKIN LYMPHOMA

Transformation of NLPHL

(Left) Diffuse large B-cell lymphoma (DLBCL) arising from NLPHL. The presence of sheets of large cells ⇨ are diagnostic of transformation. NLPHL was identified in other parts of the lymph node. *(Right)* T-cell/histiocyte-rich large B-cell lymphoma (THRLBCL) arising from NLPHL. This pattern occurred after relapses of NLPHL and multiple chemotherapies. Compared to typical cases of NLPHL, histiocytes are more abundant and and lymphocytes are less abundant in THRLBCL.

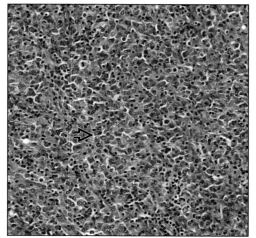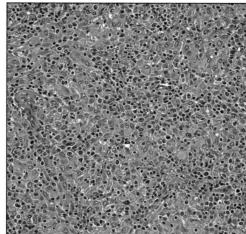

(Left) T-cell/histiocyte-rich large B-cell lymphoma (THRLBCL) arising from transformation of NLPHL. CD20 highlights the neoplastic large cells and rare small reactive B-lymphocytes. Note that the B cells are markedly depleted in comparison with typical NLPHL. *(Right)* T-cell/histiocyte-rich large B-cell lymphoma (THRLBCL) arising from NLPHL. Bone marrow involvement by THRLBCL in a patient with NLPHL indicates transformation of NLPHL.

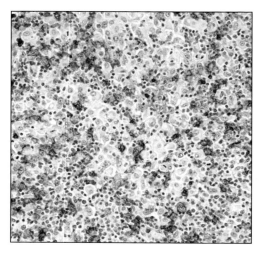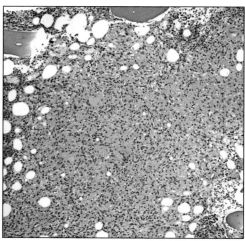

(Left) T-cell/histiocyte-rich large B-cell lymphoma (THRLBCL) in bone marrow. Bone marrow involvement by THRLBCL in a patient with NLPHL elsewhere indicates transformation of NLPHL. A large neoplastic cell ⇨ is surrounded by numerous histiocytes ⇨. *(Right)* T-cell/histiocyte-rich large B-cell lymphoma (THRLBCL) in bone marrow. A large neoplastic cell ⇨ as well as scattered small B cells ⇨ are pax-5(+).

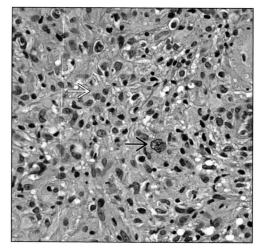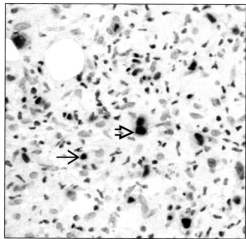

NODULAR LYMPHOCYTE PREDOMINANT HODGKIN LYMPHOMA

Differential Diagnosis

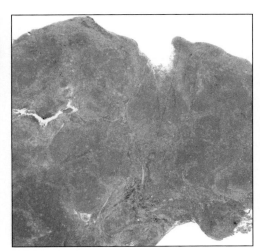
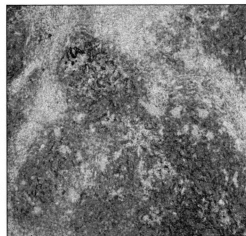

(Left) Lymph node involved by lymphocyte-rich classical Hodgkin lymphoma (LRCHL), nodular variant. This neoplasm resembles nodular lymphocyte predominant Hodgkin lymphoma (NLPHL) at low magnification. However, a "moth-eaten" pattern is not seen in this lymph node. (Right) LRCHL involving lymph node. CD21 immunohistochemistry highlights an expanded follicular dendritic cell meshwork.

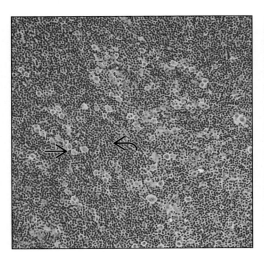
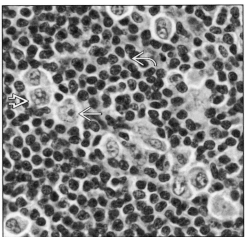

(Left) Lymphocyte-rich classical Hodgkin lymphoma (LRCHL). Hodgkin and Reed-Sternberg (HRS) cells ➡ are scattered among numerous small reactive lymphocytes ➡. Rare histiocytes are also noted. (Right) LRCHL involving lymph node. HRS cells include cells with large multilobated vesicular nuclei ➡ and large cells with prominent nucleoli ➡. The background is composed predominantly of small lymphocytes ➡.

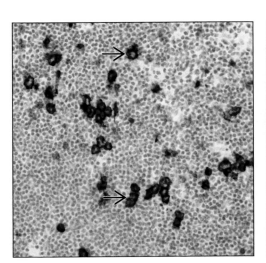
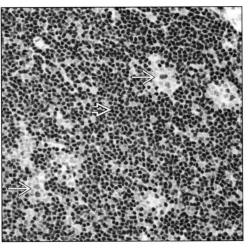

(Left) Lymphocyte-rich classical Hodgkin lymphoma (LRCHL). The neoplastic cells are strongly CD30(+) ➡, as any usual Hodgkin and Reed-Sternberg cell of classical Hodgkin lymphoma. (Right) LRCHL involving lymph node. pax-5 highlights numerous small reactive B-lymphocytes, strongly positive ➡ in the background, corresponding mainly to mantle zone lymphocytes. The neoplastic HRS cells ➡ are weakly positive.

NODULAR LYMPHOCYTE PREDOMINANT HODGKIN LYMPHOMA

Differential Diagnosis

(Left) Lymphocyte-rich classical Hodgkin lymphoma (LRCHL). A Reed-Sternberg cell ⇨ is CD45(-) whereas the surrounding small lymphocytes ⇨ are CD45/LCA(+). CD45 is almost always negative in classical Hodgkin lymphoma. (Right) LRCHL involving lymph node. In situ hybridization for EBV encoded RNA (EBER) highlights HRS cells. Approximately 20-40% of cases of LRCHL are EBV(+).

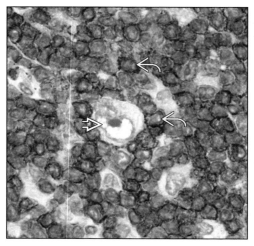
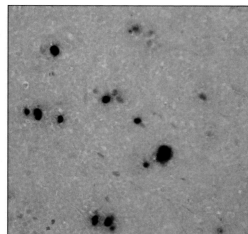

(Left) T-cell/histiocyte-rich large B-cell lymphoma (THRLBCL), involving lymph node. Diffuse infiltrate with large neoplastic cells ⇨ are scattered in a background of abundant small lymphocytes and histiocytes. (Right) THRLBCL involving lymph node. The neoplastic cells are large with prominent nucleoli ⇨ that may mimic HRS cells. Note numerous histiocytes ⇨ in the background.

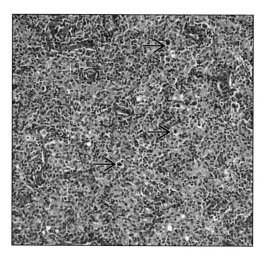
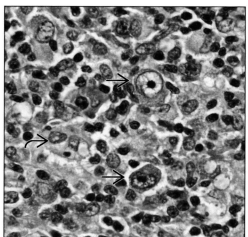

(Left) T-cell/histiocyte-rich large B-cell lymphoma (THRLBCL). Large cells are CD20(+) ⇨. The majority of cells in the background are CD20(-) and probably correspond to T cells or histiocytes. (Right) THRLBCL involving lymph node. The background is composed of abundant T cells ⇨ highlighted with CD3 that almost obscure scattered large neoplastic cells ⇨.

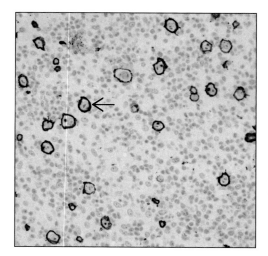
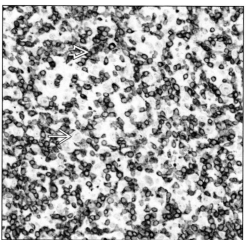

Differential Diagnosis

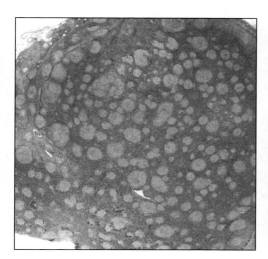
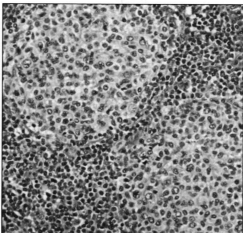

(Left) Follicular lymphoma involving lymph node. Unlike the nodules of NLPHL, the nodules of follicular lymphoma are smaller, more sharply delineated, and often lack mantle zones. *(Right)* Follicular lymphoma involving lymph node. Two neoplastic follicles are shown that are composed of centrocytes with fewer centroblasts. No lymphocyte predominant (LP) cells are identified in follicular lymphoma.

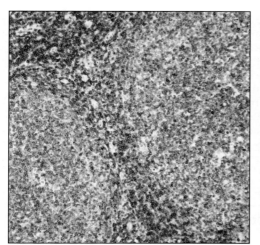
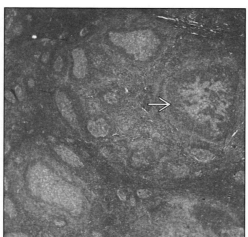

(Left) Follicular lymphoma involving lymph node. Two Bcl-2(+) neoplastic follicles are shown. *(Right)* Progressive transformation of germinal centers involving lymph node. The follicles are large and irregular with prominent germinal centers. Mantle zone lymphocytes infiltrate into germinal centers, imparting an irregular outline to the germinal centers at low-power magnification ➡.

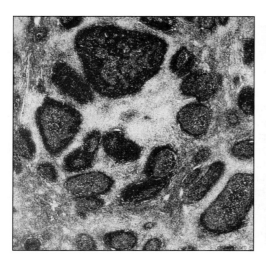
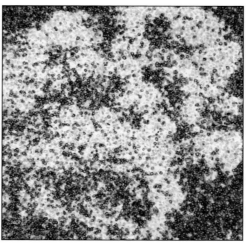

(Left) Progressive transformation of germinal centers involving lymph node. The follicles are composed of many CD20(+) B cells. The immunostain also highlights the variable, large size of transformed follicles. *(Right)* Progressive transformation of germinal centers involving lymph node. The reactive germinal center B cells in the transformed follicle are Bcl-2(-), whereas mantle zone B and T cells are Bcl-2(+).

LYMPHOCYTE-RICH CLASSICAL HODGKIN LYMPHOMA

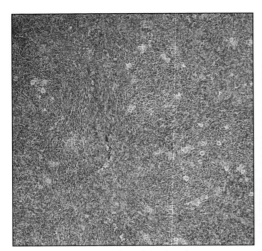

Lymphocyte-rich classical Hodgkin lymphoma (LRCHL), nodular variant, involving lymph node. The nodules are composed of many small lymphocytes and scattered Hodgkin and Reed-Sternberg (HRS) cells.

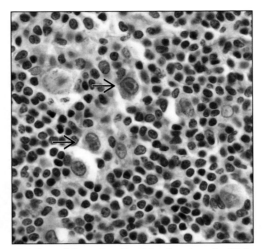

LRCHL, nodular variant, involving lymph node. High-power magnification shows HRS cells ➜ in a background of numerous small lymphocytes.

TERMINOLOGY

Abbreviations
- Lymphocyte-rich classical Hodgkin lymphoma (LRCHL)

Synonyms
- Follicular Hodgkin lymphoma
- Follicular Hodgkin disease

Definitions
- LRCHL is type of classic Hodgkin lymphoma (CHL) in which small reactive lymphocytes associated with Hodgkin and Reed-Sternberg (HRS) cells predominate
  - Neutrophils and eosinophils are rare or absent in background
  - 2 variants: Nodular and diffuse

ETIOLOGY/PATHOGENESIS

Postulated Normal Counterpart
- LRCHL may be derived from B cells in outer zone of reactive germinal centers
  - Large cells in outer zone of reactive germinal centers have immunophenotype similar to HRS cells
    - CD30(+), OCT2(+), BOB1(+), Bcl-6(+/-)
- Large cells surrounded by T-cell rosettes, as can occur in nodular lymphocyte predominant (NLP) HL
  - T cells are PD-1(+), CD57(+)

Tumorigenesis
- **HRS cells are derived from defective germinal center B cells with abnormal B-cell transcriptional program**
  - HRS cells show no immunoglobulin expression
    - Epigenetic silencing of immunoglobulin heavy chain gene (*IgH*) promoters
    - Impaired activation of Ig promoters & enhancers

- In LRCHL, B-cell transcription of HRS cells is less abnormal than in other types of CHL
  - Intermediate between NLPHL and CHL
- **NF-κB is activated in HRS cells of many cases of CHL including LRCHL**
  - c-Rel nuclear accumulation may be responsible for malignant transformation of B cells
- **HRS cells regulate host response**
  - Through expression &/or secretion of chemokines and surface ligands
  - Interplay of HRS cells and reactive cells determines tumor growth and local and systemic symptoms

CLINICAL ISSUES

Epidemiology
- Incidence
  - 4-5% of all cases of Hodgkin lymphoma
- Age
  - Most common in middle-aged persons (median age: 43 years)
- Gender
  - Male to female ratio ~ 2:1

Presentation
- Presentation of patients with LRCHL is similar to patients with NLPHL
  - B symptoms in ~ 10% of patents with LRCHL
    - Less frequent compared with other types of CHL
  - Stage I or II disease in ~ 70% of patients
  - Peripheral lymph node involvement is typical
    - Especially supradiaphragmatic lymph nodes
  - Mediastinal involvement is uncommon
    - In ~ 15% of patients; typically not bulky
  - Visceral organ involvement is relatively rare
    - Extranodal sites include: Lungs (4%), skeleton (3%), bone marrow (2%), and liver (2%)
- Although CHL is uncommon in Waldeyer ring, LRCHL is a common type in this location

LYMPHOCYTE-RICH CLASSICAL HODGKIN LYMPHOMA

Key Facts

Terminology
- Type of CHL in which small reactive lymphocytes predominate and are associated with HRS cells

Clinical Issues
- 4-5% of CHL cases
- Stage I or II disease; B symptoms uncommon
- Peripheral lymph nodes
- Survival curves of patients with LRCHL similar to patients with CHL
  - Early relapses followed by plateau
  - Unlike NLPHL patients who have late relapses without plateau

Microscopic Pathology
- Nodular variant
  - Lymph node replaced by large, often vague nodules

- Nodules are composed of expanded mantle zone small lymphocytes
- Diffuse variant, uncommon
  - Cytologic composition is similar to that seen in nodules of nodular variant

Ancillary Tests
- HRS cells have immunophenotype that supports CHL
- Small lymphocytes in background have immunophenotype of mantle zone B cells
- Loose FDC meshworks underlying nodules

Top Differential Diagnoses
- NLPHL
- Nodular sclerosis HL
- T-cell/histiocyte-rich large B-cell lymphoma
- Small B-cell lymphomas

Natural History
- Survival curves of patients with LRCHL similar to patients with CHL
  - Early relapses followed by plateau
  - Unlike patients with NLPHL who have early and late relapses without plateau

Treatment
- Drugs
  - Various chemotherapy regimens have been used for patients with LRCHL; most common are
    - Doxorubicin, bleomycin, vinblastine, and dacarbazine (ABVD) or rituximab + ABVD
    - Bleomycin, etoposide, doxorubicin, cyclophosphamide, vincristine, procarbazine, and prednisone (BEACOPP)
- Radiation
  - Patients with early and intermediate-stage disease
    - Extended-field or involved-field radiotherapy plus chemotherapy
    - Radiation alone for rare early localized disease
  - Patients with advanced-stage disease
    - Local radiotherapy to debulk tumor and for residual disease, in addition to chemotherapy

Prognosis
- Good to excellent with current treatment regimens
  - 95% complete remission rate; 17% relapse rate
  - However, not significantly better than other types of CHL that are stage-comparable
- Small subset of patients with LRCHL do poorly; fatalities due to
  - Relapsed/progressive disease ~ 9%; 2nd malignancies ~ 4%

IMAGE FINDINGS

Radiographic Findings
- Peripheral lymphadenopathy
- PET/CT scan useful for staging and helpful to assess therapeutic response

MICROSCOPIC PATHOLOGY

Histologic Features
- Nodular variant
  - Lymph node is replaced by large, often vague nodules
  - Nodules are composed of expanded mantle zone small lymphocytes
    - Small, compact, often eccentric germinal centers present in subset of cases
    - Histiocytes are present; relatively infrequent compared with lymphocytes
    - Plasma cells uncommon or absent within nodules
    - No eosinophils or neutrophils within nodules
  - Loose follicular dendritic cell (FDC) meshworks underlying nodules
    - Highlighted by FDC markers, such as CD21, CD23, and CD35
  - HRS cells are scattered among small lymphocytes
    - Predominantly found within expanded mantle zones
    - Most HRS cells have classical cytologic features
    - Subset of HRS cells can resemble lymphocyte-predominant (LP) cells seen in NLPHL
  - Eosinophils and neutrophils can be present around nodules; usually infrequent
- Diffuse variant
  - Uncommon compared with nodular variant
  - Diffuse replacement of lymph node architecture
  - Cytologic composition is similar to that seen in nodules of nodular variant

Cytologic Features
- Fine needle aspiration smears show small lymphocytes and HRS cells
  - Diagnosis of CHL can be established
  - Difficult to establish specific type of LRCHL by smear examination
- Possible to diagnose specific type of LRCHL if clot specimen contains tissue fragments of adequate size

LYMPHOCYTE-RICH CLASSICAL HODGKIN LYMPHOMA

ANCILLARY TESTS

Immunohistochemistry
- HRS cells have immunophenotype that supports CHL
  - CD15(+/-), CD30(+), CD45/LCA(-)
- Small lymphocytes in background have immunophenotype of mantle zone B cells
  - CD19(+), CD20(+), pax-5(+), IgD(+), IgM(+)
- LRCHL has some features intermediate between CHL and NLPHL
  - Features of HRS cells closer to LP cells of NLPHL
    - ~ 50-60% (+) for OCT1, OCT2, and BOB1
    - Bright pax-5(+/-); CD20(+) in ~ 30% of cases
    - Bcl-6(+) in 30% of cases
  - Features of HRS cells closer to typical cells of CHL
    - CD15(+/-), CD30(+), MUM1(+), CD45/LCA(-)
    - Expression of nuclear Rel, Rel-B, p-50, and TRAF1 consistent with NF-κB activation
    - EBV-LMP1(+) in ~ 40% of cases; EMA usually (-)
  - Microenvironment of LRCHL is similar to NLPHL
    - Numerous small B cells in background
    - FDC networks in tumor nodules
    - T cells form rosettes around HRS cells: Often PD-1(+), CD57(+), &/or CD3(+)

Flow Cytometry
- Numerous polytypic B cells
- Mature T cells with normal immunophenotype

In Situ Hybridization
- EBER(+) in HRS cells in ~ 40% of cases

PCR
- Monoclonal *Ig* gene rearrangements shown by single-cell PCR of HRS cells

DIFFERENTIAL DIAGNOSIS

Nodular Lymphocyte Predominant Hodgkin Lymphoma (NLPHL)
- NLPHL and LRCHL can closely resemble each other
- Immunohistochemical analysis is required to distinguish these entities
- LP cells of NLPHL are
  - CD45/LCA(+), CD20(+), OCT2(+), BOB1(+)
  - J chain(+), Bcl-6(+), CD30(-), CD15(-), EBER(-)
- T cells commonly form rosettes around LP cells
  - T cells have follicular T-helper cell immunophenotype
    - CD3(+), CD4(+), CD57(+), PD-1(+)

Nodular Sclerosis Hodgkin Lymphoma (NSHL)
- Some NSHL cases can exhibit prominent mantle zones with HRS cells
- Cytologic composition mixed: Granulocytes and plasma cells usually positive
- Nodules are surrounded by thick fibrous bands; polarizable

T-cell/Histiocyte-rich Large B-cell Lymphoma (TCHRLBCL)
- LRCHL and TCHRLBCL can closely resemble each other histologically
- TCHRLBCL has background composed of abundant small T cells and histiocytes
  - Small B cells are often absent in TCHRLBCL
- Neoplastic cells are CD45/LCA(+), CD20(+), CD15(-)

Small B-cell Lymphomas
- LRCHL can mimic small B-cell lymphomas including
  - Mantle cell lymphoma
  - Marginal zone lymphoma
  - Follicular lymphoma
  - Chronic lymphocytic leukemia/small lymphocytic lymphoma
- No HRS cells in small B-cell lymphomas
- Immunophenotype helpful in differential diagnosis
  - Small B-cell lymphomas are monotypic Ig(+)
  - CD5, CD10, CD23, Bcl-6, and Cyclin-D1 are useful for defining specific types

Reactive Paracortical Immunoblastic Hyperplasia
- Can mimic diffuse variant of LRCHL
  - Immunoblasts are CD30(+), CD45/LCA(+), CD15(-)

SELECTED REFERENCES

1. Muenst S et al: Increased programmed death-1+ tumor-infiltrating lymphocytes in classical Hodgkin lymphoma substantiate reduced overall survival. Hum Pathol. 40(12):1715-22, 2009
2. Nam-Cha SH et al: Lymphocyte-rich classical Hodgkin's lymphoma: distinctive tumor and microenvironment markers. Mod Pathol. 22(8):1006-15, 2009
3. de Jong D et al: Lymphocyte-rich classical Hodgkin lymphoma (LRCHL): clinico-pathological characteristics and outcome of a rare entity. Ann Oncol. 17(1):141-5, 2006
4. Shimabukuro-Vornhagen A et al: Lymphocyte-rich classical Hodgkin's lymphoma: clinical presentation and treatment outcome in 100 patients treated within German Hodgkin's Study Group trials. J Clin Oncol. 2005 Aug 20;23(24):5739-45. Epub 2005 Jul 11. Erratum in: J Clin Oncol. 24(14):2220, 2006
5. Quiñones-Avila Mdel P et al: Hodgkin lymphoma involving Waldeyer ring: a clinicopathologic study of 22 cases. Am J Clin Pathol. 123(5):651-6, 2005
6. Bräuninger A et al: Typing the histogenetic origin of the tumor cells of lymphocyte-rich classical Hodgkin's lymphoma in relation to tumor cells of classical and lymphocyte-predominance Hodgkin's lymphoma. Cancer Res. 63(7):1644-51, 2003
7. Diehl V et al: Clinical presentation, course, and prognostic factors in lymphocyte-predominant Hodgkin's disease and lymphocyte-rich classical Hodgkin's disease: report from the European Task Force on Lymphoma Project on Lymphocyte-Predominant Hodgkin's Disease. J Clin Oncol. 17(3):776-83, 1999

LYMPHOCYTE-RICH CLASSICAL HODGKIN LYMPHOMA

Microscopic and Immunohistochemical Features

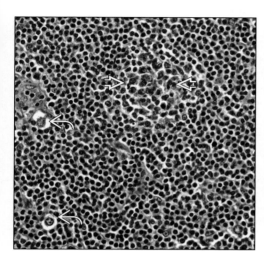
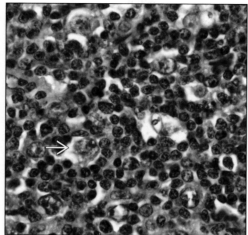

(Left) Lymphocyte-rich classical Hodgkin lymphoma (LRCHL), nodular variant, involving lymph node. A small reactive germinal center ⇨ and scattered HRS cells ⇗ are present in an expanded mantle zone composed of small lymphocytes. (Right) LRCHL, nodular variant, involving lymph node. High-power magnification shows HRS cells. One HRS cell ⇨ shows a folded nucleus that mimics a LP cell of nodular lymphocyte predominant Hodgkin lymphoma.

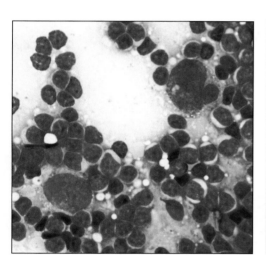
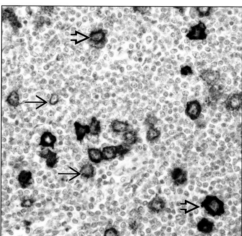

(Left) Touch imprint of a lymph node biopsy specimen involved by lymphocyte-rich classical Hodgkin lymphoma (LRCHL). Large HRS cells are present in a background of numerous small lymphocytes. (Right) LRCHL, nodular variant, involving lymph node. CD15 highlights HRS cells ⇨. Note that scattered histiocytes in the background are also CD15(+) ⇨.

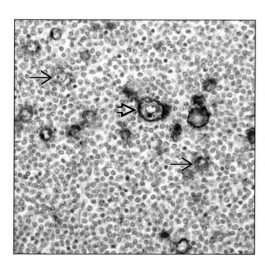
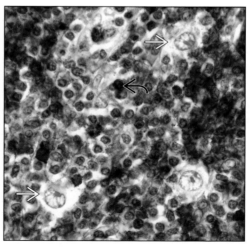

(Left) Lymphocyte-rich classical Hodgkin lymphoma, nodular variant, involving lymph node. CD30 highlights HRS cells ⇨. Note that activated intermediate-size immunoblasts ⇨ in the background are also CD30(+). (Right) LRCHL, nodular variant, involving lymph node. CD45/LCA highlights most of the cells in the background, which are lymphocytes ⇨. The HRS cells ⇨ in LRCHL are CD45(-).

LYMPHOCYTE-RICH CLASSICAL HODGKIN LYMPHOMA

Microscopic and Immunohistochemical Features

(Left) Lymphocyte-rich classical Hodgkin lymphoma (LRCHL), nodular variant, involving lymph node. CD20 shows that most cells in the background are B cells. The background cells of LRCHL are mostly mantle zone B lymphocytes. *(Right)* LRCHL, nodular variant, involving lymph node. CD3 immunohistochemistry highlights small lymphocytes forming a rosette ➡ around a Reed-Sternberg cell, similar to what occurs in nodular lymphocyte predominant Hodgkin lymphoma (NLPHL).

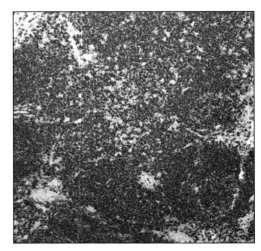

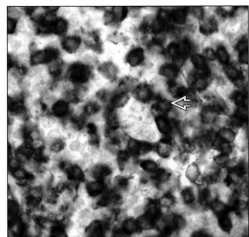

(Left) Lymphocyte-rich classical Hodgkin lymphoma, nodular variant, involving lymph node. T-cell rosettes around HRS cells are CD57(+). *(Right)* A different case of LRCH, nodular variant involving lymph node. Portions of multiple vague nodules ➡ can be seen in this field.

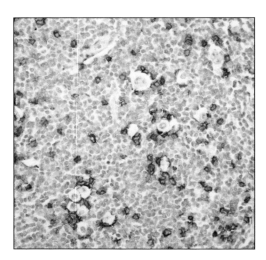

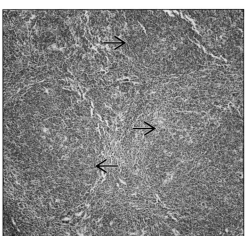

(Left) Lymphocyte-rich classical Hodgkin lymphoma, nodular variant, involving lymph node. Immunostain with anti-CD21 antibody highlights many follicular dendritic cell networks within tumor nodules. *(Right)* LRCHL, nodular variant, involving lymph node. Large HRS cells are strongly CD30(+). Smaller immunoblasts in the background are also CD30(+).

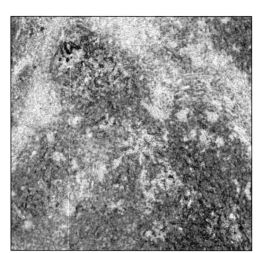

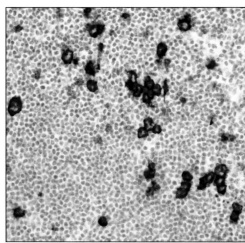

Immunohistochemical Features and Differential Diagnosis

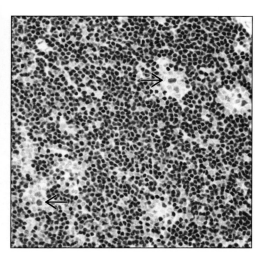

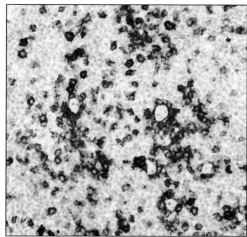

(Left) Lymphocyte-rich classical Hodgkin lymphoma (LRCHL), nodular variant, involving lymph node. Numerous small lymphocytes in the background are pax-5(+) B cells. Scattered HRS ⊇ cells are more dimly pax-5(+) and are surrounded by rosettes of T cells that are negative in this immunostain. (Right) LRCHL, nodular variant, involving lymph node. T-cell rosettes surrounding HRS cells are strongly CD43(+) in this field.

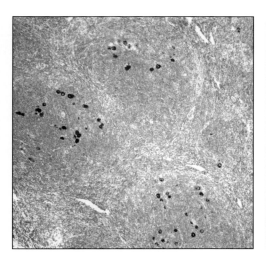

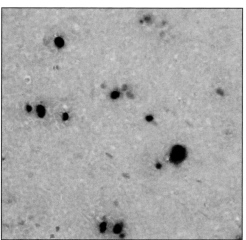

(Left) Lymphocyte-rich classical Hodgkin lymphoma, nodular variant, involving lymph node. The HRS cells are strongly EBV-LMP1(+). (Right) Lymphocyte-rich classical Hodgkin lymphoma (LRCHL), nodular variant, involving lymph node. The HRS cells in a nodule of tumor are EBER(+).

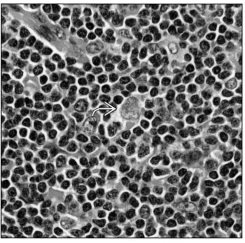

(Left) Nodular lymphocyte predominant Hodgkin lymphoma (NLPHL) involving lymph node. Low-magnification view shows a vaguely nodular pattern, mimicking a nodular variant of LRCHL. (Right) NLPHL involving lymph node. LP (formerly known as L&H) cells are often large with multilobated nuclei resembling popcorn, vesicular chromatin, and small distinct nucleoli ⊇. However, occasionally, LP cells can mimic HRS cells with prominent eosinophilic nucleoli.

Differential Diagnosis

(Left) Nodular lymphocyte predominant Hodgkin lymphoma (NLPHL) involving lymph node. The nodular pattern of NLPHL is better appreciated using anti-CD20 immunohistochemistry. The nodules are usually rich in B lymphocytes. *(Right)* NLPHL involving lymph node. The background shows that small lymphocytes ⊳ and LP cells are CD20(+) ⇨.

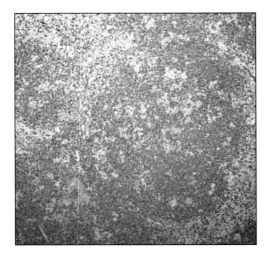 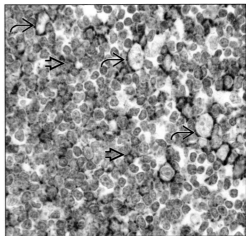

(Left) Nodular lymphocyte predominant Hodgkin lymphoma involving lymph node. CD30 immunohistochemistry highlights intermediate-sized immunoblasts ⇨ in this case. Note that LP cells ⇨ are CD30(-). *(Right)* NLPHL involving lymph node. CD3(+) T cells form rosettes around LP cells.

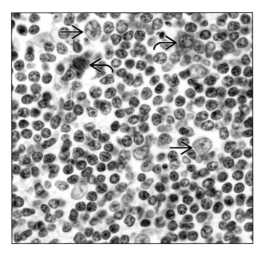 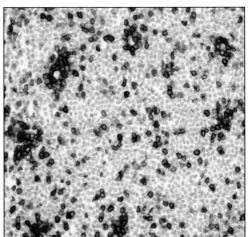

(Left) Chronic lymphocytic leukemia/small lymphocytic lymphoma (CLL/SLL) involving lymph node shows poorly circumscribed, large proliferation centers that can mimic nodules of LRCHL. However, proliferation centers do not contain HRS cells. *(Right)* CLL/SLL involving lymph node. This proliferation center contains small lymphocytes and scattered large paraimmunoblasts ⇨ with round nuclei and prominent nucleoli. No HRS cells are present in CLL/SLL.

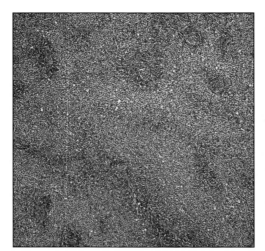 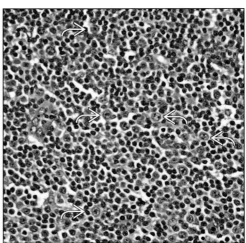

Differential Diagnosis

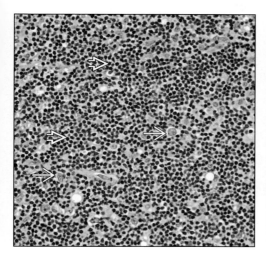

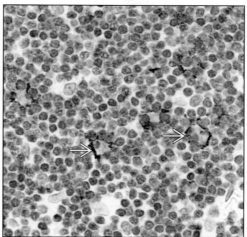

(Left) *T-cell/histiocyte-rich large B-cell lymphoma (TCHRLBCL) involving lymph node shows a diffuse growth pattern composed of few large neoplastic cells* ⮕ *surrounded by reactive lymphocytes* ⮞ *and fewer histiocytes.* **(Right)** *TCHRLBCL involving lymph node. Immunohistochemistry for CD20 shows that the large neoplastic cells* ⮕ *are strongly positive. Most of the small lymphocytes in the background are CD20(-) and represent reactive small T cells.*

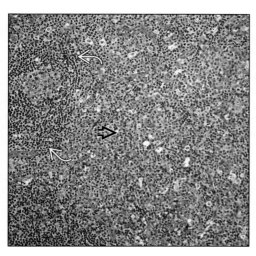

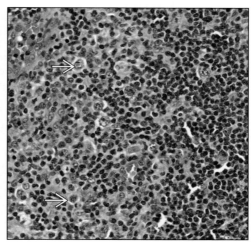

(Left) *Autoimmune lymphoproliferative syndrome. This lymph node shows paracortical expansion* ⮞ *with increased immunoblasts and a residual lymphoid follicle with regressive changes and a preserved mantle zone* ⮞. **(Right)** *Paracortical/interfollicular immunoblastic hyperplasia involving lymph node. Scattered and increased immunoblasts* ⮕ *are present that can resemble HRS cells. Immunoblasts are CD30(+), like HRS cells, but are CD15(-) and CD45/LCA(+).*

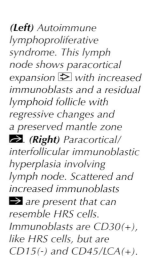

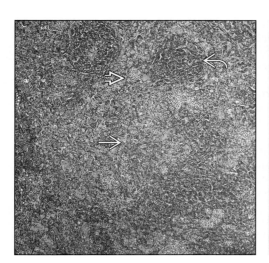

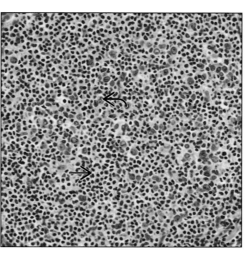

(Left) *Nodal marginal zone lymphoma (NMZL) in lymph node. This case shows an expanded marginal zone* ⮞ *with many monocytoid cells as well as an expanded interfollicular region* ⮕. *An involuted follicle is present* ⮞. **(Right)** *NMZL involving lymph node. This case shows abundant interfollicular monocytoid lymphocytes* ⮕ *with clear cytoplasm admixed with scattered large cells* ⮞. *The large cells can mimic HRS cells of LRCHL; however, they are located outside mantle zones.*

NODULAR SCLEROSIS HODGKIN LYMPHOMA

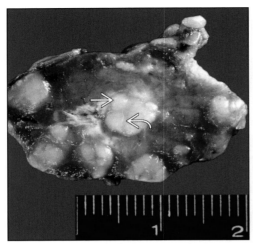

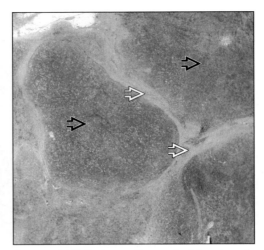

Lymph node partially effaced by nodular sclerosis Hodgkin lymphoma (NSHL). Multiple nodules ➡ are surrounded by thick fibrous bands ➡.

A case of NSHL shows effacement of lymph node architecture by neoplastic nodules ⊅ surrounded by dense fibrous bands ⊅.

TERMINOLOGY

Abbreviations
- Nodular sclerosis Hodgkin lymphoma (NSHL)

Synonyms
- Nodular sclerosis classical Hodgkin lymphoma
- Nodular sclerosis (or sclerosing) Hodgkin disease

Definitions
- Classical Hodgkin lymphoma (CHL) is a lymphoid neoplasm composed of Hodgkin and Reed-Sternberg (HRS) cells in a variable inflammatory background
- Nodular sclerosis is a type of CHL composed of lacunar-type HRS cells and inflammatory cells forming nodules surrounded by fibrous bands

ETIOLOGY/PATHOGENESIS

Infectious Agents
- Epstein-Barr virus (EBV) is present in HRS cells in ~ 20% of cases and has a probable pathogenetic role
  - Expression of EBNA1 and latent membrane proteins LMP1 and LMP2a
    - LMP1 mimics active CD40 receptor
    - LMP2a mimics B-cell receptor

Pathogenesis
- HRS cells arise from late germinal center or early post-germinal center B-cells that
  - Have undergone immunoglobulin (Ig) gene rearrangements with somatic mutations
  - Have undergone crippling Ig mutations in subset of cases
  - Lack B-cell antigen receptors
- HRS cells lose much of normal B-cell immunophenotype due to
  - Severe impairment of transcription factor network regulating B-cell gene expression
  - Low or undetectable levels of transcription factors: OCT2, BOB1, PU.1, and early B-cell factor (EBF)
    - Leads to low level of Ig transcripts in HRS cells
    - Made worse by epigenetic silencing (promoter hypermethylation) of *Ig* transcription
  - Impaired function of early B-cell development transcription factors: pax-5, E2A ,and EBF
    - pax-5 and E2A are expressed in HRS cells
    - Aberrant overexpression of NOTCH1, ABF1, and ID2 inhibit overall B-cell development
    - Also leads to decreased or absent expression of CD19, CD20, and CD79a
- Overall, these abnormalities physiologically should lead to apoptosis
  - However, HRS cells are rescued from undergoing apoptosis
- Development of antiapoptotic mechanisms to achieve survival
  - Inhibition of executors of apoptosis by expression of X-linked inhibitor of apoptosis (XIAP)
  - Expression of FLICE-like inhibitory protein
  - Deregulation of Bcl-2 family proteins
  - Protection from Fas-induced cell death
  - Deregulation of signaling pathways
    - Poorly understood causes
    - Include paracrine and autocrine feedback loops in addition to genetic lesions of HRS cells
    - Constitutive activation of NF-κB pathway: Canonical and alternative pathways
    - Activation of Janus kinase/signal transducer and activator of transcription (JAK/STAT) pathway
- Role of microenvironment
  - Reactive cellular infiltrate is induced, in part, by HRS cells
    - Protects HRS cells from apoptosis
    - Suppresses T-cell and NK-cell immune response against HRS cells
  - HRS cells produce a variety of molecules

NODULAR SCLEROSIS HODGKIN LYMPHOMA

Key Facts

Terminology
- Nodular sclerosis is type of CHL composed of lacunar-type HRS cells and inflammatory cells forming nodules surrounded by fibrous bands

Etiology/Pathogenesis
- Hodgkin and Reed-Sternberg (HRS) cells arise from late germinal center B cells
- *Ig* gene rearrangements positive; many defects in B-cell differentiation

Clinical Issues
- Represents ~ 70% of CHL cases in developed countries
- 15-34 years; mediastinal or cervical lymph nodes
- Current chemotherapy ± radiation can cure many patients

Microscopic Pathology
- Lymph node architecture effaced by nodules surrounded by broad collagen bands
- HRS cells have features of lacunar cells
- Background of inflammatory cells

Ancillary Tests
- CD30(+) in > 95%; CD15(+) ~ 70-80% of cases
- pax-5(dim +) ~ 90%, CD20(variably +) ~ 20%
- EBV(+) ~ 20%, CD45/LCA(-)

Top Differential Diagnoses
- Primary mediastinal large B-cell lymphoma
- B-cell lymphoma, unclassifiable, with features intermediate between DLBCL and CHL
- Lymphocyte-rich classical Hodgkin lymphoma
- Nodular lymphocyte predominant HL

- Th2 cytokines, chemokines, growth factors, and their receptors
  - IL-1, IL-10, TNF-α, TGF-β, and eotaxin
  - Most cytokines signal via JAK/STAT pathway
- HRS cells in NSHL show increased production of IL-13
  - May be responsible for broad bands of birefringent collagen

Possible Origin
- Thymic B cell in patients with mediastinal involvement

CLINICAL ISSUES

Epidemiology
- Incidence
  - Represents ~ 70% of CHL cases in developed countries
    - Relatively less frequent in underdeveloped nations
- Age
  - Peak at 15-34 years
- Gender
  - Slightly more prevalent in women
- Ethnicity
  - More common in whites than in African-Americans or Latino-Americans

Site
- Mediastinal or cervical lymph nodes

Presentation
- Mediastinal involvement in ~ 80% of cases
  - Bulky disease in ~ 50% of cases
- B symptoms in ~ 40% of cases
- Associated predominantly with clinical stage II

Treatment
- Current chemotherapy &/or radiation can cure disease in many patients
- Chemotherapy with or without radiation

- ABVD: Adriamycin (doxorubicin), bleomycin, vinblastine, and dacarbazine
- Chemotherapy alone or reduced cycles for early stage NSHL

Prognosis
- > 90% survival at 5 years in patients with early stage disease
- Therapy modifies prognosis
- Adverse prognostic factors
  - Advanced stage
  - Massive mediastinal involvement
  - Older age, usually > 45 years
  - Male gender
- Histologic grading of NSHL is predictive but less important than clinical factors
- Recurrent disease with multiple adverse factors results in 56% overall survival at 5 years
- Deaths mostly related to 2nd malignancy, therapeutic toxicity, and older age

IMAGE FINDINGS

General Features
- Current imaging techniques have made staging laparotomy obsolete

MACROSCOPIC FEATURES

General Features
- Nodular surface; nodules often surrounded by bands of fibrosis

MICROSCOPIC PATHOLOGY

Histologic Features
- Lymph node architecture effaced by neoplastic nodules surrounded by broad collagen bands
  - Originate in thickened capsule
  - Dissect lymph node into nodules of various sizes

- o Lacunar cells formed due to retraction artifact of HRS cells in formalin-fixed tissue sections
  - ▪ Nuclei tend to be lobated with smaller lobes, less prominent nucleoli than HRS of other CHL types
  - o Number of HRS cells and lacunar cells highly variable
    - ▪ Lacunar cells may form cell aggregates associated with necrosis and histiocytes
- Background of inflammatory cells
  - o Eosinophils, histiocytes, &/or neutrophils are often numerous
    - ▪ Occasional eosinophilic abscesses are noted

Cytologic Features
- Lacunar cells in an inflammatory background can be appreciated in fine needle aspiration smears
  - o Immunophenotype can be assessed in cell block

Syncytial Variant of NSHL
- Confluent aggregates of lacunar cells
- Cohesive appearance may resemble large cell non-Hodgkin lymphoma or metastatic carcinoma
- Limited number of birefringent collagen bands and occasional necrosis

Grading of NSHL
- British National Lymphoma Investigation (BNLI) system developed in 1989
  - o Based on amount of HRS cells, anaplasia of HRS cells, and fibrosis features
    - ▪ Grade 1 NS: Scattered HRS cells in lymphocyte-rich or mixed cellular infiltrate
    - ▪ Grade 2 NS: Aggregates of HRS cells or pleomorphic cytology in > 25% of nodules
    - ▪ Grade showed differences in outcome for patients with advanced disease only
    - ▪ Lack of prognostic significance with current chemotherapeutic regimens
- German Hodgkin Lymphoma Study Group system reported in 2003
  - o Similar to BNLI system but also includes tissue eosinophilia (> 5% of cell infiltrate)
  - o Controversial results; prognostic value for intermediate and high-stage disease

Extranodal Involvement of NSHL
- Spleen
  - o ~ 30% of patients with NSHL
  - o Usually presents as solitary or multiple nodules
  - o Tumor nodules surrounded by sclerosis that effaces splenic architecture
    - ▪ Incipient lesions are periarteriolar or at periphery of marginal zone
    - ▪ Nodules of NSHL in spleen do not necessarily show fibrous bands
- Liver
  - o ~ 10% of patients with NSHL; usually microscopic clusters
    - ▪ Mainly detected in wedge biopsies of staging laparotomy (procedure now obsolete)
  - o Infiltrates with preferential portal or portal to central vein distribution

- ▪ Associated with constitutional symptoms and biochemical abnormalities
- o Sometimes nondiagnostic inflammatory changes, without HRS cells
- Bone marrow (BM)
  - o ~ 5-10% of cases of NSHL, up to 70% in necropsies
  - o Can be detected during staging of CHL or may be presenting finding
    - ▪ CHL presenting in BM usually manifests with cytopenias
    - ▪ Unlikely involvement in young patients with normal blood counts and low-stage disease
    - ▪ Likely involvement in older patients with cytopenias, B symptoms, and high-stage disease
  - o Variable extent of involvement, amount of neoplastic cells, and stromal changes
    - ▪ Eosinophilia may be prominent including microabscesses
    - ▪ Diffuse stromal fibrosis and histiocytic infiltrate may obscure HRS cells
- Thymus
  - o NSHL is type of CHL most frequently associated with mediastinal involvement
  - o Thymus is commonly involved and may be cystic
  - o In some cases, granulomatous inflammation can obscure neoplastic cells

ANCILLARY TESTS

Immunohistochemistry
- CD30(+) in > 95%; CD15(+) in 70-80% of cases
  - o Characteristic membranous pattern with accentuation in Golgi area
- pax-5(dim +) ~ 90%, CD20(variably +) ~ 20%, CD79a(+) ~ 10-20%
- Ki-67(+), p53(+), MUM1(+)
- CCL17(+), Fascin(+/-), Bcl-2(+/-)
- CD45/LCA(-), EMA(-), Ig(-), clusterin(-)
- OCT2(-/+), BOB.1(-/+), PU.1(-)
- EBV(+) with latency type II pattern in ~ 20% of cases
  - o LMP-1(+), LMP2a(+), EBNA1(+), EBNA2(-)
- T-cell antigens can be aberrantly expressed by HRS cells in up to 15% of cases
- Background CD4(+) T cells form rosettes around HRS cells

Flow Cytometry
- Polytypic B cells and T cells with normal immunophenotype, CD4:CD8 ratio often elevated
- Useful to exclude non-Hodgkin lymphoma

Cytogenetics
- Data derived from HL cell lines and primary HRS cells
- Aneuploidy and hypertetraploidy
- Random numerical chromosomal aberrations

In Situ Hybridization
- EBER(+) in ~ 20% of cases

Array CGH
- Many recurrent chromosomal abnormalities
  - o Gains of 2p, 9q34, 12q13

- Losses of Xp21, 6q23, 13q22
- Amplification of 4p16, 4q23-24, 9p23-24

Molecular Genetics

- Monoclonal *Ig* gene rearrangements of HRS cells
- Rearranged *Ig* genes harbor somatic mutations in *IgH* variable regions
  - Rare (~ 2%) cases reported with monoclonal T-cell receptor gene rearrangements
    - Unclear if these cases are truly examples of CHL
- *REL* gene on 2p16 that encodes 1 component of NF-κB shows gains or amplifications in 50% of CHL
- Inactivating mutations of NF-κB inhibitor IκBα in 10-20% of CHL

Gene Expression Profiling

- Signature of NSHL shares features with primary mediastinal large B-cell lymphoma

DIFFERENTIAL DIAGNOSIS

Primary Mediastinal Large B-cell Lymphoma (PMBL)

- Nodal and soft tissue effacement
- Interstitial collagen deposition surrounding clusters or sheets of large lymphoma cells
  - Large cells often exhibit cytoplasmic retraction artifact
- Immunophenotype of neoplastic B cells
  - CD19(+), CD20(+), CD22(+), CD45/LCA(+), CD79a(+)
    - CD30(+/-) and often dim; MAL(+/-)
  - Surface Ig(-), CD10(-), CD15(-)

B-cell Lymphoma, Unclassifiable, with Features Intermediate Between DLBCL and CHL

- a.k.a. "gray zone lymphoma"
- Mostly located in mediastinum; men 20-40 years of age
- Morphologic &/or immunophenotypic overlap between DLBCL (often PMBL) and CHL
- Immunophenotype
  - CD45/LCA(+), CD20(+ often bright), CD15(+), CD30(+)

Lymphocyte-rich Classical Hodgkin Lymphoma (LRCHL)

- Usually nodular pattern; diffuse pattern uncommon
- Nodules composed mainly of small lymphocytes that represent expanded mantle zones
  - ± reactive germinal centers; often eccentrically located in nodules
- HRS cells located mainly within nodules
  - Some HRS cells may resemble LP cells of NLPHL cases
  - Background of small B lymphocytes; but no eosinophils or neutrophils
- Immunophenotype of HRS as seen in other types of CHL

Nodular Lymphocyte Predominant Hodgkin Lymphoma (NLPHL)

- Nodal architecture effaced by large nodules containing scattered LP cells
  - Nodules are not surrounded by birefringent collagen bands
- Immunophenotype of LP cells
  - CD20(+), CD45/LCA(+), CD79a(+)
  - pax-5(+), OCT2(+), BOB1(+), EMA(+/-)
  - CD15(-), EBV(-), CD30(-/+)
    - Scattered CD30(+) immunoblasts are usually present
- Background composed of many small B lymphocytes
- Small T lymphocytes can surround LP cells and appear as rosettes

Lymphocyte-depleted Hodgkin Lymphoma (LDHL)

- Rare subtype of CHL that has undergone extensive reclassification over the years
- Often associated with HIV-infected patients
- Histologic features
  - Diffuse replacement of architecture
  - Depletion of nonneoplastic lymphocytes
  - Variable numbers of HRS cells
    - Can be isolated or confluent, pleomorphic, sarcomatous, or multinucleated
  - ± thin, disorganized, nonbirefringent fibrosis without lacunar cells

Anaplastic Large Cell Lymphoma (ALCL), ALK(+)

- Rare variant is characterized by nodules surrounded by fibrous bands
- Common in adolescent and young adult males
- Immunophenotype
  - ALK(+); CD30(+) with membranous and paranuclear pattern
  - T-cell antigens(+), cytotoxic molecules(+), CD15(-), pax-5(-)
- Flow cytometry often shows aberrant T-cell immunophenotype
- Molecular studies usually show evidence of T-cell clonality

ALCL, ALK(-)

- Provisional WHO entity, histologically similar to ALCL, ALK(+)
- Peak incidence in adults aged 40-65 years
- Involves peripheral lymph nodes and extranodal sites
- Effacement by cohesive sheets of neoplastic cells
  - Partial nodal effacement reveals lymphoma cells within sinuses
- Immunophenotype
  - CD30(+) with membranous and paranuclear pattern
  - T-cell antigens(+), cytotoxic molecules(+/-)
  - CD15(-), pax-5(-), ALK(-)
- Flow cytometry often shows aberrant T-cell immunophenotype
- Molecular studies usually show evidence of T-cell clonality

NODULAR SCLEROSIS HODGKIN LYMPHOMA

Differential Diagnosis of Nodular Sclerosis Hodgkin lymphoma

	NSHL	MCHL	LDHL	LRCHL
Frequency of subtype	40-70%	20-25%	~ 1%	5%
Clinical Features				
Male to female ratio	1:1	2:1	4:1	2:1
Median age	15-34 years	38 years	57 years	30-50 years
Preferential sites	Mediastinal and cervical nodes	Peripheral nodes, spleen	Retroperitoneal and abdominal nodes, spleen, and bone marrow	Peripheral nodes
Stage at presentation	Stage II	Stage III or IV	Stage III or IV	Stage I or II
B symptoms	~ 40%	More common than other CHL subtypes	More common than other CHL subtypes	Rare
Histopathologic Features				
Architecture	Broad collagen bands surround cellular nodules	Diffuse growth pattern	Diffuse fibrosis and reticular variants	Nodular growth pattern more common; rare fibrosis
Cytologic features	Lacunar cells and mummified cells	Frequent HRS cells admixed with cellular inflammatory background	Many HRS cells admixed with a few inflammatory cells and a few lymphocytes	Few HRS cells in marginal and mantle zone surrounding small germinal centers
Special Markers*				
EBER association	10-40%	70%	75%	40%

LDHL = lymphocyte-depleted Hodgkin lymphoma (HL); MCHL = mixed cellularity HL; NSHL = nodular sclerosis HL; LRCHL = lymphocyte-rich classical Hodgkin lymphoma.
*Immunophenotype: All subtypes of classical HL share the following phenotype: CD30(+), CD15(+/-), pax-5(dim +), CD45/LCA(-).

Peripheral T-cell Lymphoma, Not Otherwise Specified

- Diffuse effacement; often many small reactive lymphocytes and eosinophils
- May have numerous highly atypical cells with HRS-like cells
- T-cell markers(+), CD15(-), CD30(-/+), pax-5(-)
- Flow cytometry often shows aberrant T-cell immunophenotype
- Molecular studies usually show evidence of T-cell clonality

Metastatic Carcinoma

- May present as neck lymphadenopathy and be clinically suggestive of lymphoma
- Some cases grow in nodular pattern and are associated with HRS-like cells, fibrosis, and inflammatory cells
- Cytokeratin(+), CD15(-), CD45/LCA(-), pax-5(-), EBV(-)
  - Nasopharyngeal carcinoma is usually EBV(+)

Primary Myelofibrosis

- Myeloproliferative neoplasm often associated with *JAK2* V617F mutation
- May resemble CHL because of presence of fibrosis admixed with large pleomorphic cells
- Bone marrow and hematologic findings may be necessary to establish diagnosis
  - Osteosclerosis, megakaryocytic atypia, and leukoerythroblastosis favor myelofibrosis
- Large cells in infiltrate are of myeloid, erythroid, or megakaryocytic lineage

SELECTED REFERENCES

1. Steidl C et al: Tumor-associated macrophages and survival in classic Hodgkin's lymphoma. N Engl J Med. 362(10):875-85, 2010
2. Eberle FC et al: Histopathology of Hodgkin's lymphoma. Cancer J. 15(2):129-37, 2009
3. Schmitz R et al: Pathogenesis of classical and lymphocyte-predominant Hodgkin lymphoma. Annu Rev Pathol. 4:151-74, 2009
4. Ma Y et al: The CD4+CD26- T-cell population in classical Hodgkin's lymphoma displays a distinctive regulatory T-cell profile. Lab Invest. 88(5):482-90, 2008
5. Fraga M et al: Diagnosis of Hodgkin's disease: an update on histopathological and immunophenotypical features. Histol Histopathol. 22(8):923-35, 2007
6. Savage KJ et al: The molecular signature of mediastinal large B-cell lymphoma differs from that of other diffuse large B-cell lymphomas and shares features with classical Hodgkin lymphoma. Blood. 102(12):3871-9, 2003
7. Rassidakis GZ et al: BCL-2 expression in Hodgkin and Reed-Sternberg cells of classical Hodgkin disease predicts a poorer prognosis in patients treated with ABVD or equivalent regimens. Blood. 100(12):3935-41, 2002
8. van Spronsen DJ et al: Disappearance of prognostic significance of histopathological grading of nodular sclerosing Hodgkin's disease for unselected patients, 1972-92. Br J Haematol. 96(2):322-7, 1997
9. Elenitoba-Johnson KS et al: P53 expression in Reed-Sternberg cells does not correlate with gene mutations in Hodgkin's disease. Am J Clin Pathol. 106(6):728-38, 1996
10. MacLennan KA et al: Diagnosis and grading of nodular sclerosing Hodgkin's disease: a study of 2190 patients. Int Rev Exp Pathol. 33:27-51, 1992
11. Urba WJ et al: Hodgkin's disease. N Engl J Med. 326(10):678-87, 1992

MIXED CELLULARITY HODGKIN LYMPHOMA

Microscopic Features

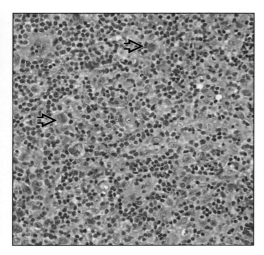
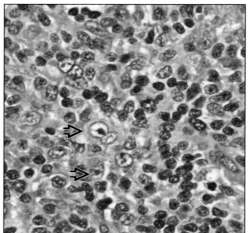

(Left) Mixed cellularity Hodgkin lymphoma (MCHL) involving lymph node shows that the architecture is effaced by a neoplastic proliferation composed of scattered HRS cells ⊳ admixed with inflammatory cells. (Right) Lymph node involved by MCHL shows a few scattered Hodgkin cells (mononuclear variant) ⊳ in a background of small lymphocytes, eosinophils, and histiocytes.

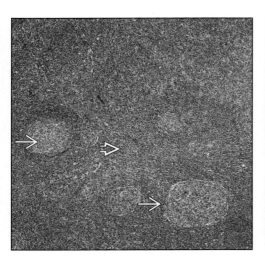
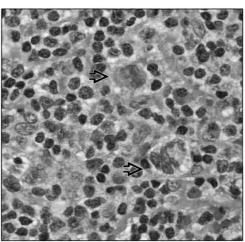

(Left) Mixed cellularity Hodgkin lymphoma (MCHL), interfollicular pattern. The overall nodal architecture is preserved. There is interfollicular expansion by MCHL ⊳ between reactive hyperplastic lymphoid follicles ➤. (Right) MCHL, interfollicular pattern, involving lymph node. Scattered HRS cells ⊳ in a background of small lymphocytes, histiocytes, and eosinophils are noted.

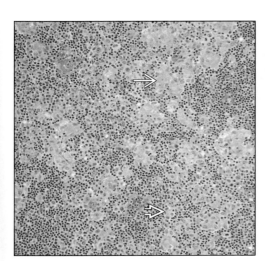
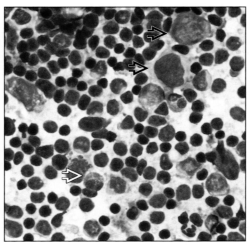

(Left) Lymph node involved by mixed cellularity Hodgkin lymphoma (MCHL) shows abundant histiocytes ➤ arranged as granulomas ➤ in the background. Increased histiocytes in classical Hodgkin lymphoma are associated with decreased disease-free survival. (Right) Touch imprint of a lymph node involved by MCHL. Scattered Hodgkin cells ⊳ are present in a mixed background of small lymphocytes, eosinophils ➤, and neutrophils.

MIXED CELLULARITY HODGKIN LYMPHOMA

Immunohistochemical Features and Ancillary Techniques

(Left) Mixed cellularity Hodgkin lymphoma (MCHL) involving lymph node. Immunohistochemistry for CD30 highlights many HRS ⇒ cells. (Right) MCHL involving lymph node. Immunohistochemistry for CD15 is dim positive →️ and highlights scattered HRS cells. In CHL, CD15 reactivity typically occurs with less intensity and in fewer cells than is observed with CD30.

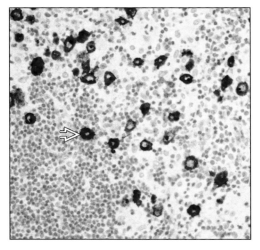
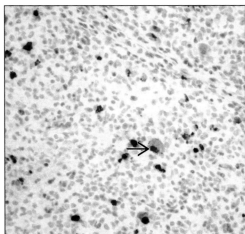

(Left) Mixed cellularity Hodgkin lymphoma (MCHL) involving lymph node. CD68 immunohistochemistry highlights abundant histiocytes in the background. (Right) MCHL involving lymph node. T-cell intracellular antigen-1 (TIA-1) immunohistochemistry highlights abundant cytotoxic lymphocytes in the background.

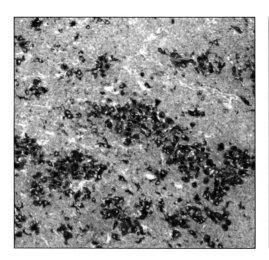
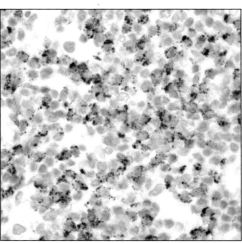

(Left) Mixed cellularity Hodgkin lymphoma (MCHL) involving lymph node. In situ hybridization for EBV encoded RNA (EBER) highlights the lymphoma cells. (Right) Gel electrophoresis of PCR products using primers specific for EBV type A in cases of CHL. The expected band size is 249 bp →️. Lanes 4, 5, 7, and 8 are cases of CHL that are positive. Lanes 3 and 6 (neither MCHL) are negative. Lanes 1 and 2 are negative and positive controls, respectively.

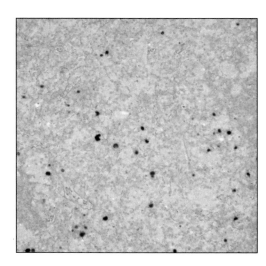
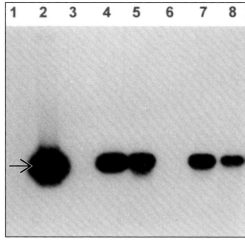

Differential Diagnosis

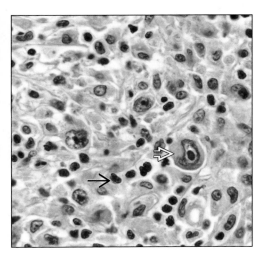

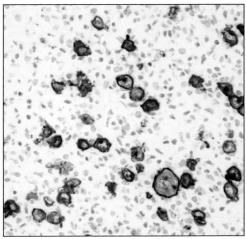

(Left) Lymphocyte-depleted Hodgkin lymphoma (LDHL) involving intraabdominal lymph node. Only scattered lymphocytes are noted ➡ in the background. Hodgkin and Reed-Sternberg (HRS) cells ⮕, the predominant cell in the infiltrate, are relatively abundant. *(Right)* LDHL involving intraabdominal lymph node. Immunohistochemical analysis for CD30 highlights many HRS cells.

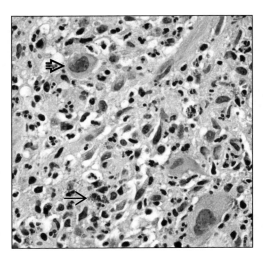

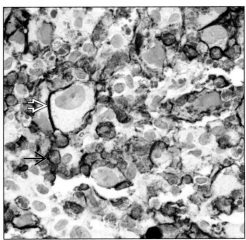

(Left) Anaplastic large cell lymphoma, ALK(-) shows abundant inflammatory cells ➡ and scattered large neoplastic cells ⮕, giving an overall resemblance to MCHL. *(Right)* ALCL, ALK(-) in which CD43 immunohistochemistry highlights large neoplastic cells ⮕ as well as smaller cells ➡ in the background. HRS cells of CHL only rarely express T-cell markers such as CD43.

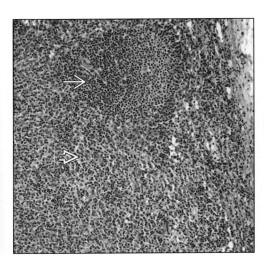

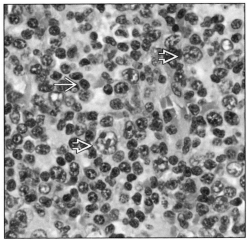

(Left) Lymph node involved by infectious mononucleosis shows interfollicular expansion ⮕. A lymphoid follicle ⮕ is present at the top of the field. *(Right)* Lymph node with reactive interfollicular expansion in a patient with infectious mononucleosis. Scattered immunoblasts ⮕ are admixed with small lymphocytes ➡. Occasionally, large immunoblasts may mimic HRS cells.

LYMPHOCYTE-DEPLETED HODGKIN LYMPHOMA

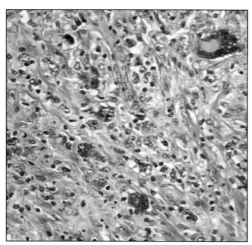

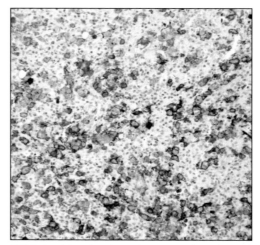

Lymphocyte-depleted Hodgkin lymphoma (LDHL) involving lymph node. Hodgkin and Reed-Sternberg (HRS) cells are numerous and highly pleomorphic, and small lymphocytes are depleted.

LDHL involving lymph node. Immunohistochemical analysis for CD30 highlights numerous HRS cells. Numerous HRS cells are a feature of the reticular morphologic variant of LDHL.

TERMINOLOGY

Abbreviations
- Lymphocyte-depleted Hodgkin lymphoma (LDHL)

Synonyms
- Lymphocyte-depleted classical Hodgkin lymphoma
- Lymphocyte-depleted (depletion) Hodgkin disease

Definitions
- Classical Hodgkin lymphoma (CHL) is lymphoid neoplasm composed of Hodgkin and Reed-Sternberg (HRS) cells in variable inflammatory background
- Lymphocyte depletion is a type of CHL characterized by depletion of small lymphocytes
  - Subset of cases has numerous &/or anaplastic HRS cells

ETIOLOGY/PATHOGENESIS

Infectious Agents
- Epstein-Barr virus (EBV) probably has a pathogenic role in a subset of cases that are EBV(+)
- HIV infection is associated with higher frequency of LDHL type

Pathogenesis
- HRS cells arise from late germinal center or early post germinal center B cells that
  - Have undergone immunoglobulin (*Ig*) gene rearrangements with somatic mutations
  - Undergo crippling *Ig* gene mutations in subset of cases
  - Do not express B-cell antigen receptors
- HRS cells lose much of normal B-cell immunophenotype due to
  - Severe impairment of transcription factor network regulating B-cell gene expression

- Low or undetectable levels of transcription factors: OCT2, BOB1, PU.1, and early B-cell factor (EBF)
  - Leads to low level of Ig transcripts in HRS cells
  - Made worse by epigenetic silencing (promoter hypermethylation) of *Ig* transcription
- Impaired function of early B cell development transcription factors: pax-5, E2A, and EBF
  - pax-5 dimly expressed or rarely absent in HRS cells
  - Aberrant overexpression of NOTCH1, ABF, and ID2 inhibit B-cell differentiation
  - Absent or dim expression of B-cell antigens: e.g., CD20
- Overall these abnormalities physiologically should lead to apoptosis
  - However HRS are rescued from undergoing apoptosis
- Development of antiapoptotic mechanisms to achieve survival
  - Inhibition of executors of apoptosis
  - Dysregulation of signaling pathways
  - Microenvironment is protective of HRS cells
- LDHL most likely represents progression from other types of CHL
  - Suggested by older patient age at onset

CLINICAL ISSUES

Epidemiology
- Incidence
  - < 1% of cases of CHL
- Age
  - Median: 4th decade (or older in some studies)
- Gender
  - M:F = 2-3:1

Site
- Lymph nodes: Retroperitoneal or abdominal > peripheral
- Abdominal organs, bone marrow

LYMPHOCYTE-DEPLETED HODGKIN LYMPHOMA

Key Facts

Clinical Issues
- < 1% of cases of CHL
- Lymph nodes: Retroperitoneal or abdominal > peripheral
- Abdominal organs, bone marrow
- B symptoms are frequent
- Clinical stage III-IV disease
- Current chemotherapy and radiation can cure disease in many patients

Microscopic Pathology
- Lymph node architecture is usually diffusely effaced
- Generalized depletion of small lymphocytes
- Eosinophils, neutrophils, and plasma cells are usually scant or absent
- ± coagulative necrosis; ± sinusoidal invasion
- ± disordered nonbirefringent fibrillary fibrosis

- 3 morphologic variants
  - Diffuse fibrosis
  - Reticular or sarcoma-like
  - Mixed cellularity-like with numerous HRS cells

Ancillary Tests
- CD30(+) in > 95%; CD15(+) in ~ 70-80% of cases
- pax-5(dim +) ~ 90%), CD20(variably +) ~ 20%
- EBV(+) with latency type II pattern in subset of cases
- CD45/LCA(-)

Top Differential Diagnoses
- Nodular sclerosis Hodgkin lymphoma, grade 2
- Anaplastic large cell lymphoma, either ALK1(+) or ALK1(-)
- Nonhematopoietic neoplasms
- Peripheral T-cell lymphoma

Presentation
- B symptoms are frequent
- Lymphadenopathy
- Clinical stage III-IV disease
- LDHL can spread contiguously (like other types of CHL) or by noncontiguous/vascular spread

Treatment
- Chemotherapy ± radiation
  - Chemotherapy ABVD: Adriamycin (doxorubicin), bleomycin, vinblastine, and dacarbazine
- Current chemotherapy and radiation can cure disease in many patients

Prognosis
- Factors relevant to prognosis and to determination of mode of therapy
  - Male sex, B symptoms, high clinical stage
  - Elevated levels of serum LDH and β2-microglobulin
- With therapy, prognosis of LDHL patients is similar to patients with other CHL types of similar stage
- Recurrent disease with multiple adverse factors results in ~ 60% overall survival at 5 years

MICROSCOPIC PATHOLOGY

Histologic Features
- Lymph node architecture is usually diffusely effaced
- Generalized depletion of small lymphocytes
- Eosinophils, neutrophils, and plasma cells are usually scant or absent
- ± coagulative necrosis; ± sinusoidal invasion
- ± disordered nonbirefringent fibrillary fibrosis
- 3 morphologic variants
  - Diffuse fibrosis
    - Scant HRS cells admixed with few or abundant fibroblasts, fibrillary stroma, and scant lymphocytes
  - Reticular or sarcoma-like
    - Abundant HRS cells, including pleomorphic, bizarre (sarcomatous) cells

- Capsular and perinodal infiltration are common
  - Mixed cellularity-like with numerous HRS cells
    - HRS cells include typical Reed-Sternberg cells and mononuclear variants

Cytologic Features
- LDHL is difficult to diagnose in fine needle aspiration smears
  - Numerous HRS cells and depleted inflammatory background lead one away from diagnosis of CHL

ANCILLARY TESTS

Immunohistochemistry
- CD30(+) in > 95%; CD15(+) in ~ 70-80% of cases
  - Characteristic membranous pattern with accentuation in Golgi area
- pax-5(dim +) ~ 90%, CD20(variably +) ~ 20%, CD79a(+) ~ 10-20%
- Ki-67(+), p53(+), MUM1(+)
- CCL17(TARC)(+), fascin(+/-), Bcl-2(+/-)
- CD45/LCA(-), EMA(-), Ig(-)
- EBV(+) with latency type II pattern in ~ 50% of cases
  - EBV-LMP(+), LMP2a(+), EBNA1(+), EBNA2(-)

Flow Cytometry
- Polytypic B cells and T cells with normal immunophenotype
- Useful to exclude non-Hodgkin lymphomas

In Situ Hybridization
- EBER(+) in ~ 50% of cases

PCR
- Monoclonal *Ig* rearrangements detected in subset of cases by standard PCR methods
  - Attributable to large number of HRS cells in these cases

Molecular Genetics
- Monoclonal *Ig* rearrangements in HRS cells shown by single-cell PCR

- Rearranged *Ig* genes harbor somatic mutations in *Ig* variable regions

DIFFERENTIAL DIAGNOSIS

Nodular Sclerosis Hodgkin Lymphoma (NSHL)
- NSHL with lymphocyte depletion (grade 2) can mimic LDHL
- Features that support NSHL over LDHL
  - Mediastinal disease; unusual in LDHL
  - Broad sclerosing bands and nodularity
  - Lacunar-type HRS cells

Classical Hodgkin Lymphoma After Therapy
- Recurrent CHL after therapy can mimic LDHL
  - Generalized lymphocyte depletion and increased HRS cells
  - HRS cells can be present in sheets
  - Fibrous bands ± lacunar-type HRS can be less prominent
- For these reasons, CHL after therapy is not further classified

Mixed Cellularity Hodgkin Lymphoma (MCHL)
- Variable number of HRS cells in MCHL; can be abundant and overlap with LDHL
- Features that support MCHL over LDHL
  - HRS cells tend to have classical cytologic features
    - Not anaplastic and not as numerous as in LDHL
  - Background inflammatory infiltrate has granulocytes &/or plasma cells

Classical Hodgkin Lymphoma-like Lesions in Patients Treated with Methotrexate
- Usually patients have autoimmune diseases; rheumatoid arthritis most common
- Clinical history is essential to establish this diagnosis
- These lesions can have numerous HRS cells that can mimic LDHL
- HRS-like cells are CD30(+), CD15(+/-), CD20(+, often bright)
- Complete resolution can occur after methotrexate therapy is discontinued

ALK(+) Anaplastic Large Cell Lymphoma (ALCL)
- Subset of cases once classified as LDHL are now classified as ALK(+) ALCL
  - Most cases were once considered reticular variant of LDHL
- Features that support ALK(+) ALCL over LDHL
  - Children and young adults; extranodal sites common
  - Marked sinusoidal involvement; hallmark cells
  - CD30(+), in target-like pattern, ALK1(+), pax-5(-), CD15(-), EBV(-)
  - Translocations involving ALK at chromosome 2p23

ALK(-) ALCL
- Subset of cases once classified as LDHL are now classified as ALK(-) ALCL
- Features that support ALK(-) ALCL over LDHL
  - No preference for retroperitoneal or abdominal lymph nodes
  - Marked sinusoidal involvement; ± hallmark cells
  - CD30(+), in target-like pattern, ALK(-), pax-5(-), CD15(-)

Peripheral T-cell Lymphoma (PTCL)
- Subset of PTCL cases can have highly pleomorphic, HRS-like cells
- Features that support PTCL over LDHL
  - Neoplastic cells with range of size and pleomorphism
  - Background usually rich in small reactive lymphocytes and eosinophils
  - T-cell antigens(+), CD30(-/+), CD15(-), pax-5(-)
  - Molecular studies show evidence of T-cell clonality

Metastatic Carcinoma
- Cases of reticular variant LDHL can overlap morphologically with carcinoma
- Features that support metastatic carcinoma over LDHL
  - Clinical history or evidence of primary site
  - Neoplastic cells are cohesive; often with well-defined cytoplasmic borders
  - Cytokeratins(+), CD30(-), pax-5(-)
  - Desmosomes or cell junctions identified by electron microscopy (EM)

Metastatic Melanoma
- Cases of reticular variant LDHL can overlap morphologically with melanoma
- Features that support metastatic melanoma over LDHL
  - Clinical history or evidence of primary site
  - Neoplastic cells are cohesive; often with abundant cytoplasm and nuclear pseudoinclusions
  - S100 protein(+), HMB-45(-), CD30(-), pax-5(-)
  - Melanin pigment; melanosomes identified by EM

Sarcoma
- Cases of diffuse fibrosis variant LDHL can overlap morphologically with sarcoma
- Features that support sarcoma over LDHL
  - Spindle-shaped cells; ± abundant cytoplasm
  - IHC or EM evidence of soft tissue origin

SELECTED REFERENCES

1. Slack GW et al: Lymphocyte depleted Hodgkin lymphoma: an evaluation with immunophenotyping and genetic analysis. Leuk Lymphoma. 50(6):937-43, 2009
2. Benharroch D et al: Lymphocyte-depleted classic Hodgkin lymphoma-a neglected entity? Virchows Arch. 453(6):611-6, 2008
3. Grosso LE et al: Lymphocyte-depleted Hodgkin's disease: diagnostic challenges by fine-needle aspiration. Diagn Cytopathol. 19(1):66-9, 1998
4. Greer JP et al: Lymphocyte-depleted Hodgkin's disease. Clinicopathologic review of 25 patients. Am J Med. 81(2):208-14, 1986

Microscopic and Immunohistochemical Features

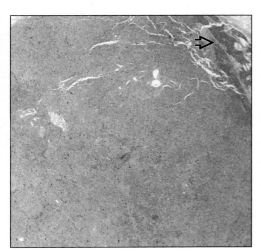

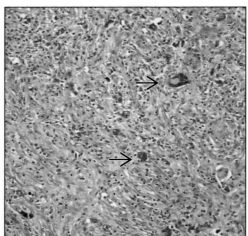

(Left) Lymphocyte-depleted Hodgkin lymphoma (LDHL) involving lymph node. At this magnification, one can appreciate the generalized depletion of small reactive lymphocytes as manifested by the pale, eosinophilic appearance. Residual uninvolved lymph node is present at the upper right of the field ➡. (Right) LDHL involving lymph node. The HRS cells are large and pleomorphic ➡. Background small, reactive lymphocytes are markedly depleted.

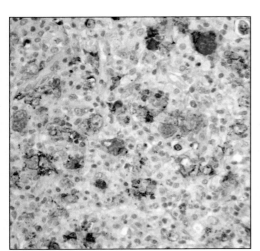

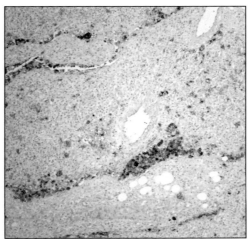

(Left) Lymphocyte-depleted Hodgkin lymphoma (LDHL) involving lymph node. The anti-CD15 antibody highlights many large and pleomorphic HRS cells. (Right) LDHL involving lymph node. The anti-CD30 antibody highlights the prominent sinusoidal involvement by HRS cells. Sinusoidal involvement can be seen in LDHL, but is unusual in other types of classical Hodgkin lymphoma.

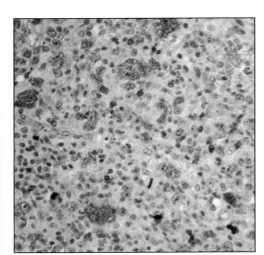

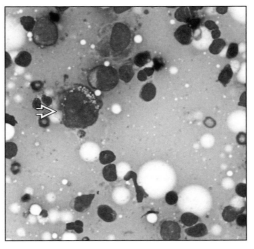

(Left) Lymphocyte-depleted Hodgkin lymphoma (LDHL) involving lymph node. The anti-CD79a highlights a subset of HRS cells with a mostly cytoplasmic pattern of staining. (Right) Touch imprint of a case of LDHL involving lymph node. The HRS cell ➡ has a large nucleus, prominent nucleoli, and abundant vacuolated basophilic cytoplasm.

Microscopic and Immunohistochemical Features

(Left) Lymphocyte-depleted Hodgkin lymphoma (LDHL) involving lymph node. Many HRS cells ⇒ are seen admixed with inflammatory cells and few lymphocytes, consistent with the reticular morphologic variant of LDHL. *(Right)* LDHL, reticular variant, involving lymph node. Many HRS cells ⇒ are seen admixed with inflammatory cells and few lymphocytes.

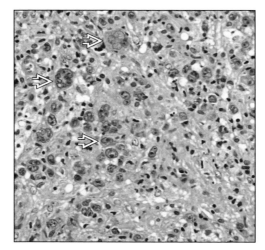
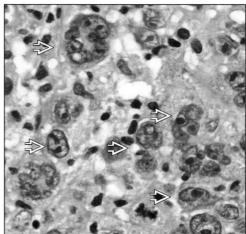

(Left) Lymphocyte-depleted Hodgkin lymphoma (LDHL) involving lymph node. Immunohistochemistry for CD30 highlights many Hodgkin ⇒ and fewer multinucleated Reed-Sternberg cells ⇒. *(Right)* LDHL involving lymph node. Immunohistochemistry for CD15 highlights many HRS cells consistent with the reticular morphologic variant.

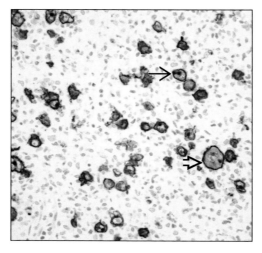
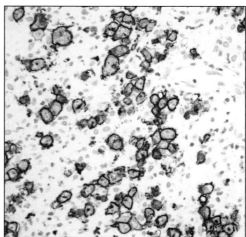

(Left) Lymphocyte-depleted Hodgkin lymphoma (LDHL) involving lymph node. Immunostain for pax-5 shows that the HRS cells ⇒ are dimly positive in comparison with small reactive B cells that are brightly positive ⇒. *(Right)* LDHL involving lymph node. Immunostain for EBV-LMP highlights many HRS cells. Based on the limited number of cases diagnosed, ~ 50% of cases of LDHL are EBV(+).

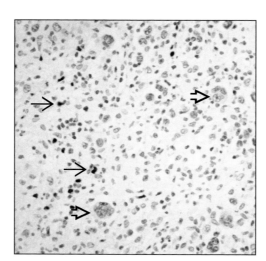
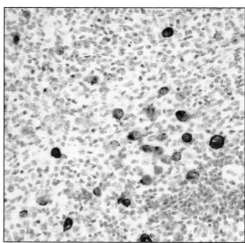

Microscopic Features and Differential Diagnosis

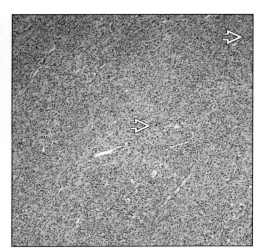 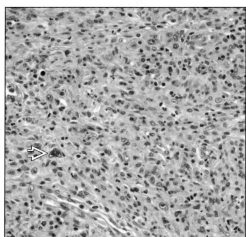

(Left) Lymphocyte-depleted Hodgkin lymphoma (LDHL) involving lymph node. Scattered HRS cells ⬭ are seen admixed with fibroblasts and scant reactive lymphocytes, consistent with the diffuse fibrosis morphologic variant of LDHL. (Right) LDHL, diffuse fibrosis morphologic variant, involving lymph node. Scattered HRS cells ⬭ are seen admixed with fibroblasts and scant background lymphocytes.

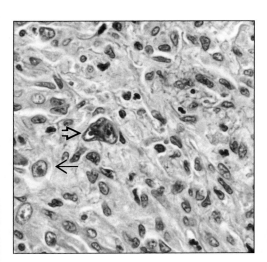 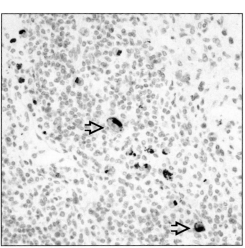

(Left) Lymphocyte-depleted Hodgkin lymphoma (LDHL) involving lymph node. A Reed-Sternberg cell ⬭ and Hodgkin cell ➔ are admixed with fibroblasts imparting a spindle cell appearance, raising the differential diagnosis with sarcoma. (Right) LDHL involving lymph node. Immunostain with anti-CD15 antibody highlights rare HRS cells ⬭ as well as smaller granulocytes.

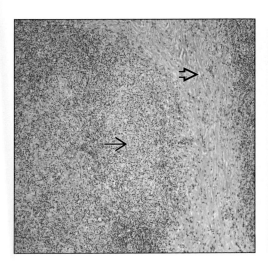 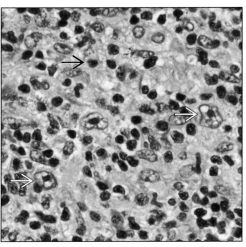

(Left) Nodular sclerosis Hodgkin lymphoma (NSHL) shows depletion of small lymphocytes ➔ resembling LDHL. However, the presence of a nodule surrounded by a thick fibrous band ⬭ supports NSHL. (Right) NSHL displays depletion of lymphocytes ➔ resembling LDHL. Frequent HRS cells ⬭ are noted.

PROTOCOL FOR EXAMINATION OF HODGKIN LYMPHOMA SPECIMENS

Hodgkin Lymphoma: Biopsy, Resection

Surgical Pathology Cancer Case Summary (Checklist)

Specimen (select all that apply)

____ Lymph node(s)

____ Other (specify): _____

____ Not specified

Procedure

____ Biopsy

____ Resection

____ Other (specify): _____

____ Not specified

Tumor Site (select all that apply)

____ Lymph node(s), site not specified

____ Lymph node(s)

 Specify site(s): _____

____ Other tissue(s) or organ(s) (specify): _____

____ Not specified

Histologic Type (based on 2008 WHO classification)

____ Hodgkin lymphoma, histologic subtype cannot be determined

____ Classical Hodgkin lymphoma, histologic subtype cannot be determined

____ Nodular lymphocyte predominant Hodgkin lymphoma

____ Nodular sclerosis classical Hodgkin lymphoma

____ Mixed cellularity classical Hodgkin lymphoma

____ Lymphocyte-rich classical Hodgkin lymphoma

____ Lymphocyte-depleted classical Hodgkin lymphoma

*Pathologic Extent of Tumor (select all that apply)

*____ Involvement of a single lymph node region

 *Specify sites: _____

*____ Involvement of ≥ 2 lymph node regions on same side of diaphragm

 *Specify sites: _____

*____ Involvement of lymph node regions on both sides of diaphragm

 *Specify sites: _____

*____ Spleen involvement

*____ Liver involvement

*____ Bone marrow involvement

*____ Other site involvement

 *Specify site(s): _____

*Additional Pathologic Findings

 *Specify: _____

Immunophenotyping (immunohistochemistry)

____ Performed, see separate report: _____

____ Performed

 Specify method(s) and results: _____

____ Not performed

*Clinical Prognostic Factors and Indices (select all that apply)

*____ International Prognostic Score (IPS) (specify): _____

*____ B symptoms present

*____ Other (specify): _____

Adapted with permission from College of American Pathologists, "Protocol for the Examination of Specimens from Patients with Hodgkin Lymphoma." Web posting date October 2009, www.cap.org.

B-LYMPHOBLASTIC LEUKEMIA/LYMPHOMA

Differential Diagnosis

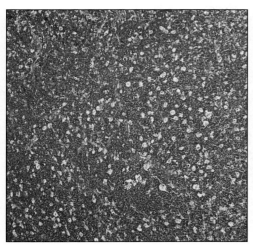 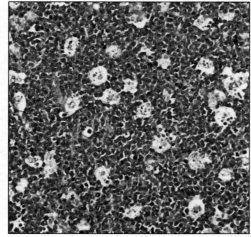

(Left) Burkitt lymphoma involving the ileocecal region. The tumor cells are medium-sized (nuclei similar or smaller to those of histiocytes) and show a diffuse monotonous pattern of growth. (Right) Burkitt lymphoma has very high proliferation fraction (many mitotic figures) as well as a high fraction of apoptosis. Note the "starry sky" pattern present in this case of BL which is imparted by numerous benign macrophages that have ingested apoptotic tumor cells.

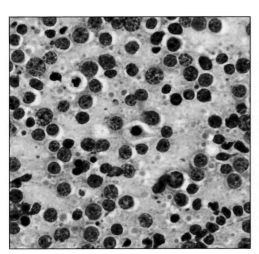 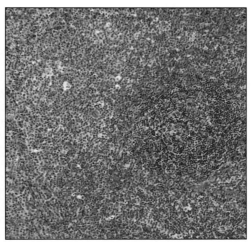

(Left) Burkitt lymphoma, touch imprint. The neoplastic cell nuclei are round to ovoid and vary relatively little in size and shape. The chromatin is coarse and irregularly distributed, and nucleoli are prominent and basophilic. Note the karyorrhexis in the background, indicating high cell turnover. (Right) Myeloid sarcoma involving lymph node. The neoplasm diffusely infiltrates the lymph node but spares lymphoid follicles.

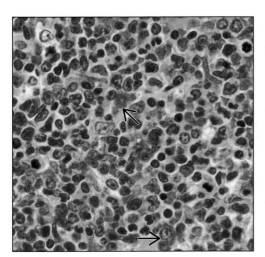 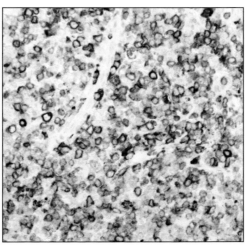

(Left) Myeloid sarcoma, poorly differentiated. The neoplastic cells have fine chromatin and irregular/folded nuclear contours suggestive of monocytic differentiation. Note the presence of scattered immature and mature eosinophilic elements ➡. (Right) Myeloid sarcoma. The neoplastic cells are positive for myeloperoxidase shown by immunohistochemical stain.

T-LYMPHOBLASTIC LEUKEMIA/LYMPHOMA

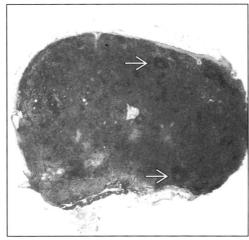

Lymph node with subtotal replacement by T-lymphoblastic lymphoma/leukemia. A few preserved lymphoid follicles ➡ can be seen.

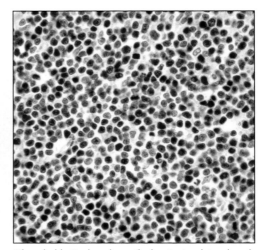

T-lymphoblastic lymphoma/leukemia involving lymph node. TdT is strongly positive in the nuclei of the neoplastic cells.

TERMINOLOGY

Abbreviations
- T-lymphoblastic leukemia/lymphoma (T-LBL)

Synonyms
- Precursor T-cell lymphoblastic lymphoma/leukemia
- T-cell lymphoblastic lymphoma/acute lymphoblastic leukemia

Definitions
- Neoplasm of lymphoblasts committed to T-cell lineage
- Distinction between lymphoma and leukemia is arbitrary; by convention
- T-lymphoblastic lymphoma
  - Presentation with involvement of thymus, lymph nodes, &/or extranodal sites
  - No or minimal involvement of peripheral blood (PB) or bone marrow (BM)
- T-lymphoblastic leukemia (T-ALL)
  - Presentation with involvement of PB and BM

ETIOLOGY/PATHOGENESIS

Genetic
- Recurrent genetic aberrations that block precursor T-cell differentiation and survival
  - T-LBL is genetically heterogeneous disease
  - Number of translocations, deletions, and gene mutations have been shown
- Possible in utero origin in subset of cases

CLINICAL ISSUES

Epidemiology
- Incidence
  - 85-90% of lymphoblastic tumors presenting as lymphoma are of T-cell lineage

- Age
  - Median: 17 years for adolescents and 25 years for adults
- Gender
  - Sex ratio: 70% male, 30% female

Presentation
- T-lymphoblastic lymphoma
  - Rapidly growing anterior mediastinal mass (~ 75% of patients)
    - ± pleural effusions
    - Superior vena cava syndrome can occur
  - Lymphadenopathy is typically supradiaphragmatic (~ 50% of patients)
  - Extranodal presentation (~ 35% of patients)
    - Frequent sites: Skin, tonsils, liver, spleen, central nervous system, and testes
  - Most patients present with stage III or IV disease (~ 75% of patients)
- T-ALL
  - High leukocyte count
  - Lymphadenopathy and hepatosplenomegaly are common

Treatment
- Drugs
  - Aggressive chemotherapy
    - Cyclophosphamide, vincristine, doxorubicin, and dexamethasone/methotrexate/ara-C (HyperCVAD regimen)
    - High rates of complete response
- Radiation
  - Mediastinal radiation for bulky disease

Prognosis
- 5-year disease-free survival
  - Children: 65-75%
  - Adults: 40-60%

T-LYMPHOBLASTIC LEUKEMIA/LYMPHOMA

Key Facts

Terminology
- T-LBL is neoplasm of lymphoblasts committed to T-cell lineage
- Distinction between lymphoma and leukemia is arbitrary; by convention
  - T-lymphoblastic lymphoma: Presentation with disease in thymus, lymph nodes, &/or extranodal sites
  - T-lymphoblastic leukemia: Presentation with involvement of PB and BM

Clinical Issues
- Median age: 17 years for adolescents and 25 years for adults
- Sex ratio: 70% male, 30% female
- Stage III or IV disease (~ 75% of patients)

- Rapidly growing anterior mediastinal mass (~ 75% of patients)
- Lymphadenopathy is typically supradiaphragmatic

Microscopic Pathology
- Diffuse pattern of infiltration
  - "Starry sky" pattern in 10-20% of cases
- Small to medium-sized lymphoblasts with fine nuclear chromatin
- Lymphoblasts can infiltrate extranodal tissues in single-file pattern

Ancillary Tests
- Immunophenotype
  - T-cell antigens(+), TdT(+)
  - CD1a(+), CD10(+) in pre-T and cortical T stages
- Monoclonal *TCR* gene rearrangements

IMAGE FINDINGS

Radiographic Findings
- Anterior mediastinal mass can be shown by various modalities
- FDG-avid PET scan

MICROSCOPIC PATHOLOGY

Histologic Features
- Lymph node
  - Diffuse pattern of involvement
  - Complete or subtotal replacement of architecture
  - In cases with subtotal effacement
    - Preferential involvement of paracortical regions
    - Preserved lymphoid follicles
  - Tumor cells can infiltrate capsule and pericapsular tissue in single-file arrangement
  - "Starry sky" pattern in 10-20% of cases
  - Fibrous bands through tumor can impart nodular appearance
- Bone marrow
  - By convention
    - Lymphoma with < 25% of bone marrow involved
    - T-ALL: Extensive bone marrow disease
- Extranodal sites
  - Tumor cells often infiltrate fibrous tissue in single-file pattern

Cytologic Features
- In PB and BM aspirate smears
  - L1 blasts: Small with high nuclear to cytoplasm ratio and visible but not prominent nucleoli
  - L2 blasts: Intermediate size with prominent nucleoli and more abundant cytoplasm
  - Lymphoblasts usually are devoid of cytoplasmic granules
- In histologic sections of lymph nodes or extranodal sites
  - Lymphoblasts are small to medium-sized with scant cytoplasm

  - High mitotic activity
  - Convoluted or round nuclear contours
  - Immature (blastic) nuclear chromatin
    - "Dusty" or "salt and pepper" chromatin
    - Usually indistinct nucleoli
    - In small subset of cases, nucleoli are distinct and visible (so-called L2 variant)
- Rare cases of T-LBL are associated with eosinophilia
  - Either in PB and BM or intermixed with lymphoma cells in tissues

Predominant Cell/Compartment Type
- Hematopoietic, lymphoid

ANCILLARY TESTS

Immunohistochemistry
- T-cell antigens(+)
  - Cytoplasmic expression precedes surface expression
    - Cytoplasmic and surface antigen expression can be detected by immunohistochemistry
    - Routine flow cytometry detects surface antigen expression
    - Therefore, potential for discordance
- TdT(+), CD1a(+), CD10(+) in pre-T and cortical T stages
- CD34(+/-), CD99(+/-), CD117/C-Kit(-/+)
- CD45/LCA(+) at later stage of differentiation, TAL-1(+ ~ 50%)
- Ig(-), CD19(-), CD20(-), CD22(-)
  - CD79a(+/-)
- Proliferation rate usually high but variable
  - Ki-67 ~ 50-90%

Immunofluorescence
- TdT(+) in nuclear pattern in most cases
- This method can be used to assess T- and B-cell antigens
  - In large part, immunofluorescence has been replaced by flow cytometry

5

T-LYMPHOBLASTIC LEUKEMIA/LYMPHOMA

Flow Cytometry
- T-cell antigens are expressed in sequence as precursor T-cells mature
  - T-LBL and T-ALL arise from precursor cell "frozen" in differentiation
  - T-ALL cases are more immature than T-LBL cases
- Pro-T (T-I)
  - CD7(+), cytoplasmic (c) CD3(+), CD34(+/-), CD2(-), CD5(-), CD4(-)/CD8(-), CD1a(-), surface(s) CD3(-)
- Pre-T (T-II)
  - TdT(+), CD7(+), cCD3(+), CD34(+/-), CD2(+), CD5(+), CD4(+/-)/CD8(+/-), CD1a(-), sCD3(-)
- Cortical T (T-III)
  - TdT(+), CD7(+), cCD3(+), CD2(+), CD5(+), CD4(+)/CD8(+), CD1a(+), sCD3(-), CD34(-)
- Mature T (T-IV)
  - CD7(+), cCD3(+), CD2(+), CD5(+), CD4(+) or CD8(+), CD1a(-), sCD3(+), CD34(-)
- Small subset of LBL may be of natural killer cell lineage
  - CD16(+), CD56(+), CD57(+), or CD94a(+)
  - CD2(+/-), CD7(+/-), CD3(-), CD5(-)
- TdT(+) in nuclear pattern in most cases
  - Cell permeabilization is required to assess by flow cytometry
- CD13(-/+) or CD33(-/+) in 20-30% of cases

Cytogenetics
- Normal karyotype in 30-40% of cases
- Common abnormalities at chromosome loci 14q11.2, 7q35, and 7p14-15
  - Location of T-cell receptors α and δ, β and γ, respectively
  - Translocations juxtapose protooncogene with *TCR* resulting in overexpression
  - 1p32 *TAL1*
    - < 1% in infants, 7% in children, 12% in adults
    - t(1;14)(p32;q11)
  - 10q24 *HOX11*
    - 7% in children, 30% in adults
    - t(10;14)(q24;q11)
    - Early cortical stage; CD4(+)/CD8(+)
    - Better prognosis than other T-LBL types
  - 5q35 *HOX11L2*
    - 20% in children, 10-15% in adults
    - Pro-T stage
  - 9q34.3 *NOTCH1*
    - Translocations involving *NOTCH1* are rare: t(7;9)(q34;q34.3)
    - t(7;9)(q34;q34.3) results in truncated and active form of gene
- Other translocations
  - *NUP214/ABL1*
    - 8% adults
    - Both are on 9q34
    - Amplification with formation of episomal elements
  - 19p13 *LYL1*
    - 1.5% children, 2.5% adults
  - *MLL/ENL*/t(11;19)(q23;p13.3)
    - 0.3% children, 0.5% adults
  - Other *ABL1* translocations

- *ETV6/ABL1*/t(9;12)(q34;p13)
- *EML1/ABL1*/t(9;14)(q34;q32)
- In vitro inhibition by ABL1 kinase inhibitors
- *BCR/ABL1*/t(9;22)(q34;q11.2) rare in T-LBL
- Deletion of chromosome 9p
  - Deleted in 70% of T-LBL
  - Corresponds to loss of tumor suppressor gene *CDKN2A* (inhibitor of CDK4)
  - Leads to loss of G1 control of cell cycle

Molecular Genetics
- Gene rearrangements
  - Monoclonal T-cell receptor (*TCR*) gene rearrangements in almost all cases
    - Rearrangement of *TCRδ* occurs first
    - Followed by rearrangements of *TCR* γ, β, and α
  - Monoclonal *IgH* gene rearrangements in 20% of cases
- 1p32 *TAL1*
  - Interstitial deletions of TAL-1 locus are more common than t(1;14)(p32;q11)
- *NOTCH1* mutations are common
  - 58% of T-LBL carry mutation
    - Heterodimerization domain (HD): 27%
    - PEST domain: 15%
    - HD and PEST domains: 16%
  - *NOTCH1* activation signal can be abrogated by inhibition of γ-secretase
  - Protein regulates T-cell development
  - *PTEN* mutated in γ-secretase-resistant T-LBL

Gene Expression Profiling
- Studies have shown that T-LBL can be subdivided into multiple molecular signatures
  - These signatures correspond to cytogenetic subgroups
  - Signatures are also present in cases with normal cytogenetics

T-LBL with Eosinophilia
- Associated with abnormalities of FGFR1
- Most common: *ZNF198-FGFR1*/t(8;13)(p11;q12)
- Patients present with
  - Peripheral blood eosinophilia
  - Bone marrow myeloid hyperplasia with eosinophilia
  - ± morphologic evidence of dysplasia
- T-LBL (and rarely B-lymphoblastic leukemia/lymphoma [B-LBL]) is common in patients with *ZNF198-FGFR1*
- Patients subsequently develop myeloid malignancy
  - Acute myeloid leukemia most common
  - Myelodysplastic syndromes or myeloproliferative neoplasms also reported

DIFFERENTIAL DIAGNOSIS

B-Lymphoblastic Leukemia/Lymphoma (B-LBL)
- Most (~ 90%) cases present as B-lymphoblastic leukemia
  - ~ 10% of B-lymphoblastic tumors present as lymphoma

T-LYMPHOBLASTIC LEUKEMIA/LYMPHOMA

- Morphologically identical to T-LBL
  - Convoluted or round nuclear contours
  - Immature (blastic) chromatin
  - Numerous mitotic figures
- Immunophenotype needed to distinguish B- from T-LBL
  - Pan-B-cell antigens(+) in B-LBL
    - CD19(+), CD20(+/-), CD22(+/-), pax-5(+)
  - ~ 10% of T-LBL are CD79a(+)
    - Potential pitfall when using limited panel
  - TdT(+), CD10(+/-): Similar to T-LBL
- Cytogenetics and molecular genetics
  - *BCR-ABL1*/t(9;22)(q34;q11.2) in approximately 30% of B-LBL cases
    - Mostly in adults
  - Monoclonal *IgH* gene rearrangements

Burkitt Lymphoma

- 3 types: Endemic (African), sporadic, and immunodeficiency-related
- Usually arises in extranodal sites
- Sporadic type occurs in Western nations
  - Ileocecal region of gastrointestinal tract very common
  - Mediastinum is rarely involved
- Morphologic features differ from T-LBL
  - Prominent "starry sky" pattern in virtually all cases
  - Monotonous, medium-sized cells with 2-5 distinct nucleoli
  - Very high mitotic and apoptotic rates
  - In smears: Moderate to abundant, deeply basophilic cytoplasm with many vacuoles
- Immunophenotype
  - Surface IgM(+), CD10(+), CD19(+)
  - CD20(+), CD22(+), CD79a(+)
  - Ki-67 > 99%, Bcl-6(+)
  - T-cell antigens(-), TdT(-), Bcl-2(-)
- Cytogenetics and molecular genetics
  - Translocations involving *MYC*
    - *MYC-IgH*/t(8;14)(q24;q32)
    - *Ig κ-MYC*/t(2;8)(p11;q24)
    - *MYC-Ig λ*/t(8;22)(q24;q11)
  - Monoclonal *IgH* gene rearrangements

Thymoma

- Presents as mediastinal mass as does T-LBL
- Lymphocyte-rich variants of thymoma are particularly troublesome
  - Many small thymic lymphocytes with immature cytologic features
  - Thymic lymphocytes are immature T cells similar to T-LBL
- Features helpful in differential diagnosis
  - Mitotic activity in thymoma is low to moderate and not high as in T-LBL
  - Thymic epithelial cells can be appreciated in lymphocyte-rich thymoma
    - Scattered intermediate to large cells with thin nuclear membranes
- Immunophenotype
  - Keratin(+) "interlocking" pattern of thymic epithelial cells in thymoma

- Molecular genetics
  - No evidence of monoclonal *TCR* gene rearrangements

Myeloid Sarcoma

- Tumor mass of myeloid blasts at extramedullary site
- Adults: Median age = 6th decade
- Can occur as
  - 1st manifestation or relapse of acute myeloid leukemia
  - Blastic transformation of myelodysplastic syndromes (MDS), myeloproliferative neoplasms (MPN), or MDS/MPN
- Mediastinum is unusual site for myeloid sarcoma
- Immunophenotype
  - CD33(+), CD68(+), CD117(+)
  - MPO(+), lysozyme(+)
  - CD3(-), CD5(-)
- Cytogenetics and molecular genetics
  - ± acute myeloid leukemia-type chromosomal changes (e.g., monosomy 7, trisomy 8, etc.)
  - Acute myeloid leukemia-type translocations can be present in myeloid sarcoma
  - No evidence of monoclonal *TCR* gene rearrangements

Blastoid Variant of Mantle Cell Lymphoma

- Tumor cells can appear lymphoblastoid with immature chromatin and high mitotic rate
- Immunophenotype
  - Surface Ig(+), CD19(+), CD20(+)
  - Cyclin-D1(+), CD5(+)
  - CD10(-), TdT(-)
- Cytogenetics and molecular genetics
  - *CCND1/IgH*/t(11;14)(q13;q32)
  - Monoclonal *IgH* gene rearrangements
  - No evidence of monoclonal *TCR* gene rearrangements

Ewing Sarcoma/Peripheral Neuroectodermal Tumor (ES/PNET)

- ES/PNET does not present as anterior superior mediastinal mass
- LBL can present as 1 or more lytic bone lesions and be misinterpreted as ES/PNET
  - More common for B-LBL than for T-LBL
- Immunophenotype
  - CD99(+) in common with T-LBL
  - ES/PNET does not express T-cell or B-cell antigens
- t(11;22)(q24;q12), t(21;22)(q22;q12), t(1;16)(q11;q11)
- Cytogenetics and molecular genetics
  - *EWS/FLI1*/t(11;22)(q24;q12) and other abnormalities involving *EWS* gene
  - No evidence of monoclonal *TCR* gene rearrangements

Small (Oat) Cell Carcinoma

- Primary lung neoplasm, but metastases can cause prominent mediastinal lymphadenopathy
- Patient population: Adults with history of smoking
- Small cell carcinoma is composed of cohesive tumor cells larger than lymphoblasts
- Immunophenotype

o Keratin(+), chromogranin(+/-), synaptophysin(+/-)
o CD3(-), CD5(-), TdT(-)

Merkel Cell Carcinoma

- Patient population: Elderly patients who present with skin lesions
- Does not present as mediastinal mass
- Merkel cell carcinoma is composed of cohesive tumor cells larger than lymphoblasts
- Immunophenotype
  o Keratin(+), cytokeratin 20(+, often perinuclear)
  o T-cell antigens(-), TdT(-)

Rhabdomyosarcoma

- Alveolar rhabdomyosarcoma is type most likely to be confused with T-LBL
- Can present initially as extensive BM disease mimicking T-ALL
- Immunophenotype
  o Muscle markers(+)
  o T-cell antigens(-), TdT(-)
- Cytogenetics and molecular genetics
  o *PAX3-FOXO1*/t(2;13)(q35;q14) or *PAX7-FOXO1*/ t(1;13)(p36;q14)
  o *PAX3-NCOA1*/t(2;2)(p23;q35) and *PAX3-NCOA2*/ t(2;8)(q35;q13)

Acute Undifferentiated Leukemia (AUL)

- Can morphologically mimic T-ALL
- Unlike T-ALL, AUL does not express lineage-specific antigens
- Immunophenotyping of AUL must be comprehensive to exclude other entities

Mixed Phenotype Acute Leukemia (MPAL)

- Diagnostic criteria for MPAL are strict
- Criteria include
  o Bilineage: 2 distinct blast populations, 1 of which would meet criteria for AML even if < 20% **or**
  o Biphenotypic: Single blast population that meets criteria for T- (or B)-ALL and also expresses myeloid/ monocytic markers
  o MPAL with t(9;22)(q34;q11.2); *BCR-ABL1*
  o MPAL with t(v;11q23), *MLL* rearranged
  o MPAL, B/myeloid or T/myeloid, not otherwise specified

Dermatofibrosarcoma Protuberans (DFSP)

- DFSP does not present as anterior mediastinal mass
- DFSP very rarely spreads to lymph nodes or BM
- DFSP involves dermis of skin
- Most patients with DFSP are adults 20-50 years of age
- DFSP in dermis infiltrates in single file similar to T-LBL
- Immunophenotype
  o DFSP and T-LBL can be CD34(+)
  o DFSP is TdT(-), T-cell antigens(-)
- Cytogenetics and molecular genetics
  o *COL1A1-PDGFRβ*/t(17;22)(q22;q13) in ~ 90% of cases

DIAGNOSTIC CHECKLIST

Clinically Relevant Pathologic Features

- T-LBL is disease that primarily affects adolescents and young adults
- Male predominance
- Presenting symptoms and signs related to
  o Anterior mediastinal mass
  o Supradiaphragmatic lymphadenopathy
  o BM and PB involvement

Pathologic Interpretation Pearls

- Important morphologic features of T-LBL
  o Preferential involvement of paracortical regions of lymph node
  o Small to medium-sized cells with immature (blastic) nuclear chromatin
  o Single file pattern of infiltration in extranodal tissues
  o High mitotic activity
- Important immunophenotypic features
  o TdT(+), T-cell antigens(+)
  o CD1a(+/-), CD10(+/-), CD34(+/-)
  o Immunophenotype corresponds to precursor T cell "frozen" in differentiation

SELECTED REFERENCES

1. Burkhardt B: Paediatric lymphoblastic T-cell leukaemia and lymphoma: one or two diseases? Br J Haematol. 149(5):653-68, 2010
2. Fortune A et al: T-lymphoblastic leukemia/lymphoma: a single center retrospective study of outcome. Leuk Lymphoma. 51(6):1035-9, 2010
3. Jackson CC et al: 8p11 myeloproliferative syndrome: a review. Hum Pathol. 41(4):461-76, 2010
4. Pieters R et al: Biology and treatment of acute lymphoblastic leukemia. Hematol Oncol Clin North Am. 24(1):1-18, 2010
5. Marks DI et al: T-cell acute lymphoblastic leukemia in adults: clinical features, immunophenotype, cytogenetics, and outcome from the large randomized prospective trial (UKALL XII/ECOG 2993). Blood. 114(25):5136-45, 2009
6. Teitell MA et al: Molecular genetics of acute lymphoblastic leukemia. Annu Rev Pathol. 4:175-98, 2009
7. Han X et al: Precursor T-cell acute lymphoblastic leukemia/ lymphoblastic lymphoma and acute biphenotypic leukemias. Am J Clin Pathol. 127(4):528-44, 2007
8. Armstrong SA et al: Molecular genetics of acute lymphoblastic leukemia. J Clin Oncol. 23(26):6306-15, 2005
9. Weng AP et al: Activating mutations of NOTCH1 in human T cell acute lymphoblastic leukemia. Science. 306(5694):269-71, 2004
10. Dabaja BS et al: The role of local radiation therapy for mediastinal disease in adults with T-cell lymphoblastic lymphoma. Cancer. 94(10):2738-44, 2002
11. Nathwani BN et al: Lymphoblastic lymphoma: a clinicopathologic study of 95 patients. Cancer. 48(11):2347-57, 1981

T-LYMPHOBLASTIC LEUKEMIA/LYMPHOMA

Microscopic Features

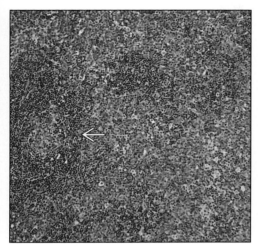

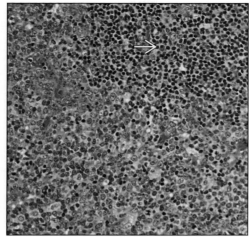

(Left) T-lymphoblastic lymphoma/leukemia involving lymph node. Hematoxylin & eosin shows lymphoblasts subtotally replacing lymph node. A residual follicle is present ➡. *(Right)* T-lymphoblastic lymphoma/leukemia subtotally replacing lymph node. The neoplastic lymphoblasts are larger than normal lymphocytes and have fine chromatin and scant cytoplasm. Note residual small lymphocytes at upper right ➡.

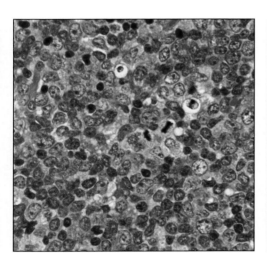

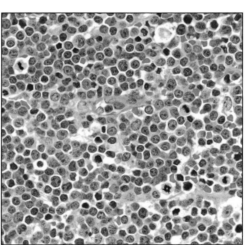

(Left) T-lymphoblastic lymphoma/leukemia involving lymph node. The neoplastic lymphoblasts have fine (immature) chromatin, small nucleoli, and a high mitotic rate. *(Right)* T-lymphoblastic lymphoma/leukemia involving lymph node. The lymphoblasts are medium-sized with irregular nuclei, fine chromatin, inconspicuous nucleoli, and a high mitotic rate.

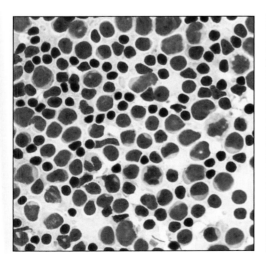

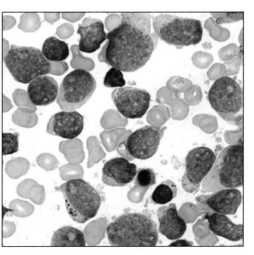

(Left) T-lymphoblastic lymphoma/leukemia involving lymph node. Touch imprint shows small to medium-sized lymphoblasts with fine chromatin and indistinct nucleoli. Mature small lymphocytes are also present in the background. *(Right)* Wright-Giemsa stain of bone marrow aspirate smear shows lymphoblasts with high nuclear to cytoplasmic ratio, fine chromatin, small nucleoli, and basophilic cytoplasm. Note that some blasts have cytoplasmic azurophilic granules.

T-LYMPHOBLASTIC LEUKEMIA/LYMPHOMA

Diagrammatic and Flow Cytometry Features

(Left) Schematic shows the sequential stages of precursor T-cell differentiation. The immunophenotype of T-lymphoblastic lymphoma/leukemia (T-LBL) corresponds to a "frozen" stage of precursor T-cell differentiation. *(Right)* Flow immunophenotypic studies show that T-LBL blasts express CD34 and CD38.

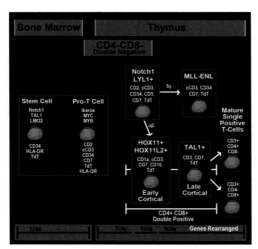
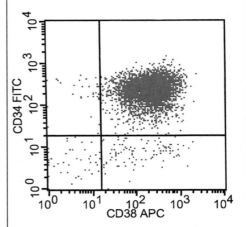

(Left) Flow immunophenotypic studies show that T-LBL blasts are negative for TdT and positive for CD34. *(Right)* Flow immunophenotypic studies show that T-LBL blasts express CD5 and partial HLA-DR.

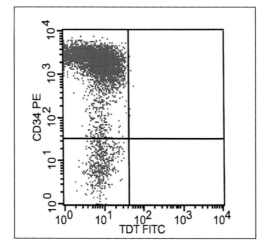
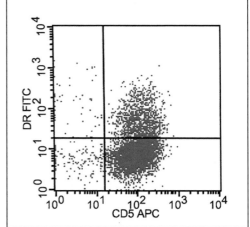

(Left) Flow immunophenotypic studies show that T-LBL blasts express CD7 and are negative for CD2. *(Right)* Flow immunophenotypic studies show that this hypodiploid T-LBL with rearrangement involving 17p/TP53 expresses CD4 and partially expresses CD1.

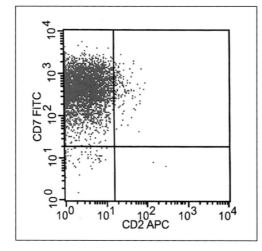
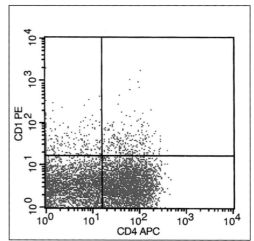

T-LYMPHOBLASTIC LEUKEMIA/LYMPHOMA

Immunohistochemistry and Differential Diagnosis

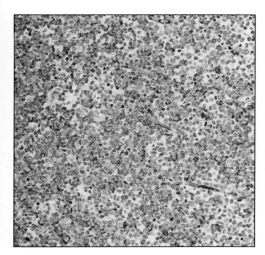

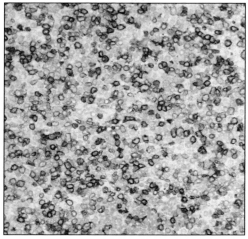

(Left) T-lymphoblastic lymphoma/leukemia involving lymph node. CD34 is expressed by a subset of lymphoblasts in this case. *(Right)* T-lymphoblastic lymphoma/leukemia involving lymph node. CD3 is positive with variable intensity in many lymphoblasts in this case.

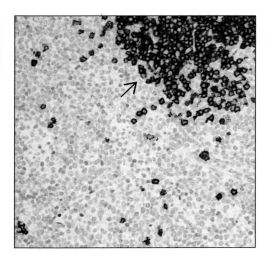

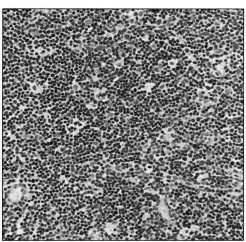

(Left) T-lymphoblastic lymphoma/leukemia involving lymph node. CD20 stain is negative in lymphoblasts in this case. A residual follicle is CD20(+) ➡. *(Right)* Thymoma composed of a high content of small lymphocytes and relatively few thymic epithelial cells that are difficult to appreciate in this field. Also note the absence of mitotic figures in this neoplasm.

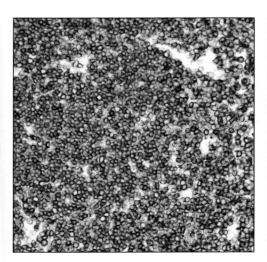

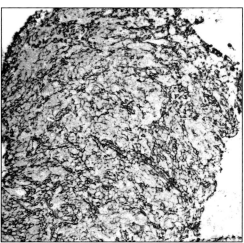

(Left) Thymoma composed of a high content of small lymphocytes. CD3 is strongly positive in the many small lymphocytes in this case. *(Right)* Thymoma composed of a high content of small lymphocytes. Keratin stain shows interlocking pattern of keratin(+) epithelial cells in this case of lymphocyte-predominant thymoma.

LYMPHOMAS ASSOCIATED WITH FGFR1 ABNORMALITIES

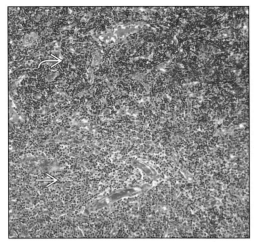

Lymphoma associated with FGFR1 rearrangement displays a biphasic pattern with a lymphoblastic ➡ component in the upper half and a myeloid ➡ component in the lower half.

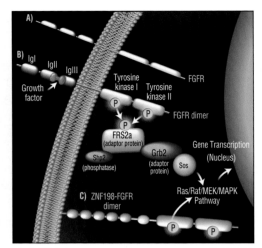

A) FGFR1 is a transmembrane monomer. B) FGFR1 dimerizes upon growth factor binding. C) The t(8;13) (p11;q12) leads to the formation of ZNF198-FGFR1 chimeric protein, which is constitutively activated.

TERMINOLOGY

Abbreviations
- Fibroblast growth factor receptor 1 (FGFR1) abnormalities
- 8p11 myeloproliferative syndrome (EMS)

Synonyms
- Bilineal lymphoma or blastic T-cell/myeloid lymphoma
- T-lymphoblastic leukemia/lymphoma ± eosinophilia
- Synonyms of 8p11 myeloproliferative syndrome
  - Myeloid and lymphoid neoplasms with *FGFR1* gene abnormalities
    - 2008 World Health Organization classification
  - 8p11 stem cell leukemia/lymphoma syndrome

Definitions
- Lymphoblastic lymphoma occurring in patients with 8p11 myeloproliferative syndrome
  - T-cell, T-cell/myeloid, or rarely B-cell lineage reported in literature
- Definition of 8p11 myeloproliferative syndrome
  - Clinically aggressive disease associated with *FGFR1* gene abnormalities
  - Diagnostic features include
    - Myeloproliferative neoplasm usually associated with dysplasia and eosinophilia
    - Lymphadenopathy usually due to T-lymphoblastic leukemia/lymphoma
    - Frequent progression to acute myeloid leukemia

ETIOLOGY/PATHOGENESIS

Cell of Origin
- Unknown but suspected to be pluripotent (lymphoid/myeloid) stem cell

CLINICAL ISSUES

Epidemiology
- Age
  - Range: 3-84 years; median: 44 years
- Gender
  - Slight male predominance

Presentation
- Patients may present with fatigue, night sweats, weight loss, or fever
  - ~ 20% of patients are asymptomatic, and disease is discovered incidentally
- Most patients present with lymphadenopathy
  - Usually generalized but can be localized
- Hepatomegaly, splenomegaly, and hepatosplenomegaly are common
- Extranodal sites of disease are uncommon
  - Sites reported: Tonsil, lung, and breast

Laboratory Tests
- Leukocytosis is common at presentation; median: 46 x 10^9/L
  - Neutrophilia, eosinophilia, and monocytosis are common
- Anemia or thrombocytopenia in ~ 50% of patients

Natural History
- Common evolution to acute leukemia of myeloid or mixed lineage

Treatment
- Various protocols for acute leukemia have been used and have not been effective
- Early stem cell transplantation may lead to long-term remission

Prognosis
- Poor despite aggressive chemotherapy
  - Most patients die of disease

LYMPHOMAS ASSOCIATED WITH FGFR1 ABNORMALITIES

Key Facts

Terminology
- Lymphoblastic lymphoma occurring in patients with 8p11 myeloproliferative syndrome
- EMS is aggressive disease associated with *FGFR1* gene abnormalities; diagnostic features include
  - Myeloproliferative neoplasm usually associated with dysplasia and eosinophilia
  - Lymphadenopathy usually due to T-LBL or bilineal T-cell/myeloid lymphoma
  - Frequent progression to acute myeloid leukemia
- Synonym of 8p11 myeloproliferative syndrome
  - Myeloid and lymphoid neoplasms with FGFR1 abnormalities (WHO, 2008)

Clinical Issues
- Lymphadenopathy is common
  - Cases associated with t(8;13)(p11;q12)

- Leukocytosis is common at presentation
- Poor prognosis despite aggressive chemotherapy
- Stem cell transplantation may lead to long-term remission

Microscopic Pathology
- Diffuse or partial effacement of architecture by blasts
- Mature eosinophils are commonly admixed within neoplasm
- In some cases, biphasic pattern can be observed
  - Sheets of lymphoblasts
  - Larger cells, often perivascular, with moderate eosinophilic cytoplasm

Ancillary Tests
- Chromosome 8p11/*FGFR1* gene abnormalities

MICROSCOPIC PATHOLOGY

Histologic Features
- Lymph node
  - Diffuse or partial effacement of architecture
    - Paracortical distribution in cases with partial involvement
  - Neoplastic cells are blasts that may show single file pattern of infiltration
  - Mature eosinophils are commonly admixed within neoplasm
  - Prominent high endothelial venules are common
  - In some cases, biphasic pattern with 2 components can be observed
    - Sheets of cells that are consistent with lymphoblasts (appear darker)
    - Larger cells with moderately abundant eosinophilic cytoplasm (appear pale)
- Bone marrow
  - Usually hypercellular, eosinophilia is common
  - Blast count usually normal or slightly increased
    - ~ 15% of cases reported had > 20% blasts
  - Blasts are usually of myeloid or myeloid/lymphoid lineage
  - Features raise suspicion for myeloproliferative or myeloproliferative/myelodysplastic neoplasm
- Peripheral blood smear
  - Leukocytosis with left shift in granulocyte maturation; ± blasts
  - Eosinophilia very common; ± monocytosis

ANCILLARY TESTS

Immunohistochemistry
- Many cases of lymphoma in EMS reported as T-lymphoblastic leukemia/lymphoma
  - T-cell antigens(+), TdT(+), CD1a(+), Ig(-), B-cell antigens(-)
- For cases of bilineal lymphoma in EMS that have 2 morphologic components

  - Myeloid cells express 1 or more myeloid-associated antigens
    - Myeloperoxidase(+/-), CD68(+/-), CD117(+/-), lysozyme(+/-), CD15(-/+)
  - Lymphoblasts: T-cell antigens(+), TdT(+), CD1a(+)

Flow Cytometry
- Suspicion of EMS is helpful to ensure analysis of lymphoid and myeloid components
- Blasts are usually positive for T-lineage markers, TdT, and CD1a

Cytogenetics
- All cases of EMS carry abnormality involving *FGFR1* gene at chromosome 8p11
  - 10 translocations and 1 insertion have been identified
  - t(8;13)(p11;q12) is most common
- Translocations are usually detected by conventional cytogenetic analysis; rarely are there cryptic translocations
- Additional cytogenetic abnormalities are associated with progression to acute leukemia
  - Trisomy 21, in particular, is linked to progression

Molecular Genetics
- As consequence of 8p11 abnormalities, *FGFR1* gene is disrupted
  - Results in creation of novel fusion genes and chimeric proteins
- Chimeric proteins include portions of N-terminal partner gene and C-terminal portion of FGFR1
  - Partner genes and proteins foster dimerization and constitutional activation of FGFR1 tyrosine kinase domain
- FISH and RT-PCR can be used to detect these translocations/gene rearrangements
  - Because of rarity of disease, these tests are not routinely available
- Most cases of lymphoma carry monoclonal T-cell receptor *(TCR)* gene rearrangements
  - Subset of cases lack *TCR* gene rearrangements

- ▪ Suggests that neoplastic transformation occurs at stem cell stage, before gene rearrangements occur
- Patients with EMS have clinicopathological manifestations that correlate with specific molecular abnormalities
  - ○ *ZNF198-FGFR1*: Lymphoma
  - ○ *FOP-FGFR1*: Polycythemia, eosinophilia, older patient age
  - ○ *CEP110-FGFR1*: Monocytosis, tonsillar involvement
  - ○ *BCR-FGFR1*: Chronic myelogenous leukemia-like syndrome

DIFFERENTIAL DIAGNOSIS

Myeloid Sarcoma (MS)

- Usually, underlying myeloproliferative neoplasm (MPN) or acute leukemia (AL)
  - ○ Less frequently, myelodysplastic syndrome (MDS) or MDS/MPN
  - ○ Association with characteristic cytogenetic or molecular abnormalities of underlying disease
- Approximately 5% of AML cases can present as MS
  - ○ MS can be nodal or extranodal
    - ▪ Nodal involvement is localized rather than generalized
- Histologically there is diffuse infiltrate of intermediate to large myeloblasts or immature myelomonocytes
- Immunophenotype: Lysozyme(+), CD68(+), myeloperoxidase(+), CD117(+)
  - ○ Frequently CD13(+) and CD33(+)
  - ○ CD34(+/-), CD99(+/-)
- Cytochemistry on touch imprints is useful to define myeloid vs. monocytic lineage

Lymphoblastic Leukemia/Lymphoma (LBL)

- Nodal or extranodal involvement is common at presentation
  - ○ T-LBL may present with mediastinal mass
  - ○ B-LBL is more frequently extranodal
- Histologically there is diffuse and uniform infiltrate of small to intermediate-sized lymphoblasts
- Immunophenotype of immature lymphoid cells; of B-cell more frequently than of T-cell lineage
- Cytogenetic abnormalities are common and define subtypes

Chronic Myelogenous Leukemia, Blast Phase (CML-BP)

- Nodal or extranodal myeloid blast proliferation occurs in ~ 15% of cases of CML
  - ○ Usually associated with blast phase in bone marrow or peripheral blood
- Karyotype and FISH are required to establish
  - ○ t(9;22)(q34;q11.2)
  - ○ Complex cytogenetic abnormalities associated with blast phase
  - ○ *BCR-ABL* fusion gene
- RT-PCR can show *BCR-ABL* and quantify levels
- Patients with t(8;22)(p11;q11) may present with leukocytosis and basophilia, simulating CML

Myeloproliferative Neoplasm (MPN) or Myelodysplastic/MPN (MDS/MPN)

- MPN or MDS/MPN may be associated with lymphadenopathy
- Lymph node involvement may be similar to lymphomas associated with *FGFR1* abnormalities
- Myeloid infiltrates may contain variable amounts of lymphoblasts, usually of T-cell lineage
- Negative for cytogenetic or molecular features that define other diseases, e.g., *BCR-ABL*, *JAK2*, *FIP1L1-PDGFRα*
- Further studies are required to define these processes

DIAGNOSTIC CHECKLIST

Clinically Relevant Pathologic Features

- Lymphadenopathy associated with leukocytosis and eosinophilia should raise suspicion of this disease

Pathologic Interpretation Pearls

- Lymphadenopathy with diffuse effacement due to lymphoblasts and myeloblasts
- Bone marrow with features of MPN or MPN/MDS and eosinophilia
- Peripheral blood may show leukocytosis and CML-like features

SELECTED REFERENCES

1. Jackson CC et al: 8p11 myeloproliferative syndrome: a review. Hum Pathol. 41(4):461-76, 2010
2. Tefferi A et al: Hypereosinophilic syndrome and clonal eosinophilia: point-of-care diagnostic algorithm and treatment update. Mayo Clin Proc. 85(2):158-64, 2010
3. Vega F et al: t(8;13)-positive bilineal lymphomas: report of 6 cases. Am J Surg Pathol. 32(1):14-20, 2008
4. Pardanani A et al: FIP1L1-PDGFRA in eosinophilic disorders: prevalence in routine clinical practice, long-term experience with imatinib therapy, and a critical review of the literature. Leuk Res. 30(8):965-70, 2006
5. Roumiantsev S et al: Distinct stem cell myeloproliferative/T lymphoma syndromes induced by ZNF198-FGFR1 and BCR-FGFR1 fusion genes from 8p11 translocations. Cancer Cell. 5(3):287-98, 2004
6. Macdonald D et al: The 8p11 myeloproliferative syndrome: a distinct clinical entity caused by constitutive activation of FGFR1. Acta Haematol. 107(2):101-7, 2002
7. Demiroglu A et al: The t(8;22) in chronic myeloid leukemia fuses BCR to FGFR1: transforming activity and specific inhibition of FGFR1 fusion proteins. Blood. 98(13):3778-83, 2001
8. Fioretos T et al: Fusion of the BCR and the fibroblast growth factor receptor-1 (FGFR1) genes as a result of t(8;22)(p11;q11) in a myeloproliferative disorder: the first fusion gene involving BCR but not ABL. Genes Chromosomes Cancer. 32(4):302-10, 2001
9. Naeem R et al: Translocation t(8;13)(p11;q11-12) in stem cell leukemia/lymphoma of T-cell and myeloid lineages. Genes Chromosomes Cancer. 12(2):148-51, 1995
10. Abruzzo LV et al: T-cell lymphoblastic lymphoma with eosinophilia associated with subsequent myeloid malignancy. Am J Surg Pathol. 16(3):236-45, 1992

LYMPHOMAS ASSOCIATED WITH FGFR1 ABNORMALITIES

Cytogenetic and Molecular Abnormalities in 8p11 Myeloproliferative Syndrome

Cytogenetic Abnormality	Partner Gene	Name of Partner Gene	Clinicopathologic Correlates
t(8;13)(p11;q12)	ZNF198	Zinc finger 198	Lymphoma
t(8;9)(p11;q33)	CEP110	Centrosome protein 110 kd	Monocytosis, tonsillar enlargement
t(6;8)(q27;p11)	FOP	FGFR1 oncogenic partner 1	Older patient age, polycythemia, eosinophilia
t(8;22)(p11;q11)	BCR	Breakpoint cluster region	Basophilia, leukocytosis, CML-like syndrome
t(8;9)(p12;q13.3)	HERV-K	Human endogen retrovirus gene	
t(7;8)(q34;p11)	TIF1	Transcription intermediary factor 1 α	
t(8;17)(p11;q23)	MYO18A	Myosin 18A	
t(8;12)(p11;q15)	CPSF6	Cleavage and polyadenylation specific factor 6	
t(8;11)(p11;p15)	NUP98	Nucleoporin 98 kd	
t(2;8)(q37;p11)	LRRFP1	Leucine-rich repeat flightless-interacting protein 1	
ins(12;8)(p11;p11p22)	FGFR1OP2	FGFR1 oncogenic partner 2	

Differential Diagnosis of Lymphomas Associated with FGFR1 Abnormalities

Characteristic	LA-FGFR1	MS	ALL	CML-BP	MPN or MDS/MPN
Clinical Features					
	Acute onset	Acute onset	Acute onset	Chronic onset followed by acute phase	Insidious, chronic onset
	Children to adults	Adults	Children and young adults	Adults	Adults to elderly
Lymphadenopathy	Generalized	Localized	Generalized or mediastinal	Localized	Localized
Lymph Node Features					
Nodal compartment	Diffuse	Paracortical or diffuse	Diffuse	Paracortical or diffuse	Paracortical or diffuse
Cytologic features	Immature myeloid cells with granular cytoplasm; lymphoblasts are small	Immature myeloid cells granular cytoplasm; sometimes with immature eosinophils	Lymphoblasts are small with immature fine chromatin; focal "starry sky" pattern	Immature myeloid or myelomonocytic cells; lymphoblasts less common	Immature myeloid or myelomonocytic cells; occasional extramedullary hematopoiesis
Myeloid component	Usually perivascular	Paracortical or diffuse	Absent	Paracortical or diffuse	Paracortical or diffuse
Immunophenotype	Myeloid cells are positive for CD117, CD34, MPO &/or lysozyme; lymphoblasts are TdT(+) and T-cell markers(+)	Positive for CD117, CD34, myeloperoxidase, CD68, lysozyme, CD13, &/or CD33	Positive for TdT, CD34, T- or B-cell markers	Positive for CD117, CD34, MPO, CD68, &/or lysozyme; lymphoblasts are TdT(+) and positive for T- or B-cell markers	(+) for CD117, CD34, myeloperoxidase, CD68, lysozyme, CD13, &/or CD33
Bone Marrow Features					
Cellularity	Usually hypercellular	Usually hypercellular	Hypercellular	Hypercellular	Variable; usually hypercellular
% blasts	Variable; may be > or < 20%	> 20%	> 25%	> 20%	Variable; may be > or < 20%
% lymphoblasts	Variable; may be > or < 25%	< 5%	> 25%	May be > 25% in lymphoid blast phase	Variable; may be > or < 25%
Laboratory Findings					
	Leukocytosis, usually neutrophilia; eosinophilia common; basophilia rare	Leukocytosis or leukopenia, blasts, anemia, thrombocytopenia	Leukocytosis with blasts and lymphocytosis	Leukocytosis, basophilia, variable eosinophilia, blasts, anemia, or thrombocytosis	Variable cytosis or cytopenias; few or no blasts
Molecular Features					
	Translocations involving 8p11 or rearrangements of FGFR1	Variable nonrandom translocations and gene rearrangements	Variable nonrandom translocations and gene rearrangements	t(9;22)(q34;q11) or BCR-ABL ± other abnormalities	Point mutations of JAK-2 or MPL

LA-FGFR1 = lymphomas associated with FGFR1 abnormalities; MS = myeloid sarcoma; ALL = acute lymphoblastic leukemia/lymphoma; CML-BP = chronic myelogenous leukemia, blast phase; MDS/MPN = myelodysplastic syndrome/myeloproliferative neoplasm.

LYMPHOMAS ASSOCIATED WITH FGFR1 ABNORMALITIES

Microscopic Features

(Left) Lymphoma associated with FGFR1 rearrangement displays complete effacement of the lymph node architecture. *(Right)* Lymphoma associated with FGFR1 rearrangement shows a predominance of small lymphoblasts ➡. Increased high endothelial venules ➡ are surrounded by intermediate-sized myeloid cells ➡, also noted in this field.

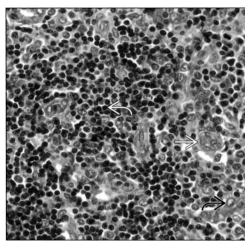

(Left) Lymphoma associated with FGFR1 rearrangement. Most of this field shows a predominance of small lymphoblasts ➡ positive for the T-cell marker CD3. A residual lymphoid follicle is at the upper right ➡. *(Right)* Lymphoma associated with FGFR1 rearrangement. This field shows many T-lymphoblasts ➡ that are CD1a(+). A residual lymphoid follicle is at the upper right ➡.

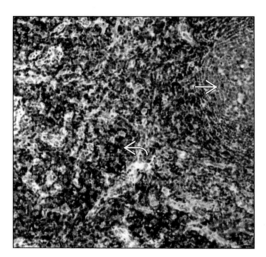
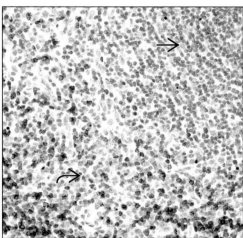

(Left) Lymphoma associated with FGFR1 rearrangement. This field shows many T-lymphoblasts ➡ that are TdT(+) with a nuclear pattern of expression. *(Right)* Lymphoma associated with FGFR1 rearrangement. This area shows a predominance of myeloid precursors ➡, eosinophils ➡, and a "starry sky" pattern ➡.

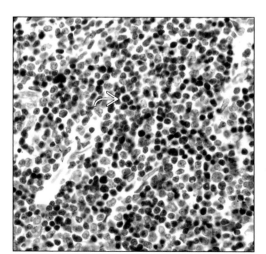
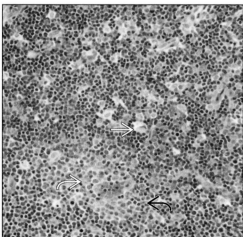

LYMPHOMAS ASSOCIATED WITH FGFR1 ABNORMALITIES

Microscopic and Diagrammatic Features

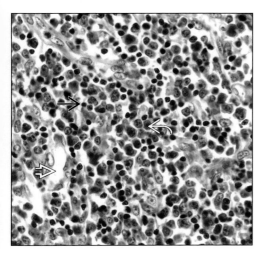

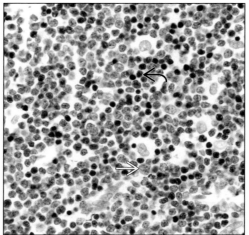

(Left) Lymphoma associated with FGFR1 rearrangement. This area shows a mixture of myeloid precursors ⇒ and lesser numbers of lymphoblasts →. It is apparent that myeloid cells tend to surround small vessels ⇒. *(Right)* Lymphoma associated with FGFR1 rearrangement. Scattered lymphoblasts are highlighted with TdT ⇒ in a portion of the lymph node where most of the cells are myeloid and TdT(-) ⇒.

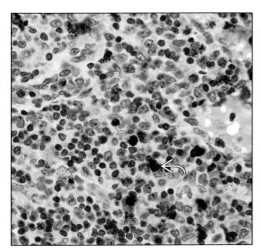

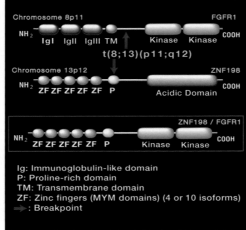

(Left) Lymphoma associated with FGFR1 rearrangement. Scattered myeloid cells are highlighted by antibody reactive for lysozyme ⇒. *(Right)* The most common translocation of lymphoma associated with FGFR1 rearrangement is t(8;13)(p11;q12). Breakpoints at 8p11 and 13p12 (upper half) lead to a chimeric gene composed of the C-terminus of FGFR1 and the N-terminus of ZNF198 (lower half).

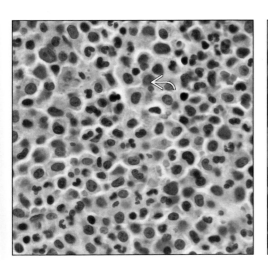

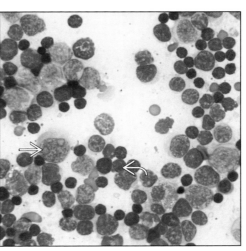

(Left) Lymphoma associated with FGFR1 rearrangement. Bone marrow clot specimen is hypercellular and shows a predominance of myeloid precursors ⇒. *(Right)* Lymphoma associated with FGFR1 rearrangement. Bone marrow aspirate smear shows immature myeloid precursors ⇒ admixed with lymphoblasts ⇒.

LYMPHOMAS ASSOCIATED WITH FGFR1 ABNORMALITIES

Differential Diagnosis

(Left) Myeloid sarcoma in a lymph node shows a diffuse infiltrate of immature myeloid cells ➡ around a residual lymphoid follicle ⮕. Bone marrow showed acute myelomonocytic leukemia. *(Right)* Myeloid sarcoma in a lymph node shows a diffuse infiltrate composed of immature myeloid cells ➡ with folded nuclei and distinct nucleoli. Bone marrow showed acute myelomonocytic leukemia. No lymphoblasts are noted.

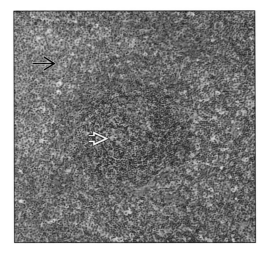
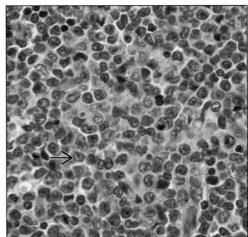

(Left) T-lymphoblastic lymphoma/leukemia in lymph node. In this case, lymphoblasts are intermediate in size with distinct nucleoli. Residual lymphoid follicle composed of small lymphocytes is displayed on the top ➡. *(Right)* T-lymphoblastic lymphoma/leukemia in lymph node shows nuclei with fine chromatin, small distinct nucleoli ➡, and numerous mitoses ➡. Closely apposed nuclei ➡ indicate the scant cytoplasm of lymphoblasts. No immature myeloid cells are noted.

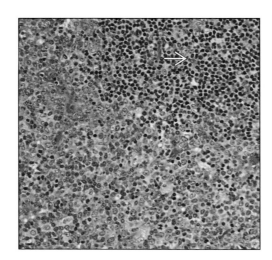
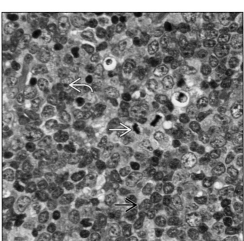

(Left) Chronic myelogenous leukemia, blast phase/myeloid sarcoma in a lymph node. There is a diffuse effacement of the lymph node architecture due to sheets of immature myeloid cells. *(Right)* Chronic myelogenous leukemia, blast phase/myeloid sarcoma in a lymph node. Intermediate to large size immature myeloid cells display oval nuclei with vesicular chromatin, occasional distinct nucleoli ➡, and moderately abundant granular cytoplasm. No lymphoblasts are noted.

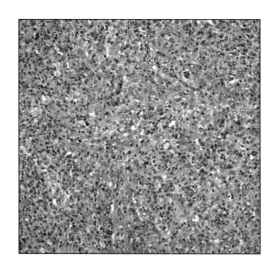
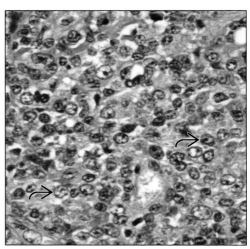

LYMPHOMAS ASSOCIATED WITH FGFR1 ABNORMALITIES

Differential Diagnosis

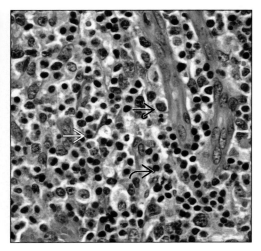

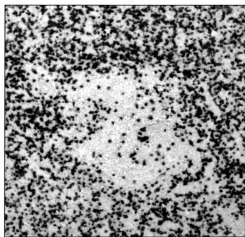

(Left) Lymph node with myeloid and lymphoid blasts similar to lymphoma associated with FGFR1 abnormalities (LA-FGFR1) is shown in a patient with a myeloproliferative neoplasm and generalized lymphadenopathy. There are immature myeloid cells ⊒ admixed with eosinophils ⊒ and small lymphoblasts ⊒. Karyotype demonstrated trisomy 8. (Right) Lymph node with myeloid and lymphoid blasts simulating LA-FGFR1 demonstrates abundant CD3(+) T-cells.

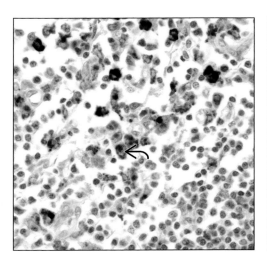

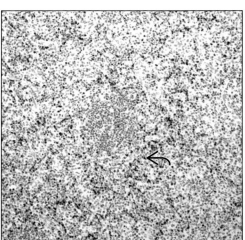

(Left) Lymph node with myeloid and lymphoid blasts simulating LA-FGFR1 demonstrates scattered immature myeloid cells positive for lysozyme ⊒. Bone marrow demonstrated hypercellularity and eosinophilia. Karyotype demonstrated trisomy 8. (Right) Lymph node with myeloid and lymphoid blasts simulating LA-FGFR1 demonstrates scattered TdT(+) lymphoblasts ⊒. Karyotype demonstrated trisomy 8.

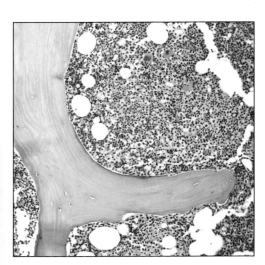

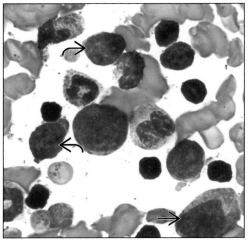

(Left) Myeloproliferative neoplasm with t(8;22)(p11;q11) that presented with leukocytosis and eosinophilia. Bone marrow biopsy shows hypercellularity with low percentage of blasts, mostly lymphoblasts. (Right) Myeloproliferative neoplasm with t(8;22)(p11;q11) that presented with leukocytosis and eosinophilia. Myeloid precursors ⊒ are admixed with lymphoblasts ⊒. FISH to determine FGFR1 gene rearrangement was not performed in this case.

Nodal B-cell Lymphomas

CHRONIC LYMPHOCYTIC LEUKEMIA/SMALL LYMPHOCYTIC LYMPHOMA

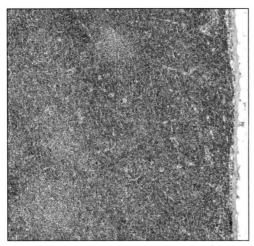

CLL/SLL involving a lymph node with proliferation centers. Note the vaguely nodular, irregularly distributed, pale-staining areas in a dark background of small cells.

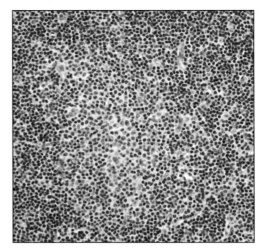

CLL/SLL involving lymph node. A central proliferation center contains a continuum of small lymphocytes, prolymphocytes, and paraimmunoblasts.

TERMINOLOGY

Abbreviations
- Chronic lymphocytic leukemia (CLL)/small lymphocytic lymphoma (SLL)

Definitions
- Neoplasm of monomorphic, small round B cells in peripheral blood, bone marrow, lymph nodes, and spleen
- CLL/SLL cells usually coexpress CD5 and CD23
- SLL is used for nonleukemic cases in which tissue infiltrate has morphology and immunophenotype of CLL
- Prolymphocytes and paraimmunoblasts form proliferation centers in tissues

CLINICAL ISSUES

Presentation
- Lymphadenopathy, generalized
  - Occurs primarily in persons older than 50 years
  - Most patients are asymptomatic
  - Patients with SLL present with lymphadenopathy and often develop lymphocytosis
  - Patients with CLL present with lymphocytosis and fatigue and may develop lymphadenopathy
  - Organ infiltration → splenomegaly, hypersplenism, and peripheral cytopenias
  - Bone marrow becomes extensively infiltrated by neoplastic cells, resulting in severe anemia, thrombocytopenia, and neutropenia
  - Patients with CLL/SLL have significantly impaired immunologic activity
  - Autoimmunity frequently seen in CLL/SLL; up to 25% of patients develop Coombs(+) autoimmune hemolytic anemia
  - Red cell aplasia is rare occurrence

  - Serum M component present in some patients

Treatment
- CLL/SLL not considered to be curable with available therapy
- Chemoimmunotherapy combinations of fludarabine, cyclophosphamide, and rituximab (FCR) result in complete response rate of 72%

Prognosis
- Median survival is 7.5 years
  - 5-year survival (79%)
  - 10-year survival (< 30%)
  - Clinical staging systems: Rai (0-IV) and Binet (A-C) are best predictors of survival

MACROSCOPIC FEATURES

Lymph Node Features
- Lymph nodes are enlarged, and cut surface usually shows diffuse replacement
- Necrosis is rare

MICROSCOPIC PATHOLOGY

Histologic Features
- Lymph nodes
  - Vaguely nodular pattern with alternating dark zones of mature CLL cells and light zones (proliferation centers)
  - Predominant cell is small lymphocyte with clumped chromatin, usually round nucleus, and occasionally small nucleolus
  - Mitotic activity usually very low
  - Proliferation centers contain continuum of small, medium, and large cells
  - Prolymphocytes are medium-sized cells with dispersed chromatin and small nucleoli

CHRONIC LYMPHOCYTIC LEUKEMIA/SMALL LYMPHOCYTIC LYMPHOMA

Key Facts

Terminology
- Chronic lymphocytic leukemia (CLL)/small lymphocytic lymphoma (SLL)

Clinical Issues
- 5-year survival (79%)
- Clinical staging systems: Rai (0-IV) and Binet (A-C) are best predictors of survival

Microscopic Pathology
- Lymph nodes
  - Vaguely nodular pattern with alternating dark zones of mature CLL cells and light zones (proliferation centers)
- Peripheral blood
  - Diagnosis requires persistent (> 1 month) peripheral blood lymphocytosis (> 5 x 10⁹ cells/L)
  - Mature-appearing lymphocytes with CLL immunophenotype in absence of other causes

Ancillary Tests
- Dim expression of sIg (IgM or IgM + IgD or, rarely, IgG) with κ or λ light chain restriction
- Dim CD20(+), CD19(+), CD5(+), CD23(+), FMC7(-)
- Expression of T-cell-associated antigen ZAP70 is associated with *Ig* gene mutational status
- ZAP70 on > 30% of cells by flow cytometry has worse prognosis than ZAP70(-) cases
- About 50% of cases have abnormal karyotypes

Top Differential Diagnoses
- Follicular lymphoma, mantle cell lymphoma
- Hairy cell leukemia, monoclonal B-lymphocytosis

- Paraimmunoblasts: Medium to large cells with round to oval nuclei, dispersed chromatin, central eosinophilic nucleoli
- In some cases, cells show moderate nuclear irregularity (atypical cytology), which can lead to differential diagnosis of mantle cell lymphoma
- Occasional cases show plasmacytoid differentiation
- CLL/SLL can involve lymph nodes with interfollicular pattern, surrounding reactive follicles
- Peripheral blood (PB)
  - Mature-appearing lymphocytes with scant agranular cytoplasm and homogeneously condensed chromatin without nucleoli
  - Characteristic "soccer ball" chromatin pattern and numerous smudge cells
  - Proportion of prolymphocytes (larger cells with prominent nucleoli) in blood films usually < 2%
  - ↑ numbers of prolymphocytes correlate with more aggressive disease course, *P53* abnormalities, and trisomy of chromosome 12
  - Variant CLL with ↑ prolymphocytes (CLL/PL) is defined by > 10% but < 55% prolymphocytes
  - Diagnosis requires persistent (> 1 month) PB lymphocytosis (> 5 x 10⁹ cells/L) of mature-appearing lymphocytes
  - Circulating lymphocytes with CLL immunophenotype
- Bone marrow (BM)
  - Involvement may be nodular, interstitial, or diffuse
  - Proliferation centers are less common in bone marrow than in lymph nodes but can be found with extensive involvement
  - Paratrabecular aggregates are not typical
  - Advanced disease and bone marrow failure are associated with diffuse pattern of infiltration
  - Examination of bone marrow is essential for staging and helpful to monitor response to therapy

Predominant Pattern/Injury Type
- Diffuse

Predominant Cell/Compartment Type
- Hematopoietic, lymphoid

ANCILLARY TESTS

Immunohistochemistry
- B-cell antigens (CD20, CD79a, and pax-5) are positive, but CD20 expression can be very weak (dim)
- Tumor cells characteristically express CD5 and CD23
- CD23 is particularly useful in distinguishing CLL/SLL from mantle cell lymphoma
  - Should be evaluated in every case, if possible
- Some cases of CLL may express CD23 only weakly or partially; some cases of mantle cell lymphoma can be dimly CD23(+)
  - Evaluation of Cyclin-D1 or t(11;14) is suggested
- P53 is expressed in ~ 10% of cases

Flow Cytometry
- Dim expression of sIg (IgM or IgM + IgD or, rarely, IgG) with κ or λ light chain restriction
- Expression of CD19, CD20 (dim), and CD79a
- CD5(+), CD23(+), CD43(+)
- CD11c(+/-), CD10(-), FMC7(-)
- Expression of CD38 on > 30% of cells is seen in about 1/2 of cases and reported to be associated with worse prognosis
- Expression of T-cell-associated antigen ZAP70 is associated with unmutated *Ig* variable genes
- Cases with ZAP70 on > 30% of cells by flow cytometry have worse prognosis than ZAP70(-) cases

Cytogenetics
- About 50% of cases have abnormal karyotypes (conventional methods); FISH is more often abnormal
- Trisomy 12 reported in 1/3 of cases with cytogenetic abnormalities
  - Correlates with atypical histology and aggressive clinical course
- Cases with trisomy 12 have predominantly unmutated *Ig* variable region genes

o Those with 13q14 abnormalities more often have mutations
- Abnormalities of 13q reported in up to 25% of cases; associated with longer survival
- Abnormalities of 11q23 are found in small subset of cases; associated with lymphadenopathy and aggressive course
- Deletions of 6q21 or 17p13 (*TP53* locus) seen in 5% and 10% of cases, respectively
- *P53* mutations or deletions are associated with worse prognosis regardless of *IgH* mutational status

DIFFERENTIAL DIAGNOSIS

Follicular Lymphoma (FL)
- Follicles can enlarge and coalesce to form large, grossly visible masses
- Neoplastic lymphocytes are centrocytes and centroblasts
  o Positive for CD10, CD19, CD20, and CD22; bright monoclonal sIg
  o Positive for Bcl-6 by immunohistochemistry
  o CD5(-), CD11c(-), CD43(-)

Mantle Cell Lymphoma (MCL)
- Lymphocytes intermediate in size with irregular nuclear contours
  o Positive for CD5, CD19, CD20, CD22, and CD43; moderate monoclonal sIg
  o CD10(-), CD23(-/+)
- Cyclin-D1(+) by immunohistochemistry; t(11;14) (q13;q32) positive by conventional cytogenetics or FISH

Hairy Cell Leukemia (HCL)
- Patients present with splenomegaly and pancytopenia
- Indented nuclei with abundant clear cytoplasm
- Lymphocytes are positive for CD11c (bright), CD19, CD20, CD22 (bright), CD25, and CD103
- CD5(-), CD10(-), CD23(-)
- Tartrate-resistant acid phosphatase stain is strongly positive in hairy cells

Monoclonal B Lymphocytosis (MBL)
- Healthy adults who have absolute increase in monoclonal B lymphocytes
- < 5 x 10^9/L B lymphocytes in peripheral blood
- Absence of lymphadenopathy or organomegaly, cytopenias, or disease-related symptoms
- May progress to frank CLL/SLL at rate of 1-2% per year

DIAGNOSTIC CHECKLIST

Pathologic Interpretation Pearls
- Dimming light during light microscopy is helpful in appreciating proliferation centers in histologic sections of lymph node
- Atypical immunophenotype occurs in ~ 10-20% of cases

SELECTED REFERENCES

1. Lin KI et al: Relevance of the immunoglobulin VH somatic mutation status in patients with chronic lymphocytic leukemia treated with fludarabine, cyclophosphamide, and rituximab (FCR) or related chemoimmunotherapy regimens. Blood. 113(14):3168-71, 2009
2. Hallek M et al: Guidelines for the diagnosis and treatment of chronic lymphocytic leukemia: a report from the International Workshop on Chronic Lymphocytic Leukemia updating the National Cancer Institute-Working Group 1996 guidelines. Blood. 111(12):5446-56, 2008
3. Kantarjian H et al: Therapeutic advances in leukemia and myelodysplastic syndrome over the past 40 years. Cancer. 113(7 Suppl):1933-52, 2008
4. Müller-Hermelink HK et al: Chronic lymphocytic leukemia/small lymphocytic lymphoma. In: WHO Classification of Tumours of Haematopoietic and Lymphoid Tissues. Lyon, France: IARC Press. 180-182, 2008
5. Rassenti LZ et al: Relative value of ZAP-70, CD38, and immunoglobulin mutation status in predicting aggressive disease in chronic lymphocytic leukemia. Blood. 112(5):1923-30, 2008
6. Huh YO et al: The t(14;19)(q32;q13)-positive small B-cell leukaemia: a clinicopathologic and cytogenetic study of seven cases. Br J Haematol. 136(2):220-8, 2007
7. Zanotti R et al: ZAP-70 expression, as detected by immunohistochemistry on bone marrow biopsies from early-phase CLL patients, is a strong adverse prognostic factor. Leukemia. 21(1):102-9, 2007
8. Marti GE et al: Diagnostic criteria for monoclonal B-cell lymphocytosis. Br J Haematol. 130(3):325-32, 2005
9. Admirand JH et al: Immunohistochemical detection of ZAP-70 in 341 cases of non-Hodgkin and Hodgkin lymphoma. Mod Pathol. 17(8):954-61, 2004
10. Crespo M et al: ZAP-70 expression as a surrogate for immunoglobulin-variable-region mutations in chronic lymphocytic leukemia. N Engl J Med. 348(18):1764-75, 2003
11. Tobin G et al: Somatically mutated Ig V(H)3-21 genes characterize a new subset of chronic lymphocytic leukemia. Blood. 99(6):2262-4, 2002
12. Rosenwald A et al: Relation of gene expression phenotype to immunoglobulin mutation genotype in B cell chronic lymphocytic leukemia. J Exp Med. 194(11):1639-47, 2001
13. Binet JL et al: A clinical staging system for chronic lymphocytic leukemia: prognostic significance. Cancer. 40(2):855-64, 1977
14. Hernandez-Nieto L et al: Bone-marrow patterns and clinical staging in chronic lymphocytic leukaemia. Lancet. 1(8024):1269, 1977
15. Rai KR et al: Clinical staging of chronic lymphocytic leukemia. Blood. 46(2):219-34, 1975

CHRONIC LYMPHOCYTIC LEUKEMIA/SMALL LYMPHOCYTIC LYMPHOMA

Microscopic and Immunohistochemical Features

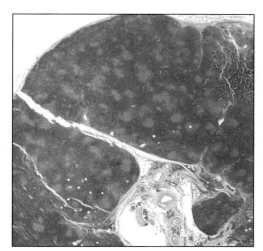
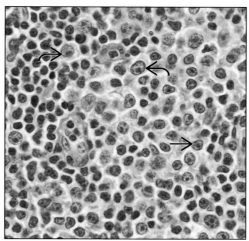

(Left) Lymph node involved by CLL/SLL with numerous proliferation centers (a.k.a. pseudofollicular growth centers or pseudofollicles). *(Right)* Hematoxylin & eosin of a lymph node shows a proliferation center of CLL/SLL. The proliferation center is composed of small lymphocytes, prolymphocytes ⇥, and paraimmunoblasts ⇨.

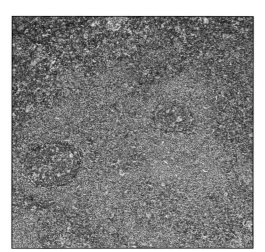
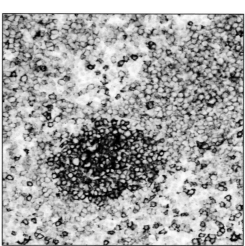

(Left) Lymph node involved by CLL/SLL with an interfollicular pattern. Darkly stained reactive follicles are surrounded by large proliferation centers of SLL/CLL. This pattern mimics marginal zone lymphoma. *(Right)* CD20 immunohistochemical stain highlights dim and variable CD20 expression in CLL/SLL, interfollicular pattern. Residual germinal center cells are brightly CD20(+).

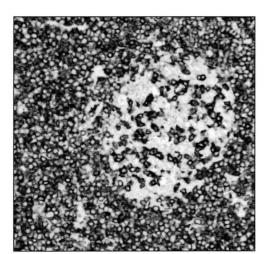
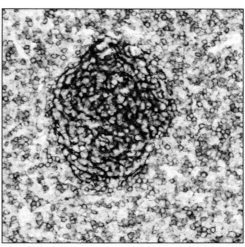

(Left) CD5 shows CLL/SLL, interfollicular pattern with aberrant staining for the T-cell-associated marker CD5. The central benign germinal center is negative for CD5. *(Right)* CD23 illustrates CD23 expression in CLL/SLL, interfollicular pattern in a lymph node. The central benign germinal center has many CD23(+) follicular dendritic cells.

CHRONIC LYMPHOCYTIC LEUKEMIA/SMALL LYMPHOCYTIC LYMPHOMA

Microscopic and Immunohistochemical Features

(Left) CLL/SLL involving a lymph node with proliferation centers. Note the vaguely nodular, irregularly distributed, pale-staining areas in a dark background of small cells. (Right) CLL/SLL involving lymph node. A central proliferation center contains a continuum of small lymphocytes, prolymphocytes, and paraimmunoblasts.

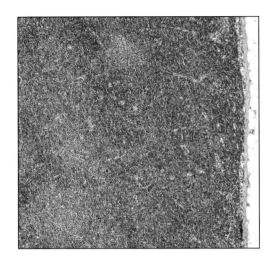
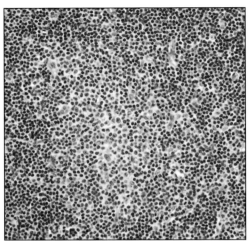

(Left) CD20 highlights CLL/SLL cells. The proliferation centers are more brightly positive than the neoplastic small lymphocytes. (Right) CD23 immunostain of CLL/SLL highlights the vaguely nodular proliferation centers as well as the small neoplastic cells.

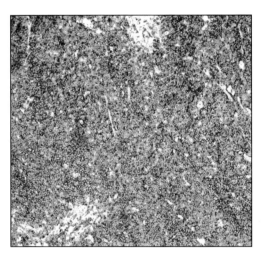
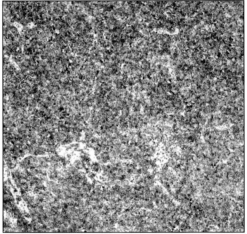

(Left) CD5 shows CLL/SLL that is weakly positive for CD5. Scattered reactive T cells are darkly stained. (Right) Cyclin-D1 is negative in CLL/SLL. Endothelial cells are positive and serve as an internal control.

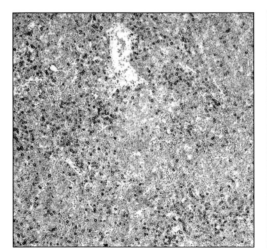
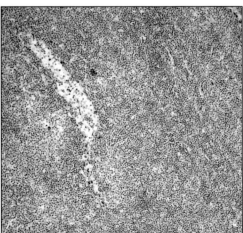

CHRONIC LYMPHOCYTIC LEUKEMIA/SMALL LYMPHOCYTIC LYMPHOMA

Microscopic and Immunophenotypic Features

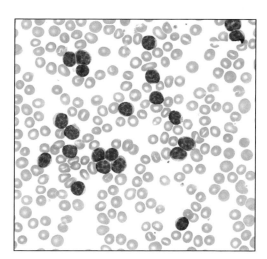
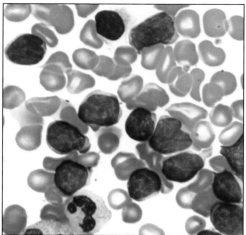

(Left) Wright-Giemsa shows CLL involving the peripheral blood. There is marked lymphocytosis, and most lymphocytes have sparse cytoplasm, round to oval nuclei, and no evident nucleoli. This morphology is characteristic of most cases of CLL. *(Right)* Wright-Giemsa shows CLL with cytologically atypical morphology in this peripheral blood smear with a population of small and medium-sized cells, some with indented nuclei.

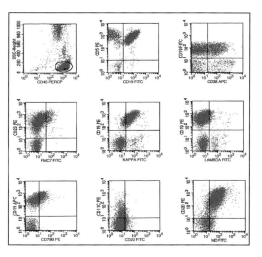
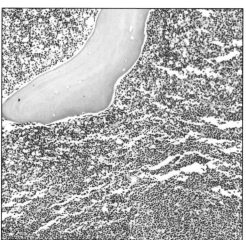

(Left) Representative immunophenotypic analysis of CLL by flow cytometry. The neoplastic cells express CD5, CD11c(partial), CD19, CD20, CD23, CD38, weak surface immunoglobulin M&D, and monotypic κ light chain. *(Right)* Bone marrow involvement by CLL with a diffuse pattern. The entire bone marrow space between bone trabeculae is replaced by small lymphocytes.

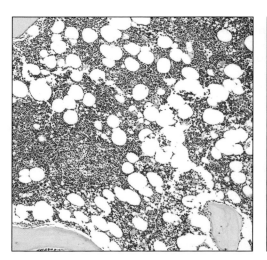
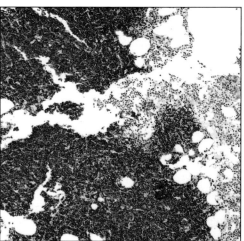

(Left) Bone marrow involvement by CLL with an interstitial pattern of lymphocytic infiltration, demonstrating preservation of the normal architecture. The mature lymphocytes infiltrate the interstitium with substantial sparing of normal hematopoietic cells. *(Right)* ZAP70 is strongly expressed in this case of CLL shown by immunohistochemistry. The expression is nuclear and cytoplasmic. ZAP70 expression in CLL is associated with a poor prognosis.

RICHTER SYNDROME

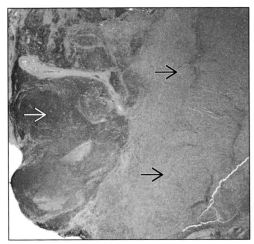

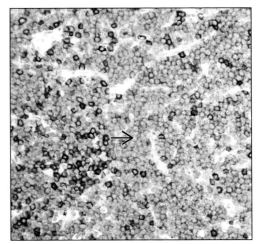

In this patient with Richter syndrome, a tonsil was involved by chronic lymphocytic leukemia/small lymphocytic lymphoma (CLL/SLL) ⇒ and diffuse large B-cell lymphoma (DLBCL) ⇒.

Diffuse large B-cell lymphoma component of Richter syndrome involving tonsil. The neoplastic large cells ⇒ express CD5 more dimly than reactive T cells.

TERMINOLOGY

Abbreviations
- Richter syndrome (RS)

Synonyms
- Richter transformation

Definitions
- Aggressive lymphoma arising in patients with chronic lymphocytic leukemia/small lymphocytic lymphoma (CLL/SLL)
- Histologic types of aggressive lymphoma
  - Diffuse large B-cell lymphoma (DLBCL), most common
  - Classical Hodgkin lymphoma (CHL)
  - Peripheral T-cell lymphoma (PTCL)
  - B-lymphoblastic lymphoma/leukemia (very rare)

ETIOLOGY/PATHOGENESIS

Clonal Relationship
- Aggressive lymphoma is clonally related to CLL/SLL in ~ 80% of cases
  - Both DLBCL and CHL can be clonally related to CLL/SLL

Other Possible Causes
- CLL/SLL may contribute to genetic instability, allowing development of additional genetic abnormalities
- *ATM* or *P53* abnormalities in CLL/SLL may impair cell response to DNA damage
- CLL/SLL is associated with immunosuppression and loss of immunosurveillance
  - Chemotherapy for CLL/SLL may contribute to immunocompromise
    - Nucleoside analogues impair host immunity

CLINICAL ISSUES

Epidemiology
- Incidence
  - 2-8% of patients with CLL/SLL develop RS
  - ~ 0.5% of patients with CLL/SLL develop CHL
  - Peripheral T-cell lymphoma in CLL/SLL patients is extremely rare
- Age
  - Median age: 7th decade
- Gender
  - Male to female ratio: ~ 2.5 to 1

Site
- Most common: Lymph nodes, bone marrow, peripheral blood, spleen
- Extranodal sites are not commonly involved
  - Skin, testes, gastrointestinal tract, liver
  - Tonsils, bones, lungs, central nervous system

Presentation
- Median time from diagnosis of CLL/SLL to RS: ~ 2-3 years
- RS can be diagnosed 1st, before presence of CLL/SLL is known
- Sudden onset of symptoms
  - B symptoms: Fever, night sweats, &/or weight loss
  - Rapidly progressive lymphadenopathy
    - Generalized more common than single site

Laboratory Tests
- Anemia, neutropenia, and thrombocytopenia
- Rapid increase in serum lactate dehydrogenase
- Serum paraprotein in subset of patients

Treatment
- Fractionated cyclophosphamide, vincristine, liposomal daunorubicin, dexamethasone, and rituximab (HyperCVXD-R)

RICHTER SYNDROME

Key Facts

Terminology
- Aggressive lymphoma arising in patient with chronic lymphocytic leukemia/small lymphocytic lymphoma (CLL/SLL)
- Subtypes
  - Common: Diffuse large B-cell lymphoma
  - Uncommon: Classical Hodgkin lymphoma
  - Rare: Peripheral T-cell lymphoma, B-lymphoblastic lymphoma

Etiology/Pathogenesis
- Aggressive lymphoma is clonally related to CLL/SLL in ~ 80% of cases
- Both DLBCL and classical Hodgkin lymphoma can be clonally related to CLL/SLL

Clinical Issues
- 2-8% of patients with CLL/SLL develop RS
- ~ 0.5% of patients with CLL/SLL develop CHL
- Sudden fever, night sweats, &/or weight loss
- Rapidly progressive lymphadenopathy
  - Generalized more common than single site
- Anemia, neutropenia, and thrombocytopenia
- Rapid rise of serum LDH
- Generally dismal prognosis
  - Median survival: ~ 20-30 months

Top Differential Diagnoses
- Lymphadenopathy secondary to infectious causes
- CLL/SLL with prominent proliferation centers
- CLL/SLL in prolymphocytoid transformation
- CD5(+) de novo DLBCL

- Oxaliplatin, fludarabine, cytarabine, and rituximab (OFAR)
- Autologous or allogeneic stem cell transplantation
  - For younger patients

Prognosis
- Generally dismal; median survival: ~ 20-30 months
  - Often, survival is < 1 year
- Prognosis relatively better for patients with CHL

Risk Factors for RS
- Lymph node size > 3 cm
- CD38 expression
- Absence of del(13q14)
- *IgVH4-39* gene usage

IMAGE FINDINGS

Radiographic Findings
- Generalized or localized lymphadenopathy
- Increased 18F-FDG uptake on PET/CT
- Increased gallium-67 uptake on single photon emission computed tomography scans (controversial)

MICROSCOPIC PATHOLOGY

Histologic Features
- DLBCL
  - Centroblastic (most common) or immunoblastic variant
  - Immunoblastic variant more common relative to de novo DLBCL
  - Rare cases resemble T-cell/histiocyte-rich large B-cell lymphoma
  - High mitotic rate; ± necrosis
- CHL
  - Hodgkin and Reed-Sternberg (HRS) cells
  - Inflammatory background of T cells, histiocytes, ± eosinophils
  - Necrosis is common
- Peripheral T-cell lymphoma, not otherwise specified

  - Mixture of intermediate-sized and large cells, or predominance of large cells
- B-lymphoblastic lymphoma/leukemia
  - Small- to intermediate-sized cells with blastic chromatin
- In all types of RS, evidence of CLL/SLL is also commonly present
  - Discrete foci of CLL/SLL and aggressive lymphoma
  - CLL/SLL cells intermixed with aggressive lymphoma

ANCILLARY TESTS

Immunohistochemistry
- DLBCL
  - Monotypic Ig(+), CD19(+), CD22(+); pan-T-cell antigens(-)
  - Clonally related cases of DLBCL share immunophenotype of CLL/SLL
    - CD20(dim+), but CD5, CD23, and ZAP-70 often negative
  - Clonally unrelated cases commonly CD5(-), CD23(-)
  - Using the Hans et al classifier (based on CD10, Bcl-6, and IRF-4/MUM1)
    - ABC phenotype in 70-80% of cases
    - GC phenotype in 20-30% of cases
- Commonly p53(+), proliferation (Ki-67) rate is usually high (> 50%)
- Epstein-Barr virus (EBV)(+) in subset of cases
- Classical Hodgkin lymphoma
  - Immunophenotype of HRS cells
    - CD30(+), CD15(-/+), pax-5(dim+), EBV(+/-), CD45/LCA(-), CD20(-)
- Peripheral T-cell lymphoma, not otherwise specified
  - Pan-T-cell antigens(+), B-cell antigens(-), EBV(-)
- B-lymphoblastic lymphoma/leukemia
  - CD10(+), CD19(+), TdT(+), T-cell antigens(-)

Flow Cytometry
- In general, agreement with immunohistochemistry findings

6

- Better suited for documenting dim expression or aberrant immunophenotypes
- CD5, CD23, &/or ZAP70 detected by flow cytometry more often than by immunohistochemistry

Cytogenetics

- Complex karyotype in subset of cases
  - Del(17p13) involved in subset of cases
- No consistent chromosomal abnormalities

PCR

- DLBCL
  - Positive for monoclonal *IgH* gene rearrangements
    - In clonally related cases, CLL/SLL and DLBCL share sequence
  - *IgVH* genes are often unmutated in clonally related cases
  - *IgVH* genes are often mutated in clonally unrelated cases
  - *IgVH3* gene family is used most often
- CHL
  - Positive for monoclonal *IgH* gene rearrangements in HRS cells
    - Can be clonally related to CLL/SLL
    - Clonally related cases usually EBV(-)
  - *IgVH* genes are often mutated
  - ~ 50% of CHL cases are clonally related to CLL/SLL
    - Clonally related cases usually EBV(-)
  - Clonally unrelated cases of CHL often EBV(+)
- Peripheral T-cell lymphoma
  - Positive for monoclonal *TCR* gene rearrangements

DIFFERENTIAL DIAGNOSIS

Lymphadenopathy Secondary to Infectious Causes

- Patients with CLL/SLL are at risk for infections
- Enlarged lymph nodes in CLL/SLL patient can show evidence of infectious etiology
  - Necrosis, neutrophilic infiltrate, organisms may be identified
  - Evidence of CLL/SLL is also present
- Herpes simplex lymphadenitis can closely mimic RS
  - Patients have rapid enlargement of lymph nodes
  - FDG-PET scan often shows high uptake
  - Necrosis (+); many immunoblasts can be present
  - HSV nuclear inclusions usually present
  - In situ hybridization for HSV(+)

CLL/SLL with Prominent Proliferation Centers

- In some cases of CLL/SLL, proliferation centers are large
- Discrete proliferation centers are evidence against RS
- Fine needle aspiration of proliferation center can be misinterpreted as DLBCL

CLL/SLL in Prolymphocytoid Transformation

- Patients with CLL/SLL can have increased prolymphocytes

- Best defined by complete blood count and differential count of peripheral blood smear
- Applying this approach to lymph node biopsy specimens is controversial
  - Prognostic significance not proven

CD5(+) de Novo DLBCL

- DLBCL/RS and de novo DLBCL can be histologically indistinguishable
- Neither immunophenotype nor molecular analysis can reliably distinguish these possibilities
- Patients with de novo CD5(+) DLBCL
  - No history of CLL/SLL; blood and bone marrow negative for CLL/SLL
  - No evidence of CLL/SLL in biopsy specimen

Lymphoproliferative Disorders (LPD) Associated with Fludarabine Therapy

- Histologically, show spectrum of small and large cells
  - Resemble, in part, immunodeficiency-associated LPDs
- Usually EBV(+)
- Can resolve after fludarabine is discontinued ± antiviral therapy

Myeloid/Monocytic Sarcoma

- Small number of CLL/SLL patients subsequently develop acute myeloid leukemia
  - Subset of patients initially 1st present with lymphadenopathy as result of myeloid/monocytic sarcoma
  - Not included as part of spectrum of RS
- Immunophenotype
  - Myeloperoxidase(+), CD43(+), other myeloid-associated antigens(+)

Metastatic Carcinoma

- Patients with CLL/SLL have increased risk of 2nd tumors
  - Carcinomas of head and neck, lungs, colon, etc.
  - Immunophenotype
    - Keratins(+), EMA(+), CD20(-), CD45/LCA(-)

SELECTED REFERENCES

1. Molica S: A systematic review on Richter syndrome: what is the published evidence? Leuk Lymphoma. 51(3):415-21, 2010
2. Rossi D et al: Richter syndrome: molecular insights and clinical perspectives. Hematol Oncol. 27(1):1-10, 2009
3. Omoti CE et al: Richter syndrome: a review of clinical, ocular, neurological and other manifestations. Br J Haematol. 142(5):709-16, 2008
4. Mao Z et al: IgVH mutational status and clonality analysis of Richter's transformation: diffuse large B-cell lymphoma and Hodgkin lymphoma in association with B-cell chronic lymphocytic leukemia (B-CLL) represent 2 different pathways of disease evolution. Am J Surg Pathol. 31(10):1605-14, 2007

RICHTER SYNDROME

Microscopic Features

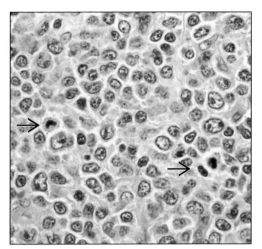

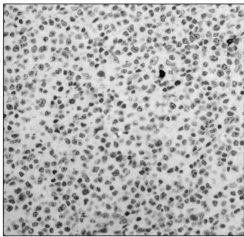

(Left) DLBCL component of Richter syndrome. The neoplastic cells are large and highly proliferative with 2 mitotic figures ➡ identified in this field. *(Right)* DLBCL component of Richter syndrome involving tonsil. The neoplastic large cells are CD23(-), unlike the cells in the CLL/SLL component, which were CD23(+).

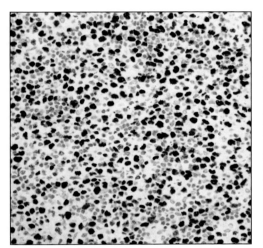

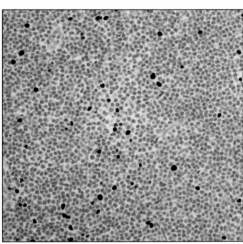

(Left) DLBCL component of Richter syndrome involving the tonsil. Ki-67 immunostain demonstrates a high proliferation rate of ~ 70-80%. *(Right)* Chronic lymphocytic leukemia/small lymphocytic lymphoma component of Richter syndrome involving the tonsil. Ki-67 immunostain demonstrates a low proliferation rate of < 5%.

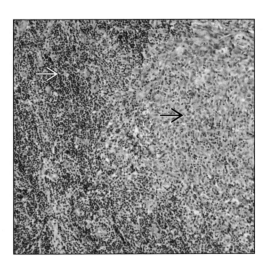

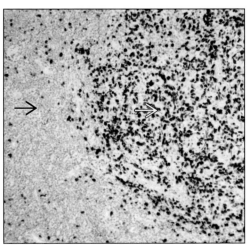

(Left) In this patient with Richter syndrome, a lymph node biopsy specimen showed chronic lymphocytic leukemia/small lymphocytic lymphoma (CLL/SLL) ➡ and diffuse large B-cell lymphoma (DLBCL) ➡. *(Right)* CLL/SLL and DLBCL consistent with Richter syndrome involving the lymph node. Ki-67 immunostain demonstrates a high (70-80%) proliferation rate in DLBCL ➡ but not in CLL/SLL ➡.

RICHTER SYNDROME

Microscopic Features

(Left) CLL/SLL and DLBCL consistent with Richter syndrome. Unlike the CLL/SLL component, the DLBCL cells are strongly Bcl-6(+) ➡. *(Right)* CLL/SLL and DLBCL consistent with Richter syndrome involving lymph node. CD5 is expressed by CLL/SLL cells ➡ but is not expressed by the neoplastic cells of DLBCL ➡.

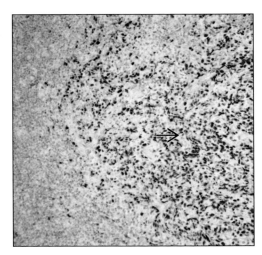
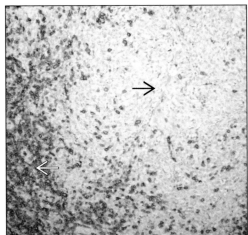

(Left) CLL/SLL and DLBCL consistent with Richter syndrome (RS) involving lymph node. CD23 is expressed by CLL/SLL cells ➡ but is not expressed by the neoplastic cells of the DLBCL component ➡. *(Right)* A cervical lymph node biopsy specimen involved by CLL/SLL ➡ and classical Hodgkin lymphoma ➡ supporting Hodgkin variant of RS.

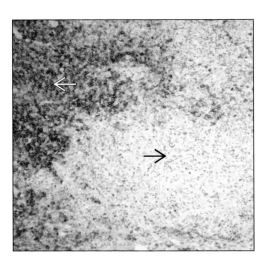
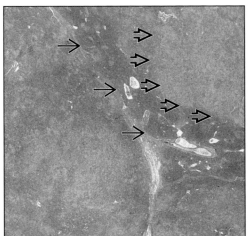

(Left) Cervical lymph node involved by CLL/SLL and classical Hodgkin lymphoma, consistent with Hodgkin type of Richter syndrome. A classical Reed-Sternberg cell is shown ➡. *(Right)* Cervical lymph node involved by CLL/SLL and classical Hodgkin lymphoma consistent with Hodgkin type of Richter syndrome. The neoplastic cells are CD30(+).

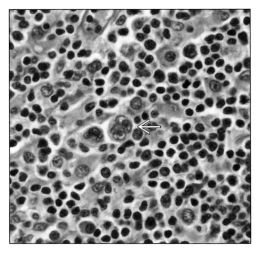
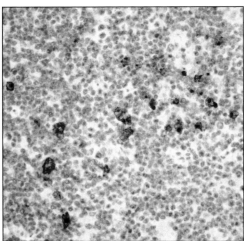

Differential Diagnosis

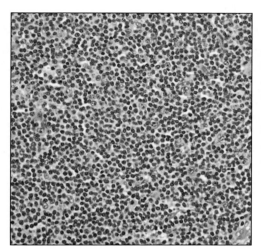 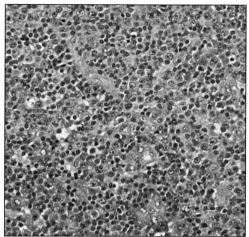

(Left) Chronic lymphocytic leukemia/small lymphocytic lymphoma (CLL/SLL) and herpes simplex infection involving lymph node. In this field, the findings are typical of CLL/SLL. *(Right)* CLL/SLL and herpes simplex infection involving the lymph node. In this field, many larger cells are present, suggesting the possibility of diffuse large B-cell lymphoma. After antiviral therapy was initiated, the patient had complete resolution of symptoms without evidence of Richter syndrome elsewhere.

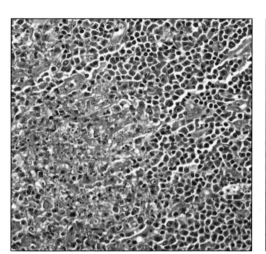 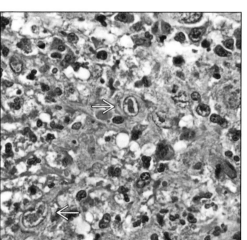

(Left) Chronic lymphocytic leukemia/small lymphocytic lymphoma (CLL/SLL) and herpes simplex infection involving lymph node. This field shows necrosis with neutrophilic exudate. Viral inclusions cannot be appreciated at this power. *(Right)* CLL/SLL and herpes simplex infection involving lymph node. High-power magnification of necrotic areas shows viral inclusions ➡ typical of herpes simplex infection.

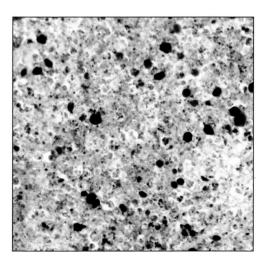 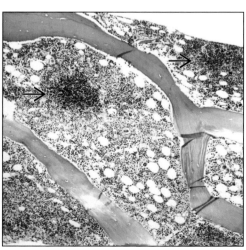

(Left) Chronic lymphocytic leukemia/small lymphocytic lymphoma (CLL/SLL) and herpes simplex virus (HSV) infection involving lymph node. Immunostain for HSV shows many positive nuclei. After antiviral therapy was initiated, there was no evidence of Richter syndrome. *(Right)* Bone marrow biopsy specimen in a patient with CLL/SLL and herpes simplex infection. The bone marrow showed only CLL/SLL present in a nodular pattern ➡ in this field.

LYMPHOPLASMACYTIC LYMPHOMA AND WALDENSTROM MACROGLOBULINEMIA

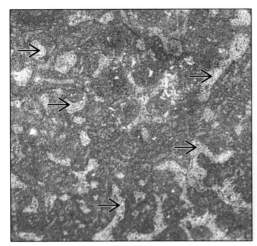

Lymphoplasmacytic lymphoma and Waldenström macroglobulinemia (LPL/WM) involving lymph node. Low-power view shows a diffuse pattern of growth with patent sinuses ⊟ that contain histiocytes.

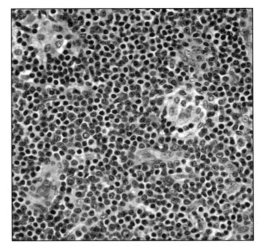

LPL/WM involving lymph node. The proliferating cells are small lymphocytes, and a subset of cells has plasmacytoid features.

TERMINOLOGY

Abbreviations
- Lymphoplasmacytic lymphoma (LPL)
- Waldenström macroglobulinemia (WM)

Synonyms
- Terms used in earlier lymphoma classification systems are not exact synonyms as the definition of LPL has been refined over the years
- Older terms that included LPL along with other B-cell lymphomas include
  - Well-differentiated lymphocytic, plasmacytoid (Rappaport classification)
  - Immunocytoma, lymphoplasmacytic type (Kiel classification)
  - Malignant lymphoma, small lymphocytic, plasmacytoid (Working Formulation)
  - Lymphoplasmacytoid lymphoma (REAL classification)
- Terms "LPL" and "WM" are often used interchangeably, but the 2 are not identical
  - WM represents great majority of LPL cases

Definitions
- LPL is a neoplasm of small B lymphocytes, plasmacytoid lymphocytes, and plasma cells that does not meet criteria for any other type of small B-cell lymphoma showing plasmacytic differentiation
  - LPL is usually associated with serum monoclonal paraprotein
    - Usually IgM; rarely IgG or IgA
    - Monoclonal paraprotein is not required for diagnosis of LPL
- WM is LPL involving bone marrow associated with an IgM paraprotein
  - No specific cutoff level of IgM is required

ETIOLOGY/PATHOGENESIS

Infectious Agents
- Hepatitis C is implicated in some cases of LPL; data are controversial

Genetic Predisposition
- Familial cases of WM are reported
  - Usually occurs in younger patients
- Monoclonal gammopathy of unknown significance (MGUS) is most likely a precursor of WM

CLINICAL ISSUES

Epidemiology
- Incidence
  - ~ 1% of non-Hodgkin lymphomas
- Age
  - Median age: 63 to 71 years
- Gender
  - Male to female ratio = 2:1
- Ethnicity
  - Whites are more frequently affected than African Americans or Asians

Presentation
- Relatively little data are available for patients with LPL that do not also have WM
- About 25% of patients with WM are asymptomatic, so-called smoldering WM
- Symptoms and signs of patients with WM are related to
  - Tissue infiltration by neoplastic cells **or**
  - Effects of elevated IgM paraprotein
- Anemia due to bone marrow infiltration is common and causes fatigue and weakness
  - Bilineage cytopenia or pancytopenia can occur if infiltration by WM is extensive

LYMPHOPLASMACYTIC LYMPHOMA AND WALDENSTROM MACROGLOBULINEMIA

Key Facts

Terminology
- LPL is a neoplasm of small B lymphocytes ± plasmacytoid features and plasma cells that does not meet criteria for any other small B-cell lymphoma showing plasmacytic differentiation
- WM is LPL involving bone marrow associated with an IgM paraprotein of any level

Clinical Issues
- Symptoms and signs of patients with WM are related to
  ○ Tissue infiltration by neoplastic cells **or**
  ○ Effects of elevated IgM paraprotein
- WM is usually indolent; median survival: 5-10 years

Microscopic Pathology
- Bone marrow involvement is constant in WM

- 3 subtypes of WM are recognized
  ○ Polymorphous subtype predicts poorer prognosis

Ancillary Tests
- LPL and WM have 2 immunophenotypic components
  ○ B cells and plasmacytoid/plasma cells
- Del6q is the most common cytogenetic aberration in WM, ~ 40% of cases
- IgH translocations are uncommon

Top Differential Diagnoses
- Marginal zone lymphoma
- Chronic lymphocytic leukemia/small lymphocytic lymphoma with plasmacytic differentiation
- Plasma cell myeloma, small cell variant
- Splenic marginal zone lymphoma

- Hepatomegaly occurs in ~ 20% and splenomegaly in ~ 15% of WM patients
  ○ WM can involve gastrointestinal tract, kidney, and other extramedullary sites
- Lymphadenopathy in ~ 15% of WM patients
  ○ Lymphadenopathy is usually mild compared with other types of non-Hodgkin lymphoma
- Elevated serum IgM paraprotein levels can cause variety of symptoms
  ○ Hyperviscosity syndrome occurs in 5-15% of cases
    ▪ Headache, vision disturbance (retinopathy), neurologic changes, and cardiac failure
    ▪ Bing-Neel syndrome is central nervous system manifestation
  ○ Cryoglobulinemia, cold agglutinin hemolysis, autoimmune thrombocytopenia
    ▪ Type II cryoglobulinemia associated with HCV may cause Raynaud phenomenon, arthralgia, skin purpura, and vasculitis
    ▪ IgM-associated neuropathy is autoimmune mediated and tends to be distal, sensory, and symmetric
  ○ Deposition of IgM in skin and gastrointestinal tract causes related symptoms
- Rare manifestations include amyloidosis or light-chain deposition disease
  ○ Any site: Most common in kidney, skin, or bone marrow

Laboratory Tests
- IgM monoclonal protein is usually present in serum
  ○ WM
    ▪ IgM paraprotein is required for diagnosis
    ▪ No cutoff level for IgM in serum
  ○ LPL
    ▪ IgM paraprotein not required for diagnosis
    ▪ Rarely, IgA or IgG paraprotein alone or coexisting with IgM in serum
- Other laboratory abnormalities well described in WM patients
  ○ Elevated erythrocyte sedimentation rate, cytopenia (usually anemia)

○ Elevated serum levels of LDH or β-2 microglobulin

Treatment
- Treatment regimens are best defined for WM patients
  ○ Alkylating agents (chlorambucil), nucleoside analogs (cladribine or fludarabine), or single-agent rituximab is used
  ○ Autologous or allogeneic stem cell transplantation in eligible candidates
  ○ Plasmapheresis for hyperviscosity syndrome, cryoglobulinemia, neuropathy, amyloidosis, and light chain nephropathy
  ○ Corticosteroids for autoimmune hemolytic anemia or thrombocytopenia
- No consensus on optimal therapy of LPL patients without WM or serum IgM paraprotein
  ○ For cases without serum paraprotein: Patients often treated with low-grade B-cell lymphoma regimens

Prognosis
- WM
  ○ Usually indolent; median overall survival: 5-10 years
  ○ International prognostic scoring system designed to stratify patients into low-, intermediate-, and high-risk groups
    ▪ Age > 65 years
    ▪ Hemoglobin ≤ 11.5 g/dL
    ▪ Platelet count ≤ 100 X 10⁹
    ▪ Serum β-2 microglobulin > 3 mg/L
    ▪ Serum M protein concentration > 7 g/dL
    ▪ 5-year survival rates are 87%, 68%, and 36%, respectively, for low-, intermediate- and high-risk groups
  ○ Poor performance status and elevated serum LDH level also predict poorer prognosis

MACROSCOPIC FEATURES

Size
- Lymph nodes are usually only modestly enlarged

MICROSCOPIC PATHOLOGY

Histologic Features

- Lymph node
  - Involvement is usually total or subtotal, extending through capsule into perinodal adipose tissue
  - Pattern of growth is diffuse, but sinuses often are patent
  - Small residual follicles, usually in subcortical areas
  - Lymphoma cells are small ± plasmacytoid differentiation; monocytoid B cells can be seen
  - Blood vessels and sinuses may appear to be markedly dilated
  - Epithelioid histiocytes may be abundant or form scattered clusters
  - Hemosiderin or amyloid deposition
  - Scattered mast cells
- Bone marrow involvement is constant in WM
  - Pattern of infiltration can be diffuse, interstitial, and nodular
- 3 subtypes of WM are recognized
  - **Lymphoplasmacytoid**: Usually composed of monotonous small mature lymphocytes with varying degrees of plasmacytoid differentiation
  - **Lymphoplasmacytic**: Usually composed of lymphocytes and plasmacytic (Marschalko) cells; ± Dutcher or Russell bodies
  - **Polymorphous**: Has increased (5-10%) large cells; likely represents initial progression to large B-cell lymphoma
  - Subtypes do not predict level of serum IgM
- Peripheral blood smear
  - Rouleaux formation is common if IgM paraprotein level is high
  - Leukemic involvement (i.e., high leukocyte count) is unusual
  - Occasional neoplastic cells can be present
- WM and LPL can be associated with so-called crystal-storing histiocytosis
- Transformation of WM to diffuse large B-cell lymphoma (DLBCL) occurs in small subset of patients
  - WM and DLBCL components are usually of identical light chain type, suggesting clonal relationship
  - Serum IgM levels may paradoxically decrease
  - EBV is not usually implicated in transformation
- Rare patients with WM can develop classical Hodgkin lymphoma (CHL)
  - Clonal relationship between WM and CHL is unknown

ANCILLARY TESTS

Immunohistochemistry

- LPL and WM have 2 components: B cells and plasmacytoid/plasma cells
- B cells
  - pax-5(+), CD19(+), CD20(+), CD22(+)
  - CD45/LCA(+), Bcl-2(+), cytoplasmic Ig(-)
  - CD5(-), CD10(-), Cyclin-D1(-), Bcl-6(-)
- Plasmacytoid/plasma cells
  - CD38(+), CD138(+), CD20(-), pax-5(-/+)
  - Monotypic cytoplasmic Ig light chain (+), IgM(+)
  - Monotypic plasma cells may not be demonstrable in lymphoplasmacytoid subtype
- Ki-67 typically low, p53(-), CD3(-)

Flow Cytometry

- B cells
  - Surface IgM(+), Ig light chain (+), CD19(+), CD20(+)
  - Usually CD5(-), CD10(-), CD23(-)
  - Subset of cases may express CD5, CD10, or CD23
    - CD5 expression can be distinct or variable
    - CD10(+) cases are usually Bcl-6(-)
    - CD23 expression is usually dim/partial
  - CD11c(+/-), CD22(+/- dim), FMC-7(+/-), CD43(+/-)
  - CD25(-/+), CD103(-)
- Plasma cells
  - Cytoplasmic IgM(+), Ig light chain (+)
  - CD19(+), CD38(+), CD138(+)
  - IgG type of LPL may not coexpress CD19 and CD138
  - Monotypic plasma cells may be only evidence of persistent disease after chemotherapy

Cytogenetics

- Cytogenetic data are available for WM
  - Deletion of 6q in 40% of cases
  - Trisomy 4 in 20% of cases
  - Deletion of 13q in subset
  - Trisomy 3 is rare
  - Frequency of these abnormalities has not been confirmed in lymph node
- IgH translocations are uncommon in WM
- *PAX5-IgH*/t(9;14) is neither specific nor common in WM

In Situ Hybridization

- EBER(-)

Array CGH

- Deletions of 6q23 and 13q14
- Gains of 3q13-q28, 6p, and 18q
- Gains of 4q and 8q occur in 12% and 10% of WM cases, respectively

Molecular Findings in WM

- IgH is hypermutated, and VH3 family is preferentially used
- Cell of origin is probably memory B cells

DIFFERENTIAL DIAGNOSIS

Nodal Marginal Zone Lymphoma (NMZL)

- Morphologic and immunophenotypic features overlap with those of LPL
- Monocytoid B cells typically seen in NMZL are not unique to this neoplasm
- Some LPL cases may have prominent residual follicles similar to NMZL
- Unlike LPL, neoplastic cells of NMZL can be centrocyte-like cells with scattered large forms
- Diagnosis of WM may not be reliably rendered without knowledge of serum protein study

o Differential diagnosis of WM vs. MZL may be offered instead

Chronic Lymphocytic Leukemia/Small Lymphocytic Lymphoma (CLL/SLL) with Plasmacytic Differentiation

- Lymphoplasmacytoid variant of WM resembles CLL/SLL
- Pseudofollicles (proliferation centers) are present in SLL but not LPL
- Neoplastic cells of CLL/SLL are sIg(+ dim), CD5(+), and CD23(+)
- Serum IgM levels rarely exceed 3 g/dL in patients with CLL/SLL

Plasma Cell Myeloma, Small Cell Variant

- Rare cases of IgM(+) myeloma overlap with rare cases of IgG(+) or IgA(+) LPL
- ± clinical features of myeloma such as lytic bone lesions and renal insufficiency
- Myeloma plasma cells may be CD20(+)/CD138(+) but are usually CD19(-)/CD45(-/+ dim)
  o Myeloma cells are rarely CD19(+) and CD138(+)
- Cyclin-D1(+/-) in a nuclear and cytoplasmic pattern; absent in LPL/WM
- IgH translocation is present in 40-60% of cases of myeloma
- Cytogenetics and FISH confirm t(11;14)(q13;q32)

Splenic Marginal Zone Lymphoma (SMZL)

- SMZL can be associated with serum IgM paraprotein and involve bone marrow
- Patients have predominantly splenic disease with low level of lymph node involvement
- CD43(-) in splenic marginal zone lymphoma

Extranodal Marginal Zone Lymphoma of Mucosa-associated Tissue (MALT Lymphoma)

- Morphology and immunophenotype overlap between CPL/WM and MALT lymphoma
- LPL/WM may spread to extranodal sites such as orbit, gastrointestinal tract, lung, and skin
  o History of LPL/WM is essential for excluding diagnosis
- MALT lymphoma may be associated with high levels of IgM: Up to 5 g/dL in rare cases
- Identification of MALT lymphoma-associated cytogenetic aberrations may help in differential diagnosis
  o t(11;18), t(14;18), t(1;14), and t(3;14) are only reported in MALT lymphoma

Follicular Lymphoma (FL) with Plasmacytic Differentiation

- Rare cases of FL exhibit prominent plasmacytoid differentiation
- FL usually has follicular growth pattern
- FL is CD10(+), Bcl-6(+), Bcl-2-IgH/t(14;18)(q32;q21) (+)

Mantle Cell Lymphoma (MCL) with Plasmacytic Differentiation

- Rare cases of MCL exhibit prominent plasmacytoid differentiation
  o Can be associated with serum monoclonal IgM
  o IgM level in MCL patients is usually low (< 1 g/dL)
- CD5(+) LPL or WM may resemble MCL
- Cyclin-D1 stain or identification of t(11;14)(q13;q32)/CCND1-IgH supports MCL

DIAGNOSTIC CHECKLIST

Pathologic Interpretation Pearls

- Distinction of LPL/WM from MZL may not be possible in all cases
- General term "small B-cell lymphoma with plasmacytic differentiation" may be necessary

SELECTED REFERENCES

1. Kastritis E et al: Validation of the International Prognostic Scoring System (IPSS) for Waldenstrom's macroglobulinemia (WM) and the importance of serum lactate dehydrogenase (LDH). Leuk Res. 34(10):1340-3, 2010
2. Morice WG et al: Novel immunophenotypic features of marrow lymphoplasmacytic lymphoma and correlation with Waldenström's macroglobulinemia. Mod Pathol. 22(6):807-16, 2009
3. Konoplev S et al: Immunophenotypic profile of lymphoplasmacytic lymphoma/Waldenström macroglobulinemia. Am J Clin Pathol. 124(3):414-20, 2005
4. Lin P et al: Lymphoplasmacytic lymphoma/waldenstrom macroglobulinemia: an evolving concept. Adv Anat Pathol. 12(5):246-55, 2005
5. Lin P et al: Diffuse large B-cell lymphoma occurring in patients with lymphoplasmacytic lymphoma/Waldenström macroglobulinemia. Clinicopathologic features of 12 cases. Am J Clin Pathol. 120(2):246-53, 2003
6. Lin P et al: Waldenstrom macroglobulinemia involving extramedullary sites: morphologic and immunophenotypic findings in 44 patients. Am J Surg Pathol. 27(8):1104-13, 2003
7. Mansoor A et al: Cytogenetic findings in lymphoplasmacytic lymphoma/Waldenström macroglobulinemia. Chromosomal abnormalities are associated with the polymorphous subtype and an aggressive clinical course. Am J Clin Pathol. 116(4):543-9, 2001
8. Rosales CM et al: Lymphoplasmacytic lymphoma/Waldenström macroglobulinemia associated with Hodgkin disease. A report of two cases. Am J Clin Pathol. 116(1):34-40, 2001

LYMPHOPLASMACYTIC LYMPHOMA AND WALDENSTROM MACROGLOBULINEMIA

Microscopic Features

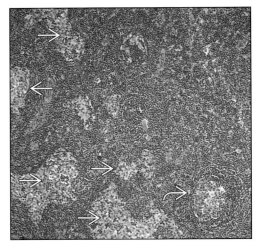

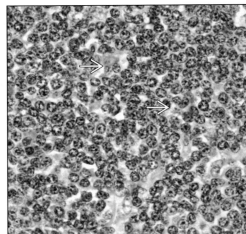

(Left) Lymphoplasmacytic lymphoma and Waldenström macroglobulinemia (LPL/WM), lymphoplasmacytoid subtype involving lymph node. The neoplasm has a diffuse pattern, but sinuses are patent ➡. A small residual germinal center ➡ is also present in this field. *(Right)* LPL/WM, lymphoplasmacytoid subtype involving lymph node. The proliferating cells are monotonous small mature lymphocytes, a subset of which has plasmacytoid differentiation ➡.

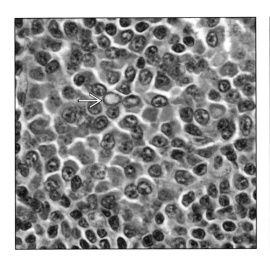

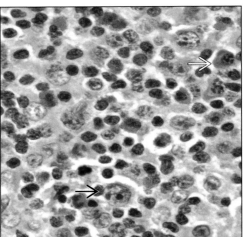

(Left) Lymphoplasmacytic lymphoma and Waldenström macroglobulinemia (LPL/WM), lymphoplasmacytic subtype involving lymph node. This field shows many plasmacytic cells and plasmacytoid lymphocytes. A Dutcher body (nuclear pseudoinclusion) is also shown ➡. *(Right)* LPL/WM, polymorphous subtype involving lymph node. Large immunoblasts ➡ are scattered among small lymphocytes, eosinophils, and plasma cells ➡.

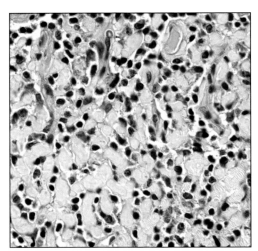

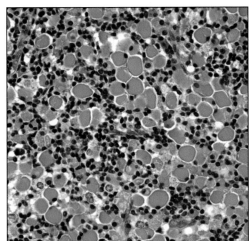

(Left) A case of lymphoplasmacytic lymphoma/Waldenström macroglobulinemia (LPL/WM). In this field, many neoplastic cells contain abundant cytoplasmic immunoglobulin and resemble signet ring cells. *(Right)* A case of LPL/WM is shown in which many plasmacytic cells contain prominent cytoplasmic inclusions of immunoglobulin (Russell bodies).

Variant Microscopic Features

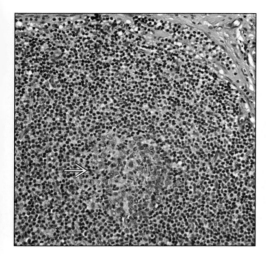

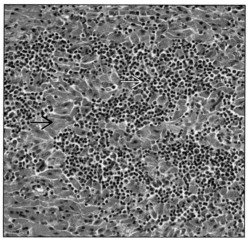

(Left) Lymphoplasmacytic lymphoma/Waldenström macroglobulinemia involving lymph node. A benign germinal center ➡ surrounded by lymphoma is shown. Residual germinal centers may be seen in the subcapsular region of lymph nodes involved by LPL/WM. *(Right)* LPL/WM associated with crystal-storing histiocytosis. Numerous histiocytes with their cytoplasm distended by crystals of immunoglobulin ➡ are present. Note the neoplastic small lymphocytes ➡.

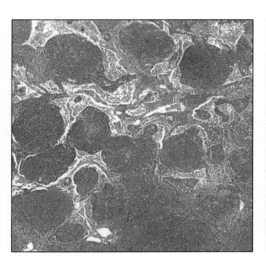

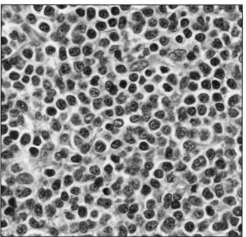

(Left) Lymphoplasmacytic lymphoma/Waldenström macroglobulinemia (LPL/WM) involving splenic hilar lymph node. In this specimen, partial involvement by lymphoma imparts a nodular pattern. *(Right)* LPL/WM involving lymph node. In this case, the neoplastic cells have a monocytoid appearance.

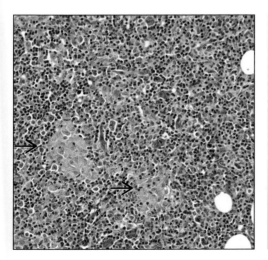

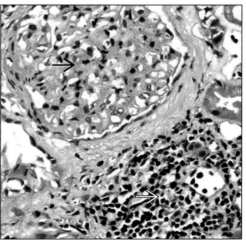

(Left) Clusters of histiocytes forming granuloma-like lesions ➡ may be observed in some cases of lymphoplasmacytic lymphoma/Waldenström macroglobulinemia (LPL/WM). *(Right)* LPL/WM involving kidney. The renal parenchyma is infiltrated by the neoplastic cells ➡. In addition, the glomerulus shown displays thickened basement membranes due to immunoglobulin deposition ➡.

Microscopic and Immunohistochemical Features

(Left) Lymphoplasmacytic lymphoma/Waldenström macroglobulinemia (LPL/WM) involving lymph node associated with amyloid deposition. A neoplastic lymphoplastic infiltrate ⮕ is surrounded by amorphous eosinophilic amyloid ⮕. Cracking artifact of the amyloid ⮒ can be seen. *(Right)* LPL/WM involving lymph node associated with amyloid deposition. Congo red stain viewed under polarized light highlights the amyloid, which shows apple-green birefringence ⮕.

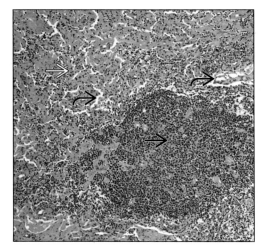
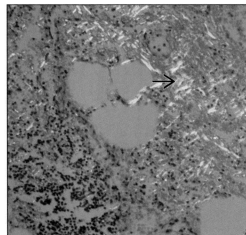

(Left) Lymphoplasmacytic lymphoma/Waldenström macroglobulinemia (LPL/WM) involving lymph node. CD20 stain highlights the neoplastic lymphocytes. *(Right)* LPL/WM involving lymph node. CD138(+) plasma cells are present and tend to be more common around blood vessels.

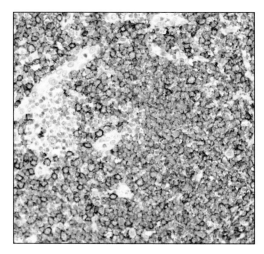
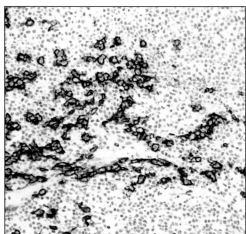

(Left) Lymphoplasmacytic lymphoma/Waldenström macroglobulinemia (LPL/WM) involving lymph node. The plasma cells express monotypic κ light chain. *(Right)* LPL/WM involving lymph node. Only rare plasma cells are positive for λ light chain.

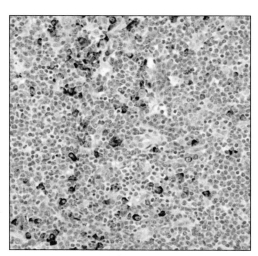
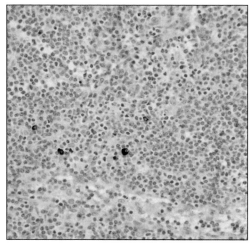

LYMPHOPLASMACYTIC LYMPHOMA AND WALDENSTROM MACROGLOBULINEMIA

Microscopic Features

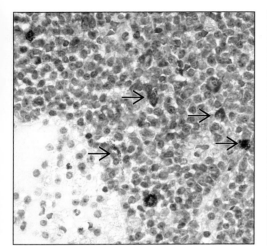

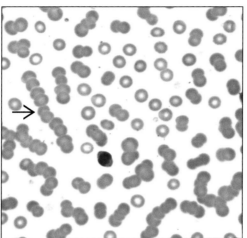

(Left) Lymphoplasmacytic lymphoma/Waldenström macroglobulinemia (LPL/WM) involving lymph node. Giemsa stain highlights mast cells admixed within the neoplasm. Note that some mast cells can have a spindled shape ➡. *(Right)* Wright-Giemsa stain of a peripheral blood smear shows rouleaux formation ➡ in a patient with LPL/WM.

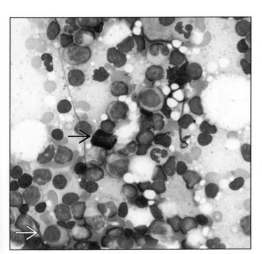

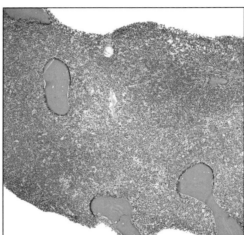

(Left) Lymphoplasmacytic lymphoma/Waldenström macroglobulinemia (LPL/WM). Bone marrow aspirate smear shows mast cells ➡, small lymphocytes, and plasma cells ➡. *(Right)* LPL/WM involving bone marrow biopsy specimen shows an extensive and diffuse infiltrate of neoplastic cells replacing the medullary space.

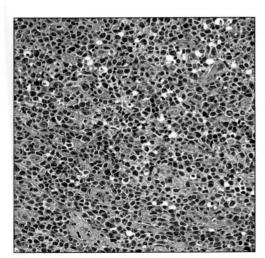

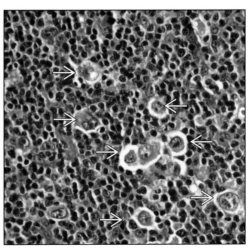

(Left) Lymphoplasmacytic lymphoma/Waldenström macroglobulinemia (LPL/WM) undergoing transformation to diffuse large B-cell lymphoma is shown. *(Right)* Classical Hodgkin lymphoma and LPL/WM involving lymph node. The large HRS cells ➡ are scattered among the background small lymphoid cells, some of which have plasmacytoid features. The HRS cells were CD15(+) and CD30(+) (not shown).

LYMPHOPLASMACYTIC LYMPHOMA AND WALDENSTROM MACROGLOBULINEMIA

Microscopic Features

(Left) LPL in a patient with an IgG paraprotein in serum. The patient also had bone marrow involvement, but based on the type of paraprotein, this case was not designated as Waldenström macroglobulinemia (WM). *(Right)* LPL in a patient with an IgG paraprotein in serum. The neoplasm surrounds a central reactive germinal center ⮞. This feature overlaps with nodal marginal zone lymphoma. This case does not meet the criteria for WM.

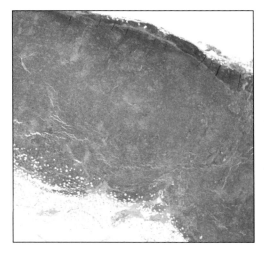
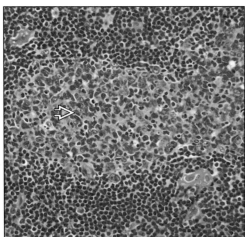

(Left) LPL in a patient with an IgG paraprotein in serum. The neoplasm had areas in which the neoplastic cells had monocytoid cytoplasm. This feature overlaps with nodal marginal zone lymphoma. This case does not meet the criteria for Waldenström macroglobulinemia (WM). *(Right)* LPL in a patient with an IgG paraprotein in serum. The neoplastic cells exhibit plasmacytoid differentiation. This case does not meet the criteria for WM.

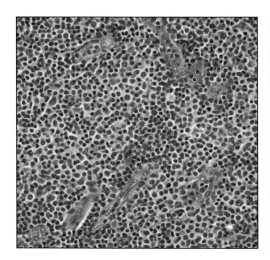
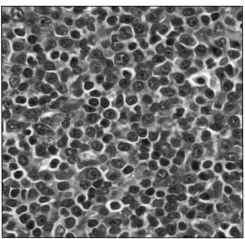

(Left) LPL involving bone marrow in a patient with a serum IgG paraprotein. This bone marrow smear shows neoplastic lymphocytes with plasmacytoid differentiation. Based on the paraprotein type, this case does not meet the criteria for Waldenström macroglobulinemia (WM). *(Right)* LPL involving bone marrow biopsy specimen in a patient with a serum IgG paraprotein. This case does not meet the criteria for WM.

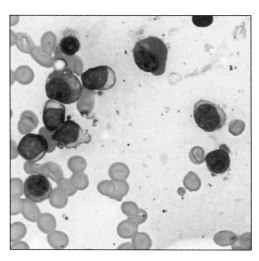
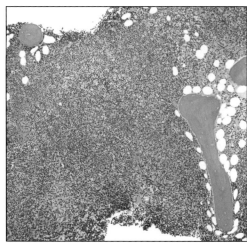

Differential Diagnosis

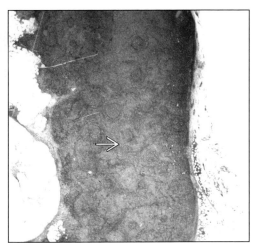

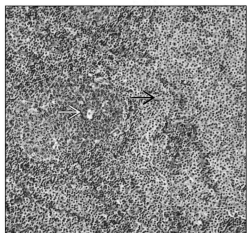

(Left) Nodal marginal zone B-cell lymphoma involving axillary lymph node. The neoplasm can be seen as pale rings ➡ around central reactive germinal centers (that appear darker). *(Right)* Nodal marginal zone B-cell lymphoma shows expansion of the marginal zone ➡. A reactive germinal center is present in this field ➡.

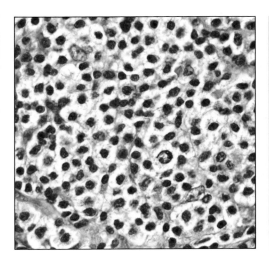

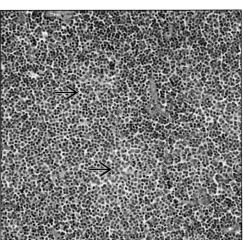

(Left) Nodal marginal zone B-cell lymphoma. The neoplastic cells in this case exhibit a marked monocytoid appearance. *(Right)* Small lymphocytic lymphoma/chronic lymphocytic leukemia (CLL/SLL) involving lymph node. Proliferation centers ➡ typical of CLL/SLL are present in this case.

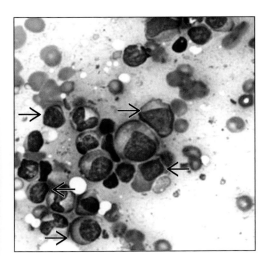

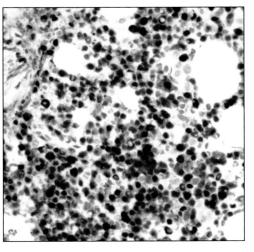

(Left) Plasma cell myeloma, small cell variant involving bone marrow. Smaller plasma cells ➡ resemble plasmacytoid lymphocytes, as can be seen in lymphoplasmacytic lymphoma. *(Right)* Plasma cell myeloma, small cell variant involving bone marrow. The neoplastic cells are Cyclin-D1(+). This finding is helpful for differential diagnosis, as lymphoplasmacytic lymphoma and Waldenström macroglobulinemia are Cyclin-D1(-).

NODAL MARGINAL ZONE B-CELL LYMPHOMA

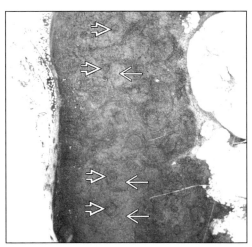

Nodal marginal zone lymphoma. The architecture is altered by nodules composed of central darker areas (germinal centers) ⮂ surrounded by peripheral pale areas (marginal zone areas) ➡.

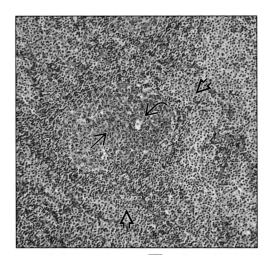

A residual germinal center ➡ with tingible body macrophages ➚ is surrounded by lymphoma cells with pale cytoplasm expanding marginal zones and interfollicular areas ⮂.

TERMINOLOGY

Abbreviations
- Nodal marginal zone B-cell lymphoma (NMZL)

Synonyms
- Nodal marginal zone lymphoma
- Monocytoid B-cell lymphoma
- Parafollicular B-cell lymphoma
- NMZL can be placed in any of 3 categories depending on large cell number (Working Formulation [1982])
  - Small lymphocytic plasmacytoid, diffuse small cleaved cell, or diffuse mixed small and large cell

Definitions
- Primary nodal B-cell lymphoma histologically resembling lymph nodes involved by MZL of extranodal or splenic types
  - There can be no evidence of extranodal or splenic disease

CLINICAL ISSUES

Epidemiology
- Incidence
  - Low, ~ 2% of all non-Hodgkin lymphomas
- Age
  - 5th-6th decades
    - Median age around 60 years
    - Can occur in children
- Gender
  - Female predominance

Presentation
- Lymphadenopathy, localized or widespread
  - Systemic (B) symptoms in 1/3 of patients
  - In patients with localized disease, head and neck region is most often affected

- Bone marrow involvement common (30-60% of patients in various studies)
- Leukemic involvement (elevated WBC) is uncommon
- Association with hepatitis C infection in Italy

Prognosis
- Clinically indolent
  - > 60% of patients have overall survival > 5 years
  - Affected children have excellent long-term survival
- Patients can undergo transformation to diffuse large B-cell lymphoma
  - Prognosis substantially worse

MICROSCOPIC PATHOLOGY

Histologic Features
- Lymph nodes can be partially or completely effaced by lymphoma
  - Marginal zones expanded in cases with partial involvement
  - Neoplasm has diffuse pattern in completely replaced lymph nodes
- Cytologically, predominant cell type is small with variably irregular nuclear contours
  - Lymphoma cells commonly have abundant pale cytoplasm (so-called monocytoid features)
  - Lymphoid cells with plasmacytoid differentiation or plasma cells are common and can be numerous
  - Large cells are always present in varying numbers; can be numerous
- Residual reactive follicles with hyperplastic germinal centers are common
  - Germinal centers often have numerous tingible body macrophages
  - Reactive follicles can be colonized by lymphoma (mimicking follicular lymphoma)
- Bone marrow shows paratrabecular and nonparatrabecular pattern of involvement

NODAL MARGINAL ZONE B-CELL LYMPHOMA

Key Facts

Clinical Issues
- Age: 5th-6th decades
- No evidence of extranodal or splenic lymphoma
- Can transform to diffuse large B-cell lymphoma

Microscopic Pathology
- Expanded marginal zones or replacement of lymph node by small cells with scattered large cells
- Small cells can be centrocyte-like or monocytoid
- Lymphoplasmacytoid or mature-appearing plasma cells can be prominent
- Residual reactive follicles with hyperplastic germinal centers

Ancillary Tests
- Positive for monotypic Ig (bright) and B-cell markers
  - In paraffin sections, only plasmacytoid cells express cytoplasmic Ig
- Aberrantly express CD43 in ~ 50% of cases
- Usually negative for CD5, CD10, and CD23

Top Differential Diagnoses
- MALT lymphoma secondarily involving lymph node
- Lymphoplasmacytic lymphoma
- Mantle cell lymphoma
- CLL/SLL with plasmacytoid differentiation
- Peripheral T-cell lymphoma

Diagnostic Checklist
- Often pale appearance at low-power magnification
- Residual germinal centers surrounded by centrocyte-like and monocytoid cells
- Scattered large cells present

- Lymphoma aggregates often associated with follicular dendritic cells, CD21(+)

Predominant Pattern/Injury Type
- Lymphoid, marginal zone

Predominant Cell/Compartment Type
- Centrocyte-like or monocytoid cells, lymphoplasmacytoid cells or plasma cells

ANCILLARY TESTS

Immunohistochemistry
- Neoplastic plasmacytoid lymphocytes and plasma cells express monotypic cytoplasmic Ig light chain
- Aberrant expression of CD43 is common (~ 50%)
- Positive for pan-B-cell antigens (e.g., CD19, CD20, pax-5)
- Bcl-2(+), CD10(-), Bcl-6(-), Cyclin-D1(-)
- Usually negative for CD5 and CD23

Flow Cytometry
- Usually express monotypic surface Ig
- Brightly positive for pan-B-cell antigens (CD19, CD20, CD22) and negative for CD10
- Negative for T-cell antigens (CD2, CD3, CD5, CD7, TCR-β)
- CD43 is commonly expressed
- Subset of cases can be CD23(+)
  - Rare cases can be CD5(+)

Cytogenetics
- No consistent translocations identified
- Trisomies of 3, 7, and 18 in subset of cases

PCR
- *Ig* gene rearrangements are present
- *Ig* genes are commonly mutated
  - May result in false-negative PCR results
- No evidence of *BCL1/IgH* or *IgH/BCL2* translocations

DIFFERENTIAL DIAGNOSIS

Extranodal Marginal Zone B-cell Lymphoma of Mucosa-associated Lymphoid Tissue (MALT Lymphoma)
- Can be associated with autoimmune diseases
- Involves extranodal sites: GI tract, lung, salivary glands, orbit, skin
  - Stomach most common site
- Cytologically, can closely resemble NMZL
- Chromosomal translocations are reported in subset of MALT lymphomas
  - t(11;18)(q21;q21)/*API2-MALT1*
  - t(14;18)(q32;q21)/*MALT1-IgH*
  - T(3;14)(p14.1;q32)/*FOXP1-IgH*
  - T(1;14)(p22;q32)/*BCL-10-IgH*

Lymphoplasmacytic Lymphoma (LPL)
- In lymph nodes, LPL can histologically resemble NMZL
- Almost all patients with LPL also have Waldenström macroglobulinemia (WM)
  - Serum IgM monoclonal gammopathy is present (any level)
  - Bone marrow is involved
- Immunophenotype of NMZL and LPL/WM overlap
- No distinctive molecular markers in either NMZL or LPL/WM
  - 6q loss is relatively common but not specific
- In lymph nodes, distinction of NMZL and LPL can be arbitrary in some cases using current criteria

Mantle Cell Lymphoma
- Clinically more aggressive disease
  - Lymphadenopathy ± involvement of spleen, liver, bone marrow, and peripheral blood
- Diffuse, nodular, or mantle zone patterns
- Cytologically, neoplastic cells are small and relatively uniform
- Intermixed large cells are usually not present

NODAL MARGINAL ZONE B-CELL LYMPHOMA

Immunohistochemistry

Antibody	Reactivity	Staining Pattern	Comment
CD45	Positive	Cell membrane	
CD43	Positive	Cell membrane	In 50% of cases
Bcl-2	Positive	Cytoplasmic	
CD5	Negative	Cell membrane	Positive in small subset of cases
CD23	Negative	Cell membrane	Positive in a subset of cases
CD10	Negative	Cell membrane	Positive in residual germinal centers
Bcl-6	Negative	Nuclear	Positive in residual germinal centers

- Epithelioid histiocytes and "naked" germinal centers often present
- Neoplastic cells are CD5(+) and Cyclin-D1(+)
- t(11;14)(q13;q32)/BCL1-JH is present

Chronic Lymphocytic Leukemia/Small Lymphocytic Lymphoma (CLL/SLL)
- Lymphadenopathy often generalized
- Bone marrow and peripheral blood involvement very common
- Histologic assessment of lymph nodes shows proliferation centers
  - Small cells tend to be round with little cytoplasm
  - Large cells have cytologic features of prolymphocytes and paraimmunoblasts
  - Plasmacytoid differentiation can occur but is unusual
- Interfollicular variant of CLL/SLL can closely mimic NMZL
  - Immunophenotyping important
- Flow cytometry of CLL/SLL: Dim monotypic surface Ig; CD5(+), CD23(+), dim CD20(+)

Follicular Lymphoma (FL)
- Most cases show a follicular pattern of replacement
- Composed of centrocytes and centroblasts
- CD10(+), Bcl-6(+), CD5(-)
- t(14;18)(q32;q21)/IgH-BCL2 is present
- Rare cases of FL exhibit monocytoid differentiation
  - Monocytoid B cells are only subset of neoplasm; at periphery of neoplastic follicles

Peripheral T-cell Lymphoma (PTCL)
- Interfollicular pattern of PTCL can mimic marginal zone and interfollicular pattern of NMZL
- In PTCL, neoplastic cells express T-cell markers
- Eosinophils and histiocytes may be abundant in PTCL
- Monoclonal T-cell receptor gene rearrangements

Reactive Follicular and Interfollicular Hyperplasia
- Preserved overall architecture of lymph node
- Spectrum of reactive lymphoid cells in interfollicular zones
- B-cells express polytypic Ig light chains
- No evidence of monoclonal Ig gene rearrangements; no translocations

DIAGNOSTIC CHECKLIST

Clinically Relevant Pathologic Features
- Lymphadenopathy without extranodal or splenic involvement

Pathologic Interpretation Pearls
- Residual lymphoid follicles with hyperplastic germinal centers surrounded by lymphoma
- Cytologically, lymphoma cells can be centrocyte-like or monocytoid
  - Large cells usually present in variable numbers

SELECTED REFERENCES

1. Inamdar KV et al: Bone marrow involvement by marginal zone B-cell lymphomas of different types. Am J Clin Pathol. 129(5):714-22, 2008
2. Naresh KN: Nodal marginal zone B-cell lymphoma with prominent follicular colonization - difficulties in diagnosis: a study of 15 cases. Histopathology. 52(3):331-9, 2008
3. Arcaini L et al: Primary nodal marginal zone B-cell lymphoma: clinical features and prognostic assessment of a rare disease. Br J Haematol. 136(2):301-4, 2007
4. Kim WS et al: Genome-wide array-based comparative genomic hybridization of ocular marginal zone B cell lymphoma: comparison with pulmonary and nodal marginal zone B cell lymphoma. Genes Chromosomes Cancer. 46(8):776-83, 2007
5. Kojima M et al: Clinical implications of nodal marginal zone B-cell lymphoma among Japanese: study of 65 cases. Cancer Sci. 98(1):44-9, 2007
6. Oh SY et al: Nodal marginal zone B-cell lymphoma: Analysis of 36 cases. Clinical presentation and treatment outcomes of nodal marginal zone B-cell lymphoma. Ann Hematol. 85(11):781-6, 2006
7. Camacho FI et al: Nodal marginal zone lymphoma: a heterogeneous tumor: a comprehensive analysis of a series of 27 cases. Am J Surg Pathol. 27(6):762-71, 2003
8. Berger F et al: Non-MALT marginal zone B-cell lymphomas: a description of clinical presentation and outcome in 124 patients. Blood. 95(6):1950-6, 2000
9. Gupta D et al: Small lymphocytic lymphoma with perifollicular, marginal zone, or interfollicular distribution. Mod Pathol. 13(11):1161-6, 2000
10. Nathwani BN et al: Marginal zone B-cell lymphoma: A clinical comparison of nodal and mucosa-associated lymphoid tissue types. Non-Hodgkin's Lymphoma Classification Project. J Clin Oncol. 17(8):2486-92, 1999
11. Brynes RK et al: Numerical cytogenetic abnormalities of chromosomes 3, 7, and 12 in marginal zone B-cell lymphomas. Mod Pathol. 9(10):995-1000, 1996

NODAL MARGINAL ZONE B-CELL LYMPHOMA

Microscopic Features

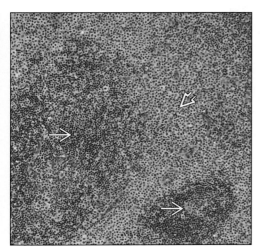

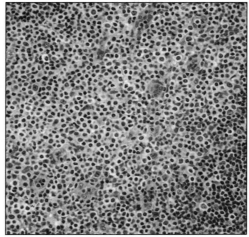

(Left) Nodal marginal zone B-cell lymphoma (NMZL). Neoplastic monocytoid (pale) cells expand interfollicular areas ⮞. Two residual germinal centers are present ⮞; 1 is nearly replaced by the neoplasm while the other shows marked follicular colonization by the neoplastic cells. *(Right)* NMZL. Hematoxylin & eosin shows neoplastic cells that are predominantly small with abundant, pale cytoplasm imparting a monocytoid appearance.

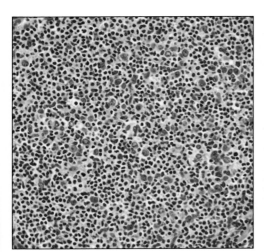

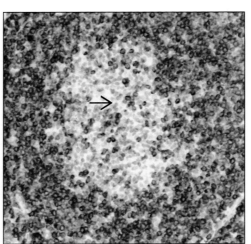

(Left) NMZL. Hematoxylin & eosin shows scattered, larger cells in a background of mostly small centrocyte-like cells. Many of the neoplastic cells have pale or monocytoid cytoplasm. *(Right)* NMZL. Bcl-2 immunostain shows that the neoplastic cells surrounding the residual reactive germinal center ⮞ are positive whereas the nonneoplastic germinal center B cells are negative for Bcl-2.

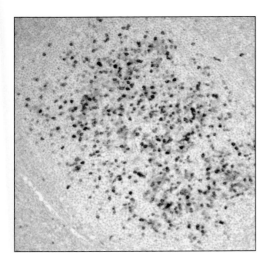

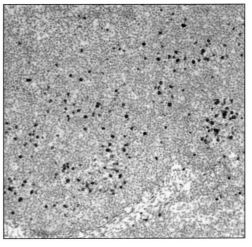

(Left) NMZL. This immunostain shows that the neoplastic cells are negative for CD10. The residual germinal center B cells are positive. *(Right)* Ki-67 (MIB1) highlights the proliferating residual germinal center B cells in a lymphoid follicle that is almost completely replaced by NMZL. The neoplastic cells are largely negative for Ki-67, indicating that this lymphoma is low grade with a low proliferation fraction.

NODAL MARGINAL ZONE B-CELL LYMPHOMA

Microscopic Features and Differential Diagnosis

(Left) NMZL with a nodular pattern simulating follicular lymphoma at low power. This pattern can be seen when follicular colonization of the reactive follicles by neoplastic cells does not completely disrupt the follicular architecture. *(Right)* Wright-Giemsa shows lymphoma cells in the peripheral blood smear of a patient with NMZL.

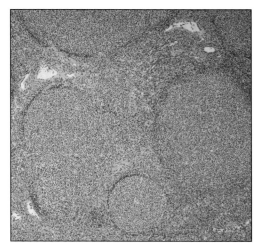
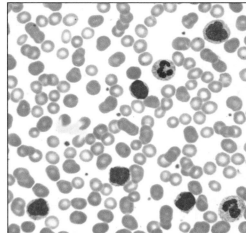

(Left) Hematoxylin & eosin shows a residual, benign germinal center ⇨ surrounded by mantle cell lymphoma. In this case, mantle cell lymphoma expanded the mantle and marginal zones, simulating nodal marginal zone lymphoma. *(Right)* A case of mantle cell lymphoma in which a residual germinal center ⇨ is surrounded by small lymphoma cells with slightly irregular nuclei.

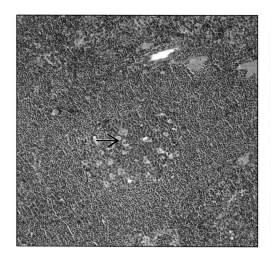
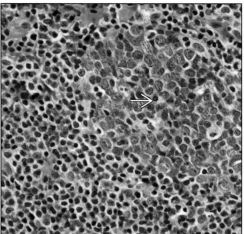

(Left) Cyclin-D1 immunostain of mantle cell lymphoma highlights the neoplastic cells that confirm the diagnosis. The residual germinal center B cells ⇨ are negative for Cyclin-D1. *(Right)* CLL/SLL shows a central, pale area rich in paraimmunoblasts consistent with a proliferation center ⇨. The pale cells can simulate the monocytoid B cells in NMZL at low power.

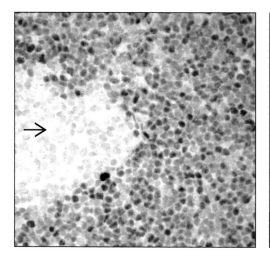
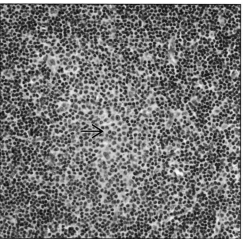

NODAL MARGINAL ZONE B-CELL LYMPHOMA

Differential Diagnosis

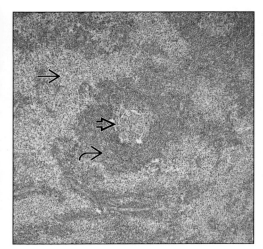

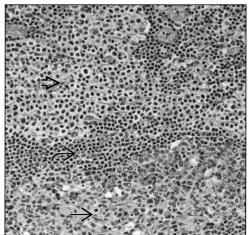

(Left) At low power, angioimmunoblastic T-cell lymphoma (AITL) can resemble NMZL. The interfollicular zone is expanded by T cells with clear cytoplasm ➡. A residual germinal center ⊡ and surrounding mantle zone ➡ are still visible. *(Right)* High-power view of AITL shows a residual reactive germinal center ➡ and preserved mantle zone ➡ bordered by sheets of cytologically atypical neoplastic T cells with enlarged nuclei and clear cytoplasm ⊡.

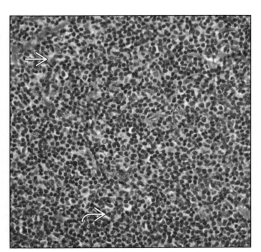

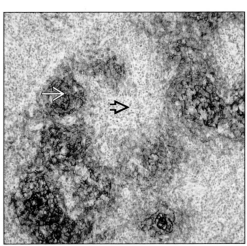

(Left) The neoplastic cells in AITL are atypical with enlarged nuclei and irregular nucleoli. There are mixed small and large cells as well as rare plasma cells ➡ and eosinophils ➡. *(Right)* CD21 highlights disrupted follicular dendritic cell meshworks ➡ in AITL caused by infiltration of neoplastic T cells ⊡.

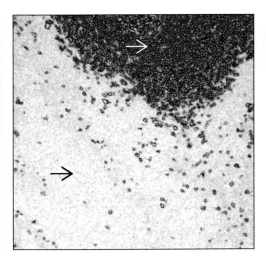

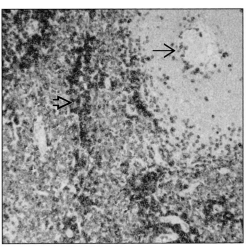

(Left) A case of AITL in which CD20 highlights a residual germinal center ➡. The interfollicular zones are populated by neoplastic T cells ➡ negative for CD20. *(Right)* In AITL, the B cells in a residual germinal center and mantle zone ➡ are negative for CD3 whereas the interfollicular zone is populated by neoplastic CD3(+) T cells ⊡.

NODAL FOLLICULAR LYMPHOMA

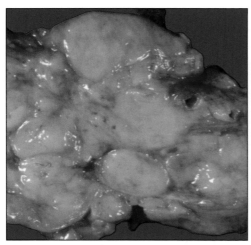

Gross photograph shows matted mesenteric lymph nodes involved by low-grade follicular lymphoma (FL). This specimen was obtained at time of autopsy.

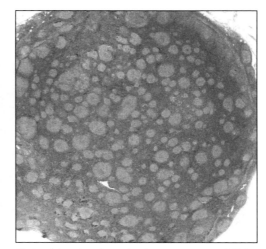

FL involving lymph node shows numerous follicles throughout the cortex and medulla. The large number and random distribution of follicles supports lymphoma.

TERMINOLOGY

Abbreviations
- Follicular lymphoma (FL)

Synonyms
- Follicle (germinal) center cell lymphoma
- Centroblastic/centrocytic lymphoma

Definitions
- B-cell neoplasm composed of germinal center B cells (centrocytes and centroblasts)
  - Follicular, follicular and diffuse, and diffuse growth patterns

ETIOLOGY/PATHOGENESIS

t(14;18)(q32;q21) Resulting in Overexpression of Bcl-2
- Bcl-2 is antiapoptotic and confers survival advantage
- t(14;18) is considered initiating molecular event of FL
  - Insufficient to induce lymphomagenesis by itself
  - Other molecular changes necessary for development of lymphoma

Imbalance of Other Proteins Involved in Apoptosis
- Overexpression of cell death suppressor proteins BCL-xL and MCL1
- Decreased expression of cell death promoting proteins BAX and BAD
- Overexpression of inhibitors of apoptosis proteins (IAP)

Germline Susceptibility Factors
- Genotypic analysis has identified novel susceptibility locus at 6p21.3
  - Contains single gene, chromosome 6 open reading frame 15 (C6orf15)

- 4-fold increased lymphoma risk in 1st-degree relatives of patients with FL
- Association of single nucleotide polymorphisms of estrogen receptor gene with reduced risk of FL

Immunologic Microenvironment
- CD40L(+) T cells in secondary follicles inhibit FL cell death
- Follicular dendritic cells contribute to preventing apoptosis of FL cells

CLINICAL ISSUES

Epidemiology
- Incidence
  - ~ 20% of NHL; 2nd most common NHL in USA and Europe
  - Uncommon in Asia and underdeveloped countries
- Age
  - Median = 59 years
- Gender
  - M:F = 1:1.7

Site
- Cervical and inguinal lymph nodes are more frequently affected
- Commonly affected extranodal sites
  - Bone marrow, spleen, liver, and peripheral blood
- FL uncommonly arises at extranodal sites
  - Skin, gastrointestinal tract, thyroid gland, testis

Presentation
- Insidious onset
- Often asymptomatic at time of initial diagnosis
- Almost always disseminated (stages III-IV)

Natural History
- Indolent clinical course but frequent relapses
- Some cases progress to diffuse large B-cell lymphoma (DLBCL)

Key Facts

Terminology
- B-cell neoplasm composed of germinal center B cells (centrocytes and centroblasts)

Etiology/Pathogenesis
- Overexpression of antiapoptotic Bcl-2 due to t(14;18)(q32;q21)
- Susceptibility locus at 6p21.3 and higher risk in 1st-degree relatives of patients with FL

Clinical Issues
- ~ 20% of NHL, 2nd overall, in USA and Western Europe
- Usually asymptomatic although disseminated at presentation
- Overall 10-year survival is up to ~ 80%

Microscopic Pathology
- Closely packed neoplastic follicles, fairly uniform in size and shape
- Neoplastic follicles composed of variable amounts of centrocytes and large centroblasts
- Grading has prognostic and therapeutic significance

Ancillary Tests
- B cells positive for Bcl-2, Bcl-6, and CD10
- Bcl-2(+) in 85-90% of FL grade 1 and grade 2; 50% in FL grade 3

Top Differential Diagnoses
- Reactive follicular hyperplasia
- Nodular lymphocyte predominant HL
- Mantle cell lymphoma
- Nodal marginal zone lymphoma

Treatment
- In the past, "watch and wait" strategy was usually employed for asymptomatic patients
- Chemotherapy is currently used upfront more often for patients with stage III-IV disease
  - Rituximab, cyclophosphamide, adriamycin (doxorubicin), vincristine, and prednisone (R-CHOP)
  - Bulky disease or signs of progression necessitate chemotherapy
- Radiation has value for subset of patients with stage I and II disease

Prognosis
- Overall 10-year survival is up to ~ 80%
- Adverse prognostic factors summarized in FL International Prognostic Index 2 (FLIPI 2)
  - High serum β2-microglobulin
  - Bulky lymph nodes > 6 cm
  - Bone marrow involvement
  - Hemoglobin < 12 g/dL
  - Age > 60 years
- FLIPI 2 prognostic model stratifies patients into different prognostic risk groups
  - Model developed in post rituximab era using prospective analysis
- Pathologic adverse prognostic factors include
  - High histologic grade and diffuse areas > 25% with predominance of large cells
    - These areas are designated as DLBCL
  - High proliferation index
  - Complex karyotype
  - Del6q23-26; del17p and mutation of TP53

IMAGE FINDINGS

General Features
- Widespread lymphadenopathy; often small lymph nodes

MACROSCOPIC FEATURES

General Features
- Replacement of nodal parenchyma by "fish-flesh" tumor; ± nodularity

MICROSCOPIC PATHOLOGY

Histologic Features
- Lymph node
  - Partial or complete effacement of architecture
  - Closely packed neoplastic follicles, fairly uniform in size and shape
  - Follicles usually poorly circumscribed with faint or absent mantle zones
  - "Cracking" artifact may surround neoplastic follicles
  - Neoplastic follicles are composed of centrocytes and centroblasts
    - Cells randomly distributed throughout individual follicles, without polarity
    - Infrequent mitoses and absent or scanty tingible body macrophages
    - Centrocytes: Small to large with angulated, elongated, or twisted nuclei, with dark chromatin and scant cytoplasm
    - Centroblasts: Large cells with oval or multilobated nuclei, vesicular chromatin, 1-3 nucleoli, and moderate cytoplasm
  - Diffuse areas with or without sclerosis
    - More frequent in mesenteric and retroperitoneal lymph nodes
    - Scattered interfollicular neoplastic lymphocytes are not considered as diffuse growth pattern
    - Follicular dendritic cell meshworks are absent in diffuse areas
- Bone marrow
  - Paratrabecular aggregates of centrocytes and, less frequently, centroblasts in bone marrow
    - Aspirate smears may have scant lymphoma cells or are negative

NODAL FOLLICULAR LYMPHOMA

- o Interstitial &/or diffuse patterns in advanced disease
- Peripheral blood
  - o Marked leukemic involvement in 5-10% of patients
  - o Neoplastic cells have highly cleaved nuclei and are known as "buttock cells"
  - o Low-level involvement is detected by molecular methods in ~ 90% of patients
- Liver
  - o Portal tracts are preferentially involved
  - o Large mass lesions usually indicate transformation to DLBCL
- Spleen
  - o Preferential involvement of white pulp
- Unusual morphologic variants of FL
  - o Floral variant
    - Mantle zone lymphocytes penetrate into neoplastic follicles, imparting irregular shapes
    - Better highlighted with follicular dendritic cell markers, e.g., CD21
    - Often grade 3
  - o Plasmacytic differentiation
    - Focal plasmacytic differentiation can occur rarely in FL, intrafollicular or interfollicular
    - Extreme degrees with intracytoplasmic inclusions appear as "signet ring cells"
  - o Marginal zone differentiation
    - Monocytoid cells with clear cytoplasm at periphery of neoplastic follicles
    - Has been correlated with poorer prognosis

Cytologic Features

- Diagnosis of FL can be established by FNA with ancillary support
  - o In smears, aggregates of cells bound by follicular dendritic cells
  - o Variable mixture of centrocytes and centroblasts
  - o Usually, absence of tingible body macrophages

Grading of FL

- Grading has prognostic and therapeutic significance
- Most reliably performed on lymph node biopsy specimen
- System is based on mean number of centroblasts per high power field (HPF)
  - o Count 10 HPFs and divide by 10
- Grade 1: 0-5 centroblasts/HPF
- Grade 2: 6-15 centroblasts/HPF
- Grade 3: > 15 centroblasts/HPF
  - o Grade 3A: Centrocytes admixed with centroblasts
  - o Grade 3B: Sheets of centroblasts with rare or no centrocytes
- Remember: Cutoff values are based on 40x objective and 18 mm field-of-view ocular
  - o Many microscopes have larger field-of-view ocular
    - 20 mm field-of-view ocular: Divide 10 HPF count by 12
    - 22 mm field-of-view ocular: Divide 10 HPF count by 15
- 2008 WHO classification recommends lumping cases of FL 1-2 together as low grade
  - o Minimal differences in outcome between patients with FL grade 1 vs. 2

- o Diffuse areas > 25% of grade 3 FL should be diagnosed as DLBCL

Histologic Discordance (Discrepant Histology) in Patients with FL

- FL involving different lymph node groups may show different grades
  - o Occurs in up to 1/3 of patients who undergo staging laparotomy
- Lymph node can be involved by grade 3 FL or DLBCL with bone marrow showing grade 1 FL
  - o Occurs in ~ 10-20% of patients with grade 3 FL or DLBCL
  - o Low-grade bone marrow involvement does not affect prognosis

Reporting Pattern in FL

- Most reliably performed on lymph node biopsy specimen
- Follicular: > 75% follicular
- Follicular and diffuse: 25-75% follicular
- Focally follicular: 1-25% follicular
- Diffuse: 0% follicular

Diffuse Follicular Lymphoma

- Diffuse growth of small centrocytes with few or absent centroblasts
  - o Immunophenotype: CD10(+), Bcl-6(+), Bcl-2(+)
  - o *IgH-BCL2* fusion gene or t(14;18)(q32;q21) present
- Rare diagnosis; more common in core needle biopsy specimens
  - o Extensive sampling may reveal focal follicular pattern

Intrafollicular Neoplasia/In Situ Follicular Lymphoma

- Lymph node with widely spaced follicles of which a subset have Bcl-2(+) germinal centers
  - o Bcl-2 expression by germinal centers is characteristically bright
  - o Bcl-2(+) follicles have immunophenotype of FL and t(14;18)
  - o Using histologic criteria alone, diagnosis of FL can be difficult or not possible
- Patients with intrafollicular neoplasia may
  - o Have FL elsewhere simultaneously or develop FL subsequently
  - o Have other types of non-Hodgkin lymphoma or Hodgkin lymphoma simultaneously or subsequently
  - o Not develop lymphoma on clinical follow-up

Clinically Aggressive B-cell Lymphoma

- FL transformation to more clinically aggressive B-cell lymphomas occurs in ~ 30% of FL patients
- Usually transforms into DLBCL
  - o Accounts for most disease-related deaths
- Transformed tumor less often resembles Burkitt lymphoma (BL) or tumor with features intermediate between BL and DLBCL
- Transformation is commonly associated with
  - o Resistance to therapy and median survival ~ 1 year
  - o Inactivation of *P53* or *P16*; activation of *MYC*

NODAL FOLLICULAR LYMPHOMA

Pediatric FL
- Localized disease, usually involves neck lymph nodes
- Extranodal sites also affected: testis, Waldeyer ring
- High histological grade; usually with large follicles
- Usually Bcl-2(-) and lacks t(14;18)(q32;q21) or *IgH-BCL2*
- Most patients have good prognosis without disease progression

ANCILLARY TESTS

Immunohistochemistry
- Monotypic surface Ig(+); pan-B-cell markers(+)
- CD10(+), Bcl-6(+)
  - CD10 and Bcl-6 more brightly expressed within follicles than in interfollicular regions
- HGAL(+), LMO2(+)
- Bcl-2(+) in 85-90% of FL grade 1 and grade 2; 50% in FL grade 3
  - Bcl-2(+) is useful to distinguish FL from reactive follicles that are Bcl-2(-)
- Follicular dendritic cell meshworks are present in follicles
  - Variable expression of CD21, CD23, or CD35
- CD23(+/-), IRF-4/MUM1(-)
- FLs are usually CD5(-), CD43(-)
  - Small subset (< 5%) can be CD5(+) or CD43(+)
- CD2(-), CD3(-), CD4(-), CD7(-), CD8(-)
- Proliferation rate of FLs assessed by Ki-67
  - Percentage of Ki-67(+) cells correlates with grade
    - Most low-grade FLs show low proliferation rate (< 20%)
    - High-grade FLs show moderate to high proliferation rate (> 40%)
  - Approximately 20% of low-grade FLs have moderate/high proliferation rate
    - These FLs appear to behave more aggressively, similar to grade 3A FL
- Grade 3 FLs
  - Can be CD10(-), Bcl-2(-), IRF-4/MUM1(+)

Cytogenetics
- 80-90% of cases have t(14;18)(q32;q21)
  - Juxtaposes *BCL2* at 18q21 adjacent to *IgH* on derivative chromosome 14
  - Is rarely (10%) the only karyotypic abnormality
- Other common chromosomal aberrations in FL include
  - Deletions of 1p, 6q, 10q, 17p
  - Gains of 1, 6p, 7, 8, 12q, 18q, X
- Complex karyotype correlates with poorer prognosis

In Situ Hybridization
- FISH can detect t(14;18)(q32;q21) in up to 90% of FL cases
  - Large probes can detect multiple breakpoints

PCR
- Monoclonal *IgH* and *Ig* light chain gene rearrangements
  - Variable regions of *Ig* genes undergo extensive and ongoing mutations

- Mutations can cause false-negative result when using PCR to assess for *Ig* gene rearrangements
  - Multiple primer sets are therefore required for analysis
- There are multiple breakpoints in Bcl-2 that must be individually assessed by PCR
  - Major breakpoint cluster region (MBR): ~ 50-60% of FLs with t(14;18)
  - Minor breakpoint cluster region (MCR): ~ 5-10% of FLs
  - Intermediate cluster region (ICR): ~ 10-15% of FLs
  - 5' breakpoint region: ~ 5% of FLs

Array CGH
- ~ 90% of FLs have abnormalities detected by CGH or array CGH
  - Gains: 2p15, 7p, 7q, 8q, 12q, 18p, 18q
  - Losses: 1p36, 3q, 6q, 9p, 11q, 13q, 17p
- Abnormalities associated with worse prognosis
  - Loss of 6q or 9p21
  - Gain of chromosome X
- Abnormalities associated with transformation to DLBCL
  - Gains of 2, 3q, and 5

Molecular Genetics
- *IgH-BCL2*/t(14;18)(q32;q21) is insufficient to induce lymphomagenesis
  - *IgH-BCL2* fusion gene can be detected in blood of 50% of healthy individuals by using sensitive nested PCR methods
- *BCL6/3q27* rearrangement occurs in ~ 15% of FLs
  - More common in grade 3B tumors
- Inactivation of tumor suppressor genes *P53*, *P15*, *P16*
  - Occurs in FLs but is more common at time of transformation to DLBCL
- *MYC* rearrangement is associated with transformation to DLBCL

Gene Expression Profiling
- Initial study from Leukemia/Lymphoma Molecular Profiling Project showed
  - Host response in FLs has prognostic importance
  - 2 gene expression profiles: Immune response (IR) 1 and IR2
    - IR1: Good prognosis: Genes related to T cells and macrophages
    - IR2: Poor prognosis: Genes related to monocytes and dendritic cells
  - These studies included FLs ± t(14;18)(q32;q21)
- Other groups have shown importance of host response but emphasize different gene signatures
- Recent studies have analyzed t(14;18)(+) FL and t(14;18)(-) FL separately
  - FL with t(14;18)(q32;q21)
    - Enriched germinal center B-cell genes
  - FL without t(14;18)(q32;q21)
    - Enriched activated B-cell-like, NF-κB, and proliferation genes

NODAL FOLLICULAR LYMPHOMA

DIFFERENTIAL DIAGNOSIS

Reactive Follicular Hyperplasia (RFH)

- Children and young adults; patients with autoimmune disease
- Features that distinguish RFH from FL
  - Lymph node architecture preserved with follicles located mostly in cortex
  - Follicles vary in size and shape; widely spaced
  - Polarization of germinal centers into light and dark zones
  - Frequent mitoses and tingible body macrophages in germinal centers
  - Sharply demarcated mantle zones surround germinal centers
  - Immunophenotype: Polytypic B cells; Bcl-2(-)
  - No evidence of monoclonal *Ig* gene rearrangements

Progressive Transformation of Germinal Centers

- Partial lymph node replacement
- Nodules are 3-4 times larger than background reactive follicles
- Small lymphocytes with mantle cell immunophenotype infiltrate and eventually replace germinal centers
- Immunophenotype: Polytypic B cells; Bcl-2(-)
- No evidence of monoclonal *Ig* gene rearrangements

Nodular Lymphocyte Predominant Hodgkin Lymphoma

- Large, vague nodules
- Most cells in nodules are small round lymphocytes
  - Admixed with fewer LP ("popcorn") cells
- LP cells are CD20(+), CD45(+), CD10(-), Bcl-2(-)
- Small cells in tumor nodules are mostly reactive B cells
- CD4(+) and CD57(+) T cells commonly form rosettes around LP cells

Lymphocyte-rich Classical Hodgkin Lymphoma

- Large vague nodules
- Most cells in nodules are small round lymphocytes
  - Admixed with Hodgkin and Reed-Sternberg (HRS) cells
  - HRS cells are CD15(+), CD30(+), CD45/LCA(-)
- No evidence of monotypic B cells or monoclonal *Ig* gene rearrangements

Mantle Cell Lymphoma (MCL)

- Usually MCL completely effaces lymph node architecture
  - Nodular pattern can resemble FL
- MCL cells are small with irregular nuclear contours; no centroblasts
- Hyalinized blood vessels and histiocytes with eosinophilic cytoplasm are common
- Immunophenotype
  - Monotypic B-cell population
  - CD5(+), CD43(+), Cyclin-D1(+)

- Detection of t(11;14)(q13;q32) by cytogenetics, FISH, or PCR

Nodal Marginal Zone Lymphoma

- Partial effacement of lymph node architecture with marginal zone expansion
- Neoplastic lymphocytes include small lymphocytes, lymphocytes with monocytoid nuclei, and large cells
  - Frequent plasmacytic differentiation
  - Neoplastic lymphocytes colonize and may replace germinal centers
- Bcl-2(-) in residual centrocytes of germinal centers
- Bcl-2(+) in marginal zone lymphocytes
- Immunophenotype
  - Monotypic B-cell population; Bcl-2(+)
  - CD5(-), CD10(-), Cyclin-D1(-), Bcl-6(-)
  - No evidence of t(14;18)(q32;q21)

SELECTED REFERENCES

1. Cheung KJ et al: High resolution analysis of follicular lymphoma genomes reveals somatic recurrent sites of copy-neutral loss of heterozygosity and copy number alterations that target single genes. Genes Chromosomes Cancer. 49(8):669-81, 2010
2. Eide MB et al: Genomic alterations reveal potential for higher grade transformation in follicular lymphoma and confirm parallel evolution of tumor cell clones. Blood. 116(9):1489-97, 2010
3. Gradowski JF et al: Follicular lymphomas with plasmacytic differentiation include two subtypes. Mod Pathol. 23(1):71-9, 2010
4. Montes-Moreno S et al: Intrafollicular neoplasia/in situ follicular lymphoma: review of a series of 13 cases. Histopathology. 56(5):658-62, 2010
5. Wrench D et al: Molecular signatures in the diagnosis and management of follicular lymphoma. Curr Opin Hematol. 17(4):333-40, 2010
6. Carlotti E et al: Transformation of follicular lymphoma to diffuse large B-cell lymphoma may occur by divergent evolution from a common progenitor cell or by direct evolution from the follicular lymphoma clone. Blood. 113(15):3553-7, 2009
7. Cheung KJ et al: Genome-wide profiling of follicular lymphoma by array comparative genomic hybridization reveals prognostically significant DNA copy number imbalances. Blood. 113(1):137-48, 2009
8. Federico M et al: Follicular lymphoma international prognostic index 2: a new prognostic index for follicular lymphoma developed by the international follicular lymphoma prognostic factor project. J Clin Oncol. 27(27):4555-62, 2009
9. Leich E et al: Follicular lymphomas with and without translocation t(14;18) differ in gene expression profiles and genetic alterations. Blood. 114(4):826-34, 2009
10. Schwaenen C et al: Microarray-based genomic profiling reveals novel genomic aberrations in follicular lymphoma which associate with patient survival and gene expression status. Genes Chromosomes Cancer. 48(1):39-54, 2009
11. Ghia P et al: Unbalanced expression of bcl-2 family proteins in follicular lymphoma: contribution of CD40 signaling in promoting survival. Blood. 91(1):244-51, 1998

Microscopic Features

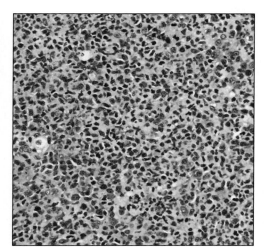
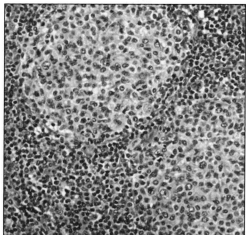

(Left) Follicular lymphoma (FL) involving lymph node. The follicles are composed of numerous centrocytes and fewer centroblasts, supporting grade 2. *(Right)* FL, grade 3A, follicular pattern. The follicles are composed of many centroblasts, but centrocytes are also present.

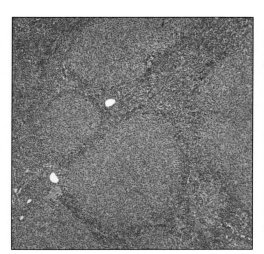
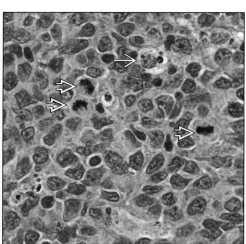

(Left) Follicular lymphoma (FL), grade 3B, replacing lymph node. The neoplastic follicles are composed of numerous large cells, many of which are consistent with centroblasts. *(Right)* FL, grade 3B, replacing lymph node. The architecture is replaced by neoplastic follicles composed of numerous centroblasts. In this neoplastic follicle, mitotic figures ⇒ and tingible body macrophages ⇒ are seen. No small centrocytes are noted.

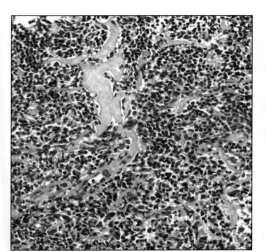
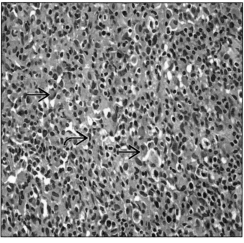

(Left) Follicular lymphoma, low grade involving a retroperitoneal lymph node. This field shows sclerosis that is associated with the neoplastic lymphoid infiltrate. *(Right)* FL with plasmacytic differentiation involving lymph node. Scattered plasma cells ⇒ admixed with centrocytes ⇒ are noted. Flow cytometric immunophenotyping demonstrated a population of CD10(+) B cells, and FISH revealed the IgH/BCL2 fusion gene.

NODAL FOLLICULAR LYMPHOMA

Microscopic and Immunohistochemical Features

(Left) Initial sections of this core needle biopsy revealed FL with a diffuse growth pattern. Subsequent deeper levels of the block showed rare follicles. The diagnosis of FL was further confirmed by reactivity of the neoplastic cells with CD10, Bcl-6, and Bcl-2. *(Right)* Diffuse FL involving lymph node. The neoplasm had a diffuse growth pattern and was composed predominantly of centrocytes, supporting grade 1. The proliferation rate was less than 5%.

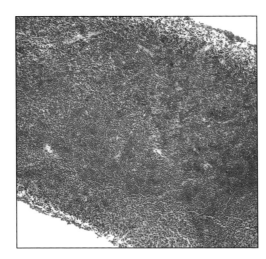
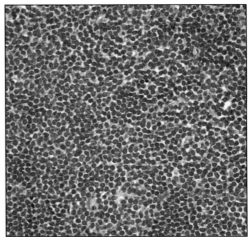

(Left) Floral variant of follicular lymphoma (FL) involving lymph node. The fused or fragmented follicles have the appearance of flower petals ➹. *(Right)* Immunohistochemical stain for Bcl-2 reveals a single positive germinal center ➦ showing intrafollicular neoplasia. A nearby hyperplastic germinal center is Bcl-2(-) ➦. Routine histologic examination revealed a benign-appearing germinal center with a predominance of small centrocytes.

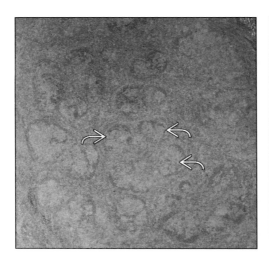
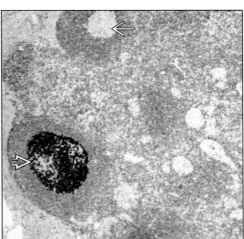

(Left) Fine needle aspiration of a lymph node from a patient with follicular lymphoma (FL), grade 2 shows aggregates of monotonous lymphoid cells bound by follicular dendritic cells. *(Right)* Fine needle aspiration of a lymph node from a patient with FL, grade 2 demonstrates a mixture of centrocytes and centroblasts.

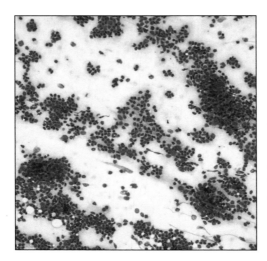
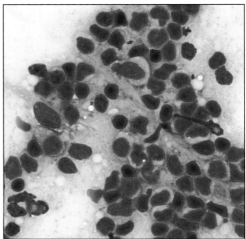

MANTLE CELL LYMPHOMA

Key Facts

Terminology
- Clinically aggressive B-cell lymphoma associated with t(11;14)(q13;q32) and Cyclin-D1 overexpression

Clinical Issues
- Elderly people; male predominance
- Most patients present with clinical stage III/IV disease
- B symptoms, lymphadenopathy, extranodal involvement
- Currently considered incurable with median survival of 2-5 years

Microscopic Pathology
- Architectural effacement by lymphoma with nodular, diffuse, or mantle zone growth pattern
- Monotonous population of small/medium-sized cells with variably irregular nuclear contours

Ancillary Tests
- Immunohistochemistry: Cyclin-D1(+)
- Flow cytometry: CD5(+), CD19(+), CD20(+), CD43(+/-), FMC-7(+), CD10(-), CD23(-)
- Cytogenetics: t(11;14)(q13;q32) or *CCND1-IgH* (FISH)
- Gene expression profiling
  - Unique profile
  - Proliferation predicts prognosis

Top Differential Diagnoses
- Chronic lymphocytic leukemia/small lymphocytic lymphoma
- Follicular lymphoma
- Nodal marginal zone B-cell lymphoma

- Rare Cyclin-D1(-) variants described, but this entity is controversial

Flow Cytometry
- CD5(+), CD19(+), CD20(+), CD22(+), CD79b(+), FMC-7(+), Sox11(+/-), and monotypic Ig
- Bcl-2(+), CD11c(+/-)
- CD3(-), CD10(-), CD23(-), CD43(+/-)
- Rare cases have atypical immunophenotype: CD5(-) or CD10(+) or CD23(+) (dim ~ 10%)

Cytogenetics
- Numerous methods can be used for demonstrating t(11;14)(q13;q32)
  - FISH is convenient because it can be performed on fixed tissue sections
  - Conventional cytogenetics if fresh material available

Molecular Genetics
- PCR detects 1 major breakpoint (MTC) in 30-50% of cases

Gene Expression Profiling
- MCL has proliferation signature that can be used to divide patients into prognostic subgroups

DIFFERENTIAL DIAGNOSIS

Chronic Lymphocytic Leukemia/Small Lymphocytic Lymphoma
- Proliferation centers; mixture of small lymphocytes, prolymphocytes, and paraimmunoblasts
- Cells express dim surface Ig, CD5, and CD23, but not Cyclin-D1

Follicular Lymphoma
- Sharply circumscribed nodules composed of centrocytes and centroblasts
- Cells express CD10 but not CD5, CD43, or Cyclin-D1

Nodal Marginal Zone B-cell Lymphoma
- Neoplastic B cells ± monocytoid cytoplasm; reactive germinal centers are common; CD5(-) and Cyclin-D1(-)

Lymphoblastic Lymphoma
- Mimics classic blastoid variant of MCL
- Younger patients; TdT(+) and Cyclin-D1(-)

Diffuse Large B-cell Lymphoma
- Mimics pleomorphic blastoid variant of MCL
- CD5(-) and Cyclin-D1(-)

Reactive Follicular Hyperplasia
- Thinner mantle zones composed of small, round, mature lymphocytes surrounding prominent germinal centers
- No evidence of monoclonality

Castleman Disease, Hyaline Vascular Type
- Large localized mass in young person
- Architecture not entirely effaced
- Hyaline-vascular follicles, "onion skin" lymphocytes concentrically layered around germinal centers

SELECTED REFERENCES

1. Dictor M et al: Strong lymphoid nuclear expression of SOX11 transcription factor defines lymphoblastic neoplasms, mantle cell lymphoma and Burkitt's lymphoma. Haematologica. 94(11):1563-8, 2009
2. Jares P et al: Genetic and molecular pathogenesis of mantle cell lymphoma: perspectives for new targeted therapeutics. Nat Rev Cancer. 7(10):750-62, 2007
3. Rosenwald A et al: The proliferation gene expression signature is a quantitative integrator of oncogenic events that predicts survival in mantle cell lymphoma. Cancer Cell. 3(2):185-97, 2003

MANTLE CELL LYMPHOMA

Microscopic and Immunohistochemical Features

(Left) A case of mantle cell lymphoma (MCL) with a completely diffuse pattern. *(Right)* Mantle cell lymphoma with a nodular pattern. This pattern, in part, resembles follicular lymphoma at low-power magnification, but the neoplastic nodules lack centroblasts.

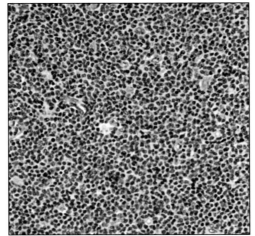 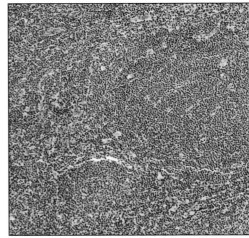

(Left) Mantle cell lymphoma with a mantle zone pattern. In this pattern, the neoplasm surrounds reactive germinal centers. *(Right)* A case of mantle cell lymphoma shows "naked" reactive germinal centers and many benign histiocytes with eosinophilic cytoplasm (so-called pink histiocytes). Pink histiocytes are a helpful clue for the diagnosis of MCL but are not specific.

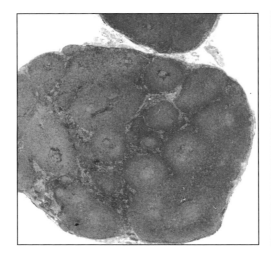 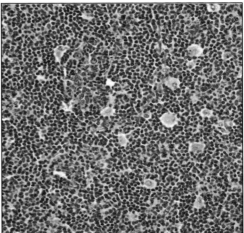

(Left) Smear of a lymph node prepared at the time of a frozen section shows mantle cell lymphoma. In addition to the neoplastic lymphoid cells, a benign pink histiocyte is shown in this field. *(Right)* Cyclin-D1 immunostain shows nuclear expression in the cells of mantle cell lymphoma. This immunostain is helpful for recognizing MCL at extranodal sites, especially in small biopsy specimens.

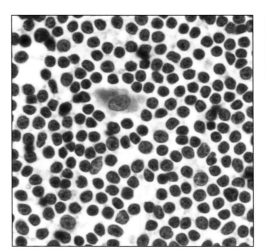 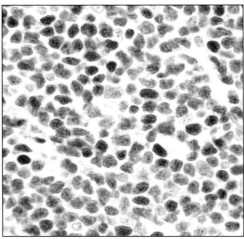

MANTLE CELL LYMPHOMA

Microscopic and Immunohistochemical Features

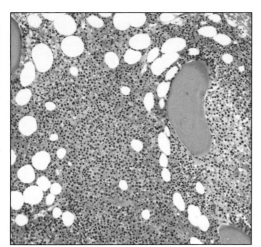

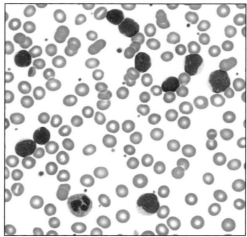

(Left) MCL involving bone marrow. In this case, the neoplastic cells had relatively abundant "monocytoid" cytoplasm mimicking marginal zone lymphoma. However, the neoplastic cells expressed Cyclin-D1, and conventional cytogenetics showed the t(11;14) (q13;q32). *(Right)* Wright-Giemsa stain shows a case of MCL in the leukemic phase. The neoplastic lymphocytes of MCL often show variation in size and shape in a blood smear, as seen in this case.

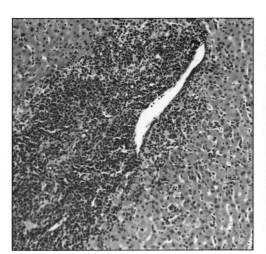

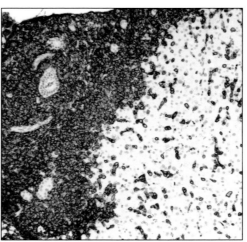

(Left) Mantle cell lymphoma involving the liver. The neoplasm fills a portal tract and infiltrates sinusoids. *(Right)* CD20 immunostain highlights mantle cell lymphoma cells within a portal tract and sinusoids.

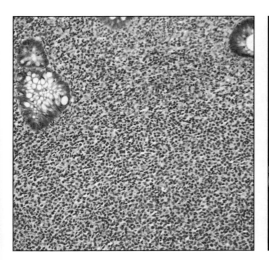

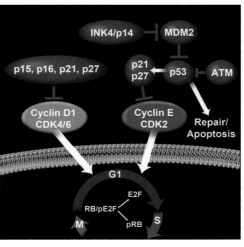

(Left) Mantle cell lymphoma involving the colonic mucosa. MCL has a tropism for the gastrointestinal tract and commonly involves this site at the time of diagnosis. However, GI symptoms occur in only 10-20% of patients. *(Right)* Schematic of the cell cycle shows the G1 to S transition and the role of Cyclin-D1-cyclin dependent kinase complexes. Some of the genes of interest in the pathogenesis of mantle cell lymphoma are also shown.

MANTLE CELL LYMPHOMA, BLASTOID VARIANT

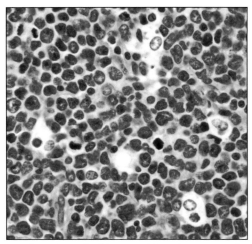

Lymph node involved by MCL, blastoid variant. In this case, a "starry sky" pattern is present and the neoplastic cells resemble, in part, lymphoblasts. This case carried the t(11;14)(q13;q32).

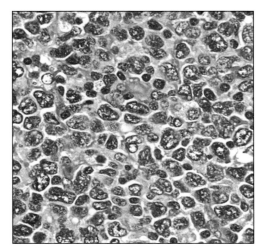

Lymph node involved by MCL, pleomorphic variant. In this case, the neoplastic cells are large and resemble, in part, large B-cell lymphoma. This case carried the t(11;14)(q13;q32).

TERMINOLOGY

Abbreviations
- Mantle cell lymphoma (MCL), blastoid variant (BV)

Synonyms
- Mantle cell lymphoma, lymphoblastoid variant
- Mantle cell lymphoma, large cell variant
- Mantle cell lymphoma, blastic

Definitions
- Clinically aggressive type of MCL with high-grade cytologic features: 2 major variants
- 2 variants of MCL as stated in 2001 WHO classification
  - Classical and pleomorphic
- 2 aggressive variants of MCL as stated in 2008 WHO classification
  - Blastoid and pleomorphic

ETIOLOGY/PATHOGENESIS

t(11;14)(q13;q32)
- Virtually all cases of MCL carry t(11;14)(q13;q32)
- Juxtaposes *CCND1* at 11q13 with *IgH* at 14q32 and results in Cyclin-D1 overexpression, Rb phosphorylation, and release of E2F
- Facilitates cell cycle progression from G1 to S phase

Other Cytogenetic and Molecular Genetic Abnormalities
- *P53* overexpression and mutations
- *P16/INK4a* deletions and mutations

CLINICAL ISSUES

Epidemiology
- Incidence

  - MCL represents approximately 6% of all non-Hodgkin lymphomas
  - MCL-BV represents at least 10-15% of all MCL cases
    - Frequency is probably higher in patients who are followed for long periods of time

Presentation
- Median age: 6th to 7th decades
- Clinical features of MCL-BV are comparable to those of typical MCL
- Male predominance (M:F = 2-3:1)
- B symptoms in 30-50%; may be more common in patients with MCL-BV
- Lymphadenopathy, generalized
- Extranodal involvement is common
  - Gastrointestinal tract is most common site
  - Unusual extranodal sites can be involved in patients with MCL-BV
- Most patients present with Ann Arbor clinical stage III/IV
- MCL International Prognostic Index (MIPI) often high
  - Based on: Age, ECOG performance status, serum lactate dehydrogenase (LDH), blood leukocyte count
- Rare prolymphocytoid variant of MCL is probably a form of MCL-BV
  - Patients present with high leukocyte count (often > 100 K/uL) and poor prognostic features
    - Extensive bone marrow involvement
    - Prominent splenomegaly
    - Often short survival

Treatment
- Aggressive chemotherapy &/or stem cell transplantation
  - R-HyperCVAD used at many institutions
    - Rituximab, hyperfractionated cyclophosphamide, vincristine, doxorubicin, dexamethasone alternating with methotrexate and cytosine arabinoside
  - R-CHOP is inadequate therapy for long-term cure

MANTLE CELL LYMPHOMA, BLASTOID VARIANT

Key Facts

Terminology

- Highly aggressive subtype of mantle cell lymphoma composed of cells that resemble lymphoblasts (classic variant) or are large, atypical, and pleomorphic (pleomorphic variant)
- Clinically aggressive type of MCL with high-grade cytologic features: 2 major variants

Etiology/Pathogenesis

- t(11;14)(q13;q32) juxtaposes *CCND1* with *IGH* and results in Cyclin-D1 overexpression and cell cycle progression
- Other molecular genetic abnormalities
  - *P53, P21, P16, MYC*

Clinical Issues

- Clinical and biological features are comparable to those of typical MCL
- Associated with particularly short durations of response after chemotherapy and poorer overall survival

Microscopic Pathology

- 2 variants are recognized: Classic and pleomorphic

Top Differential Diagnoses

- Lymphoblastic lymphoma
- Myeloid sarcoma
- Diffuse large B-cell lymphoma
- Burkitt lymphoma

  - Rituximab, cyclophosphamide, doxorubicin, vincristine, and prednisone

Prognosis

- Short durations of clinical response after chemotherapy and poorer overall survival
- MCL-BV patients have poor overall survival
  - Reported to be 14.5 months in 1 study

IMAGE FINDINGS

Radiographic Findings

- Widespread lymphadenopathy

MICROSCOPIC PATHOLOGY

Histologic Features

- Blastoid variant
  - Resembles, in part, lymphoblastic lymphoma
  - Small to intermediate-sized cells with immature chromatin and high mitotic rate
  - At least 10 mitoses per 10 high-power (400x) fields (hpf), and often much higher rates (20-30/10 hpf)
  - Often presents in patients de novo
- Pleomorphic variant
  - Resembles, in part, large B-cell lymphoma
  - Heterogeneous cell population including large cleaved or noncleaved cells ± prominent nucleoli
  - At least 10 mitoses per 10 high-power fields, and often higher rates
  - Can occur in patients with history of typical MCL or in patients with other sites involved by typical MCL
- Prolymphocytoid variant of MCL
  - Peripheral blood lymphocytes are intermediate-sized with prominent nucleoli
  - Marked splenomegaly

ANCILLARY TESTS

Immunohistochemistry

- Similar to typical MCL cases
  - Cyclin-D1 virtually always positive
  - Sox11 usually (+)
  - Ki-67 shows high (> 60%) proliferation rate
    - Proliferation rate predicts prognosis
  - CD10 or Bcl-6 can be expressed in MCL-BV
  - p53 expressed in subset; intense expression correlates with *P53* gene mutation

Flow Cytometry

- Surface Ig(+), λ > κ, IgM(+), IgD(+)
- Pan-B-cell antigens(+), FMC7(+), CD5(+), CD10(-), CD11c(-), CD23(-)
  - MCL-BV can be CD5(-) or CD10(+)

Cytogenetics

- Conventional cytogenetic or FISH analysis shows t(11;14)(q13;q32)
  - Both MCL and MCL-BV are typically associated with many other abnormalities
  - Karyotypes of MCL-BV are more often complex (≥ 3 abnormalities)
  - Some abnormalities may be specifically involved in pathogenesis of MCL-BV
    - Chromosome 17p deletions (*P53*)
    - Chromosome 9p deletions (*P16*)
    - Chromosome 8q24 translocations or amplification (*MYC*)
    - Chromosome 3q27/*BCL6* translocations (these cases express Bcl-6)
    - *BMI-1* polycomb amplification, *CDK4* amplification
    - *P18/INK4c* deletions, *RB1* gene microdeletions
- Some correlation between type of MCL-BV and cytogenetic abnormalities
  - Blastoid: Chromosomes 8, 13, and 18 more often abnormal
  - Pleomorphic: Chromosomes 3, 13, and 17

MANTLE CELL LYMPHOMA, BLASTOID VARIANT

- o Prolymphocytoid: High frequency of chromosome 17p abnormalities and *P53* gene mutation

PCR
- Monoclonal *Ig* gene rearrangements; T-cell receptor genes germline
  - o Somatic mutations in *Ig* variable genes ~ 25% (lower mutation load than CLL/SLL)
- Clonal identity shown in patients with both typical MCL and MCL-BV
- t(11;14)(q13;q32) shown by PCR in 30-50% of cases
  - o Can only detect major translocation cluster (MTC) by PCR
- *P53* or *P16/INK4a/ARF* gene mutations have been shown in MCL in ~ 25%
  - o Presence correlates well with MCL-BV
- Truncated Cyclin-D1 transcripts more common in MCL-BV
  - o These transcripts have longer half-life; correlated with increased proliferation

Array CGH
- Multiple gains and losses of chromosomal material reported in both MCL and MCL-BV
  - o Correlations with typical versus MCL-BV currently not well understood

Gene Expression Profiling
- Group of 42 genes involved in characteristic gene expression signature for MCL
- Expression abnormalities can be simplified into 3 general types
  - o Cell cycle dysregulation
  - o Impaired DNA repair (e.g., *ATM*, *p53*)
  - o Impaired apoptosis
- Proliferation signature high in MCL-BV

DIFFERENTIAL DIAGNOSIS

Lymphoblastic Lymphoma (LBL)
- Can resemble classical variant of MCL-BV
- Most LBLs occur in younger patients (children or adults < 40 years)
- Most LBLs are TdT(+), and all are Cyclin-D1(-)
- B-LBLs commonly involve extranodal sites
  - o CD10(+), surface Ig(-), CD5(-), t(11;14)(q13;q32)(-)
- T-LBLs commonly involve mediastinum
  - o T-cell lineage

Diffuse Large B-cell Lymphoma (DLBCL)
- Pleomorphic variant of MCL-BV can resemble DLBCL
- Usually CD5(-) and Cyclin-D1(-)
  - o ~ 5% of DLBCL can be Cyclin-D1(+) but no evidence of t(11;14)(q13;q32)
- Less commonly involves peripheral blood or bone marrow

Myeloid Sarcoma
- Often associated with history of or simultaneous acute myeloid leukemia
- Neoplastic cells can have eosinophilic cytoplasmic granules

- Myeloperoxidase(+), lysozyme(+), CD117(+), B-cell antigens(-), Cyclin-D1(-)

B-cell Prolymphocytic Leukemia (B-PLL)
- Irregular lymphocytes are more often present in background of prolymphocytoid MCL
- B-PLL is negative for Cyclin-D1 and t(11;14)(q13;q32)

Burkitt Lymphoma
- "Starry sky" pattern can occur in MCL-BV mimicking Burkitt lymphoma
- Rarely t(8;14)(q24;q32) occurs in MCL-BV (as routinely occurs in Burkitt lymphoma)
- Burkitt lymphoma is CD10(+), Bcl-6(+), CD5(-), and Cyclin-D1(-)

Blastic Plasma Cell Myeloma (PCM)
- Approximately 30-40% of PCM can express Cyclin-D1; can be bright (+)
- Typically in bone and associated with lytic lesions and serum paraprotein
- Cytoplasmic Ig(+), CD138(+), CD5(-), CD20(-)

DIAGNOSTIC CHECKLIST

Pathologic Interpretation Pearls
- High-grade B-cell lymphoma that is sIg, CD5, and Cyclin-D1(+)
- t(11;14)(q13;q32) virtually constant in MCL-BV

SELECTED REFERENCES

1. Garcia M et al: Proliferation predicts failure-free survival in mantle cell lymphoma patients treated with rituximab plus hyperfractionated cyclophosphamide, vincristine, doxorubicin, and dexamethasone alternating with rituximab plus high-dose methotrexate and cytarabine. Cancer. 115(5):1041-8, 2009
2. Jares P et al: Advances in the understanding of mantle cell lymphoma. Br J Haematol. 142(2):149-65, 2008
3. Yin CC et al: Sequence analysis proves clonal identity in five patients with typical and blastoid mantle cell lymphoma. Mod Pathol. 20(1):1-7, 2007
4. Khoury JD et al: Cytogenetic findings in blastoid mantle cell lymphoma. Hum Pathol. 34(10):1022-9, 2003
5. Onciu M et al: Cytogenetic findings in mantle cell lymphoma cases with a high level of peripheral blood involvement have a distinct pattern of abnormalities. Am J Clin Pathol. 116(6):886-92, 2001
6. Schlette E et al: Mature B-cell leukemias with more than 55% prolymphocytes. A heterogeneous group that includes an unusual variant of mantle cell lymphoma. Am J Clin Pathol. 115(4):571-81, 2001

MANTLE CELL LYMPHOMA, BLASTOID VARIANT

Microscopic and Immunohistochemical Features

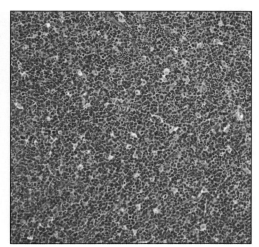 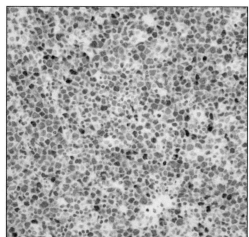

(Left) Low-power view of a lymph node involved by MCL, blastoid variant. A "starry sky" pattern is present, and the neoplastic cells resemble, in part, lymphoblasts. *(Right)* Immunohistochemical stain for Cyclin-D1 in a case of MCL-BV shows the neoplastic cells are Cyclin-D1 positive with variable intensity from cell to cell.

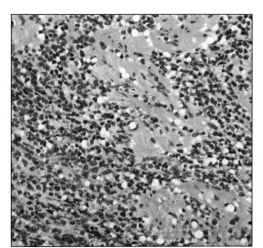 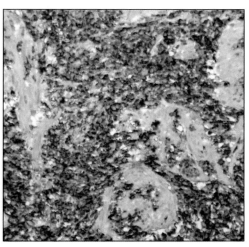

(Left) Blastoid variants of MCL can involve unusual extranodal sites, as was the case in this patient with MCL-BV diffusely involving bladder wall. *(Right)* Immunohistochemical stain for CD20 highlights the neoplastic cells in a case of MCL-BV involving the bladder wall.

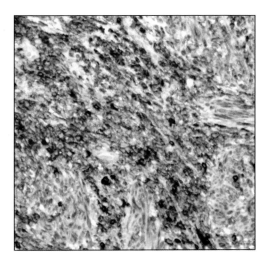 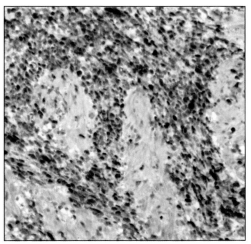

(Left) Immunohistochemical stain for CD5 highlights the neoplastic cells in a case of MCL-BV involving the bladder wall. MCL, including blastoid variants, commonly express CD5 with B-cell antigens. The CD5 expression level is usually dim compared with reactive T cells. *(Right)* Immunohistochemical stain for Cyclin-D1 highlights the neoplastic cells in a case of MCL-BV involving the bladder wall.

MANTLE CELL LYMPHOMA, BLASTOID VARIANT

Microscopic and Immunohistochemical Features

(Left) MCL, blastoid variant involving nasal mucosa. This is an example of an anatomic site involved by MCL-BV that is uncommonly involved in typical MCL. This neoplasm was Cyclin-D1 positive but had an unusual immunophenotype (CD5[-], Bcl-6[+]). *(Right)* High-power view of MCL, blastoid variant involving nasal mucosa. The neoplastic cells have immature ("blastic") chromatin and a high mitotic rate.

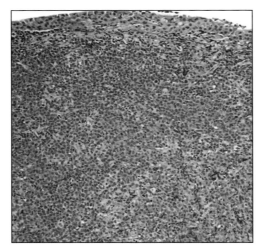 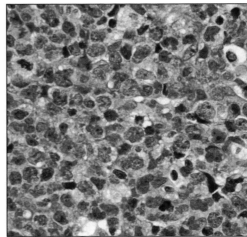

(Left) Immunohistochemical stain for CD20 in a case of MCL, blastoid variant involving nasal mucosa shows the lymphoma cells are positive for CD20. *(Right)* Immunohistochemical stain for CD5 in a case of MCL, blastoid variant involving nasal mucosa. The neoplastic cells are negative with positive reactive T cells. Most cases of MCL are CD5(+), but blastoid variants can be negative in ~ 10% of cases.

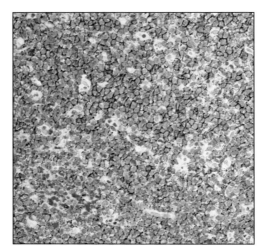 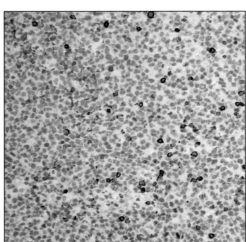

(Left) Immunohistochemical stain for Cyclin-D1 in a case of MCL, blastoid variant. Nasal mucosa was shown to carry the CCND1/IgH fusion gene, consistent with the t(11;14)(q13;q32). *(Right)* Immunohistochemical stain for Bcl-6 in a case of MCL, blastoid variant involving nasal mucosa, shows that the neoplastic cells are positive. Bcl-6 is typically expressed in lymphomas of follicle center cell lineage and is negative in typical MCL. However, 5-10% of MCL-BV can be Bcl-6(+).

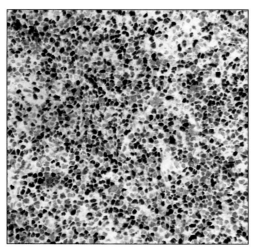 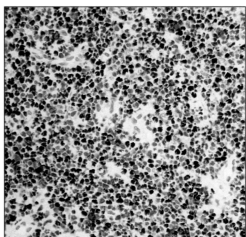

MANTLE CELL LYMPHOMA, BLASTOID VARIANT

Microscopic and Immunohistochemical Features

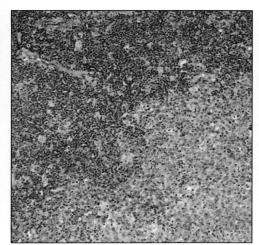

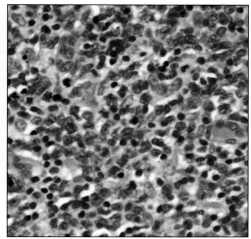

(Left) Light microscopy shows a colon resection specimen involved by MCL with typical (upper left) and pleomorphic blastoid variant (lower right) components. IgH sequence analysis proved that both components were clonally related. (Right) High-power view of a case of MCL-BV, pleomorphic variant. The neoplastic cells are large with a high mitotic rate.

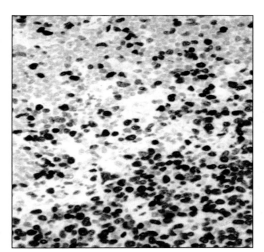

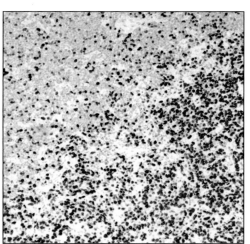

(Left) Immunohistochemical stain for p53 shows lower number of cells positive in typical MCL (upper left) and many positive cells in MCL-BV (lower right). (Right) Immunohistochemical stain for Ki-67 (MIB-1) shows lower proliferative activity in typical MCL (upper left) and higher proliferative activity in MCL-BV (lower right).

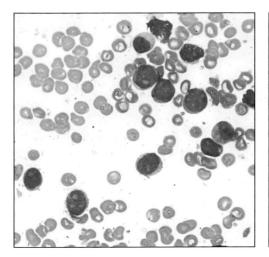

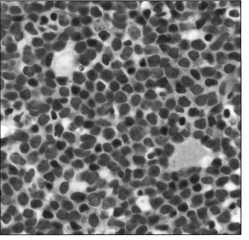

(Left) Peripheral blood smear involved by MCL, prolymphocytoid variant. The patient presented with a leukocyte count > 100K. Conventional cytogenetic karyotyping showed the t(11;14)(q13;q32). Many prolymphocytoid MCL carry P53 gene mutations or deletions. (Right) Bone marrow biopsy involved by MCL, prolymphocytoid variant. The prominent nucleoli in MCL cells are more difficult to discern as compared with the peripheral blood smear.

DIFFUSE LARGE B-CELL LYMPHOMA, NOS, CENTROBLASTIC

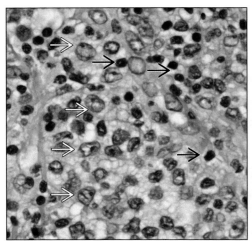

Diffuse large B-cell lymphoma (DLBCL). Typical centroblasts ➡ are large, noncleaved with vesicular chromatin and have membrane-bound nucleoli. Reactive small lymphocytes are also present ➡.

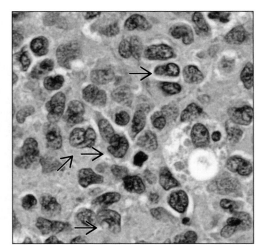

DLBCL composed of multilobated centroblasts ➡. The tumor cells are large, and some have deeply lobated nuclei.

TERMINOLOGY

Abbreviations
- Diffuse large B-cell lymphoma (DLBCL), centroblastic

Synonyms
- Centroblastic lymphoma

Definitions
- Diffuse proliferation of large neoplastic B cells composed predominantly of centroblasts
  - Centroblasts
    - Typical: Medium to large cells (10-14 μm) with fine chromatin, 2-3 small nucleoli often closely apposed to nuclear membrane, and scant basophilic cytoplasm
    - Multilobated: Medium to large cells with lobated nuclei (> 3 lobes)

CLINICAL ISSUES

Epidemiology
- Incidence
  - Predominantly disease of adults and elderly but also occurs in children and young adults
  - Most frequent morphologic variant of DLBCL

Presentation
- Enlarging mass in nodal or extranodal sites
- Gastrointestinal tract is frequent extranodal site
- Stage IV in at least 1/3 of cases
- Bone marrow involvement occurs less frequently than in patients with low-grade B-cell lymphomas
- Certain morphologic variants more prevalent at particular extranodal sites
  - Cells with multilobated nuclei in cases involving bone

Treatment
- R-CHOP regimen (rituximab + cyclophosphamide, doxorubicin, vincristine, prednisone)

Prognosis
- 5-year survival: Overall, 75%

MICROSCOPIC PATHOLOGY

Histologic Features
- Diffuse growth pattern
  - Neoplasm replaces normal architecture with diffuse and usually dense lymphoid infiltrate
  - Sometimes present as vague nodules
  - Sclerosis is frequent in extranodal sites
- Centroblastic morphology
  - Composed predominantly of centroblasts (large noncleaved cells); immunoblast-like cells can be seen
  - Polymorphic variant: Mixture of centroblasts, immunoblasts, multilobated cells, and cells with overlapping cytologic features

ANCILLARY TESTS

Immunohistochemistry
- Pan-B cell antigens(+)
- Germinal center (GC) markers positive in subset
  - CD10(+), Bcl-6(+), CM02(+)
  - Centerin/GCET1(+), HGAL/GCET2(+)
- Bcl-2(+/-), CD30(-/+)
- Proliferation fraction (Ki-67) usually high (> 30-40%)
- Algorithms proposed to identify GC and non-GC types
  - Hans et al
  - Choi et al

DIFFUSE LARGE B-CELL LYMPHOMA, NOS, CENTROBLASTIC

Key Facts

Terminology
- Diffuse proliferation of large neoplastic B cells composed predominantly of centroblasts
- Typical: Medium to large cells (10-14 μm) with fine chromatin, 2-3 small nucleoli often apposed to nuclear membrane, and scant basophilic cytoplasm

Clinical Issues
- Most frequent morphologic variant of DLBCL

Microscopic Pathology
- Diffuse growth pattern and predominantly composed of centroblasts
- Sclerosis is frequent in extranodal sites
- Usually express pan-B markers: CD20, CD22, CD79a, PAX5
- Germinal center markers, CD10 and Bcl-6, expressed in variable proportion of cases

Ancillary Tests
- t(14;18) is detected in almost 30% of cases; translocations involving 3q27 are also common
- 2 major molecular groups of DLBCL
  - GC type
  - ABC type
  - Patients with DLBCL of GC type have better prognosis than those with ABC type

Top Differential Diagnoses
- DLBCL, immunoblastic variant
- DLBCL, anaplastic variant
- Plasmablastic lymphoma
- Follicular lymphoma (grade 3B)

Cytogenetics
- t(14;18) is 1 of most frequent translocations, detected in almost 30% of cases
- Translocations involving 3q27 are also common

Gene Expression Profiling
- Expression microarray studies have established 2 major groups of DLBCL
  - GC type (gene expression profile similar to GC B cells)
  - Activated B-cell (ABC) type (gene expression profile similar to activated B cells)
- Patients with DLBCL with GC signature have better prognosis than patients with DLBCL with ABC signature when treated with CHOP or R-CHOP therapies

DIFFERENTIAL DIAGNOSIS

DLBCL, Immunoblastic Variant
- Distinction can be arbitrary, reducing diagnostic reproducibility
- Most cells (90%) are immunoblasts (large cells with single, centrally located nucleolus and moderate amounts of basophilic cytoplasm)
- Subtle features supporting centroblastic variant
  - More peripheral location of nucleoli (i.e., apposed to nuclear membrane)
  - Absence of plasmacytoid differentiation
  - Residual follicular pattern

DLBCL, Anaplastic Variant
- Neoplastic cells are large with bizarre and anaplastic morphology and may resemble Hodgkin &/or Reed-Sternberg cells
- CD30 can be positive

Plasmablastic Lymphoma
- Large neoplastic cells, most of which resemble immunoblasts
- Expression of CD138 and CD38 and negativity for CD20 and pax-5

Burkitt Lymphoma
- Monomorphic medium-sized cells with multiple small nucleoli
- Numerous mitoses and "starry sky" pattern
- Characteristic immunophenotype: Positive for CD10, Bcl-6 (strong), and CD20; negative for Bcl-2
- Ki-67 positive in virtually 100% of tumor cells (uniformly strong)
- Chromosomal translocations involving MYC gene at 8q24 are characteristic

Follicular Lymphoma (Grade 3B)
- CD21, CD23, or CD35 highlights follicular dendritic cells in follicular areas

SELECTED REFERENCES

1. Meyer PN et al: Immunohistochemical methods for predicting cell of origin and survival in patients with diffuse large B-cell lymphoma treated with rituximab. J Clin Oncol. 29(2):200-7, 2011
2. Fu K et al: Addition of rituximab to standard chemotherapy improves the survival of both the germinal center B-cell-like and non-germinal center B-cell-like subtypes of diffuse large B-cell lymphoma. J Clin Oncol. 26(28):4587-94, 2008
3. Lossos IS et al: Prognostic biomarkers in diffuse large B-cell lymphoma. J Clin Oncol. 24(6):995-1007, 2006

Microscopic Features

(Left) Nonneoplastic centroblasts inside a reactive germinal center show centroblasts that are intermediate to large in size with small nucleoli apposed to the nuclear membrane ➡. *(Right)* DLBCL, centroblastic variant shows the diffuse growth pattern and the loss of normal nodal architecture. The neoplasm extends into the fibroadipose tissue.

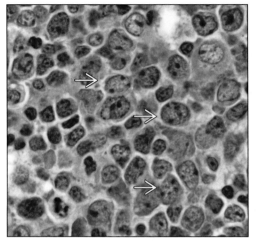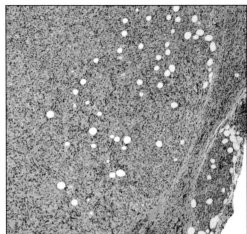

(Left) DLBCL, centroblastic variant shows that this lymph node involved by lymphoma has a prominent capsular fibrosis ➡. *(Right)* Hematoxylin & eosin of touch imprint shows medium to large lymphoid cells, some with small nucleoli apposed to the nuclear membrane. Few multilobated cells are also seen ➡.

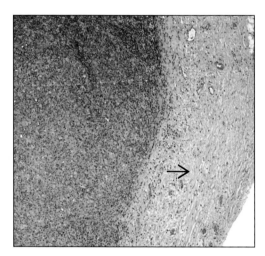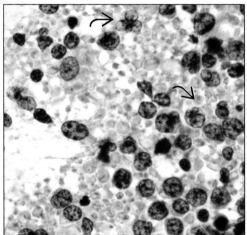

(Left) DLBCL, centroblastic variant. Centroblasts ➡ admixed with small reactive lymphocytes and occasional eosinophils. Some of the centroblasts are large and have cleaved nuclei. *(Right)* DLBCL, centroblastic variant shows marked sclerosis. The centroblasts are large with vesicular nuclear chromatin and cleaved nuclei. Sclerosis is frequently seen in cases of DLBCL involving extranodal sites and retroperitoneum.

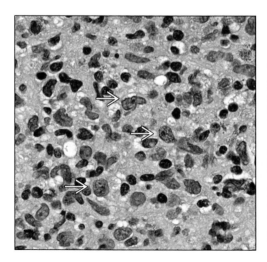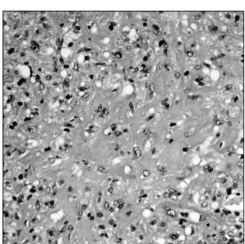

Ancillary Techniques and Differential Diagnosis

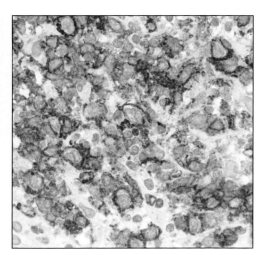
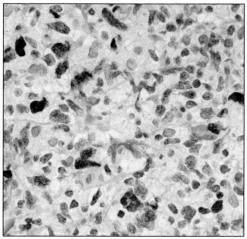

(Left) CD10(+) DLBCL, centroblastic variant. The large tumor cells are positive for CD10. (Right) DLBCL centroblastic variant shows a subset of large neoplastic cells that are positive for Bcl-6. Expression of CD10 and Bcl-6 are consistent with a germinal center cell phenotype. DLBCL cells, when positive for Bcl-6, usually show variable degrees of nuclear positivity. However, Burkitt lymphoma cells are usually strongly and uniformly positive for Bcl-6.

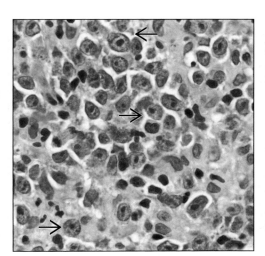
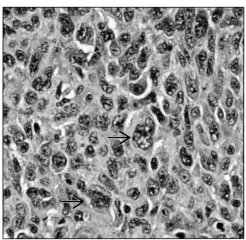

(Left) DLBCL, immunoblastic variant demonstrates a monotonous population of large cells with central prominent nucleoli ➡. (Right) DLBCL, anaplastic variant shows the malignant cells are very pleomorphic ➡, mostly large with irregular nuclei, vesicular chromatin, and distinct nucleoli. The tumor cells were positive for CD20 and CD30 and negative for CD10, CD5, and CD3.

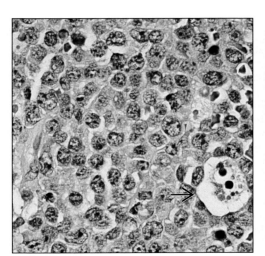
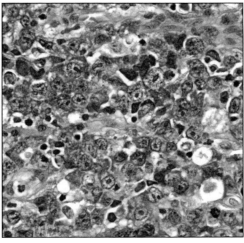

(Left) Characteristic morphologic features of Burkitt lymphoma: The tumor cells are fairly monotonous, medium in size, with nuclear molding, high mitotic rate, and macrophages ➡ ("starry sky" pattern). (Right) A case of plasmablastic lymphoma shows the tumor cells are large & pleomorphic, some with features of immunoblasts. The tumor cells were positive for CD38, CD138, & CD10 and negative for CD20 & PAX5/ BSAP.

DIFFUSE LARGE B-CELL LYMPHOMA, NOS, IMMUNOBLASTIC

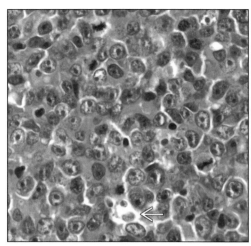

DLBCL-IB shows large immunoblasts compared with the size of histiocyte nuclei ➡. Immunoblasts have a single, central, prominent nucleolus.

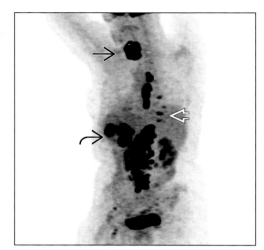

PET/CT scan of a patient with DLBCL-IB shows bulky lymphoma of the left neck ➡, right paratracheal space, retroperitoneum, spleen ➡, and vertebral bodies ➡.

TERMINOLOGY

Abbreviations
- Diffuse large B-cell lymphoma, immunoblastic variant (DLBCL-IB)

Synonyms
- Immunoblastic lymphoma
- Immunoblastic sarcoma

Definitions
- Diffuse proliferation of large neoplastic B cells with immunoblastic cytologic features
  - By definition, immunoblasts must be > 90% of all cells
- Immunoblast
  - Large lymphocyte with centrally located nucleolus and moderate basophilic cytoplasm
- DLBCL-IB variant superseded by specific types of DLBCL as defined in WHO classification

CLINICAL ISSUES

Epidemiology
- Incidence
  - Predominantly disease of older adults
    - Children and young adults can be affected

Presentation
- Enlarging mass in nodal or extranodal sites
- Gastrointestinal tract is frequent extranodal site
- ~ 1/3 of patients have stage IV disease
- Bone marrow involvement less frequent than in patients with low-grade B-cell lymphomas
- Frequent B symptoms (fever, night sweats, or weight loss)

Treatment
- R-CHOP regimen (rituximab + cyclophosphamide, doxorubicin, vincristine, and prednisone)

Prognosis
- Some studies have identified immunoblastic variant as being clinically more aggressive than centroblastic variant
- 5-year overall survival for patients with DLBCL ranges from 25-75% depending on prognostic factors present at diagnosis

MICROSCOPIC PATHOLOGY

Histologic Features
- Diffuse growth pattern
  - Irrespective of location, DLBCL-IB diffusely replaces normal architecture
- Immunoblastic morphology
- Plasmacytoid differentiation is common

ANCILLARY TESTS

Immunohistochemistry
- Pan-B cell antigens(+)
  - CD20 can be dim, attributable to plasmacytoid differentiation
- CD10(+), Bcl-6(+), LM02(+), HGAL(+) in subset
- MUM1(+) in cases with plasmacytoid differentiation
- FoxP1(+/-), Bcl-2(+/-), CD30(-/+), and usually weak and partial
- Proliferation fraction (Ki-67) is usually high
- Algorithms proposed to identify GC and non-GC types
  - Hans et al
  - Choi et al

DIFFUSE LARGE B-CELL LYMPHOMA, NOS, IMMUNOBLASTIC

Key Facts

Terminology
- Diffuse proliferation of large neoplastic B cells with immunoblastic cytologic features
- Immunoblasts must be > 90% of all cells
- DLBCL-IB variant superseded by specific types of DLBCL as defined in WHO classification

Clinical Issues
- Some studies identified immunoblastic variant as being more clinically aggressive than centroblastic variant
- Stage IV in at least 1/3 of cases
- Bone marrow involvement less frequent than low-grade B-cell lymphomas

Microscopic Pathology
- Diffuse growth pattern

- Composed predominantly of immunoblasts
- Express pan-B cell markers

Ancillary Tests
- 2 major molecular groups
  - GC type
  - ABC type

Top Differential Diagnoses
- DLBCL, centroblastic variant
- DLBCL, anaplastic variant
- Plasmablastic lymphoma
- Primary cutaneous DLBCL, leg type
- ALK(+) large B-cell lymphoma
- B-cell lymphoma, unclassifiable, with features between DLBCL and Burkitt lymphoma

DIFFERENTIAL DIAGNOSIS

DLBCL, Centroblastic Variant
- Centroblastic and immunoblastic variants can be difficult to distinguish reliably
  - Justifies their inclusion into DLBCL as variants
- By definition, at least a significant number (> 10%) of neoplastic cells are centroblasts
- Subtle morphologic features supporting centroblastic variant
  - 2-3 nucleoli with 1 central and 1-2 apposed to nuclear membrane
  - Absence of plasmacytoid differentiation
  - Presence of small and large cleaved cells
  - Residual follicular pattern

DLBCL, Anaplastic Variant
- Large neoplastic cells with bizarre morphology; may resemble Hodgkin &/or Reed-Sternberg cells
- These neoplasms may have intrasinusoidal growth pattern
- CD30 often positive

Plasmablastic Lymphoma
- Large neoplastic cells, most of which resemble immunoblasts or plasmablasts
- Plasma cell-associated markers expressed (CD138, CD38, Vs38c, and EMA)
- CD56 frequently positive
  - CD56 expression is rare in DLBCL
- Almost always negative for CD20 and pax-5
- CD45 (LCA) weak or negative
- Some cases positive for some T-cell markers, including CD4 and CD7
- EBV frequently positive (~ 75%)

Primary Cutaneous DLBCL, Leg Type
- Not limited to lower extremities
- Multiple tumors frequent, sometimes ulcerated
- Large monotonous lymphoid cells (immunoblastic morphology)
- No epidermotropism

- Positive for CD20, Bcl-2, Bcl-6, MUM-1, and FOXP1
- CD10 usually negative

Lymphomatoid Granulomatosis
- Patients may have underlying immunodeficiency disorder
- Lung is most common site of involvement (almost essential for diagnosis)
  - Other extranodal sites: Skin, kidney, liver, and central nervous system
- Angiocentric and angiodestructive polymorphic lymphoid infiltrate with necrosis
- Positive for CD20, CD30 (variable), and EBV (LMP-1 and EBER)
- Monotonous population of EBV(+) large B cells without polymorphous background should be classified as DLBCL, not as lymphomatoid granulomatosis (WHO)

ALK(+) Large B-cell Lymphoma
- ~ 80 cases reported
- More commonly reported in children
- Immunoblastic/plasmablastic morphology
- Intrasinusoidal growth pattern
- Positive for ALK, EMA, CD138, Vs38c, and monotypic cytoplasmic light chain
  - ALK less often nuclear and cytoplasmic, corresponding to t(2;5)
  - ALK often coarsely granular and cytoplasmic, corresponding to t(2;17)
- T-cell antigens are negative except CD4, which is often expressed
- CD30 is usually negative
- EBV is frequently negative
- *ALK* gene at 2p23 can be involved in translocations with
  - Clathrin (*CTCL*) gene on 17p23, resulting in CTCL-ALK fusion protein
  - Nucleophosmin (*NPM*) gene on 5q35, resulting in NPM-ALK fusion protein

DIFFUSE LARGE B-CELL LYMPHOMA, NOS, IMMUNOBLASTIC

Primary Mediastinal (Thymic) Large B-cell Lymphoma

- Young females
- Anterosuperior mediastinal mass
- Locally aggressive with local compressive effects
- Large cells with pale cytoplasm (often is retraction artifact) and sclerosis (compartmentalization)
- Thymic components, such as Hassall corpuscles, may be identified
- Positive for pan-B-cell markers
- CD30 often (+) but usually weak &/or focal (~ 75%)
- CD23 (70%), Bcl-6, and MUM-1 (most cases)
- From practical point of view, difficult to diagnose by histologic findings alone
  o Clinical correlation is essential for diagnosis

Primary DLBCL of Central Nervous System

- Is recognized as distinct subtype in 2008 WHO classification
- All primary or intraocular lymphomas are considered in this category
- Bcl-6 and MUM-1 positive in most cases
- CD10(+) in up to 20% of cases
- EBV(-) in immunocompetent patients
- Patients may have sporadic systemic relapses, in particular, in testis and breast

EBV(+) DLBCL of Elderly

- > 50 years of age
- No history of chronic inflammation, immunodeficiency, or previous lymphoma
- Believed to be related to senescence of immune system
- Frequent extranodal involvement
- Epstein-Barr virus always positive (EBER and LMP-1)
- MUM-1(+) in most cases
- CD10 and Bcl-6 usually negative

DLBCL Associated with Chronic Inflammation

- History of longstanding chronic inflammation
- Associated with EBV (EBER and LMP-1 positive)
- Pleural cavity, bone (femur), and periarticular joint tissues
- CD30 may be positive

Primary Effusion Lymphoma

- Serous effusions (pleural, pericardial, and peritoneal cavities) without tumor masses
- Usually in context of HIV infection
- Positive for CD45 (LCA) and plasma cell markers
- Negative for B-cell markers
- EBV infection common (EBER[+], LMP-1[-])
- Usually associated with human herpes virus 8 (HHV8)

B-cell Lymphoma, Unclassifiable, with Features between DLBCL and Burkitt Lymphoma (BL)

- Features of high-grade lymphoma
  o High proliferation rate
  o Apoptosis/necrosis
  o "Starry sky" pattern
- Morphology intermediate between BL and DLBCL
- Immunophenotype can be suggestive of BL
- Bcl-2 can be strongly positive
- Subset of cases has translocations involving *MYC*, *BCL-2*, &/or *BCL-6* (double- and triple-hit lymphomas)

SELECTED REFERENCES

1. Meyer PN et al: Immunohistochemical methods for predicting cell of origin and survival in patients with diffuse large B-cell lymphoma treated with rituximab. J Clin Oncol. 29(2):200-7, 2011
2. Ott G et al: Immunoblastic morphology but not the immunohistochemical GCB/nonGCB classifier predicts outcome in diffuse large B-cell lymphoma in the RICOVER-60 trial of the DSHNHL. Blood. 116(23):4916-25, 2010
3. Gibson SE et al: Epstein-Barr virus-positive B-cell lymphoma of the elderly at a United States tertiary medical center: an uncommon aggressive lymphoma with a nongerminal center B-cell phenotype. Hum Pathol. 40(5):653-61, 2009
4. Johnson NA et al: Lymphomas with concurrent BCL2 and MYC translocations: the critical factors associated with survival. Blood. 114(11):2273-9, 2009
5. Niitsu N et al: Clinical features and prognosis of de novo diffuse large B-cell lymphoma with t(14;18) and 8q24/c-MYC translocations. Leukemia. 23(4):777-83, 2009
6. Saito M et al: BCL6 suppression of BCL2 via Miz1 and its disruption in diffuse large B cell lymphoma. Proc Natl Acad Sci U S A. 106(27):11294-9, 2009
7. Tilly H et al: Diffuse large B-cell non-Hodgkin's lymphoma: ESMO clinical recommendations for diagnosis, treatment and follow-up. Ann Oncol. 20 Suppl 4:110-2, 2009
8. Camara DA et al: Immunoblastic morphology in diffuse large B-cell lymphoma is associated with a nongerminal center immunophenotypic profile. Leuk Lymphoma. 48(5):892-6, 2007
9. Le Gouill S et al: The clinical presentation and prognosis of diffuse large B-cell lymphoma with t(14;18) and 8q24/c-MYC rearrangement. Haematologica. 92(10):1335-42, 2007
10. Lin P et al: High-grade B-cell lymphoma/leukemia associated with t(14;18) and 8q24/MYC rearrangement: a neoplasm of germinal center immunophenotype with poor prognosis. Haematologica. 92(10):1297-301, 2007
11. Vega F et al: Plasmablastic lymphomas and plasmablastic plasma cell myelomas have nearly identical immunophenotypic profiles. Mod Pathol. 2005 Jun;18(6):806-15. Erratum in: Mod Pathol. 18(6):873, 2005
12. Onciu M et al: ALK-positive anaplastic large cell lymphoma with leukemic peripheral blood involvement is a clinicopathologic entity with an unfavorable prognosis. Report of three cases and review of the literature. Am J Clin Pathol. 120(4):617-25, 2003
13. Lim MS et al: T-cell/histiocyte-rich large B-cell lymphoma: a heterogeneous entity with derivation from germinal center B cells. Am J Surg Pathol. 26(11):1458-66, 2002
14. Lazzarino M et al: Primary mediastinal B-cell lymphoma with sclerosis: an aggressive tumor with distinctive clinical and pathologic features. J Clin Oncol. 11(12):2306-13, 1993

DIFFUSE LARGE B-CELL LYMPHOMA, NOS, IMMUNOBLASTIC

Microscopic Features

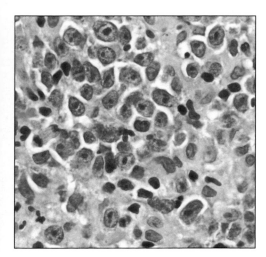

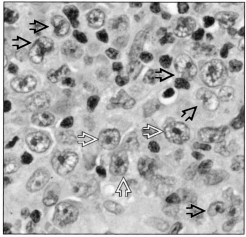

(Left) DLBCL-IB variant composed of a monotonous population of large cells with central nucleoli and a plasmacytoid appearance. *(Right)* DLBCL-IB shows a mixture of many immunoblasts ➡ and fewer large cells with features of centroblasts ➡.

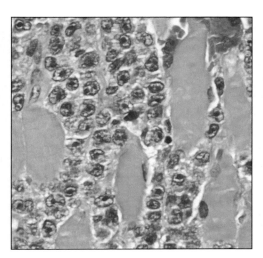

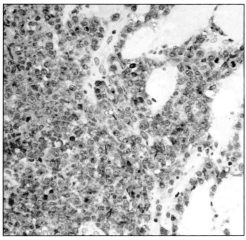

(Left) DLBCL-IB infiltrating skeletal muscle. Note the central prominent nucleoli. *(Right)* DLBCL-IB. The tumor cells are infiltrating skeletal muscle and are positive for CD10. DLBCL positive for CD10 are considered of germinal center cell origin.

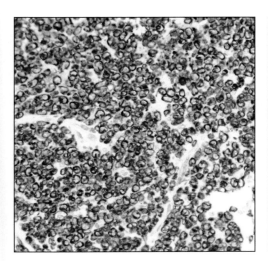

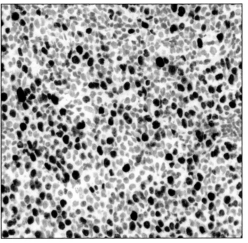

(Left) DLBCL-IB. The neoplastic cells are strongly positive for Bcl-2. *(Right)* DLBCL-IB shows a proliferation rate, as measured by MIB-1 (Ki-67), of 40-50%.

DIFFUSE LARGE B-CELL LYMPHOMA, NOS, IMMUNOBLASTIC

Differential Diagnosis

(Left) DLBCL, centroblastic variant composed of large cells with noncleaved nuclear contours, vesicular nuclear chromatin, and 2-3 nucleoli apposed to the nuclear membrane ➡. *(Right)* Hematoxylin & eosin of touch imprint shows a DLBCL centroblastic variant composed of medium to large lymphoid cells, some with small nucleoli apposed to the nuclear membrane. Few multilobated cells are also seen ➡.

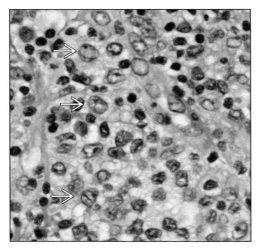
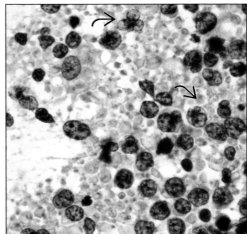

(Left) DLBCL, anaplastic variant is characterized by pleomorphic neoplastic cells, mostly large with irregular nuclei, vesicular chromatin, and distinct nucleoli ➡. This neoplasm was positive for CD20 and CD30. *(Right)* Note the presence of large tumor cells within the sinuses ➡ in this case of DLBCL, anaplastic variant. The neoplasm was positive for CD20, CD30, and CD45 (LCA) and was negative for CD3 and CD15.

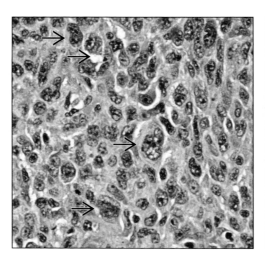
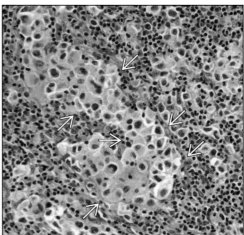

(Left) A case of plasmablastic lymphoma showing a diffuse neoplasm with a prominent "starry sky" pattern. *(Right)* Plasmablastic lymphoma. The tumor cells are large and pleomorphic; some cells have features of immunoblasts ➡.

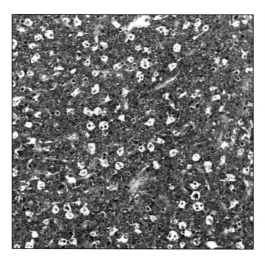
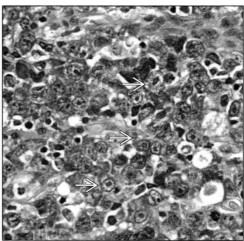

DIFFUSE LARGE B-CELL LYMPHOMA, NOS, IMMUNOBLASTIC

Differential Diagnosis

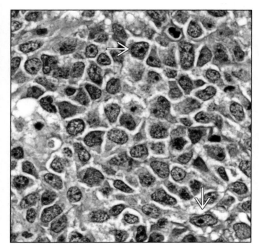

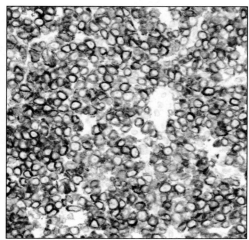

(Left) Primary cutaneous DLBCL, leg type extensively involving the dermis and subcutaneous tissue and composed of large cells, some with immunoblastic features ➡. *(Right)* Primary cutaneous DLBCL, leg type. The tumor cells were strongly positive for Bcl-2. In addition, they were positive for CD20, Bcl-6, and MUM-1 and negative for CD10 (not shown).

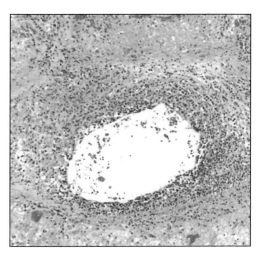

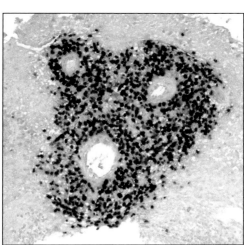

(Left) Lymphomatoid granulomatosis in the lung showing extensive necrosis and an angiocentric pattern of the lymphoid infiltrate. These are characteristic features of these neoplasms. *(Right)* Lymphomatoid granulomatosis. The large neoplastic cells are positive for Epstein-Barr virus as detected by in situ hybridization for EBV-encoded RNA (EBER).

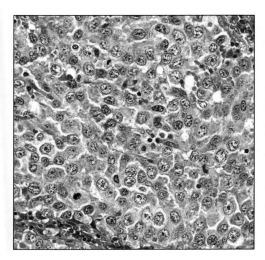

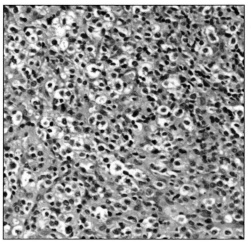

(Left) DLBCL ALK(+) is a diffuse neoplasm composed of immunoblasts with plasmacytic appearance. The tumor cells were focally positive for CD79a and ALK (cytoplasmic and coarsely granular) and negative for CD30. *(Right)* DLBCL presenting as an anterosuperior mass. The tumor is composed of large cells with pale cytoplasm and sclerosis (features of primary mediastinal large B-cell lymphoma). The tumor cells were positive for CD20, CD30 (focal), and MUM-1 and were negative for CD10.

T-CELL/HISTIOCYTE-RICH LARGE B-CELL LYMPHOMA

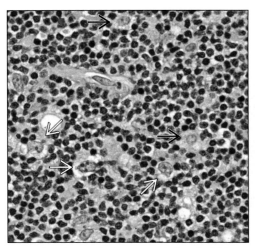

THRLBCL. Scattered, large, atypical cells ⮕ are surrounded by numerous small lymphocytes and occasional histiocytes ⮕.

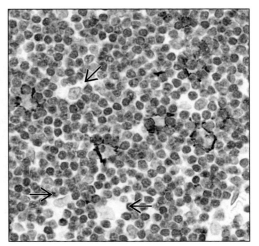

THRLBCL. Large neoplastic cells show membranous reactivity for CD20. Histiocytes ⮕ are negative for CD20.

TERMINOLOGY

Abbreviations
- T-cell/histiocyte-rich large B-cell lymphoma (THRLBCL)

Synonyms
- T-cell-rich B-cell lymphoma
- Large B-cell lymphoma rich in T-cells and simulating Hodgkin disease
- Histiocyte-rich T-cell-rich B-cell lymphoma
- Histiocyte-rich B-cell lymphoma

Definitions
- Large B-cell lymphoma characterized by scattered large cells representing < 10% of total cell population

CLINICAL ISSUES

Presentation
- Young to middle-aged males
- Advanced clinical stage at diagnosis
  - Commonly involves liver, spleen, and bone marrow

Treatment
- Rituximab, cyclophosphamide, doxorubicin, vincristine, and prednisone (R-CHOP) is standard

Prognosis
- Clinically aggressive and often refractory to chemotherapy

MICROSCOPIC PATHOLOGY

Histologic Features
- Diffuse pattern of growth replacing lymph node parenchyma
- Small number of large lymphoma cells
  - May resemble centroblasts, immunoblasts, or Hodgkin cells including LP (a.k.a. L&H or "popcorn" cells)
  - By definition, < 10% of total cell population
- Numerous reactive small lymphocytes often associated with histiocytes
  - 90% or more of cell population
- Cases with histiocytes represent more homogeneous group of patients with very aggressive course
  - According to 2008 WHO classification, absence of histiocytes should be reported

ANCILLARY TESTS

Immunohistochemistry
- Large neoplastic cells
  - Positive for CD45/LCA and pan-B antigens CD20, CD79a, and pax-5
  - Bcl-6 is often positive; CD10 can be positive
  - Bcl-2(+/-)
  - CD30 is usually, but not invariably, negative
  - CD15(+), T-cell antigens(-)
  - EBV rarely (+)
- Reactive cells
  - CD3(+) T cells (either CD4[+] or CD8[+])
  - T-cells often have cytotoxic immunophenotype
  - CD68(+) histiocytes
  - Few numbers of small B cells
  - Networks of CD21(+) follicular dendritic cells are usually absent

PCR
- Monoclonal *IgH* gene rearrangements with high number of somatic mutations and intraclonal diversity
- No monoclonal *TCR*γ or *TCR*β gene rearrangements
- No specific chromosomal translocations

T-CELL/HISTIOCYTE-RICH LARGE B-CELL LYMPHOMA

Key Facts

Terminology
- Large B-cell lymphoma characterized by scattered large lymphoma cells representing < 10% of total cell population

Clinical Issues
- Young to middle-aged males
- Usually aggressive and often refractory to chemotherapy
- Liver, spleen, and bone marrow often involved

Microscopic Pathology
- Diffuse pattern
- Large lymphoma cells have variable cytologic features
  - Centroblasts, immunoblasts, or HRS-like
- Reactive cells are small lymphocytes and histiocytes
  - Histiocyte number can be variable

Ancillary Tests
- Large lymphoma cells are B cells
  - Positive for CD20, CD79a, pax-5, and other pan-B-cell markers
  - CD45/LCA positive; CD15 negative
  - Bcl-6 usually positive; CD10 variable
  - CD30 often negative but can be positive in subset
  - Negative for T-cell antigens
- Reactive lymphocytes are T cells and histiocytes

Top Differential Diagnoses
- Classical Hodgkin lymphoma
- Nodular lymphocyte-predominant Hodgkin lymphoma
- Diffuse large B-cell lymphoma, NOS
- Angioimmunoblastic T-cell lymphoma

Differential Diagnosis: THRLBCL and NLPHL (Microenvironment)

Background	THRLBCL	NLPHL
Small B cells	-/+	+
Cytotoxic TIA1(+) T cells	+	-/+
GZM-B(+) T cells	+	-/+
CD4(+) rosetting T cells	-	+
CD8(+) rosetting T cells	-	+
CD57(+) rosetting T cells	-	-/+
MUM1/IRF4(+) rosetting T cells	-	+
Follicular dendritic cells	-	+

DIFFERENTIAL DIAGNOSIS

Classical Hodgkin Lymphoma
- Tumor cells are negative for CD45/LCA and usually (~ 75%) negative for CD20 and CD79a
- CD30(+) and CD15(+/-)
- Background of mixed inflammatory cells
  - Granulocytes and plasma cells common
- No *IgH* gene rearrangements using standard PCR

Nodular Lymphocyte Predominant Hodgkin Lymphoma (NLPHL)
- Nodular pattern with many small reactive B cells
- Preservation of CD21(+) follicular dendritic cells in nodules
- CD3(+) T-cell rosettes and to lesser extent CD57(+) T-cell rosettes surrounding LP cells

Diffuse Large B-cell Lymphoma, Not Otherwise Specified
- Subset of DLBCL can be rich in T cells
- Large B cells far greater than 10%
- Variable morphology and growth pattern with clusters or sheets of large B cells

Angioimmunoblastic T-cell Lymphoma
- T-cell lymphoma associated with abundant polymorphous reactive cells
- Extensive high endothelial venule and follicular dendritic cell proliferation
- T-cells are CD10(+), Bcl-6(+), CXCL13(+), or PD-1(+)
- Frequent large B immunoblasts
  - Often EBV(+)

SELECTED REFERENCES

1. Nam-Cha SH et al: PD-1, a follicular T-cell marker useful for recognizing nodular lymphocyte-predominant Hodgkin lymphoma. Am J Surg Pathol. 32(8):1252-7, 2008
2. El Weshi A et al: T-cell/histiocyte-rich B-cell lymphoma: Clinical presentation, management and prognostic factors: report on 61 patients and review of literature. Leuk Lymphoma. 48(9):1764-73, 2007
3. Boudová L et al: Nodular lymphocyte-predominant Hodgkin lymphoma with nodules resembling T-cell/histiocyte-rich B-cell lymphoma: differential diagnosis between nodular lymphocyte-predominant Hodgkin lymphoma and T-cell/histiocyte-rich B-cell lymphoma. Blood. 102(10):3753-8, 2003
4. Achten R et al: Histiocyte-rich, T-cell-rich B-cell lymphoma: a distinct diffuse large B-cell lymphoma subtype showing characteristic morphologic and immunophenotypic features. Histopathology. 40(1):31-45, 2002
5. Lim MS et al: T-cell/histiocyte-rich large B-cell lymphoma: a heterogeneous entity with derivation from germinal center B cells. Am J Surg Pathol. 26(11):1458-66, 2002

6

T-CELL/HISTIOCYTE-RICH LARGE B-CELL LYMPHOMA

Microscopic Features

(Left) THRLBCL is diffuse and composed of scattered large cells, histiocytes, and numerous small lymphocytes. Note that the large atypical cells are difficult to recognize at low magnification. *(Right)* Higher magnification reveals the presence of histiocytes, some with foamy cytoplasm ➡, in a background of small lymphocytes with rare and scattered large cells.

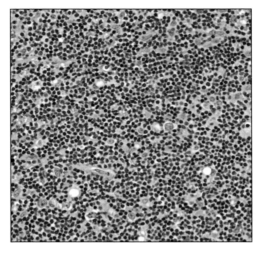
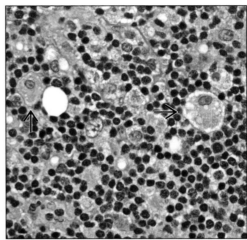

(Left) THRLBCL shows scattered tumor cells positive for CD20. *(Right)* THRLBCL. The tumor cells can also be highlighted using antibodies specific for transcription factor pax-5 ➡. Note that only rare small lymphoid cells are also positive for pax-5 ➡.

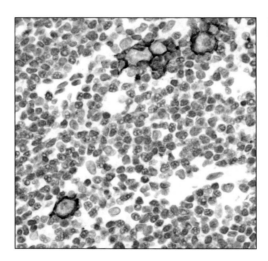
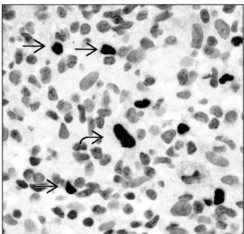

(Left) In THRLBCL, most of the small lymphocytes seen in the background are T cells, here highlighted by reactivity for the T-cell marker CD3. *(Right)* The large neoplastic cells are positive for CD45/LCA. Note the membranous positivity of the neoplastic cells ➡. The histiocytes are negative ➡. This is helpful in distinguishing THRLBCL from classical Hodgkin lymphoma.

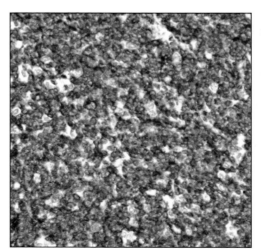
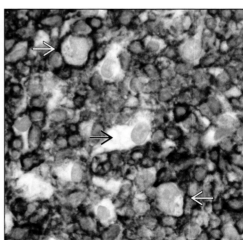

T-CELL/HISTIOCYTE-RICH LARGE B-CELL LYMPHOMA

Differential Diagnosis

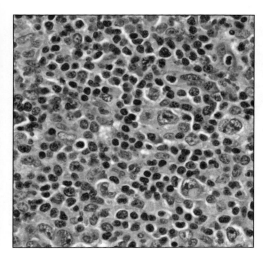
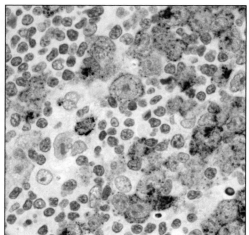

(Left) This case of classical Hodgkin lymphoma shows scattered and small clusters of large HRS cells in a background rich in small lymphocytes, eosinophils, and plasma cells. *(Right)* Classical Hodgkin lymphoma. Most of the HRS cells were positive for CD15. They were also strongly and uniformly positive for CD30, weakly positive for pax-5, and negative for CD45/LCA and CD20.

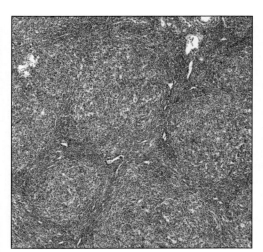
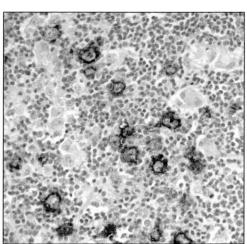

(Left) NLPHL shows a nodular pattern of growth. Scattered large atypical cells, some with LP morphology, were identified inside of the nodules. They are difficult to recognize at low magnification. *(Right)* In NLPHL, the LP cells are usually positive for epithelial membrane antigen. In addition, they were positive for CD45, CD20, and CD79a, focally positive for CD30, and negative for CD3, CD10, and CD15. Most of the LP cells were ringed by CD3 positive T cells.

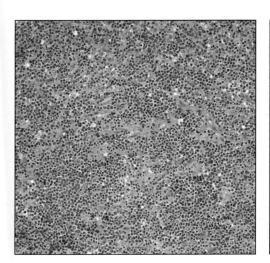
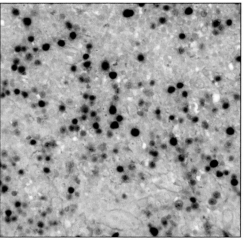

(Left) Angioimmunoblastic T-cell lymphoma shows effacement of lymph node architecture associated with vascular proliferation and with a polymorphic infiltrate composed of small lymphocytes and occasional large immunoblastic cells. *(Right)* B immunoblasts and some small lymphoid cells were EBER positive in this case of angioimmunoblastic T-cell lymphoma. The neoplastic T cells were positive for CD3 and negative for CD5. The B immunoblasts were variably positive for CD30.

ALK+ DIFFUSE LARGE B-CELL LYMPHOMA

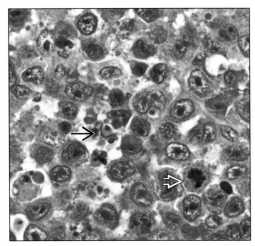

ALK(+) diffuse large B-cell lymphoma involving lymph node. The neoplastic cells have large nuclei with prominent central nucleoli. Apoptotic cells ⇒ and a mitotic figure ⧐ are present.

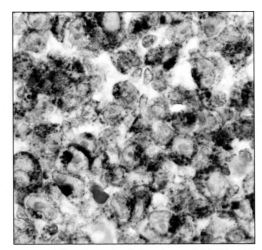

ALK(+) diffuse large B-cell lymphoma (DLBCL). ALK is expressed in a granular and cytoplasmic pattern consistent with t(2;17)(p23;q23)/CLTC-ALK.

TERMINOLOGY

Abbreviations
- Diffuse large B-cell lymphoma (DLBCL), anaplastic lymphoma kinase (ALK)

Definitions
- Diffuse large B-cell lymphoma expressing ALK protein and associated with ALK gene abnormalities

ETIOLOGY/PATHOGENESIS

Etiology
- No known association with infectious or environmental factors

Genetics
- ALK gene abnormalities at chromosome 2p23 appear to be key transforming event
  - Result in formation of fusion genes
    - Clathrin heavy-chain gene (CLTC)-ALK
    - Nucleophosmin (NPM)-ALK
    - SEC31A-ALK
  - Overexpression of ALK protein

CLINICAL ISSUES

Epidemiology
- Incidence
  - < 1% of all cases of DLBCL
  - Approximately 80 cases reported to date
- Age
  - Range: 9-85 years
    - Median: ~ 40 years
- Gender
  - Male to female ratio: ~ 5 to 1
- Ethnicity
  - No apparent ethnic predisposition

Site
- Lymph nodes are most commonly involved and biopsied (~ 75%)
- Extranodal sites of involvement include
  - Bone marrow in ~ 25% of patients
  - Nasal cavity, nasopharynx, oral cavity
  - Stomach, small intestine
  - Spleen, ovary
  - Bones, soft tissues
  - Epidural mass, brain
- Enlarged mediastinal lymph nodes can present as mediastinal mass
- Patients can present with leukemic involvement

Presentation
- Systemic (B-type) symptoms common
- 60-70% of patients have stage III or IV disease
  - Widespread lymphadenopathy
- Aggressive clinical course

Laboratory Tests
- Serum lactate dehydrogenase (LDH) levels elevated in ~ 50% of patients
- HIV serology is (-)

Treatment
- Drugs
  - Most patients have been treated with cyclophosphamide, doxorubicin, vincristine, and prednisone (CHOP) regimen
    - Based on survival data, this therapeutic approach is not optimal

Prognosis
- 5-year overall survival is ~ 25%
  - ~ 50% of patients die within 1 year
- Survival is shorter for patients with advanced-stage disease
- Children appear to have better prognosis

ALK+ DIFFUSE LARGE B-CELL LYMPHOMA

Key Facts

Etiology/Pathogenesis
- *ALK* gene abnormalities at chromosome 2p23 appear to be key transforming event
  - Result in formation of fusion genes and ALK overexpression

Clinical Issues
- Rare; ~ 80 cases reported
- Lymph nodes are most commonly involved and biopsied (~ 75%)
- 60-70% of patients have stage III or IV disease
- Aggressive clinical course and poor survival

Microscopic Pathology
- Partial or diffuse effacement of lymph node architecture
- Lymphoma cells infiltrate sinusoids in many cases

- Monomorphic, large immunoblast-like cells; ± plasmacytoid differentiation

Ancillary Tests
- ALK strongly positive
- EMA(+), CD138(+), VS38c(+)
- Cytoplasmic IgA(+) in > 95% of cases
- CD30 usually (-), EBER(-)
- Pan-B- and pan-T-cell markers negative
- *ALK* gene abnormalities in all cases
  - Most common: *CLTC-ALK*

Top Differential Diagnoses
- Plasmablastic lymphoma
- DLBCL immunoblastic variant
- Plasmacytoma/plasma cell myeloma
- ALK(+) anaplastic large cell lymphoma

  - Prolonged survival (> 156 months) has been reported

MICROSCOPIC PATHOLOGY

Histologic Features
- Lymph node
  - Partial or diffuse effacement of lymph node architecture
  - Lymphoma cells infiltrate sinusoids in many cases
  - ± focal necrosis
  - ± binucleated HRS–like cells
  - ± multinucleated giant lymphoma cells
  - Mitotic figures easily identified
- Extranodal sites
  - Similar morphologic features
  - Sinusoidal infiltration usually not appreciated at extranodal sites
- Bone marrow
  - Variable degree of involvement
  - Sinusoidal involvement is uncommon in bone marrow

Cytologic Features
- Monomorphic, large, immunoblast-like cells
- Plasmablastic differentiation in most cases
- Round pale nuclei, large central nucleoli, and abundant basophilic cytoplasm

ANCILLARY TESTS

Immunohistochemistry
- ALK strongly positive
  - Pattern of ALK expression predicts *ALK* partner in fusion gene
    - Granular and cytoplasmic: *CLTC* and *SEC31A*
    - Nuclear, nucleolar, and cytoplasmic: *NPM*
- CD138 and VS38 strongly positive in all cases
- EMA strongly positive in all cases
- ~ 90% of cases express cytoplasmic Ig

  - IgA expressed in > 95% of Ig(+) cases; rare cases express IgG
- CD45/LCA(+) in ~ 80% of cases; expression often weak
- OCT2(-/+), pax-5(-/+)
- CD30(-) except in rare cases showing focal weakly positive cells
  - < 5% of cases can exhibit weak CD30 expression in small subset of cells
- CD57(+) in ~ 10% of cases
- Cytokeratin expression in ~ 10% of cases
  - Dot-like paranuclear pattern in subset of cells
- T-cell antigens
  - CD4(+) in ~ 40% of cases
  - CD43 can be focally (+) in small subset of cases
  - Pan-T-cell antigens(-); CD8(-)
- B-cell antigens
  - CD20 and CD79a are usually negative
    - ~ 10% of cases exhibit weak expression of CD20 or CD79a by small subset of cells
    - CD10(-), Bcl-6(-)
- IRF-4/MUM1(-), cytotoxic proteins(-), Cyclin-D1(-)
- HHV8(-); EBV-LMP(-)

Cytogenetics
- Data available in limited number of cases
- Karyotypes have been complex with translocations involving chromosome 2p23

In Situ Hybridization
- EBV small-encoded RNA (EBER)(-)

PCR
- *CLTC-ALK* or *NPM-ALK* transcripts detected by reverse transcriptase (RT)-PCR

Molecular Genetics
- t(2;17)(p23;q23) resulting in clathrin heavy-chain gene (*CLTC*)-ALK fusion protein most common rearrangement
- t(2;5)(p23;q35) present in occasional cases
- Cryptic insertion of 3'*ALK* gene sequences into chromosome 4q22-24 in rare cases

• Monoclonal *Ig* gene rearrangements

DIFFERENTIAL DIAGNOSIS

Plasmablastic Lymphoma (PBL)
• Morphologic and immunophenotypic overlap between PBL and DLBCL ALK(+)
  ○ Immunoblastic/plasmablastic cytologic features
  ○ CD138(+), VS38c(+), CD20(-)
• Patients with PBL often present differently from patients with DLBCL ALK(+)
  ○ PBL usually associated with
    ▪ HIV infection (most common)
    ▪ Other immunodeficiency states
  ○ PBL more commonly involves extranodal sites
• Immunohistochemistry of PBL
  ○ ALK(-)
  ○ CD79a(+) in 50-85% of cases
  ○ IRF-4/MUM1 usually (+)
  ○ CD30(+/-)
  ○ CD4(-/+), CD57(-)
• ISH for EBER is positive in 60-75% of cases of PBL
• No abnormalities of *ALK* gene

DLBCL Immunoblastic Variant
• These neoplasms usually exhibit plasmacytoid differentiation that can overlap with ALK(+) DLBCL
• Immunohistochemistry of DLBCL immunoblastic variant
  ○ CD20(+), CD79a(+), pax-5(+)
  ○ CD30(-), ALK(-)
  ○ CD4(-), CD5(-)
• ISH for EBER is negative
• No abnormalities of *ALK* gene

Plasmacytoma/Plasma Cell Myeloma
• Subset of ALK(+) DLBCL exhibits marked plasmacytoid features overlapping with plasma cell tumors
• Immunohistochemistry of plasmacytoma/plasma cell myeloma
  ○ ALK(-), CD45/LCA(-), pax-5(-)
  ○ Cytoplasmic IgG > IgA; Cyclin-D1(-/+)
• ISH for EBER is negative
• No abnormalities of *ALK* gene

ALK(+) Anaplastic Large Cell Lymphoma (ALCL)
• Predominantly in 1st 3 decades of life
• Hallmark cells are usually present in ALK(+) ALCL but not in ALK(+) DLBCL
• CD30 strongly and uniformly positive
  ○ Paranuclear (Golgi zone) and membranous pattern
• ALK(+) in nuclear and cytoplasmic pattern in cases with *NPM-ALK*
• All cases have *ALK* gene abnormalities
  ○ t(2;5)(p23;q35)/*NPM-ALK* in ~ 80% of cases; *CLTC-ALK* rare
• T-cell lineage(+); cytotoxic proteins(+)
• Monoclonal T-cell receptor gene rearrangements

ALK(-) ALCL
• Hallmark cells are usually present in ALK(-) ALCL but not in ALK(+) DLBCL
• CD30 strongly and uniformly (+)
  ○ Paranuclear (Golgi zone) and membranous pattern
• T-cell lineage(+); cytotoxic proteins(+/-)
• Monoclonal T-cell receptor gene rearrangements

Poorly Differentiated Carcinoma
• ALK(+) DLBCL can be misdiagnosed as carcinoma
  ○ Small subset of cases can be keratin(+) and CD45/LCA(-)
  ○ Carcinomas can be CD138(+)
• ALK(+) is key to correct diagnosis
• No *Ig* gene rearrangements and no *ALK* gene abnormalities

DIAGNOSTIC CHECKLIST

Clinically Relevant Pathologic Features
• HIV serology is negative
• Aggressive clinical course with poor prognosis

Pathologic Interpretation Pearls
• Consider performing ALK immunostaining on all tumors with immunoblastic/plasmablastic features
• ALK immunostaining may be necessary for identifying scattered cells in bone marrow

SELECTED REFERENCES

1. Laurent C et al: Anaplastic lymphoma kinase-positive diffuse large B-cell lymphoma: a rare clinicopathologic entity with poor prognosis. J Clin Oncol. 2009 Sep 1;27(25):4211-6. Epub 2009 Jul 27. Erratum in: J Clin Oncol. 28(1):182, 2010
2. Van Roosbroeck K et al: ALK-positive large B-cell lymphomas with cryptic SEC31A-ALK and NPM1-ALK fusions. Haematologica. 95(3):509-13, 2010
3. Beltran B et al: ALK-positive diffuse large B-cell lymphoma: report of four cases and review of the literature. J Hematol Oncol. 2:11, 2009
4. Lee HW et al: ALK-positive diffuse large B-cell lymphoma: report of three cases. Hematol Oncol. 26(2):108-13, 2008
5. Reichard KK et al: ALK-positive diffuse large B-cell lymphoma: report of four cases and review of the literature. Mod Pathol. 20(3):310-9, 2007
6. Stachurski D et al: Anaplastic lymphoma kinase-positive diffuse large B-cell lymphoma with a complex karyotype and cryptic 3' ALK gene insertion to chromosome 4 q22-24. Hum Pathol. 38(6):940-5, 2007
7. Gascoyne RD et al: ALK-positive diffuse large B-cell lymphoma is associated with Clathrin-ALK rearrangements: report of 6 cases. Blood. 102(7):2568-73, 2003
8. Onciu M et al: ALK-positive anaplastic large cell lymphoma with leukemic peripheral blood involvement is a clinicopathologic entity with an unfavorable prognosis. Report of three cases and review of the literature. Am J Clin Pathol. 120(4):617-25, 2003
9. Onciu M et al: ALK-positive plasmablastic B-cell lymphoma with expression of the NPM-ALK fusion transcript: report of 2 cases. Blood. 102(7):2642-4, 2003

ALK+ DIFFUSE LARGE B-CELL LYMPHOMA

Microscopic and Immunohistochemical Features

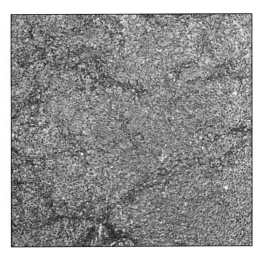
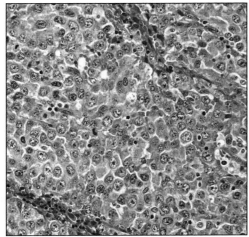

(Left) Lymph node biopsy specimen involved by ALK(+) DLBCL demonstrates sheets of large, monotonous lymphoma cells totally effacing lymph node architecture. *(Right)* Lymph node biopsy specimen involved by ALK(+) DLBCL demonstrates sheets of large immunoblast-like cells with round nuclei, open chromatin, and large central nucleoli. There is prominent plasmablastic differentiation with eccentric nuclei and abundant basophilic cytoplasm.

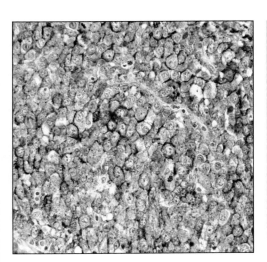
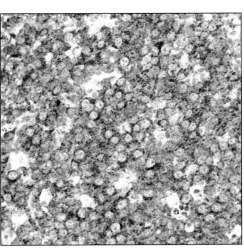

(Left) Lymph node biopsy specimen involved by ALK(+) DLBCL demonstrates strong membranous expression of epithelial membrane antigen (EMA). Virtually all cases of ALK(+) DLBCL are positive for EMA. *(Right)* Lymph node biopsy specimen involved by ALK(+) DLBCL demonstrates strong granular ALK expression limited to cytoplasm of lymphoma cells. This indicates clathrin heavy-chain gene (CLTC-ALK) protein resulting from t(2;17)(p23;q23).

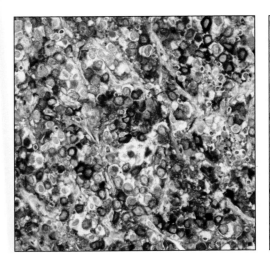
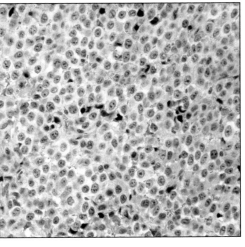

(Left) Lymph node biopsy specimen involved by ALK(+) DLBCL demonstrates strong cytoplasmic IgA expression. In > 90% of cases, IgA is expressed in these neoplasms. Rare neoplasms express cytoplasmic IgG. *(Right)* Lymph node biopsy specimen involved by ALK(+) DLBCL demonstrates that the lymphoma cells are CD30(-). The absence of CD30 distinguishes this neoplasm from anaplastic large cell lymphoma.

ALK+ DIFFUSE LARGE B-CELL LYMPHOMA

Differential Diagnosis

(Left) ALK(+) diffuse large B-cell lymphoma (DLBCL). The neoplastic cells in this case are focally CD4(+). Approximately 40% of cases express CD4, often in a focal manner. (Right) Plasmablastic lymphoma involving lymph node in a patient with human immunodeficiency virus (HIV). The neoplasm has a diffuse pattern, is composed of large cells, and has a "starry sky" pattern in areas. Histiocytes are highlighted ➡.

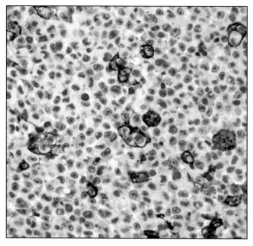
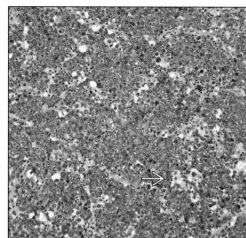

(Left) Plasmablastic lymphoma involving lymph node in an HIV(+) patient. The neoplastic cells show a range in size and variable plasmacytoid differentiation, with some cells looking more like immunoblasts ➡ and other cells more closely resembling plasma cells ➡. (Right) Plasmablastic lymphoma involving lymph node in an HIV(+) patient. The neoplastic cells show abundant Epstein-Barr virus (EBV) encoded RNA (EBER). EBV is present in most cases of plasmablastic lymphoma.

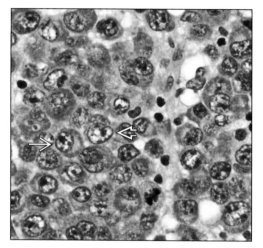
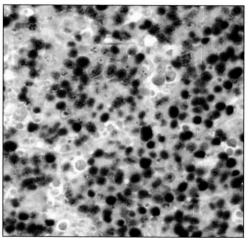

(Left) Diffuse large B-cell lymphoma, immunoblastic variant involving skin. The neoplastic cells are large with large nuclei and prominent central nucleoli. This patient had a history of DLBCL involving lymph nodes and breast. (Right) Diffuse large B-cell lymphoma, immunoblastic variant involving skin. Most of the neoplastic cells are CD20(+), which distinguishes this neoplasm from ALK(+) DLBCL. This patient had a history of DLBCL involving lymph nodes and breast.

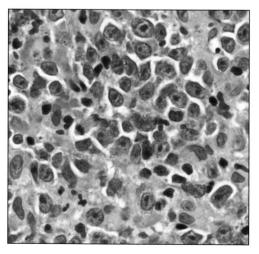
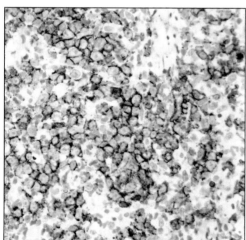

ALK+ DIFFUSE LARGE B-CELL LYMPHOMA

Differential Diagnosis

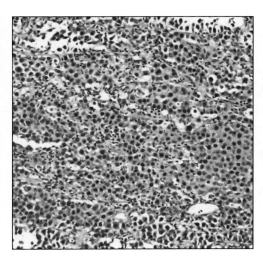 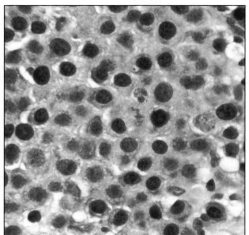

(Left) Anaplastic plasmacytoma presenting as a right shoulder mass in a patient with a history of plasma cell myeloma. Even at this low magnification, abundant cytoplasm is seen in the neoplastic cells, consistent with plasmacytoid differentiation. *(Right)* Anaplastic plasmacytoma presenting as a right shoulder mass in a patient with a history of plasma cell myeloma. The nuclei are eccentrically located in abundant cytoplasm, consistent with plasmacytoid differentiation.

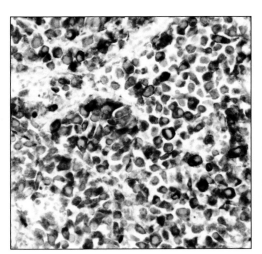 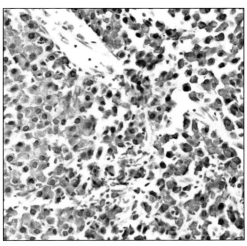

(Left) Anaplastic plasmacytoma presenting as a right shoulder mass in a patient with a history of plasma cell myeloma. The neoplastic cells are strongly CD138(+). *(Right)* Anaplastic plasmacytoma presenting as a right shoulder mass in a patient with a history of plasma cell myeloma. The neoplastic cells express cytoplasmic monotypic Ig λ light chain.

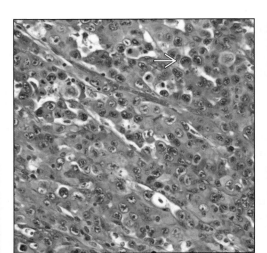 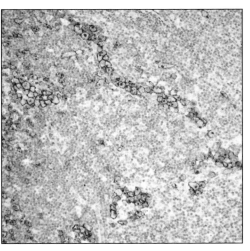

(Left) Lymph node involved by ALK(+) anaplastic large cell lymphoma (ALCL) demonstrates architectural effacement by sheets of large pleomorphic cells with vesicular nuclei, prominent nucleoli, and abundant basophilic cytoplasm. Numerous cells with horseshoe-shaped nuclei ➡ consistent with hallmark cells are identified. *(Right)* Lymph node involved by ALK(+) ALCL demonstrates large pleomorphic, strongly CD30(+) lymphoid cells infiltrating lymph node sinuses.

EBV+ DIFFUSE LARGE B-CELL LYMPHOMA OF THE ELDERLY

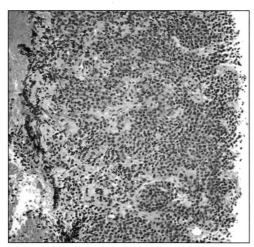

EBV(+) diffuse large B-cell lymphoma of the elderly (EBV[+] DLBCL-E) involving needle biopsy of thigh mass. This neoplasm is the monomorphous subtype and is composed of sheets of lymphoma cells.

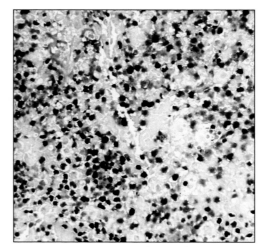

EBV(+) DLBCL-E, monomorphous subtype involving needle biopsy of thigh mass. In situ hybridization analysis shows that the lymphoma cells are strongly positive for EBV small encoded RNA (EBER).

TERMINOLOGY

Abbreviations
- Epstein-Barr virus(EBV) diffuse large B-cell lymphoma of the elderly (DLBCL-E)

Synonyms
- Senile EBV(+) B-cell lymphoproliferative disorder
- Age-related EBV(+) lymphoproliferative disorder
- EBV-associated B-cell lymphoproliferative disorder of the elderly

Definitions
- DLBCL infected by EBV occurring in patients > 50 years old without history of immunodeficiency or lymphoma
- These tumors exhibit a broad morphologic spectrum from polymorphous and Hodgkin-like lesions to monotonous DLBCL

ETIOLOGY/PATHOGENESIS

Epstein-Barr Virus (EBV) Drives B-cell Transformation and Lymphoproliferation
- EBV: γ-herpes virus ubiquitous in humans
- > 90% of humans are infected
  - Most have lifelong asymptomatic infection
- EBV can infect B, T, and NK cells as well as epithelial cells
- Increased risk for EBV-associated lymphomas in patients with
  - Congenital immunodeficiency
  - Acquired immunodeficiency
    - Human immunodeficiency virus infection
    - Iatrogenic causes
  - Elderly adults in apparent good health recently identified as at-risk group
    - Impaired immunity associated with aging is implicated
    - In particular, impaired host T-cell surveillance
- When EBV infects B cells, the virus will
  - Upregulate and activate multiple cell signaling pathways and antiapoptotic proteins
  - Induce B-cell proliferation and transformation
- In EBV(+) DLBCL-E, virus shows type III EBV latency pattern
  - All EBV nuclear antigens (EBNAs), EBER, and latent membrane proteins (LMPs) are expressed

CLINICAL ISSUES

Epidemiology
- Incidence
  - In Asian countries, EBV(+) DLBCL-E represents up to 10% of all DLBCL cases in patients without apparent immunodeficiency
  - Apparently less common in Western nations; little data available
- Age
  - Median: ~ 70 years (range: 45–92 years)
  - ~ 25% of patients ≥ 90 years
- Gender
  - M:F = 1.4:1

Site
- Extranodal sites involved in 70% of patients
  - Skin, lung, tonsil, and stomach most common
  - Bone marrow or blood involved in ~ 10% of patients
- Lymph nodes

Presentation
- Affected patients are relatively healthy prior to diagnosis
- Extranodal mass ± lymphadenopathy in ~ 70% of patients
  - Only lymphadenopathy in ~ 30% of patients

EBV+ DIFFUSE LARGE B-CELL LYMPHOMA OF THE ELDERLY

Key Facts

Terminology
- DLBCL infected by EBV occurring in patients > 50 years old without history of immunodeficiency or lymphoma

Clinical Issues
- Median age: ~ 70 years (range: 45–92 years)
- Affected patients are relatively healthy prior to diagnosis
- Extranodal mass ± lymphadenopathy in ~ 70%
  - Only lymphadenopathy in ~ 30%
- Median survival is 2 years

Microscopic Pathology
- EBV(+) DLBCL-E effaces architecture of extranodal site &/or lymph node

- 2 subtypes: Polymorphous and large cell lymphoma (monomorphous)
  - Represent a morphologic spectrum
  - No clinical or prognostic relevance
- Sheets of necrosis; often with geographic pattern

Ancillary Tests
- CD20(+), CD22(+), CD79α(+), pax-5(+)
- IRF-4/MUM1(+), CD30(+/-)
- Ki-67 (MIB1) shows high proliferation index
- Lymphoma cells have EBV type III latency pattern
- EBV present in monoclonal episomal form

Top Differential Diagnoses
- DLBCL, not otherwise specified
- Plasmablastic lymphoma
- Classical Hodgkin lymphoma

- B symptoms in ~ 60% of patients
- High International Prognostic Index (IPI) score in ~ 60% of patients
- Ann Arbor stage III-IV in ~ 60% of patients

Laboratory Tests
- ~ 50% of patients have elevated lactate dehydrogenase (LDH) level

Treatment
- Drugs
  - Consensus for specific chemotherapy regimen has not been established
  - Cyclophosphamide, adriamycin, vincristine, and prednisone (CHOP) regimen has been used
  - Clinical remission achieved in 63%
    - Response worse than in patients with EBV(-) DLBCL
  - Role of rituximab has not been determined

Prognosis
- Median survival is 2 years
- Presence of B symptoms and age > 70 years indicate worse prognosis

MICROSCOPIC PATHOLOGY

Histologic Features
- EBV(+) DLBCL-E effaces architecture of extranodal site &/or lymph node
- 2 subtypes: Polymorphous and large cell lymphoma (monomorphous)
  - Represent a morphologic spectrum
  - Distinguishing these subtypes histologically can be arbitrary in some cases
  - No clinical or prognostic relevance
- Both types demonstrate
  - Large lymphoma cells and Hodgkin and Reed-Sternberg (HRS)-like cells
  - Increased mitotic activity
  - Sheets of necrosis; often with geographic pattern
- Polymorphous subtype

  - Broad spectrum of B-cell maturation
  - Polymorphous reactive infiltrate in background: Small lymphocytes, plasma cells, and histiocytes
- Monomorphous subtype
  - Sheets of large monomorphous cells resembling DLBCL

Cytologic Features
- Large lymphoma cells can be centroblastic, immunoblastic, or plasmablastic

ANCILLARY TESTS

Immunohistochemistry
- CD20(+), CD22(+), CD79a(+), pax-5(+)
- IRF4/MUM1(+), CD30(+/-)
- ± monotypic cytoplasmic immunoglobulin light chain in cells with plasmacytoid differentiation
- Ki-67 (MIB1) shows high proliferation index
- CD10(-), CD15(-), Bcl-6(-)
- T-cell antigens(-), myeloid-associated antigens(-)
  - Reactive T cells often have memory/effector immunophenotype
    - CD45RO(+), CCR4(+), and FOX3(+)
  - Cytotoxic T cells are TIA-1(+)
- Lymphoma cells have EBV type III latency pattern
  - LMP-1(+) ~ 95%
  - EBNA2(+) ~ 30%
- EBV chemokines (CCL17, CCL22)(+); NF-κB(+)

In Situ Hybridization
- EBER(+)

PCR
- EBV present in monoclonal episomal form
- Monoclonal IgH gene rearrangements
- No evidence of monoclonal T-cell receptor rearrangements

6

73

EBV+ DIFFUSE LARGE B-CELL LYMPHOMA OF THE ELDERLY

DIFFERENTIAL DIAGNOSIS

Diffuse Large B-cell Lymphoma (DLBCL), Not Otherwise Specified

- DLBCL resembles monomorphous subtype of EBV(+) DLBCL-E
- These tumors are rarely EBV(+) at initial diagnosis; EBV can be positive
  - In relapsed DLBCL
  - In DLBCL arising in patients with history of therapy for other tumor types
    - Different types of lymphoma or solid tumors
- DLBCL occurs in younger patients relative to EBV(+) DLBCL-E
- Prognosis of patients with DLBCL is better than patients with EBV(+) DLBCL-E

Plasmablastic Lymphoma (PBL)

- PBL can resemble monomorphous subtype of EBV(+) DLBCL-E
- PBL is strongly associated with HIV infection
- Diffuse pattern; spectrum with immunoblastic and plasmablastic cells
- Immunophenotype
  - MUM1(+), CD38(+), CD138(+), VS38/p63(+)
  - EMA(+/-); CD30(+) in subset
  - CD79a(+/-, often dim), CD20(-), CD22(-), pax-5(-)
  - Monotypic cytoplasmic light chain positive in 50%-70% of cases
- EBER usually positive

Classical Hodgkin Lymphoma (CHL)

- CHL, particularly mixed cellularity type, can resemble polymorphous subtype of EBV(+) DLBCL-E
- Features that support CHL over EBV(+) DLBCL-E
  - Background inflammatory cells include many granulocytes
  - Geographic necrosis is less common in CHL
  - HRS cells have typical cytologic and immunophenotypic features
    - CD15(+), CD20(-), CD45/LCA(-)
  - EBV(+) in HRS cells of CHL exhibit type II latency pattern
    - EBER(+), EBNA-1(+), LMP-1(+), and LMP-2A(+)
  - Relatively few T cells in background of CHL are cytotoxic
    - Unlike EBV(+) DLBCL-E in which > 30% of T cells are often cytotoxic

B-cell Post-transplant Lymphoproliferative Disorder (PTLD)

- Lymphoproliferative disorder due to immunosuppression arising in recipients of organ allografts
- Lymphoma cells express EBV in most PTLD with type III latency pattern
- Polymorphous PTLD
  - Clinically and morphologically can resemble EBV(+) DLBCL-E, polymorphous type
    - Extranodal sites or lymph nodes involved; necrosis common
    - Infiltrate of plasma cells, small lymphocytes, large lymphoid cells, ± HRS-like cells
- Monomorphous PTLD
  - Sheets of atypical large B cells effacing architecture
  - Centroblastic or immunoblastic morphology is most common, ± HRS-like cells
  - Plasmacytoid or plasmacytic differentiation may be present

Methotrexate-associated B-cell Lymphoproliferative Disorder (LPD)

- B-cell LPDs associated with methotrexate therapy can resemble monomorphous or polymorphous subtype of EBV(+) DLBCL-E
  - Extranodal sites or lymph nodes involved; necrosis common
  - Infiltrate plasma cells, small lymphocytes, large lymphoid cells, and ± HRS-like cells

Burkitt Lymphoma

- "Starry sky" pattern, monomorphous medium-sized lymphoma cells, many mitoses and apoptotic cells
- Pan-B-cell antigens(+), CD10(+), Bcl-6(+); Ki-67 high
- *MYC* translocations are characteristic
  - Partners: IgH at 14q32, Igκ at 2p11, and Igλ at 22q11
- Endemic
  - Africa or other endemic regions; children; EBV(+) > 95%
- Sporadic type
  - Worldwide; adolescents and young adults mostly affected; EBV(+) ~ 30%
- Immunodeficiency associated
  - Generally seen in setting of HIV infection; EBV(+) ~ 25-40%

Angioimmunoblastic T-cell Lymphoma (AITL)

- Lymph node architecture effaced by polymorphous infiltrate composed of
  - Lymphoma cells: Small to medium-sized; ± clear to pale cytoplasm and distinct cell borders
  - Admixed small reactive lymphocytes, eosinophils, plasma cells, and histiocytes
- Marked proliferation of arborizing high endothelial venules (HEV)
- Prominent follicular dendritic cell (FDC) meshwork surrounds HEV
- Immunophenotype
  - CD3(+), CD4(+), CD5(+), CD8(-)
  - ± aberrant loss or decrease of CD7 expression
  - T cells have T-follicular helper cell immunophenotype
    - CD10 (+/-), BCL6, CXCL13, &/or PD-1 in ~ 60%-100% of cases
- FDC are CD21(+), CD23(+), CD35(+), EGFR(+/-)
- B-immunoblasts admixed within neoplasm, often numerous
  - Express pan-B-cell markers; often EBV(+)
  - May progress to DLBCL

Infectious Mononucleosis

- Clinical course is usually acute

EBV+ DIFFUSE LARGE B-CELL LYMPHOMA OF THE ELDERLY

EBV-associated B-cell Lymphoproliferative Disorders

Disorder Name

Burkitt lymphoma

Classical Hodgkin lymphoma

Post-transplant lymphoproliferative disorders

Lymphomas associated with HIV infection

Primary diffuse large B-cell lymphoma of the central nervous system

EBV(+) diffuse large B-cell lymphoma of the elderly

HHV8(+) primary effusion lymphoma and its solid variant

Plasmablastic lymphoma

EBV-associated T-/NK-cell Lymphoproliferative Disorders

Disorder Name

Peripheral T-cell lymphoma, not otherwise specified

Angioimmunoblastic T-cell lymphoma

Extranodal T-/NK-cell lymphoma, nasal type

EBV = Epstein–Barr virus; NK = natural killer.

Latent EBV-encoded Genes

EBV-encoded Genes	Location
EBNA-1	Nucleus
EBNA-2	Nucleus
EBNA-3	Nucleus
LMP-1	Membrane
LMP-2	Membrane
EBER-1 and EBER-2	Nucleus

EBV = Epstein–Barr virus; EBNA = Epstein–Barr nuclear antigen; LMP = latent membrane protein; EBER = Epstein–Barr encoded small RNA.

- Lymphadenopathy and splenomegaly; other extranodal sites are uncommonly involved
- Serology studies show acute rise in EBV antibody titers
- Histologically, lymph node architecture is not usually effaced

Chronic Active Epstein-Barr Virus (CAEBV) Infection

- Occurs in minority of EBV-infected subjects
- Pathogenesis unclear; impaired T-cell response implicated
- Onset with acute EBV infection; markedly elevated
  o IgG titers against EBV; EBV DNA(+) in blood
- Histologic evidence of organ infiltration with virus-infected cells
- Clonal, oligoclonal, or polyclonal disease
- Fever, liver dysfunction, and splenomegaly in most patients
- Lymphadenopathy, thrombocytopenia, and anemia in ~ 50% of patients
- Rash, hypersensitivity to mosquito bites, hemophagocytic syndrome in 20–40% of patients
- May progress to overt lymphoma
- EBV(+) cells have
  o B-phenotype in cases identified in USA and Europe
  o T-/NK-phenotype in Japan

DIAGNOSTIC CHECKLIST

Clinically Relevant Pathologic Features

- EBV(+) DLBCL-E can only be diagnosed in patients without history of
  o Immunodeficiency or lymphoma
- Must exclude other well-defined EBV(+) lymphoproliferative diseases

Pathologic Interpretation Pearls

- In past, EBV(+) DLBCL-E was divided into 2 histological subtypes
  o Polymorphous and monomorphous
  o These subtypes represent continuum of disease without differences in
    ▪ Pathogenesis
    ▪ Clinical presentation or prognosis

SELECTED REFERENCES

1. Asano N et al: Age-related Epstein-Barr virus (EBV)-associated B-cell lymphoproliferative disorders: comparison with EBV-positive classic Hodgkin lymphoma in elderly patients. Blood. 113(12):2629-36, 2009

EBV+ DIFFUSE LARGE B-CELL LYMPHOMA OF THE ELDERLY

Microscopic and Immunohistochemical Features

(Left) EBV(+) diffuse large B-cell lymphoma of the elderly, monomorphous subtype shows sheets of centroblasts that are intermediate to large, have finely dispersed chromatin, and 2-3 small nucleoli ➡ *often closely apposed to the nuclear membrane. (Right) EBV(+) DLBCL-E, monomorphous subtype. The neoplastic cells are strongly CD20(+), supporting B-cell lineage.*

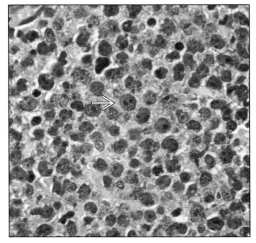
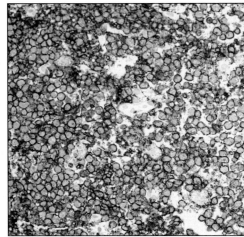

(Left) EBV(+) diffuse large B-cell lymphoma of the elderly, monomorphous subtype. The neoplastic cells express CD10. The cells were also Bcl-6(+) and Bcl-2(-) (not shown). (Right) EBV(+) DLBCL-E, monomorphous subtype. Immunohistochemical analysis for Ki-67 (MIB1) showed a high proliferation index of approximately 90-100%.

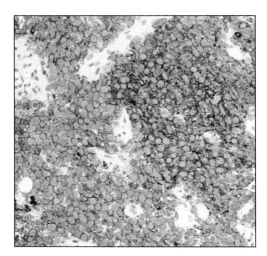
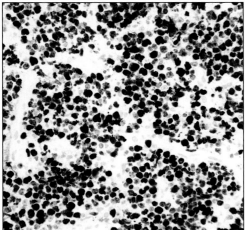

(Left) EBV(+) diffuse large B-cell lymphoma of the elderly, polymorphous subtype involving retroperitoneal lymph node. The lymph node architecture is effaced by scattered large atypical lymphoid cells and numerous intermixed reactive histiocytes, small granulomas ➡*, and giant cells* ➡*. (Right) EBV(+) DLBCL-E, polymorphous subtype. Foci of coagulative necrosis* ➡ *are surrounded by scattered centroblasts* ➡ *and intermixed histiocytes.*

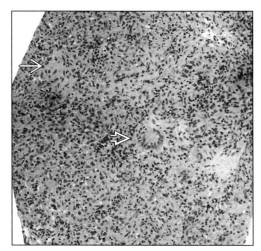
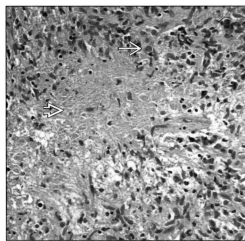

EBV+ DIFFUSE LARGE B-CELL LYMPHOMA OF THE ELDERLY

Differential Diagnosis

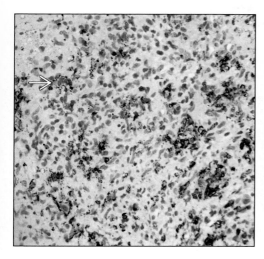

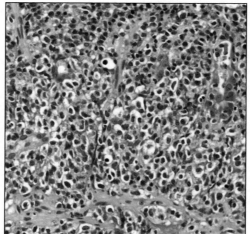

(Left) EBV(+) diffuse B-cell lymphoma of the elderly, polymorphous subtype, involving retroperitoneal lymph node, in which the large lymphoma cells are CD20(+) ➡. The cells also expressed pax-5 (bright), CD30, and CD45/LCA but were CD15(-) (not shown). (Right) Diffuse large B-cell lymphoma, EBV(+), involving the intestine of a patient with a history of T-cell prolymphocytic leukemia (T-PLL) treated with chemotherapy including anti-CD52 antibody (Campath-1H) is shown.

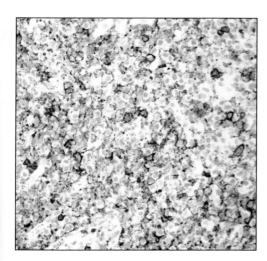

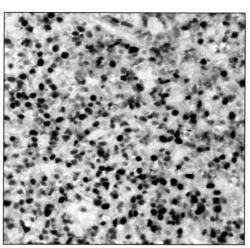

(Left) Diffuse large B-cell lymphoma (DLBCL), EBV(+) involving the intestine of a patient with a history of T-PLL treated with chemotherapy including anti-CD52 antibody (Campath-1H). The neoplastic cells are variably CD20(+). (Right) DLBCL, EBV(+) involving the intestine of a patient with a history of T-PLL treated with chemotherapy including anti-CD52 antibody (Campath-1H). In situ hybridization shows that many neoplastic cells were EBER(+).

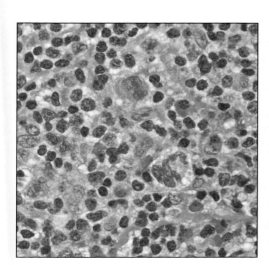

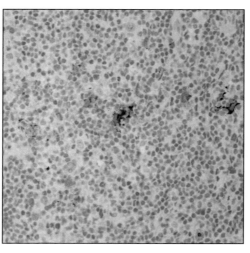

(Left) Classical Hodgkin lymphoma (CHL), mixed cellularity type involving lymph node. The presence of eosinophils in the background, common in CHL, is less common in EBV(+) DLBCL of the elderly, polymorphous type. (Right) CHL, mixed cellularity type involving lymph node. Neoplastic cells are CD15(+). Expression of CD15 by Hodgkin and Reed-Sternberg cells is common in CHL and is unusual in EBV(+) DLBCL of the elderly, polymorphous type.

PLASMABLASTIC LYMPHOMA ARISING IN HHV8+ MULTICENTRIC CASTLEMAN DISEASE

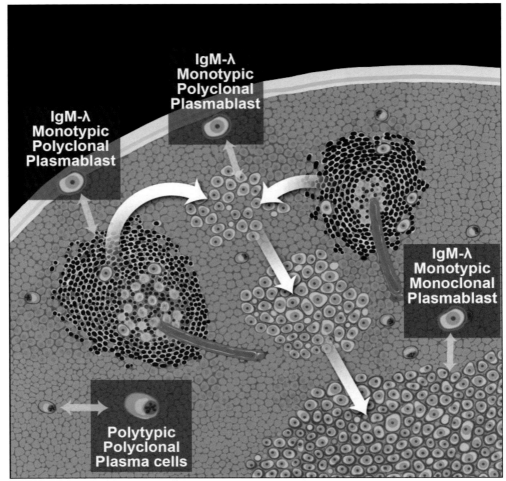

Schematic of the pathogenesis of plasmablastic lymphoma (PBL) arising in human herpes virus 8 (HHV8) (+) multicentric Castleman disease (MCD). HHV8 initially infects polyclonal IgMλ(+) plasmablasts that reside in the mantle zones of lymphoid follicles. These plasmablasts are polyclonal, lack Ig somatic mutations, and correspond to naïve B-cells. Plasmablasts subsequently coalesce into microlymphomas that are IgMλ(+) but polyclonal. Microlymphomas further coalesce and progress to monotypic and monoclonal PBL. HHV8 infection drives this sequence of events, most likely combined with other genetic alterations. Plasma cells in the MCD component are polytypic and IgA or IgG(+).

TERMINOLOGY

Abbreviations
- Plasmablastic lymphoma (PBL) arising in HHV8(+) multicentric Castleman disease (MCD)

Synonyms
- Large B-cell lymphoma arising in HHV8(+) MCD
  - Terminology of World Health Organization Classification, 2008
- HHV8(+) plasmablastic lymphoma
- KSHV(+) plasmablastic lymphoma

Definitions
- PBL-MCD is a monoclonal proliferation of HHV8(+) plasmablasts that express IgMλ and arise in MCD

ETIOLOGY/PATHOGENESIS

Infectious Agents
- Human herpes virus 8 (HHV8) is involved in pathogenesis
  - a.k.a. Kaposi sarcoma herpes virus (KSHV)
- HHV8 initially infects singly scattered plasmablasts in mantle zones of follicles
  - These plasmablasts are naive B cells that express IgM
    - Plasmablasts express λ light chain but are polyclonal at molecular level
    - Plasmablasts lack evidence of immunoglobulin (Ig) somatic hypermutation
  - HHV8 encodes at least 10 homologues of cellular genes
    - Inhibit cell apoptosis, promote cell proliferation, and drive infected B cells to differentiate into plasmablasts
    - HHV8 encodes for viral homologue of IL-6, which is thought to induce many features of MCD

PLASMABLASTIC LYMPHOMA ARISING IN HHV8+ MULTICENTRIC CASTLEMAN DISEASE

Key Facts

Terminology
- PBL-MCD is a monoclonal proliferation of HHV8(+) plasmablasts that express IgMλ and arise in MCD

Etiology/Pathogenesis
- HHV8 initially infects singly scattered plasmablasts in mantle zones of follicles
- HHV8(+) plasmablasts expand to form so-called microlymphomas
- HHV8(+) "microlymphomas" expand into histologically overt lymphoma
- Most patients with PBL-MCD have profound immunosuppression

Clinical Issues
- Lymph nodes, spleen
- Leukemic involvement as part of a terminal phase

- Poor; survival often < 1 year

Microscopic Pathology
- Plasmablastic lymphoma
  ○ Sheets of plasmablasts (or immunoblasts)
  ○ Mitotic figures common

Ancillary Tests
- HHV8(+), IgM(+), λ(+)
- CD45/LCA(+/-), CD20(-/+), CD79a(-), EBV(-)
- Single-cell PCR studies show monoclonal IgH rearrangements in PBL

Top Differential Diagnoses
- Primary effusion lymphoma (PEL)
- Extracavitary PEL
- HHV8(+) germinotropic lymphoproliferative disorder

- HHV8(+) plasmablasts expand to form so-called microlymphomas
  ○ Polyclonal or monoclonal associated with HHV8(-) polyclonal cells
- HHV8(+) "microlymphomas" expand into histologically overt lymphoma
  ○ Cells in overt lymphoma are monoclonal
  ○ Analysis of HHV8 episomes shows virus is monoclonal
    ▪ Indicates HHV8 is present prior to clonal expansion

Immunosuppression
- Most patients with PBL-MCD have profound immunosuppression
  ○ HIV infection is very common
- Patients with MCD and HIV have 15x increased risk of non-Hodgkin lymphoma

CLINICAL ISSUES

Epidemiology
- Incidence
  ○ Rare
- Age
  ○ Depends in part on presence or absence of HIV infection
    ▪ HIV(+): Age mirrors that of HIV(+) patients in general
    ▪ HIV(-): Older patients
- Ethnicity
  ○ In HIV(-) patients, PBL-MCD is more common in regions endemic for HHV8 infection
    ▪ Mediterranean basin, Africa

Site
- Lymph nodes, spleen
- Leukemic involvement as part of a terminal phase
- Extranodal sites not (or rarely) involved

Presentation
- Evidence of profound immunosuppression

- Lymphadenopathy; ± splenomegaly
- ± Kaposi sarcoma

Treatment
- No consensus
- Therapeutic choices often limited by marked immunosuppression

Prognosis
- Poor; survival often < 1 year

IMAGE FINDINGS

General Features
- Lymphadenopathy and splenomegaly are most common

MICROSCOPIC PATHOLOGY

Histologic Features
- Multicentric Castleman disease is characterized by
  ○ Hyaline-vascular &/or lymphocyte-depleted follicles
  ○ Scattered plasmablasts/immunoblasts in mantle zones of follicles
  ○ Marked interfollicular plasmacytosis without atypia
  ○ Vascular proliferation
- Microlymphomas
  ○ Small clusters of atypical cells arising in mantle zone ± surrounding germinal centers
  ○ Large cells with plasmablastic or (less likely) immunoblastic features
    ▪ Abundant cytoplasm, vesicular nucleus, prominent nucleoli
- Plasmablastic lymphoma
  ○ Large sheets of plasmablasts (or immunoblasts)
  ○ Mitotic figures common

Cytologic Features
- Very few cases of PBL-MCD assessed by fine needle aspiration are reported

6

PLASMABLASTIC LYMPHOMA ARISING IN HHV8+ MULTICENTRIC CASTLEMAN DISEASE

ANCILLARY TESTS

Immunohistochemistry
- Cytoplasmic (cyt) IgM(+), cyt λ(+), EBV(-)
- CD27(+), CD45/LCA(+/-), CD20(-/+)
- CD30(-/+), CD38(-/+), CD79a(-), CD138(-)
- T-cell antigens(-); rare cases with aberrant T-cell antigen expression
- Human or viral IL-6(+) in subset of plasmablasts in most cases
- Interfollicular plasma cells
  ○ Polytypic Ig light chain expression
  ○ Cyt IgA(+), cyt IgM(-), HHV8(-)

Cytogenetics
- Very little (if any) cytogenetic or CGH data available in literature

In Situ Hybridization
- HHV8(+), EBER(-)

Molecular Genetics
- Single-cell PCR studies show monoclonal *IgH* rearrangements in PBL
- *Ig* variable genes usually lack evidence of somatic hypermutation
  ○ Supports concept that PBL-MCD arises from naive B cell
- Analysis of HHV8 episomes shows virus is monoclonal
  ○ Suggests virus is present prior to monoclonal expansion

DIFFERENTIAL DIAGNOSIS

Primary Effusion Lymphoma (PEL)
- Arises in setting of profound immunosuppression; usually HIV infection
- Can arise in patients with MCD and HIV infection
- PEL involves body cavities without tissue masses
- Immunophenotype
  ○ Usually Ig(-); subset of cases are κ light chain(+)
  ○ CD45/LCA(+), CD138(+), CD30(+/-)
  ○ CD38(+/-), EMA(+/-), IRF-4/MUM1(+/-)
  ○ CD20(-), CD79a(-), Bcl-6(-)
- HHV8(+), EBV(+)
- Monoclonal *IgH* rearrangements
- *Ig* variable genes show high number of somatic hypermutations
  ○ Supports late germinal center or post-germinal center B-cell origin

Extracavitary PEL
- Arises in setting of profound immunosuppression; usually HIV infection
- Can arise in patients with MCD and HIV infection
- These tumors form tissue-based masses
  ○ Usually involve lymph nodes or extranodal sites
- Immunophenotype and molecular findings similar to PEL
- HHV8(+), EBV(-/+)

HHV8(+) Germinotropic Lymphoproliferative Disorder
- Occurs in HIV(-) patients; no evidence of MCD
- Patients present with localized lymphadenopathy
- Patients often respond well to chemotherapy
- HHV8(+) plasmablasts infiltrate germinal centers
- Immunophenotype
  ○ κ or λ light chain restriction; EBV(+)
  ○ CD10(-), CD20(-), CD27(-)
  ○ CD79a(-), CD138(-), Bcl-6(-)
- *Ig* genes show polyclonal or oligoclonal pattern of rearrangement

Plasmablastic Lymphoma Not Associated with MCD
- Commonly occurs in setting of profound immunosuppression
- Extranodal sites of disease are common
- Immunophenotype
  ○ CD138(+), CD38(+), CD79a(+/-)
  ○ CD20(-), pax-5(-)
  ○ T-cell antigens usually negative, but CD3 can be aberrantly expressed
- EBER(+) in most cases; HHV8(-)

Diffuse Large B-cell Lymphoma
- Most cases arise in patients without evidence of immunosuppression
- Neoplastic cells resemble centroblasts or immunoblasts
- Immunophenotype
  ○ κ or λ light chain(+)
  ○ CD20(+), CD22(+), CD79a(+), pax-5(+)
- HHV8(-); EBV infection uncommon (< 10%)

Plasmacytoma
- Uncommonly associated with HIV infection
- Patients can present with lymphadenopathy or extranodal mass
- Sheets of monotonous plasma cells ± atypia that replace architecture
- Immunophenotype
  ○ κ or λ light chain (+)
  ○ CD138(+), CD38(+), CD79a(+/-)
  ○ CD20(-), pax-5(-)

SELECTED REFERENCES
1. Carbone A et al: HIV-associated lymphomas and gamma-herpesviruses. Blood. 113(6):1213-24, 2009
2. Oksenhendler E et al: High incidence of Kaposi sarcoma-associated herpesvirus-related non-Hodgkin lymphoma in patients with HIV infection and multicentric Castleman disease. Blood. 99(7):2331-6, 2002
3. Dupin N et al: HHV-8 is associated with a plasmablastic variant of Castleman disease that is linked to HHV-8-positive plasmablastic lymphoma. Blood. 95(4):1406-12, 2000

PLASMABLASTIC LYMPHOMA ARISING IN HHV8+ MULTICENTRIC CASTLEMAN DISEASE

Microscopic and Immunohistochemical Features

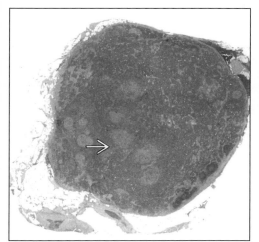

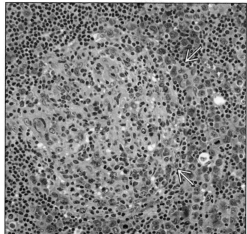

(Left) Plasmablastic lymphoma (PBL) arising in HHV8(+) multicentric Castleman disease (MCD). Paler nodules of PBL ➡ are present in a purple-pink background of MCD. *(Right)* PBL arising in HHV8(+) MCD. Large plasmablasts ➡ are seen surrounding and encroaching into a reactive germinal center.

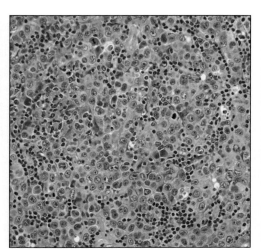

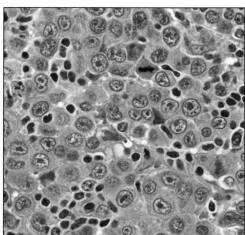

(Left) PBL arising in HHV8(+) MCD. PBL is composed of large cells with abundant cytoplasm. *(Right)* PBL arising in HHV8(+) MCD. Plasmablasts have prominent central nucleoli and abundant eosinophilic cytoplasm. This patient was HIV(-).

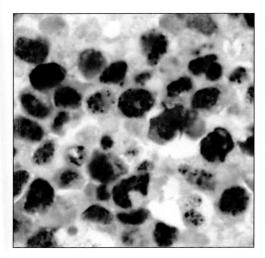

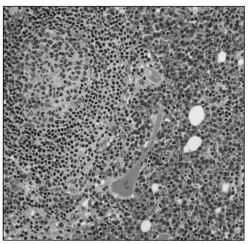

(Left) PBL arising in HHV8(+) MCD. The plasmablasts are HHV8(+). *(Right)* PBL arising in HHV8(+) MCD. This field shows the background of MCD with sheets of mature plasma cells surrounding a reactive follicle with a lymphocyte-depleted germinal center. The PBL is not shown.

BURKITT LYMPHOMA

Microscopic and Immunohistochemical Features

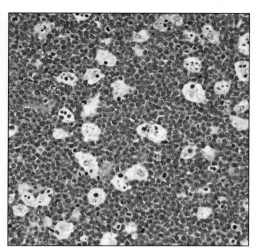

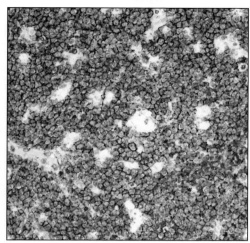

(Left) *Burkitt lymphoma. At high-power magnification, the lymphoma cells are of intermediate size, similar to the size of benign histiocyte nuclei. The lymphoma cells have round nuclear contours, multiple nucleoli, and basophilic cytoplasm. Macrophages with engulfed pyknotic nuclei are also present.* *(Right)* *Burkitt lymphoma. The neoplastic cells are strongly CD20(+). This neoplasm was also positive for CD19, CD38, CD43, and Bcl-6 (not shown).*

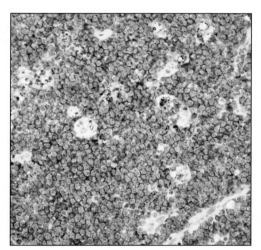

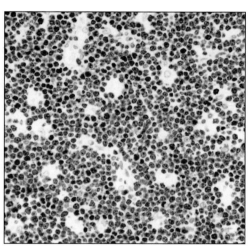

(Left) *Burkitt lymphoma. The neoplastic cells are strongly CD10(+).* *(Right)* *Burkitt lymphoma. MIB-1 (Ki-67) antibody shows that virtually all of the lymphoma cells are strongly positive and are therefore proliferating. Typically, Burkitt lymphoma cases have a very high proliferation rate (Ki-67 index > 95%).*

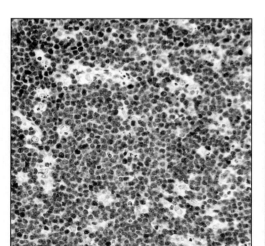

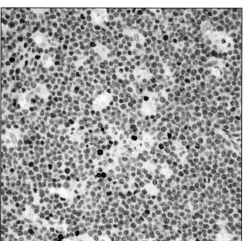

(Left) *Burkitt lymphoma. The lymphoma cells are strongly positive for T-cell leukemia 1 (TCL1). Burkitt lymphoma is the only germinal center-derived tumor with uniformly high TCL-1 expression.* *(Right)* *Burkitt lymphoma. The lymphoma cells are Bcl-2(-). Burkitt lymphoma is usually Bcl-2(-) although a subset of cases (~ 20%) may be weakly positive. Cases of Burkitt lymphoma are also usually positive for CD10 and Bcl-6 (not shown).*

BURKITT LYMPHOMA

Microscopic and Immunohistochemical Features

(Left) Touch imprint of a lymph node involved by Burkitt lymphoma. The lymphoma cells show round nuclei, stippled chromatin, 2-5 nucleoli, and a well-defined narrow rim of basophilic cytoplasm. *(Right)* Burkitt lymphoma in a blood smear. The cytologic features of a Burkitt lymphoma cell in blood are somewhat similar to those of lymphoblasts and were designated as the L3 type of acute lymphoblastic leukemia in the French-American-British classification.

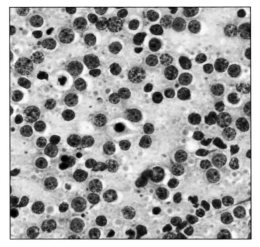
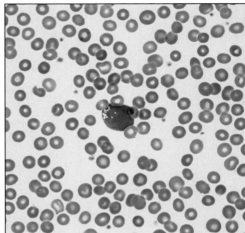

(Left) Burkitt lymphoma in touch imprint of bone marrow biopsy specimen. The lymphoma cells are intermediate-sized and possess a basophilic cytoplasm containing numerous vacuoles. *(Right)* Burkitt lymphoma involving bone marrow biopsy specimen. The Burkitt lymphoma cells have round to oval uniform nuclei. Note the nuclei with 2 or more nucleoli and cell cytoplasm that tends to "square off" with that of other cells.

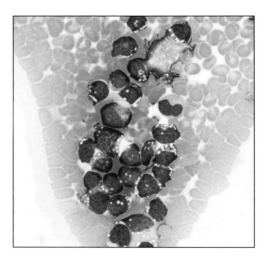
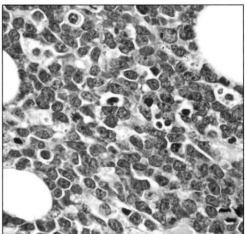

(Left) Burkitt lymphoma involving a bone marrow aspirate smear. The cytoplasmic vacuoles in Burkitt lymphoma cells are positive for lipid as shown in this oil red O stain. The lipid in this field appears as red droplets ➡. *(Right)* Bone marrow aspirate smear involved by Burkitt lymphoma. Note that the lymphoma cells in this case are slightly larger and more variable. This patient had relapsed disease, and the cytological features may be altered by exposure to chemotherapy.

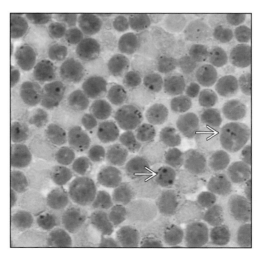
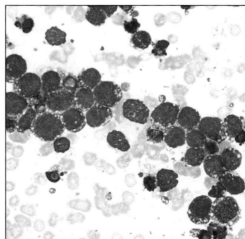

Microscopic and Diagrammatic Features

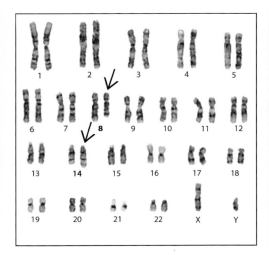

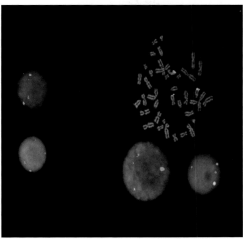

(Left) Conventional cytogenetic analysis reveals a karyotype showing the t(8;14)(q24;q32) ⮕. (Courtesy L. Abruzzo, MD.) *(Right)* Fluorescence in situ hybridization (FISH) using a MYC break-apart probe shows 1 allele with colocalization of red and green signals (normal) and 1 allele with segregation of both probes (rearranged allele). (Courtesy L. Abruzzo, MD.)

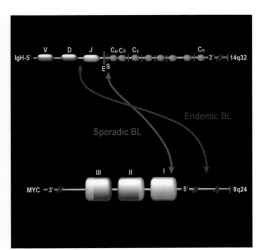

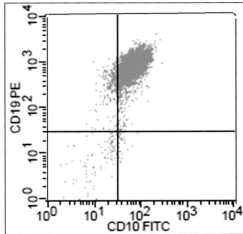

(Left) t(8;14)(q24;q32) in BL. MYC exons are rectangles with roman numerals. MYC coding regions are solid rectangles. V) variable; D) diversity; J) joining; E) enhancer; S) switch; C) constant regions of IgH gene; ALL) acute lymphoblastic leukemia; e) endemic; s) sporadic; AIDS-ML) AIDS-related lymphoma; +++) most cases; +) minority of cases. *(Right)* Flow cytometric immunophenotyping results in a case of BL. The lymphoma cells express CD19 and CD10.

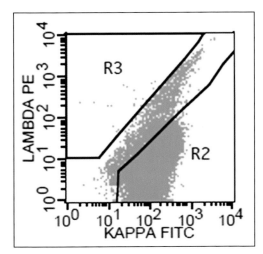

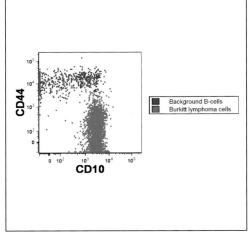

(Left) Flow cytometric immunophenotyping results in a case of Burkitt lymphoma. The Burkitt lymphoma cells demonstrate surface immunoglobulin κ light-chain restriction. *(Right)* Flow cytometric immunophenotyping results in a case of Burkitt lymphoma. Expression of CD44 is negative in Burkitt lymphoma. Expression levels of CD44 and CD54 are decreased in Burkitt lymphoma compared with CD10(+) diffuse large B-cell lymphoma. (Courtesy J. Jorgensen, MD.)

Extranodal B-cell Lymphomas

EXTRANODAL MARGINAL ZONE B-CELL LYMPHOMA (MALT LYMPHOMA)

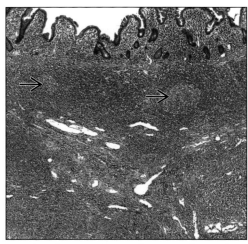

MALT lymphoma involving small intestine. The neoplastic infiltrate is diffuse. A few residual germinal centers ⮕ are present. The villi are blunted.

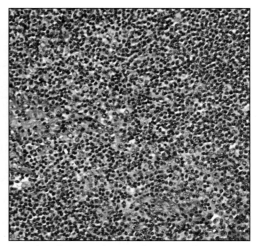

MALT lymphoma involving small intestine. The neoplastic cells are predominantly small, and many cells have pale, monocytoid cytoplasm.

TERMINOLOGY

Abbreviations
- Extranodal marginal zone B-cell lymphoma of mucosa-associated lymphoid tissue (MALT lymphoma)

Synonyms
- Low-grade B-cell lymphoma of MALT
- MALToma

Definitions
- Low-grade B-cell lymphoma arising at extranodal sites, presumably in marginal zone of reactive follicles

ETIOLOGY/PATHOGENESIS

Infectious Agents
- Implicated in pathogenesis of MALT lymphomas
  - *Helicobacter pylori*
    - Gastric marginal zone lymphoma
  - *Campylobacter jejuni*
    - Immunoproliferative small intestinal disease; also known as α heavy chain disease
  - *Chlamydia psittaci*
    - Ocular adnexal marginal zone lymphoma
  - *Borrelia burgdorferi*
    - Cutaneous marginal zone lymphoma
    - More common in Europe

Autoimmune Disorders
- 2 autoimmune diseases have been implicated in pathogenesis of MALT lymphomas
  - Sjögren syndrome
    - MALT lymphomas of parotid gland and lung
  - Hashimoto thyroiditis
    - Thyroid MALT lymphoma

Chromosomal Translocations
- Identified in 30-40% of MALT lymphomas

- Result in NF-κB pathway activation resulting in enhanced cell survival and proliferation and impaired apoptosis

MALT Lymphomas Without Chromosomal Translocations
- Possible role for antigen drive
  - Chronic antigen stimulation via infection or autoimmune disease
    - Leads to accumulation of extranodal lymphoid tissue
    - Polyclonal B-cell population evolves to oligoclonal and then monoclonal B-cell population
- No central role for NF-κB activation

CLINICAL ISSUES

Epidemiology
- Incidence
  - 7-8% of all B-cell non-Hodgkin lymphomas
- Age
  - Median: 61 years
- Gender
  - Female predominance

Presentation
- Subset of patients are asymptomatic
- Symptoms are related to organ involved
  - Stomach: Anemia, weight loss, and pain are common
  - Lung: ± cough and dyspnea
  - Mass and related symptoms in other locations

Treatment
- Stomach MALT lymphoma: Antibiotics to eradicate *H. pylori*
  - Chemotherapy ± radiation if transformed to large B-cell lymphoma or disseminated
- Ocular adnexa

EXTRANODAL MARGINAL ZONE B-CELL LYMPHOMA (MALT LYMPHOMA)

Key Facts

Etiology/Pathogenesis

- Infectious agents are implicated in pathogenesis of MALT lymphomas at specific sites
  - *Helicobacter pylori*: Stomach
  - *Campylobacter jejuni*: Intestine
  - *Chlamydia psittaci*: Ocular adnexa
  - *Borrelia burgdorferi*: Skin
- Autoimmune diseases are implicated in pathogenesis of MALT lymphomas at specific sites
  - Sjögren syndrome: Salivary glands and lung
  - Hashimoto thyroiditis: Thyroid gland

Microscopic Pathology

- MALT lymphomas share common features
  - Marginal zone pattern surrounding reactive follicles
  - Heterogeneous cell population
  - ± lymphoepithelial lesions

Ancillary Tests

- CD20(+), CD22(+), CD79a(+), pax-5(+)
- Monotypic Ig(+), Bcl-2(+), CD43(+/-), Ki-67 low
- Recurrent translocations identified in 30-40% of MALT lymphomas
- 4 common translocations
  - *IAP2-MALT1*/t(11;18)(q21;q21)
  - *IgH-MALT1*/t(14;18)(q32;q21)
  - *FOXP1-IgH*/t(3;14)(p14.1;q32)
  - *BCL10-IgH*/t(1;14)(p22;q32)

Top Differential Diagnoses

- Reactive hyperplasia
- Mantle cell lymphoma
- Follicular lymphoma
- Plasmacytoma

- MALT lymphoma often stage IE and is treated by radiation alone
- Other sites
  - Chemotherapy &/or radiation therapy depending on
    - Site, size, and stage

Prognosis

- Stomach MALT lymphoma
  - Lymphoma can regress after eradication of *H. pylori* by antibiotics; true in ~ 75% of cases
  - t(11;18)(q21;q21) is associated with resistance to antibiotics
  - < 10% of cases transform to diffuse large B-cell lymphoma
  - 5-year overall survival is ~ 90%
  - 25-35% relapse rate in stomach or other extranodal sites
- Other sites of MALT lymphoma
  - Disseminated disease is more common
  - Higher relapse rate

IMAGE FINDINGS

Radiographic Findings

- Single or multiple masses
- Lung(s) involved by MALT lymphoma ± consolidation

Endoscopic Findings

- Gastric or intestinal MALT lymphoma: ± mass, ulcer, or bleeding

MICROSCOPIC PATHOLOGY

Histologic Features

- Diffuse or nodular pattern of growth
- Expansion of marginal zone by cytologically heterogeneous cell population
  - Predominantly centrocyte-like cells with small irregular nuclei

- Monocytoid appearance with distinct rim of clear cytoplasm
- Scattered large cells (centroblasts or immunoblasts) are present; up to 10% of all cells
- ± plasmacytoid differentiation; ± Dutcher bodies
- Hyperplastic lymphoid follicles are common
  - ± colonized by lymphoma imparting nodular pattern
- Lymphoepithelial lesions are common in epithelial tissues involved by MALT lymphoma
  - Infiltration and distortion of epithelial structures by 3 or more neoplastic lymphoid cells
  - Epithelial degeneration and glandular structure destruction
  - Most prominent in thyroid and parotid glands
- Transformation to diffuse large B-cell lymphoma
  - Large cells form sheets or large clusters of > 20 cells
  - May coexist with MALT lymphoma at initial presentation
- Multifocal disease
  - ~ 25% of patients have > 1 extranodal site of involvement

Cytologic Features

- FNA smears show polymorphous cell population
  - Small round or irregular lymphocytes, variable numbers of large cells &/or plasma cells

Lymph Nodes

- Involvement is indistinguishable from nodal marginal zone B-cell lymphoma
  - Usually lymph nodes draining primary site of disease are involved
  - Distant lymph nodes involved in < 10% of patients

Bone Marrow

- 10-20% of patients with MALT lymphoma have bone marrow disease at staging
- Paratrabecular &/or nonparatrabecular aggregates
  - Follicular dendritic cells commonly present in aggregates
- Sinusoidal pattern highly unusual

EXTRANODAL MARGINAL ZONE B-CELL LYMPHOMA (MALT LYMPHOMA)

Skin
- Most common B-cell lymphoma of skin
- Follicular colonization can be prominent; these lesions closely mimic follicular lymphoma

Ocular Adnexal Region
- Includes orbital soft tissue, conjunctiva, and lacrimal gland
- MALT is most common type of lymphoma at this location

Lung
- Lymphoepithelial lesions common in MALT lymphoma and lymphocytic interstitial pneumonitis
- Circumscribed mass supports diagnosis of MALT lymphoma

Salivary Gland
- Arises in background of myoepithelial sialadenitis (MESA)
- Lymphoepithelial lesions (epithelial-myoepithelial islands) common in MALT lymphoma and MESA
- Concentric zones of pale cells around ducts are helpful clue for MALT lymphoma

Thyroid Gland
- Arises in background of Hashimoto thyroiditis
- Lymphoepithelial lesions common in both MALT lymphoma and Hashimoto thyroiditis
- Lymphoma cells within follicles tend to be centrocyte-like cells
- Lymphoma cells outside follicles often are extremely plasmacytic

Breast
- Lymphoepithelial lesions are uncommon at this site
- Can arise in or be disseminated to breast

Other MALT Lymphoma Sites
- Very wide range of body sites can be involved
  - Dura, soft tissues, thymus, gallbladder, kidney, bladder

ANCILLARY TESTS

Immunohistochemistry
- CD19(+), CD20(+), CD22(+), CD79a(+), pax-5(+)
- IgM(+) > IgA(+) > IgG(+)
- Monotypic Ig light chain(+); best seen in plasmacytoid cells
- Bcl-2(+), CD43(+/-), Bcl-10(+/-)
- Ki-67(MIB-1) is low; high in residual reactive germinal centers
- IgD(-) but demonstrates intact follicular IgD(+) mantle zones
- CD21 highlights follicular dendritic cell (FDC) meshworks in follicles
  - Meshworks are disrupted by follicular colonization
- Cytokeratin(-); useful for highlighting lymphoepithelial lesions
- CD10(-), Bcl-6(-), Cyclin-D1(-)
- T-cell antigens(-), EBV-LMP1(-)

Flow Cytometry
- Monotypic surface Ig light chain(+)
- FMC7(+), CD11c(+/-), CD23(-/+), CD25(-), CD103(-)

Cytogenetics
- Recurrent translocations have been identified in 30-40% of MALT lymphomas
  - Generally specific for MALT lymphomas; translocations are mutually exclusive
  - 4 common translocations; additional translocations recently described but not fully characterized
    - Frequency of translocations shows geographic variation; also correlates with site of MALT lymphoma
  - *API2-MALT1*/t(11;18)(q21;q21)
    - Most common in stomach, lung, and intestine
  - *IgH-MALT1*/t(14;18)(q32;q21)
    - Most common in ocular adnexa, skin, salivary glands, and liver
  - *FOXP1-IgH*/t(3;14)(p14.1;q32)
    - Most common in ocular adnexa, thyroid gland, and skin
  - *BCL10-IgH*/t(1;14)(p22;q32)
    - Rare overall frequency; more common in intestine, salivary glands, and lung
  - Recent study has identified 5 or 6 new translocations in MALT lymphomas
    - Currently poorly defined; genes not cloned for subset of translocations
- Trisomies 3 and 18 are frequently present in MALT lymphomas at various sites
  - Nonspecific; can be seen in other types of lymphoma
- Homozygous deletions of chromosome 6p23 in ~ 20% of cases
  - Location of tumor necrosis factor α induced protein 3 (TNFFAIP3; also known as A20)

In Situ Hybridization
- FISH can be used to detect MALT lymphoma-associated translocations
- EBER(-)

PCR
- Monoclonal *IgH* rearrangements
  - Rearrangements can persist for years after therapy and complete clinical remission
- RT-PCR and PCR assays developed to detect translocations

Molecular Genetics
- Inactivating mutations of *TNFFAIP3*/A20
  - ~ 20% of MALT lymphomas
  - Mutations also occur in other types of marginal zone lymphoma

Gene Expression Profiling
- NF-κB pathway activation a shared feature of MALT lymphomas with t(11;18), t(14;18), and t(1;14)
- 2nd distinct subset of MALT lymphomas
  - T-cell or memory B-cell signature reported in one study

EXTRANODAL MARGINAL ZONE B-CELL LYMPHOMA (MALT LYMPHOMA)

Immunohistochemistry

Antibody	Reactivity	Staining Pattern	Comment
CD45	Positive	Cell membrane	
CD20	Positive	Cell membrane	
CD79-α	Positive	Cell membrane	
pax-5	Positive	Nuclear	
CD43	Positive	Cell membrane	
Bcl-2	Positive	Cell membrane	
CD5	Negative		May be occasionally positive
Cyclin-D1	Negative		

- o Plasma cell gene signature identified in another study
- o No NF-κB pathway activation

DIFFERENTIAL DIAGNOSIS

Reactive Inflammatory Diseases
- Florid gastritis or inflammatory lung diseases can show lymphoepithelial lesions
- Do not form expansile destructive mass as observed in MALT lymphoma
- Plasma cells are polytypic; B cells are CD43(+)

Lymphoepithelial/Myoepithelial Sialadenitis (LESA/MESA)
- Occurs as a result of autoimmune process (e.g., Sjögren syndrome) or HIV-related changes
- Nests of ductal epithelial cells extensively infiltrated by small lymphoid cells
- No concentric rings of monocytoid cells around ducts
- No evidence of monotypic B-cell population or monoclonal *Ig* gene rearrangements

Mantle Cell Lymphoma
- Has tropism for gastrointestinal tract; can involve other extranodal sites
- Monotonous neoplastic cells without intermixed large cells or plasma cells
- ± mantle zone pattern; no follicular colonization
- Results of ancillary studies helpful
  - o B-cell antigens(+), CD5(+), Cyclin-D1(+)
  - o *CCND1-IgH*/t(11;14)(q13;q32)

Follicular Lymphoma
- Can arise at extranodal sites and mimic, in part, MALT lymphoma with colonization of follicles
- Results of ancillary studies helpful
  - o B-cell antigens(+), CD10(+), Bcl-6(+)
  - o *IgH-BCL2*/t(14;18)(q32;q21)

Plasmacytoma
- Plasmacytoma at extranodal sites may be closely related to MALT lymphoma
  - o Patients can present with plasmacytoma and relapse as MALT lymphoma
  - o Patients may present with MALT lymphoma and relapse as plasmacytoma
  - o Extranodal plasmacytoma is clinically indolent

- Results of ancillary studies helpful
  - o No component of neoplastic/monotypic B-lymphocytes
  - o Usually IgA(+) or IgG(+)

SELECTED REFERENCES

1. Edinger JT et al: Cutaneous marginal zone lymphomas have distinctive features and include 2 subsets. Am J Surg Pathol. 34(12):1830-41, 2010
2. Hamoudi RA et al: Differential expression of NF-kappaB target genes in MALT lymphoma with and without chromosome translocation: insights into molecular mechanism. Leukemia. 24(8):1487-97, 2010
3. McKelvie PA: Ocular adnexal lymphomas: a review. Adv Anat Pathol. 17(4):251-61, 2010
4. Sagaert X et al: Comparative expressed sequence hybridization studies of t(11;18)(q21;q21)-positive and -negative gastric MALT lymphomas reveal both unique and overlapping gene programs. Mod Pathol. 23(3):458-69, 2010
5. Chng WJ et al: Gene expression profiling of pulmonary mucosa-associated lymphoid tissue lymphoma identifies new biologic insights with potential diagnostic and therapeutic applications. Blood. 113(3):635-45, 2009
6. Kaba S et al: Cytologic findings of primary thyroid MALT lymphoma with extreme plasma cell differentiation: FNA cytology of two cases. Diagn Cytopathol. 37(11):815-9, 2009
7. Novak U et al: The NF-{kappa}B negative regulator TNFAIP3 (A20) is inactivated by somatic mutations and genomic deletions in marginal zone lymphomas. Blood. 113(20):4918-21, 2009
8. Vinatzer U et al: Mucosa-associated lymphoid tissue lymphoma: novel translocations including rearrangements of ODZ2, JMJD2C, and CNN3. Clin Cancer Res. 14(20):6426-31, 2008
9. Bacon CM et al: Mucosa-associated lymphoid tissue (MALT) lymphoma: a practical guide for pathologists. J Clin Pathol. 60(4):361-72, 2007
10. Talwalkar SS et al: MALT1 gene rearrangements and NF-kappaB activation involving p65 and p50 are absent or rare in primary MALT lymphomas of the breast. Mod Pathol. 19(11):1402-8, 2006

Microscopic and Immunohistochemical Features

(Left) MALT lymphoma involving stomach. Note the mucosal ulceration. (Right) MALT lymphoma involving stomach. A lymphoepithelial lesion ➡ is shown characterized by atypical lymphocytes infiltrating the glandular structure.

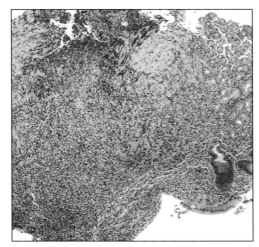
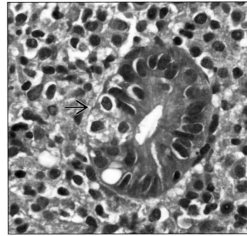

(Left) MALT lymphoma involving stomach. Giemsa stain shows numerous H. pylori-like organisms in the lumen ➡. (Right) MALT lymphoma involving stomach. The neoplastic cells in this case are CD20(+).

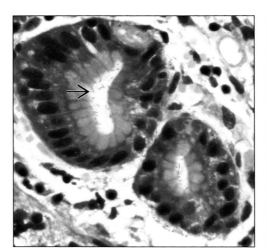
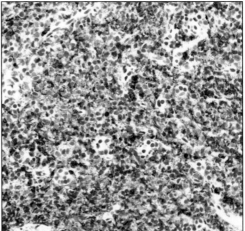

(Left) MALT lymphoma involving kidney. The infiltrate is diffuse and predominantly involves the interstitium. (Right) MALT lymphoma involving kidney. The infiltrating cells are small mature lymphocytes with marked plasmacytoid features. Residual renal tubules ➡ are shown.

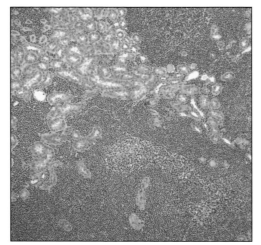
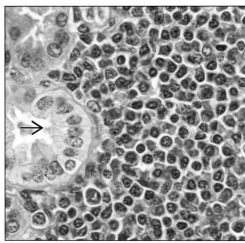

EXTRANODAL MARGINAL ZONE B-CELL LYMPHOMA (MALT LYMPHOMA)

Microscopic and Immunohistochemical Features

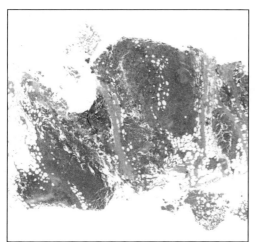

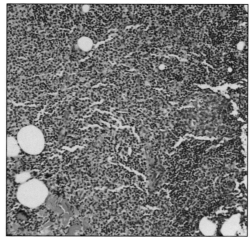

(Left) MALT lymphoma involving breast. The infiltrate forms a mass lesion. *(Right)* MALT lymphoma involving breast. Many neoplastic cells have monocytoid features.

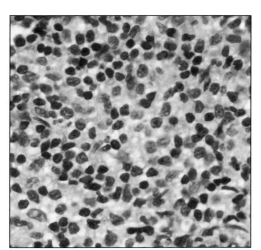

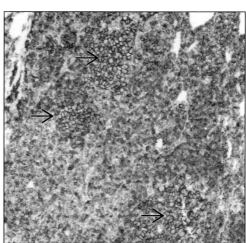

(Left) MALT lymphoma involving breast. The monocytoid cells have ample pale cytoplasm. The nuclei of the infiltrating cells are slightly irregular. *(Right)* MALT lymphoma involving breast. CD20 highlights the residual germinal center B cells ➡ (brighter CD20 positive) and the surrounding neoplastic cells (dim CD20 positive).

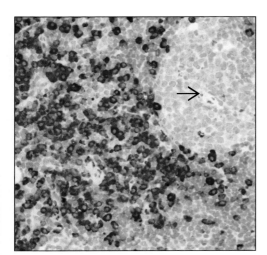

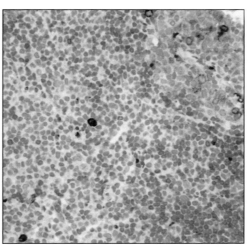

(Left) MALT lymphoma involving breast. Note the large reactive germinal center ➡. Numerous λ light chain-restricted plasma cells or plasmacytoid lymphocytes are present. *(Right)* MALT lymphoma involving breast. κ light chain stain shows only rare positive cells in the neoplastic infiltrate.

EXTRANODAL MARGINAL ZONE B-CELL LYMPHOMA (MALT LYMPHOMA)

Microscopic and Immunohistochemical Features

(Left) MALT lymphoma involving orbit. Between numerous residual reactive germinal centers are expanded marginal zone-like areas ➔. (Right) MALT lymphoma involving orbit. Note the residual germinal center ➔ surrounded by the mantle zone ➔ and markedly expanded marginal zone ➔.

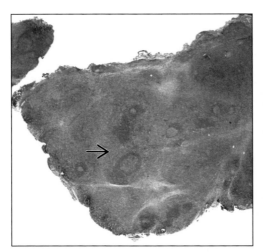
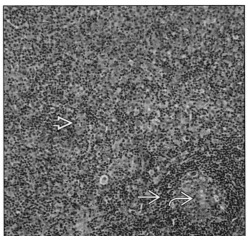

(Left) MALT lymphoma involving orbit. The infiltrating cells are a mixed population of small mature lymphocytes, plasmacytoid cells, and scattered large cells. (Right) MALT lymphoma involving orbit. Mature plasma cells with ample immunoglobulin cytoplasmic inclusions (Russell bodies) ➔ are present in this field.

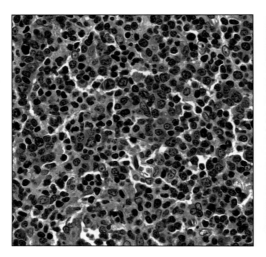
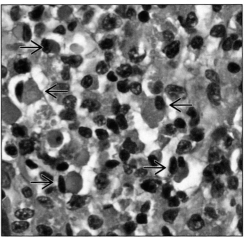

(Left) MALT lymphoma involving orbit. The plasma cells are predominantly positive for κ light chain. (Right) MALT lymphoma involving orbit. Only rare plasma cells are positive for λ light chain.

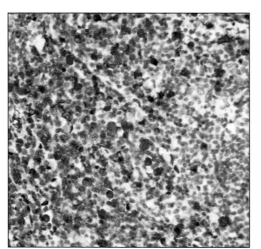
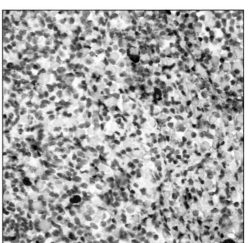

EXTRANODAL MARGINAL ZONE B-CELL LYMPHOMA (MALT LYMPHOMA)

Microscopic Features

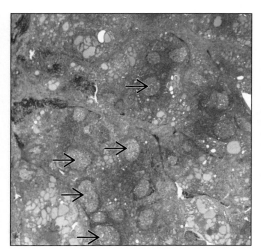

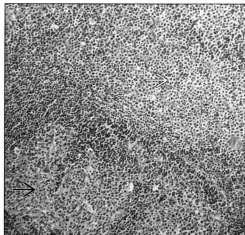

(Left) MALT lymphoma involving thyroid gland. Note the many hyperplastic germinal centers ➡ also present. *(Right)* MALT lymphoma involving thyroid gland. High-power view depicts a residual germinal center ➡ that is hyperplastic and colonized by plasmacytoid cells. The marginal zone ➡ is expanded and populated by monocytoid cells.

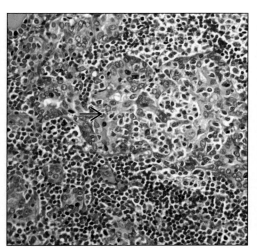

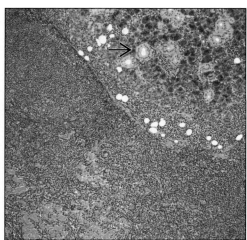

(Left) MALT lymphoma involving thyroid gland. The follicles are infiltrated by the neoplastic cells ➡ forming the so-called "MALT ball." *(Right)* MALT lymphoma extensively involving parotid gland. Note the residual salivary gland tissue ➡.

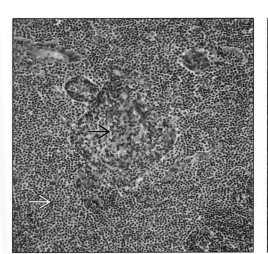

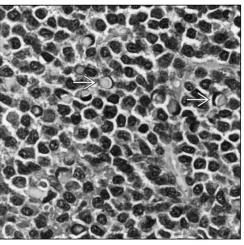

(Left) MALT lymphoma involving parotid gland. Note the lymphoepithelial lesion ➡ and monocytoid cells in the markedly expanded marginal zones ➡. *(Right)* MALT lymphoma involving parotid gland. Numerous plasmacytoid/plasmacytic cells with prominent nuclear pseudoinclusions (Dutcher bodies) ➡ are present.

EXTRANODAL MARGINAL ZONE B-CELL LYMPHOMA (MALT LYMPHOMA)

Immunohistochemistry and Differential Diagnosis

(Left) MALT lymphoma involving thyroid gland. The neoplastic cells are mostly CD20(-) because they exhibit plasmacytoid differentiation. Lymphoid follicles in the field are CD20(+). *(Right)* MALT lymphoma involving thyroid gland. The neoplastic B cells are CD3(-).

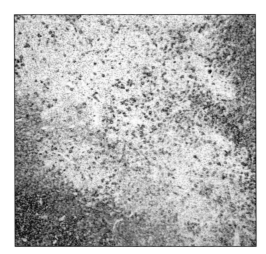
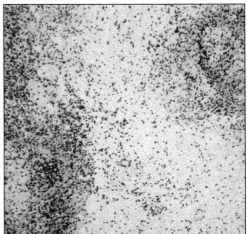

(Left) MALT lymphoma involving thyroid gland. The κ immunohistochemical stain highlights neoplastic plasmacytoid lymphocytes and plasma cells that surround follicles and colonize germinal centers. *(Right)* MALT lymphoma involving thyroid gland. CD10 highlights the residual germinal center B cells. Note the intact mantle zone ⇥ and the expanded marginal zone and interfollicular areas ⇨.

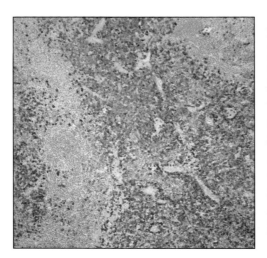
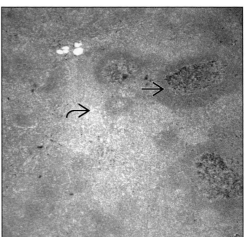

(Left) Mantle cell lymphoma involving colon. The neoplasm forms a polyp grossly, and patients can have multiple polyps known as multiple lymphomatous polyposis. *(Right)* Mantle cell lymphoma involving colon. Cyclin-D1 stain highlights the neoplastic cells in mantle cell lymphoma.

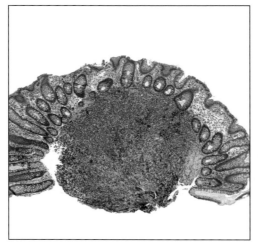
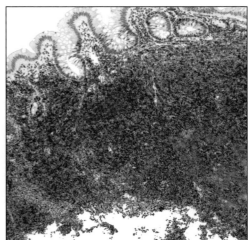

EXTRANODAL MARGINAL ZONE B-CELL LYMPHOMA (MALT LYMPHOMA)

Differential Diagnosis

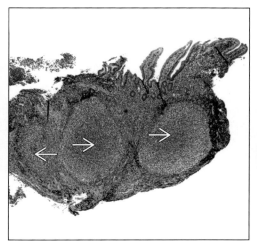 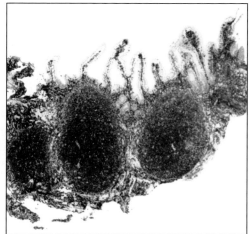

(Left) Low-grade follicular lymphoma involving small intestine. Note 3 neoplastic follicles ➡. (Right) Low-grade follicular lymphoma involving small intestine. The neoplastic cells in follicular lymphoma are Bcl-2(+).

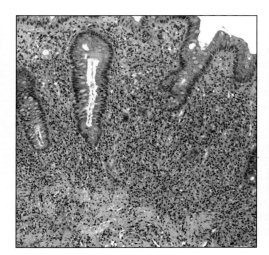 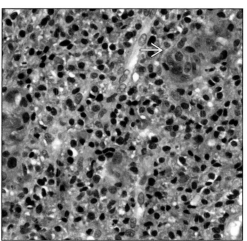

(Left) Plasmacytoma involving colon. Mature plasma cells fill and distend the lamina propria of the colonic mucosa. Plasmacytoma involving extranodal sites and MALT lymphoma appear to be closely related. (Right) Plasmacytoma involving colon. The infiltrating cells are mature plasma cells with ample cytoplasm. A residual colonic gland is seen at the upper right corner ➡.

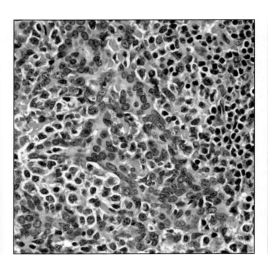 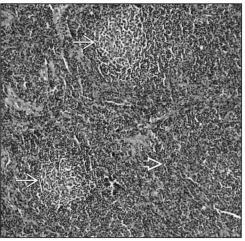

(Left) Salivary gland involved by myoepithelial sialadenitis (MESA). Lymphoepithelial lesions are prominent in MESA and therefore not helpful in establishing the diagnosis of MALT lymphoma at this site. (Right) Lung involved by plasma cell granuloma that can mimic MALT lymphoma. Two large residual germinal centers ➡ are noted. The plasma cells ➡ in this case were polytypic and there was no evidence of clonality by molecular methods; evidence against MALT lymphoma.

EXTRANODAL FOLLICULAR LYMPHOMA

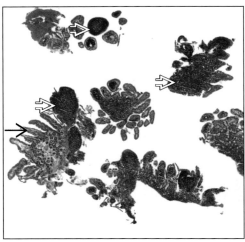

Follicular lymphoma (FL) forming polyps involving the small intestine. Well-preserved villi ➡ alternate with expanded villi due to intramucosal FL ⇒.

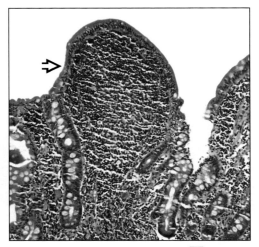

FL, grade 1, expanding a small bowel villus ⇒. This villus appears as a polyp when viewed by endoscopy.

TERMINOLOGY

Abbreviations
- Follicular lymphoma (FL)

Synonyms
- Follicle (germinal) center cell lymphoma
- Centroblastic/centrocytic lymphoma

Definitions
- Lymphoma composed of follicle center B cells that arises in extranodal sites
- FL involving extranodal sites as manifestation of systemic disease is excluded

ETIOLOGY/PATHOGENESIS

Predisposing Medical Conditions
- Poorly understood in patients with extranodal FL
  - Antigen drive may have a role; depends on site

Dysregulation of Apoptosis
- t(14;18)(q32;q21) is present in subset of cases
  - Frequency is lower than in nodal FL
  - Frequency depends, in part, on site of disease

CLINICAL ISSUES

Epidemiology
- Incidence
  - Primary cutaneous FL
    - Most common site of extranodal FL
  - Gastrointestinal (GI) tract FL
    - < 1% of all GI tract NHL are gastric FL
    - 2% of all GI tract NHL are intestinal FL
  - Thyroid FL
    - Rare; MALT lymphoma far more common at this site
  - Testicular FL
    - Rare; much less frequent than testicular diffuse large B-cell lymphoma
  - Ocular adnexal FL
    - Primary FL at this site is rare
    - FL commonly involves ocular adnexa as part of disseminated disease
    - Ocular adnexa involvement can be 1st manifestation of systemic FL
- Age
  - GI tract FL
    - Gastric: Median age: 52 years
    - Intestinal: Median age: 52 years
  - Thyroid FL
    - Median age: 60 years
  - Testicular FL
    - Children and young adults
  - Ocular adnexal FL
    - Median age: 60 years
- Gender
  - GI tract FL: M:F ratio is ~ equal
  - Thyroid FL: M:F ~ 1:3
  - Ocular adnexa: M:F ~ 1:2
- Ethnicity
  - GI tract FL
    - More common in Japan
    - May be related to systematic GI screening

Site
- GI tract FL
  - Gastric FL usually appears as discrete mass
  - Most cases of primary intestinal FL occur in small intestine
    - Particularly in 2nd portion of duodenum
    - Endoscopic capsule may detect asymptomatic multifocal tumors
- Thyroid FL
  - Single or multinodular mass
- Testicular FL

EXTRANODAL FOLLICULAR LYMPHOMA

Key Facts

Clinical Issues
- Common sites of extranodal FL
  - Skin, GI tract, thyroid gland, testis
- Extranodal FL is usually localized
  - Systemic relapses are uncommon
- Clinical approach to patients with extranodal FL is similar to that for patients with nodal FL
- Management of extranodal FL is controversial
- Local radiation and chemotherapy are tailored according to staging

Microscopic Pathology
- Extranodal FL similar to nodal FL
- Grading criteria designed for nodal FL are applied to extranodal FLs
  - Grade 1-2 (low grade)
  - Grades 3A and 3B

- Prognostic importance of diffuse pattern is controversial at some extranodal sites

Ancillary Tests
- Monotypic Ig(+), pan-B-cell antigens (+)
- Bcl-6(+), Bcl-2(+), CD10(±)
- Monoclonal *Ig* gene rearrangements
- Frequency of t(14;18)(q32;q21) varies by site
  - ~ 50% up to 80-90%
- Relatively little data on cytogenetic abnormalities other than t(14;18) in extranodal FLs

Top Differential Diagnoses
- Reactive follicular hyperplasia
- MALT lymphoma
- Mantle cell lymphoma
- Diffuse large B-cell lymphoma

  - Tumor involves testicular parenchyma as well as adnexa
  - Unilateral
- Ocular adnexal FL
  - Lacrimal gland most frequent site of primary FL

Presentation
- Extranodal FL is usually localized, and systemic relapses are uncommon
- GI tract FL
  - Duodenum
    - Usually incidentally found during endoscopic procedures
  - Jejunum and proximal ileum
    - Usually present with abdominal pain
  - Distal ileum or ileocecal valve
    - Intussusception can be 1st manifestation of disease
  - Colon/rectum
    - Bleeding common
- Thyroid FL
  - Most primary FL are grade 3
    - Present as mass; stage IE disease
    - ± hoarseness, dysphagia, or dyspnea
  - Patients with Hashimoto thyroiditis have up to 60x increased risk of thyroid lymphoma
    - Mostly associated with increased risk of MALT lymphoma or DLBCL
    - Relationship of Hashimoto thyroiditis to FL is unknown
- Testicular FL
  - Painless discrete mass or diffuse testicular enlargement
- Ocular adnexal FL
  - Small nodule or mass without impairment; clinically indolent

Treatment
- Management of extranodal FL is controversial due to rarity of diseases
- Many reported cases had diagnostic or therapeutic resection for extranodal FL

- Local radiation and chemotherapy are tailored according to staging
  - Cyclophosphamide, doxorubicin (Adriamycin), vincristine, prednisone (CHOP) chemotherapy
  - Rituximab added more recently to regimen
- Gastrointestinal FL
  - Intestinal FL requires surgery more frequently than gastric FL
  - "Watch and wait" for asymptomatic stage I intestinal FL
- Thyroid FL
  - Many reported cases had resection with or without subsequent chemotherapy
- Testicular FL
  - Reported cases were usually resected and subsequently received chemotherapy
- Ocular adnexal FL
  - Excision ± local irradiation

Prognosis
- Clinical approach to patients with extranodal FL is similar to that for patients with nodal FL
  - Stage and international prognostic index (IPI) are important
    - Recently proposed IPI for patients with FL: So-called FLIPI
  - Histologic grade of FL has some prognostic value
    - Cases of grade 1 or 2 extranodal FL are clinically indolent
    - Predicting behavior of grade 3 extranodal FL is more controversial
    - Chemotherapy may obscure significance of grading
  - Complex karyotype correlates with poor prognosis
  - Worse prognosis associated with del6q23-26, del17p, and mutations of *TP53*
  - Transformation to high-grade lymphoma can occur in small subset of patients with extranodal FL
    - Most transformed tumors meet criteria for diagnosis of DLBCL
- GI tract FL

7

EXTRANODAL FOLLICULAR LYMPHOMA

- o Patients with stage I and II disease have better survival than patients with systemic disease
  - ▪ Use of Lugano staging system is recommended for GI lymphomas
  - o Patients with FL of duodenum have excellent prognosis and survival with low-stage disease
- Thyroid FL
  - o Complete remission and no deaths in patients with grade 3 FL
- Testicular FL
  - o Excellent prognosis for children and young adults with stage IE FL of testis
- Ocular adnexal FL
  - o If truly stage IE, excellent prognosis

MACROSCOPIC FEATURES

Gastrointestinal FL

- Gastric FL usually appears as multiple nodular lesions or mass ± ulcer
- Duodenal FL usually appears as multiple nodular lesions
  - o Multifocality detected with pan-endoscopic staging
- Jejunum, ileum, and colonic FL usually appear as multiple nodular lesions, 1-2 mm in diameter
  - o Less frequently as mass ± ulcer
    - ▪ Median tumor size: 4.5 cm (range: 0.3-10 cm)

Thyroid FL

- Single or multinodular mass

Testicular FL

- Distinct nodule, 1.2-4 cm in diameter; tan or pink
- FL can also entirely replace testis

Ocular Adnexal FL

- Friable, fleshy appearance

MICROSCOPIC PATHOLOGY

Histologic Features

- Histologic features of extranodal FL are similar to nodal FL
  - o Closely-packed neoplastic follicles that efface architecture
  - o Attenuated or absent mantle zones
  - o Tingible body macrophages usually decreased or absent
  - o Follicle centers composed of randomly distributed centrocytes and centroblasts
    - ▪ Polarization into dark and light zones is unusual
    - ▪ Monomorphic appearance (compared with reactive germinal centers)
    - ▪ ± monocytoid/marginal zone or plasmacytic differentiation
- GI tract FL
  - o Usually grade 1-2; rarely (~ 5%) grade 3
  - o Bcl-2 (+) is essential for diagnosing FL in small lesions confined to mucosa
  - o Neoplastic follicles expand villi, without destroying glandular epithelium

- Thyroid FL
  - o Grade 3 thyroid FL; interfollicular diffuse pattern common
    - ▪ Occasionally DLBCL areas
  - o Lymphoepithelial lesions detected in most cases (similar to MALT lymphomas)
    - ▪ Contained within thyroid follicles or admixed with epithelial cell clusters
  - o ± Hashimoto thyroiditis
- Testicular FL
  - o FL involves mainly testicular parenchyma, and secondarily adnexa
    - ▪ Neoplastic follicles grow amidst tubules or completely replace parenchyma
  - o Reported cases are predominantly grade 3A
    - ▪ Occasionally focal areas of diffuse growth support focal DLBCL
- Ocular adnexal FL
  - o Most FL at this site are grade 1-2
  - o Cannot distinguish stage IE tumor from systemic involvement; staging mandatory

Cytologic Features

- Extranodal FLs are rarely assessed by fine needle aspiration

Grading in Extranodal FLs

- Grading criteria designed for nodal FL are applied to extranodal FLs
  - o Grade 1-2 (low grade)
  - o Grades 3A and 3B
  - o Report diffuse areas > 25% composed predominantly of large cells as DLBCL
- No rigorous studies have been performed to prove scientific merit of this approach in extranodal FLs

Reporting Pattern in Extranodal FLs

- Pattern criteria designed for nodal FL are applied to extranodal FLs
- Report percentage of follicular pattern
  - o Follicular pattern (> 75%)
  - o Follicular and diffuse pattern (25-75%)
  - o Focally follicular pattern (1-24%)
  - o Diffuse pattern (0%)
- Prognostic importance of diffuse pattern is controversial at some extranodal sites

ANCILLARY TESTS

Immunohistochemistry

- Immunophenotype similar to nodal FL
- Monotypic Ig(+), pan-B-cell antigens(+)
- CD10(+/-)
  - o Tends to be stronger within follicles and dim or negative in interfollicular areas
  - o CD10 can be negative in FL grade 3
- Bcl-6(+); often downregulated in interfollicular areas
- Bcl-2(+)
  - o Positive in ~ 85-90% of grade 1 FL
  - o Positive in ~ 50% of grade 3 FL
- IRF-4/MUM1(-/+)

EXTRANODAL FOLLICULAR LYMPHOMA

- Usually negative in low-grade FL; can be positive in grade 3 FL
- MUM1(+) in up to half of cases with DLBCL areas
- Follicles are highlighted by antibodies reactive with follicular dendritic cell markers
  - CD21, CD23, CD35, others
- Pan-T-cell antigens (-), Cyclin-D1(-)
- Gastrointestinal FL
  - Most cases CD20(+), CD10(+), and Bcl-2(+)
  - CD10(+) in ~ 60% of FL of GI tract
  - Expression of IgA and integrin α4β7, a mucosal homing receptor, has been suggested
- Thyroid FL
  - Subset of grade 3A FL are Bcl-2(-); frequently CD10(-)
- Testicular FL
  - Usually Bcl-2(-)
- Ocular adnexa FL
  - Most cases CD20(+), CD10(+), Bcl-6(+), and Bcl-2(+)

Flow Cytometry
- Monotypic sIg(+), with IgM > IgG > IgA
- CD19(+), CD20(+), CD22(+)
- CD10(+/-), pan-T-cell antigens (-)

Cytogenetics
- Variable frequency of t(14;18)(q32;q21) depending on site
  - Frequency ranges from ~ 50% up to 80-90%
  - FISH is most sensitive technique to detect this translocation
  - FL 3B often not associated with t(14;18)(q32;q21)
- Relatively little data on cytogenetic abnormalities other than t(14;18) in extranodal FLs
- Translocations involving 3q27/*BCL6* reported

PCR
- *IgH* and *Ig* light chain genes are clonally rearranged
  - Extensive and ongoing somatic mutations of variable regions of *IgH* and light chain genes
  - Result in 10-40% false negative rate of detection by PCR
    - Can be reduced by expanding primer sets
- Thyroid FL
  - PCR can detect monoclonality in ~ 80% of cases

Molecular Genetics
- *BCL2* gene rearrangements detected by Southern blot analysis in ~ 60%
- ~ 70% detection of *IgH-BCL2* fusion gene by FISH
- *BCL6* gene rearrangements in ~ 20% of cases
- Thyroid FL
  - *IgH-BCL2* fusion gene rare in grade 3 FL
- Testicular FL
  - By either PCR or FISH, *IgH-BCL2* fusion gene is uncommon
  - ± *BCL6* translocations

DIFFERENTIAL DIAGNOSIS

Reactive Follicular Hyperplasia (RFH)
- Pattern and cytology can simulate FL
- Features that support RFH over extranodal FL

- Follicles show polarization; surrounded by distinct mantle zones
- Follicles have polymorphic appearance, with tingible body macrophages
- Immunophenotype: B-cell antigens (+), CD10(+), Bcl-6(+), Bcl-2(-)
- No evidence of monoclonal *Ig* gene rearrangements

Extranodal Marginal Zone B-cell Lymphoma of Mucosa-associated Lymphoid Tissue (MALT Lymphoma)
- MALT lymphoma is common entity in differential diagnosis of extranodal FLs
- MALT lymphoma can display nodular or diffuse pattern
  - Predominance of small round and monocytoid lymphocytes
  - Lymphoepithelial lesions are common; often prominent
  - Immunophenotype: B-cell antigens (+), Bcl-2(+), CD10(-), Bcl-6(-)
- GI tract FL
  - Features that support MALT lymphoma over GI tract FL
    - Association with other extranodal sites of MALT lymphoma
    - MALT lymphoma common in stomach
    - MALT lymphoma is commonly associated with *Helicobacter pylori* infection
    - MALT lymphoma associated with t(11;18)(q21;q21)/*API2-MALT1* or t(1;14)(p22;q32)/*BCL10-IgH*
- Thyroid FL
  - MALT lymphoma far more common than FL at this site
  - Features that support MALT lymphoma over thyroid FL
    - Usually associated with Hashimoto thyroiditis
    - History of hypothyroidism in some patients
    - Diffuse or nodular thyroid enlargement
    - Reactive lymphoid follicles; many plasma cells
    - Interspersed with atrophic thyroid follicles with Hürthle cell changes
    - MALT lymphoma associated with t(3;14)(p14.1;q32)/*FOXP1-IgH*
- Ocular adnexal FL
  - MALT lymphoma far more common than stage IE FL at this site
  - Features that support MALT lymphoma over ocular adnexal FL
    - Association with autoimmune disease or other extranodal sites of MALT lymphoma
    - MALT lymphoma associated with t(14;18)(q32;q21)/*IgH-MALT1*

Mantle Cell Lymphoma (MCL)
- Commonly involves GI tract and can involve other extranodal sites
  - Usually as part of disseminated disease
- In GI tract, MCL can present as multiple lymphomatous polyposis
- Features that support MCL over extranodal FL

EXTRANODAL FOLLICULAR LYMPHOMA

Differential Diagnosis of Extranodal Follicular Lymphoma

	Stomach	Intestine	Thyroid	Testis	Ocular Adnexa
Clinical Features					
Age (median)	Adults	Adults (52 years)	Adults (60 years)	Children and young adults	Adults (60 years)
Gender (M:F)	1:1	1:1	1:3	Males only	1:2
Site	Antrum or body	Duodenum, small bowel	Any lobe	Testicle and adnexa	Lacrimal gland, conjunctiva
Symptoms	Abdominal pain	Asymptomatic; found on gastrointestinal screening	Mass	Painless mass	Mass
Stage	IE	IE-IIE	Stage IE in grade 3 FL; stage 2E-4E in grade 1-2 FL	IE	IE-IVE
Pathologic Features					
Gross appearance	Nodule or tumor	Polypoid mucosa or nodule	Single or multinodular mass	Discrete mass or diffuse involvement	Mass
Histologic grading	Low or high grade	Low grade	Subset with grade 1-2 FL; subset with grade 3a FL	Grade 3	Low grade predominant
Immunophenotype					
CD10	(+)	(+)	(-) in grade 3A FL subset	(+/-)	(+)
Bcl-2	(+)	(+)	(-) in grade 3A FL subset	(-)	(+)
Molecular Features					
BCL2 gene rearrangements	(+)	(+)	(+) in grade 1-2 FL subset; (-) in grade 3A FL subset	(-)	(+)

FL = follicular lymphoma.

- o Uniform population of small neoplastic lymphocytes
- o No centroblasts
- o Immunophenotype: B-cell antigens (+), Bcl-2(+), CD5(+), Cyclin-D1(+), CD10(-), Bcl-6(-)
- o Presence of t(11;14)(q13;q32)/*CCND1-IgH*

Diffuse Large B-cell Lymphoma (DLBCL)
- DLBCL is most common lymphoma involving testes
  - o Can arise in testis or be manifestation of disseminated disease
- Histologically, extranodal FL of testis can be grade 3 and predominantly diffuse
- Features supporting DLBCL over extranodal FL
  - o Evidence of other disease sites in patients with systemic DLBCL
  - o No areas of follicular pattern in primary DLBCL of testis
  - o Immunophenotype: DLBCL often CD10(-), Bcl-6(-)

DIAGNOSTIC CHECKLIST

Pathologic Interpretation Pearls
- Reporting FL as truly extranodal is often problematic in real time
  - o Staging may not have been performed prior to biopsy
  - o Important to not commit to extranodal diagnosis until information is known
  - o Addendum to report is often needed to subsequently include relevant data

SELECTED REFERENCES

1. Akamatsu T et al: Usefulness of double balloon enteroscopy and video capsule endoscopy for the diagnosis and management of primary follicular lymphoma of the gastrointestinal tract in its early stages. Dig Endosc. 22(1):33-8, 2010
2. Yamamoto S et al: Gastrointestinal follicular lymphoma: review of the literature. J Gastroenterol. 45(4):370-88, 2010
3. Bacon CM et al: Follicular lymphoma of the thyroid gland. Am J Surg Pathol. 33(1):22-34, 2009
4. Sentani K et al: Follicular lymphoma of the duodenum: a clinicopathologic analysis of 26 cases. Jpn J Clin Oncol. 38(8):547-52, 2008
5. Bacon CM et al: Primary follicular lymphoma of the testis and epididymis in adults. Am J Surg Pathol. 31(7):1050-8, 2007
6. Waisberg J et al: Curative resection plus adjuvant chemotherapy for early stage primary gastric non-Hodgkin's lymphoma: a retrospective study with emphasis on prognostic factors and treatment outcome. Arq Gastroenterol. 43(1):30-6, 2006
7. Lu D et al: Primary follicular large cell lymphoma of the testis in a child. Arch Pathol Lab Med. 125(4):551-4, 2001
8. Medeiros LJ et al: Lymphoid infiltrates of the orbit and conjunctiva. A morphologic and immunophenotypic study of 99 cases. Am J Surg Pathol. 13(6):459-71, 1989
9. Otter R et al: Primary gastrointestinal non-Hodgkin's lymphoma in a population-based registry. Br J Cancer. 60(5):745-50, 1989

Extranodal FL of Gastrointestinal Tract

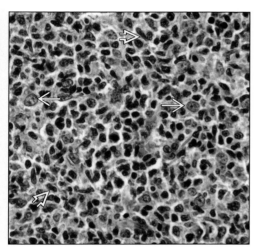

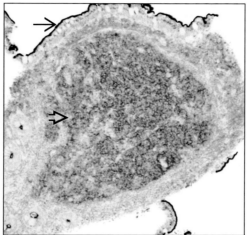

(Left) High magnification of follicular lymphoma (FL), grade 1, involving small intestine. Cells are mostly small centrocytes ⇒ with only rare large centroblasts ⇒. *(Right)* FL, grade 1, of the small intestine shows neoplastic lymphocytes ⇒ that are CD10(+) in a pattern similar to nodal FL. CD10 also highlights the intestinal absorptive epithelium ⇒, which is an internal control.

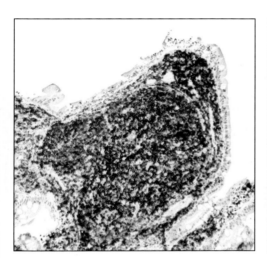

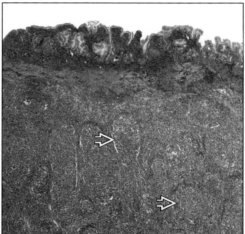

(Left) This case of follicular lymphoma, grade 1, involves the duodenum and is limited to the mucosa. Immunohistochemistry for Bcl-2 demonstrates that cells are positive, which supports the diagnosis. Bcl-2 immunohistochemistry is essential to the diagnosis of intramucosal FL. *(Right)* Resection specimen of small bowel demonstrated transmural involvement by FL. Neoplastic follicles ⇒ are noted through the intestinal wall.

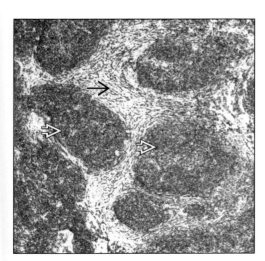

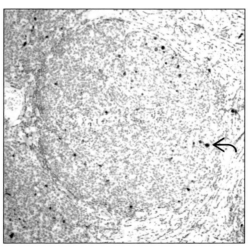

(Left) This segmental resection specimen of the small intestine shows follicular lymphoma highlighted with the B-cell marker pax-5 ⇒. Interfollicular lymphocytes ⇒ are also highlighted. *(Right)* Intestinal FL assessed for Ki-67 by immunohistochemistry shows rare positive cells ⇒, consistent with a low proliferation rate. The neoplastic follicles of most low-grade FLs show a low proliferation rate.

EXTRANODAL FOLLICULAR LYMPHOMA

Extranodal FL of Orbit and Thyroid Gland

(Left) Follicular lymphoma, grade 1, involving orbital soft tissue. Axial T1 magnetic resonance (MR) shows an infiltrating mass ➡ in the medial anterior extraconal orbit that "points" into the nasolacrimal duct ⮞. For this patient, staging is mandatory as most patients with orbital FL have systemic disease. *(Right)* FL, grade 1, follicular pattern, involving the orbit. Large neoplastic follicles are focally confluent ⮞. These follicles lack mantle zones ➡.

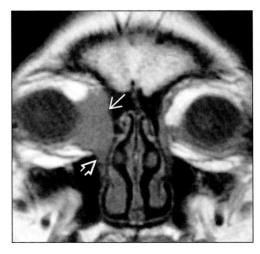
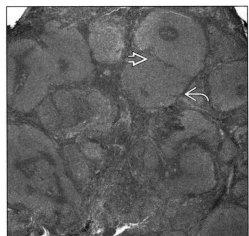

(Left) Follicular lymphoma, grade 1, involving the orbit. This neoplastic follicle is composed of a uniform population of small centrocytes. *(Right)* FL, grade 3A, involving thyroid gland as shown by the formation of neoplastic follicles ⮞. Residual thyroid follicles ➡ are noted. FL, grade 3A, is usually associated with stage IE disease and patients have a good prognosis.

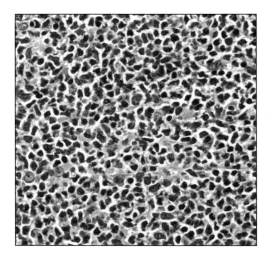
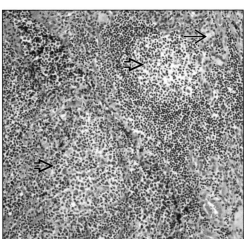

(Left) In this case of follicular lymphoma, grade 3A, involving thyroid gland, Bcl-6 immunohistochemistry highlights confluent neoplastic follicles ⮞. *(Right)* FL involving thyroid gland. Immunohistochemistry for CD20 highlights a lymphoepithelial lesion in which neoplastic lymphocytes ➡ infiltrate a thyroid follicle ⮞. Lymphoepithelial lesions are common in thyroid gland involved by FL, and do not distinguish FL from MALT lymphoma.

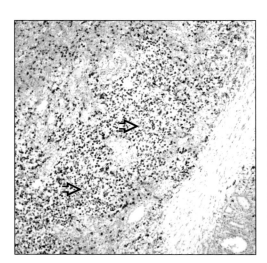
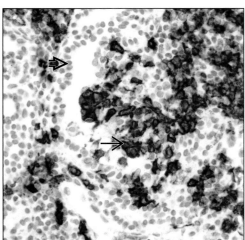

Extranodal FL of Testis

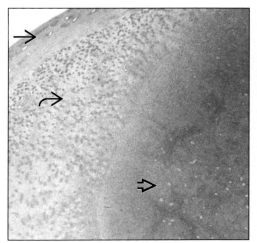

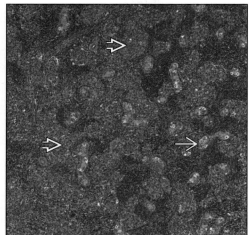

(**Left**) Panoramic view of a painless testicular mass in a 4-year-old boy revealed follicular lymphoma, grade 3A. Neoplastic follicles ⊳ are noted deep in the parenchyma. Remnants of seminiferous tubules ⇒ are noted under the albuginea ⊟. (**Right**) FL, grade 3A, involving the testis in a 2-year-old boy. This field shows confluent neoplastic follicles ⊳ admixed with seminiferous tubules ⇒. This tumor affects mainly children and young adults.

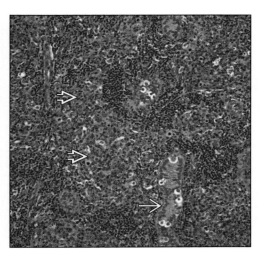

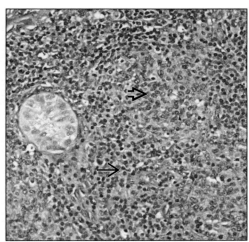

(**Left**) Follicular lymphoma, grade 3A, involving the testis in a 2-year-old boy. This field shows confluent neoplastic follicles ⊳ admixed with seminiferous tubules ⇒. Like most testicular FL, this tumor was Bcl-2(-). (**Right**) FL, grade 3A, presenting as a testicular mass in a 3-year-old boy. A neoplastic follicle is composed predominantly of large centroblasts ⊳ admixed with small lymphocytes ⇒.

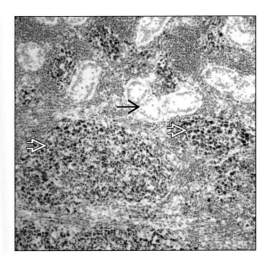

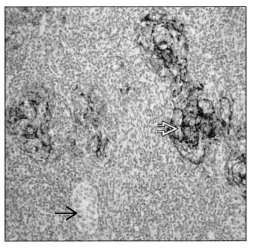

(**Left**) Follicular lymphoma, grade 3A, presenting as a testicular mass in a 3-year-old boy. Bcl-6 immunohistochemistry highlights confluent neoplastic follicles ⊳ admixed with seminiferous tubules ⇒. (**Right**) FL, grade 3A, presenting as a testicular mass in a 3-year-old boy. CD21 immunohistochemistry highlights follicular dendritic cell meshworks ⊳. Remnants of seminiferous tubules ⇒ are noted.

EXTRANODAL FOLLICULAR LYMPHOMA

Differential Diagnosis of FL of the GI Tract

(Left) Extranodal marginal zone B-cell lymphoma of mucosa-associated lymphoid tissue (MALT lymphoma) in the stomach. The mucosa is destroyed by an extensive infiltrate, which is focally nodular ➡. The infiltrate extends through the gastric glands ➡. *(Right)* MALT lymphoma involving the stomach. A lymphoepithelial lesion is depicted in which gastric glands are infiltrated by monocytoid lymphocytes ➡.

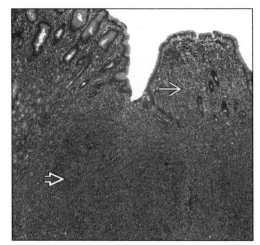
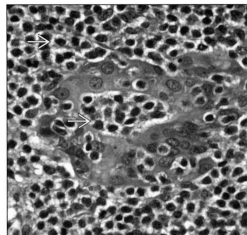

(Left) MALT lymphoma involving the stomach. Neoplastic lymphocytes ➡ colonize and disrupt germinal centers. Bcl-6 immunohistochemistry highlights follicular center cells of disrupted residual germinal centers ➡. *(Right)* MALT lymphoma involving the stomach. Most lymphocytes in this lymphoid follicle are Bcl-2(+) ➡, consistent with follicular colonization by MALT lymphoma. Few residual Bcl-2(-) germinal center cells remain ➡.

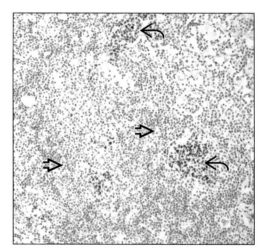
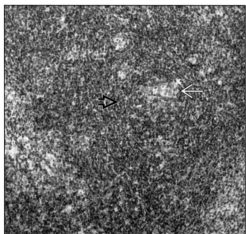

(Left) Panoramic view of distal ileum involved by mantle cell lymphoma (MCL) displays a multiple lymphomatous polyposis pattern. Tumor is confined to mucosa and submucosa ➡, sparing muscularis propria ➡. *(Right)* Low magnification of distal ileum with MCL forming a polypoid nodule. The tumor is confined to mucosa and causes a nodule that is similar to follicular lymphoma.

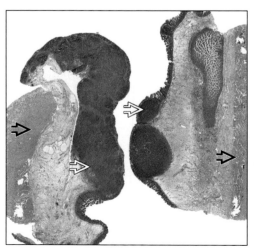
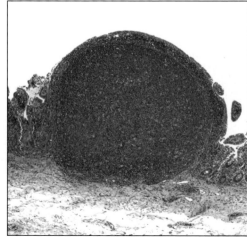

EXTRANODAL FOLLICULAR LYMPHOMA

Differential Diagnosis

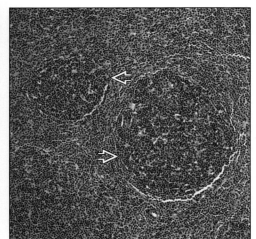

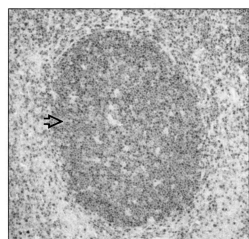

(Left) Distal ileum involved by mantle cell lymphoma (MCL) presents as multiple lymphomatous polyposis. The tumor displays a nodular pattern, and the nodules ⮕ can be confused with follicular lymphoma. *(Right)* Intermediate magnification of distal ileum involved by MCL. Cyclin-D1 immunohistochemistry supports the diagnosis by highlighting the tumor nodule ⮞.

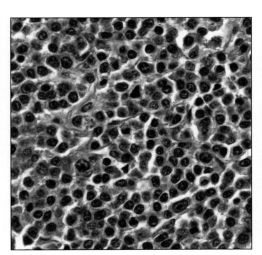

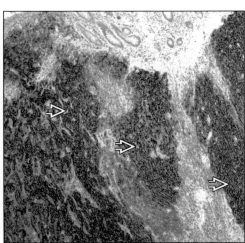

(Left) Patient with distal ileum involved by diffuse large B-cell lymphoma (DLBCL) presented with intussusception. Some areas showed low-grade B-cell lymphoma, consistent with MALT lymphoma, suggesting transformation. *(Right)* CD21 immunohistochemistry in a patient with distal ileum DLBCL shows abundant, confluent follicular dendritic cell meshworks ⮕ that raise the suspicion of underlying follicular lymphoma or marginal zone lymphoma.

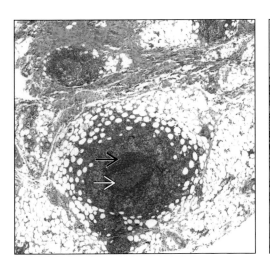

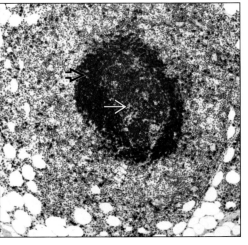

(Left) Patient presented with mass in the orbit. This biopsy demonstrates follicular lymphoid hyperplasia. Sections show soft tissue with scattered lymphoid follicles with well-circumscribed germinal centers ⮕ and mantle zones ⮕. *(Right)* Patient presented with mass in the orbit, diagnosed with follicular lymphoid hyperplasia. Immunohistochemistry for CD20 highlights a benign lymphoid follicle with germinal center ⮕; lymphocytes of the mantle zone are darker ⮞.

EXTRANODAL FOLLICULAR LYMPHOMA

Differential Diagnosis of Thyroid FL

(Left) MALT lymphoma involving the thyroid gland. There are ill-defined nodules ⇨ admixed with remnants of thyroid follicles. This lymphoma is much more common in thyroid gland than is FL. (Right) MALT lymphoma involving the thyroid gland. Increased large cells ➡ are noted. It is common that this tumor displays increased large cells and evidence of histologic transformation to diffuse large B-cell lymphoma.

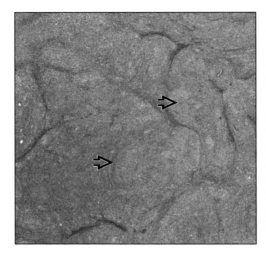
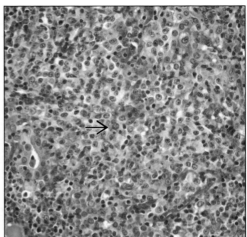

(Left) In this case of MALT lymphoma involving the thyroid gland, Bcl-6 immunohistochemistry highlights residual and disrupted germinal center cells ➡ due to colonization by marginal zone lymphoma cells ➡. (Right) Hashimoto thyroiditis. Multiple reactive follicles ➡ displace thyroid parenchyma ➡. Patients with Hashimoto thyroiditis can present with diffuse thyroid enlargement or as nodular growth.

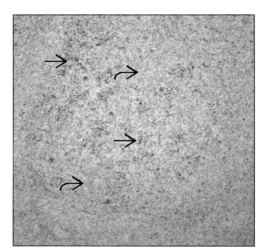
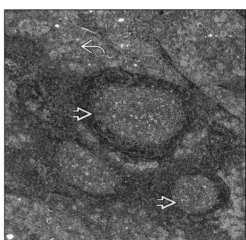

(Left) In this case of Hashimoto thyroiditis, a reactive lymphoid follicle shows a distinct mantle zone ➡, and the germinal center has tingible body macrophages ➡. This lymphoid follicle is partially surrounded by thyroid follicles ➡. (Right) This lymphoid follicle in Hashimoto thyroiditis shows that the germinal center ➡ is Bcl-2(-), supporting a reactive follicle. Caution is recommended since most cases of FL grade 3 of the thyroid are also Bcl-2(-).

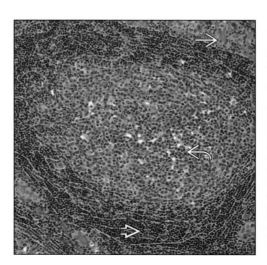
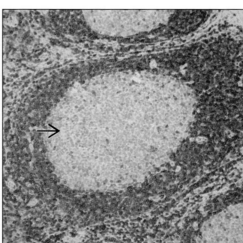

EXTRANODAL FOLLICULAR LYMPHOMA

Differential Diagnosis of Testicular FL

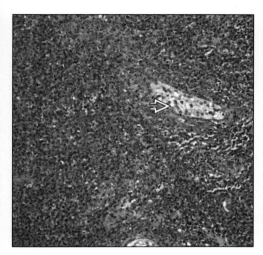

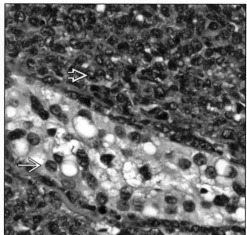

(Left) Elderly patient who presented with a testicular mass involved by diffuse large B-cell lymphoma (DLBCL). The neoplasm infiltrates through testicular parenchyma. Note the residual seminiferous tubule ➡. (Right) DLBCL infiltrating testicular parenchyma. A dense large cell infiltrate ➡ surrounds a seminiferous tubule ➡. DLBCL is the most common primary lymphoma of the testis and affects the elderly population.

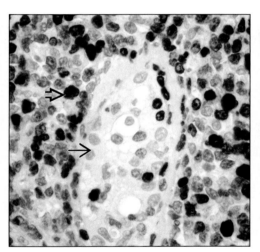

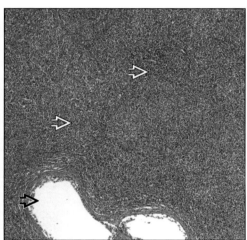

(Left) Diffuse large B-cell lymphoma of the testicle. The proliferation marker Ki-67 shows that most of the neoplastic lymphocytes are positive ➡. A seminiferous tubule ➡ is almost negative. (Right) Testis involved by small lymphocytic lymphoma/chronic lymphocytic leukemia (SLL/CLL). This field shows dilated ducts ➡ of epididymis surrounded by SLL/CLL with proliferation centers ➡ that may suggest FL.

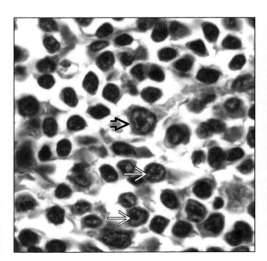

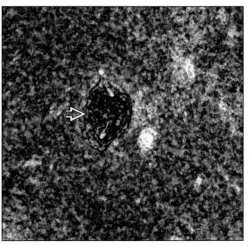

(Left) Testis involved in SLL/CLL is shown in this high-power view of a proliferation center. A paraimmunoblast ➡ is surrounded by small lymphocytes ➡. Retraction artifact is present, accounting for the space around the cells. (Right) Testis involved by SLL/CLL. CD23 immunohistochemistry highlights neoplastic lymphocytes, as well as the follicular dendritic cell meshwork of a benign follicle ➡.

PRIMARY CUTANEOUS FOLLICLE CENTER LYMPHOMA

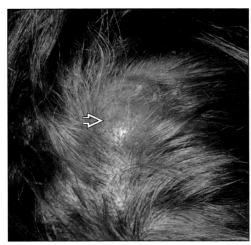

Primary cutaneous follicle center lymphoma (PCFCL) presenting as a 1 cm erythematous nodule ⇨ in the scalp. Most cases of PCFCL are found in the head and neck region.

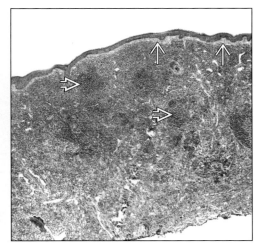

PCFCL displaying a dense lymphocytic infiltrate in the dermis, sparing the subepidermal layer (grenz zone ⇨). The neoplasm contains ill-defined follicles ⇨.

TERMINOLOGY

Abbreviations
- Primary cutaneous follicle center lymphoma (PCFCL)

Synonyms
- Follicular lymphoma (FL) of skin
- Follicular center cell lymphoma
- Centroblastic/centrocytic lymphoma
- PCFCL on back previously referred to as
  - Reticulohistiocytoma of the dorsum
  - Crosti disease

Definitions
- Lymphoma arising in skin composed of follicular center cells
  - Confined to skin for at least 6 months upon staging
  - Mainly centrocytes (small cleaved cells); less frequently centroblasts (large cleaved and noncleaved cells)
  - Follicular or diffuse growth pattern
- Recently defined as entity; diagnostic criteria may require further refinement
  - Some published cases with diagnosis based on clinicopathologic findings; lack evidence of clonality
- Subset of cases appear to be clinically and genetically distinct from nodal FL
  - *BCL2* gene rearrangements less frequent than in nodal FL

ETIOLOGY/PATHOGENESIS

Etiology
- Unknown

Cell of Origin
- Mature germinal center B lymphocyte

CLINICAL ISSUES

Epidemiology
- Incidence
  - 2nd most common extranodal B-cell lymphoma after gastrointestinal lymphomas
  - 0.1-0.2 per 100,000 persons per year
- Age
  - Affects adults; median 60 years (range 33-88 years)
- Gender
  - Male to female ratio is 1.5:1

Site
- Usually in head and neck
  - Affects mainly scalp and forehead
- Less frequent on trunk
- Legs affected in 5% of cases

Presentation
- Usually solitary, firm, and erythematous to violaceous lesion
  - May be plaques, nodules, or tumor masses of variable size
  - Lesions range from < 1 cm to large, confluent nodules > 40 cm in diameter
- Multifocal in 15% of patients
- Presentation on trunk is usually preceded by erythematous papules or figurate plaques
  - This form was designated in past as "reticulohistiocytoma of the dorsum"

Natural History
- Lesions gradually increase in size if left untreated
- Dissemination to extracutaneous sites is uncommon (~ 10%)
- Recurrences occur at proximal site compared with initial site of presentation
  - Recurrences occur in 30-40% of patients

PRIMARY CUTANEOUS FOLLICLE CENTER LYMPHOMA

Key Facts

Terminology
- Lymphoma arising in skin composed of follicular center cells
- Subset of cases appear to be clinically and genetically distinct from nodal FL

Clinical Issues
- Usually solitary, erythematous lesion in head and neck
- Therapy with local radiation or surgical excision
- Prognosis favorable, even in patients with multiple skin lesions
- 5-year survival rate is 95%

Microscopic Pathology
- Dermal lymphoid follicular infiltrate that spares epidermis

Ancillary Tests
- CD10(+) in cases with follicular pattern
- Bcl-6(+); Bcl-2(+/-) in up to 60% of cases
- PCFCL that is CD10(+), Bcl-2(+) likely carries t(14;18)(q32;q21)
- ~ 30% of PCFCL cases have t(14;18) by FISH

Top Differential Diagnoses
- Secondary follicular lymphoma of skin
  - Usually strongly CD10(+) and Bcl-2(+)
  - *BCL2* gene rearrangements in ~ 80-90% of cases
- Cutaneous marginal zone B-cell lymphoma
- Primary cutaneous diffuse large B-cell lymphoma (PCLBCL), leg type
- PCLBCL, other (non-leg type)
- Cutaneous follicular hyperplasia

Treatment
- Local radiation or surgical excision of lesions
- Systemic therapy required for patients with
  - Extensive disease, very thick skin tumors, or extracutaneous disease

Prognosis
- Favorable, even in patients with multiple skin lesions
  - Most patients achieve complete remission with therapy
- Survival is 95% at 5 years; not affected by presence of
  - Follicular or diffuse growth pattern or cytologic grade
  - t(14;18) or *BCL2* gene rearrangements
  - Extent or relapse of disease

MICROSCOPIC PATHOLOGY

Histologic Features
- Dermal infiltrate that spares epidermis (grenz zone)
- Growth patterns
  - Pure follicular
  - Mixed follicular and diffuse
  - Pure diffuse
- Cell composition
  - Small- to intermediate-sized centrocytes admixed with variable amount of large centroblasts
  - Grading is not recommended for PCFCL
    - Amount of large cells in follicles does not influence prognosis in patients with PCFCL
- Lymphoid follicles and germinal centers are better appreciated in small or incipient lesions
  - Follicles are ill defined and composed of rather monotonous lymphoid population
    - Usually, tingible body macrophages are absent
    - Attenuated or absent mantle zones
- Variable amounts of sclerosis
- Infiltrate may reach subcutaneous tissue in ~ 75% of cases
  - Most follicles in deep dermis ('bottom heavy')
- Advanced lesions show less conspicuous follicles, if present
  - Usually composed of multilobated, cleaved, or spindle-shaped lymphocytes
  - Remnants of follicular dendritic cells (FDCs)
- Extreme cases with many centroblasts simulate DLBCL
  - Should be considered as PCFCL if follicular component
    - Considered to share excellent prognosis of other, more typical PCFCL
  - DLBCL is diagnosed when large cells grow in pure diffuse pattern

ANCILLARY TESTS

Immunohistochemistry
- Pan-B-cell antigens(+), pax-5(+)
- CD10 is typically positive but can be negative in cases with diffuse pattern
  - CD10(+) cell clusters may be found in interfollicular areas
- Bcl-6(+) consistently found in follicles
- Bcl-2(+/-) in up to 60% of cases
  - When positive, Bcl-2 is often dim
    - (+) more frequently in cases with follicular pattern
- PCFCL that are CD10(+) and Bcl-2(+) likely carry t(14;18)(q32;q21)
- Monotypic B lymphocytes can be detected in fixed, paraffin-embedded tissue sections
  - ~ 1-20% using routine immunohistochemistry
  - Role of mRNA expression of κ and λ in cutaneous infiltrates not established
- IRF-4/MUM1 and FOXP1 are usually (-)
- Cytoplasmic IgM(-), IgD(-)
- Underlying FDC network: CD21(+), CD23(+), &/or CD35(+)
- T-cell antigens(-)
  - Variable number of reactive small T-lymphocytes

Flow Cytometry
- Monotypic surface Ig(+), pan-B-cell antigens(+)

PRIMARY CUTANEOUS FOLLICLE CENTER LYMPHOMA

• CD10(+), CD19(+ dim), CD20(+ bright), FMC-7(+)

In Situ Hybridization
• ~ 30% of PCFCL cases have t(14;18) by FISH

Array CGH
• Chromosomal imbalances in minority of cases

Molecular Genetics
• Monoclonal *Ig* gene rearrangements
  ○ Detected by PCR in 40-50% of cases
  ○ Somatic hypermutation of *Ig* genes is common
• *IgH-BCL2* fusion occurs at variable frequency in PCFCL

Gene Expression Profiling
• Gene expression profile similar to germinal center-like large B-cell lymphoma
  ○ *REL* gene amplification is common

DIFFERENTIAL DIAGNOSIS

Secondary Follicular Lymphoma (FL) of Skin
• Evidence of systemic FL elsewhere
  ○ Head and neck are most frequent sites
• Immunophenotype
  ○ Bcl-6(+), CD10(+), Bcl-2(+)
• *IgH-BCL2*/t(14;18)(q32;q21) in ~ 80-90% of cases

Marginal Zone B-cell Lymphoma of Skin
• Usually multifocal
  ○ Previous nomenclature included
    ▪ B-cell lymphoma of mucosa-associated lymphoid tissue (MALT lymphoma)
    ▪ Cutaneous immunocytoma
    ▪ Cutaneous follicular lymphoid hyperplasia with monotypic plasma cells
• Indolent low-grade lymphoma, 99% 5-year survival
• Association with *Borrelia burgdorferi*, mostly in Europe
• Marginal zone and interfollicular distribution
• Mixed cell composition
  ○ Marginal zone (centrocyte-like) cells
  ○ Monocytoid cells or small round lymphocytes
  ○ Scattered large cells, centroblast-like
  ○ ± plasma cell differentiation
    ▪ Subepidermal or at advancing edge of tumor
• Immunophenotype
  ○ B-cell antigens(+), CD10(-), Bcl-6(-)
  ○ Monotypic cytoplasmic Ig in cases with plasmacytoid differentiation
  ○ Clusters of reactive CD123(+) plasmacytoid dendritic cells are common
• Underlying disrupted and colonized germinal centers highlighted by FDC markers
  ○ Residual germinal center cells are CD10(+) and Bcl-6(+)

Primary Cutaneous Diffuse Large B-cell Lymphoma (PCLBCL), Leg Type
• Disease of elderly
• Rapidly growing tumors with 50% 5-year survival
• Primarily affects lower extremities; occasionally occurs at other body sites

• Diffuse and monotonous infiltrate composed of large centroblasts or immunoblasts
  ○ Absence of neoplastic follicles and small or large centrocytes
  ○ Distinct from DLBCL with centrocytes or neoplastic follicles
• Non-germinal center cell (activated B-cell) immunophenotype
  ○ B-cell antigens(+), cytoplasmic IgM(+), Bcl-6(+)
  ○ Bcl-2(+), IRF-4/MUM1(+), FOXP1(+)
  ○ CD10(-), CD138(-)

Primary Cutaneous Diffuse Large B-cell Lymphoma (PCLBCL), Other (Non-Leg Type)
• Includes DLBCL that does not fit with
  ○ PCLBCL leg type
  ○ PCFCL with diffuse large cells
  ○ Also encompasses T cell-rich large B-cell lymphoma and plasmablastic lymphoma
• Large neoplastic cells are admixed with inflammatory reactive infiltrate
• Phenotype may be germinal and non-germinal center type
• Lymphoma of adults with slightly better prognosis than PCLBCL leg type

Cutaneous Follicular Hyperplasia
• Lesions of variable ages; may be associated with
  ○ Insect or tick bites
  ○ Hair follicle inflammation
• Well-defined follicles with distinct germinal centers and mantle zones
  ○ Most follicles are in superficial dermis ('top heavy')
• Frequent tingible body macrophages
• Immunophenotype
  ○ Mixture of B cells and T cells; often in compartments
  ○ Germinal centers are Bcl-6(+), Bcl-2(-)
• No evidence of monoclonal *Ig* gene rearrangements

DIAGNOSTIC CHECKLIST

Clinically Relevant Pathologic Features
• FL confined to skin for at least 6 months upon staging

Pathologic Interpretation Pearls
• Grading is not recommended for PCFCL
• Lower frequency of t(14;18)/IgH-*BCL2* than in nodal FL

SELECTED REFERENCES

1. Koens L et al: IgM expression on paraffin sections distinguishes primary cutaneous large B-cell lymphoma, leg type from primary cutaneous follicle center lymphoma. Am J Surg Pathol. 34(7):1043-8, 2010
2. Dijkman R et al: Array-based comparative genomic hybridization analysis reveals recurrent chromosomal alterations and prognostic parameters in primary cutaneous large B-cell lymphoma. J Clin Oncol. 24(2):296-305, 2006

PRIMARY CUTANEOUS FOLLICLE CENTER LYMPHOMA

Differential Diagnosis of Primary Cutaneous Follicle Center Lymphoma

	PCFCL	Secondary FL of Skin	MZL	PCLBCL Leg Type	FH
Clinical Appearance					
	Erythematous plaques, nodules, or tumors	Nodular	Erythematous plaques or nodules	Multiple dome-shaped red tumors	Papules or nodules
Preferential Sites					
	Head and neck and trunk	Head and neck	Upper extremities, multiple sites	Lower extremities; unusual non-leg sites	Head and neck; upper extremities
Clinical Stage					
	Stage I	High stage	Stage I	Stage I with rapid progression to higher stages	NA
Histopathology					
	Follicular, follicular and diffuse, or diffuse; superficial or deep-seated	Follicular, follicular and diffuse, or diffuse; deep-seated in dermis or subcutaneous	Follicular or diffuse; superficial or deep-seated in dermis	Diffuse growth pattern only; deep in dermis and subcutaneous tissue	Follicular; upper dermis > deep dermis or subcutaneous
Lymphoid Follicles Appearance					
	Poorly defined germinal centers and attenuated mantle zones	Poorly defined germinal centers and attenuated mantle zones	Residual germinal centers colonized by monocytoid cells	Absent lymphoid follicular structures	Well-circumscribed lymphoid follicles with distinct germinal centers
Cell Type					
	Small centrocyte predominance; less centroblasts; grading not recommended	Centrocytes and centroblasts; grading is required	Mixture of small and monocytoid lymphocytes and plasma cells	Large centroblasts or immunoblasts; monomorphic	Mixture of small and large centrocytes, and centroblasts with tingible bodies
Useful Markers					
	Bcl-6(+), Bcl-2(dim +/-); CD10(+/-); CD21(+) meshworks; low Ki-67	Bcl-6(+), Bcl-2(strong +); CD10(+/-); CD21(+) meshworks; low Ki-67	Bcl-6(-), Bcl-2(+), CD10(-); CD21(+) FDC meshworks; monotypic plasma cells	IRF-4/MUM1(+), cIgM(+), FOXP1(+), Bcl-6(+), Bcl-2(+), CD10(-)	Bcl-6(+), Bcl-2(-); CD10(+); CD21(+) meshworks; high Ki-67
Cytogenetic or Molecular Markers					
	IgH R(+), Bcl-2 R(-/+), Bcl-6 R(-)	IgH R(+), Bcl-2 R(+), Bcl-6 R(+)	IgH R(+), Bcl-2 R(-), Bcl-6 R(-)	IgH R(+), Bcl-2 R(-), Bcl-6 R(-)	IgH R(-), Bcl-2 R(-), Bcl-6 R(-)
Prognosis					
	Excellent; local recurrences 30%; 95% 5-year survival	Variable; recurrences; 60-70% 5-year survival	Excellent; recurrences; ≥ 95% 5-year survival	Fair; 55% 5-year survival	Excellent; non-death related

PCFCL = primary cutaneous follicle center lymphoma; FL = follicular lymphoma; MZL = primary cutaneous marginal B-cell lymphoma; PCLBCL = primary cutaneous diffuse large B-cell lymphoma; FH = cutaneous lymphoid follicular hyperplasia; R = monoclonal gene rearrangements; NA = not applicable.

3. Hoefnagel JJ et al: Distinct types of primary cutaneous large B-cell lymphoma identified by gene expression profiling. Blood. 105(9):3671-8, 2005
4. Kim BK et al: Clinicopathologic, immunophenotypic, and molecular cytogenetic fluorescence in situ hybridization analysis of primary and secondary cutaneous follicular lymphomas. Am J Surg Pathol. 29(1):69-82, 2005
5. Kodama K et al: Primary cutaneous large B-cell lymphomas: clinicopathologic features, classification, and prognostic factors in a large series of patients. Blood. 106(7):2491-7, 2005
6. Willemze R et al: WHO-EORTC classification for cutaneous lymphomas. Blood. 105(10):3768-85, 2005
7. Goodlad JR et al: Primary cutaneous diffuse large B-cell lymphoma: prognostic significance of clinicopathological subtypes. Am J Surg Pathol. 27(12):1538-45, 2003
8. Goodlad JR et al: Primary cutaneous follicular lymphoma: a clinicopathologic and molecular study of 16 cases in support of a distinct entity. Am J Surg Pathol. 26(6):733-41, 2002
9. Mirza I et al: Primary cutaneous follicular lymphoma: an assessment of clinical, histopathologic, immunophenotypic, and molecular features. J Clin Oncol. 20(3):647-55, 2002
10. Aguilera NS et al: Cutaneous follicle center lymphoma: a clinicopathologic study of 19 cases. Mod Pathol. 14(9):828-35, 2001
11. Cerroni L et al: Primary cutaneous follicle center cell lymphoma with follicular growth pattern. Blood. 95(12):3922-8, 2000

PRIMARY CUTANEOUS FOLLICLE CENTER LYMPHOMA

Imaging and Microscopic Features

(Left) Positron emission tomography shows primary cutaneous follicle center lymphoma (PCFCL) involving the scalp ➡. A 4 units standard uptake value (SUV) was reported. Note the high activity elicited by the normal brain. *(Right)* Primary cutaneous follicle center lymphoma displaying a dense lymphocytic infiltrate in the dermis, sparing the subepidermal layer (grenz zone ➡). There are several ill-defined follicles ➡.

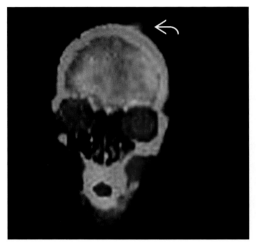
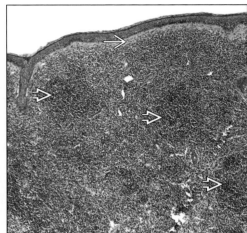

(Left) A case of PCFCL in which neoplastic follicles are composed predominantly of centrocytes ➡. There are no tingible body macrophages. This is the most common cell composition of PCFCL. *(Right)* PCFCL displaying a follicle with a predominance of large cells (centroblasts) ➡. Currently, the World Health Organization (WHO) classification recommends that PCFCL should not be graded. Similar features in a lymph node would warrant the designation of grade 3.

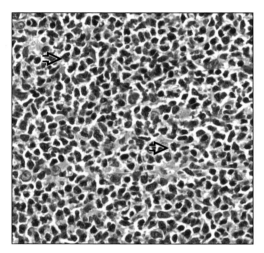
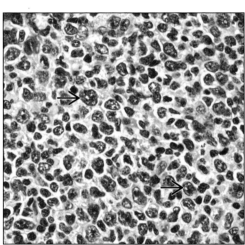

(Left) PCFCL composed of centrocytes ➡ and centroblasts ➡. This is the 2nd most common cell composition found in cases of PCFCL. *(Right)* In this case of PCFCL, reactive lymphocytes are strongly Bcl-2(+) ➡ whereas PCFCL cells are dimly Bcl-2(+) ➡. This pattern is opposite to that in nodal follicular lymphoma, where follicular lymphoma lymphocytes are strongly Bcl-2(+). PCFCL expresses Bcl-2 in ~ 60% of cases.

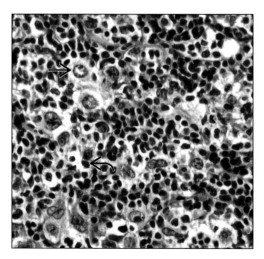
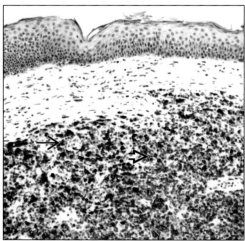

PRIMARY CUTANEOUS FOLLICLE CENTER LYMPHOMA

Microscopic Features

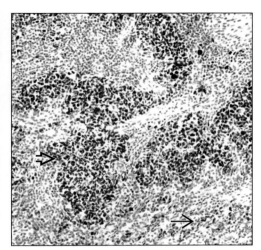
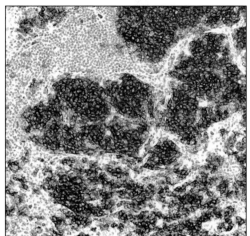

(Left) Primary cutaneous follicle center lymphoma (PCFCL). The neoplastic lymphocytes express Bcl-6, and the reactivity highlights irregular follicular structures ⮕. Note that Bcl-6 is strong in follicles and dim in diffuse areas ⮕. (Right) Primary cutaneous follicle center lymphoma (PCFCL). Anti-CD10 highlights a follicular pattern in this case. CD10 is usually reactive in PCFCL with a follicular pattern and tends to be negative in diffuse areas.

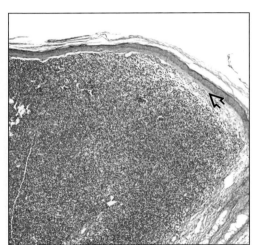
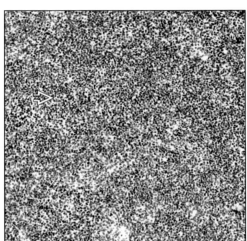

(Left) PCFCL displays a diffuse pattern, sparing the subepidermal layer (grenz zone ⮕). (Right) Primary cutaneous follicle center lymphoma displaying a diffuse pattern highlighted by immunohistochemistry for Bcl-6 ⮕. Bcl-6 is consistently expressed in cases of PCFCL whereas CD10 can be negative in diffuse areas.

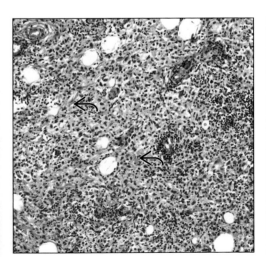
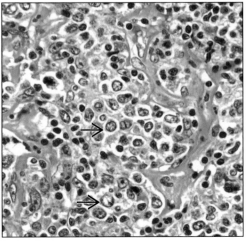

(Left) PCFCL displaying a diffuse pattern with sclerosis ⮕. Neoplastic cells are infiltrating among collagen fibers and adipose tissue. (Right) Primary cutaneous follicle center lymphoma. This area of diffuse growth is composed predominantly of large cells ⮕. The WHO classification recommends diagnosis as PCFCL and not as diffuse large B-cell lymphoma if an area of follicular pattern is detected elsewhere in the lesion.

Secondary Follicular Lymphoma of Skin

(Left) Secondary follicular lymphoma of the skin displays a deep-seated neoplastic follicle ⮆. Follicles deep in the dermis or subcutaneous tissue support the diagnosis of lymphoma but do not distinguish between primary and secondary follicular lymphoma. *(Right)* Secondary follicular lymphoma of the skin. In this case, the neoplastic follicles ⮆ are deep-seated. This field shows extensive infiltration of the nerve bundles ➡.

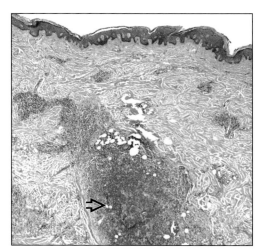
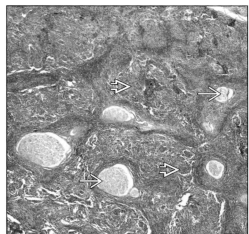

(Left) Secondary follicular lymphoma of the skin displays deep-seated neoplastic follicles ⮆ infiltrating the subcutaneous tissue ➡. *(Right)* Secondary follicular lymphoma of the skin displays deep-seated neoplastic follicles ⮆.

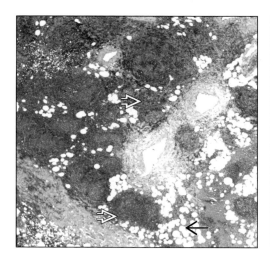
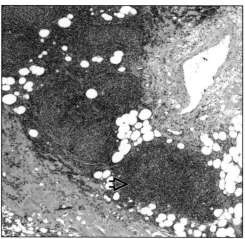

(Left) Secondary follicular lymphoma (FL) of the skin. CD21 immunohistochemistry highlights follicular dendritic cell meshworks within neoplastic follicles ⮆. The appearance of dendritic meshworks ranges from well-defined to remnant fibers. *(Right)* Secondary follicular lymphoma of the skin. Immunohistochemistry highlights strongly Bcl-2(+) follicular center lymphocytes ⮆, contrary to PCFCL where neoplastic lymphocytes may be dim positive.

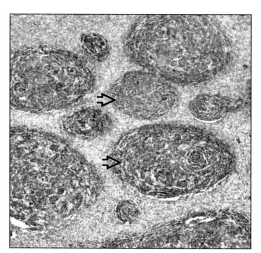
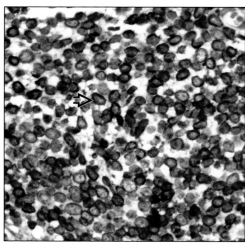

PRIMARY CUTANEOUS FOLLICLE CENTER LYMPHOMA

Cutaneous Marginal Zone B-cell Lymphoma

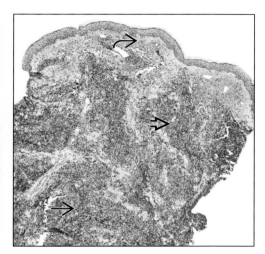

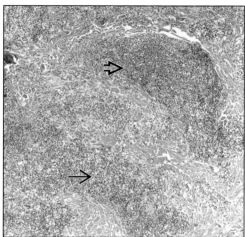

(Left) Cutaneous marginal zone B-cell lymphoma displays diffuse ⇨ and vaguely nodular ⇨ patterns. The lesion is deep in the dermis, and a grenz zone ⇨ separates the tumor from the epidermis. *(Right)* Cutaneous marginal zone B-cell lymphoma displays a vaguely nodular ⇨ pattern in the dermis. Diffuse areas ⇨ are common in cutaneous marginal zone B-cell lymphoma.

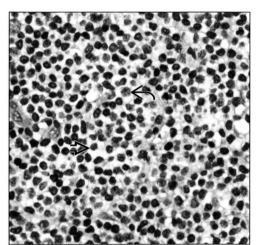

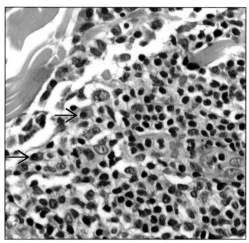

(Left) Cutaneous marginal zone B-cell lymphoma composed of monocytoid small lymphocytes characterized by slightly irregular nuclei surrounded by pale or clear cytoplasm ⇨. Scattered large cells ⇨ are also noted. *(Right)* Cutaneous marginal zone B-cell lymphoma displays focal plasmacytic differentiation. Plasma cells ⇨ are usually found at the advancing edge of the tumor or in the subepidermis and are often monotypic as shown by immunohistochemistry.

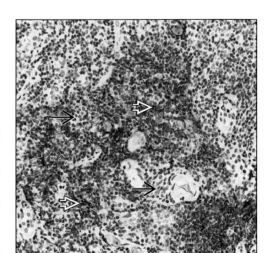

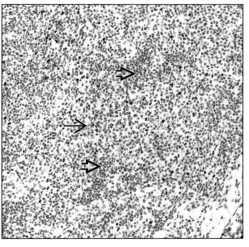

(Left) Cutaneous marginal zone B-cell lymphoma. CD21 immunohistochemistry highlights a disrupted follicular dendritic cell meshwork ⇨. This change is due to colonization of a reactive germinal center by neoplastic marginal zone lymphocytes ⇨. *(Right)* Cutaneous marginal zone B-cell lymphoma. Bcl-6 immunohistochemistry highlights residual follicular center cells ⇨ in a lymphoid follicle partially colonized by marginal zone lymphocytes ⇨.

PRIMARY CUTANEOUS FOLLICLE CENTER LYMPHOMA

Cutaneous DLBCL Leg Type

(Left) Cutaneous diffuse large B-cell lymphoma, leg type. The tumor is confined to the dermis and separated from the epidermis by a narrow grenz zone ⊡. The tumor appears monomorphic. (Right) Cutaneous diffuse large B-cell lymphoma, leg type. The tumor is monomorphic and composed of large cells. In this field, the neoplastic cells are immunoblasts with central prominent nucleoli ⊡. No centrocytes are noted, and reactive small lymphocytes are very scant ⊡.

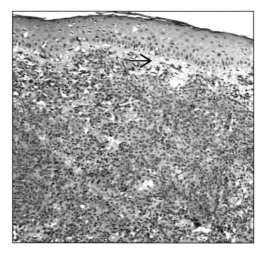
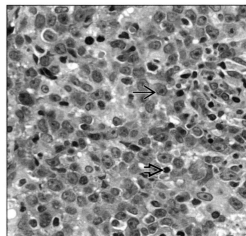

(Left) Cutaneous diffuse large B-cell lymphoma, leg type. CD20 immunohistochemistry highlights the presence of monomorphic large neoplastic cells ⊡. Note the scarcity of reactive cells, a feature characteristic of this tumor. (Right) Cutaneous diffuse large B-cell lymphoma, leg type. IRF-4/MUM1 immunohistochemistry shows that a subset (> 30%) of neoplastic cells ⊡ is positive, which is characteristic of this tumor and consistent with a non-germinal center phenotype.

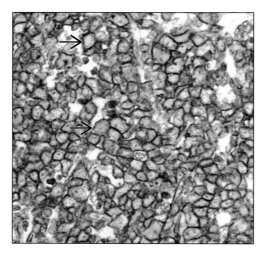
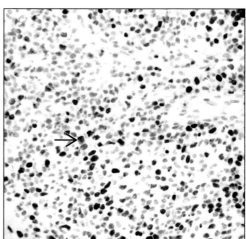

(Left) Cutaneous diffuse large B-cell lymphoma, leg type. Ki-67 immunohistochemistry shows that ~ 80-90% of the neoplastic cells ⊡ are positive, which is consistent with the high proliferation rate common in these tumors. (Right) Cutaneous diffuse large B-cell lymphoma, leg type. The neoplastic cells are CD10(-) ⊡, which is characteristic of this tumor and consistent with a non-germinal center phenotype. Rare stromal cells are positive ⊡.

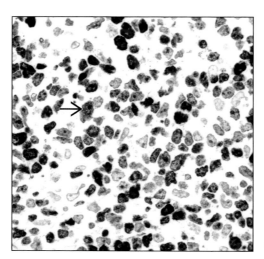
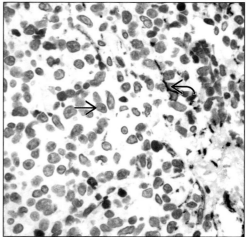

PRIMARY CUTANEOUS FOLLICLE CENTER LYMPHOMA

Differential Diagnosis

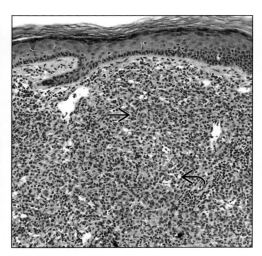
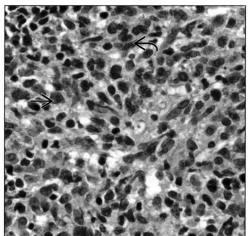

(Left) Cutaneous diffuse large B-cell lymphoma, other (non-leg type). The infiltrate appears polymorphic, with a mixture of large neoplastic cells ➡ and smaller neoplastic and nonneoplastic cells ➘. *(Right)* Cutaneous diffuse large B-cell lymphoma, non-leg type. In this diffuse infiltrate, the large neoplastic cells ➡ are admixed with intermediate-sized centrocytes ➘, and the infiltrate is polymorphic rather than monotonous.

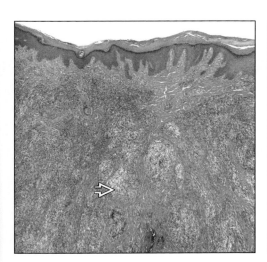
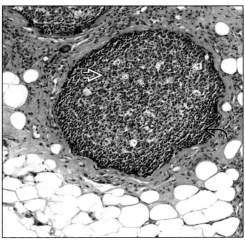

(Left) Reactive lymphoid hyperplasia of the skin. There is a dense dermal infiltrate with a nodular pattern ➡. This lesion appeared a few weeks after a tick bite. *(Right)* Reactive lymphoid hyperplasia of the skin. A representative deep-seated lymphoid follicle shows a reactive germinal center ➡ with tingible body macrophages and a distinct mantle zone ➘. This lesion appeared a few weeks after a tick bite.

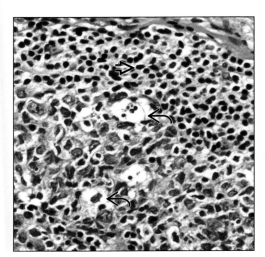
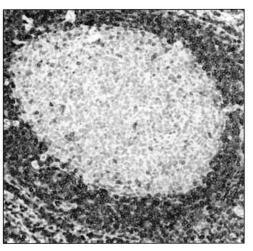

(Left) Reactive lymphoid hyperplasia of the skin. A prominent germinal center with tingible body macrophages ➘, surrounded by a distinct mantle zone ➘ is shown. This lesion appeared a few weeks after a tick bite. *(Right)* Bcl-2 immunohistochemistry in a reactive lymphoid follicle. Germinal center is negative for Bcl-2 and supports the morphologic impression of a reactive/nonneoplastic follicle.

PRIMARY MEDIASTINAL (THYMIC) LARGE B-CELL LYMPHOMA

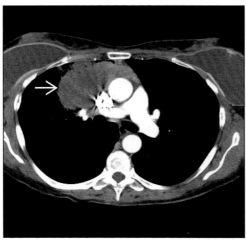

CT scan of a young woman who presented with a large anterior mediastinal mass ➡ shows an example of primary mediastinal large B-cell lymphoma (PMLBCL).

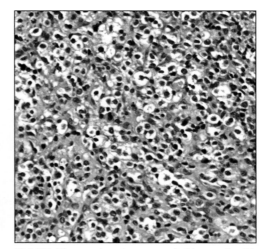

PMLBCL. The neoplasm is composed of large cells with pale cytoplasm (retraction artifact) and fine sclerosis compartmentalizing the tumor cells. The neoplastic cells were CD20(+) (not shown).

TERMINOLOGY

Abbreviations
- Primary mediastinal (thymic) large B-cell lymphoma (PMLBCL)

Synonyms
- Mediastinal large B-cell lymphoma
- Thymic large B-cell lymphoma

Definitions
- Diffuse large B-cell lymphoma (DLBCL) arising in mediastinum of putative thymic B-cell origin

ETIOLOGY/PATHOGENESIS

Cell of Origin
- Thymic B cell is presumed

CLINICAL ISSUES

Epidemiology
- Incidence
  - 2% of all non-Hodgkin lymphomas
- Age
  - Most frequent from 20-35 years
- Gender
  - M:F ratio = 1:2

Presentation
- Enlarging mass in anterior-superior mediastinum
- Often manifests as bulky disease defined as > 10 cm in diameter
  - ~ 75% of patients
- B symptoms in 20-30%
- PMLBCL patients have distinctive serum chemistry profile
  - Low serum β2 microglobulin and high lactate dehydrogenase (LDH) levels
- Locally aggressive with compression of contiguous organs
  - Superior vena cava syndrome occurs in up to 30% of patients
- Frequent infiltration of local structures and organs
  - Lung parenchyma, chest wall, pleura, and pericardium
- Extrathoracic disease at diagnosis is rare
- Bone marrow infiltration at presentation is also rare
- Extrathoracic sites are often involved at relapse
  - Central nervous system, liver, adrenals, ovaries, and kidneys

Treatment
- Drugs
  - Systemic chemotherapy is required; many regimens can be used
    - R-CHOP, rituximab, cyclophosphamide, hydroxydaunorubicin (doxorubicin), Oncovin (vincristine), prednisone
    - MACOPB, methotrexate, leucovorin, doxorubicin, cyclophosphamide, vincristine, prednisone, bleomycin
    - DA-EPOCH+R, etoposide, prednisone, vincristine, cyclophosphamide, doxorubicin plus rituximab
    - HyperCVAD-R, high-dose cyclophosphamide, vincristine, doxorubicin, cytarabine, methotrexate, rituximab
  - If risk factors are present, central nervous system prophylaxis is recommended
    - High-dose methotrexate therapy
- Radiation
  - Involved field therapy can be used for patients with bulky disease

Prognosis
- 60-70% chance of cure with appropriate therapy

PRIMARY MEDIASTINAL (THYMIC) LARGE B-CELL LYMPHOMA

Key Facts

Terminology
- Diffuse large B-cell lymphoma (DLBCL) arising in mediastinum of putative thymic B-cell origin

Clinical Issues
- Most frequent from 20-35 years
- M:F ratio = 1:2
- Enlarging mass in anterior-superior mediastinum
- Frequent infiltration of mediastinal structures and organs
- Prognosis is similar to patients with other types of DLBCL
  - 60-70% chance of cure with appropriate therapy

Microscopic Pathology
- Diffuse to vaguely nodular growth pattern usually associated with variable degrees of sclerosis
- Interstitial sclerosis with compartmentalization of tumor cells
- Hodgkin-like or Reed-Sternberg-like cells can be present

Ancillary Tests
- CD20(+), CD45/LCA(+), IRF-4/MUM1(+/-)
- CD30(+) ~ 75%, usually weak &/or focal
- CD10(-), CD15(-), Cyclin-E(-)
- Monoclonal *Ig* gene rearrangements

Top Differential Diagnoses
- Nodular sclerosis Hodgkin lymphoma
- B-cell lymphoma, unclassifiable, with features intermediate between DLBCL and CHL
- Diffuse large B-cell lymphoma
- T-lymphoblastic leukemia/lymphoma

  - Outcome similar to that of patients with nodal DLBCL
- Recurrences are almost always seen in 1st 2 years of follow-up

IMAGE FINDINGS

Radiographic Findings
- Large mass in anterior-superior mediastinum
- Often FDG-PET scan positive

MACROSCOPIC FEATURES

General Features
- Unusual for mass to be resected based on size and location
- In resection specimens, residual thymus gland may be identified
- Currently, diagnosis is often established by needle biopsy

MICROSCOPIC PATHOLOGY

Histologic Features
- Diffuse to vaguely nodular growth pattern usually associated with variable degrees of sclerosis
- Interstitial sclerosis surrounds and compartmentalizes small groups of tumor cells
- Broad collagenous bands divide tumor into large nodules
- Intermediate to large lymphoid cells
  - Pale cytoplasm, often result of retraction artifact
  - HRS-like cells can be present
- Reactive infiltrate of small T lymphocytes and histiocytes
  - ± plasma cells and eosinophils
- Thymic components, such as Hassall corpuscles, may be identified
  - If present, supports thymic involvement and diagnosis of PMLBCL

Cytologic Features
- Large lymphoma cells are present in fine needle aspiration smears
  - Not readily distinguishable from other types of large B-cell lymphoma
  - Extensive sclerosis can reduce yield of neoplastic cells aspirated

ANCILLARY TESTS

Immunohistochemistry
- Positive for common pan-B-cell markers
  - CD19, CD20, CD22, CD79a
- Positive for B-cell transcription factors
  - BOB1, OCT2, PU.1, pax-5
- CD45/LCA(+), p63(+) in ~ 95%
- CD30(+/-), in ~ 75% of cases
  - Expression is usually weak &/or focal
- IRF-4/MUM-1(+) in ~ 75%
- CD23(+/-), MAL(+/-)
- Bcl-2(+/-), Bcl-6(+/-); staining intensity can be variable
- CD10(-), CD15(-)
- T-cell antigens(-)
- EBV LMP is usually negative
- Cyclin-D1(-), Cyclin-E(-)

Flow Cytometry
- B-cell immunophenotype
- Discordance in B-cell receptor expression is common in PMLBCL
  - Surface Ig(-) and CD79a(+)
- Variable loss of HLA class I and II (HLA-DR) molecules

Cytogenetics
- Comparative genomic hybridization
  - Common regions of gain
    - Gains in 9p24 ~ 75% and 2p15 ~ 50%
    - Gains in chromosome X and in 12q31
    - *JAK2* at 9p24 is not mutated
  - Common regions of loss
    - 1p, 3p, 13q, 15q, and 17p

PRIMARY MEDIASTINAL (THYMIC) LARGE B-CELL LYMPHOMA

- Well-characterized chromosomal translocations are rare/absent in PMLBCL
  - *CCND1, BCL2, BCL6*, and *MYC*

In Situ Hybridization
- EBER(-)

Molecular Genetics
- Monoclonal *Ig* gene rearrangements
- No monoclonal T-cell receptor gene rearrangements
- High frequency of *BCL6* gene mutations
- *SOCS1* mutations in subset of cases
- High levels of expression of
  - IL-13 receptor
  - JAK2 and STAT1

Gene Expression Profiling
- Studies have shown overlap in gene expression profile between PMLBCL and classical Hodgkin lymphoma
  - Signature is distinct from nodal DLBCLs
    - Either germinal center B-cell or activated B-cell types

Activation of NF-κB
- Nuclear location of c-REL
- Cytoplasmic expression of TRAF1
- Combination of nuclear c-REL with expression of TRAF1 is highly specific for PMLBCL

DIFFERENTIAL DIAGNOSIS

Nodular Sclerosis (NS) Classical Hodgkin Lymphoma (CHL)
- Usually young patients
- Slight female predominance
- Mediastinal involvement in ~ 80%
- Histologic features
  - Nodular growth pattern with fibrosis
    - Dense collagenous bands surround nodules
    - Collagenous bands are polarizable
  - Variable numbers of large Hodgkin/lacunar and Reed-Sternberg (HRS) cells
  - Many inflammatory cells present
    - Eosinophils, neutrophils, plasma cells
- Many histologic variants of nodular sclerosis CHL have been described
  - Based on number of neoplastic cells, extent and nature of fibrosis, and inflammatory background
  - Syncytial variant is most relevant
    - Sheets of large HRS cells can mimic DLBCL
    - Often large areas of necrosis
    - Immunophenotype typical of CHL
- Immunophenotype of CHL
  - CD30(+), CD15(+/-)
  - pax-5 (+) with characteristic weaker (dim) expression than reactive B cells
  - CD20(-/+), CD79a(-/+)
    - Weakly &/or variably positive in 20% of cases
  - Other B-cell transcription factors absent or dimly expressed
  - CD45/LCA(-), EMA usually negative

- Small subset (~ 5%) of CHL can express T-cell antigens
- Molecular genetic features
  - Monoclonal *IgH* gene rearrangements (+)
    - Best detected by single cell PCR analysis
    - Can be positive by standard PCR methods in cases with many HRS cells
  - No evidence of monoclonal *TCR* gene rearrangements

B-cell Lymphoma with Features Intermediate Between DLBCL and CHL
- Lymphoma with clinical, morphologic, &/or immunophenotypic features between DLBCL and CHL
- Usually young patients
- Male predominance
- Mediastinum is most commonly involved
  - Supraclavicular lymph nodes can be involved
- Histologic features
  - Areas of confluent sheets of pleomorphic large tumor cells resembling DLBCL
  - Other areas can show scattered large cells resembling HRS cells in CHL
- Mixed immunophenotype
  - Expression of common markers of CHL
    - CD30(+) all cases &/or CD15(+/-)
    - pax-5(+) and IRF-4/MUM-1(+)
  - Expression of markers usually absent in CHL
    - CD45/LCA(+), CD20(+) uniform and strong, and C79a(+)
    - OCT-2(+), BOB1(+)
  - Cells with this "mixed immunophenotype" constitute predominant neoplastic cell population
- Molecular genetic features
  - Most cases have monoclonal *IgH* gene rearrangements
  - Few cases reported have *BCL6* rearrangements

Diffuse Large B-cell Lymphoma
- Older adults, but it also occurs in children and young adults
- Histologic features
  - Diffuse growth pattern
  - Large neoplastic cells (centroblasts &/or immunoblasts)
  - Large anaplastic cells can be present; known as anaplastic variant
    - These neoplasms may have intrasinusoidal growth pattern
    - CD30(+/-)
  - Large pleomorphic cells with features of HRS-like cells can be present
  - Sclerosis is frequent in extranodal sites
- Immunophenotype
  - CD19(+), CD20(+), CD22(+), CD79a(+)
  - pax-5(+), OCT2(+), BOB1(+)
  - CD10(+) and Bcl-6(+) in variable proportion of cases
  - CD30(-/+); if positive, often weak and focal except anaplastic variant
  - CD45/LCA(+), CD15(-)
  - Monotypic Ig(+)

- Cytoplasmic, in cases with plasmacytoid differentiation
  - Surface; best shown by flow cytometry
- Molecular genetic features
  - Monoclonal *IgH* gene rearrangements positive
  - t(14;18)(q32;q21)/*IgH-BCL2*(+) in ~ 20-30%
  - t(3;14)(q27;q32) or other partners with *BCL6* in ~ 20-30%
  - *MYC* translocations or gene rearrangements in ~ 10-15%
- Gene expression profiling has shown 2 subsets
  - Germinal center B cell
  - Activated B cell
    - This subset has poorer prognosis

T-Lymphoblastic Leukemia/Lymphoma
- Adolescents and young adults
- Male predominance
- High leukocyte count and bone marrow involvement common
- Large mediastinal mass in ~ 75% of patients
- Histologic features
  - Diffuse pattern
    - "Starry sky" appearance is present in 10-20% of cases
  - Small to medium-sized lymphoblasts with fine ("dusty") nuclear chromatin
  - High mitotic activity
  - Sclerosis can be present compartmentalizing lymphoma cells in groups
    - This feature can mimic PMLBCL
- Immunophenotype
  - Immature T-cell lineage
    - TdT(+) in almost all cases
    - Variable expression of CD1a, CD2, CD3, CD4, CD5, CD7, and CD8
    - CD34(+/-), CD99(-/+)
- Molecular genetics
  - Monoclonal T-cell receptor gene rearrangements
  - Monoclonal *IgH* gene rearrangements also common
    - Known as "lineage infidelity"

DIAGNOSTIC CHECKLIST

Clinically Relevant Pathologic Features
- Age: 20-35 years
- Gender: Female predominance
- Localization: Anterior mediastinum
- No systemic lymphadenopathy at presentation

Pathologic Interpretation Pearls
- Morphology: Sclerosis
- Immunophenotype characteristic
  - CD45/LCA(+), CD20(+)
  - CD30(+) variable and weak
  - IRF-4/MUM1(+/-), Bcl-2(+/-), Bcl-6(+/-)
  - EBV(-), CD10(-), T-cell markers(-)

Current Definition of PMLBCL is Problematic
- Criteria for diagnosis are in large part clinical in patients with DLBCL

- Location of disease
- Age and sex of patient
- Cases of nodal DLBCL can involve mediastinal lymph nodes
  - In small biopsy specimens, PMLBCL and nodal DLBCL can be indistinguishable
- In effect, this makes the category of PMLBCL somewhat impure
  - ~ 25% of all cases classified as PMLBCL may instead be nodal DLBCL
- Immunophenotypic or molecular makers that specifically recognize PMLBCL and can be assessed routinely in clinical laboratories are needed

SELECTED REFERENCES

1. Hoeller S et al: BOB.1, CD79a and cyclin E are the most appropriate markers to discriminate classical Hodgkin's lymphoma from primary mediastinal large B-cell lymphoma. Histopathology. 56(2):217-28, 2010
2. Pervez S et al: Mediastinal lymphomas: Primary Mediastinal (Thymic) Large B-cell Lymphoma versus classical Hodgkin lymphoma, histopathologic dilemma solved? Pathol Res Pract. Epub ahead of print, 2010
3. Salama ME et al: The value of CD23 expression as an additional marker in distinguishing mediastinal (thymic) large B-cell lymphoma from Hodgkin lymphoma. Int J Surg Pathol. 18(2):121-8, 2010
4. Faris JE et al: Primary mediastinal large B-cell lymphoma. Clin Adv Hematol Oncol. 7(2):125-33, 2009
5. Mottok A et al: Inactivating SOCS1 mutations are caused by aberrant somatic hypermutation and restricted to a subset of B-cell lymphoma entities. Blood. 114(20):4503-6, 2009
6. Zinzani PL et al: Rituximab combined with MACOP-B or VACOP-B and radiation therapy in primary mediastinal large B-cell lymphoma: a retrospective study. Clin Lymphoma Myeloma. 9(5):381-5, 2009
7. Rodríguez J et al: Primary mediastinal B-cell lymphoma: treatment and therapeutic targets. Leuk Lymphoma. 49(6):1050-61, 2008
8. Rodig SJ et al: Expression of TRAF1 and nuclear c-Rel distinguishes primary mediastinal large cell lymphoma from other types of diffuse large B-cell lymphoma. Am J Surg Pathol. 31(1):106-12, 2007
9. Weniger MA et al: Gains of REL in primary mediastinal B-cell lymphoma coincide with nuclear accumulation of REL protein. Genes Chromosomes Cancer. 46(4):406-15, 2007
10. Calaminici M et al: CD23 expression in mediastinal large B-cell lymphomas. Histopathology. 45(6):619-24, 2004
11. Pileri SA et al: Primary mediastinal B-cell lymphoma: high frequency of BCL-6 mutations and consistent expression of the transcription factors OCT-2, BOB.1, and PU.1 in the absence of immunoglobulins. Am J Pathol. 162(1):243-53, 2003
12. Lamarre L et al: Primary large cell lymphoma of the mediastinum. A histologic and immunophenotypic study of 29 cases. Am J Surg Pathol. 13(9):730-9, 1989

PRIMARY MEDIASTINAL (THYMIC) LARGE B-CELL LYMPHOMA

Radiographic and Microscopic Features

(Left) Chest radiograph shows a large mediastinal mass in this case of primary mediastinal large B-cell lymphoma. *(Right)* Primary mediastinal large B-cell lymphoma. Residual thymic tissue ➡ can be associated with PMLBCL ➡ in excisional biopsy specimens. The identification of thymic tissue is helpful as it supports PMLBCL and is evidence against systemic nodal diffuse large B-cell lymphoma at this site.

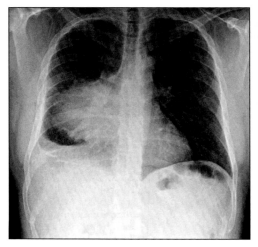
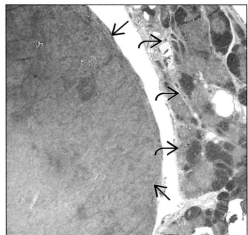

(Left) Primary mediastinal large B-cell lymphoma. The neoplasm has a nodular pattern with nodules partially surrounded by fibrosis ➡. The neoplastic cells were CD20(+), focally CD30(+), CD3(-), and CD10(-) (not shown). *(Right)* Primary mediastinal large B-cell lymphoma. This case is composed of a relatively homogeneous population of medium-sized tumor cells with scattered large and pleomorphic tumor cells ➡.

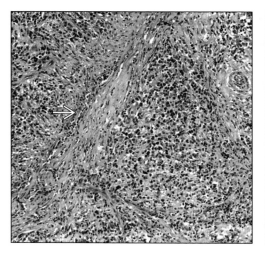
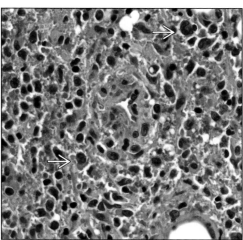

(Left) PMLBCL. Scattered large neoplastic cells are present in a background of small lymphocytes resembling T-cell/histiocyte-rich large B-cell lymphoma. In other areas, sheets of large tumor cells were present (not shown). *(Right)* Primary mediastinal large B-cell lymphoma. This case of PMLBCL is composed of medium-sized tumor cells with angulated nuclei and scattered large pleomorphic tumor cells ➡ in a background of interstitial fibrosis.

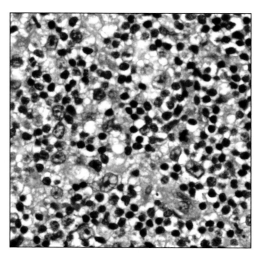
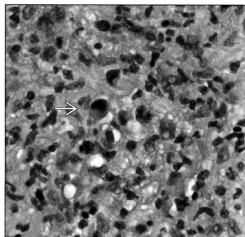

PRIMARY MEDIASTINAL (THYMIC) LARGE B-CELL LYMPHOMA

Microscopic Features

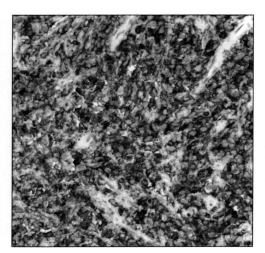

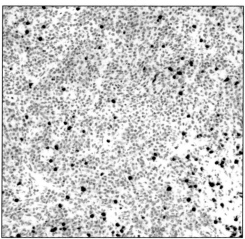

(Left) Primary mediastinal large B-cell lymphoma. The tumor cells are strongly and uniformly positive for CD20 as well as other B-cell markers (not shown). *(Right)* Primary mediastinal large B-cell lymphoma. The tumor cells are usually negative for T-cell markers, including CD3. PMLBCL are also usually negative for CD10, CD15, and EBER (not shown).

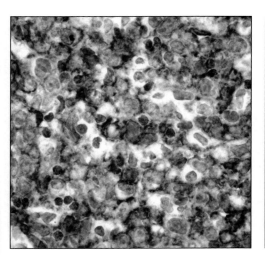

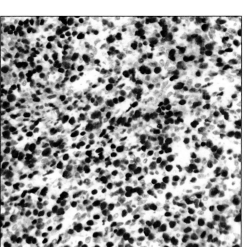

(Left) Primary mediastinal large B-cell lymphoma. The tumor cells in this case are focally and weakly CD30(+). The quality of this positivity is different from that found in classical Hodgkin lymphoma (bright and homogeneous). *(Right)* Primary mediastinal large B-cell lymphoma. The tumor cells in this case are brightly and uniformly IRF-4/ MUM1(+). This antigen is expressed in most cases (~ 75%) of PMLBCL.

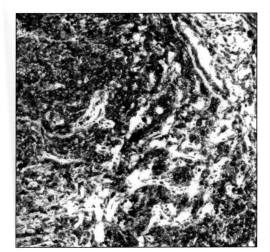

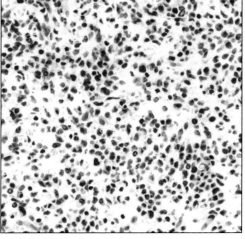

(Left) Primary mediastinal large B-cell lymphoma. The tumor cells are strongly CD45/LCA positive in this case. *(Right)* Primary mediastinal large B-cell lymphoma. The tumor cells are negative for TdT. TdT is positive in lymphoblastic lymphomas/leukemias of B- and T-cell lineages. T-cell lymphoblastic lymphoma/ leukemia typically occurs as a mediastinal mass, often with superior vena caval obstruction in adolescents and young adult men.

Microscopic Features

(Left) Primary mediastinal large B-cell lymphoma (PMLBCL). Needle biopsy specimen shows 2 cores of tissue. Needle biopsy, often performed with fine needle aspiration and flow cytometry immunophenotyping, is a very common method for establishing the diagnosis of PMLBCL. *(Right)* Primary mediastinal large B-cell lymphoma. This field shows abundant thin strands of sclerosis ➡ that partially surround and compartmentalize the neoplastic cells.

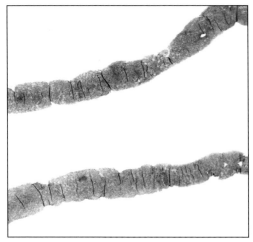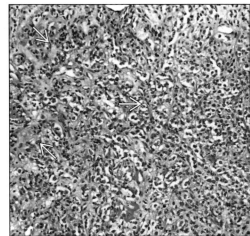

(Left) Primary mediastinal large B-cell lymphoma. In this field, the neoplastic cells are large and exhibit artifactual retraction of the cytoplasm imparting a clear appearance. A thin band of sclerosis ➡ is also present in this field. *(Right)* Primary mediastinal large B-cell lymphoma. The neoplastic cells are brightly CD20(+). CD20 expression in classical Hodgkin lymphoma is usually dim and variable, unlike the pattern shown here.

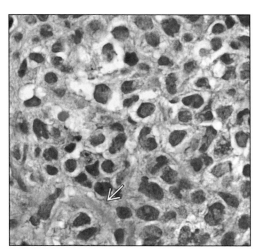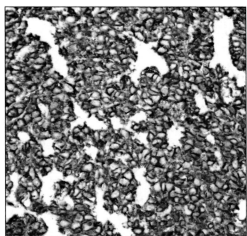

(Left) Primary mediastinal large B-cell lymphoma. The neoplastic cells are dimly CD30(+). This pattern of CD30 expression is common in PMLBCL and not seen in most cases of classical Hodgkin lymphoma. *(Right)* Primary mediastinal large B-cell lymphoma. The neoplastic cells are CD3(-). Small reactive T cells are CD3(+) and serve as an internal control for this immunostain.

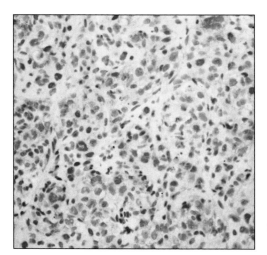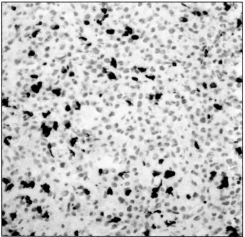

PRIMARY MEDIASTINAL (THYMIC) LARGE B-CELL LYMPHOMA

Differential Diagnosis

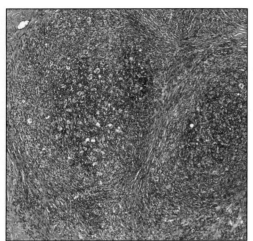

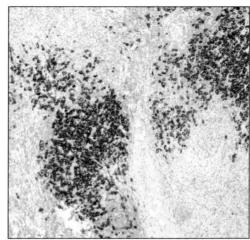

(Left) A case of nodular sclerosis Hodgkin lymphoma (NSHL). The neoplasm is nodular with nodules surrounded by collagen bands. *(Right)* Inside the nodules of NSHL, the large tumor cells are uniformly and strongly CD30(+) (shown). The neoplastic cells were also pax-5(+) and CD15(+), and were CD20(-) and CD45/LCA(-) (not shown). This immunophenotype supports the diagnosis of NSHL.

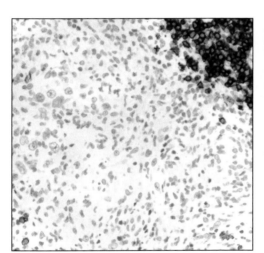

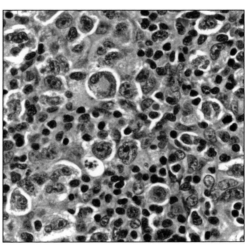

(Left) In classical Hodgkin lymphoma, tumor cells are characteristically negative for CD45/LCA. Note presence of reactive lymphoid cells (right upper corner) that are CD45/LCA(+). *(Right)* This case of syncytial variant NSHL shows sheets of large neoplastic cells with few eosinophils in the background. Note presence of many large pleomorphic tumor cells. Tumor cells were CD30(+), CD15(+), pax-5(+) and EBER(+), and CD3(-), CD20(-), and CD45/LCA(-) (not shown).

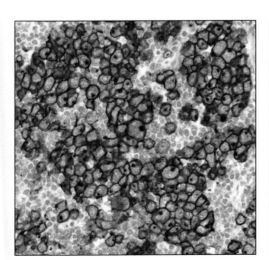

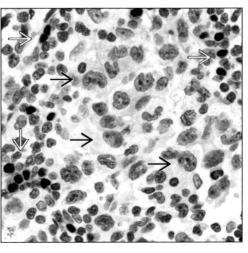

(Left) Syncytial variant of NSHL shows sheets of large neoplastic cells strongly and uniformly CD30(+). *(Right)* In classical Hodgkin lymphoma (CHL), the tumor cells are characteristically weakly positive for pax-5 ➔. Note the presence of reactive small B cells strongly pax-5(+) ➔.

PRIMARY MEDIASTINAL (THYMIC) LARGE B-CELL LYMPHOMA

Differential Diagnosis

(Left) A case of B-cell lymphoma, unclassifiable, with features intermediate between diffuse large B-cell lymphoma and classical Hodgkin lymphoma (DLBCL/CHL) is characterized by scattered large tumor cells with large eosinophilic nucleoli ➡ in a background of numerous small lymphocytes. *(Right)* This case of DLBCL/CHL shows areas of scattered large neoplastic cells in a background of small lymphocytes resembling CHL. In other areas, there are sheets of large tumor cells resembling DLBCL.

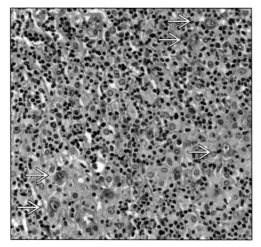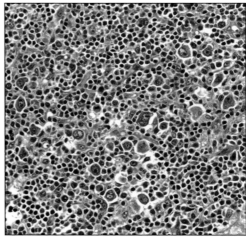

(Left) This case of DLBCL/CHL is composed of large and very pleomorphic tumor cells, some of which are multinucleated ➡. *(Right)* The tumor cells in this case of DLBCL/CHL are brightly CD20(+). Although CD20 may be weakly and focally positive in a subset of CHL, strong and uniform expression is unusual. This case also has diffuse areas of tumor cells resembling DLBCL.

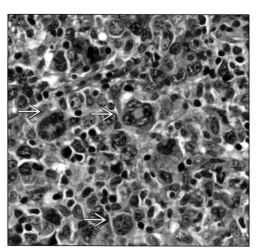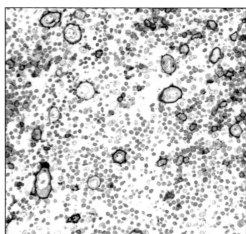

(Left) In this case of DLBCL/CHL, the tumor cells are brightly CD79a(+). CD79a is uncommonly expressed in CHL. This case also has diffuse areas resembling DLBCL. *(Right)* DLBCL/CHL shows focal positivity for CD30. Note that the tumor cells show variable degrees of CD30 expression, and the variable size of the neoplastic cells is also highlighted by CD30. CHL is usually characterized by a strong and uniform positivity for CD30. The tumor cells are also usually large in size.

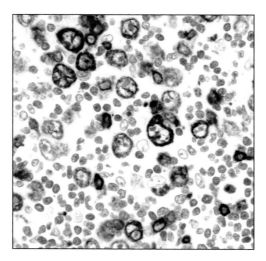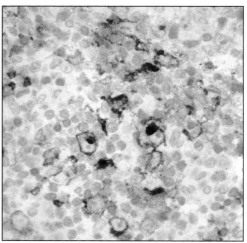

PRIMARY MEDIASTINAL (THYMIC) LARGE B-CELL LYMPHOMA

Differential Diagnosis

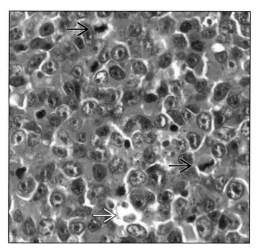

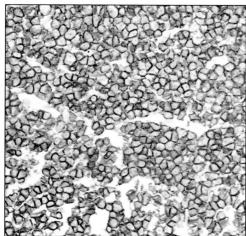

(Left) Diffuse large B-cell lymphoma (DLBCL), immunoblastic variant, shows large immunoblasts compared with the size of histiocyte nuclei ➡. Immunoblasts have a single, central, prominent nucleolus. Note the presence of several mitoses ➡. *(Right)* In this case of DLBCL, immunoblastic variant, the neoplastic cells are strongly CD20(+).

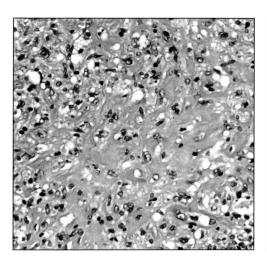

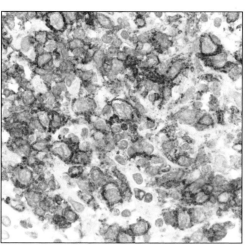

(Left) DLBCL, centroblastic variant, associated with marked sclerosis. The centroblasts are large with vesicular nuclear chromatin and cleaved nuclei. Sclerosis is frequently seen in cases of DLBCL involving extranodal sites. *(Right)* Nodal DLBCL, centroblastic variant, with large tumor cells that are CD10(+). PMLBCL is characteristically negative for CD10.

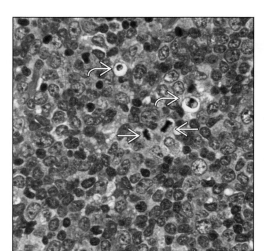

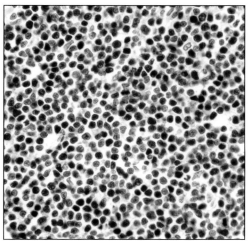

(Left) T-lymphoblastic leukemia/lymphoma is composed of lymphoblasts with irregular nuclear contours, fine chromatin (blastic appearance), small nucleoli, and a high mitotic rate. Note presence of several mitoses ➡ and apoptotic bodies ➡. *(Right)* TdT shows T-lymphoblastic leukemia/lymphoma. The lymphoblasts are usually TdT(+). Tumor cells also express T-cell antigens, such as CD1a, CD2, CD3, CD4, CD5, CD7, and CD8 in accord with their stage of differentiation.

PRIMARY DIFFUSE LARGE B-CELL LYMPHOMA OF THE CNS

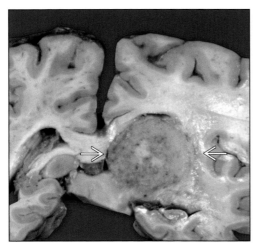

Gross photograph of brain involved by primary diffuse large B-cell lymphoma (DLBCL) demonstrates a well-circumscribed mass ➡ involving basal ganglia. The cut surface is heterogeneous and granular.

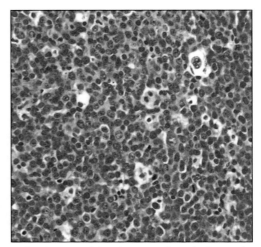

Diffuse large B-cell lymphoma involving the brain. The neoplasm has a "starry sky" pattern, indicating high proliferation and cell turnover.

TERMINOLOGY

Abbreviations
- Primary diffuse large B-cell lymphoma of CNS (DLBCL-CNS)

Synonyms
- Primary central nervous system lymphoma

Definitions
- Diffuse large B-cell lymphoma confined to central nervous system &/or intraocular location
- Immunocompromised patients are excluded from this category of disease
- Distinct entity in World Health Organization (WHO) 2008 classification

ETIOLOGY/PATHOGENESIS

Infectious Agents
- In immunocompetent patients, there is no etiologic relationship with known viruses

Origin of Lymphoma-initiating Cells
- Unknown; possibilities include
  - Benign systemic B cells entering CNS under physiologic conditions
  - Dissemination of systemic lymphoma
    - Extra-CNS disease eliminated by immune response, but lymphoma cells survive in immune-privileged CNS

Molecular Heterogeneity
- Features encompass spectrum of systemic DLBCL subtypes: Germinal center (GC) and activated B cell (ABC)
- Germinal center origin supported by following features
  - Immunophenotype: CD10 &/or Bcl-6(+)
  - Very high load of somatic mutations of *Ig* genes
    - Mutations ongoing
    - May be caused by reactive T cells and antigen-presenting cells in presence of unknown antigen
- ABC origin supported by following features
  - IgM expression
  - Lack of class switch recombination
  - Activation of NF-κB pathway
- Suggested pathogenesis
  - Lymphoma originates from germinal center B cells destined to become IgM-expressing memory B cells
  - Subsequent maturation steps blocked

Possible Transforming Events
- Chromosomal translocations
  - *BCL-6* gene at chromosome locus 3q27
    - Correlated with shorter overall survival
  - Recurrent *Ig* gene translocations
    - Present in ~ 15% of cases
- Ongoing aberrant somatic hypermutation (SHM)
  - Increased 2-5x compared with DLBCL
- 6q deletions
  - Correlated with shorter overall survival
  - *PRDM1* gene on 6q22–23 locus may function as tumor suppressor gene in subset of cases
    - Belongs to protein tyrosine phosphatase superfamily
    - Involved in cell contact and adhesion
    - Loss of protein expression in 76% of cases
- Gene inactivation by DNA methylation
  - *DAPK* or *MGMT*
  - *CDKN2A* (*P14ARF* and *P16INK4a*)
- Mutations of tumor suppressor genes
  - *MYC, PAX-5, PIM1, Rho/TTF*
  - Due to aberrant and ongoing somatic hypermutation

Other Factors
- Role of CNS microenvironment

PRIMARY DIFFUSE LARGE B-CELL LYMPHOMA OF THE CNS

Key Facts

Clinical Issues
- Neuropsychiatric signs and symptoms
- Raised intracranial pressure
- Intraocular involvement: blurred vision and floaters

Image Findings
- Single or multiple bilateral, symmetric, periventricular lesions
- Homogeneous contrast enhancement

Macroscopic Features
- Circumscribed masses; may be ill-defined infiltrates
- Gray; granular appearing; soft consistency

Microscopic Pathology
- Diffuse pattern; may be patchy
- Angiocentric and angioinvasive pattern
- High-grade centroblastic morphology

- Single-cell apoptosis and geographic necrosis
- Intermixed cells: Small reactive lymphocytes, reactive astrocytes, foamy histiocytes
- Corticosteroid effects
  - Extensive necrosis, sheets of macrophages

Ancillary Tests
- Pan-B-cell antigens(+)
- Bcl-6(+), IRF-4/MUM1(+), Bcl-2(+)
- Proliferation index (Ki-67) > 50%
- Monoclonal *Ig* gene rearrangements

Top Differential Diagnoses
- Primary DLBCL of CNS associated with HIV infection
- Primary intravascular lymphoma
- High-grade astrocytoma
- Poorly differentiated carcinoma

- Not known whether B cells enter CNS as benign reactive cells or as malignant lymphoma cells
- Extracerebral relapse rare
- Lymphoma cell angiotropism may be due to
  - Interactions between homing receptors and ligands expressed by CNS endothelial cells
- *IGHV4-34* gene segment shows preferential usage in DLBCL-CNS
  - Open reading frame maintained
  - CNS microenvironment may favor development of lymphomas with specific *Ig* genes; or
  - Neurotropic viruses or superantigens may elicit antibodies encoded by *IgHV4-34* gene segment
    - B cells may expand and persist in CNS

CLINICAL ISSUES

Epidemiology
- Incidence
  - Less than 1% of all non-Hodgkin lymphomas
  - Approximately 2-3% of brain tumors
  - Incidence is reported to be increasing
- Age
  - Median: 60 years
- Gender
  - Slight male preponderance
- Ethnicity
  - No ethnic predisposition

Site
- In descending order: Cerebrum, cerebellum, and brainstem
  - Supratentorial in 60% of patients
- Spinal cord in 1%
- Intraocular
  - ~ 20% of patients with DLBCL-CNS have intraocular involvement at diagnosis
  - ~ 80% of patients with intraocular lymphoma develop contralateral and parenchymal CNS lesions
  - Ocular disease may precede clinically detectable brain lesions

- Multifocal in 20-40%
- Extraneural sites rarely involved

Presentation
- Focal neurologic symptoms and signs in 50-80%
- Psychiatric symptoms and signs in 20-30%
- Seizures less frequent than in other brain tumors due to deep location
- Symptoms and signs of raised intracranial pressure in ~ 30%
- Asymmetric cranial neuropathies in leptomeningeal involvement
- Presents with intraocular involvement in ~ 5%
  - Blurred vision and floaters
  - Ocular slit-lamp examination
    - Lymphoma cells in vitreous or retina
- B symptoms (fever, night sweats, weight loss) rare

Laboratory Tests
- Human immunodeficiency virus (HIV) serology is negative in DLBCL-CNS
  - DLBCL-CNS in HIV(+) patients is considered as separate category
- Cerebrospinal fluid (CSF) analysis
  - Lymphoma cells identified by cytology in ~ 25% of cases
  - Assessment for B-cell clonality
    - Flow cytometry
    - PCR
- Serum lactate dehydrogenase (LDH) levels may be elevated
- Ocular interleukin (IL)-10 levels elevated in patients with ocular involvement

Natural History
- Disappearance of lesions ("ghost tumors") can occur
  - Rarely spontaneous
  - More often corticosteroid-induced

Treatment
- Options, risks, complications
  - Patients ≥ 60 years

PRIMARY DIFFUSE LARGE B-CELL LYMPHOMA OF THE CNS

- Tumors demonstrate low radiosensitivity
- High incidence of delayed neurotoxicity
- Radiotherapy (RT) may be deferred
  - Refractory disease
    - Intensive chemotherapy (ICT) with autologous stem cell transplantation (ASCT)
  - Salvage treatment
    - ICT–ASCT may be useful
    - 2nd-line chemotherapeutic agents
  - Primary intraocular lymphoma
    - Initial treatment similar to that for other DLBCL-CNS cases
    - Goal is to eradicate reservoir of disease in eye and decrease risk of recurrence
    - Dedicated ocular radiotherapy, intraocular chemotherapy
- Surgical approaches
  - CNS
    - Biopsy for pathologic diagnosis
    - Resection performed only for herniation due to mass effect
    - Median survival following surgery alone: 1-4 months
  - Ocular
    - Biopsy of vitreous, choroid, or retina for diagnosis
- Drugs
  - High-dose methotrexate (MTX)-based chemotherapy only as initial treatment
    - Highly chemosensitive tumor
    - Used infrequently
    - Combined with blood-brain barrier disruption
    - Delayed neurotoxicity less common
- Radiation
  - Whole-brain radiotherapy (WBRT) alone
    - DLBCL-CNS is usually radiosensitive
    - Microscopic diffuse lesions present even in radiologically localized disease
    - Delayed neurotoxicity frequent
    - Limited survival benefit
- High-dose MTX-based chemotherapy + WBRT
  - Median survival time: 2–4 years
  - 5-year survival rate: 20–40%
- Anti-CD20 antibodies (rituximab)
  - Direct intraventricular/intrathecal administration
  - May be useful for leptomeningeal and ocular disease
  - Intravenous rituximab used in combination with high-dose MTX-based chemotherapy

Prognosis

- Poor prognosis of DLBCL-CNS compared with patients with systemic DLBCL may be due to
  - Immune-privileged location
  - Intrinsic aggressive biologic behavior
- Several prognostic scoring systems proposed
  - International Extranodal Lymphoma Study Group prognostic index (0–5 scale)
    - Age, performance status, lactate dehydrogenase level, CSF protein, and involvement of deep structures
  - Nottingham/Barcelona score (0–3 scale)
    - Age, performance status, and extent of brain disease

  - Memorial Sloan Kettering Cancer Center prognostic score
    - Age and Karnofsky performance status score
- Ocular involvement is not independent risk factor
- Response to corticosteroids is favorable prognostic marker
- Bcl-6 expression reported to be associated with better prognosis

IMAGE FINDINGS

General Features

- Location
  - Single lesion in ~ 50%
  - Periventricular lesions common
  - Subependymal infiltration may be present
  - Spans corpus callosum occasionally
  - Leptomeninges involved in ~ 5%
  - Intraocular lesions in ~ 20%
- General considerations
  - CT and MR findings not specific
  - Findings overlap with inflammatory and infectious causes as well as with other brain tumors

MR Findings

- Contrast-enhanced MR modality of choice
- Homogeneous contrast enhancement
- Contrast-enhancing single (45%) or multiple (35%) focal lesions
- Ring enhancement in 5-10% of patients

CT Findings

- Contrast-enhanced CT if MR contraindicated or cannot be performed
- Homogeneous contrast enhancement
- Negative findings do not rule out diagnosis

Positron Emission Tomography (PET)

- 7% of patients demonstrate evidence of systemic disease with full-body scan in presence of
  - Negative full-body CT scans and bone marrow examination

MACROSCOPIC FEATURES

General Features

- White matter in brain parenchyma affected
- ~ 15% of cases involve leptomeninges
- Deep location
  - Periventricular
  - Corpus callosum
  - Leptomeninges in ~ 15% of cases
  - Subependymal extension in occasional cases
- Circumscribed masses usually; may be ill-defined infiltrates
  - Less circumscribed than metastatic carcinomas
  - Surrounding brain parenchyma relatively preserved
- Gray; granular appearing
- Soft consistency

PRIMARY DIFFUSE LARGE B-CELL LYMPHOMA OF THE CNS

MICROSCOPIC PATHOLOGY

Histologic Features
- Infiltrative pattern
  o Diffuse pattern with sheets of lymphoma cells
  o May be patchy
  o Poorly demarcated infiltrates merging into less cellular zones
- Perivascular pattern
  o Concentric rings around blood vessel walls
  o Angiocentric and angioinvasive pattern typical
  o Circumferential bands of reticulin
    ▪ Within and around vessels
    ▪ Alternate with rings of lymphoma cells
    ▪ May extend into surrounding parenchyma
- High-grade centroblastic morphology
- Neoplastic cells larger and rounder than in most glioblastomas
- Single-cell apoptosis and geographic necrosis prominent
  o No pseudopalisading as seen in glioblastomas
- Smaller cells with less pleomorphism in subset of cases
- Plasmacytoid features may be prominent
- Intermixed cells include
  o Small reactive lymphocytes
    ▪ May be prominent in some cases
  o Normal entrapped and reactive astrocytes
  o Activated microglial cells
  o Foamy histiocytes
- Lack microvascular proliferation
- Corticosteroid effect
  o Extremely lymphotoxic
  o Response lasts weeks to months; relapse inevitable
  o Marked apoptosis and extensive necrosis
  o Sheets of macrophages identified on biopsy
  o Definitive pathologic diagnosis may not be possible
  o Repeat biopsy may be necessary
  o Has been referred to as "ghost cell tumor" or "disappearing tumor"

Cytologic Features
- Lymphoma cells are dispersed
- Large nuclei; round nuclear contours
- Coarse chromatin; prominent nucleoli
- No nuclear molding as in metastatic carcinoma
- No fibrillary processes as in malignant astrocytoma

ANCILLARY TESTS

Frozen Sections
- Useful technique but with limitations
  o Loss of cytologic details
  o Nuclear angulation artifact
  o Cellular distortion
- Helpful features to differentiate from malignant astrocytoma
  o Patchy involvement
  o Angiocentric and angioinvasive pattern
  o Single-cell apoptosis more prominent
  o Nuclei larger, rounder; nucleoli more prominent
- Cytologic examination (i.e., squash preparation) helpful as complementary intraoperative technique

Immunohistochemistry
- B-cell antigens(+)
  o CD19, CD20, CD22
  o CD79a, pax-5
- CD10(+) in 10-20% of cases
- Bcl-6(+) in 60-80% of cases
- IRF-4/MUM1(+) in 90% of cases
- CD45/LCA(+), Bcl-2 usually (+)
- Proliferation index (Ki-67) usually high (> 50%)
- MALT1(+/-), Bcl-10(+/-)
- Myeloid-associated antigens(-)
- T-cell antigens(-)
  o CD3, CD5, CD43, CD45RO
  o Reactive T cells are interspersed within tumor
- EBV-LMP1(-)
- Simian virus (SV40[-]), HHV6(-), HHV8(-)

Flow Cytometry
- May demonstrate
  o Ig light chain restriction
  o ± aberrant immunophenotype
- Particularly helpful to confirm diagnosis in
  o Ocular specimen
  o CSF

Cytogenetics
- *BCL-6* locus (3q27) translocated in ~ 20%
- *Ig* gene translocations in ~ 15%
  o Most partners of *Ig* genes unknown
- 6q deletions in 60–75% (FISH)

In Situ Hybridization
- EBV small-encoded RNA (EBER)(-)

Array CGH
- 18q21 gains, including both *BCL-2* and *MALT1* genes, are very common genetic abnormality
  o Corresponds to activation of NF-κB pathway

Molecular Genetics
- Monoclonal *Ig* gene rearrangements
- No evidence of monoclonal *TCR* gene rearrangements
- *BCL-6* translocations
  o In ~ 20%
  o Numerous translocation partners
- *MYC* translocations infrequent (~ 5%)
- *BCL-2* translocations infrequent

Gene Expression Profiling
- Gene expression profile studies indicate specific signature distinct from systemic DLBCL

DIFFERENTIAL DIAGNOSIS

Primary DLBCL of CNS Associated with HIV Infection
- Long history and advanced stage of AIDS
  o Very low CD4(+) count
- Immunoblastic morphology common
- EBV(+) in 80-100% of cases

PRIMARY DIFFUSE LARGE B-CELL LYMPHOMA OF THE CNS

Post-transplant Lymphoproliferative Disorder (PTLD) Involving CNS
- CNS involved in ~ 5% of PTLD cases
- Median time from transplantation to diagnosis is 4.4 years
- Most commonly located in subcortical white matter of cerebri or basal ganglia
  - Often multifocal
- Imaging: Lesions enhance homogeneously or in ring-enhancing pattern
- Histologic findings
  - Usually monomorphic, angiocentric, and angioinvasive
  - Extensive necrosis common
- EBV(+) in most cases
- Median survival: ~ 50 months

Anaplastic Large Cell Lymphoma, ALK(+)
- Clinical features may mimic infectious or connective tissue disease
- Prominent reactive cellular infiltrate may suggest reactive condition
- ~ 75% of cases involve leptomeninges and dura in addition to brain parenchyma
- Hallmark cells, high proliferation rate
- Immunophenotype
  - T-cell antigens(+), CD30(+), ALK(+)
- Most patients with ALCL, ALK(+) of brain have rapidly fatal course

Intravascular Large B-cell Lymphoma
- Lymphoma cells infiltrate within lumina of small vessels, especially capillaries
- Minimal extravascular infiltration
- ± fibrin thrombi, hemorrhage, and necrosis
- Widely disseminated at diagnosis
- ± hemophagocytic syndrome and multiorgan failure

Solitary Plasmacytoma
- Rare intracerebral cases reported
- Most adjacent to dura
  - Imaging studies suggest meningioma
- Occasional cases are intrasellar
  - Imaging studies suggest pituitary adenoma
- Immunophenotype
  - CD138(+), Ig light chain restriction(+)

High-Grade Astrocytoma
- Tissue infiltration more marked
- Cell size smaller than DLBCL cells; more nuclear pleomorphism
- No angioinvasion identified

Poorly Differentiated Carcinoma
- Cells are cohesive; nuclear molding present
- Prominent nucleoli in adenocarcinoma
- No angioinvasion
- Sharp demarcation at interface with normal brain parenchyma
- Immunophenotype
  - Cytokeratins(+)
  - TTF-1(+) in metastatic lung carcinoma
  - Tissue-specific markers helpful in determining site of origin
    - e.g., thyroglobulin, PSA, calcitonin, carcinoembryonic antigen

Metastatic Melanoma
- Prominent nucleoli
- Hemorrhagic background common
- Melanin deposition should be diligently sought within neoplastic cells or macrophages
- Immunophenotype
  - S100(+), HMB-45(+), Melan-A(+), tyrosinase(+)

Demyelinating Disease
- Macrophage-rich lesion after steroid treatment may simulate demyelinating disease
- Imaging studies helpful

Idiopathic Inflammatory Lesions
- Dense lymphoplasmacytic infiltrate; ± mild atypia
- Immunophenotype
  - Mixed infiltrate with polytypic plasma cells

DIAGNOSTIC CHECKLIST

Clinically Relevant Pathologic Features
- Brain biopsy can be avoided if lymphoma cells identified in
  - CSF (~ 10-30% of patients)
  - Ocular vitrectomy (~ 40% of patients)

Pathologic Interpretation Pearls
- If lesion appears neoplastic, need to exclude other tumors
- If lesion appears lymphoid, need to exclude inflammatory lesions
- Lymphoma cells may be obscured by reactive T cells
- Diagnosis often made by stereotactic biopsy
  - Material may be limited or not representative
  - Frozen section should be performed to ensure tissue adequacy
  - Cytologic smears are very helpful in frozen section interpretation

SELECTED REFERENCES

1. Haldorsen IS et al: CT and MR imaging features of primary central nervous system lymphoma in Norway, 1989-2003. AJNR Am J Neuroradiol. 30(4):744-51, 2009
2. Montesinos-Rongen M et al: Primary lymphoma of the central nervous system: just DLBCL or not? Blood. 113(1):7-10, 2009

PRIMARY DIFFUSE LARGE B-CELL LYMPHOMA OF THE CNS

Microscopic and Immunohistochemical Features

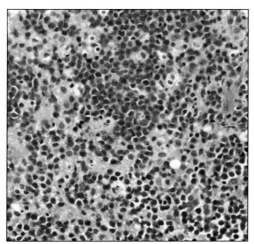

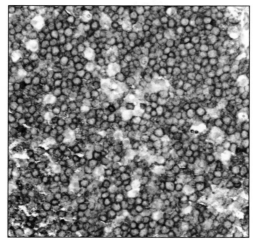

(Left) Brain biopsy of primary diffuse large B-cell lymphoma (DLBCL) demonstrates a diffuse infiltrate of intermediate to large atypical lymphoid cells with round to slightly irregular nuclei, moderately dispersed chromatin, occasionally prominent nucleoli, and scant to moderate amounts of cytoplasm. Frequent mitotic figures and apoptotic cells are identified. *(Right)* Brain biopsy of primary DLBCL demonstrates that the lymphoma cells are CD20(+) in a membranous pattern.

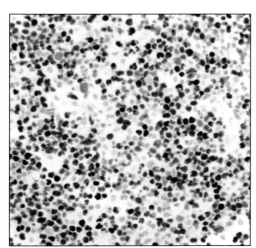

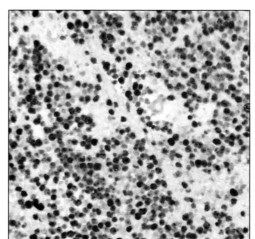

(Left) Brain biopsy of primary DLBCL of central nervous system (CNS) demonstrates that the lymphoma cells express Bcl-6 (nuclear stain). *(Right)* Brain biopsy of primary DLBCL of CNS demonstrates a proliferation index of 80-90% using Ki-67 antibody.

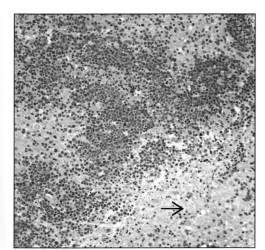

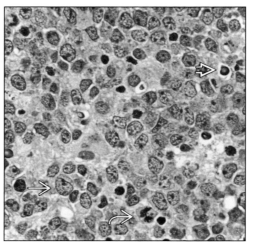

(Left) Brain biopsy of primary DLBCL of parietooccipital lobe demonstrates sheets of large atypical lymphoma cells and necrosis ➡. *(Right)* Brain biopsy of primary DLBCL of parietooccipital lobe demonstrates sheets of large atypical centroblastic lymphoma cells ➡. The cells are round to oval, have vesicular chromatin, 1-3 peripheral nucleoli, and abundant basophilic cytoplasm. Numerous mitotic figures ➡ and occasional apoptotic bodies ➡ are present.

Microscopic and Immunohistochemical Features

(Left) Biopsy of frontal lobe demonstrates primary diffuse large B-cell lymphoma (DLBCL) involving brain parenchyma. The atypical lymphoma cells are intermediate to large in size and show prominent perivascular distribution with numerous scattered isolated neoplastic cells ➡️ also present. *(Right)* Biopsy of frontal lobe demonstrates primary DLBCL involving brain parenchyma. The lymphoma cells express CD20 in a membranous pattern.

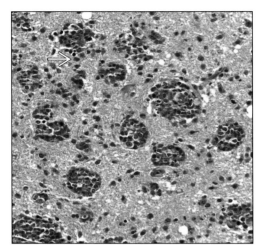 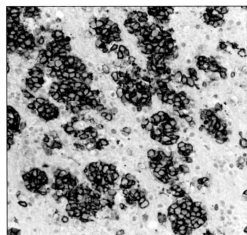

(Left) Brain biopsy of primary DLBCL of CNS involving a blood vessel demonstrates large atypical lymphoma cells with irregular nuclear contours and hyperchromatic nuclei infiltrating the vascular wall and occluding the lumen. *(Right)* Brain biopsy of primary DLBCL of CNS involving a blood vessel demonstrates that the large atypical lymphoma cells are CD20(+). The vascular outline is well demarcated.

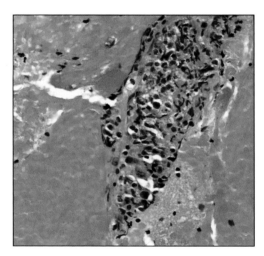 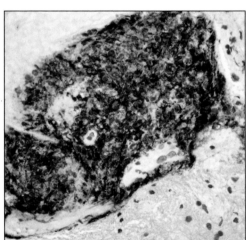

(Left) Brain biopsy of primary DLBCL of CNS demonstrates sheets of intermediate to large lymphoma cells ➡️ infiltrating brain parenchyma. Intermixed are scattered reactive small lymphocytes ➡️ and plasma cells ➡️ as well as reactive glial cells. *(Right)* Brain biopsy of primary DLBCL of CNS demonstrates that the large lymphoma cells express pax-5 (nuclear stain). The stain highlights nuclear pleomorphism ➡️. Numerous macrophages with bean-shaped nuclei are negative for pax-5 ➡️.

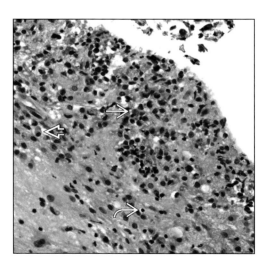 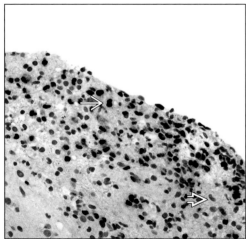

PRIMARY DIFFUSE LARGE B-CELL LYMPHOMA OF THE CNS

Microscopic and Immunohistochemical Features

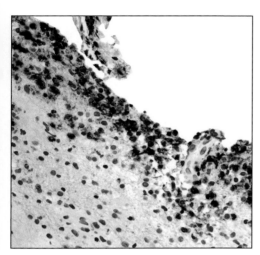
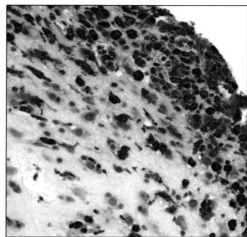

(Left) Brain biopsy of primary diffuse large B-cell lymphoma (DLBCL) of CNS demonstrates that the large lymphoma cells express CD20. *(Right)* Brain biopsy of primary DLBCL of CNS demonstrates a dense infiltrate of macrophages expressing CD68 that obscures the sheets of lymphoma cells.

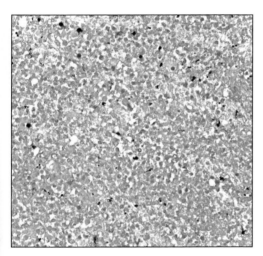
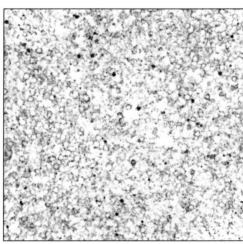

(Left) Brain biopsy of primary DLBCL of CNS demonstrates sheets of necrotic large cells with well-demarcated nuclear outlines as well as karyorrhectic debris. No viable tumor is present in this field. *(Right)* Brain biopsy of primary DLBCL of CNS demonstrates sheets of necrotic large cells expressing CD20. The CD20 antigen is often preserved in necrotic tissue and is very useful in determining the lineage of a necrotic tumor suspected of being a lymphoma.

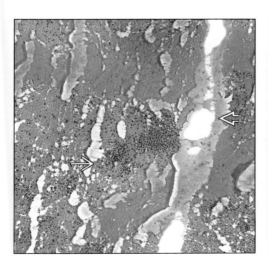
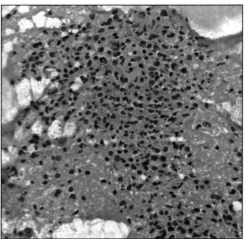

(Left) Brain biopsy (frozen section) of primary DLBCL of CNS demonstrates patchy sheets of atypical large lymphoma cells ➡ infiltrating the brain parenchyma. Note prominent edema ⇗ and hemorrhage contributing to the frozen artifact. *(Right)* Brain biopsy (frozen section) of primary DLBCL demonstrates sheets of atypical large lymphoma cells. The cells have irregular nuclear contours, heterogeneous chromatin, and distinct nucleoli.

PRIMARY DIFFUSE LARGE B-CELL LYMPHOMA OF THE CNS

Differential Diagnosis

(Left) Systemic diffuse large B-cell lymphoma (DLBCL) involving the brain. This field shows a diffuse infiltrate of intermediate to large atypical lymphoid cells with frequent mitotic figures ➡ and apoptotic cells ⇒ identified. *(Right)* Brain temporal lobe involved by systemic diffuse large B-cell lymphoma. The neoplastic cells in this case are CD10(+).

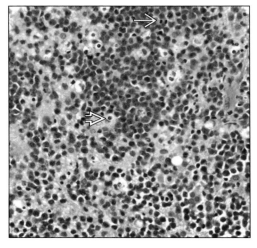
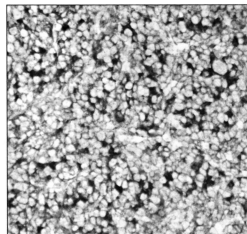

(Left) Brain temporal lobe involved by systemic diffuse large B-cell lymphoma. The neoplastic cells are Bcl-6(+) with a nuclear pattern of staining. *(Right)* Biopsy of splenium of the corpus callosum of brain involved by relapsed systemic DLBCL demonstrates sheets of atypical large lymphoid cells infiltrating white matter parenchyma in a patchy distribution. Prominent vascular cuffing ➡ is present.

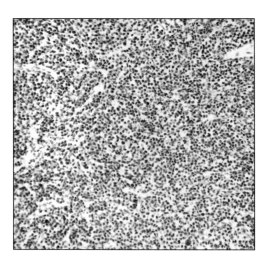
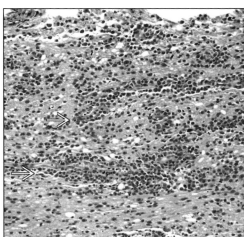

(Left) Splenium of the corpus callosum of the brain involved by relapsed systemic DLBCL demonstrates large atypical lymphoma cells with prominent centroblastic morphology surrounding a vessel. *(Right)* Splenium of the corpus callosum of the brain involved by relapsed systemic DLBCL involving the brain. The neoplastic cells express CD20 with prominent perivascular cuffing.

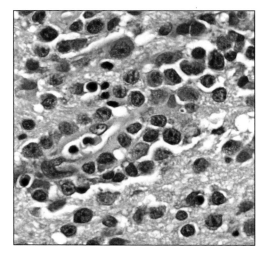
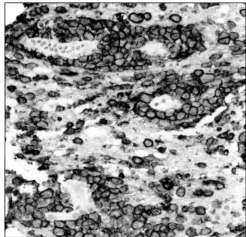

7

PRIMARY DIFFUSE LARGE B-CELL LYMPHOMA OF THE CNS

Differential Diagnosis

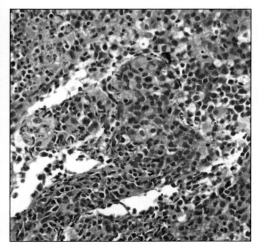

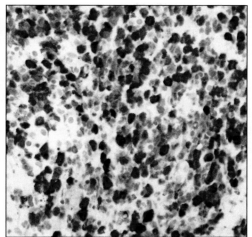

(Left) Anaplastic large cell lymphoma, ALK(+) involving brain. The neoplastic cells are intermixed with inflammatory cells and necrosis in this field. *(Right)* Anaplastic large cell lymphoma, ALK(+) involving brain. The neoplastic cells express anaplastic lymphoma kinase (ALK) in a nuclear and cytoplasmic pattern consistent with t(2;5) (p23;q35)/NPM-ALK.

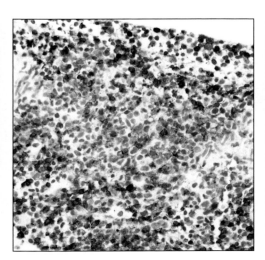

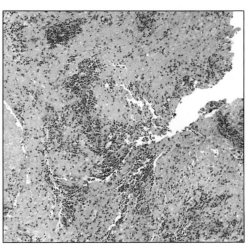

(Left) Anaplastic large cell lymphoma, ALK(+) involving brain. The neoplastic cells express CD2, supporting T-cell lineage. *(Right)* Polymorphic post-transplant B-cell lymphoproliferative disorder involving brain. The lesions were multifocal in this patient.

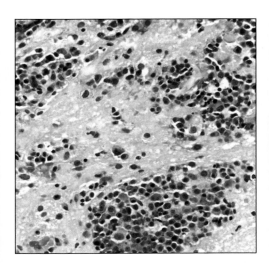

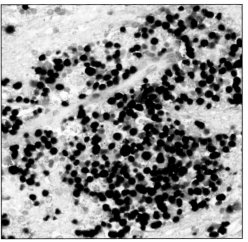

(Left) Polymorphic post-transplant B-cell lymphoproliferative disorder involving brain. This lesion is composed of small and large lymphoid cells, some with plasmacytoid features associated with histiocytes. *(Right)* Polymorphic post-transplant B-cell lymphoproliferative disorder involving brain. In situ hybridization shows that many cells are strongly EBER(+).

DIFFUSE LARGE B-CELL LYMPHOMA ASSOCIATED WITH CHRONIC INFLAMMATION

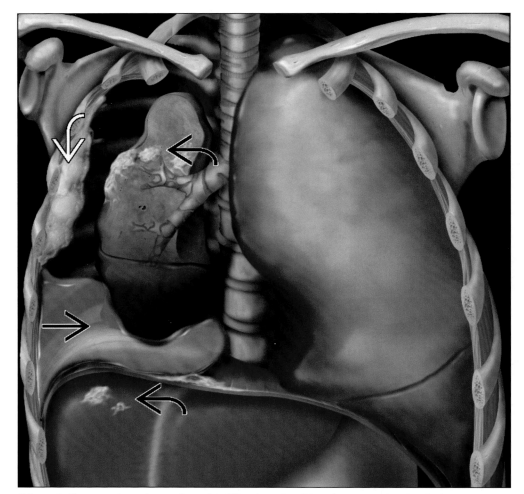

Schematic illustrates thorax in a patient with diffuse large B-cell lymphoma associated with chronic inflammation, also known as pyothorax-associated lymphoma (PAL). The neoplasm ⤳ involves the pleura and can encase the lung &/or invade locally into contiguous organs. Spread to the surface of lung and liver ⇲ is shown. A pleural effusion ⇥ is typically associated with the tumor. PAL occurs mainly in Japan and is highly associated with artificial pneumothorax, which was commonly used in Japan to treat patients with tuberculosis in the past. Typically, there is a long latency interval between artificial pneumothorax and onset of PAL.

TERMINOLOGY

Abbreviations
- Diffuse large B-cell lymphoma associated with chronic inflammation (DLBCL-CI)

Synonyms
- Pyothorax-associated lymphoma (PAL)
  - PAL is not true synonym but represents > 90% of cases of DLBCL-CI

Definitions
- DLBCL-CI is large B-cell neoplasm that occurs in context of longstanding chronic inflammation
  - Most cases occur in body cavities or narrow spaces
- Pyothorax-associated lymphoma (PAL)
  - Most common form of DLBCL-CI and prototype
  - Develops in pleural cavity of patients with longstanding pyothorax

ETIOLOGY/PATHOGENESIS

Infectious Agents
- Epstein-Barr virus (EBV) is present in most cases of DLBCL-CI reported
  - EBV(+) in type III latency pattern in most cases

Chronic Inflammation
- Chronic pyothorax precedes PAL type of DLBCL-CI in most cases
  - Very long latency period from onset of pyothorax until PAL
    - 19-67 years; median 43 years
- Other causes of DLBCL-CI are rare including
  - Metallic implants in bones and joints; surgical mesh implant
  - Chronic osteomyelitis; longstanding hydrocele
  - False cyst within spleen; atrial myxoma
- Causes of pyothorax in patients who develop PAL type of DLBCL-CI

DIFFUSE LARGE B-CELL LYMPHOMA ASSOCIATED WITH CHRONIC INFLAMMATION

Key Facts

Terminology
- DLBCL-CI is large B-cell neoplasm that occurs in context of longstanding chronic inflammation
  - Most cases occur in body cavities or narrow spaces
- Pyothorax-associated lymphoma (PAL) is most common and prototype

Etiology/Pathogenesis
- Chronic pyothorax precedes PAL type of DLBCL-CI
  - Very long latency period from onset of pyothorax until PAL
- Other causes of DLBCL-CI are rare and include
  - Metallic implants in bones/joints, surgical mesh implant, longstanding hydrocele
  - Chronic osteomyelitis; splenic false cyst, atrial myxoma

Clinical Issues
- Patients with PAL present with
  - Chest/back pain, tumor/swelling of chest wall
  - B symptoms, cough, dyspnea, hemoptysis
- Other types of DLBCL-CI can present incidentally

Microscopic Pathology
- Diffuse large B-cell lymphoma
  - Centroblastic, immunoblastic, or plasmablastic

Ancillary Tests
- Nongerminal center B-cell immunophenotype
- EBV(+), HHV8(-)

Top Differential Diagnoses
- Primary effusion lymphoma
- Systemic lymphomas involving body cavity lining

- Result of surgical use of artificial pneumothorax to treat pulmonary tuberculosis
  - Widely performed in Japan, especially from 1930s through 1950s
  - ~ 15-20% of patients with PAL have no history of artificial pneumothorax
  - Tuberculous pleuritis is another cause of chronic pyothorax
- Possible roles of chronic inflammation in pathogenesis
  - Generation of reactive oxygen species
  - "Local immunosuppression"
    - EBV(+) B cells can secrete various cytokines; e.g., interleukin-10 inhibits T-cell proliferation
    - Fibrosis surrounding area may limit access by cells involved in immunosurveillance
  - Autocrine growth
    - Interleukin-6 is autocrine growth factor that may be involved
- Patients with DLBCL-CI also may have systemic immunosuppression
  - Not obvious clinically in most patients but possibility not excluded

Possible Role of Gender
- PAL type of DLBCL-CI is much more common in men
  - Men have substantially worse prognosis
- Unknown if related to hormonal status, environmental factors, patient behavior, or genetic component

Genetic Factors
- PAL type of DLBCL-CI appears to arise from post-germinal center B cells, often with crippling *Ig* gene mutations
  - EBV may rescue cells from apoptosis (which would be expected physiologically)

CLINICAL ISSUES

Epidemiology
- Incidence

- Rare
  - Most cases of PAL type of DLBCL-CI are reported from Japan; rare in Western countries
  - 2% of patients with chronic pyothorax develop PAL in Japan
  - Non-PAL types of DLBCL-CI are exceptionally rare, mostly case reports
- Age
  - Adults
    - Median 65-70 years; range 29-88 years
- Gender
  - Marked male predominance
    - In various PAL studies, M:F = 8-12:1
  - Male predominance true in non-PAL types of DLBCL-CI
- Ethnicity
  - PAL type of DLBCL-CI most common in Japanese patients
    - In part, related to clinical practice (e.g., artificial pneumothorax)
    - Genetic factors also may be involved

Site
- Depends on underlying cause of DLBCL-CI
- Pleural cavity is most common
  - Invasion of contiguous lung, bone, soft tissues, mediastinum
- Other sites
  - Bones (especially femur) and periarticular soft tissue
    - Related to chronic osteomyelitis or metallic implants
  - Rare reported sites
    - Site of surgical mesh implant, splenic false cyst, atrial myxoma

Presentation
- Patients with PAL type of DLBCL-CI present with
  - Chest/back pain in ~ 50-60%
    - Shoulder, limb, or abdominal pain in smaller subsets of patients
  - ~ 40% present with tumor or swelling in chest wall
  - B symptoms, especially fever, in ~ 50%

DIFFUSE LARGE B-CELL LYMPHOMA ASSOCIATED WITH CHRONIC INFLAMMATION

- o Cough, dyspnea, or hemoptysis in ~ 25%
- o Lymph node or bone marrow involvement are uncommon at initial diagnosis
- o Leukemic phase is very rare
- Stage of PAL patients
  - o Stage I or II: ~ 70%
  - o Stage III or IV: ~ 30%
- Some patients with DLBCL-CI of non-PAL type are asymptomatic and detected incidentally
  - o Stage I
  - o No gross mass; only microscopic disease

Laboratory Tests
- Leukocytosis (> 10 x 10³/mm³) is frequent
- Elevated serum levels
  - o C-reactive protein (CRP)
  - o Lactate dehydrogenase (LDH)
- Mildly elevated serum neuron-specific enolase (NSE) in subset of patients
  - o Mechanism is unexplained

Natural History
- With progression, widespread disease dissemination can occur
- Sites of distant disease (in order of frequency)
  - o Lymph nodes (~ 45%)
  - o Contralateral lung (~ 19%)
  - o Liver, bones, or gastrointestinal tract (~ 13%)
  - o Central nervous system, skin, or bone marrow (~ 12%)
  - o Other sites (each < 10%)
    - ▪ Spleen, kidney, diaphragm, pancreas, heart, bladder, prostate, testes

Treatment
- Surgical approaches
  - o Complete surgical excision is effective in many PAL patients with localized disease
  - o Inadequate for high-stage disease
- Drugs
  - o Combination chemotherapy regimens for DLBCL
- Radiation
  - o Radiation therapy is often included in therapeutic regimen
- Incidental DLBCL-CI of non-PAL type
  - o No therapy other than excision may be needed in patients without gross disease

Prognosis
- Poor for patients with PAL
  - o 5-year survival ranges from 20-35%

IMAGE FINDINGS

PAL Type of DLBCL-CI
- Pleural-based mass seen by chest radiograph or CT
  - o Tends to be confined to thoracic cavity at time of diagnosis
  - o Size
    - ▪ < 5 cm: ~ 20%
    - ▪ > 5 cm: ~ 80%
    - ▪ Tumors can be massive (> 10 cm)

- Effusions commonly present

MACROSCOPIC FEATURES

General Features
- Pleural-based mass that can surround or locally invade lung

MICROSCOPIC PATHOLOGY

Histologic Features
- Diffuse growth pattern composed of sheets of large cells
- ± massive necrosis; ± angiocentric growth pattern
- High mitotic rate common

Cytologic Features
- Large cells can exhibit centroblastic or immunoblastic features
  - o ± plasmacytoid differentiation
  - o Rare cases exhibit anaplastic features

ANCILLARY TESTS

Immunohistochemistry
- Non-germinal center B-cell immunophenotype
  - o CD20(+), CD79a(+), pax-5(+), IRF-4/MUM1(+)
  - o CD10(-), Bcl-6(-)
  - o Cases with plasmacytoid differentiation can be CD138(+), monotypic Ig(+/-)
- Monotypic cytoplasmic Ig(+) in subset
- Evidence of EBV infection is very common
  - o EBNA-2(+), LMP1(+/-)
- CD43 commonly positive; Ki-67 usually high; ~ 70% up to 100%
- Pan-T-cell antigens usually negative, but rare cases show aberrant expression
  - o CD2, CD3, CD4, CD5, or CD7
  - o Aberrant expression may be related to immunosuppression
- CD30(-/+), CD33(-), CD34(-), CD56(-)
- Human herpesvirus 8 (HHV8)

Cytogenetics
- Complex karyotype common
- No recurrent chromosomal translocations identified

In Situ Hybridization
- EBER(+) in most cases

Molecular Genetics
- Monoclonal *Ig* gene rearrangements
- *P53* gene mutations in ~ 70% of PAL cases

Gene Expression Profiling
- Only PAL type of DLBCL-CI has been assessed
- PAL is distinct from nodal DLBCL
  - o 348 genes expressed with 2x difference between PAL and nodal DLBCL
    - ▪ 71 genes expressed with 5x difference

DIFFUSE LARGE B-CELL LYMPHOMA ASSOCIATED WITH CHRONIC INFLAMMATION

- ▪ Genes involved in apoptosis, signal transduction, and interferon response
  - ○ Very high interferon-α-inducible protein 27 (IFI27) in PAL
    - ▪ Induced in B cells by interferon-α stimulation
  - ○ Interferon-inducible protein 56 (IFI56) increased
    - ▪ EBV regulates this gene suggesting that EBV infection influences gene expression
  - ○ PAL has gene signature similar to nodal DLBCL of activated B-cell type

DIFFERENTIAL DIAGNOSIS

Primary Effusion Lymphoma (PEL)
- • Occurs in setting of immunodeficiency
  - ○ Human immunodeficiency virus (HIV) infection most common
- • Commonly presents as serous effusion without detectable tumor masses
  - ○ Small subset of tumors can present as solid masses in lymph nodes or other organs
    - ▪ Designated as extracavitary PEL
- • Neoplastic cells have immunoblastic, plasmablastic, or anaplastic cytologic features
- • All cases are associated with HHV8 infection
- • Immunophenotype
  - ○ CD45/LCA(+), CD138(+), EMA(+)
  - ○ Pan-B-cell markers(-), CD10(-), Bcl-6(-)
- • Coinfection with EBV very common

Systemic Lymphomas Involving Lining of Body Cavities
- • Variety of types of systemic lymphoma can involve lining of body cavities
  - ○ Stage IV disease; often associated with poor prognosis
  - ○ Tissue-based mass; effusion usually present
- • Diffuse large B-cell lymphoma (DLBCL) is most common type of B-cell lymphoma
  - ○ Pan-B-cell antigens(+), pan-T-cell antigens(-)
  - ○ CD10(+/-) and/or Bcl-6(+/-)
  - ○ EBV(-), HHV8(-)
- • Peripheral T-cell lymphoma NOS is most common type of T-cell lymphoma
  - ○ T-cell antigens(+); aberrant immunophenotype common

EBV(+) DLBCL of Elderly
- • Occurs in patients > 50 years without known immunodeficiency or prior lymphoma
- • Patients present with extranodal masses without involvement of body cavities
  - ○ Common sites: Tonsils, skin, lung, stomach
- • Neoplastic cells have immunoblastic &/or plasmablastic cytologic features
  - ○ 2 subtypes: Polymorphous and large B-cell lymphoma
- • Immunophenotype
  - ○ CD20(+), CD79a(+), CD45/LCA(+)
  - ○ IRF-4/MUM1(+/-), CD30(-/+), CD15(-)
  - ○ CD10(-), Bcl-6(-), T-cell antigens(-)

- • EBV(+)
  - ○ EBER(+) by in situ hybridization
  - ○ LMP1(+) and EBNA-2(-/+) by immunohistochemistry

DLBCL Arising in Periarticular Soft Tissues of Patients with Rheumatoid Arthritis
- • Affected patients have longstanding history of severe rheumatoid arthritis
- • Not associated with implants; do not involve body cavities; EBV(-)

Lymphomatoid Granulomatosis
- • Most commonly presents as bilateral lung nodules
  - ○ Nodules often have central necrosis and cavitation
- • Angiocentric and angiodestructive polymorphous lymphoid infiltrate
- • Does not involve body cavities
- • Immunophenotype
  - ○ Pan-B cell antigens(+)
- • EBV(+)

DIAGNOSTIC CHECKLIST

Clinically Relevant Pathologic Features
- • Occurrence in enclosed environment, such as pleural cavity or joint space
- • Longstanding history of chronic inflammation

SELECTED REFERENCES

1. Loong F et al: Diffuse large B-cell lymphoma associated with chronic inflammation as an incidental finding and new clinical scenarios. Mod Pathol. 23(4):493-501, 2010
2. Takakuwa T et al: Cell origin of pyothorax-associated lymphoma: a lymphoma strongly associated with Epstein-Barr virus infection. Leukemia. 22(3):620-7, 2008
3. Narimatsu H et al: Clinicopathological features of pyothorax-associated lymphoma; a retrospective survey involving 98 patients. Ann Oncol. 18(1):122-8, 2007
4. Vega F et al: Lymphomas involving the pleura: a clinicopathologic study of 34 cases diagnosed by pleural biopsy. Arch Pathol Lab Med. 130(10):1497-502, 2006
5. Aozasa K et al: Pyothorax-associated lymphoma: a lymphoma developing in chronic inflammation. Adv Anat Pathol. 12(6):324-31, 2005
6. Cheuk W et al: Metallic implant-associated lymphoma: a distinct subgroup of large B-cell lymphoma related to pyothorax-associated lymphoma? Am J Surg Pathol. 29(6):832-6, 2005
7. Nishiu M et al: Distinct pattern of gene expression in pyothorax-associated lymphoma (PAL), a lymphoma developing in long-standing inflammation. Cancer Sci. 95(10):828-34, 2004
8. Nakatsuka S et al: Pyothorax-associated lymphoma: a review of 106 cases. J Clin Oncol. 20(20):4255-60, 2002
9. Petitjean B et al: Pyothorax-associated lymphoma: a peculiar clinicopathologic entity derived from B cells at late stage of differentiation and with occasional aberrant dual B- and T-cell phenotype. Am J Surg Pathol. 26(6):724-32, 2002

DIFFUSE LARGE B-CELL LYMPHOMA ASSOCIATED WITH CHRONIC INFLAMMATION

Microscopic Features

(Left) Diffuse large B-cell lymphoma associated with chronic inflammation (DLBCL-CI) of PAL type. The large cells in this case were a mixture of centroblasts and immunoblasts. (Courtesy S. Nakamura, MD.) (Right) DLBCL-CI of PAL type with anaplastic cytologic features. This tumor was pax-5(+) and CD30(+) and aberrantly expressed T-cell antigens. (Courtesy S. Nakamura, MD.)

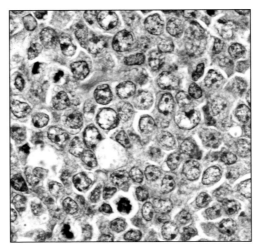 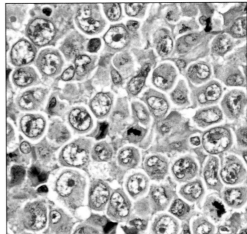

(Left) Diffuse large B-cell lymphoma associated with chronic inflammation (DLBCL-CI) of PAL type. Large areas of this neoplasm showed apoptosis &/or necrosis, as can be seen in this field. (Courtesy E. Drakos, MD, PhD.) (Right) DLBCL-CI of PAL type. In this case the neoplastic cells are large with relatively abundant, retracted cytoplasm due to fixation artifact or poor preservation. (Courtesy E. Drakos, MD, PhD.)

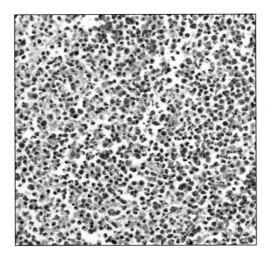 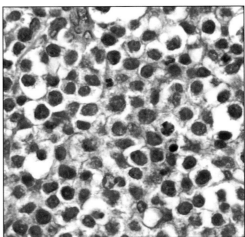

(Left) Diffuse large B-cell lymphoma associated with chronic inflammation (DLBCL-CI) of PAL type. The neoplastic cells are pax-5(+), supporting B-cell lineage. (Right) DLBCL-CI of PAL type. The neoplasm is EBNA2(+). Most cases of DLBCL-CI are EBV(+) with a type III latency pattern. (Courtesy S. Nakamura, MD.)

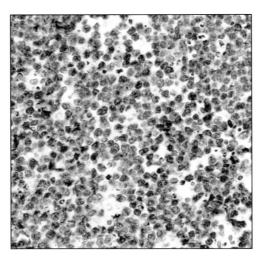 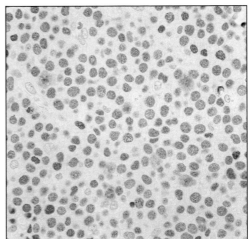

DIFFUSE LARGE B-CELL LYMPHOMA ASSOCIATED WITH CHRONIC INFLAMMATION

Differential Diagnosis

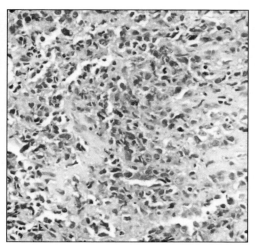
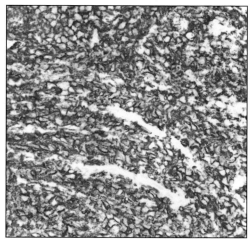

(Left) Systemic diffuse large B-cell lymphoma (DLBCL) involving the pleura. The neoplasm is associated with sclerosis. This patient had widespread disease and a pleural effusion with respiratory symptoms. (Right) Systemic DLBCL involving the pleura. The neoplastic cells are brightly CD20(+) supporting B-cell lineage.

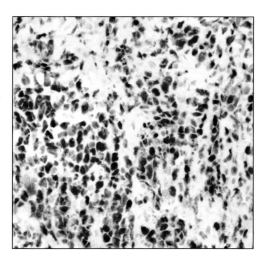
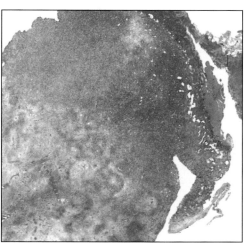

(Left) Systemic diffuse large B-cell lymphoma (DLBCL) involving the pleura. The neoplastic cells are Bcl-6(+) and were also CD10(+) (not shown) supporting a germinal center B-cell immunophenotype. (Right) Systemic peripheral T-cell lymphoma (PTCL) involving the pleura. This 43-year-old man presented with dyspnea, shoulder pain, a pleural-based mass, and increased eosinophils in the blood and bone marrow.

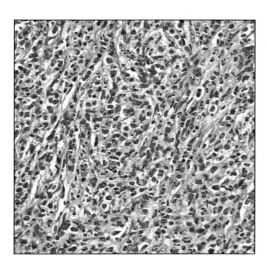
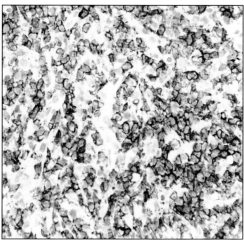

(Left) Systemic peripheral T-cell lymphoma (PTCL) involving the pleura. The neoplastic cells exhibit cytologic atypia, and there are many admixed eosinophils. (Right) Systemic PTCL involving the pleura. The neoplastic cells are CD43(+). These cells were also CD4(+) and CD45RO(+) (not shown) and carried monoclonal T-cell receptor γ-chain gene rearrangements.

PRIMARY CUTANEOUS DIFFUSE LARGE B-CELL LYMPHOMA, LEG TYPE

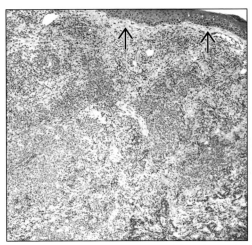

Primary cutaneous diffuse large B-cell lymphoma, leg type (PCDLBCL-LT). This field shows a diffuse infiltrate replacing the dermis with sparing of the epidermis ➡.

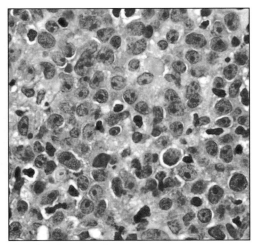

The lymphoma cells in PCDLBCL-LT are large and strikingly round with centrally located nucleoli (immunoblasts).

TERMINOLOGY

Abbreviations
- Primary cutaneous diffuse large B-cell lymphoma, leg type (PCDLBCL-LT)

Synonyms
- Primary cutaneous large B-cell lymphoma, leg type
- Primary cutaneous diffuse large B-cell lymphoma

Definitions
- Primary cutaneous diffuse large B-cell lymphoma composed exclusively of large transformed B cells
  - Often occurs in lower leg(s) but can arise at other skin sites

ETIOLOGY/PATHOGENESIS

Cell of Origin
- Peripheral B cell of post-germinal center cell origin
  - Immunophenotype: IRF-4/MUM1(+), FOXP1(+)
  - High frequency of somatic mutations of *IgH* variable (V)-region genes

Possible Role of Antigen Selection
- Preferential use of certain *IgH* V gene segments
  - Suggests that antigen stimulation may be involved in pathogenesis

Role of Molecular Abnormalities
- Number of genetic rearrangements and deletions reported
- No abnormality consistently present

CLINICAL ISSUES

Epidemiology
- Incidence
  - Rare
    - 4% of all cutaneous lymphomas
    - 20% of primary cutaneous B-cell lymphomas
- Age
  - Elderly patients; median age: 7th decade
- Gender
  - More common in women
    - Male to female ratio: 1:1.6; as high as 1:4 in some studies

Site
- Most cases arise in skin of lower leg; 1 or both legs
  - ~ 85% of all cases
- Subset of cases arise in skin of other sites (trunk, arms, head and neck)
  - ~ 15% of cases
  - Similar morphologic and immunophenotypic characteristics
- Single or multiple lesions at time of presentation
  - Some patients have dissemination at initial diagnosis

Presentation
- Red or blue-red lesions on skin
  - Plaque, verrucous plaques, or deep plaques
  - Nodular, tumoral lesions
  - Often associated with ulcer
  - Multiple lesions are common
- B symptoms in 10-20% of patients

Treatment
- Anthracycline-containing systemic chemotherapy plus rituximab (R-CHOP)
- Radiotherapy has role for localized lesions in elderly patients

Prognosis
- Relapse is common
- 40-50% 5-year survival rate
  - Factors adversely correlated with prognosis
    - Older age

PRIMARY CUTANEOUS DIFFUSE LARGE B-CELL LYMPHOMA, LEG TYPE

Key Facts

Terminology
- Primary cutaneous DLBCL composed exclusively of large transformed cells

Clinical Issues
- 20% of primary cutaneous B-cell lymphomas
- Most cases arise in skin of lower leg(s)
  ○ ~ 85% of all cases
- Subset of cases arise in skin of other sites (trunk, arms, head and neck)
  ○ ~ 15% of cases
- Single or multiple lesions at time of presentation
- Relapse is common; 50% 5-year survival
- Treated with systemic R-CHOP

Microscopic Pathology
- Diffuse pattern of involvement in dermis
- Monotonous sheets of large immunoblasts or centroblasts
- Few small reactive T cells in background
- No centrocytes (or small B cells) present
- No epidermotropism

Ancillary Tests
- Pan-B-cell antigens(+), Bcl-2(+), Bcl-6(+)
- MUM1(+), FOXP1(+), IgM(+), CD10(-)

Top Differential Diagnoses
- Primary cutaneous follicle center lymphoma
- Systemic DLBCL involving skin
- Plasmablastic lymphoma involving skin
- EBV(+) DLBCL of elderly
- Monomorphic post-transplant lymphoproliferative disorder

- Multiple lesions at presentation
- Inactivation of *CDKN2A*
○ Factors not correlated with prognosis
  - Duration of lesions before diagnosis
  - Gender, B symptoms, performance status or serum lactate dehydrogenase level
  - Bcl-2 or IRF-4/MUM1 expression

MICROSCOPIC PATHOLOGY

Histologic Features
- Diffuse pattern of involvement in dermis
  ○ Infiltrate can be deep
- Cohesive, monotonous sheets of large cells
  ○ Centroblasts or immunoblasts
  ○ Often very round nuclei
- Mitotic figures numerous
- Few small reactive T cells in background
- No centrocytes (or small B cells) present
- No epidermotropism

ANCILLARY TESTS

Immunohistochemistry
- Pan-B-cell antigens(+)
- Cytoplasmic IgM(+), IgD(+/-)
- Bcl-2(+), IRF-4/MUM1(+), FOXP1(+)
- Bcl-6(+), CD10(-)
- No follicular dendritic cell (FDC) meshworks
  ○ CD21(-), CD23(-), CD35(-)
- T-cell antigens(-), LMP1(-), HHV8(-)

In Situ Hybridization
- FISH often shows rearrangements of *MYC*, *BCL-6*, or *IgH* genes
  ○ No evidence of *IgH-BCL-2*/t(14;18) or *BCL-2* rearrangements
- EBER(-)

Array CGH
- Amplification of 18q21.31-33 involving *BCL-2* and *MALT1* genes

Molecular Genetics
- Monoclonal *IgH* gene rearrangements
- No evidence of *IgH-BCL-2*/t(14;18)

Gene Expression Profiling
- Profile is consistent with activated B-cell phenotype

DIFFERENTIAL DIAGNOSIS

Primary Cutaneous Follicle Center Cell Lymphoma (PCFCL)
- Most PCFCL have follicular pattern and can therefore be distinguished from PCDLBCL-LT
- PCFCL cases with diffuse pattern and predominance of large centrocytes or centroblasts are challenging
  ○ Used to be designated as diffuse large B-cell lymphoma (DLBCL)
    - However, clinically it is confined to skin, and prognosis is good
    - Could lead to over-treatment with multiagent chemotherapy
- Sites of skin involvement
  ○ Mostly in head and neck, trunk, back, arms
  ○ Some cases of PCFCL can present on leg
    - Patients with PCFCL on leg often have worse prognosis than patients with PCFCL at other sites
    - Prognosis of PCFCL of leg is similar to, or slightly better than, PCDLBCL-LT
- Histologic features of PCFCL
  ○ Areas of follicular pattern can be predominant, focal, or absent
  ○ Often, perivascular &/or periadnexal pattern in dermis is present
  ○ Mixture of centrocytes and centroblasts
    - Cells can be polylobated or spindle-shaped
  ○ Stromal reaction with fibrosis and sclerosis is common

PRIMARY CUTANEOUS DIFFUSE LARGE B-CELL LYMPHOMA, LEG TYPE

- Immunophenotype
  - CD10(+), Bcl-6(+)
  - Bcl-2 often negative; if positive, often weak and focal
  - FDC meshwork is present
    - CD21, CD23, CD35, or other markers
  - IRF-4/MUM1(-), FOXP1(-)
  - Small B cells/centrocytes positive (absent in PCDLBCL-LT)
  - CD3(+) reactive T cells relatively numerous (compared with PCDLBCL-LT)
  - Cases of PCFCL with diffuse pattern
    - CD10 often negative in areas of diffuse pattern
    - Residual FDC meshwork usually can be identified

Systemic DLBCL Involving Skin

- Systemic DLBCL can involve skin
  - Can be difficult to distinguish from PCDLBCL-LT based on morphology and immunophenotype
- Clinical history of systemic disease is key for differential diagnosis
- If patient has systemic and skin involvement at time of initial presentation
  - It can be difficult to distinguish systemic DLBCL from PCDLBCL-LT
  - Large tumors on lower leg(s) support PCDLBCL-LT

Plasmablastic Lymphoma Involving Skin

- Most patients have high-stage disease at time of presentation
  - Mucosal involvement is common
- Any skin site can be involved; leg uncommon
- Histologic features
  - Cohesive sheets of monomorphic plasmablasts can closely mimic PCDLBCL-LT
  - Some cases may show plasmacytic differentiation
- Immunophenotype
  - CD138(+), CD38(+)
  - Cytoplasmic monotypic Ig light chain (+)
  - EBER(+)

EBV(+) DLBCL of Elderly

- Cutaneous involvement can be initial presentation
- Histologic features
  - Tumor cells are often more polymorphic than PCDLBCL-LT
    - Plasmacytoid or plasmacytic differentiation positive
    - Large transformed cells, Reed-Sternberg-like cells
    - Background often has small lymphocytes, neutrophils, plasma cells, and histiocytes
  - Necrosis is common
- Immunophenotype is similar to PCDLBCL-LT; EBER(+)

Monomorphic Post-Transplant Lymphoproliferative Disorder (PTLD)

- Monomorphic PTLD can involve skin
- Histologic features
  - Tumor cells are often more polymorphic than PCDLBCL-LT
    - Plasmacytoid or plasmacytic differentiation positive
    - Large transformed cells, Reed-Sternberg-like cells

  - Necrosis is common, often with geographic pattern
- Immunophenotype is similar to PCDLBCL-LT; EBER(+)
- Clinical history of organ transplantation

DIAGNOSTIC CHECKLIST

Clinically Relevant Pathologic Features

- PCDLBCL-LT usually involves lower leg(s) but can present at other sites
  - Leg location is adverse prognostic factor

Pathologic Interpretation Pearls

- Diffuse involvement of dermis by sheets of round immunoblasts or centroblasts
  - Very few or absent small B cells
  - Relatively few reactive T cells (compared with PCFCL)
- Immunophenotype
  - Bcl-2(+), Bcl-6(+), MUM1(+), FOXP1(+), IgM(+)

SELECTED REFERENCES

1. Gokdemir G et al: Primary cutaneous diffuse large B-cell lymphoma of the leg, with an atypical clinical picture of verrucous plaques associated with stasis dermatitis. Clin Exp Dermatol. 35(3):e87-9, 2010
2. Guyot A et al: Combined treatment with rituximab and anthracycline-containing chemotherapy for primary cutaneous large B-cell lymphomas, leg type, in elderly patients. Arch Dermatol. 146(1):89-91, 2010
3. Koens L et al: IgM expression on paraffin sections distinguishes primary cutaneous large B-cell lymphoma, leg type from primary cutaneous follicle center lymphoma. Am J Surg Pathol. 34(7):1043-8, 2010
4. Perez M et al: Primary cutaneous B-cell lymphoma is associated with somatically hypermutated immunoglobulin variable genes and frequent use of VH1-69 and VH4-59 segments. Br J Dermatol. 162(3):611-8, 2010
5. Pham-Ledard A et al: IRF4 expression without IRF4 rearrangement is a general feature of primary cutaneous diffuse large B-cell lymphoma, leg type. J Invest Dermatol. 130(5):1470-2, 2010
6. Grange F et al: Primary cutaneous diffuse large B-cell lymphoma, leg type: clinicopathologic features and prognostic analysis in 60 cases. Arch Dermatol. 143(9):1144-50, 2007
7. Senff NJ et al: Reclassification of 300 primary cutaneous B-Cell lymphomas according to the new WHO-EORTC classification for cutaneous lymphomas: comparison with previous classifications and identification of prognostic markers. J Clin Oncol. 25(12):1581-7, 2007
8. Zinzani PL et al: Prognostic factors in primary cutaneous B-cell lymphoma: the Italian Study Group for Cutaneous Lymphomas. J Clin Oncol. 24(9):1376-82, 2006
9. Kodama K et al: Primary cutaneous large B-cell lymphomas: clinicopathologic features, classification, and prognostic factors in a large series of patients. Blood. 106(7):2491-7, 2005
10. Wiesner T et al: Genetic aberrations in primary cutaneous large B-cell lymphoma: a fluorescence in situ hybridization study of 25 cases. Am J Surg Pathol. 29(5):666-73, 2005
11. Grange F et al: Prognostic factors in primary cutaneous large B-cell lymphomas: a European multicenter study. J Clin Oncol. 19(16):3602-10, 2001

PRIMARY CUTANEOUS DIFFUSE LARGE B-CELL LYMPHOMA, LEG TYPE

Comparison of PCDLBCL-LT with PCFCL with Diffuse Pattern and Increased Large Cells

Parameter	PCDLBCL-LT	PCFCL with Diffuse Pattern and Increased Large Cells
Demographic Information		
Age	Older, 7th decade	6th decade
Gender	Female preponderance	Slight male preponderance
Sites of Involvement		
Location	Leg, 1 or both	Head and neck most frequent, followed by trunk or arms
	15% involving other sites, e.g., trunk, arm, head and neck	Rarely on leg, which has worse prognosis than PCFCL on other sites
	Multiple lesions common, some with deep plaques	Multiple sites of involvement are common
Risk for developing extracutaneous disease	~ 50%	~ 10%
Disseminated	~ 30%	~ 10%
Morphologic Features		
	Cohesive sheets of centroblasts or immunoblasts	Diffuse growth pattern with predominance of large centrocytes or centroblasts
	Cells often have strikingly round nuclei with many mitoses	Often cleaved, polylobated, irregular, or spindle-shaped
	No centrocytes (or small B cells) present	Often have admixed small centrocytes
Small reactive T cells	Very few, often in perivascular areas	Less pronounced, but more than PCDLBCL-LT
Epidermotropism	Not present	Not present
Perivascular/periadnexal	Not present	Often
Follicular dendritic cell (FDC) meshwork	Not present	Small broken clusters of FDC may be present
Immunohistochemistry		
Bcl-6	Mostly positive	Positive
Bcl-2	Positive ~ 90%	Often negative; if positive, often weak or focal
CD10	Negative	Often negative in diffuse areas; often positive in follicular areas
MUM1	(+, 50-80%)	Negative
FOXP1	Positive	Negative
IgM &/or IgD	Positive	Negative
Molecular Genetics		
	Similar to systemic DLBCL	Different from nodal follicular lymphoma
MYC, BCL6, and IgH rearrangement by FISH	Can be present	Often absent
Amplification of *BCL2* and *MALT1* genes	Can be present	Absent
Deletions of chromosome 9p21.3 (containing *CDKN2a* and *CDKN2b*)	Reported in 67% of cases	Absent
t(14;18)(q32;q21)	Absent	Reported in 10-40% of cases
Treatment		
	Anthracycline-containing chemotherapy plus rituximab	If single lesion, radiation therapy or surgical excision
	Radiation therapy for localized lesion in elderly	If multiple lesions, systemic chemotherapy may be used
Prognosis		
Relapse	Yes, frequent	Yes, ~ 30% of patients
5-year survival rate	50%	85-100%

PRIMARY CUTANEOUS DIFFUSE LARGE B-CELL LYMPHOMA, LEG TYPE

Microscopic Features

(Left) This case of PCDLBCL-LT almost completely fills the dermis. The neoplasm has a diffuse pattern with a grenz zone ⇨ between the neoplasm and the uninvolved epidermis. (Right) PCDLBCL-LT often appears confluent at low-power magnification. Small reactive T cells can be seen in 1 corner ⇒ of the field, but relatively few are admixed with the lymphoma cells.

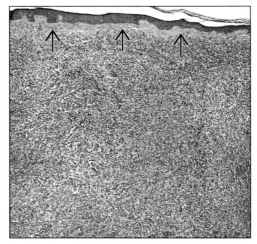
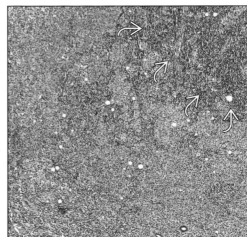

(Left) In PCDLBCL-LT, the lymphoma cells often have a striking round cell morphology and grow in sheets that appear cohesive. (Right) In this case of PCDLBCL-LT, the lymphoma cells are centroblasts that are very similar to each other, imparting a monotonous appearance.

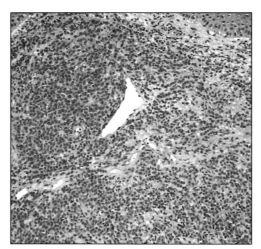
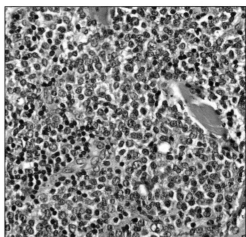

(Left) In this case of PCDLBCL-LT, the lymphoma cells are strongly CD20(+) and form cohesive-appearing sheets. The epidermis ⇨ is not involved, and a grenz zone is present ⇨. (Right) Most cases of PCDLBCL-LT are strongly Bcl-2(+), as shown in this case.

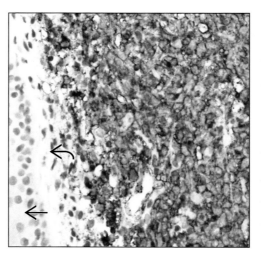
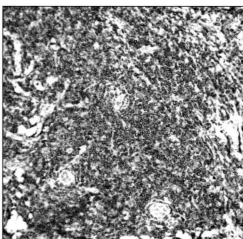

PRIMARY CUTANEOUS DIFFUSE LARGE B-CELL LYMPHOMA, LEG TYPE

Immunohistochemical Features of PCDLBCL-LT

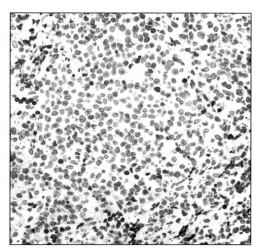
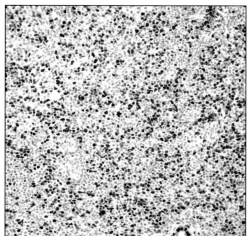

(Left) In PCDLBCL-LT, the lymphoma cells are usually CD10(-), consistent with a post-germinal center origin of lymphoma cells. (Right) In PCDLBCL-LT, the lymphoma cells are often Bcl-6(+).

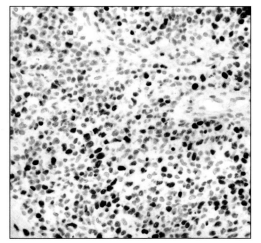
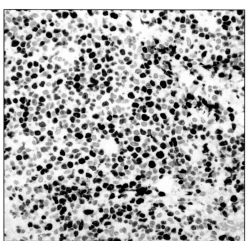

(Left) Approximately 50-80% of cases of PCDLBCL-LT are IRF-4/MUM1(+), a marker indicating a post-germinal center origin. (Right) In PCDLBCL-LT, Ki-67 shows a high proliferation fraction in lymphoma cells.

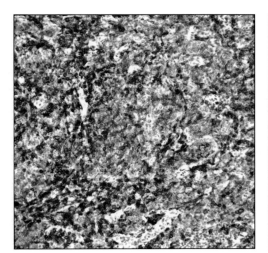
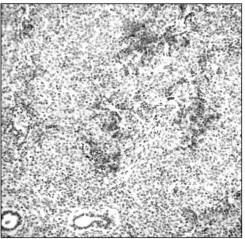

(Left) This case of PCDLBCL-LT is strongly CD23(+). A subset of these tumors is CD23(+), unlike primary cutaneous follicle center lymphoma. Also note that no CD23(+) follicular dendritic cells are present, confirming the presence of a diffuse growth pattern. (Right) In this case of PCDLBCL-LT, a CD21 immunostain does not highlight any follicular dendritic cells, supporting a diffuse growth pattern. A small subset of lymphoma cells is CD21(+) in this field.

Differential Diagnosis

(Left) Primary cutaneous follicular center cell lymphoma with a diffuse pattern. The lymphoma cells spare the epidermis, leaving a grenz zone ➡. *(Right)* This case of PCFCL also shows a predominance of large cells. In contrast with PCDLBCL-LT, the tumor cells are cleaved, polylobated, irregular, spindle-shaped (large centrocytes and centroblasts), and admixed with many small lymphocytes.

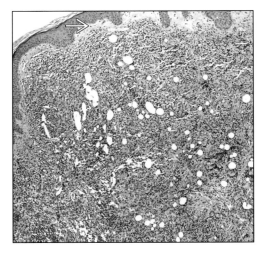
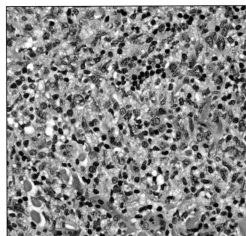

(Left) PCFCL with a predominance of large cells. The infiltrate appears to be noncohesive and is associated with stromal reaction, unlike cases of PCDLBCL-LT. *(Right)* PCFCL often shows vascular invasion or has a perivascular pattern of infiltration. These features are uncommon in PCDLBCL-LT.

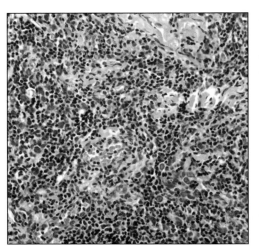
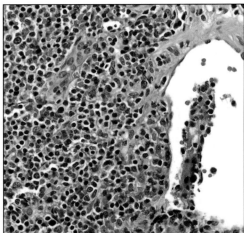

(Left) This case of PCFCL with a diffuse pattern was CD10(-). It needs to be remembered that CD10 is commonly expressed in follicular areas but can be negative in diffuse areas of PCFCL. *(Right)* Many cases of PCFCL are negative for Bcl-2. In some cases of PCFCL, the lymphoma cells can be Bcl-2(+), but expression is often weak or present in only a subset of cells, as shown in this field. Small reactive T cells are strongly Bcl-2(+).

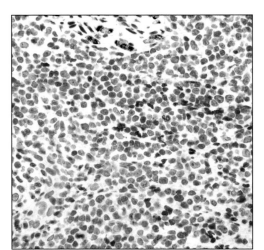
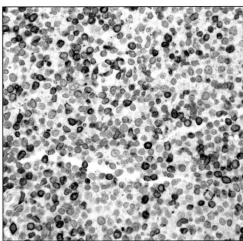

PRIMARY CUTANEOUS DIFFUSE LARGE B-CELL LYMPHOMA, LEG TYPE

Differential Diagnosis

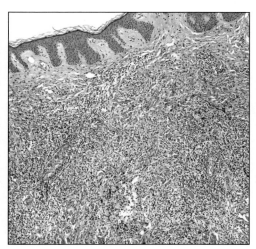
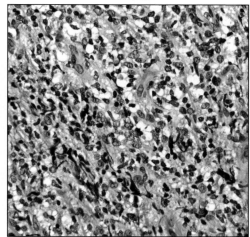

(Left) A case of primary mediastinal (thymic) large B-cell lymphoma disseminated to skin. The pattern of infiltration mimics primary cutaneous lymphoma under low-power magnification. *(Right)* Primary mediastinal (thymic) large B-cell lymphoma disseminated to skin. The lymphoma cells are polylobated and spindle-shaped.

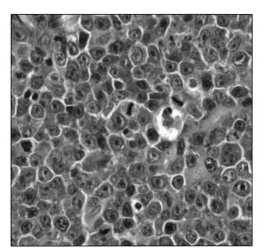
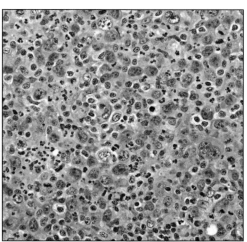

(Left) A case of systemic diffuse large B-cell lymphoma, immunoblastic variant, involving the skin. The lymphoma cells resemble the immunoblasts observed in some cases of PCDLBCL-LT. *(Right)* EBV(+) diffuse large B-cell lymphoma of the elderly involving skin. The lymphoma cells are large and polymorphous, with Reed-Sternberg-like cells and plasmacytoid cells. Many neutrophils as well as eosinophils are present in the background.

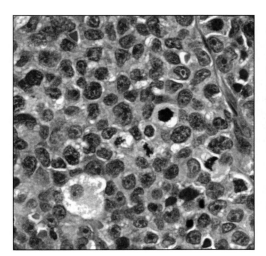
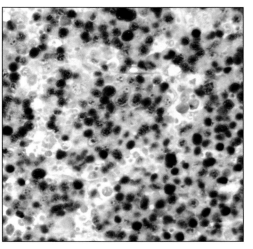

(Left) Plasmablastic lymphoma involving the skin. Plasmablastic lymphoma usually shows a cohesive proliferation of plasmablasts or immunoblasts, and these features overlap with PCDLBCL-LT. *(Right)* Plasmablastic lymphoma involving the skin. In situ hybridization for Epstein-Barr virus small-encoded RNA (EBER) is usually positive in plasmablastic lymphoma, unlike in PCDLBCL-LT.

PLASMABLASTIC LYMPHOMA

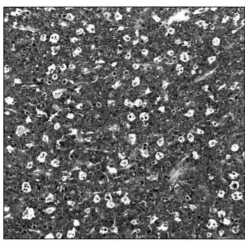

This case of plasmablastic lymphoma (PBL) is characterized by diffuse infiltrate of large atypical lymphoid cells with a "starry sky" pattern.

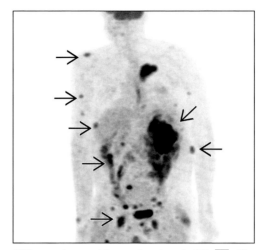

PET scan shows widespread metastatic PBL ➡. The patient was HIV positive and initially presented with PBL of the left jaw.

TERMINOLOGY

Abbreviations
- Plasmablastic lymphoma (PBL)

Definitions
- PBL was initially described as rare variant of diffuse large B-cell lymphoma (DLBCL) involving oral cavity
  - 15 of 16 patients were immunodeficient as a result of human immunodeficiency virus (HIV) infection
- PBL is currently defined as diffuse proliferation of large neoplastic cells
  - Immunoblastic or plasmablastic cytologic features
  - Plasma cell immunophenotype: CD38(+), CD138(+), CD20(-)

ETIOLOGY/PATHOGENESIS

Infectious Agents
- EBV positive
- Strongly associated with HIV infection
- Has been reported in patients with immunodeficiency due to other causes
  - Example: Post-transplantation

CLINICAL ISSUES

Epidemiology
- Incidence
  - Unknown
    - Frequency: PBL represents < 1% of all non-Hodgkin lymphomas
- Age
  - Depends on clinical setting
    - HIV(+) patients: Median age = 40 years
    - HIV(-) patients: Children or elderly
- Gender
  - Male predominance: 7:1

- Related to HIV(+) population affected

Presentation
- PBL most often originates in mucosal extranodal sites
  - 2 general groups: Oral and nonoral sites
  - Rapidly growing and often painful mass
- Oral cavity is most common site
  - 90% of patients are HIV(+)
    - Patients have very low CD4(+) counts
  - Mean duration of HIV(+) prior to PBL: 5 years
  - 60% have localized disease (stage I) at diagnosis
  - PBL frequently arises near mucosa
    - Often involves gingiva
    - Frequently infiltrates adjacent bone
- Nonoral type PBL
  - Less frequently HIV(+)
  - 60% are disseminated disease (stage IV) at diagnosis
  - Most common nonoral sites
    - Maxillary sinus, nasopharynx, gastrointestinal tract
  - Less common nonoral sites
    - Orbit, skin, lung, gastrointestinal tract, soft tissues
  - Rare sites of PBL (case reports)
    - Mediastinum, vulva, bone marrow
- PBL uncommonly involves lymph nodes
- PBL can widely disseminate during course of disease
- International prognostic Index (IPI): Usually intermediate or high score
- Some cases are reported in patients with history of myeloma or lymphoma
  - Better considered as plasmablastic transformation of underlying neoplasm

Treatment
- CHOP (cyclophosphamide, doxorubicin, vincristine, and prednisone)
  - Some regimens have included rituximab &/or radiotherapy
- More aggressive chemotherapy regimens have been employed without benefit

PLASMABLASTIC LYMPHOMA

Key Facts

Terminology
- Diffuse neoplasm with immunoblastic or plasmablastic features and plasma cell immunophenotype
- Aggressive clinical course
- Poor prognosis

Etiology/Pathogenesis
- Associated with immunodeficiency
  - HIV infection most common

Clinical Issues
- Frequently originates in mucosa of oral cavity
- Nonoral cases also occur

Microscopic Pathology
- Large neoplastic cells with variable degree of immunoblastic or plasmablastic features

- "Starry sky" pattern frequent
- High mitotic and apoptotic rates

Ancillary Tests
- Pan-B-cell antigens: Weak or absent
- Plasma cell markers(+)
- EBER(+), HHV8(-)
- Monoclonal *IgH* gene rearrangements
- High proliferation index (Ki-67)

Top Differential Diagnoses
- Diffuse large B-cell lymphoma, immunoblastic variant
- Plasmablastic plasma cell myeloma
- Multicentric Castleman disease, HHV8 positive
- ALK(+) large B-cell lymphoma

- Addition of antiretroviral therapy (HAART) improves prognosis

Prognosis
- Poor prognosis
- Most patients die within 1st year after diagnosis
- In large review, prognosis did not correlate with
  - Age, sex, CD4(+) count, HIV load
  - Stage, anatomic site of PBL, EBV status
  - Use of CHOP chemotherapy

IMAGE FINDINGS

Radiographic Findings
- PBL is PET scan positive
- PET or CT scan can show widespread bone involvement

MICROSCOPIC PATHOLOGY

Histologic Features
- Diffuse growth pattern
- Frequent "starry sky" pattern with tingible body macrophages
- Apoptotic bodies and mitoses are usually numerous
- Confluent areas of necrosis are common

Cytologic Features
- Monotonous proliferation of large neoplastic cells in histologic sections
  - More cytologic variability in smear/imprint preparations
- PBL cases can exhibit cytologic spectrum
  - Immunoblastic
    - Cells have prominent central nucleoli
    - More common in oral cavity and in HIV(+) patients
  - Plasmablastic
    - Cells have more abundant cytoplasm and eccentrically located nuclei
    - More common in nonoral sites

- Binucleation or multinucleation is common in PBL
- Cytoplasm of PBL cells is usually deeply basophilic
  - Dutcher and Russell bodies are usually absent in PBL

ANCILLARY TESTS

Immunohistochemistry
- Immunophenotype is essential to establish diagnosis of PBL
- Common pan-B-cell markers commonly absent
  - CD20, CD22, and pax-5
  - Weak expression reported in small subset of cases
  - CD79a is more often positive; also often weak intensity
- Strong positivity for plasma cell-associated markers
  - IRF-4/MUM1(+), CD38(+), CD138/syndecan-1(+), VS38/p63(+)
  - PRMD1/BLIMP1(+), XBP1(+)
- Ki-67 is high: > 70% in most cases
- Monotypic cytoplasmic light chain positive in 50-70% of cases
- EMA is often positive; CD30(+) in subset
- Aberrant expression of T-cell markers in some cases
  - CD3, CD4, CD43, CD7
- Germinal center B-cell antigens positive in subset of PBL
  - Bcl-6 uncommon; CD10 (+ in ~ 50%)
- CD56 can be positive in cases with plasmablastic cytologic features
  - Must exclude plasma cell myeloma
- Bcl-2 is usually negative
- CD45/LCA is negative or weakly positive in subset of cases
- ALK1(-), CD117(-), Cyclin-D1(-)
- HHV8(-)
- EBV-LMP 1 and 2 are not expressed
  - Consistent with restricted latency
  - In contrast to AIDS-related immunoblastic lymphomas that usually express EBV-LMP 1

PLASMABLASTIC LYMPHOMA

- No significant differences in frequency of expression of any immunohistochemical marker between PBL and plasmablastic plasma cell myeloma

Cytogenetics
- t(8;14)(q24;q32) or *MYC-IgH* fusion identified in subset of PBL
  - HIV(+) patients

In Situ Hybridization
- EBV small encoded RNA (EBER) is positive in ~ 75% of cases
  - EBER useful for distinguishing PBL from plasmablastic plasma cell myeloma (EBER[-])

PCR
- Monoclonal *IgH* gene rearrangements
- *T-cell receptor* genes usually in germline configuration
  - Single case reports showing both *IgH* and *TCR* gene rearrangements
- *IgH* genes commonly show somatic mutations of *IgH* variable regions

DIFFERENTIAL DIAGNOSIS

Diffuse Large B-cell Lymphoma, Not Otherwise Specified (DLBCL)
- DLBCL often has centroblastic cytologic features
  - Plasmacytoid differentiation is uncommon
- Immunophenotype of DLBCL is distinct from PBL
  - CD19(+), CD20(+), CD22(+), pax-5(+)
  - CD45/LCA is usually positive
  - Large subset is strongly positive for CD10 &/or Bcl-6

Diffuse Large B-cell Lymphoma, Immunoblastic Variant (DLBCL-IB)
- Morphologic overlap between DLBCL-IB and PBL
  - Immunophenotype is needed to make this distinction
  - DLBCL-IB is usually CD20(+) &/or pax-5(+)
  - CD45/LCA often positive
  - CD10(+/-), Bcl-6(+/-)
  - CD4(+) is extremely rare in DLBCL-IB
- By contrast, PBL is CD20(-), CD38(+), CD138/syndecan-1(+), and VS38/p63(+)
  - CD4 or CD56 can be positive

Plasma Cell Myeloma (PCM)
- Clinically important to distinguish between PCM and PBL
  - Treatment regimens for these 2 diseases are different
- Usually, cytologic features of PCM are obviously those of plasma cells
  - Not blastic; lower number of mitoses or proliferation rate
- Plasmablastic PCM can closely resemble PBL
  - Clinical features of plasmablastic PCM also apply to PCM in general

Plasmablastic PCM
- Plasmablastic PCM and PBL greatly overlap histologically
  - Clinical correlation often needed to distinguish
  - Plasmablastic PCM and PBL can have virtually identical immunophenotypic profile
- Features that favor diagnosis of plasmablastic PCM
  - Presence of serum monoclonal protein (paraprotein)
  - Detection of paraproteinemia in blood &/or excess light chains (Bence Jones protein) in urine
  - Bone marrow involvement with radiologic evidence of lytic lesions
  - EBER (-)
- Positivity for HIV does not favor diagnosis of PBL over plasmablastic plasma cell myeloma
- Presence of atypical but more mature plasma cells supports diagnosis of plasmablastic PCM

Multicentric Castleman Disease, HHV8(+)
- Patients have clinical and histologic features of multicentric Castleman disease
  - Usually HIV(+)
- Characteristically involves lymph nodes &/or spleen
- Immunophenotype is helpful
  - HHV8(+) in all cases
  - Ig λ(+), CD20(+/-)
  - CD138/syndecan-1(-), EBER(-)

ALK(+) Diffuse Large B-cell Lymphoma
- Most common in children
- Immunoblastic/plasmablastic cytology
- Intrasinusoidal growth pattern common
- Immunophenotype is distinctive
  - ALK(+) in all cases
  - CD138/syndecan-1(+), VS38/p63(+), and monotypic cytoplasmic light chain
  - CD4(+) and CD45/LCA(+) common
  - CD79a(-/+), CD20(-), CD30(-)
- ALK pattern correlates with cytogenetic abnormalities
  - Most cases carry t(2;17)(p23;q23)/clathrin-ALK
    - Pattern is cytoplasmic and granular
    - Correlates with location of clathrin in cytoplasmic vesicles
  - Some cases carry t(2;5)(p23;q35)/nucleophosmin-ALK
    - Pattern is nuclear and cytoplasmic
    - Correlates with location of nucleophosmin

Myeloid Sarcoma
- a.k.a. extramedullary myeloid cell tumor or granulocytic sarcoma
- Cells have immature (blastic) chromatin and thin nuclear membranes
- Eosinophilic metamyelocytes in ~ 50% of cases
- Immunophenotype helpful
  - MPO(+), lysozyme(+), CD68(+), CD117(+)
  - TdT(+/-), CD34(+/-)
  - Plasma cell markers(-)

Burkitt Lymphoma (BL)
- BL and PBL can share extranodal location, "starry sky" pattern, and high proliferation rate
- BL can occur in HIV(+) patients and rarely shows plasmacytoid differentiation
- Immunophenotype is helpful

PLASMABLASTIC LYMPHOMA

Differential Diagnosis of PBL with DLBCL and Plasma Cell Myeloma

	Plasmablastic Lymphoma	DLBCL, Immunoblastic Variant	Plasmablastic Plasma Cell Myeloma
CD20	-	+	-
pax-5	-/+	+	-/+
CD79a	-/+	+	-
CD45/LCA	-/+	+	-/+
Bcl-6	-/+	-/+	-
ALK1	-	-	-
Bcl-2	-/+	-/+	-/+
CD138	+	-	+
CD38	+	-	+
IRF-4/MUM1	+	-/+	+
CD30	-	-/+	-
CD56	+/-	-	+/-
CD10	+/-	+/-	-/+
EBER	+	-/+	-
EBV-LMP	-	-	-
HHV8	-	-	-
p53	+/-	+/-	+/-

Lymphomas Occurring in HIV Patients

Description

Burkitt lymphoma ± plasmacytoid differentiation (30% of HIV-associated lymphomas)

DLBCL immunoblastic (usually exhibiting plasmacytoid differentiation) (10% of HIV-associated lymphomas)

Classical Hodgkin lymphomas (mixed cellularity or lymphocyte depleted)

MALT lymphomas (rare)

Primary effusion lymphoma

Plasmablastic lymphoma

Lymphoma arising in HHV8-associated multicentric Castleman disease

- BL is positive for pan-B-cell antigens (CD19, CD20, pax-5)
- CD10(+), Bcl-6(+), CD45/LCA(+)

Poorly Differentiated or Undifferentiated Carcinoma

- Diffuse or sinusoidal pattern and high mitotic rate may partially mimic PBL
- Carcinomas can express CD138/syndecan-1
- Immunophenotype helpful
  - Carcinomas are cytokeratin(+), CD38(-), IRF-4/MUM1(-)
- Electron microscopy often shows desmosomes or cellular junctions

Malignant Melanoma

- Melanoma cells can have abundant eosinophilic cytoplasm resembling plasmacytoid features
- Immunophenotype helpful
  - S100(+), HMB-45(+), Melan-A(+)
  - Melanomas are CD38(-), IRF-4/MUM1(-)
- Electron microscopy often shows melanosomes

SELECTED REFERENCES

1. Bogusz AM et al: Plasmablastic lymphomas with MYC/IgH rearrangement: report of three cases and review of the literature. Am J Clin Pathol. 132(4):597-605, 2009
2. Rafaniello Raviele P et al: Plasmablastic lymphoma: a review. Oral Dis. 15(1):38-45, 2009
3. Carbone A et al: Plasmablastic lymphoma: one or more entities? Am J Hematol. 83(10):763-4, 2008
4. Castillo J et al: HIV-associated plasmablastic lymphoma: lessons learned from 112 published cases. Am J Hematol. 83(10):804-9, 2008
5. Reid-Nicholson M et al: Plasmablastic lymphoma: Cytologic findings in 5 cases with unusual presentation. Cancer. 114(5):333-41, 2008
6. Borenstein J et al: Plasmablastic lymphomas may occur as post-transplant lymphoproliferative disorders. Histopathology. 51(6):774-7, 2007
7. Vega F et al: Plasmablastic lymphomas and plasmablastic plasma cell myelomas have nearly identical immunophenotypic profiles. Mod Pathol. 2005 Jun;18(6):806-15. Erratum in: Mod Pathol. 18(6):873, 2005
8. Delecluse HJ et al: Plasmablastic lymphomas of the oral cavity: a new entity associated with the human immunodeficiency virus infection. Blood. 89(4):1413-20, 1997

PLASMABLASTIC LYMPHOMA

Microscopic Features

(Left) This case of plasmablastic lymphoma (PBL) is characterized by sheets of large cells with a relatively monotonous appearance and focal "starry sky" pattern ➡. The tumor involved the mucosa of the oral cavity and infiltrated the maxillary bone. *(Right)* PBL involving the oral mucosa. Some neoplastic cells have immunoblastic features (prominent and centrally located nucleoli). Mitoses are easily seen ➡. A tingible body macrophage is also seen ➡.

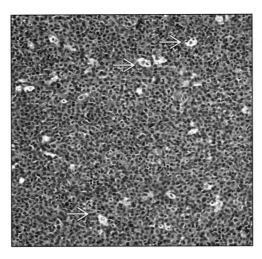
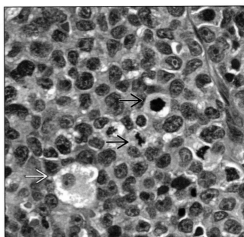

(Left) PBL characterized by diffuse infiltrate of large tumor cells with a relatively monotonous appearance and prominent vascularity. In this case, the tumor cells exhibited a higher degree of plasmacytic differentiation. A prominent "starry sky" pattern was not present. *(Right)* PBL. The tumor cells exhibit variable degrees of plasmacytoid differentiation ➡; some cells had relatively abundant cytoplasm and eccentrically placed nuclei resembling immature plasma cells.

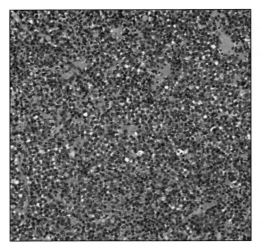
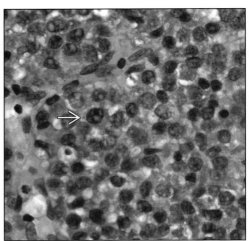

(Left) PBL composed of large and very pleomorphic tumor cells. Note that some tumor cells have features of immunoblasts (vesicular nuclear chromatin and prominent central nucleoli) ➡. Tingible body macrophages are noted ➡. *(Right)* Areas of necrosis and frequent karyorrhexis (nuclear and cellular fragmentation due to apoptosis) are frequently seen in PBL, illustrating the high grade of this neoplasm.

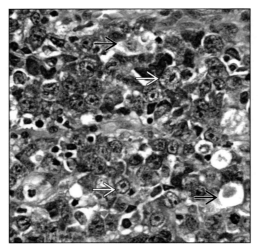
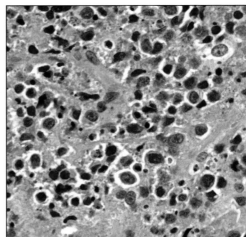

Microscopic Features and Ancillary Techniques

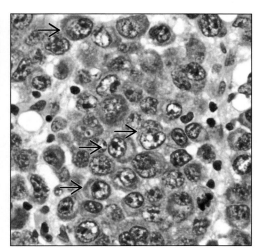

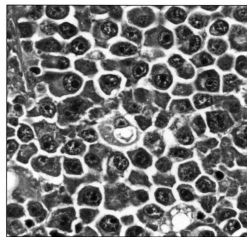

(Left) PBL composed of large tumor cells, some with features of immunoblasts with a variable degree of plasmacytic differentiation ➡️. *(Right)* In another case of PBL, the tumor cells are less pleomorphic and have a marked plasmacytic differentiation. Note the eosinophilic cytoplasm, the presence of a paranuclear Golgi area, and the eccentric nuclei. This raises the differential diagnosis with plasmablastic plasma cell neoplasm.

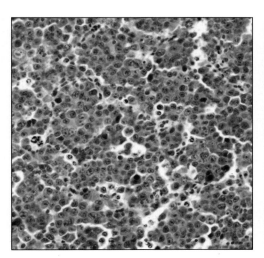

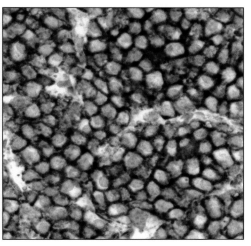

(Left) PBL composed of tumor cells that resemble small immunoblasts and exhibit plasmacytic differentiation. This morphology also raises the differential diagnosis of plasmablastic plasma cell neoplasm. *(Right)* In PBL, the neoplastic cells show strong expression of CD138/syndecan (shown). Other plasma cell-associated antigens that are usually strongly expressed in PBL cases include IRF-4/MUM1, Vs38/p63, and CD38.

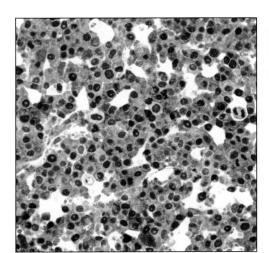

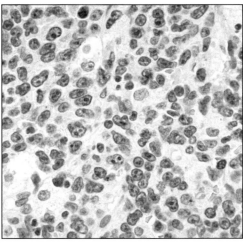

(Left) In PBL, the neoplastic cells show strong expression of IRF-4/MUM1. *(Right)* The tumor cells in PBL are negative for pax-5. Strong expression of B-cell markers supports the diagnosis of diffuse large B-cell lymphoma over PBL.

PLASMABLASTIC LYMPHOMA

Ancillary Techniques

(Left) The tumor cells in PBL are negative for CD20 (shown). Strong expression of B-cell markers supports the diagnosis of diffuse large B-cell lymphoma over PBL. However, similar to plasmablastic plasma cell myeloma, the tumor cells in PBL are usually negative for B-cell markers. *(Right)* The tumor cells in PBL can express cytoplasmic light chains, in this case κ light chain.

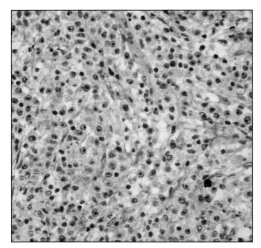
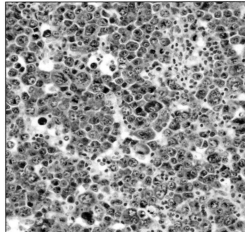

(Left) The tumor cells in PBL are positive for CD56 in almost 1/2 of cases. CD56 is also positive in a subset of plasma cell myelomas, and thus it does not allow the distinction between PBL and a plasma cell neoplasm. *(Right)* The tumor cells in PBL are positive for CD10 in almost 1/2 of cases. CD10 is also positive in a subset of plasma cell myelomas, and thus it does not allow the distinction between PBL and plasma cell neoplasm.

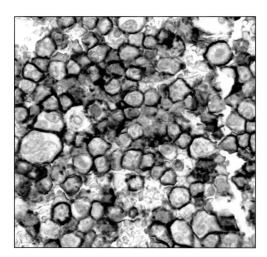
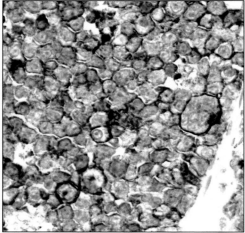

(Left) The proliferative index, as determined by Ki-67/MIB-1 staining, is usually greater than 70% in cases of PBL. *(Right)* In situ hybridization for Epstein-Barr virus small-encoded RNA (EBER) is usually positive in PBL. Note that positivity for EBER has been reported to be rare in plasma cell myeloma. Thus, a positive EBER result makes the diagnosis of plasma cell myeloma unlikely.

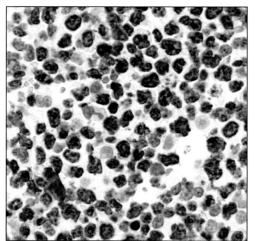
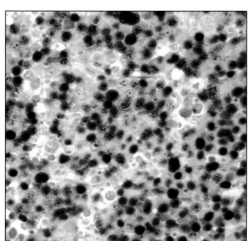

PLASMABLASTIC LYMPHOMA

Differential Diagnosis

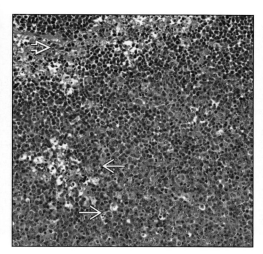

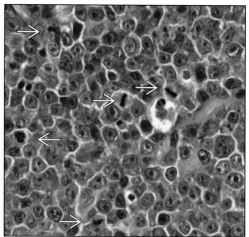

(Left) Diffuse large B-cell lymphoma (DLBCL), immunoblastic variant involving the oral cavity. The neoplasm is diffuse and composed of intermediate- to large-sized atypical cells. Note the presence of a focal "starry sky" pattern ➡ and necrosis ⇛. *(Right)* DLBCL, immunoblastic variant involving the oral cavity composed of intermediate- to large-sized lymphoid cells with immunoblastic features and plasmacytic differentiation. Mitoses are frequent ➡.

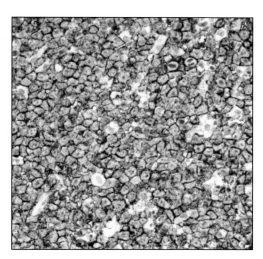

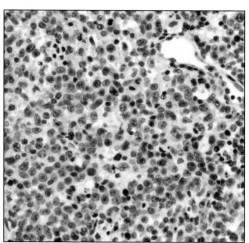

(Left) The diagnosis of DLBCL, immunoblastic variant is supported by the strong positivity for CD20. In addition, the tumor cells were negative for plasma cell marker including CD138/syndecan-1. *(Right)* DLBCL, immunoblastic variant with plasmacytic differentiation. The neoplastic cells are negative for CD138/syndecan-1. These cells were strongly positive for CD20.

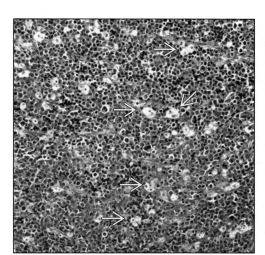

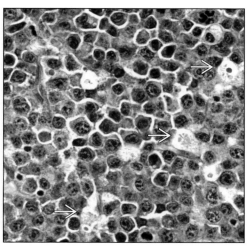

(Left) Plasmablastic plasma cell myeloma shows a diffuse infiltrate of neoplastic plasma cells. Note the presence of a "starry sky" background ➡. *(Right)* Plasmablastic plasma cell myeloma shows a diffuse infiltrate of neoplastic plasma cells. The tumor cells exhibit marked plasmacytic differentiation. Note the presence of a "starry sky" background ➡.

PLASMABLASTIC LYMPHOMA

Differential Diagnosis

*(Left) Plasmablastic plasma cell myeloma showing CD4 expression. Expression of CD56, CD10, and CD4 are frequently detected in cases of plasmablastic plasma cell myeloma. Note that these markers are not specific and can be also be detected in PBL. **(Right)** Plasmablastic plasma cell myeloma is pax-5(-).*

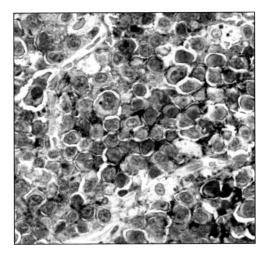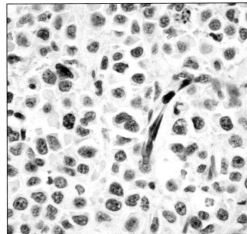

*(Left) The proliferative index, as determined by Ki-67/ MIB-1staining, is usually high in PBL. In this case of PBL, virtually all the cells are positive for Ki-67. **(Right)** Plasmablastic plasma cell myeloma is usually negative for EBER. A positive EBER result makes the diagnosis of plasma cell myeloma unlikely.*

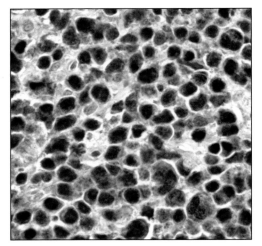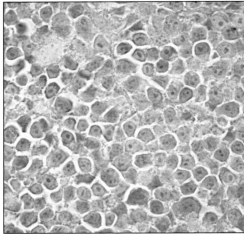

*(Left) Extramedullary plasmacytoma involving the large intestine. In this case, the degree of plasma cell differentiation shown in this field is unusual for PBL and thereby supports plasmacytoma. **(Right)** Extramedullary plasmacytoma involving the large intestine. The tumor cells are strongly positive for CD138. In addition, they were negative for CD20 and pax-5.*

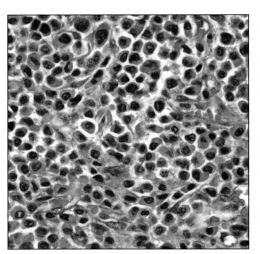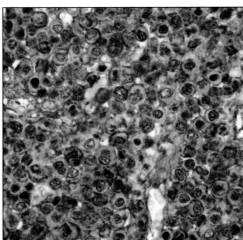

PLASMABLASTIC LYMPHOMA

Differential Diagnosis

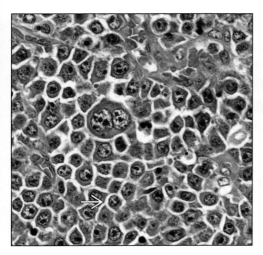

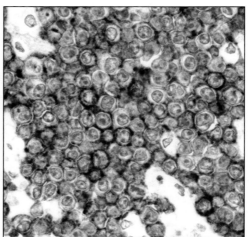

(Left) Multifocal high-grade plasmablastic neoplasm involving the small intestine in a patient with Crohn disease. The neoplasm was positive for CD138/syndecan-1 and negative for pax-5. The differential diagnosis includes plasmablastic plasmacytoma and PBL. The presence of small neoplastic plasma cells supports the diagnosis of plasmacytoma ➡. **(Right)** Plasmablastic neoplasm involving the small intestine. The tumor cells were positive for CD7.

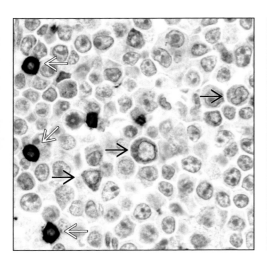

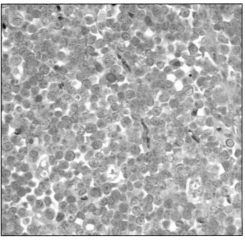

(Left) Plasmablastic neoplasm involving the small intestine. The tumor cells were focally and weakly positive for CD3 (cytoplasmic) ➡. Note the strong positivity for CD3 in the small T cells ➡. **(Right)** Plasmablastic neoplasm involving the small intestine morphologically is most consistent with plasmablastic plasmacytoma. The tumor cells were negative for EBER. A positive EBER result makes the diagnosis of plasma cell myeloma unlikely.

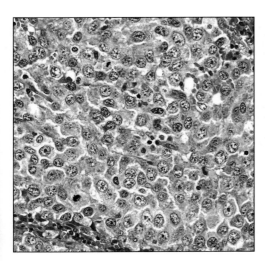

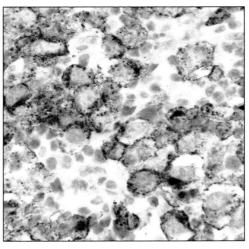

(Left) Hematoxylin & eosin shows a case of ALK(+) diffuse large B-cell lymphoma. The neoplasm has a diffuse pattern and is composed of immunoblasts with a plasmacytic appearance. The tumor cells were focally positive for CD79a and ALK (not shown) and were negative for CD30. **(Right)** ALK(+) DLBCL showing ALK positivity, which is cytoplasmic and coarsely granular, consistent with t(2;17)(p23;q23)/clathrin-ALK.

PRIMARY EFFUSION LYMPHOMA (PEL) AND SOLID VARIANT OF PEL

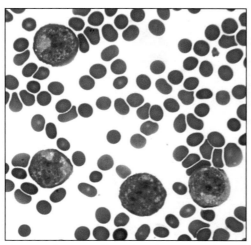

Cytospin of primary effusion lymphoma (PEL) showing medium- to large-sized lymphoid cells with abundant finely vacuolated cytoplasm and irregular nuclei. (Courtesy W. Chen, MD.)

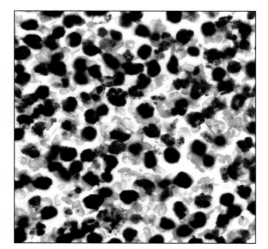

Cell block of primary effusion lymphoma (PEL) showing that virtually all neoplastic cells strongly HHV8(+). The neoplastic cells were CD20(-). Detecting evidence of HHV8 infection is essential for the diagnosis of PEL.

TERMINOLOGY

Abbreviations
- Primary effusion lymphoma (PEL)

Synonyms
- Body cavity-based lymphoma
- Kaposi sarcoma-associated herpesvirus (KSHV)-associated lymphoma

Definitions
- Human herpes virus 8 (HHV8)-associated large B-cell neoplasm most often involving body cavities
  - Pleural, pericardial, or peritoneal cavity
- HHV8(+) lymphomas indistinguishable from PEL rarely present as solid tumor mass
  - These tumors are designated as extracavitary or solid variants of PEL

ETIOLOGY/PATHOGENESIS

Infectious Agents
- PEL arises from HHV8-infected B cells that are frequently coinfected by Epstein-Barr virus (EBV)
- HHV8 virus
  - γ herpes double-stranded DNA lymphotropic virus
  - Endemic in sub-Saharan Africa and Mediterranean region
  - In addition to PEL, HHV8 is associated with
    - Kaposi sarcoma
    - Multicentric Castleman disease (MCD)
    - MCD-associated plasmablastic lymphoma
  - Encodes number of homologues of cellular genes
    - Involved in cell proliferation and apoptosis

Clinical Associations
- HIV infection or other severe acquired immunodeficiencies

- Preexisting acquired immunodeficiency syndrome (AIDS) is very common
- PEL also can occur in patients without immunodeficiency
  - Elderly patients in 8th to 9th decades in HHV8 endemic areas
    - Usually these tumors are EBV(-)
- Rare cases of PEL are associated with hepatitis C &/or B

Pathogenesis
- In PEL, B-cell differentiation program is blocked
  - In part due to overexpression of activated B-cell factor 1 (ABF-1) and inhibitor of differentiation 2 (ID2)
    - These molecules inhibit E2A (B-cell transcription factor)
    - E2A inhibition downregulates B-cell specific genes
  - Restoration of E2A activity in PEL induces apoptosis of tumor cells

CLINICAL ISSUES

Epidemiology
- Incidence
  - Rare
    - 0.3% of all aggressive lymphomas in HIV(-) patients
    - 4% of all HIV-related lymphomas

Presentation
- Lymphoma cells grow in pleural, peritoneal, &/or pericardial effusions
- Usually no distinct extracavitary tumor masses &/or organomegaly
- Frequent B symptoms
- Symptoms commonly result from massive malignant effusion
  - Dyspnea is frequent (from pleural or pericardial disease)

PRIMARY EFFUSION LYMPHOMA (PEL) AND SOLID VARIANT OF PEL

Key Facts

Etiology/Pathogenesis
- PEL arises from HHV8-infected B cells frequently coinfected by EBV
- Associated with HIV infection or other severe acquired immunodeficiencies

Clinical Issues
- 4% of all HIV-related lymphomas
- Presentation as lymphomatous growth in pleural, peritoneal, &/or pericardial effusions
- Extracavitary presentation has been described
  ○ Solid variant of PEL
- Some patients have coexistent Kaposi sarcoma

Microscopic Pathology
- Diagnosis is usually made on cytological preparations
- Cytologic features range from immunoblastic to anaplastic; plasmablastic differentiation common

Ancillary Tests
- Plasma cell-associated markers(+)
- Pan-B-cell markers(-)
- HHV8(+) is essential for diagnosis

Top Differential Diagnoses
- Diffuse large B-cell lymphoma associated with chronic inflammation
- Body cavity involvement by diffuse large B-cell lymphoma, NOS
- Large B-cell lymphoma arising in HHV8-associated multicentric Castleman disease
- Plasmablastic lymphoma
- Plasmablastic plasma cell myeloma

  ○ Abdominal distension (from peritoneal disease)
- Systemic dissemination can occur during course of disease
- Associated with clinical and laboratory findings of severe immunosuppression
  ○ Marked depletion of CD4(+) T cells
- Involvement of central nervous system and bone marrow is rare
- Standard Ann Arbor staging is not useful as, by definition, all PEL cases are stage IV
- Some patients have coexistent Kaposi sarcoma
- HHV8(+) lymphomas can present as masses involving organs (extracavitary or solid variant of PEL)
  ○ Gastrointestinal tract most frequently involved
  ○ Lymph nodes can be involved
  ○ Patients with extracavitary mass often develop malignant effusion over disease course

Treatment
- Highly active antiretroviral therapy (HAART) improves prognosis
- Intracavitary cidofovir (antiviral agent that inhibits replication of HHV8) with interferon-α
- Traditional chemotherapy, usually cyclophosphamide, doxorubicin, vincristine, and prednisone (CHOP)
- Bortezomib, a proteosome inhibitor that inhibits NF-kB pathway
- Antivirals (valganciclovir)
- Rituximab probably has no role in patients with PEL
  ○ CD20 is usually negative

Prognosis
- Usually poor; median survival < 6 months

IMAGE FINDINGS

Radiographic Findings
- Bilateral or unilateral pleural effusion
- Pericardial effusion, peritoneal effusion
- Slight thickening of parietal pleura, pericardium, or peritoneum
- Absence of solid tumor masses, parenchymal abnormalities, or mediastinal enlargement

MICROSCOPIC PATHOLOGY

Histologic Features
- Diagnosis is usually made on cytological preparations of involved effusion fluid
- Biopsy specimens of cavity lining tissue also may show small number of neoplastic cells adherent to mesothelial surfaces
- Large lymphoid cells with round to irregular nuclei, prominent nucleoli, and variable morphology
  ○ Immunoblastic
    ▪ Round nuclei with centrally located nucleoli
  ○ Plasmablastic
    ▪ Eccentric nuclei with abundant cytoplasm, sometimes with perinuclear hof
  ○ Anaplastic
    ▪ Multinucleated and Reed-Sternberg-like cells

Cytologic Features
- Medium- to large-sized atypical cells, many with irregular nuclear contours, prominent nucleoli, and abundant cytoplasm (± vacuolated)
- Cytomorphologic appearances ranging from immunoblastic to anaplastic and exhibiting frequent plasmablastic differentiation

ANCILLARY TESTS

Immunohistochemistry
- HHV8(+) is essential for diagnosis
- Plasma cell-associated markers(+)
  ○ CD138, VS38c, IRF-4/MUM1
  ○ CD38, EMA
- Cytoplasmic Ig λ light chain(+/-)
- CD30(+), CD45/LCA(+/-)
- Notch(+) in most cases
  ○ Nuclear and cytoplasmic pattern of expression

PRIMARY EFFUSION LYMPHOMA (PEL) AND SOLID VARIANT OF PEL

- Pan-B-cell markers(-)
  - CD19, CD20, CD79a, pax-5
- CD15(-), LMP-1(-)
- CD10(-), Bcl-6(-)

Flow Cytometry
- Similar immunophenotype to that observed by immunohistochemistry
- Results
  - CD45/LCA(+), CD71(+)
  - HLA-DR(+); CD23(+) in ~ 20%
  - Surface Ig light chain expression is rare
  - CD19(-), CD20(-), CD22(-)
    - ~ 10% of cases have dim CD20 expression
  - CD10(-), FMC7(-)
  - Aberrant T-cell markers are positive in subset of cases
    - CD45RO (~ 90%), CD7 (~ 30%), CD4 (~ 20%)
    - CD2(-), CD3(-), CD5(-), CD8(-)

Cytogenetics
- Usually complex karyotype
- No recurrent chromosomal abnormalities identified

In Situ Hybridization
- EBER(+) in ~ 80% of cases

Array CGH
- Gains of Iq21-41, 4q28-35, 7q, 8q, 11, 12, 17q, 19p, 20q
- Losses of 4q, 11q25, 14q32
  - Amplification of selectin-P ligand (12q24.11)

Molecular Genetics
- Monoclonal IgH gene rearrangements
- Frequent somatic hypermutation of IgH variable regions
- Monoclonal TCR rearrangements in subset

Gene Expression Profiling
- PEL in HIV(+) patients has been assessed
  - Profile is distinctive
    - Features of plasma cells and EBV-transformed lymphocytes

DIFFERENTIAL DIAGNOSIS

Diffuse Large B-cell Lymphoma Associated with Chronic Inflammation
- a.k.a. pyothorax-associated lymphoma
- Lymphoma occurring in setting of longstanding chronic inflammation
- Pyothorax-associated lymphoma is prototype
  - History of chronic pleural inflammation
    - M. tuberculosis infection &/or pyothorax
    - Artificial pneumothorax as part of therapy
- More common in Japan
- Usually in elderly men
- Usually presents as large pleural mass
  - Direct invasion of adjacent structures and organs
- Large atypical B cells
  - Immunoblastic morphology is most common
- CD20(+), CD79a(+)

- Small subset of cases exhibits plasmacytoid differentiation
  - CD20(-) or CD79a(-)
  - IRF-4/MUM1(+) or CD138(+)
- EBER(+), LMP-1(+)
- HHV8(-)
- P53 gene mutations in ~ 70%

Body Cavity Involvement by Systemic Diffuse Large B-cell Lymphoma, Not Otherwise Specified (NOS)
- Patients with non-Hodgkin lymphoma present with or subsequently develop body cavity involvement during course of disease
- Any systemic lymphoma may involve any serosal cavities
  - Most frequent type is diffuse large B-cell lymphoma, NOS
- Pleural involvement can be unilateral or bilateral
  - Unilateral involvement is more common on left side
- Immunophenotypic and molecular findings similar to DLBCL, NOS elsewhere
- HHV8(-)

Plasmablastic Lymphoma Arising in HHV8-associated Multicentric Castleman Disease
- Patients usually have clinical and histologic features of multicentric Castleman disease
  - Usually HIV(+), EBER(+)
- Characteristically involves lymph nodes &/or spleen
- Immunophenotype
  - HHV8(+) in all cases
  - Igλ(+), CD20(+/-), CD79a(-)
  - CD38(-/+), CD138(-)

Plasmablastic Lymphoma (PBL)
- Oral and nonoral types
- Associated with HIV(+) and EBV(+)
- PBL exhibits cytologic spectrum
  - Immunoblastic
    - Cells have prominent central nucleoli
    - More common in oral cavity and in HIV(+) patients
  - Plasmablastic
    - More common in nonoral sites
    - Cells have more abundant cytoplasm and eccentrically located nuclei
- Immunophenotype
  - Plasma cell-associated markers strongly positive
    - IRF-4/MUM1, CD38, CD138, VS38/p63
  - Cytoplasmic Ig(+) ~ 60-70%
  - CD79a(+) ~ 70-80%
  - Other pan-B-cell markers negative
    - CD19, CD20, CD22, and pax-5
  - CD45/LCA(-) or weakly positive in subset of cases
  - HHV8(-)

Plasmablastic Plasma Cell Myeloma (PCM)
- Evidence of plasma cell myeloma is usually present
  - Paraprotein in blood &/or excess light chains (Bence Jones protein) in urine
  - Bone marrow involvement

PRIMARY EFFUSION LYMPHOMA (PEL) AND SOLID VARIANT OF PEL

Differential Diagnosis of Primary Effusion Lymphoma

	PEL	DLBCL-NOS	Plasmablastic Lymphoma	DLBCL Associated with Chronic Inflammation
Age	Young or middle-aged	Median: 60-70 years	Any age	Median: 37 years
Associated diseases	HIV(+), Kaposi sarcoma, multicentric Castleman disease	None	HIV(+), other immunodeficiency diseases	Pyothorax or other cause of chronic inflammation
Anatomic site	Body cavities	Systemic disease; ± body cavity involved	Extranodal; body cavities rarely involved	Pleural cavity
HHV8	(+)	(-)	(-)	(-)
EBV	(+)	(-)	(+/-)	(+)
Immunophenotype	CD30(+), CD38(+), CD45/LCA(+/-), CD138(+), CD79a(-), CD19(-), CD20(-)	CD19(+), CD20(+), CD30(-/+), CD138(-/+)	CD38(+), CD138(+), CD19(-), CD20(-), CD45/LCA(-)	CD19(+), CD20(+), CD138(-)
Cytogenetic findings	Complex karyotype; no recurrent abnormalities	Subset with t(14;18)(q32;q21) or 3q27/BCL-6 translocations	Subset with t(8;14)(q24;q32)/*MYC*	Complex karyotype; *P53* mutations in ~ 70%
Prognosis	Poor; median survival < 6 months	Variable; depends on clinical parameters and biologic features	Poor; median survival < 1 year	5-year survival ~ 20-35%

- o Radiologic evidence of lytic bone lesions
- Presence of atypical but more mature plasma cells
- EBER(-)

Burkitt Lymphoma (BL)

- BL and PEL can share extranodal location and high proliferation rate
- BL can occur in HIV(+) patients but rarely shows plasmacytoid differentiation
- Immunophenotype
  - o Pan-B-cell antigens(+)
    - CD19, CD20, and pax-5
  - o Bcl-6(+), CD10(-), Bcl-2(-)
  - o MIB-1/Ki-67 high (~ 100%)
- *MYC*-associated translocations in almost all cases
  - o t(8;14)(q24;q32) ~ in 80%
  - o t(2;8)(p12;q24) or t(8;22)(q24;q11) ~ in 20%

Malignant Melanoma

- Melanoma cells can have abundant eosinophilic cytoplasm resembling plasmacytoid differentiation
- Immunophenotype helpful
  - o S100(+), HMB-45(+), Melan-A(+)
- Electron microscopy often shows melanosomes

Poorly Differentiated or Undifferentiated Carcinoma

- Carcinomas can be CD138(+)
- Immunophenotype helpful
  - o Cytokeratin(+), CD38(-), IRF-4/MUM1(-)
- Electron microscopy often shows desmosomes or cellular junctions

DIAGNOSTIC CHECKLIST

Pathologic Interpretation Pearls

- Diagnosis is usually based on cytological examination of body fluids
- Many lymphomas, mostly aggressive types, can present with neoplastic serous effusion

- PEL is associated with immunodeficiency and has
  - o Evidence of HHV8 infection

SELECTED REFERENCES

1. Luan SL et al: Primary effusion lymphoma: genomic profiling revealed amplification of SELPLG and CORO1C encoding for proteins important for cell migration. J Pathol. 222(2):166-79, 2010
2. Sunil M et al: Update on HHV-8-Associated Malignancies. Curr Infect Dis Rep. 12(2):147-154, 2010
3. Wang HY et al: Notch1 in primary effusion lymphoma: a clinicopathological study. Mod Pathol. 23(6):773-80, 2010
4. Carbone A et al: HIV-associated lymphomas and gamma-herpesviruses. Blood. 113(6):1213-24, 2009
5. Sullivan RJ et al: HIV/AIDS: epidemiology, pathophysiology, and treatment of Kaposi sarcoma-associated herpesvirus disease: Kaposi sarcoma, primary effusion lymphoma, and multicentric Castleman disease. Clin Infect Dis. 47(9):1209-15, 2008
6. Brimo F et al: Primary effusion lymphoma: a series of 4 cases and review of the literature with emphasis on cytomorphologic and immunocytochemical differential diagnosis. Cancer. 111(4):224-33, 2007
7. Chen YB et al: Primary effusion lymphoma. Oncologist. 12(5):569-76, 2007
8. Lietz A et al: Loss of bHLH transcription factor E2A activity in primary effusion lymphoma confers resistance to apoptosis. Br J Haematol. 137(4):342-8, 2007
9. Vega F et al: Lymphomas involving the pleura: a clinicopathologic study of 34 cases diagnosed by pleural biopsy. Arch Pathol Lab Med. 130(10):1497-502, 2006
10. Carbone A et al: Kaposi's sarcoma-associated herpesvirus/human herpesvirus type 8-positive solid lymphomas: a tissue-based variant of primary effusion lymphoma. J Mol Diagn. 7(1):17-27, 2005
11. Klein U et al: Gene expression profile analysis of AIDS-related primary effusion lymphoma (PEL) suggests a plasmablastic derivation and identifies PEL-specific transcripts. Blood. 101(10):4115-21, 2003

PRIMARY EFFUSION LYMPHOMA (PEL) AND SOLID VARIANT OF PEL

Microscopic Features

(Left) PEL cells are medium to large in size with oval to markedly irregular nuclear contours, slightly open chromatin, and relatively abundant and slightly vacuolated cytoplasm. Note the presence of apoptotic cells ➡. *(Right)* Histologic section of a cell block of PEL. The neoplasm is composed of medium- to large-sized cells, some with eccentric nuclei and a plasmablastic &/ or anaplastic appearance, in a hemorrhagic background.

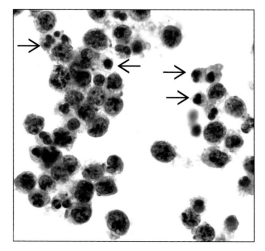
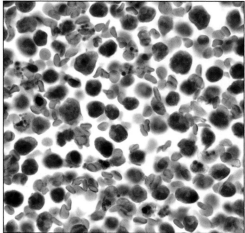

(Left) Histologic section of a cell block of PEL. The neoplastic cells in PEL are CD38(+). In this case, they were also CD45/LCA(+), CD30(+), HHV8(+), and CD20(-) (not shown). *(Right)* Histiologic section of a cell block of PEL. In PEL, the neoplastic cells are usually weakly and variably CD45/ LCA(+). They were also CD3(+) and negative for Pan-B-cell markers. PEL cells usually display a "null" immunophenotype: CD45/ LCA(+) but negative for B-, T-, and NK-cell markers.

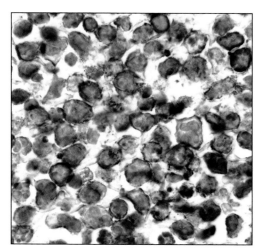
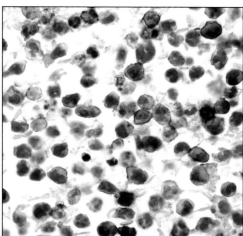

(Left) Histologic section of a cell block of PEL. The neoplastic cells are usually strongly CD30(+). The neoplastic cells in this case were negative for CD20 and CD15 (not shown). *(Right)* Histologic section of cell block of PEL. In PEL, in situ hybridization for Epstein-Barr virus small-encoded RNA (EBER) is usually positive in the neoplastic cells. Immunohistochemical staining for EBV latent membrane protein (LMP-1) can be positive (often focal) or negative.

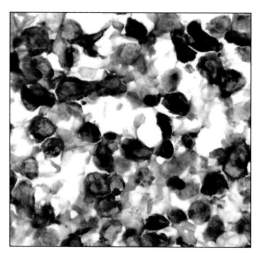
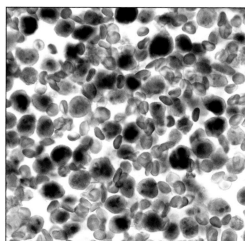

PRIMARY EFFUSION LYMPHOMA (PEL) AND SOLID VARIANT OF PEL

Microscopic Features

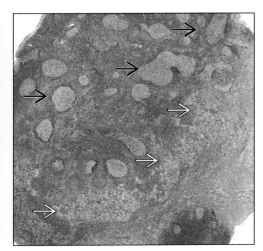

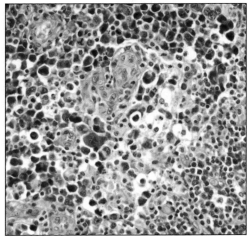

(Left) PEL, solid variant involving lymph node in an HIV(+) patient. The tumor predominantly involves sinuses ➡️. The tumor cells were CD138(+), IRF-4/MUM1(+), CD30(+, subset), CD79a(+, subset), EBER(+), HHV8(+), and CD20(-) (not shown). Note the presence of follicular hyperplasia ➡️. *(Right)* PEL, solid variant involving lymph node. The tumor cells were anaplastic, large to giant, with irregular-shaped nuclei, some with multiple nucleoli and abundant cytoplasm.

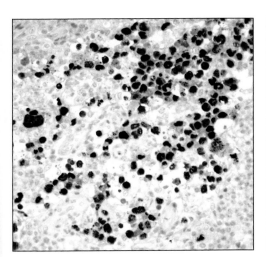

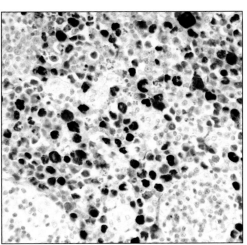

(Left) PEL, solid variant involving lymph node. It is essential to demonstrate evidence of HHV8 infection to establish the diagnosis of PEL. Note that the tumor cells are scattered and are not forming sheets as seen in diffuse large B-cell lymphoma. *(Right)* PEL, solid variant involving lymph node. In most cases of PEL, the tumor cells are coinfected with EBV. In this case, EBV infection was demonstrated by in situ hybridization for EBER.

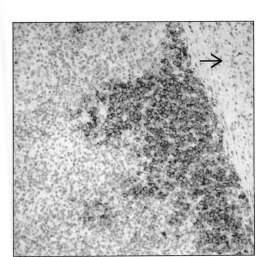

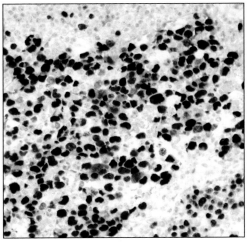

(Left) PEL, solid variant involving lymph node. The tumor cells are positive for plasma cell markers including CD138 (shown) and negative for pan-B-cell markers. Note the subcapsular sinusoidal distribution of the neoplastic cells. The lymph node capsule is fibrotic ➡️. *(Right)* PEL, solid variant involving lymph node. The tumor cells in PEL are usually positive for IRF-4/MUM1 and other plasma cell markers such as EMA and CD38 (not shown).

PRIMARY EFFUSION LYMPHOMA (PEL) AND SOLID VARIANT OF PEL

Differential Diagnosis

(Left) This pleural needle biopsy specimen shows a diffuse infiltrate of large lymphoid cells in a patient with a history of diffuse large B-cell lymphoma (DLBCL). Immunohistochemical studies revealed that the tumor cells had a B-cell phenotype and confirmed the diagnosis of DLBCL. (Right) Pleural needle biopsy specimen of DLBCL. Note the presence of clusters of large lymphoid cells in sclerotic stroma. This invasive pattern of infiltration with sclerosis is not seen in PEL.

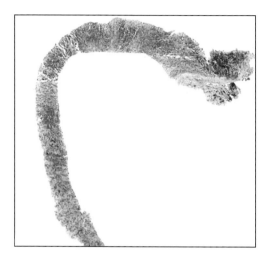 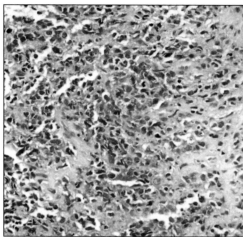

(Left) This case of diffuse large B-cell lymphoma, immunoblastic variant, is composed of intermediate-sized to large lymphoid cells with round nuclei, central nucleoli, and plasmacytic differentiation (slightly eccentric nuclei and perinuclear hof). Mitoses are frequent ➡. (Right) The diagnosis of diffuse large B-cell lymphoma, immunoblastic variant is supported by the strong CD20 positivity. In addition, the tumor cells were CD138(-) (not shown).

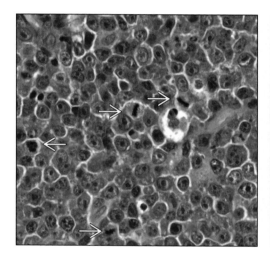 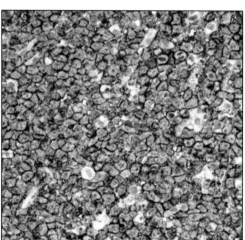

(Left) Plasmablastic lymphoma composed of large tumor cells, some with features of immunoblasts with a variable degree of plasmacytic differentiation (eccentric nuclei, abundant basophilic cytoplasm, and perinuclear hof) ➡. (Right) Similar to PEL, the tumor cells in plasmablastic lymphoma show strong expression of CD138 (shown) and are usually negative for B-cell markers. However, the tumor cells in plasmablastic lymphoma are negative for HHV8.

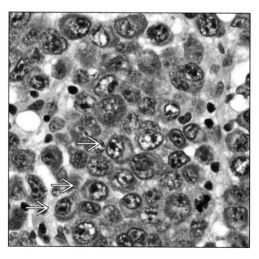 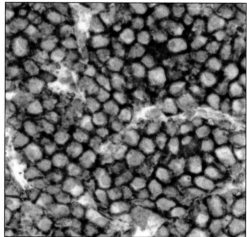

Differential Diagnosis

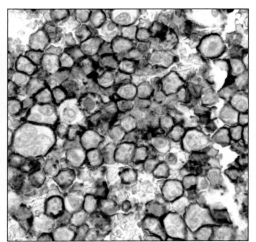
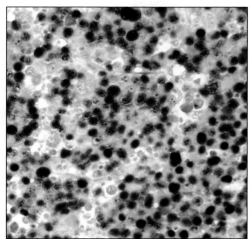

(Left) The tumor cells in plasmablastic lymphoma are CD56(+) in almost 50% of cases. CD56 is also positive in a subset of plasma cell myelomas. The expression of this marker in PEL is not well known as it has not been included in most published studies of this neoplasm. *(Right)* Similar to PEL, the tumor cells in plasmablastic lymphoma are positive for Epstein-Barr virus small-encoded RNA (EBER).

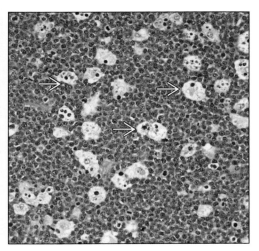
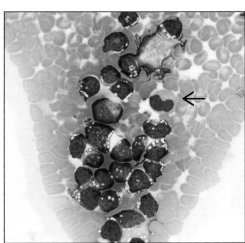

(Left) In Burkitt lymphoma, the neoplastic cells are of intermediate size, similar to the size of benign histiocyte nuclei, and have round nuclear contours, multiple small nucleoli, and basophilic cytoplasm. Macrophages with engulfed pyknotic nuclei ➡ impart a "starry sky" pattern. *(Right)* Touch imprint of Burkitt lymphoma. Lymphoma cells are intermediate in size with a scant to moderate amount of basophilic vacuolated cytoplasm. A macrophage is also shown ➡.

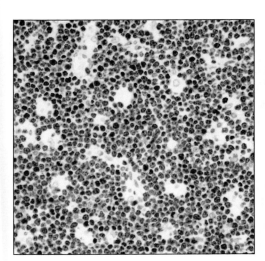
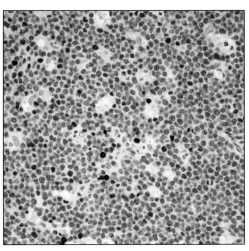

(Left) Burkitt lymphoma typically shows a high proliferation rate with virtually all tumor cells being positive for MIB-1 (Ki-67). In addition, the intensity of expression of MIB-1 is similar in all the tumor cells. *(Right)* Burkitt lymphoma cells are characteristically negative for Bcl-2. Weak Bcl-2 expression can occur in a small subset of Burkitt lymphomas, but strong Bcl-2 expression argues against the diagnosis of Burkitt lymphoma.

LYMPHOMATOID GRANULOMATOSIS

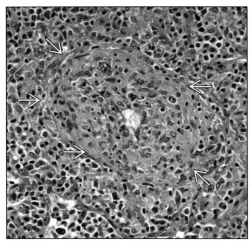

The morphologic hallmark of LYG is the presence of vessel walls with a transmural infiltrate of small lymphocytes, large atypical lymphoid cells, and histiocytes with angiodestruction ➡.

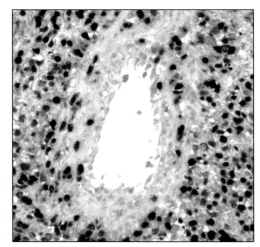

Case of LYG with numerous EBV(+) cells as shown by in situ hybridization for EBV-encoded RNA. The number of EBV(+) cells correlates with prognosis. This case was LYG grade 3.

TERMINOLOGY

Abbreviations
- Lymphomatoid granulomatosis (LYG)

Synonyms
- Angiocentric lymphoma

Definitions
- Extranodal angiocentric &/or angiodestructive B-cell lymphoproliferative disorder composed of numerous T cells and a variable number of neoplastic EBV(+) B cells

ETIOLOGY/PATHOGENESIS

Infectious Agents
- LYG presumably arises from EBV-immortalized B cells that have escaped immune surveillance
- Relationship between LYG and post-transplant lymphoproliferative disorders is unclear

Clinical Associations
- Congenital and acquired immunodeficiencies
  - Wiskott-Aldrich syndrome
  - HIV infection
  - High-dose chemotherapy

CLINICAL ISSUES

Epidemiology
- Incidence
  - Rare
- Age
  - Wide age range
  - Most frequent in young adults (~ 30-40 years)
- Gender
  - M:F ratio = > 2:1
- Ethnicity
  - No clear ethnic susceptibility; more common in Western countries

Presentation
- Generalized symptoms that suggest infection
- Lung is most frequent site of involvement
  - Multiple bilateral pulmonary nodules (most frequent)
    - Lower lobes involved most often
    - Cavitation in large nodules; ~ 25% of cases
  - Rare forms of lung involvement
    - Interstitial &/or reticulonodular patterns
    - Single &/or unilateral nodules
  - Lesions can disappear or migrate spontaneously ("wax and wane")
- Other sites of involvement
  - Skin (~ 40-50%); particularly lower extremities
  - Central nervous system (~ 30%)
  - Kidney (~ 30%) and liver (~ 30%)
  - Upper aerodigestive and gastrointestinal tracts uncommonly involved
  - Lymph nodes and spleen are involved rarely

Laboratory Tests
- Peripheral blood
  - High levels of EBV DNA

Treatment
- Interferon-α 2b is reported to be effective for LYG with few EBV(+) large cells (low-grade)
- Aggressive chemotherapy plus rituximab for LYG with numerous EBV(+) large cells

Prognosis
- Number of large EBV(+) B cells correlates with prognosis
  - Also influences choice of therapy
- Most patients have progressive course
  - Median survival: 14 months

LYMPHOMATOID GRANULOMATOSIS

Key Facts

Terminology
- Extranodal angiocentric &/or angiodestructive EBV(+) B-cell lymphoproliferative disorder

Clinical Issues
- Most frequent in young adults (~ 30-40 years)
- Lung is most frequent site of involvement
- Number of large EBV(+) large B cells correlates with prognosis

Microscopic Pathology
- Angiocentric, nodular lymphohistiocytic infiltrate
- Small lymphocytes, histiocytes, plasma cells, and variable number of large lymphoid cells
- Lymphocytic "vasculitis" with transmural invasion; ± necrosis; no granulocytes

- Grading based on number of EBV(+) large B cells and extent of necrosis

Ancillary Tests
- Large cells are B cells
  - CD45/LCA(+), EBER(+), CD30(+/-), CD15(-)
- Smaller reactive cells are T cells: CD4 > CD8
- Monoclonal *IgH* rearrangements

Top Differential Diagnoses
- Fungal or mycobacterial infections
- Necrotizing sarcoidosis
- Wegener granulomatosis
- Diffuse large B-cell lymphoma
- Classical Hodgkin lymphoma
- Peripheral T-cell lymphoma
- Extranodal NK-/T-cell lymphoma, nasal type

- Up to ~ 25% of patients may have spontaneous remission(s)

MICROSCOPIC PATHOLOGY

Histologic Features
- Angiocentric & angiodestructive lymphohistiocytic infiltrate
  - Invasion of blood vessel walls
    - Lymphocytic "vasculitis" with transmural invasion
- Small lymphocytes admixed with histiocytes, plasma cells, and variable numbers of large atypical lymphoid cells
  - Granulocytes are rare or absent
- Variable areas of necrosis
  - Vascular occlusion
  - Fibrinoid necrosis of blood vessels mediated by chemokines
- Granulomas or multinucleated giant cells are not usually seen
  - Except in skin
- Grading is based on number of EBV(+) large B cells and extent of necrosis
  - Grade 1 and 2 are considered B-cell lymphoproliferative disorder of uncertain malignant potential
    - Some cases may regress spontaneously or respond to interferon-α 2b therapy
  - Grade 3 is equivalent to diffuse large B-cell lymphoma (DLBCL)

Cytologic Features
- Larger atypical cells have round to oval nuclei and prominent nucleoli
- Binucleated cells are commonly seen

ANCILLARY TESTS

Immunohistochemistry
- Positive for common pan-B-cell markers

- CD19, CD20, CD22, CD79a, pax-5
- CD45/LCA(+), CD30(+/-)
- EBV-LMP1(+/-), CD15(-)
- Rarely can show cytoplasmic monotypic Ig light chain in large B cells
- Smaller reactive cells are T cells: CD3(+), CD4 > CD8

In Situ Hybridization
- Large B cells are EBER(+)

Molecular Genetics
- Monoclonal *IgH* gene rearrangements in grade 2 and 3 cases of LYG

DIFFERENTIAL DIAGNOSIS

Fungal or Mycobacterial Infections
- Pulmonary histoplasmosis
  - Acute form
    - Flu symptoms, pulmonary infiltrates, and serologic evidence of *Histoplasma* infection
    - Lymphohistiocytic infiltrate with parenchymal necrosis and vasculitis (differential diagnosis with LYG grade 1)
    - Small necrotizing granulomas; granulocytes(+)
    - GMS(+), EBER(-)
  - Chronic form and histoplasmoma
    - Well-formed necrotizing granulomas; granulocytes(+)
- Tuberculosis
  - Granulomatous inflammation with caseating necrosis; variable number of Langhans giant cells
  - *M. tuberculosis* organisms can be found in areas of necrosis
    - Acid-fast by Ziehl-Neelsen stain
- Atypical mycobacteriosis
  - Immunocompromised patients &/or preexisting lung disease
  - Granulomatous inflammation with caseating necrosis; variable number of Langhans giant cells
  - Culture is required for diagnosis

LYMPHOMATOID GRANULOMATOSIS

Histologic Grading Scheme

Grade	Infiltrate	Necrosis	EBER
Grade 1	Polymorphic lymphoid infiltrate	Usually small and focal	< 5 positive cells per HPF
Grade 2	Large atypical cells prominent	Necrosis is common	5-20 positive cells per HPF
Grade 3	Large atypical cells easily seen	Extensive necrosis	> 20 positive cells per HPF

Necrotizing Sarcoidosis
- Adult females; frequently asymptomatic
- Unilateral or bilateral lung lesions
- Histologic features
  o Vascular granulomas surrounding, infiltrating, and destroying pulmonary arteries and veins; necrosis(+)

Wegener Granulomatosis
- Systemic necrotizing vasculitis that primarily involves upper and lower respiratory tracts and kidneys
- Clinical criteria
  o Nasal or oral inflammation
  o Pulmonary nodules, infiltrates, or cavities
  o Abnormal urinary sediment (usually microscopic hematuria)
  o Necrotizing granulomatous inflammation involving small arteries (by biopsy)
- Limited Wegener granulomatosis
  o Female predominance; disease confined to lungs
- Hallmark histologic features
  o Liquefactive &/or coagulative necrosis, geographic-shaped
  o Eosinophils(+); multinucleated giant cells without forming well-defined granulomas
  o Destructive, leukocytolytic angiitis involving arteries and veins

Diffuse Large B-cell Lymphoma
- Primary DLBCL of lung represents < 1% of all lung neoplasms
- Histologic features
  o Sheets of large neoplastic cells (centroblasts &/or immunoblasts)
  o ± areas of coagulative necrosis
  o Invasion of normal pulmonary structures, such as bronchial wall and pleura, is common
- Immunophenotype
  o B-cell antigens(+), CD10(+/-), Bcl-6(+/-), EBV(-)
- DLBCL differs from grade 3 LYG in 2 ways
  o Grade 3 LYG resembles DLBCL but usually maintains some inflammatory background
  o Grade 3 LYG is EBV(+) unlike most cases of DLBCL

Primary Mediastinal Large B-cell Lymphoma (PMLBCL)
- Clinical features
  o Enlarging mass in anterior-superior mediastinum
  o Frequent infiltration of local organs and structures
- Histologic features
  o Diffuse to vaguely nodular growth pattern associated with variable sclerosis
  o Intermediate to large lymphoid cells
    ▪ Pale cytoplasm, often result of retraction artifact
    ▪ ± Reed-Sternberg-like or Hodgkin-like cells
  o Immunophenotype
    ▪ B-cell antigens(+)
    ▪ CD30(+/-) in ~ 75% of cases (weak and focal)
    ▪ p63(+), CD23(+/-), MAL(+/-)
    ▪ CD10(-), EBV(-)

Classical Hodgkin Lymphoma (CHL)
- When CHL involves lung, it is usually by contiguous spread from lymph nodes
- Single pulmonary mass or multiple bilateral nodules
- Same histologic features and immunophenotypic features as nodal CHL
  o Hodgkin and Reed-Sternberg cells
  o Immunophenotype
    ▪ CD30(+), CD15(+/-)
    ▪ pax-5(+); dimmer expression than reactive B cells

Peripheral T-cell Lymphoma (PTCL)
- Up to 20% of patients with PTCL have pulmonary involvement at presentation
  o In another 20%, pulmonary involvement will develop during clinical course
- Usually diffuse growth pattern with atypical lymphoid cells
- Immunophenotype
  o Aberrant T-cell phenotype with frequent downregulation of CD5 and CD7
  o CD4(+/-), CD8(-/+)

Extranodal NK-/T-cell Lymphoma, Nasal Type
- Upper aerodigestive tract
- Necrosis & vascular invasion
- Diffuse infiltrate by atypical lymphoid cells
- Immunophenotype
  o CD2(+), CD56(+), surface CD3(-)
  o EBV(+), cytotoxic markers(+)

SELECTED REFERENCES
1. Rao R et al: Lymphomatoid granulomatosis treated with rituximab and chemotherapy. Clin Adv Hematol Oncol. 1(11):658-60; discussion 660, 2003
2. Haque AK et al: Pulmonary lymphomatoid granulomatosis in acquired immunodeficiency syndrome: lesions with Epstein-Barr virus infection. Mod Pathol. 11(4):347-56, 1998
3. Jaffe ES et al: Lymphomatoid granulomatosis: pathogenesis, pathology and clinical implications. Cancer Surv. 30:233-48, 1997
4. McNiff JM et al: Lymphomatoid granulomatosis of the skin and lung. An angiocentric T-cell-rich B-cell lymphoproliferative disorder. Arch Dermatol. 132(12):1464-70, 1996

LYMPHOMATOID GRANULOMATOSIS

Imaging and Microscopic Features

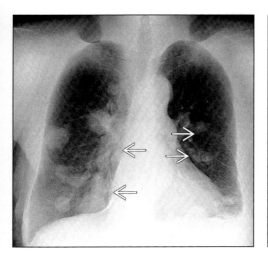

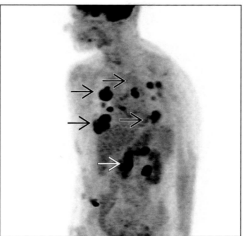

(Left) Chest radiograph shows bilateral pulmonary nodules that are larger and confluent in the middle and lower lobes ➡. A CT-guided biopsy confirmed the diagnosis of LYG. *(Right)* PET/CT scan of the same patient with LYG shows bilateral hypermetabolic pulmonary masses ➡. A 3.5 cm mass involving the left adrenal gland is also noted ➡. Fluorodeoxyglucose uptake in the liver and spleen appears normal. There are no hypermetabolic abdominal lymph nodes.

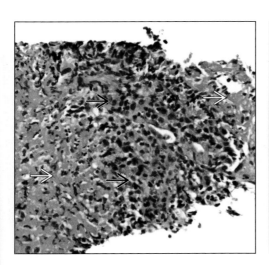

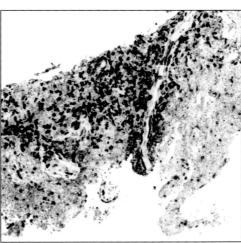

(Left) CT-guided 20-gauge core needle biopsy specimen of LYG involving the lung shows necrosis ➡ and an angiocentric lymphohistiocytic infiltrate ➡. *(Right)* CT-guided 20-gauge core needle biopsy specimen of LYG shows that the angiocentric lymphohistiocytic infiltrate was composed predominantly of small CD3(+) reactive T cells.

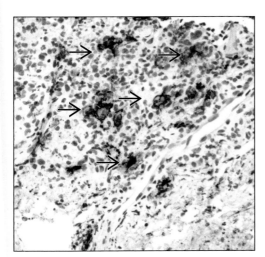

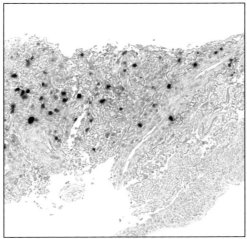

(Left) CT-guided 20-gauge core needle biopsy specimen of LYG shows that the angiocentric lymphohistiocytic infiltrate contained scattered, large CD20(+) B cells ➡. *(Right)* CT-guided 20-gauge core needle biopsy specimen of LYG shows an angiocentric lymphohistiocytic infiltrate with scattered large tumor cells that were EBER(+). Presence of EBV is an important hallmark for the diagnosis of LYG.

LYMPHOMATOID GRANULOMATOSIS

Imaging and Microscopic Features

(Left) A percutaneous guided biopsy was performed and revealed LYG grade 2 in this CT-scan of a 64-year-old woman who presented with a 5 cm left upper lobe lung mass ➡. *(Right)* CT-guided 19-gauge core needle biopsy specimen of LYG involving lung shows extensive necrosis ➡ associated with a lymphohistiocytic infiltrate ➡.

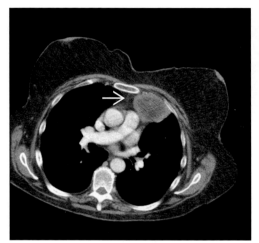
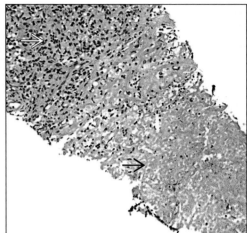

(Left) In this case of LYG, the neoplasm is composed of scattered large cells admixed with numerous small lymphocytes and histiocytes and few eosinophils. An angiocentric pattern is not noted in this field. *(Right)* LYG shows clusters of atypical large lymphoid cells that are CD20(+). Although an angiocentric pattern was not recognized in the H&E slide, this pattern was highlighted with CD20 immunostain ➡.

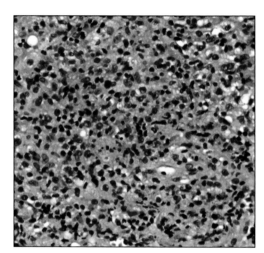
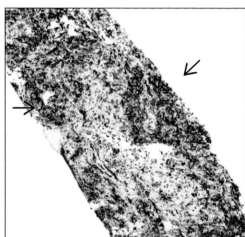

(Left) CT-guided 19-gauge core needle biopsy specimen of LYG shows that the lymphohistiocytic infiltrate was composed predominantly of CD3(+) T cells. Clusters of perivascular large atypical EBV(+) B cells were also noted (not shown). *(Right)* This case of LYG involving lung shows approximately 5-10 large cells positive for EBER per high-power field.

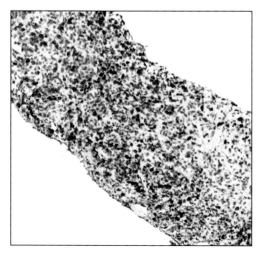
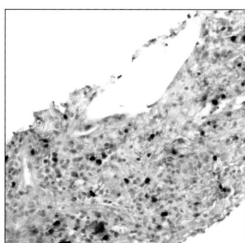

LYMPHOMATOID GRANULOMATOSIS

Microscopic Features

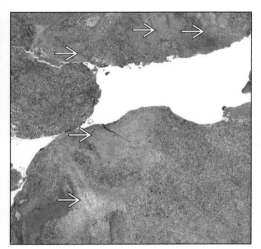

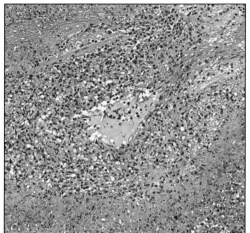

(Left) Open lung biopsy of a 29-year-old man with pulmonary LYG grade 3. There are large areas of geographic necrosis ➡ as well as a dense lymphohistiocytic infiltrate. This infiltrate is diffuse in some areas but maintained an angiocentric pattern in others. *(Right)* LYG grade 3 in a 29-year-old man shows a lymphohistiocytic infiltrate with an angiocentric growth pattern and necrosis. There are large atypical cells admixed with numerous small lymphocytes and histiocytes.

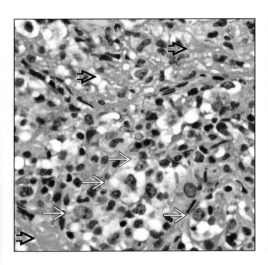

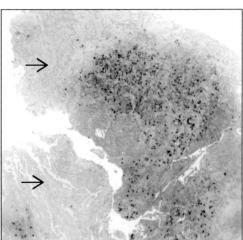

(Left) Open lung biopsy of a 29-year-old man with pulmonary LYG grade 3 shows the presence of clusters of large neoplastic cells ➡ admixed with small lymphocytes and fibrinoid necrosis ➡. *(Right)* Open lung biopsy of a 29-year-old man with pulmonary LYG grade 3 has > 20 EBER(+) large cells per high-power field, supporting LYG grade 3. Note also the presence of necrosis ➡. Grade 3 lesions are considered a subtype of diffuse large B-cell lymphoma.

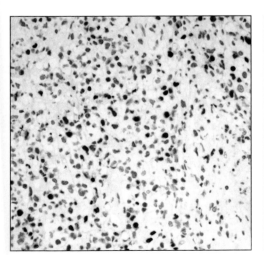

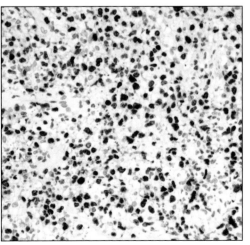

(Left) Open lung biopsy of a 29-year-old man with pulmonary LYG grade 3 shows large neoplastic cells positive for Bcl-6. *(Right)* Open lung biopsy of a 29-year-old man shows pulmonary LYG grade 3. The tumor proliferation index, as measured by MIB-1 (Ki-67), is high, approximately 80-90%.

Microscopic Features

(Left) Skin biopsy of a patient with LYG involving the lung who developed subcutaneous nodules shows an extensive lymphohistiocytic infiltrate in the dermis and subcutaneous adipose tissue. The infiltrate was composed of numerous T cells and histiocytes with a lesser number of large atypical B cells positive for CD20, CD30, LMP1, and EBER (not shown). *(Right)* Higher magnification shows a case of LYG involving skin. Note the presence of scattered large atypical cells ➡.

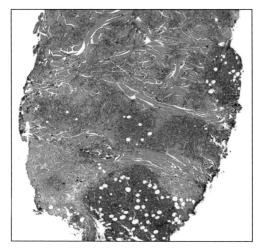 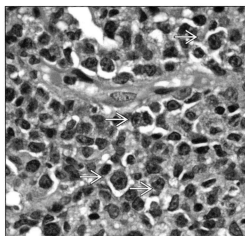

(Left) Skin biopsy of a patient with a history of LYG involving the lung who developed subcutaneous nodules shows CD20 immunohistochemical stain highlighting B cells. *(Right)* Skin biopsy of a patient with a history of LYG involving the lung who developed subcutaneous nodules. In situ hybridization for EBER shows that this neoplasm has numerous positive tumor cells supporting the diagnosis of LYG grade 3.

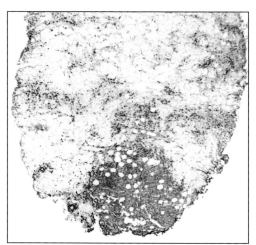 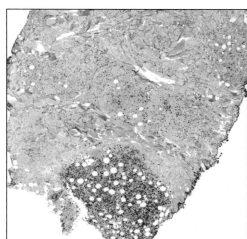

(Left) Gastric biopsy of a patient with a history of LYG involving the lung who developed multiple gastric ulcers shows large neoplastic cells present in a background rich in histiocytes and small lymphocytes, consistent with LYG. *(Right)* Gastric biopsy from a patient with history of LYG involving the lung who developed multiple gastric ulcers. The large neoplastic cells were positive for CD20 (shown), CD30, CD79a, CD45/LCA, and EBER. Numerous CD3(+) cells were seen in the background.

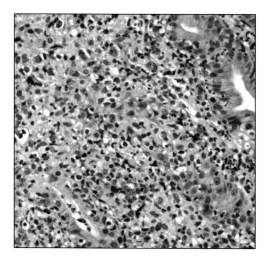 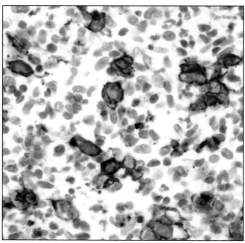

Differential Diagnosis

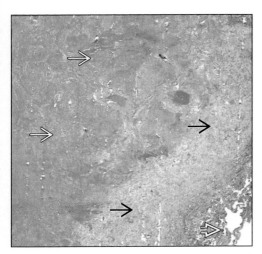
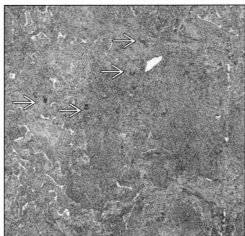

(Left) Wegener granulomatosis involving the lung with extensive areas of coagulative necrosis ➡. The necrosis is surrounded and separated from lung parenchyma ➡ by a band of granulation tissue ➡. *(Right)* Wegener granulomatosis involving the lung shows a dense lymphoid infiltrate with multinucleated giant cells ➡ obliterating the lung architecture.

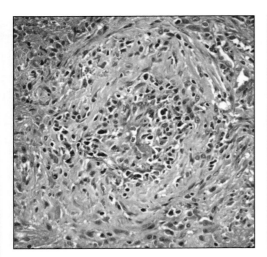
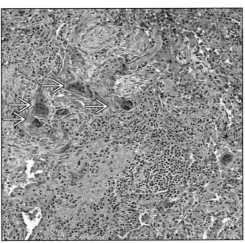

(Left) Wegener granulomatosis involving the lung shows leukocytolytic angiitis. Note the presence of scattered large lymphoid cells admixed with small lymphocytes and plasma cells infiltrating the vessel wall. *(Right)* Wegener granulomatosis involving the lung shows a lymphoid infiltrate associated with fibrosis and clusters of multinucleated giant cells ➡. Well-defined granulomas are not a characteristic of Wegener granulomatosis.

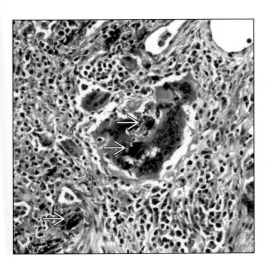
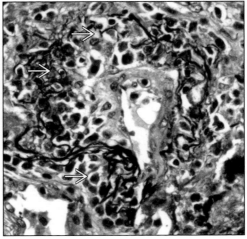

(Left) In Wegener granulomatosis the multinucleated giant cells contain elastic fibers (elastophagocytosis) ➡. A Verhoeff-van Gieson (VVG) stain outlines elastic fibers with a strong black color. *(Right)* The destructive character of the leukocytolytic angiitis seen in Wegener granulomatosis is outlined by the disruption of the network of elastic fibers of the vessel wall ➡. A Verhoeff-van Gieson (VVG) stain outlines elastic fibers with a strong black color.

Differential Diagnosis

(Left) Classical Hodgkin lymphoma involving the lung. The biopsy shows a dense lymphohistiocytic infiltrate with large neoplastic cells admixed with small lymphocytes. *(Right)* Classical Hodgkin lymphoma involving the lung. Note that the tumor cells are surrounding a medium-sized blood vessel similar to what is observed in LYG.

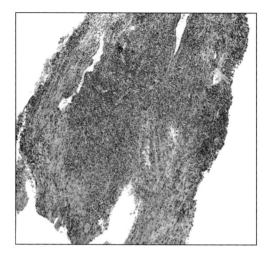 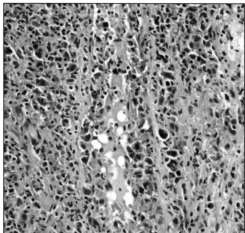

(Left) This case of classical Hodgkin lymphoma involving the lung contains areas of necrosis ➡. *(Right)* Classical Hodgkin lymphoma involving the lung. The large tumor cells are weakly positive for pax-5. They were also CD30(+), EBER(+), and CD15 (focal +), and were CD45/LCA(-), OCT2(-), and BOB1(-).

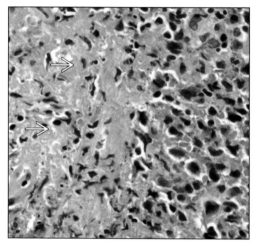 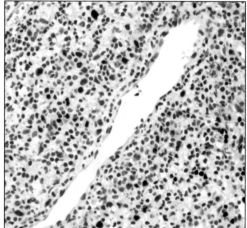

(Left) Classical Hodgkin lymphoma involving the lung. The large tumor cells are CD15(+). These cells were also CD30(+), pax-5(+), and EBER(+), and were CD45/LCA(-), OCT2(-), and BOB1(-) (not shown). *(Right)* Classical Hodgkin lymphoma involving the lung. The large tumor cells are CD45/LCA(-) (shown). They were CD30(+), pax-5(+), EBER(+), focally CD15(+), and OCT-2(-) and BOB1(-).

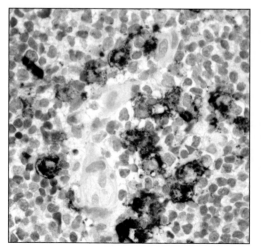 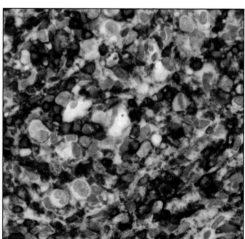

LYMPHOMATOID GRANULOMATOSIS

Differential Diagnosis

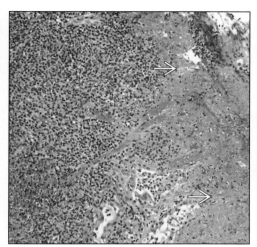

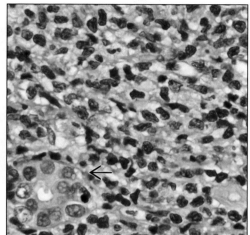

(Left) Peripheral T-cell lymphoma, not otherwise specified (PTCL, NOS) shows some necrosis ➡ and vascular involvement, features in common with LYG. However, the atypical cells have a T-cell phenotype and were EBER(-) by in situ hybridization. *(Right)* High magnification of a PTCL, NOS shows that the neoplastic cells are medium-sized and atypical. Residual epithelium is also present in this field ➡.

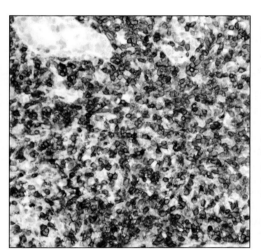

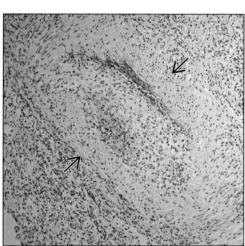

(Left) The neoplastic cells in this case of PTCL-NOS express CD3-ε. Large atypical CD20(+) cells were not seen. *(Right)* A case of PTCL-NOS. A blood vessel invaded by neoplasm is shown in this field ➡.

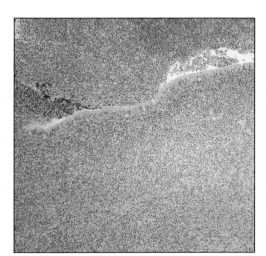

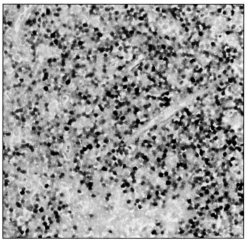

(Left) Extranodal NK-/T-cell lymphoma, nasal type, of T-cell lineage. The neoplastic cells in this case are predominantly small. T-cell lineage was shown by expression of CD8 and monoclonal T-cell receptor γ chain gene rearrangement.s *(Right)* Extranodal NK-/T-cell lymphoma, nasal type, of T-cell lineage. In situ hybridization for EBER shows that this neoplasm has numerous positive cells.

INTRAVASCULAR LARGE B-CELL LYMPHOMA

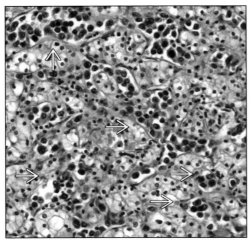

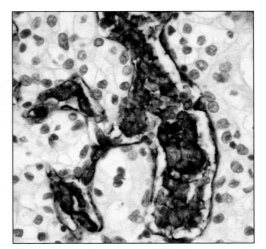

Intravascular large B-cell lymphoma (IVLBCL) in nephrectomy specimen of a patient with renal clear cell carcinoma. Large atypical lymphoid cells are seen inside of small sinusoid-like vessels ➡.

The intravascular large cells are CD20(+) and negative for T-cell antigens (not shown), which supports a B-cell lineage and the diagnosis of IVLBCL.

TERMINOLOGY

Abbreviations
- Intravascular large B-cell lymphoma (IVLBCL)

Synonyms
- Angiotropic large cell lymphoma
- Angioendotheliotropic (intravascular) lymphoma
- Intravascular lymphomatosis

Definitions
- Large B-cell lymphoma characterized by selective intravascular growth
- Preferential intravascular growth is a *conditio sine qua non* for diagnosing IVLBCL
  - Concomitant and minimal extravascular location of neoplastic cells, usually surrounding involved vessels, can be seen

CLINICAL ISSUES

Site
- Selective tumor growth within lumina of small blood vessels, particularly capillaries
- Widely disseminated
- Any organ can be involved
- Absence of marked lymphadenopathy
- Mechanisms responsible for selective growth of neoplastic cells within blood vessel lumina are unknown
- Possible explanations include
  - Chemokine-chemokine receptor interactions
    - e.g., CXCL9 (expressed in endothelium) and CXCR3 (expressed in IVLBCL)
  - Decreased expression of adhesion molecules on surface of IVLBCL cells
    - e.g., CD29 and CD54

Presentation
- Middle-aged or elderly patients; median: 67 years
- M:F ratio = 1.3:1
- IVLBCL can involve any organ with heterogeneous, often nonspecific symptoms
  - Fever of unknown origin
  - General fatigue
  - Deterioration in performance status
- Diagnosis can be clinically difficult and some cases are diagnosed postmortem
- 2 major patterns of clinical presentation
  - Western IVLBCL
    - Predominant neurologic and dermatologic manifestations
    - Central nervous system is involved in most patients
  - Asian IVLBCL
    - Hemophagocytic syndrome
    - Fever and B symptoms
    - Pancytopenia and bone marrow infiltration
    - Skin and central nervous system involvement are uncommon
- Skin lesions
  - Heterogeneous clinical presentation: Plaques, telangiectatic patches, cellulitis, ulcerated nodules
  - Skin involvement is sometimes detected by random skin biopsy of grossly unremarkable skin
  - Cutaneous variant
    - Most frequent in females
    - Younger than other IVLBCL patients
    - Better prognosis
- Kidney
  - Increased creatinine
  - Proteinuria
  - Renal insufficiency
- Liver
  - Hepatomegaly
  - Increased bilirubin and liver enzymes
- Central nervous system

INTRAVASCULAR LARGE B-CELL LYMPHOMA

Key Facts

Terminology
- Rare large B-cell lymphoma characterized by selective intravascular growth

Clinical Issues
- Absence of marked lymphadenopathy
- Middle-aged or elderly patients
- Predominant neurologic and dermatologic manifestations (Western countries)
- Patients from Asia (mainly Japan) preferentially show hemophagocytic syndrome (Asian variant)

Microscopic Pathology
- IVLBCL cells are large, with vesicular nuclear chromatin, distinct nucleoli, and frequent mitoses
- Lymphoma cells are mainly located in lumina of small vessels

- Sinusoidal involvement of liver, spleen, and bone marrow

Ancillary Tests
- Pan-B-cell markers(+), Bcl-2(+), MUM1(+)
- CD5([+] 30%); other T-cell markers(-)
- Ki-67 high

Top Differential Diagnoses
- Peripheral T- or NK-cell lymphomas with intravascular pattern
- Hepatosplenic T-cell lymphoma
- T-cell large granular lymphocytic leukemia
- Aggressive NK-cell leukemia/lymphoma
- Splenic B-cell marginal zone lymphoma
- Diffuse large B-cell lymphoma

- o Alteration of consciousness
- o Motor and sensory deficits
- o Seizure
- o Dementia
- Lungs
  - o Dyspnea and hypoxia
- Hematopoietic system
  - o Splenomegaly
  - o Hemophagocytosis
  - o Anemia, thrombocytopenia, and leukopenia
- Other
  - o Increased LDH
  - o Ascites
  - o Endocrine dysfunction (hypopituitarism)
  - o Multiorgan failure

Treatment
- Rituximab-containing chemotherapy plus central nervous system-oriented therapy
  - o R-CHOP plus high-dose methotrexate

Prognosis
- Aggressive behavior and often fatal course
- Predictive factors that are useful for risk-stratification are not established

MICROSCOPIC PATHOLOGY

Histologic Features
- Lymphoma cells are mainly located in lumina of small vessels
- Minimal extravascular location of tumor cells can be seen
  - o Usually surrounding involved vessels
  - o Extravascular masses can be detected at autopsy in some patients
- Sinusoidal involvement of liver, spleen, and bone marrow
- Spleen: Red pulp involvement
- Kidney: Neoplastic cells within glomerular capillaries and peritubular capillaries

- Brain: Neoplastic cells within small vessels
- Circulating lymphoma cells can be occasionally seen in peripheral blood
- Fibrin thrombi, hemorrhage, and necrosis

Cytologic Features
- Usually tumor cells are large, with vesicular nuclear chromatin with distinct nucleoli
- In some cases, tumor cells have coarse nuclear chromatin and irregular or indented nuclei
- Mitoses are frequent
- IVLBCL cell size may be smaller than usual in some cases

ANCILLARY TESTS

Immunohistochemistry
- Pan-B-cell markers(+)
  - o CD19, CD20, CD22, CD79a, and pax-5
- CD5([+] 30%), CD10([+] 10%), Bcl-6([+] 25%)
- Bcl-2([+] 90%), MUM1([+] 95%)
- Ki-67 reveals high proliferative activity
- CD2(-), CD3(-)

Cytogenetics
- Pathognomonic cytogenetic abnormalities have not been reported

Molecular Genetics
- Monoclonal rearrangements of the *IgH* gene can be detected by PCR
- *TCR* genes in germline configuration

DIFFERENTIAL DIAGNOSIS

Peripheral T- or NK-cell Lymphomas with Intravascular Pattern
- Rare cases of T-cell lymphoma or NK-cell lymphoma can be intravascular
- Positive for T-cell or NK markers

INTRAVASCULAR LARGE B-CELL LYMPHOMA

Lymphomas with Intravascular Pattern of Growth

Lymphoma/Leukemia Type	Immunophenotype
Intravascular large B-cell lymphoma	CD19(+), CD20(+), CD22(+), CD79(+), CD5(-/+), CD10(-/+), MUM1(+/-), CD3(-)
Peripheral T- or NK-cell lymphomas with intravascular pattern	Positive for T-cell (CD2, CD3, CD43, CD5, CD7) &/or NK markers (CD16, CD56, CD57)
Hepatosplenic T-cell lymphoma	CD2(+), CD3(+), TIA(+), GZM-M(+), GZM-B(-), perforin(-), CD4(-), CD5(-), CD16(+/-), CD56(+), CD20(-)
T-cell large granular lymphocytic leukemia	CD3(-), CD8(+), CD4(-), CD56(+), CD57(-), TIA(+), GZM-B(+), GZM-M(+), perforin(+), CD20(-)
Aggressive NK-cell leukemia/lymphoma	CD2(+), surface CD3(-), CD3-ε(+), CD4(-), CD8(-), CD16(+), CD56(+), TIA(+), GZM-B(+), CD57(-), EBV(+/-)
Splenic marginal zone B-cell lymphoma	pax-5(+), CD19(+), CD20(+), CD22(+), CD43(-), CD5(-), CD10(-), CD23(-), annexin-A1(-)
Diffuse large B-cell lymphoma	Similar immunophenotype to IVLBCL

- These rare lymphomas do not exist as diagnostic categories in 2008 WHO classification

Hepatosplenic T-cell Lymphoma
- Some reported cases of intravascular T-cell lymphomas are probably
  - γ-δ T-cell lymphoma or hepatosplenic T-cell lymphoma
- More frequent in young men
- Splenomegaly and hepatomegaly
- Bone marrow biopsy
  - Early stage disease: Small to intermediate in size lymphoma cells; intrasinusoidal pattern
  - Late stage disease: Large blastic lymphoma cells; interstitial or diffuse pattern
- T-cell markers: CD2(+), CD3(+), and cytotoxic markers TIA(+), GZM-B(+)
- B-cell markers(-)
- Isochromosome 7q is consistent abnormality

T-cell Large Granular Lymphocytic Leukemia (T-LGL)
- Indolent clinical course with long survival
- Commonly associated with infections
- Peripheral blood: Increased large granular lymphocytes
- Bone marrow, usually interstitial pattern, but sinusoidal pattern can be seen
- CD8(+), GZM-B(+), perforin(+), CD16(+), CD57(+), CD5([+]dim)

Aggressive NK-cell Leukemia/Lymphoma
- Leukemic cells can have cytoplasmic azurophilic granules
- NK-cell markers(+), GZM-B(+), perforin(+), EBV(+/-)
- Surface CD3(-), CD5(-)
- No TCR gene rearrangements

Splenic B-cell Marginal Zone Lymphoma
- Spleen: Infiltration of white and red pulp
- Small neoplastic cells with abundant pale cytoplasm
- Patients often present with cytopenias
  - Villous lymphocytes in peripheral blood smear
- Pan-B-cell markers(+), CD3(-), CD10(-)
- Allelic loss of chromosome 7q22-36 (40%)

Diffuse Large B-cell Lymphoma (DLBCL)
- Tumor cells are cytologically (and can be immunophenotypically) identical
  - IVLBCL does not present with lymphadenopathy or mass, unlike DLBCL
- Cases of nodal DLBCL can relapse with the appearance of IVLBCL
- Rare cases of IVLBCL may have derived from low-grade B-cell lymphomas
  - Identical *IgH* gene rearrangements in low-grade and IVLBCL (in some cases)

DIAGNOSTIC CHECKLIST

Pathologic Interpretation Pearls
- Large lymphoid cells in intravascular spaces
  - B-cell immunophenotype

SELECTED REFERENCES

1. Kong YY et al: Intravascular large B-cell lymphoma with cutaneous manifestations: a clinicopathologic, immunophenotypic and molecular study of three cases. J Cutan Pathol. 36(8):865-70, 2009
2. Shimada K et al: Presentation and management of intravascular large B-cell lymphoma. Lancet Oncol. 10(9):895-902, 2009
3. Ferreri AJ et al: The addition of rituximab to anthracycline-based chemotherapy significantly improves outcome in 'Western' patients with intravascular large B-cell lymphoma. Br J Haematol. 143(2):253-7, 2008
4. Gleason BC et al: Intravascular cytotoxic T-cell lymphoma: A case report and review of the literature. J Am Acad Dermatol. 58(2):290-4, 2008
5. Nakamichi N et al: NK-cell intravascular lymphomatosis--a mini-review. Eur J Haematol. 81(1):1-7, 2008
6. Ponzoni M et al: Definition, diagnosis, and management of intravascular large B-cell lymphoma: proposals and perspectives from an international consensus meeting. J Clin Oncol. 25(21):3168-73, 2007
7. Shimizu I et al: Asian variant of intravascular lymphoma: aspects of diagnosis and the role of rituximab. Intern Med. 46(17):1381-6, 2007
8. Estalilla OC et al: Intravascular large B-cell lymphoma. A report of five cases initially diagnosed by bone marrow biopsy. Am J Clin Pathol. 112(2):248-55, 1999

INTRAVASCULAR LARGE B-CELL LYMPHOMA

Microscopic Features

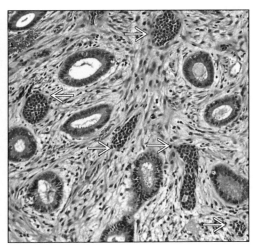

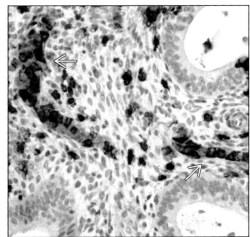

(Left) Endometrium shows involvement by IVLBCL with classical morphologic features. Small blood vessels in the endometrial mucosa are filled with large atypical neoplastic cells ➡. The endometrial glands are unremarkable. *(Right)* CD20 highlights the intravascular large neoplastic cells supporting B-cell lineage and the diagnosis of IVLBCL ➡.

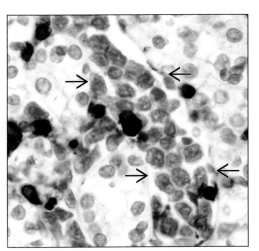

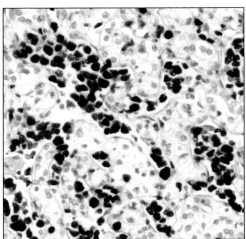

(Left) This IVLBCL was diagnosed in a nephrectomy specimen. The patient underwent nephrectomy, which revealed renal clear cell carcinoma and IVLBCL. Lymphoma cells within a capillary ➡ were positive for CD20 (not shown) and negative for CD3. *(Right)* IVLBCL is usually characterized by a high proliferation rate as shown by reactivity with the Ki-67 (MIB-1) antibody in this field.

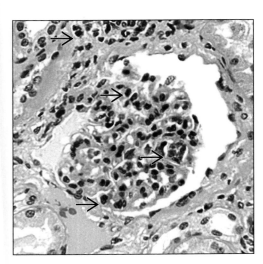

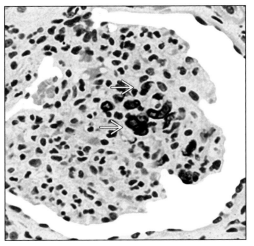

(Left) IVLBCL diagnosed in a nephrectomy specimen. The kidney was removed for transitional cell carcinoma of the renal pelvis. In this glomerulus, small clusters and single neoplastic cells highlighted by CD20 are seen within capillaries ➡. *(Right)* IVLBCL diagnosed in a nephrectomy specimen. Note few clusters of large neoplastic cells inside the glomerular capillary. The neoplastic cells are positive for CD20 (shown) ➡ and negative for CD3 (not shown).

INTRAVASCULAR LARGE B-CELL LYMPHOMA

Microscopic Features

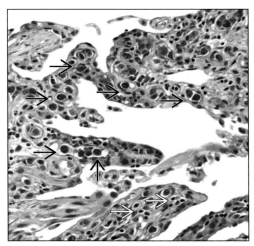 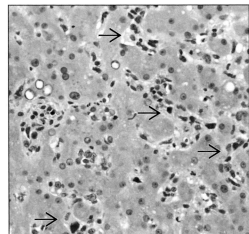

(Left) IVLBCL involving a lung biopsy specimen. The tumor cells are large and located within the alveolar capillaries. Some of the tumor cells are highlighted ➡. Note the size of the neoplastic cells compared with that of reactive lymphocytes ➡. (Right) IVLBCL involving liver. Large neoplastic cells are present within the sinusoids ➡. The tumor cells were CD20(+), Bcl-2(+), and CD3(-) (not shown), supporting B-cell lineage.

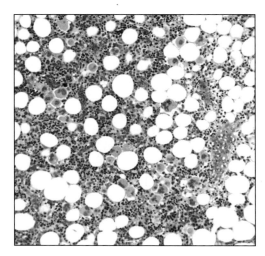 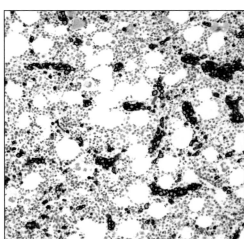

(Left) Hypercellular bone marrow in a patient with IVLBCL. Note the subtle intrasinusoidal infiltration by neoplastic cells difficult to recognize in this low-power field. Megakaryocytic hyperplasia is also present. (Right) IVLBCL involving bone marrow. The intrasinusoidal infiltrate is easily recognized using immunostains specific for B-cell markers, such as CD20.

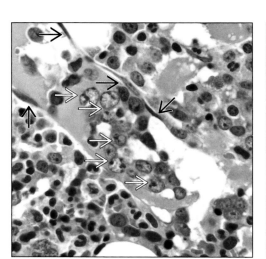 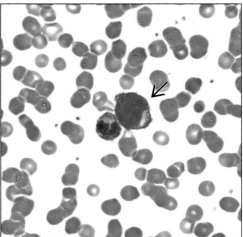

(Left) IVLBCL involving bone marrow. Note the presence of large atypical lymphoid cells inside this small blood vessel. The neoplastic cells characteristically have open nuclear chromatin, distinct nucleoli ➡, and are larger than adjacent endothelial cells ➡. (Right) IVLBCL in peripheral blood smear. In this field, large neoplastic cells can be seen ➡.

INTRAVASCULAR LARGE B-CELL LYMPHOMA

Differential Diagnosis

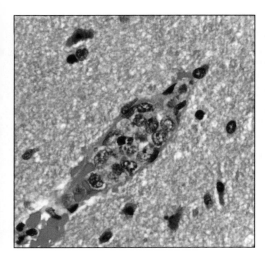

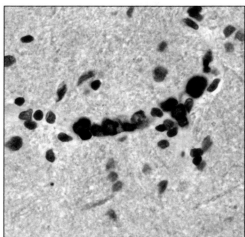

(Left) Brain biopsy shows intravascular T-cell lymphoma. Large lymphoma cells are located within a small capillary lumen. The neoplastic cells had an aberrant cytotoxic T-cell immunophenotype. *(Right)* Intravascular T-cell lymphoma diagnosed in a brain biopsy specimen. The neoplastic cells were positive for CD3 (shown), CD8, CD56, TIA-1, granzyme B, and CD56, and were negative for BF1 (TCR framework) and B-cell markers.

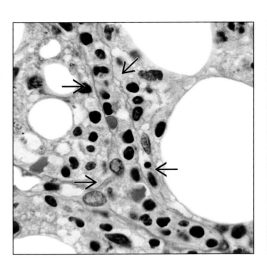

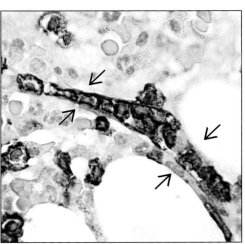

(Left) Hepatosplenic T-cell lymphoma (HSTCL) involving bone marrow. The neoplastic cells are mostly small and are located predominantly within the sinusoids ➡. *(Right)* HSTCL involving bone marrow. The intrasinusoidal neoplastic cells are highlighted by the anti-CD3 antibody ➡.

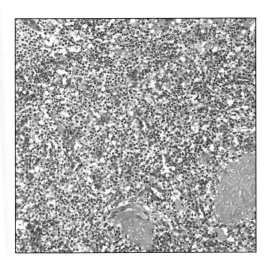

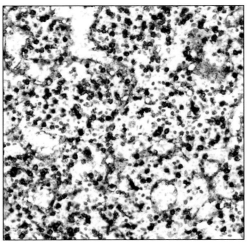

(Left) Splenic involvement by T-cell large granular lymphocytic leukemia (T-LGL). The cords and sinusoids within the red pulp are expanded by neoplastic cells. The white pulp is often spared and can be hyperplastic (not shown in this field). *(Right)* CD8(+) neoplastic T-LGL cells involving cords in splenic red pulp. The neoplastic cells were also CD3(+), TIA(+), and GZM-B(+). Note that endothelial cells lining the splenic sinusoids are also CD8(+).

PLASMACYTOMA

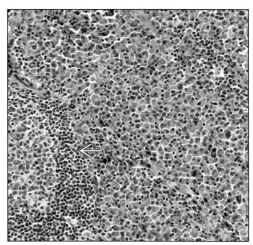

Plasmacytoma involving lymph node. The neoplasm has a parafollicular pattern and is composed of mature plasma cells. Note the presence of a lymphoid follicle with a hyperplastic germinal center ➡.

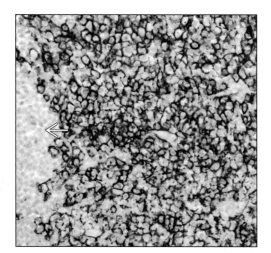

Plasmacytoma involving lymph node. The neoplasm is strongly CD138(+). A hyperplastic lymphoid follicle that is CD138(-) is at the left of the field ➡.

TERMINOLOGY

Abbreviations
- Extramedullary plasmacytoma (EP)
- Solitary plasmacytoma of bone (SPB)

Synonyms
- Extraosseous or osseous plasmacytoma

Definitions
- Neoplasm composed of monoclonal plasma cells that involves tissues
  - No evidence of bone marrow involvement
  - No clinical features of plasma cell myeloma
  - Small or absent M-component in urine or serum

ETIOLOGY/PATHOGENESIS

Immune Dysfunction
- T- or B-cell deficiency or autoimmune disorders may play a role in some cases

CLINICAL ISSUES

Epidemiology
- Incidence
  - Rare
    - < 5% of all plasma cell malignancies
  - SPB is more frequent than EP
- Age
  - Median age ~ 55 years
    - IgA(+) extramedullary plasmacytomas occur at a younger age
- Gender
  - Male:female: ~ 2-3:1

Presentation
- Extramedullary plasmacytoma
  - Head and neck is most common site of disease (90%)
    - Upper respiratory tract: Nasopharynx, sinuses, and tonsils
    - ~ 4% of all nonepithelial tumors of this area
    - Nasal obstruction, epistaxis, mass
    - May spread to cervical lymph nodes in ~ 15% of cases
  - Gastrointestinal (GI) tract is 2nd most common site
  - Other rare sites of disease
    - Lymph node, bladder, breast, thyroid, testis, brain, skin
- Solitary plasmacytoma of bone
  - Bone pain, severe back pain, spinal cord compression, pathological fracture
  - Thoracic vertebrae are most common site of disease
  - Lumbar or cervical vertebrae are 2nd most common locations
  - Involvement of distal extremities, below knees or elbow, is rare

Laboratory Tests
- Small M-component in up to 50% of SPB and in < 25% of EP cases
  - ~ 20% of EP cases have paraprotein of IgA type
- Levels of uninvolved Ig are usually normal
- No anemia or elevated creatinine
- Serum free light chain ratio may be abnormal

Treatment
- Radiation
- Surgery

Prognosis
- Prognosis of EP is significantly better than that of SPB
  - ~ 2/3 are alive for > 10 years
  - Only 15% of EP progress to plasma cell myeloma
- Survival of SPB is better than that of myeloma patients
  - 50% of SPB patients are alive at 10 years
  - 25-40% are disease free at 10 years

PLASMACYTOMA

Key Facts

Terminology
- Plasmacytoma is a neoplasm composed of monoclonal plasma cells that involves tissues
  - No evidence of bone marrow involvement
  - No clinical or laboratory evidence of myeloma
- 2 general types of plasmacytoma
  - EP: Neoplasm composed of plasma cells, which arises in tissues other than bone
  - SPB: Localized (single) bone tumor composed of plasma cells

Clinical Issues
- Small M-component in ~ 50% of SPB, < 25% of EP
- No anemia or elevated creatinine

Microscopic Pathology
- Plasma cells show a spectrum of maturation

Ancillary Tests
- CD138(+), CD38(+), MUM1/IRF-4(+), and cytoplasmic light chain restriction
- Usually pax-5(-), CD20(-)

Top Differential Diagnoses
- MALT lymphoma with marked plasmacytic differentiation
- Castleman disease, plasma cell variant
- Plasmablastic lymphoma
- ALK(+) diffuse large B-cell lymphoma

Diagnostic Checklist
- SPB has high risk of progression to myeloma; much less for EP
  - Persistent paraprotein signifies higher risk of progression

- 50% of SPB progress to plasma cell myeloma
  - Progression usually occurs within 3-4 years of diagnosis; risk is higher in patients with
    - Large mass (> 5 cm)
    - Persistent M-protein
    - Rising free Ig light chain ratio
- Recurrences are frequent in SPB and EP

IMAGE FINDINGS

General Features
- Extramedullary plasmacytoma
  - No evidence of bone involvement
- Solitary plasmacytoma of bone
  - Single lytic bone lesion
  - No additional lesions by MRI

MICROSCOPIC PATHOLOGY

Histologic Features
- Diffuse infiltrate of plasma cells
- EP of head and neck and GI tract more often show mature cytology
- Plasma cells may show spectrum of maturation from well to poorly differentiated
- Mature plasma cells
  - Round eccentric nuclei, clumped peripheral nuclear chromatin, and cytoplasmic perinuclear hof
  - Nucleoli absent or inconspicuous
- Immature plasma cells
  - Pleomorphic nuclei, fine and immature nuclear chromatin
  - Prominent nucleoli
- Plasmablastic or anaplastic morphology
  - Large nuclei with centrally located nucleoli (immunoblast-like)

Lymph Nodes
- Plasma cells present in diffuse sheets

- Partially involved cases have parafollicular or paracortical pattern
  - ± residual lymphoid follicles

ANCILLARY TESTS

Immunohistochemistry
- Plasmacytoma shows an immunophenotype similar to plasma cell myeloma
  - CD138(+), CD38(+), MUM1/IRF-4(+), and cytoplasmic light chain restricted
  - CD79a(+), usually IgG(+) or IgA(+)
  - CD56 is more frequently positive in SPB (~ 50%) than in EP (~ 10%)
  - Cyclin-D1(+) small subset
    - Some cases express Cyclin-D1 due to CCND1 gene amplification
  - CD19(-), usually pax-5(-), CD20(-), CD45/LCA(-)
    - Small subset: CD45/LCA(+) &/or CD20(+)

Flow Cytometry
- Cell permeabilization methods are required to assess cytoplasmic Ig
- Immunophenotype similar to that reported by immunohistochemistry

Cytogenetics
- EP and SPB show cytogenetic abnormalities similar to plasma cell myeloma
  - Chromosome gains ~ 80%
  - Loss of 13q ~ 40%
  - t(4;14)(FGFR3/IGH) may occur
  - IGH rearrangements in ~ 30-40%
  - t(11;14)(CCND1/IGH) is usually negative
    - Cases with amplification of CCND1 gene has been identified
  - MYC rearrangements are common in extramedullary spread of plasma cell myeloma but uncommon in EP
  - IgH rearrangements involving MALT1, BCL6, and FOXP1 have not been described

In Situ Hybridization
- EBER usually negative

DIFFERENTIAL DIAGNOSIS

MALT Lymphoma and Other Low-Grade Lymphomas with Marked Plasmacytic Differentiation
- Morphologic overlap
  - Presence of B-lymphocyte component supports diagnosis of MALT lymphoma
- Immunophenotype
  - B cells are monoclonal
  - B cells are CD20(+), CD43(+/-)
  - Usually IgM(+)
- Genetics
  - MALT-related translocations do not occur in plasmacytoma
    - IAP2-MALT1/t(11;18)(q21;q21), BCL10-IgH/t(1;14)(p22;q32)
    - MALT1-IgH/t(14;18)(q32q21), FOXP1-IgH/t(3;14)(p14.1;q32), others
- Some cases of EP may in fact be MALT lymphoma with extreme plasmacytic differentiation
  - Clinical data support this idea
    - Patients present with MALT lymphoma and recur as EP
    - Patients present with EP and recur as MALT lymphoma

Castleman Disease, Plasma Cell Variant
- Patients present with lymphadenopathy
- Morphology
  - Sheets of plasma cells expanding interfollicular areas
  - Prominent vascular proliferation
  - Small lymphoid follicles with
    - Lymphocyte-depleted germinal centers
    - Expanded mantle zones ("onion skin")
- Immunophenotype
  - Plasma cells are polytypic
  - HHV8(+) in a subset of cases; usually HIV(+)

Plasmablastic Lymphoma
- Overlap in clinical presentation
  - Oral cavity, sinuses and nasopharynx
  - Often seen in HIV(+) patients
- Immunohistochemical profile between plasmablastic lymphoma and EP is similar
- EBER usually positive in plasmablastic lymphoma and usually negative in EP or SPB

ALK(+) Diffuse Large B-cell Lymphoma
- Patients with ALK(+) large B-cell lymphoma are usually children or young adults
- Morphology
  - Immunoblastic appearance
- Typical immunophenotype
  - CD138(+), ALK(+) and CD30(-)

Plasmacytoma Arising in Setting of Immunosuppression
- Plasmacytoma is rare type of PTLD
- Plasmacytoma can rarely occur in patients treated with immunomodulator agents
- Usually extranodal; bone rarely involved
- Can be EBV-LMP1(+) or EBER(+)
- History is important to establishing diagnosis

Poorly Differentiated Carcinoma
- CD138(+) in both carcinomas and plasmacytoma
- Carcinomas are cytokeratin(+) and Ig light chain(-)

Reactive Plasma Cell Proliferation (Plasma Cell Granuloma)
- Lung is common site
- Plasma cells lack cytologic atypia and are polytypic

DIAGNOSTIC CHECKLIST

Clinically Relevant Pathologic Features
- EP is common in aerodigestive tract
- SPB often involves axial skeleton
- Persistent paraprotein (M protein) implies higher risk of progression to plasma cell myeloma
- Bone marrow biopsy and imaging studies (MRI) are essential to exclude plasma cell myeloma
- Extramedullary spread of plasma cell myeloma is biologically different from EP

Pathologic Interpretation Pearls
- Neoplastic cells in EP and SPB are morphologically indistinguishable from those of myeloma

SELECTED REFERENCES

1. Parkins E et al: Extramedullary plasmacytoma with a t(11;14)(q13;q32) and aggressive clinical course. Leuk Lymphoma. 51(7):1360-2, 2010
2. Shao H et al: Nodal and extranodal plasmacytomas expressing immunoglobulin a: an indolent lymphoproliferative disorder with a low risk of clinical progression. Am J Surg Pathol. 34(10):1425-35, 2010
3. Dores GM et al: Plasmacytoma of bone, extramedullary plasmacytoma, and multiple myeloma: incidence and survival in the United States, 1992-2004. Br J Haematol. 144(1):86-94, 2009
4. Bink K et al: Primary extramedullary plasmacytoma: similarities with and differences from multiple myeloma revealed by interphase cytogenetics. Haematologica. 93(4):623-6, 2008
5. Soutar R et al: Guidelines on the diagnosis and management of solitary plasmacytoma of bone and solitary extramedullary plasmacytoma. Clin Oncol (R Coll Radiol). 16(6):405-13, 2004
6. Hedvat CV et al: Insights into extramedullary tumour cell growth revealed by expression profiling of human plasmacytomas and multiple myeloma. Br J Haematol. 2003 Sep;122(5):728-44. Erratum in: Br J Haematol. 123(3):563, 2003
7. Hussong JW et al: Extramedullary plasmacytoma. A form of marginal zone cell lymphoma? Am J Clin Pathol. 111(1):111-6, 1999

Microscopic Features

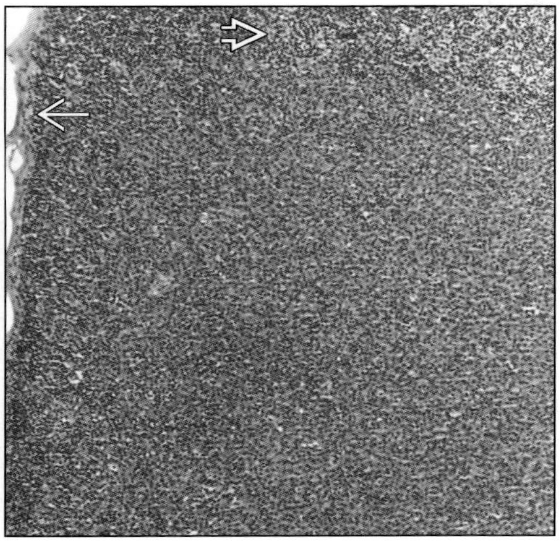

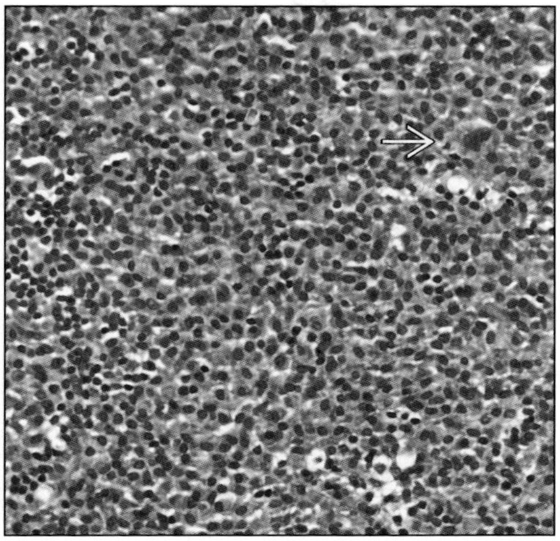

(Left) *Plasmacytoma involving lymph node. Sheets of well-differentiated plasma cells replace the lymph node, imparting a purple-pink hue at low-power magnification. Lymph node capsule ➡ and uninvolved lymph node parenchyma ⇨ are also present in this field.* ***(Right)*** *Plasmacytoma involving lymph node. Sheets of well-differentiated plasma cells replace the lymph node. Scattered multinucleated plasma cells ➡ are present in this field.*

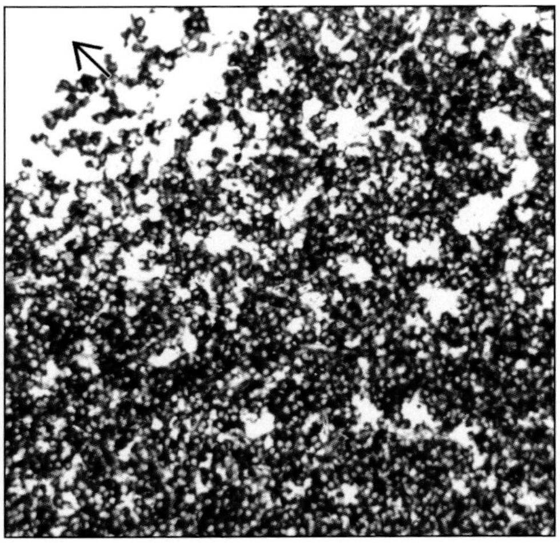

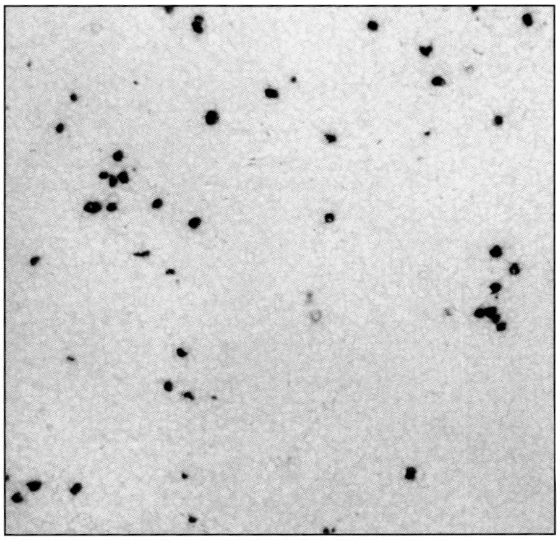

(Left) *Plasmacytoma involving lymph node. In situ hybridization shows that the plasma cells express cytoplasmic monotypic κ light chain RNA. Uninvolved lymph node is present at upper left ⇨.* ***(Right)*** *Plasmacytoma involving lymph node. In situ hybridization shows that the plasma cells are negative for lambda light chain RNA. A few reactive plasma cells are positive in this field.*

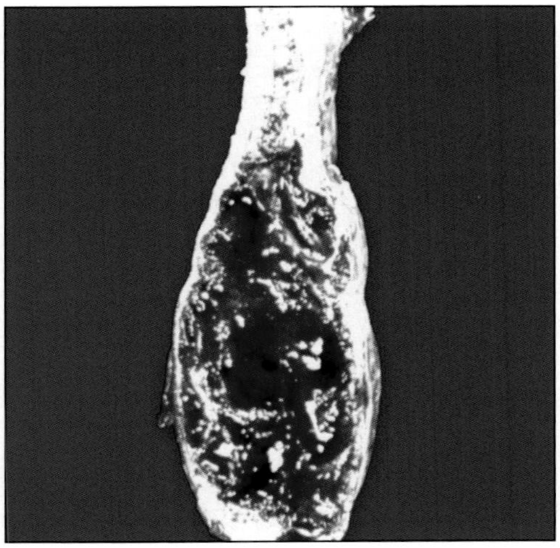

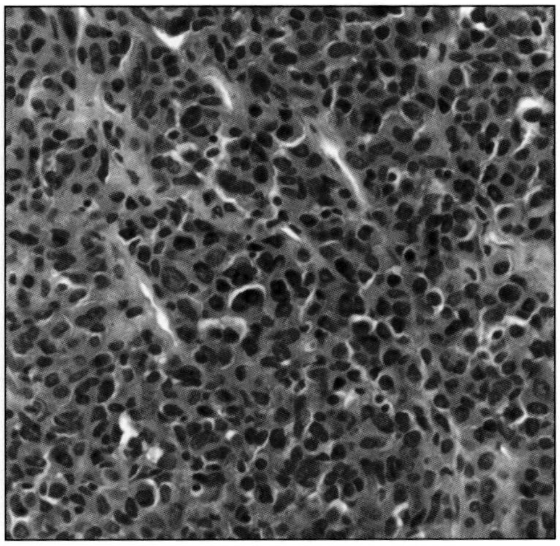

(Left) *Solitary plasmacytoma of bone (rib). The rib is expanded by a hemorrhagic plasma cell neoplasm. Staging bone marrow was negative for plasma cell neoplasm at the time this rib was resected but plasma cell myeloma developed 9 months later.* ***(Right)*** *Solitary plasmacytoma of bone (rib). The plasma cells are easily recognized as neoplastic as they have enlarged and pleomorphic nuclei.*

Microscopic Features and Differential Diagnosis

(Left) Plasmacytoma involving colon. The neoplastic cells infiltrate between the colonic glands ➡. *(Right)* Plasmacytoma involving colon. Most of the neoplastic cells in this image are small and mature appearing (well differentiated) with scattered large forms.

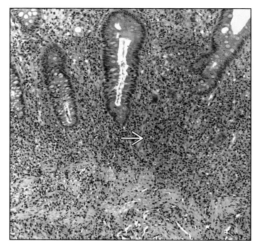
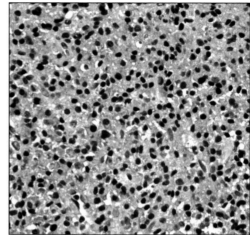

(Left) Extramedullary plasmacytoma involving the gallbladder. The neoplasm partially replaces the gallbladder mucosa and permeates between residual glands ➡. The plasma cells are small and mature with occasional hyperchromatic and enlarged forms ➡. *(Right)* High-power magnification shows a plasmacytoma involving lung (needle biopsy specimen). The plasma cells are small and mature (well differentiated).

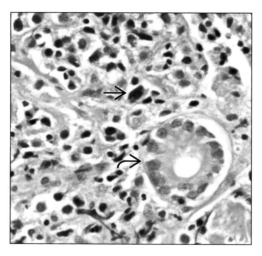
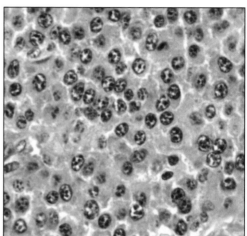

(Left) Plasma cell neoplasm involving the skin. The patient had a history of plasma cell myeloma; therefore, this neoplasm cannot be considered as an extramedullary plasmacytoma. The tumor involves the dermis and is associated with mild fibrosis. *(Right)* Plasma cell neoplasm involving the skin. The patient had a history of plasma cell myeloma; therefore, this neoplasm cannot be considered an extramedullary plasmacytoma. Note the large and anaplastic appearing plasma cells.

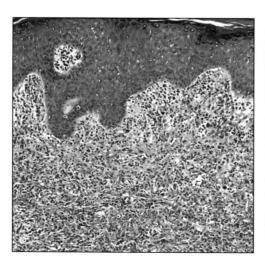
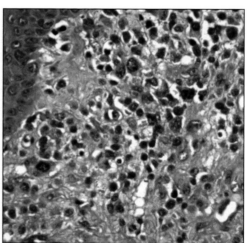

PLASMACYTOMA

Differential Diagnosis

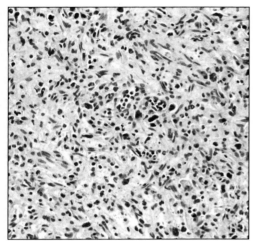
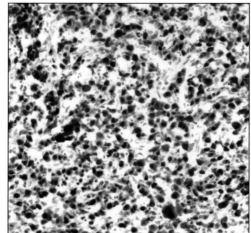

(Left) Plasma cell neoplasm involving the nasal region. The patient had a history of plasma cell myeloma and this neoplasm is therefore not an extramedullary plasmacytoma. **(Right)** Plasma cell neoplasm involving the nasal region. The patient had a history of plasma cell myeloma and therefore this neoplasm is not an extramedullary plasmacytoma. The neoplastic cells in this case expressed Cyclin-D1 in a nuclear & cytoplasmic pattern.

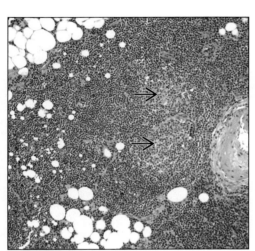
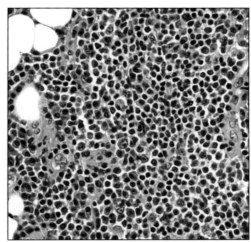

(Left) Mucosa-associated lymphoid tissue (MALT) lymphoma with plasmacytic differentiation involving subcutaneous adipose tissue. Note the 2 small germinal centers surrounded by the neoplasm ⊡. The presence of a lymphoid component justified the diagnosis of MALT lymphoma over plasmacytoma. **(Right)** MALT lymphoma with plasmacytic differentiation. The tumor cells are a mixture of small lymphocytes, plasmacytoid lymphocytes, plasma cells, and rare scattered large lymphoid cells.

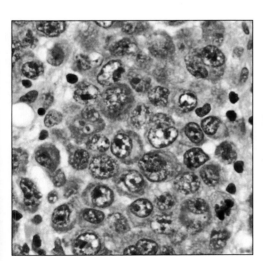
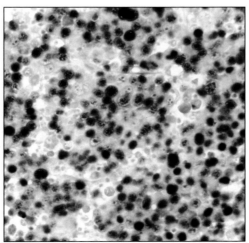

(Left) Plasmablastic lymphoma involving a lymph node. The neoplastic cells are large and highly atypical with obvious plasmacytic differentiation. **(Right)** Plasmablastic lymphoma (PBL) involving a lymph node. EBER is usually positive in PBL. Positivity for EBER is rare in plasma cell neoplasms and therefore EBER positivity makes the diagnosis of plasma cell myeloma unlikely.

PLASMACYTOMA

Differential Diagnosis

(Left) Plasmablastic lymphoma (PBL) involving lymph node. The neoplastic cells in PBL can express cytoplasmic monotypic light chain, in this case κ. (Right) Plasmablastic lymphoma (PBL) involving lymph node. The neoplastic cells in PBL are CD56(+) in ~ 50% of cases. CD56 is also positive in a subset of plasma cell myeloma cases and thus does not allow the distinction between PBL and plasma cell myeloma.

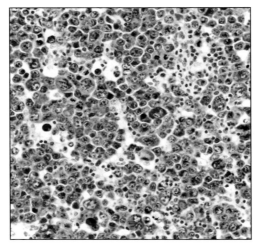
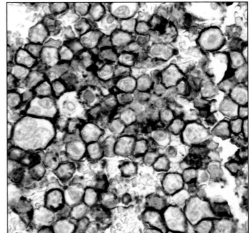

(Left) The proliferative index, as determined by Ki-67/MIB-1 staining, is usually high (> 70%) in cases of plasmablastic lymphoma. (Right) Anaplastic lymphoma kinase positive (ALK+) diffuse large B-cell lymphoma (DLBCL) involving a lymph node shows neoplastic cells having large nuclei with prominent central nucleoli. Apoptotic cells ➡ and a mitotic figure ➡ are present.

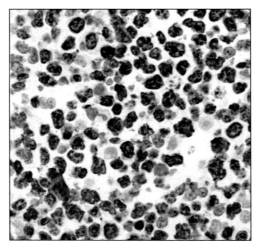
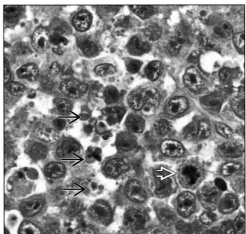

(Left) ALK(+) DLBCL involving a lymph node. The neoplastic cells show strong granular ALK expression limited to the cytoplasm of the lymphoma cells. This indicates clathrin heavy-chain gene (CLTC)-ALK protein resulting from t(2;17) (p23;q23). (Right) ALK(+) DLBCL involving lymph node. The neoplastic cells exhibit strong membranous expression of epithelial membrane antigen (EMA). Virtually all cases of ALK(+) DLBCL are positive for EMA.

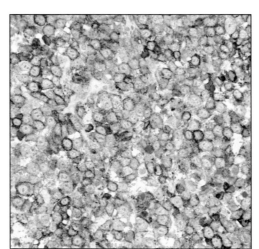
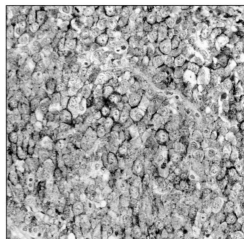

PLASMACYTOMA

Differential Diagnosis

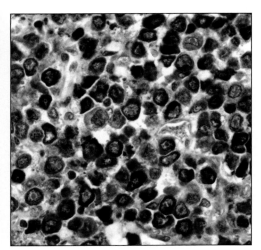
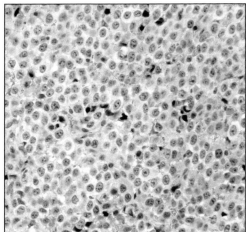

(Left) ALK(+) DLBCL involving a lymph node. The neoplastic cells are strongly IgA(+) with a cytoplasmic pattern. In > 90% of cases, IgA is expressed in these neoplasms. Rare neoplasms express cytoplasmic IgG. *(Right)* ALK(+) DLBCL involving a lymph node. The lymphoma cells are CD30(-). The absence of CD30 distinguishes this neoplasm from anaplastic large cell lymphoma.

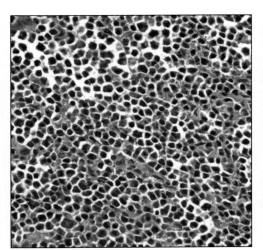
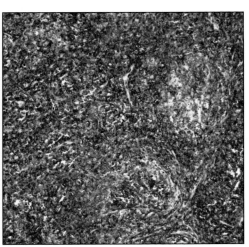

(Left) DLBCL with plasmacytic differentiation involving testis. The tumor cells are large with plasmacytoid differentiation (eccentric nuclei and moderate amounts of cytoplasm). *(Right)* DLBCL with plasmacytic differentiation involving testis. The tumor cells are strongly CD45/LCA(+) (shown). They were also CD20(+) and CD138(-).

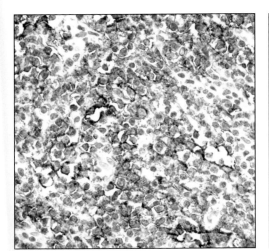

(Left) DLBCL with plasmacytic differentiation involving testis. The neoplastic cells are focally CD20(+) (shown). They are also CD45/LCA(+) and CD138(-). *(Right)* DLBCL with plasmacytic differentiation involving testis. A subset of neoplastic cells express monotypic κ light chain.

"Gray Zone" B-cell Lymphomas

B-CELL LYMPHOMA, UNCLASSIFIABLE, WITH FEATURES INTERMEDIATE BETWEEN DIFFUSE LARGE B-CELL LYMPHOMA AND BURKITT LYMPHOMA

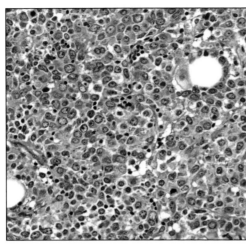

B-cell lymphoma, unclassifiable, with features intermediate between DLBCL and BL (DLBCL/BL). Note the high number of apoptotic cells and the mixture of intermediate and large-sized cells.

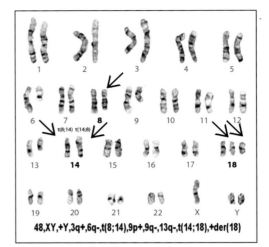

48,XY,+Y,3q+,6q-,t(8;14),9p+,9q-,13q-,t(14;18),+der(18)

Conventional cytogenetic analysis of a case of DCBCL/BL shows a complex karyotype. The presence of t(8;14)(q24;q32) ➡ and t(14;18)(q32;q21) ➡ supports further classification as a "double-hit" lymphoma.

TERMINOLOGY

Abbreviations
- B-cell lymphoma, unclassifiable, with features intermediate between diffuse large B-cell lymphoma (DLBCL) and Burkitt lymphoma (BL)

Synonyms
- Burkitt-like lymphoma
- High-grade B-cell lymphoma, Burkitt-like (Revised European American Lymphoma [REAL] classification)
- Small noncleaved cell lymphoma, non-Burkitt (Working Formulation)

Definitions
- Aggressive B-cell lymphoma with morphological and genetic features of both DLBCL and BL
- World Health Organization (WHO) classification considers this category
  - Heterogeneous and not distinct entity
  - Useful as "parking lot" for unclassifiable high-grade B-cell lymphomas

ETIOLOGY/PATHOGENESIS

Unknown
- Subset of DLBCL/BL cases includes "double-hit" or "triple-hit" lymphomas
  - "Hit" in this context refers to translocations involving MYC, BCL2, or BCL6 genes

CLINICAL ISSUES

Epidemiology
- Incidence
  - Uncommon, but true frequency not yet known
    - Frequency increases with patient age
- Age

  - Adults; median: 6th decade
- Gender
  - Males > females

Site
- > 50% of patients present with disseminated disease
  - Lymph nodes
  - Extranodal sites common and include
    - Bone marrow (~ 50%) and brain (~ 33%)

Presentation
- Patients present with lymphadenopathy &/or extranodal masses
- ~ 10-20% of patients have history of follicular lymphoma
- B-type symptoms common
- Leukemic presentation uncommon but can occur

Laboratory Tests
- Elevated serum lactate dehydrogenase &/or β-2-microglobulin levels
- Elevated leukocyte count with lymphoma cells in patients with leukemic presentation

Natural History
- Aggressive clinical course for most patients
- Poor prognostic factors
  - High clinical stage
  - Central nervous system involvement
  - History of follicular lymphoma
  - Double- or triple-hit lymphoma

Treatment
- Drugs
  - No consensus on optimal therapeutic approach
  - Rituximab, cyclophosphamide, doxorubicin, vincristine, and prednisone (R-CHOP) usually not effective
  - Rituximab, hyperfractionated cyclophosphamide, vincristine, doxorubicin, and dexamethasone (R-HyperCVAD) effective for subset of patients

B-CELL LYMPHOMA, UNCLASSIFIABLE, WITH FEATURES INTERMEDIATE BETWEEN DIFFUSE LARGE B-CELL LYMPHOMA AND BURKITT LYMPHOMA

Key Facts

Terminology

- Aggressive B-cell lymphoma with morphological and genetic features of both DLBCL and BL
- WHO classification considers this category
  - Heterogeneous and not distinct entity

Clinical Issues

- Median age: 6th decade
- Patients present with lymphadenopathy &/or extranodal masses; high stage in > 50%
- Aggressive clinical course for most patients
- Current chemotherapy regimens are ineffective

Microscopic Pathology

- Diffuse growth pattern; "starry sky" pattern is common
- High mitotic and apoptotic rates

- Intermediate-sized cells or a spectrum of cell sizes

Ancillary Tests

- Pan-B-cell antigens(+): TCL1(+/-), Ki-67 high
- In cases with immunophenotype consistent with BL
  - CD10(+), Bcl-6(+), IRF-4/MUM1(-), Bcl-2(-)
- In double-/triple-hit lymphomas, Bcl-2 is strongly (+)
- Complex karyotype is common
- *MYC* translocations in up to 50% of all cases
  - Associated with *BCL2* &/or *BCL6* rearrangements in double-/triple-hit lymphomas

Top Differential Diagnoses

- Burkitt lymphoma
- Diffuse large B-cell lymphoma
- Lymphoblastic leukemia/lymphoma
- Mantle cell lymphoma, blastoid variant

Prognosis

- DLBCL/BL is heterogeneous and therefore prognosis is also heterogeneous
- Large subset of patients have poor clinical outcome despite rigorous chemotherapy regimen

IMAGE FINDINGS

CT Findings

- F-18 fluorodeoxyglucose (FDG) positron emission tomography (PET)/computed tomography (CT)
  - DLBCL/BL is highly FDG avid

MICROSCOPIC PATHOLOGY

Histologic Features

- Diffuse growth pattern; "starry sky" is common
- High mitotic and apoptotic rates
- Intermediate-sized cells or spectrum of intermediate-sized and large cells
- Relatively few admixed small reactive lymphocytes; sclerosis uncommon
- 4 possible scenarios for diagnosis as described in WHO classification
  - Neoplasm resembles BL but too much variation in cell size and nuclear contours
  - Neoplasm resembles BL but atypical immunophenotype &/or genetic findings
  - Neoplasm has cells intermediate between DLBCL and BL with immunophenotype typical of BL
  - Rare cases with blastic chromatin with lymphoblastic lymphoma-like appearance
    - TdT(-) and Cyclin-D1(-)
- Most double-hit or triple-hit lymphomas are also classified as DLBCL/BL
  - These tumors can morphologically resemble DLBCL, BL, or have intermediate cytologic appearance

ANCILLARY TESTS

Immunohistochemistry

- In keeping with definition of DLBCL/BL, immunophenotype is variable
- All cases
  - Pan-B-cell antigens(+), TCL1(+/-), IRF-4/MUM1(+/-)
  - Ki-67 high; CD43(+/-), pan-T-cell antigens(-)
- In cases with immunophenotype consistent with BL
  - CD10(+), Bcl-6(+), IRF-4/MUM1(-), Bcl-2(-), TCL1(+)
- In double-hit lymphomas
  - Bcl-2 strongly (+), Ki-67 can range from ~ 70-100%

Flow Cytometry

- Surface Ig(+), pan-B-cell antigens(+); pan-T-cell antigens(-)
  - Except double-hit lymphomas: Surface Ig(-) and CD20(dim +)
- CD38(+), CD71(+), HLA-DR(+/-)

Cytogenetics

- Complex karyotype (> 3 abnormalities) is common
- *MYC* translocations in up to 50% of all cases
  - ~ 60% of cases with 8q24/*MYC*, translocations involve *Ig* gene loci
  - ~ 40% of cases with 8q24/*MYC*, other translocation partners are involved
- Double- or triple-hit lymphomas
  - 8q24/*MYC* translocations along with either *BCL2* &/or *BCL6* rearrangements
    - t(14;18)(q32;q21)/*IgH-BCL2*
    - Chromosome 3q27/*BCL6* translocations

In Situ Hybridization

- FISH is useful for detecting *MYC* translocation
  - *MYC* break-apart probe is used commonly
- FISH probes available to detect
  - *Ig* genes that are translocation partners of *MYC*
  - *IgH-BCL2* and *BCL6* gene rearrangements
- EBER is usually (-)

B-CELL LYMPHOMA, UNCLASSIFIABLE, WITH FEATURES INTERMEDIATE BETWEEN DIFFUSE LARGE B-CELL LYMPHOMA AND BURKITT LYMPHOMA

Array CGH
- Many chromosomal gains and losses
  - Gains: 1cen-25, 1q31-35, 7/7q, 8q24-qter, 13q11-q13, 13q31-q33
  - Losses: 13q14, 17p12-pter

Molecular Genetics
- Monoclonal *Ig* gene rearrangements (+)
- In double- or triple-hit tumors
  - *MYC* rearrangements in most cases
    - t(8;22)(q24;q11) relatively common (as compared with BL)
  - *BCL2* rearrangements common; *BCL6* rearrangements in subset

Gene Expression Profiling
- Gene expression profile is either intermediate between DLBCL and BL or very similar to BL

DIFFERENTIAL DIAGNOSIS

Burkitt Lymphoma (BL)
- Intermediate-sized cells, "squared-off" cytoplasmic borders
- Thick nuclear membranes, multiple (2-4) nucleoli
- Immunophenotype of BL
  - Surface Ig(+), CD10(+), CD20(+), Bcl-6(+), Ki-67 100%, Bcl-2(-)
- *MYC*/8q24 translocations are characteristic but not specific
- Simple karyotype relative to DLBCL/BL cases

Diffuse Large B-cell Lymphoma
- Large cells with vesicular chromatin
- Proliferation rate is usually lower than 90%; *MYC* translocation occurs in ~ 10% of cases
- Some double-hit lymphomas closely resemble DLBCL
  - Classifying these cases as DLBCL or DLBCL/BL is controversial

T- or B-Lymphoblastic Leukemia/Lymphoma
- Small- to medium-sized blasts with "dusty" chromatin
- Immunophenotype supports immature lymphoid lineage: TdT(+), CD34(+)

Mantle Cell Lymphoma (MCL), Blastoid Variant
- MCL, blastoid variant, can have prominent starry sky pattern and is composed of intermediate-sized cells
- Subset of these cases is associated with *MYC* translocation
- CD5(+), Cyclin-D1(+), and t(11;14)(q13;q32) support diagnosis of MCL

Peripheral T-cell Lymphoma (PTCL)
- Small subset of PTCL cases has prominent starry sky pattern
- Cell size can be intermediate-sized or spectrum of intermediate and large cells
- T-cell immunophenotype supports diagnosis of PTCL

Myeloid Sarcoma
- Myeloid sarcoma cells have immature chromatin and thin nuclear membranes
- Eosinophilic myelocytes are present in subset of cases
- Myeloid-associated antigens(+), B-cell antigens(-)

Ewing Sarcoma/Peripheral Neuroectodermal Tumor
- At extranodal locations, neoplasm can resemble, in part, lymphoma
- Intracytoplasmic glycogen(+), CD99(+/-), keratin(+/-); B-cell antigens(-)

Embryonal Rhabdomyosarcoma
- Nuclei are spindle-shaped, and intracytoplasmic striations are sometimes visible
- No starry sky pattern; muscle-associated markers(+), B-cell antigens(-)

Neuroblastoma
- Deposits of hematoxyphilic DNA material, rosettes, intracytoplasmic neurosecretory granules
- No starry sky pattern; neuroendocrine markers(+), B-cell antigens(-)

DIAGNOSTIC CHECKLIST

Clinically Relevant Pathologic Features
- Aggressive clinical course and poor prognosis
  - Patients with double- or triple-hit lymphoma have worst prognosis
- No consensus on optimal therapy

Pathologic Interpretation Pearls
- Definition of DLBCL/BL is currently vague and needs to be refined

SELECTED REFERENCES

1. Carbone A et al: B-cell lymphomas with features intermediate between distinct pathologic entities. From pathogenesis to pathology. Hum Pathol. 41(5):621-31, 2010
2. Snuderl M et al: B-cell lymphomas with concurrent IGH-BCL2 and MYC rearrangements are aggressive neoplasms with clinical and pathologic features distinct from Burkitt lymphoma and diffuse large B-cell lymphoma. Am J Surg Pathol. 34(3):327-40, 2010
3. Wu D et al: "Double-Hit" mature B-cell lymphomas show a common immunophenotype by flow cytometry that includes decreased CD20 expression. Am J Clin Pathol. 134(2):258-65, 2010
4. Johnson NA et al: Lymphomas with concurrent BCL2 and MYC translocations: the critical factors associated with survival. Blood. 114(11):2273-9, 2009
5. Said J: Diffuse aggressive B-cell lymphomas. Adv Anat Pathol. 16(4):216-35, 2009
6. Kluin PM et al: B-cell lymphoma, unclassifiable, with features intermediate between diffuse large B-cell lymphoma and Burkitt lymphoma. In Swerdlow SH et al: WHO classification of tumours of haematopoietic and lymphoid tissues. Lyon: IARC. 265-6, 2008

B-CELL LYMPHOMA, UNCLASSIFIABLE, WITH FEATURES INTERMEDIATE BETWEEN DIFFUSE LARGE B-CELL LYMPHOMA AND BURKITT LYMPHOMA

Microscopic and Immunophenotypic Features

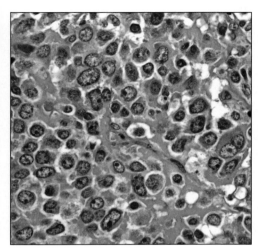
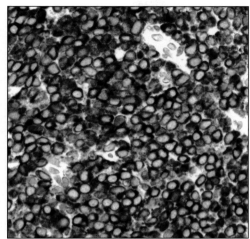

(Left) B-cell lymphoma, unclassifiable, with features intermediate between DLBCL and BL (DLBCL/BL). In this field, there is a mixture of intermediate and large-sized neoplastic cells. Immunohistochemical analysis showed CD20(+) and CD3(-) (not shown). *(Right)* DLBCL/BL. The lymphoma cells are strongly Bcl-2(+). Strong Bcl-2 expression in a neoplasm with features that resemble Burkitt lymphoma suggests a "double-hit" tumor, as was true in this case.

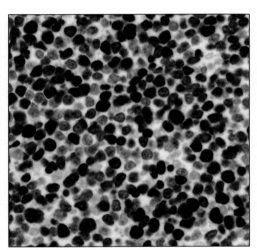
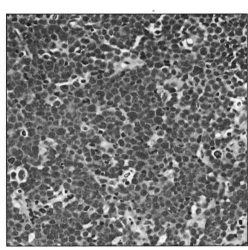

(Left) B-cell lymphoma, unclassifiable, with features intermediate between DLBCL and BL. MIB-1 (Ki-67) antibody shows a proliferation rate of virtually 100%. *(Right)* DLBCL/BL. The lymphoma cells are of intermediate size, and some of the lymphoma cells have a single prominent nucleolus. Immunohistochemistry showed CD20(+), CD5(-), CD43 (partial +) (not shown). This was a "double-hit" lymphoma with t(8;22)(q24.1;q11.2) and t(14;18)(q32;q21).

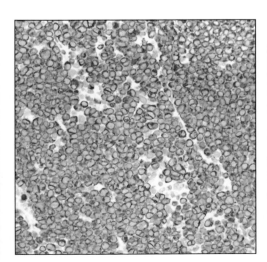
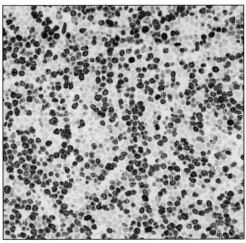

(Left) B-cell lymphoma, unclassifiable, with features intermediate between diffuse large B-cell lymphoma and Burkitt lymphoma. The lymphoma cells are strongly Bcl-2(+). *(Right)* DLBCL/BL. The MIB-1 (Ki-67) antibody shows a proliferation rate of approximately 60-70%.

B-CELL LYMPHOMA, UNCLASSIFIABLE, WITH FEATURES INTERMEDIATE BETWEEN DIFFUSE LARGE B-CELL LYMPHOMA AND BURKITT LYMPHOMA

Microscopic and Immunophenotypic Features

(Left) B-cell lymphoma, unclassifiable, with features intermediate between diffuse large B-cell lymphoma and Burkitt lymphoma. The neoplasm is composed of intermediate-sized cells with frequent mitoses ➡. Histiocytes of a "starry sky" pattern can be appreciated ➡. Fluorescence in situ hybridization analysis showed MYC gene rearrangement and IgH-BCL-2 fusion gene. *(Right)* DLBCL/BL. The lymphoma cells are strongly CD20(+).

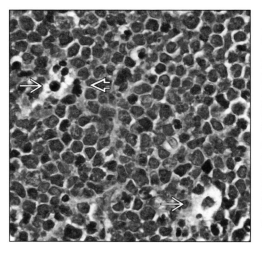

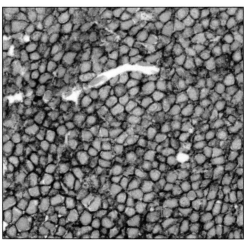

(Left) B-cell lymphoma, unclassifiable, with features intermediate between diffuse large B-cell lymphoma and Burkitt lymphoma. Most of the lymphoma cells are strongly Bcl-6(+). *(Right)* DLBCL/BL. Immunostain for CD10 is strongly positive. Flow immunophenotypic analysis showed a B-cell neoplasm, cytoplasmic monotypic immunoglobulin λ(+), CD10(+), and CD19(+).

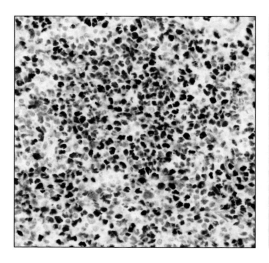

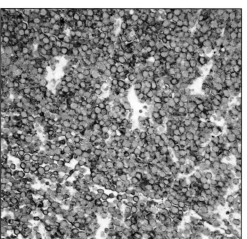

(Left) B-cell lymphoma, unclassifiable, with features intermediate between diffuse large B-cell lymphoma and Burkitt lymphoma. The neoplastic cells are strongly Bcl-2(+). *(Right)* DLBCL/BL. The Ki-67 antibody demonstrates a proliferation rate of approximately 90%.

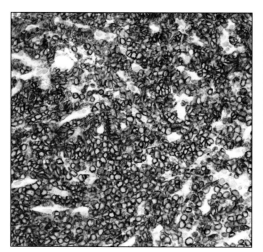

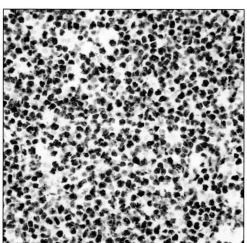

B-CELL LYMPHOMA, UNCLASSIFIABLE, WITH FEATURES INTERMEDIATE BETWEEN DIFFUSE LARGE B-CELL LYMPHOMA AND BURKITT LYMPHOMA

Differential Diagnosis

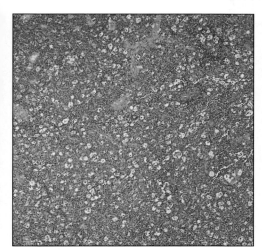
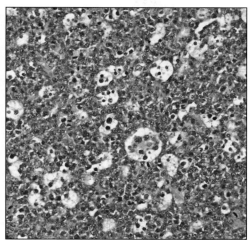

(Left) Burkitt lymphoma (BL) presenting as a mass involving an extranodal site. The neoplasm has a prominent "starry sky" pattern, a finding that is characteristic of BL but also can be seen in other highly proliferative neoplasms. (Right) BL presents here as a mass involving an extranodal site. Tingible body macrophages represent the "stars" in the starry sky pattern. The lymphoma cells are intermediate in size with 2-4 small nucleoli and numerous mitotic figures.

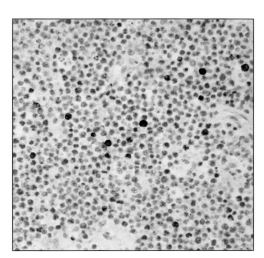
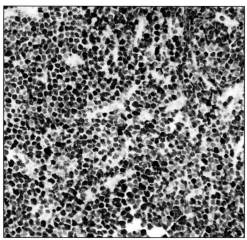

(Left) Burkitt lymphoma presenting as a mass involving an extranodal site. The neoplastic cells are Bcl-2(-). Reactive lymphocytes in the field are Bcl-2(+). (Right) BL presenting as a mass involving an extranodal site. The MIB-1 (Ki-67) antibody shows a proliferation rate of virtually 100%. An extremely high proliferation rate with uniform staining intensity is characteristic of BL.

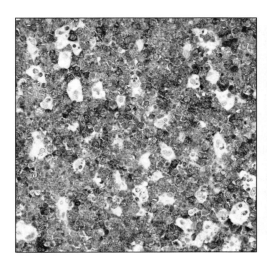
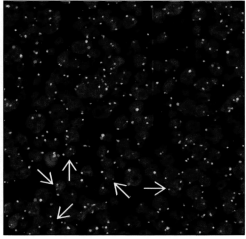

(Left) Burkitt lymphoma presenting as a mass involving an extranodal site. The neoplastic cells are TCL1(+). (Right) BL involving an extranodal site. FISH was performed using a MYC break-apart probe. This case showed 1 allele with colocalization of both probes (red and green together appear as yellow) and 1 allele that is split with segregation of the probes (separate red and green signals) ➡. The split signals support MYC gene rearrangement.

B-CELL LYMPHOMA, UNCLASSIFIABLE, WITH FEATURES INTERMEDIATE BETWEEN DIFFUSE LARGE B-CELL LYMPHOMA AND CLASSICAL HODGKIN LYMPHOMA

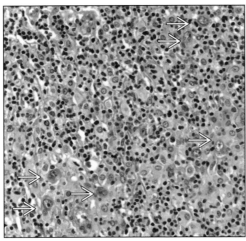

A case of DLBCL/CHL characterized by scattered large tumor cells with large eosinophilic nucleoli ➡ in a background of numerous small lymphocytes. These histologic features suggest CHL.

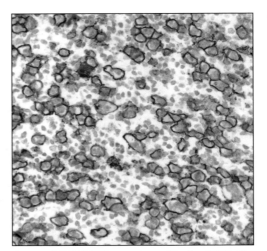

A case of DLBCL/CHL strongly positive for CD20. The tumor cells were also positive for CD30 (variable) and EBV-LMP1, as well as negative for CD15, CD45/LCA, and CD79a (not shown).

TERMINOLOGY

Abbreviations
- B-cell lymphoma, unclassifiable, with features intermediate between diffuse large B-cell lymphoma and classical Hodgkin lymphoma (DLBCL/CHL)

Synonyms
- Gray zone lymphoma
- Mediastinal gray zone lymphoma
- Large B-cell lymphoma with Hodgkin features
- Hodgkin-like anaplastic large cell lymphoma

Definitions
- Lymphoma with clinical, morphologic, &/or immunophenotypic features between diffuse large B-cell lymphoma (DLBCL) and classical Hodgkin lymphoma (CHL)

CLINICAL ISSUES

Epidemiology
- Age
  - Most common in patients 20-40 years or age (range: 13-70 years)
- Gender
  - Male predominance
- Ethnicity
  - Most common in Western countries
  - Less common in Asians and blacks

Presentation
- Most frequently patients present with anterior mediastinal mass
  - Often direct extension into lungs
  - Supraclavicular lymph nodes can be involved
- Advanced clinical stage (III or IV)
- Other peripheral lymph node groups are rarely involved

Treatment
- No consensus on optimum treatment protocol
- Some patients treated with CHL protocols have failed to respond completely
- Some groups have recommended treating DLBCL/CHL cases as aggressive DLBCL

Prognosis
- Patients have aggressive clinical course and poorer outcome than patients with either CHL or primary mediastinal B-cell lymphoma

MICROSCOPIC PATHOLOGY

Histologic Features
- Areas of confluent sheets of pleomorphic large tumor cells resembling DLBCL
- Other areas can show scattered large cells, resembling Hodgkin and Reed-Sternberg (HRS) cells in CHL
- Supraclavicular lymph nodes, if involved, can show morphologic features of either CHL or DLBCL or both
- Variable inflammatory infiltrate in background
- Mild stromal fibrosis and focal necrosis
  - Necrosis is usually not associated with neutrophils (unlike CHL)
- Nonnecrotizing granulomas and histiocytes

Cytologic Features
- Broad spectrum of cytologic appearance including
  - Centroblasts, immunoblasts, &/or HRS-like cells
- Cells with cytoplasmic retraction, resembling lacunar cells, can be seen
- Mummified cells (apoptotic large cells) are frequent

ANCILLARY TESTS

Immunohistochemistry
- "Mixed immunophenotype" with

B-CELL LYMPHOMA, UNCLASSIFIABLE, WITH FEATURES INTERMEDIATE BETWEEN DIFFUSE LARGE B-CELL LYMPHOMA AND CLASSICAL HODGKIN LYMPHOMA

Key Facts

Terminology
- B-cell lymphoma, unclassifiable, with features intermediate between DLBCL and CHL (DLBCL/CHL)

Clinical Issues
- Most frequently presents as mediastinal mass
- More aggressive clinical course than either CHL and PMLBCL

Microscopic Pathology
- Overlapping histologic features that make classification difficult
  ○ Can exhibit confluent sheets of large cells resembling DLBCL
  ○ Can have scattered HRS-like cells resembling CHL

Ancillary Tests
- Immunophenotype
  ○ Strong and uniform expression of B-cell antigens
  ○ CD30(+), CD45/LCA(+)
  ○ CD15 usually (-), EBV usually (-)

Top Differential Diagnoses
- PMLBCL
- Nodular sclerosis CHL

Diagnostic Checklist
- In cases that morphologically resemble CHL
  ○ Uniform and strong expression of B-cell markers and absence of CD15 suggest DLBCL/CHL
- In cases that morphologically resemble DLBCL
  ○ CD15(+), EBV(+), &/or CD20(-) suggest DLBCL/CHL

○ Expression of common markers of classical HL
  ▪ CD30([+] all cases) &/or CD15([+] in most cases)
  ▪ pax-5(+) and IRF-4/MUM-1(+)
○ And expression of markers usually absent in CHL
  ▪ CD45/LCA(+), CD20 ([+]; uniformly strong), and CD79a(+)
  ▪ OCT2(+), BOB1(+)
- Cells with this "mixed immunophenotype" constitute predominant neoplastic cell population
- Usually high proliferation rate, as measured by MIB-1 (Ki-67)
- MAL(+) in ~ 60% of cases
- Bcl-6([+] variable), CD10 is usually (-)
- Negative for T-cell markers, ALK(-)
- Epstein-Barr virus (EBV) is usually (-)
  ○ Few cases reported were EBV(+); EBER &/or LMP1
- Like CHL, lymphoid infiltrate in background is predominantly composed of T cells, CD3(+) and CD4(+)
- These cases show immunohistochemical features supporting activation of NF-κB pathway
  ○ Nuclear location of c-REL/p65
  ○ Overexpression of phosphorylated IκBa
  ○ Overexpression of NF-κB targets, Bcl-XL, and c-FLIP

Molecular Genetics
- Most cases have monoclonal *IgH* gene rearrangement
- Few cases have rearrangements involving *BCL6*
- Most cases lack t(14;18)(q32;q21)
- In almost all cases assessed, *P53* was in germline configuration

Gene Expression Profiling
- Studies have shown similarity between CHL and primary mediastinal large B-cell lymphoma
  ○ This is theoretical support for category of DLBCL/CHL
  ○ However, few cases of DLBCL/CHL have been analyzed by gene expression profiling

DIFFERENTIAL DIAGNOSIS

Primary Mediastinal (Thymic) Large B-cell Lymphoma (PMLBCL)
- Usually young women
- Anterosuperior mediastinal mass (rapidly progressive)
- Patients can have extrathoracic disease
  ○ Rare at time of diagnosis
  ○ More common at time of relapse
  ○ Usually extranodal: CNS, liver, adrenals, ovaries, and kidneys
  ○ Lymph nodes are often not involved at relapse
- Histologic features
  ○ Diffuse growth pattern
  ○ Large cells with pale cytoplasm (often is retraction artifact)
  ○ Sclerosis
    ▪ Often compartmentalizes tumor cells mimicking cohesive clusters
  ○ Reed-Sternberg-like or Hodgkin-like cells can be present
- Immunophenotype
  ○ Positive for common pan B-cell markers
    ▪ CD20(+), CD79a(+), pax-5(+)
  ○ CD45/LCA(+), IRF-4/MUM-1(+)
  ○ CD30([+] 80%), usually weak &/or focal
  ○ CD23([+] 70%), MAL([+] 70%)
  ○ Often surface immunoglobulin(-); best shown by flow cytometry
  ○ CD10(-), CD15(-)
  ○ EBV is usually (-)
  ○ T-cell antigens(-)
- Molecular genetic features
  ○ Monoclonal *Ig* gene rearrangements are present
  ○ No evidence of monoclonal *TCR* gene rearrangements
  ○ Array CGH shows amplification at 9p24 (~ 75%) and 2p15 (~ 50%)
  ○ These neoplasms show a number of deletions

B-CELL LYMPHOMA, UNCLASSIFIABLE, WITH FEATURES INTERMEDIATE BETWEEN DIFFUSE LARGE B-CELL LYMPHOMA AND CLASSICAL HODGKIN LYMPHOMA

Nodular Sclerosis Classical Hodgkin Lymphoma
- Usually young patients
- Slight female predominance
- Mediastinal involvement (~ 80%)
- Histologic features
  - Nodular growth pattern with fibrosis
    - Dense collagenous bands surround nodules
    - Collagenous bands are polarizable
  - Variable number of large HRS cells
- Many histological variants of nodular sclerosis CHL have been described
  - Based on number of neoplastic cells, extent and nature of fibrosis, and inflammatory background
  - Of these, syncytial variant is particularly relevant in differential diagnosis
    - Sheets of large tumor cells that can mimic DLBCL
    - Often large areas of necrosis
    - Immunophenotype is typical of CHL
- Immunophenotype
  - CD30(+), CD15(+) in most cases
  - pax-5(+) with characteristic weaker (dimmer) expression than reactive B-cells
  - CD20(-/+), CD79a(-/+)
    - Weakly &/or variably (+) in ~ 20% of cases
  - Small subset (~ 5%) of CHL can express T-cell antigens
    - These cases also express pax-5 or other B-cell antigens
  - CD45/LCA(-), EMA usually (-)
- Molecular genetic features
  - Monoclonal IgH gene rearrangements usually only detected by single cell PCR
  - Usually no evidence of monoclonal Ig or TCR gene rearrangements by routine analysis
    - Standard PCR performed on whole tissue sections
    - Southern blot analysis

Diffuse Large B-cell Lymphoma
- Older adults, but also occurs in children and young adults
- Histologic features
  - Diffuse growth pattern
  - Large neoplastic cells (centroblasts &/or immunoblasts)
  - Large anaplastic cells can be present; known as anaplastic variant
    - These neoplasms may have intrasinusoidal growth pattern
    - CD30 often (+)
  - Large pleomorphic cells with features of HRS-like cells can be present
  - Sclerosis is frequent in extranodal sites
  - Areas of coagulative necrosis are common
- Immunophenotype
  - CD20(+), CD22(+), CD79a(+)
  - pax-5(+), OCT2(+), BOB1(+)
  - CD10(+) and Bcl-6(+) in variable proportion of cases
  - CD30(-/+); if positive, often weak and focal except anaplastic variant
  - CD45/LCA(+), CD15(-)

- Monotypic immunoglobulin(+)
  - Cytoplasmic; in cases with plasmacytoid differentiation
  - Surface; best shown by flow cytometry
- Molecular genetic features
  - Monoclonal Ig gene rearrangements(+)
  - No evidence of monoclonal TCR gene rearrangements
  - t(14;18)(q32;q21)/IgH-BCL2 (+) in ~ 20-30%
  - BCL6 rearrangements in ~ 10-20%
- Gene expression profiling has shown 2 subsets
  - Germinal center cell
  - Activated B cell
    - Poorer prognosis

ALK(+) Anaplastic Large Cell Lymphoma (ALCL)
- Children and young adults
- Male predominance
- Mediastinal involvement is rare
- Histologic features
  - Diffuse &/or sinusoidal growth pattern
  - Large, irregular neoplastic cells and "hallmark cells"
  - "Hallmark cells"
    - Large cells with eccentric horseshoe-shaped nuclei
    - Prominent paranuclear eosinophilic Golgi region
- Immunophenotype
  - ALK(+); pattern correlates with molecular abnormalities involving ALK gene
    - Nuclear and cytoplasmic pattern correlates with t(2;5)(p23;q35)
  - CD30(+) strong and uniform
    - Membranous and paranuclear (target-like) pattern
  - Aberrant T-cell immunophenotype is common
    - Most tumors do not express CD3, CD5, or T-cell receptors
  - EMA(+/-), CD45/LCA(+/-), Bcl-2(-)
  - Negative for B-cell markers
- Molecular genetic features
  - There are 9 known molecular abnormalities that involve ALK gene
  - Monoclonal T-cell receptor gene rearrangements

ALK(-) Anaplastic Large Cell Lymphoma
- Considered provisional entity in 2008 World Health Organization classification
- No age or sex preferences
- Histologic features closely resemble ALK(+) ALCL
- Immunophenotype
  - CD30(+) strong and uniform; similar to ALK(+) ALCL
  - Aberrant T-cell immunophenotype
  - EMA(+/-), Bcl-2(+/-)
- Molecular genetic features
  - Monoclonal T-cell receptor gene rearrangements
  - No abnormalities involving ALK gene

Composite Lymphoma
- PMLBCL (&/or DLBCL) and CHL may coexist
- Composite lymphoma = 2 lymphomas involving same anatomic site that can be
  - Simultaneous (synchronous)

B-CELL LYMPHOMA, UNCLASSIFIABLE, WITH FEATURES INTERMEDIATE BETWEEN DIFFUSE LARGE B-CELL LYMPHOMA AND CLASSICAL HODGKIN LYMPHOMA

Differential Diagnosis between CHL, PMBCL, DLBCL, and CHL/DLBCL

Marker	CHL	PMBCL	DLBCL	DLBCL/CHL
CD30	+	+/-	-/+	+
CD15	+/-	-	-	+/-
CD45 (LCA)	-	+	+	+ (at least focally)
CD20	-/+	+	+	+ (at least focally)
CD79a	-/+	+	+	+/-
pax-5	+ (weak)	+ (strong)	+ (strong)	+ (usually strong)
IRF-4/MUM-1	+	+	+/-	+
CD10	-	-/+	+/-	-
CD43	-	-	-/+	NA
OCT2	-/+	+	+	+
BOB1	-	+	+	+
LMP1	+/-	-/+	-/+	-/+

PMBCL = primary mediastinal B-cell lymphoma; NA = not available. + all cases are positive; +/- majority of cases positive; -/+ minority of cases positive; - all cases negative.

- o Sequential (metachronous)
- Sequential tumors (metachronous lymphomas)
  - o Typically, CHL occurs 1st followed by PMLBCL or DLBCL
    - If lymphomas < 10 years apart, usually clonally related
    - If lymphomas > 10 years apart, usually clonally unrelated

Carcinomas, Sarcomas, and Melanomas
- Rarely these neoplasms contain HRS-like cells that mimic CHL
- Clinical history is often helpful in differential diagnosis
- Immunophenotypic studies distinguish DLBCL/CHL from nonhematopoietic neoplasms
- These conditions do not represent true biological overlap

DIAGNOSTIC CHECKLIST

Clinically Relevant Pathologic Features
- Young men
- Usually present with large anterior mediastinal mass
- No consensus on best therapy for patients with these neoplasms

Pathologic Interpretation Pearls
- These neoplasms are difficult to classify
- In general, there is discordance between morphologic features and immunophenotype
- Cases that morphologically resemble CHL
  - o Uniform and strong expression of B-cell markers (e.g., CD20) and absence of CD15 support DLBCL/CHL
  - o CD45/LCA(+) supports DLBCL/CHL
- Cases that morphologically resemble DLBCL
  - o CD15(+) and/or CD20(-) support DLBCL/CHL
  - o EBV(+) supports DLBCL/CHL

SELECTED REFERENCES

1. Hoeller S et al: BOB.1, CD79a and cyclin E are the most appropriate markers to discriminate classical Hodgkin's lymphoma from primary mediastinal large B-cell lymphoma. Histopathology. 56(2):217-28, 2010
2. Hasserjian RP et al: Commentary on the WHO classification of tumors of lymphoid tissues (2008): "Gray zone" lymphomas overlapping with Burkitt lymphoma or classical Hodgkin lymphoma. J Hematop. Epub ahead of print, 2009
3. Mani H et al: Hodgkin lymphoma: an update on its biology with new insights into classification. Clin Lymphoma Myeloma. 9(3):206-16, 2009
4. Dogan A: Gray zone lymphomas. Hematology. 10 Suppl 1:190-2, 2005
5. García JF et al: Large B-cell lymphoma with Hodgkin's features. Histopathology. 47(1):101-10, 2005
6. Traverse-Glehen A et al: Mediastinal gray zone lymphoma: the missing link between classic Hodgkin's lymphoma and mediastinal large B-cell lymphoma. Am J Surg Pathol. 29(11):1411-21, 2005
7. Calvo KR et al: Molecular profiling provides evidence of primary mediastinal large B-cell lymphoma as a distinct entity related to classic Hodgkin lymphoma: implications for mediastinal gray zone lymphomas as an intermediate form of B-cell lymphoma. Adv Anat Pathol. 11(5):227-38, 2004
8. Rosenwald A et al: Molecular diagnosis of primary mediastinal B cell lymphoma identifies a clinically favorable subgroup of diffuse large B cell lymphoma related to Hodgkin lymphoma. J Exp Med. 198(6):851-62, 2003
9. Chadburn A et al: Mediastinal large B-cell lymphoma vs classic Hodgkin lymphoma. Am J Clin Pathol. 112(2):155-8, 1999
10. Lamarre L et al: Primary large cell lymphoma of the mediastinum. A histologic and immunophenotypic study of 29 cases. Am J Surg Pathol. 13(9):730-9, 1989

B-CELL LYMPHOMA, UNCLASSIFIABLE, WITH FEATURES INTERMEDIATE BETWEEN DIFFUSE LARGE B-CELL LYMPHOMA AND CLASSICAL HODGKIN LYMPHOMA

Imaging and Microscopic Features

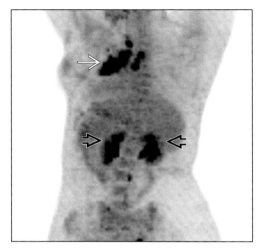

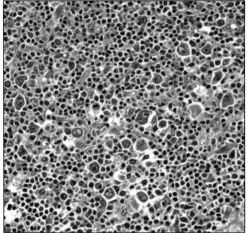

(Left) PET scan in a patient with DLBCL/CHL shows metabolically active lymphadenopathy in the anterior mediastinum and right and left paratracheal regions ➡. There is no evidence of lymphadenopathy below the diaphragm. Fludeoxyglucose (FDG) uptake in the liver and spleen appears normal ➡. *(Right)* DLBCL/CHL shows areas with scattered atypical large neoplastic cells in a background of small lymphocytes resembling CHL. In other areas, there are sheets of large tumor cells resembling DLBCL.

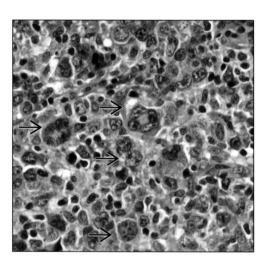

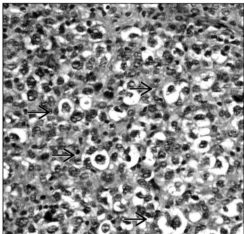

(Left) This case of DLBCL/CHL is composed of large and very pleomorphic tumor cells ➡. *(Right)* DLBCL/CHL shows clusters of atypical large tumor cells with retracted cytoplasm resembling lacunar-type HRS cells ➡. Note also the presence of fibrosis in the background.

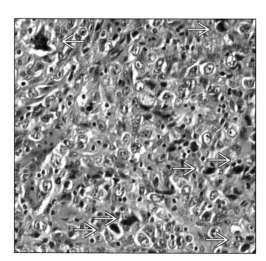

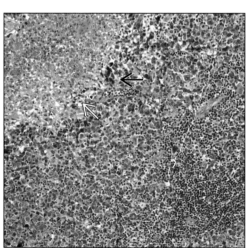

(Left) Mummified cells ➡, apoptotic large tumor cells similar to those seen in CHL, are frequently seen in DLBCL/CHL illustrating another similarity with CHL. *(Right)* Areas of necrosis can be seen ➡. Unlike CHL, the areas of necrosis usually do not have neutrophils. Note the presence of scattered large tumor cells in a background enriched with small lymphocytes. Clusters of mummified cells are also present ➡.

B-CELL LYMPHOMA, UNCLASSIFIABLE, WITH FEATURES INTERMEDIATE BETWEEN DIFFUSE LARGE B-CELL LYMPHOMA AND CLASSICAL HODGKIN LYMPHOMA

Immunohistochemical Features

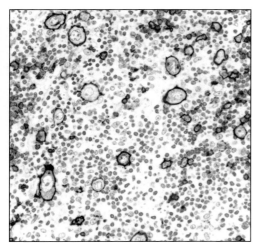
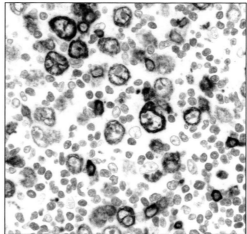

(Left) The tumor cells in this case of DLBCL/CHL are positive for CD20. Although CD20 may be weakly and focally positive in a subset of CHL, a strong and uniform expression is unusual. This case has also diffuse areas of tumor cells resembling DLBCL. *(Right)* In this case of DLBCL/CHL, the tumor cells are positive for CD79a. CD79a is rarely expressed in CHL. This case has also diffuse areas of tumor cells resembling DLBCL.

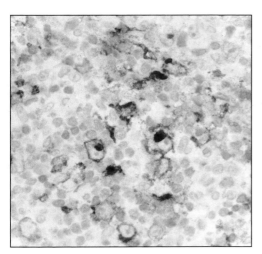
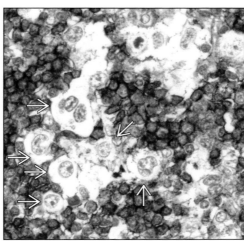

(Left) DLBCL/CHL shows focal positivity for CD30. Note that the tumor cells show variable degrees of expression of CD30 and the variable size of the neoplastic cells is also highlighted by CD30. CHL is usually characterized by a strong and uniform positivity for CD30. The tumor cells are also usually large in size. *(Right)* DLBCL/CHL shows tumor cells lacking expression of CD45/LCA ➡. The small reactive lymphocytes in the background are positive for CD45/LCA.

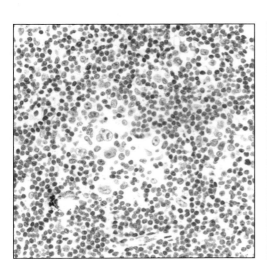
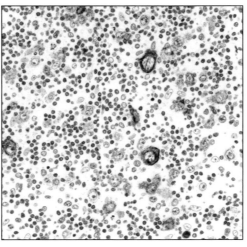

(Left) CD15 may be positive in some cases of DLBCL/CHL. However, in this case the tumor cells are negative. CD15 is one of the markers, when strong and uniformly expressed, that may support the diagnosis of DLBCL/CHL in cases morphologically resembling DLBCL. *(Right)* The tumor cells in this case of DLBCL/CHL are positive for EBV-LMP1. This case also has diffuse areas of tumor cells resembling DLBCL. Expression of EBV-LMP1 is unusual in DLBCL.

B-CELL LYMPHOMA, UNCLASSIFIABLE, WITH FEATURES INTERMEDIATE BETWEEN DIFFUSE LARGE B-CELL LYMPHOMA AND CLASSICAL HODGKIN LYMPHOMA

Microscopic Features

(Left) DLBCL/CHL involving supraclavicular lymph node of a 42-year-old woman. At this magnification, the neoplasm subtotally replaces lymph node parenchyma. *(Right)* Paraffin section of a case of DLBCL/CHL involving supraclavicular lymph node. Large, pleomorphic cells with HRS-like features ➡ are present. Small lymphocytes, histiocytes, and eosinophils are abundant in the background. These histologic findings support CHL.

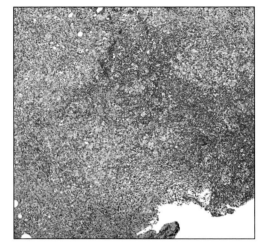
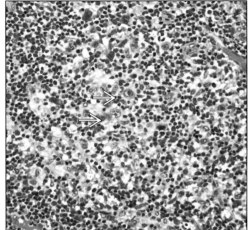

(Left) DLBCL/CHL involving supraclavicular lymph node. The large neoplastic cells are moderately and uniformly positive for CD20. *(Right)* DLBCL/CHL involving supraclavicular lymph node. The neoplastic cells are strongly and uniformly positive for pax-5. This degree of B-cell antigen expression is evidence against CHL and more in keeping with DLBCL/CHL.

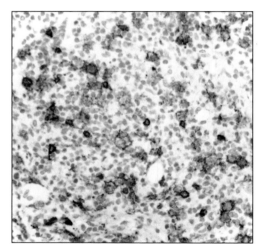
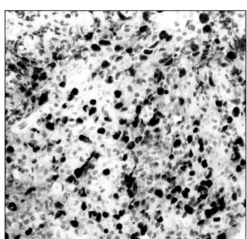

(Left) DLBCL/CHL involving supraclavicular lymph node. The neoplastic cells are positive for CD45/LCA. This finding is evidence against CHL and supports DLBCL/CHL in this case. *(Right)* DLBCL/CHL involving supraclavicular lymph node. The neoplastic cells are positive for CD30. The tumor cells were also positive for CD20 and CD45/LCA supporting the diagnosis of DLBCL/CHL in this case.

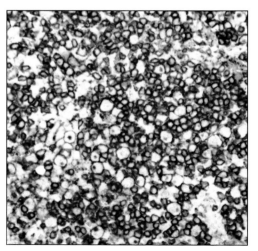
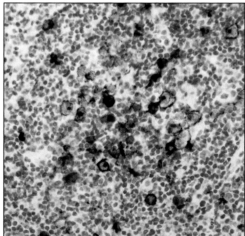

B-CELL LYMPHOMA, UNCLASSIFIABLE, WITH FEATURES INTERMEDIATE BETWEEN DIFFUSE LARGE B-CELL LYMPHOMA AND CLASSICAL HODGKIN LYMPHOMA

"Gray Zone" B-cell Lymphomas

Differential Diagnosis

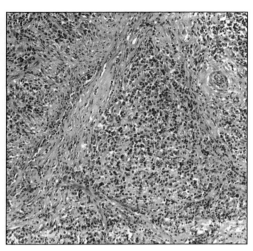

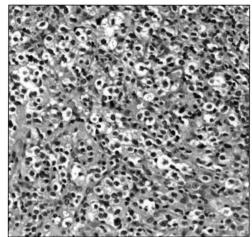

(Left) Hematoxylin & eosin stain of primary mediastinal large B-cell lymphoma. The neoplasm has a nodular pattern & fibrosis. Neoplastic cells were positive for CD20, CD30 (focal), and IRF-4/MUM-1, and were negative for CD10 (immunohistochemical stains not shown). *(Right)* Hematoxylin & eosin stain shows primary mediastinal large B-cell lymphoma. Neoplastic cells are large with pale cytoplasm & sclerosis. Tumor cells were positive for CD20, CD30 (focal), & IRF-4/MUM-1.

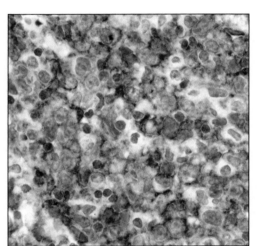

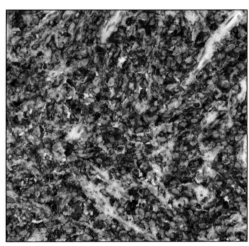

(Left) Primary mediastinal large B-cell lymphoma with tumor cells that are focally and weakly positive for CD30. *(Right)* Primary mediastinal large B-cell lymphoma shows tumor cells that are strongly and uniformly positive for B-cell markers including CD20.

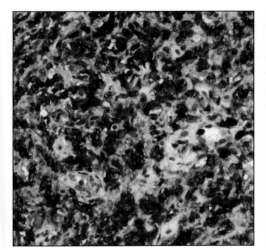

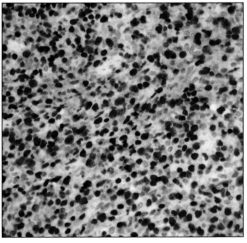

(Left) The tumor cells in this case of primary mediastinal large B-cell lymphoma are strongly positive for CD45/LCA. The tumor cells were also positive for CD20 and CD23, and were focally CD30 positive (not shown). *(Right)* Primary mediastinal large B-cell lymphoma is frequently positive for IRF-4/MUM-1 (shown). In this case, the tumor cells were also positive for CD20, CD23, and CD30 (focal) and negative for CD10 and CD15 (not shown).

B-CELL LYMPHOMA, UNCLASSIFIABLE, WITH FEATURES INTERMEDIATE BETWEEN DIFFUSE LARGE B-CELL LYMPHOMA AND CLASSICAL HODGKIN LYMPHOMA

Differential Diagnosis

(Left) Hematoxylin & eosin stain shows a case of nodular sclerosis classical Hodgkin lymphoma (NSHL). The neoplasm is nodular with nodules surrounded by collagen bands. Note the presence of many eosinophils (upper part). *(Right)* Inside the nodules of NSHL, the HRS cells are uniformly and strongly positive for CD30. They were also positive for pax-5 and CD15, and were negative for CD20 and CD45/LCA (not shown). This immunophenotype supports the diagnosis of NSHL.

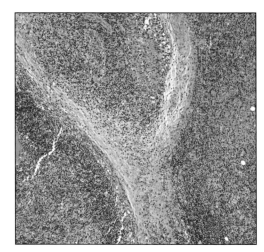
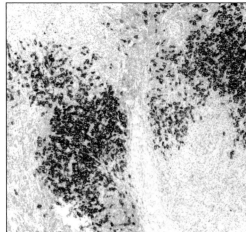

(Left) In classical Hodgkin lymphoma, the HRS cells are characteristically negative for CD45/LCA. Note the presence of reactive lymphoid cells (right upper corner), positive for CD45/LCA. *(Right)* A case of NSHL in which the HRS cells are negative for CD20. However, the presence of tumor cells positive for this B-cell marker is not unusual and may be seen in 20% of cases.

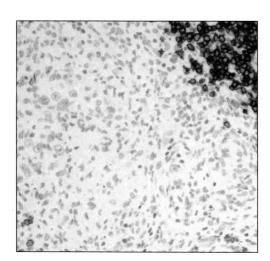
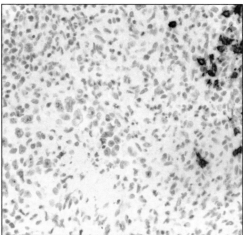

(Left) This case of syncytial variant of NSHL shows sheets of large HRS cells with few eosinophils in the background. Note the presence of large pleomorphic tumor cells ➡. The tumor cells were positive for CD30, CD15, pax-5 and EBER, and were negative for CD3, CD20, and CD45/LCA (not shown). *(Right)* Syncytial variant of NSHL showing sheets of large HRS cells strongly and uniformly positive for CD30.

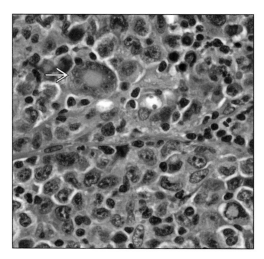
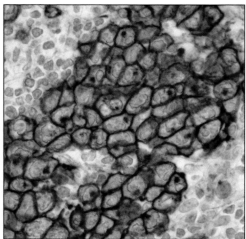

B-CELL LYMPHOMA, UNCLASSIFIABLE, WITH FEATURES INTERMEDIATE BETWEEN DIFFUSE LARGE B-CELL LYMPHOMA AND CLASSICAL HODGKIN LYMPHOMA

Differential Diagnosis

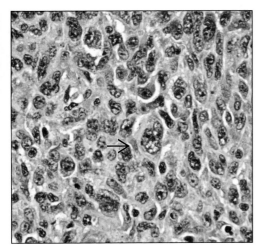

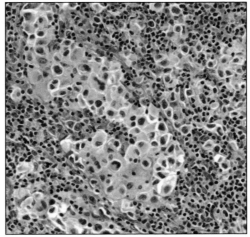

(Left) DLBCL, anaplastic variant, shows pleomorphic malignant cells ⟹ that are mostly large with irregular nuclei, vesicular chromatin, and distinct nucleoli. These cells were positive for CD20, CD30, and CD45/LCA and negative for CD15 (not shown). (Right) This case of DLBCL, anaplastic variant shows large tumor cells within sinuses. The neoplasm was positive for CD20, CD30, and CD45/LCA and was negative for CD15 (not shown).

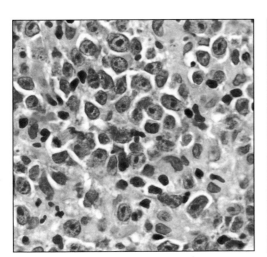

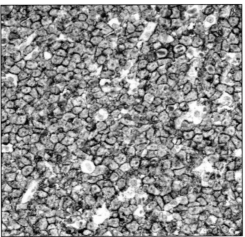

(Left) DLBCL, immunoblastic variant, composed of a monotonous population of large cells with central nucleoli. The tumor cells were positive for CD20 and CD45/LCA and were negative for CD15 and CD30 (not shown). (Right) DLBCL, immunoblastic variant, showing strong positivity for CD20. In addition, the tumor cells were positive for CD45/LCA and were negative for CD15 and CD30 (not shown).

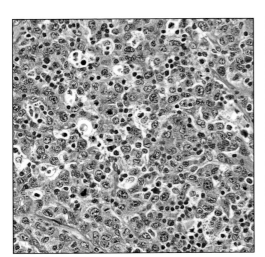

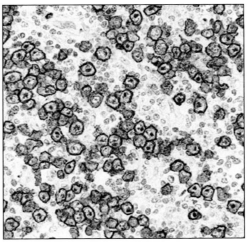

(Left) ALK(+) ALCL shows intermediate to large, monomorphic tumor cells and a starry sky pattern. The neoplastic cells were strongly positive for ALK and CD30. (Right) CD30 is strongly expressed by the tumor cells in ALK(+) ALCL. Note the characteristic membranous and paranuclear (Golgi) pattern (target-like appearance) that is seen in ALCL. This pattern is also seen in the neoplastic cells of CHL.

Nodal T-cell Lymphomas

PERIPHERAL T-CELL LYMPHOMA, NOT OTHERWISE SPECIFIED

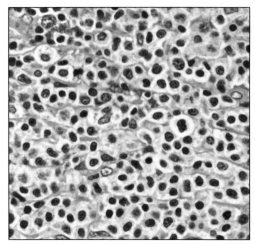

Peripheral T-cell lymphoma (PTCL) involving lymph node. The neoplastic cells in this case show abundant clear cytoplasm.

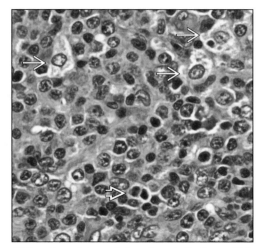

PTCL with a "starry sky" pattern indicating a high proliferation rate. The histiocytes corresponding to the "stars" are indicated ➡. Eosinophils are also present ➡.

TERMINOLOGY

Abbreviations
- Peripheral T-cell lymphoma, not otherwise specified (PTCL-NOS)

Synonyms
- Peripheral T-cell lymphoma (PTCL)
- Peripheral T-cell lymphomas, unspecified
  - Term used in 2001 World Health Organization (WHO) classification
- Post-thymic T-cell lymphoma
- Immunoblastic sarcoma of T-cell lineage

Definitions
- Mature T-cell lymphomas that cannot be classified into specific T-cell categories
  - Heterogeneous group in current WHO classification
  - PTCL is, in part, diagnosis of exclusion

ETIOLOGY/PATHOGENESIS

Etiology and Pathogenesis
- Evidence that aberrant T-cell signaling drives T-cell lymphoproliferation
- The specific etiology of PTCL is unknown
  - Once etiology or pathogenesis of a subgroup is defined, this subset is likely to be reclassified

Cell of Origin
- Activated mature T-lymphocyte, either CD4(+) or CD8(+)

CLINICAL ISSUES

Epidemiology
- Incidence
  - PTCL represents approximately 6% of all non-Hodgkin lymphomas

  - ~ 50% of all NK/T-cell neoplasms
- Age
  - Mainly arises in middle-aged adults; rare in children
- Gender
  - Male to female ratio ~ 2:1

Site
- Lymph nodes are usually involved
- Involvement of extranodal sites is common, including
  - Bone marrow, spleen, liver, lung, and skin

Presentation
- Most patients have advanced-stage disease with B symptoms
- Bulky disease in ~ 10% of patients
- Leukemic phase is rare at presentation
- Cytokine-related paraneoplastic phenomena can occur, including
  - Pruritus &/or eosinophilia
  - Hemophagocytic syndrome
- Prior to onset of PTCL, immune-mediated disorders can occur, including
  - Hashimoto thyroiditis, rheumatoid arthritis
  - Immune thrombocytopenic purpura

Laboratory Tests
- Elevated serum lactate dehydrogenase (LDH) level is common

Treatment
- Aggressive combination chemotherapy ± consolidation therapy
  - Induction combination chemotherapy regimens combine anthracycline with alkylating agent
  - Consolidation therapy
    - Hematopoietic stem cell transplantation
    - Radiation therapy
- Treatment for refractory or relapsed PTCL
  - Combination chemotherapy but there is no consensus on optimal regimen

PERIPHERAL T-CELL LYMPHOMA, NOT OTHERWISE SPECIFIED

Key Facts

Clinical Issues
- PTCL represents approximately 6.0% of all non-Hodgkin lymphomas
- Mainly arises in middle-aged adults; rare in children
- Advanced-stage disease with B symptoms
- Poor prognosis with frequent relapses
- Lymphadenopathy; extranodal sites often involved

Microscopic Pathology
- Paracortical infiltrate or diffuse effacement of lymph node architecture
- Wide cytological spectrum
- Background inflammatory cells often numerous
- ± postcapillary venules in arborizing fashion
- ± high rates of proliferation and apoptosis

Ancillary Tests
- Pan-T-cell antigens(+)
- CD4(+) CD8(-) or CD4(-) CD8(+)
- Aberrant T-cell immunophenotypes in ~ 80% of cases
- CD30 can be positive, exceptionally CD15(+)
- ± cytotoxic molecules
- Monoclonal *TCR* gene rearrangements
- No consistent chromosomal/molecular abnormality

Top Differential Diagnoses
- Angioimmunoblastic T-cell lymphoma
- Adult T-cell leukemia/lymphoma
- Anaplastic large cell lymphoma
- Classical Hodgkin lymphoma
- T-cell/histiocyte-rich large B-cell lymphoma

---

  o Participation in clinical trials is encouraged

Prognosis
- Overall response to therapy is poor with frequent relapses
- 5-year overall survival and failure-free survival (20-30%)
- Poor prognosis has been associated with
  o High stage
  o High international prognostic index (IPI)
  o Features suggested but need to be confirmed
    - Epstein-Barr virus (EBV)(+)
    - Gene expression profile showing NF-κB dysregulation or high proliferation signature
    - Cytotoxic immunophenotype
- Small subset of patients with localized disease and low IPI have better outcome

IMAGE FINDINGS

Radiographic Findings
- Lymphadenopathy
- FDG-PET is often positive

MICROSCOPIC PATHOLOGY

Histologic Features
- Lymph node
  o Paracortical infiltrate or diffuse effacement of architecture
  o Proliferation of postcapillary venules in interweaving (arborizing) fashion can be present
  o High rates of proliferation and apoptosis
  o Background inflammatory cells usually present, including:
    - Eosinophils, plasma cells, small lymphocytes
    - Epithelioid histiocytes, large B cells
  o In subset of cases, there is preferential involvement of T-zones
  o In some cases, neoplasm is associated with fibrosis

    - Fibrous bands can compartmentalize neoplasm, simulating nodular pattern
- Skin
  o PTCL commonly infiltrates dermis and subcutis; can produce nodules with central ulceration
  o Angiocentricity and adnexal involvement may be seen
  o Epidermotropism is rare
- Spleen
  o Solitary or multiple fleshy nodules involving white pulp with colonization of periarteriolar sheath
  o Predominant infiltration of red pulp in some cases

Cytologic Features
- Wide spectrum of neoplastic T-cells of small, intermediate, or large size
  o Numerous intermediate-sized &/or large cells, most common
- Neoplastic cells have sparse or abundant cytoplasm
  o Clear, eosinophilic, or basophilic
- Nuclei of neoplastic cells show wide spectrum
  o Vesicular, hyperchromatic, or pleomorphic
  o Multinucleated or Reed-Sternberg-like nuclei can occur

Morphologic Variants of PTCL
- Lymphoepithelioid (Lennert lymphoma)
  o Diffuse replacement of lymph node architecture
  o Predominantly small lymphoid cells with slight nuclear irregularities
  o Confluent clusters of epithelioid histiocytes
  o Scattered, larger, more atypical cells, including occasional Reed-Sternberg-like cells (usually EBV[+])
  o Occasional admixed inflammatory cells, including eosinophils and plasma cells
  o Neoplastic cells are often CD8(+)
- PTCL with "follicular" pattern
  o Also reported as perifollicular, intrafollicular, or paracortical nodular variants of PTCL
  o Intrafollicular aggregates of T-cell lymphoma that mimic follicular lymphoma at low-power magnification

PERIPHERAL T-CELL LYMPHOMA, NOT OTHERWISE SPECIFIED

- o Enlarged perifollicular zones surrounding hyperplastic follicles mimicking nodal marginal zone B-cell lymphoma
- o Small nodular aggregates of PTCL in background of progressively transformed germinal centers
  - ▪ Can mimic nodular lymphocyte-predominant Hodgkin lymphoma
- o Neoplastic cells are T cells, usually CD4(+)
- • T zone
  - o Predominantly perifollicular or interfollicular growth pattern
  - o Reactive follicles are preserved and can be hyperplastic
  - o Small or intermediate-sized neoplastic cells with clear or eosinophilic cytoplasm
    - ▪ Minimal nuclear pleomorphism
  - o Commonly associated with vascular proliferation and heterogeneous mixture of reactive cells

PTCL with Associated B-cell Proliferation
- • Approximately 10% (or less) of PTCL cases can be associated with numerous B cells
- • B-cells are small mature plasma cells, plasmacytoid large B-lymphocytes, or plasmablasts
- • B cells are often EBV(+)

ANCILLARY TESTS

Immunohistochemistry
- • Mature T-cell immunophenotype
  - o Pan-T-cell antigens(+)
  - o CD4(+)/CD8(-) or CD4(-)/CD8(+)
  - o TdT(-), CD1a(-), CD99(-)
  - o Pan-B-cell antigens(-), LMP1 usually negative
- • Expression patterns of T-cell receptor (TCR) are similar to normal T cells
  - o TCR-αβ(+) in 95% of cases
  - o Small subset of PTCL-U are TCR-γδ(+)
- • Aberrant T-cell immunophenotypes in ~ 80% of cases
  - o "Loss" or "deletion" of 1 or more pan-T-cell antigens
    - ▪ Frequent absence of CD2, CD3, CD5, CD7, or TCR
    - ▪ Decreased (dim) intensity of antigen expression compared with normal T cells
  - o Coexpression or absence of both CD4 and CD8
  - o Rarely B-cell antigens are aberrantly expressed
    - ▪ CD20 most frequent
- • CD30 can be positive, exceptionally with CD15(+)
  - o CD30 is usually expressed only by subset of neoplastic cells in PTCL
  - o Usually highlights large cells and with variable staining intensity
- • Cytotoxic molecules can be expressed in subset of PTCL
  - o TIA-1, granzyme B, and perforin
  - o More common in extranodal versus nodal PTCL
  - o Cytotoxic immunophenotype more common in Japan than in United States or Europe
    - ▪ These tumors are commonly EBV(+)
- • Proliferation rate (Ki-67) of PTCLs is highly variable
  - o Lower in neoplasms composed of small cells

- o Usually substantial or very high in large-cell neoplasms

Flow Cytometry
- • Immunophenotype as stated under immunohistochemistry
- • Aberrant immunophenotypes more reliably assessed by flow cytometry

Cytogenetics
- • PTCL composed of large cells have high frequency of
  - o Abnormal clones, triploid or tetraploid clones, and complex clones (> 4 abnormalities)
- • Trisomy 3 is associated with lymphoepithelioid variant of PTCL
- • Chromosomal rearrangements involving 7p15, 7q35, and 14q11 (TCR loci) are uncommon

In Situ Hybridization
- • EBER(+) in small subset of PTCL
  - o ~ 5-10% of cases

Array CGH
- • Recurrent gains in chromosomes 7q, 8q, 17q, and 22q
- • Recurrent losses in chromosomes 4q, 5q, 6q, 9p, 10q, 12q, and 13q

Molecular Genetics
- • Monoclonal TCR gene rearrangements
- • IgH gene rearrangements in approximately 1/3 of PTCLs
  - o Regardless of presence of associated B-cell proliferation
- • No known recurrent molecular abnormalities in most cases of PTCL
- • Occasional translocations present
  - o t(5;9)(q33;q22) in 5 of 30 cases of PTCL resulting in
    - ▪ Disruption of IL-2 inducible kinase (ITK) and spleen tyrosine kinase (SYK) genes
    - ▪ Novel ITK-SYK chimeric gene and overexpression of SYK
  - o t(14;19)(q11;q13) has been identified in 2 cases of PTCL
    - ▪ Results in juxtaposition of PVRL2 on chromosome 19q13 with TCRα/δ locus

Gene Expression Profiling
- • Heterogeneous profiles in accord with variability of neoplastic and inflammatory cells in PTCLs
  - o NF-κB dysregulation in subset
  - o Proliferation signature has been identified

DIFFERENTIAL DIAGNOSIS

Granulomatous Lymphadenitis
- • PTCL can present with associated chronic granulomatous inflammation
- • Presence of cytological atypia supports PTCL
- • Aberrant T-cell immunophenotype or monoclonal TCR gene rearrangements supports PTCL

PERIPHERAL T-CELL LYMPHOMA, NOT OTHERWISE SPECIFIED

Angioimmunoblastic T-cell Lymphoma (AITL)
- Patients present with advanced-stage disease similar to PTCL
- Unlike PTCL, patients with AITL often also have
  - Immunodeficiency associated with neoplasm
  - Polyclonal hypergammaglobulinemia
- Histologically, AITL is polymorphous infiltrate of small and large cells
- Prominent arborizing high endothelial venules
- Immunophenotype
  - Follicular T-helper cell (CD4[+])-associated markers
    - CD10, Bcl-6, CXCL13, PD-1
  - Expanded populations of follicular dendritic cells usually surround HEV
    - CD21(+), CD23(+), &/or CD35(+)
- EBV(+) B cells are present in most cases of AITL
  - EBV(+) immunoblastic proliferation may progress to
    - Diffuse large B-cell lymphoma
    - Classical Hodgkin lymphoma
- Most frequent cytogenetic abnormalities are
  - Trisomy 3, trisomy 5, and additional X chromosome
- Monoclonal *TCR* gene rearrangements
  - Monoclonal *Ig* gene rearrangements in 25-35% of cases by PCR

Adult T-cell Leukemia/Lymphoma (ATLL)
- Histologically and immunophenotypically, PTCL and ATLL can be indistinguishable
- ATLL is caused by infection by human T-cell leukemia virus type 1 (HTLV-1)
  - HTLV-1 is integrated into genome of neoplastic cells
- Patients with ATLL often present with hypercalcemia
- Leukemic phase is common in ATLL patients
  - Cells in blood smear are multilobated and flower-shaped

ALK(+) Anaplastic Large Cell Lymphoma (ALCL)
- ALCL occurs more often in children or young adults
- Sinuses are preferentially involved
- Cohesive and usually anaplastic neoplastic cells
- Distinctive immunophenotype of ALK(+) ALCL
  - Uniform CD30(+) in membranous and paranuclear pattern
  - ALK(+) in nuclear and cytoplasmic or cytoplasmic or membranous pattern
- *ALK* locus abnormalities(+); t(2;5)(p23;q35) is most common

ALK(-) ALCL
- PTCL can overlap with ALK(-) ALCL histologically
  - Sinus involvement and anaplastic cytologic features support ALCL
- ALK(-) and no evidence of *ALK* locus abnormalities
- In ALCL, uniform CD30(+) in membranous and paranuclear pattern

Mycosis Fungoides (MF) Involving Lymph Node
- Histologically and immunophenotypically, MF in lymph node can closely mimic PTCL
- Clinically, patients with MF involving lymph node have
  - Skin lesions
  - ± Sézary cells in peripheral blood
- MF in lymph node is associated with dermatopathic changes

Hepatosplenic T-cell Lymphoma (HSTCL)
- Most patients with HSTCL do not present as do PTCL patients
- HSTCL patients have marked splenomegaly and usually hepatomegaly
  - No lymphadenopathy
- HSTCL involves sinusoids of liver, spleen, and bone marrow
- HSTCL cells are monotonous with
  - Medium-sized nuclei and inconspicuous nucleoli
  - Rim of pale cytoplasm
- Immunophenotypically, HSTCL cells are
  - CD2(+), surface CD3(+), CD7(+), usually TCR-γ/δ(+)
  - TIA-1(+), granzyme M(+), CD4(-), CD5(-), usually CD8(-)
- Isochromosome 7q is present in large subset of cases

Extranodal NK/T-cell Lymphoma, Nasal Type
- Typically, patients present only with extranodal disease
  - Upper aerodigestive tract
  - Extranasal sites: Skin, soft tissue, gastrointestinal, and testes
- Polymorphous lymphoid infiltrate of variable morphology
  - ± angioinvasion, often associated with extensive fibrinoid necrosis
- Immunophenotype
  - Cytoplasmic CD3(+), surface CD3(-)
  - CD2(+), CD56(+), cytotoxic proteins(+)
- EBV(+) and monoclonal
- Usually germline TCR genes, unlike PTCL
  - ~ 1/3 of cases with surface CD3(+) and *TCR* gene rearrangements

Enteropathy-associated T-cell Lymphoma (EATL)
- It is unusual for PTCL to present only with intestinal disease
  - EATL is usually restricted to small intestine
- 2 types: Type I (classical) and type II EATL
- Classical EATL (80-90% of cases)
  - Intestinal tumor of intraepithelial T-lymphocytes
  - Usually composed of large cells
    - Celiac disease in adjacent small intestinal mucosa with villous atrophy and crypt hyperplasia
- Type II EATL (10-20% of cases)
  - Monomorphic medium-sized cells
  - Sporadic, without risk factors for celiac disease
- Immunophenotype
  - Classical EATL
    - CD3(+), CD7(+), CD103(+)
    - CD4(-), CD5(-), CD56(-/+)
  - Type II EATL
    - CD3(+), CD8(+), CD56(+)

9

PERIPHERAL T-CELL LYMPHOMA, NOT OTHERWISE SPECIFIED

- Frequent (up to 70%) complex segmental amplification of chromosomal 9q31.3-qter or deletion of 16q12.1

Subcutaneous Panniculitis-like T-cell Lymphoma

- Patients present with subcutaneous nodules, usually without other sites of disease
- Atypical lymphoid infiltrate in subcutaneous tissue
  o Involves fat lobules
  o Typically spares septae, overlying dermis, and epidermis
- Immunophenotype
  o CD3(+), CD8(+), TCR-αβ(+), cytotoxic proteins(+)

Classical Hodgkin Lymphoma (CHL)

- HRS-like cells can occur in PTCL and mimic CHL
  o CD45/LCA(+), T-cell antigens(+), CD30(+/-), CD15(-/+), CD45/LCA(-)
- In CHL, background cells show no cytologic atypia
- Immunophenotype of HRS cells
  o CD15(+), CD30(+), pax-5(dim +)
- No evidence of monoclonal *TCR* gene rearrangements in CHL

T-cell/Histiocyte-rich Large B-cell Lymphoma (THRLBCL)

- PTCL is usually composed of many neoplastic cells forming sheets
- In THRLBCL, neoplastic cells represent < 10% of cells within biopsy specimen
  o Neoplastic cells are B cells
  o Monoclonal *Ig* gene rearrangements
  o No evidence of monoclonal *TCR* gene rearrangements

Marginal Zone B-cell Lymphomas (MZL)

- PTCL-NOS cases can have abundant neoplastic cells with pale or clear cytoplasm
  o Resemble marginal zone (monocytoid) B cells
  o Paracortical distribution can mimic marginal zone pattern
- Histologically, PTCL cases show
  o More frequent cytological atypia than MZL
  o Higher mitotic rate than MZL
- Immunophenotype of MZL
  o Monotypic Ig(+), pan-B-cell antigens(+), T-cell antigens(-)

Follicular Lymphoma (FL)

- PTCL with "follicular pattern" can mimic FL
- Immunophenotype and genotype
  o Neoplastic cells in PTCL with "follicular pattern"
    ▪ Pan-T-cell antigens(+), CD4(+)
  o Monoclonal *TCR* gene rearrangements(+)
- In contrast, FL is B-cell neoplasm characterized by
  o Monotypic Ig(+), pan-B-cell antigens(+), CD10 &/or Bcl-6(+)
  o *IGH-BCL2*(14;18)(q32;q21)

DIAGNOSTIC CHECKLIST

Clinically Relevant Pathologic Features

- Most patients present with lymphadenopathy
- Extranodal involvement is common
- Advanced clinical stage at presentation
- PTCL is aggressive neoplasm associated with poor prognosis
- Innovative therapeutic approaches are needed

Pathologic Interpretation Pearls

- Paracortical or diffuse effacement of lymph nodes
- Wide cytological spectrum
- Vascular proliferation common
- Numerous reactive inflammatory cells in background
- Mature T-cell immunophenotype; often aberrant
- Monoclonal *TCR* gene rearrangements

SELECTED REFERENCES

1. Feeney J et al: Characterization of T-cell lymphomas by FDG PET/CT. AJR Am J Roentgenol. 195(2):333-40, 2010
2. Hartmann S et al: High resolution SNP array genomic profiling of peripheral T cell lymphomas, not otherwise specified, identifies a subgroup with chromosomal aberrations affecting the REL locus. Br J Haematol. 148(3):402-12, 2010
3. Savage K et al: Peripheral T-cell lymphoma - Not otherwise specified. Crit Rev Oncol Hematol. Epub ahead of print, 2010
4. Schmitz N et al: Treatment and prognosis of mature T-cell and NK-cell lymphoma: an analysis of patients with T-cell lymphoma treated in studies of the German High-Grade Non-Hodgkin Lymphoma Study Group. Blood. 116(18):3418-25, 2010
5. Serwold T et al: T-cell receptor-driven lymphomagenesis in mice derived from a reprogrammed T cell. Proc Natl Acad Sci U S A. 107(44):18939-43, 2010
6. Tripodo C et al: Mast cells and Th17 cells contribute to the lymphoma-associated pro-inflammatory microenvironment of angioimmunoblastic T-cell lymphoma. Am J Pathol. 177(2):792-802, 2010
7. O'Leary HM et al: Update on the World Health Organization classification of peripheral T-cell lymphomas. Curr Hematol Malig Rep. 4(4):227-35, 2009
8. Agostinelli C et al: Peripheral T cell lymphoma, not otherwise specified: the stuff of genes, dreams and therapies. J Clin Pathol. 61(11):1160-7, 2008
9. Piccaluga PP et al: Gene expression analysis of peripheral T cell lymphoma, unspecified, reveals distinct profiles and new potential therapeutic targets. J Clin Invest. 117(3):823-34, 2007
10. Warnke RA et al: Morphologic and immunophenotypic variants of nodal T-cell lymphomas and T-cell lymphoma mimics. Am J Clin Pathol. 127(4):511-27, 2007
11. Rizvi MA et al: T-cell non-Hodgkin lymphoma. Blood. 107(4):1255-64, 2006
12. Went P et al: Marker expression in peripheral T-cell lymphoma: a proposed clinical-pathologic prognostic score. J Clin Oncol. 24(16):2472-9, 2006

PERIPHERAL T-CELL LYMPHOMA, NOT OTHERWISE SPECIFIED

Microscopic and Immunohistochemical Features

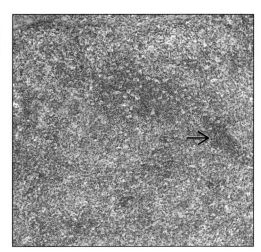
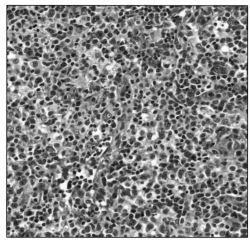

(Left) Peripheral T-cell lymphoma involving lymph node. The lymph node architecture is almost completely replaced by lymphoma showing a paracortical and diffuse pattern. A few residual lymphoid follicles ➡ are present. *(Right)* PTCL involving lymph node. The neoplasm is composed of small- and intermediate-sized cells with relatively abundant cytoplasm. Reactive eosinophils and vascular proliferation were also present.

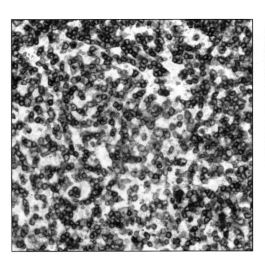
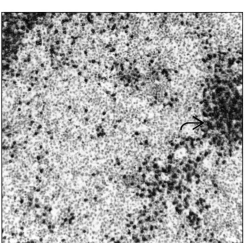

(Left) Peripheral T-cell lymphoma involving lymph node. Most of the lymphoid cells in this case are CD3(+), supporting T-cell lineage. *(Right)* PTCL involving lymph node. The neoplastic cells are CD20(-). CD20 highlights cells in the residual lymphoid follicles ➡.

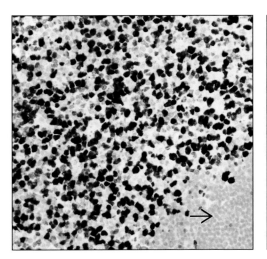
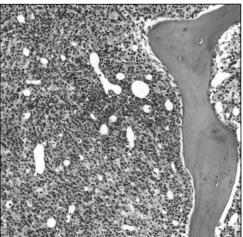

(Left) Peripheral T-cell lymphoma involving lymph node. The neoplastic cells in this case showed a high proliferation rate as shown by Ki-67 immunostain. A benign follicle is also present ➡. *(Right)* PTCL involving bone marrow biopsy specimen. Patients with PTCL usually present with systemic disease, and the bone marrow is commonly involved.

Microscopic Features

(Left) Peripheral T-cell lymphoma, not otherwise specified (PTCL) involving a skin biopsy specimen. The neoplasm filled the dermis without epidermotropism. Note the grenz zone between the neoplasm and the epidermis ➡. *(Right)* PTCL involving skin. Most of the neoplastic cells in this case were of intermediate size, but some large, multinucleated cells were also present ➡. These large cells were CD3(+).

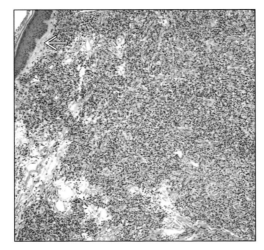
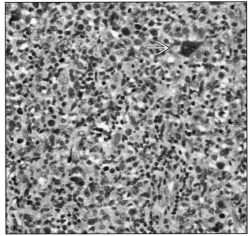

(Left) Peripheral T-cell lymphoma involving skin. The neoplastic cells in this case had an aberrant T-cell immunophenotype, being CD3(+) and CD5(-) (not shown). This aberrant immunophenotype does not occur in normal T cells; therefore, its presence supports T-cell lymphoma. *(Right)* PTCL involving skin. The neoplastic cells in this case had an aberrant T-cell immunophenotype, being CD3(+) (not shown) and CD5(-). Aberrant immunophenotypes occur in ~ 80% of PTCLs.

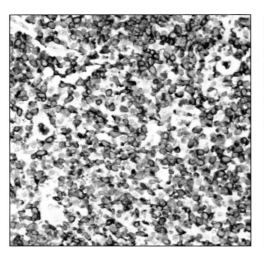
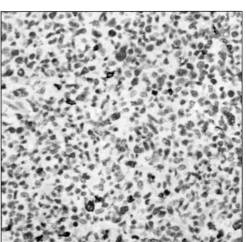

(Left) Peripheral T-cell lymphoma, not otherwise specified (PTCL) involving lymph node. The neoplastic cells were predominantly small in this neoplasm and had a low proliferation rate (not shown). *(Right)* PTCL involving lymph node. Most of the neoplastic cells in this case were large and had a high proliferation rate (not shown).

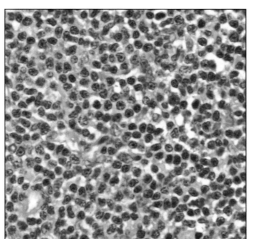
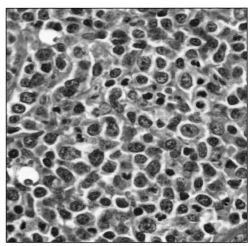

PERIPHERAL T-CELL LYMPHOMA, NOT OTHERWISE SPECIFIED

Microscopic and Immunohistochemical Features

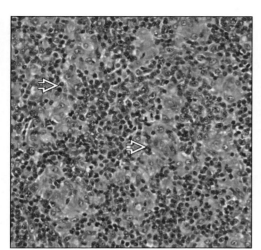
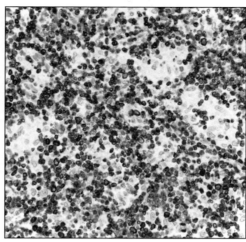

(Left) PTCL, lymphoepithelioid variant (Lennert lymphoma) involving lymph node. The neoplastic T-cells are associated with clusters of epithelioid histiocytes ⇒. (Right) PTCL, lymphoepithelioid variant (Lennert lymphoma) involving a lymph node. CD3 immunostain highlights T cells.

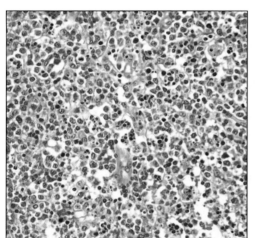
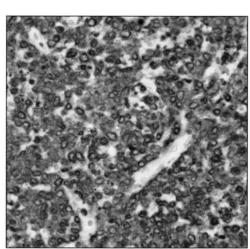

(Left) PTCL involving lymph node. Note the abundant apoptosis shown in this field. The neoplastic cells were CD8(+) and expressed cytotoxic proteins (cytotoxic immunophenotype). (Right) PTCL with a cytotoxic immunophenotype involving a lymph node. Most of the lymphoid cells are CD3(+), supporting T-cell lineage.

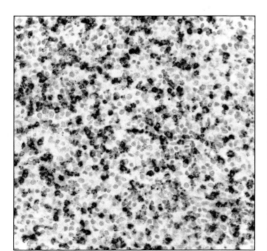
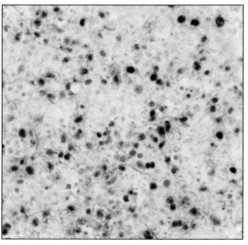

(Left) Peripheral T-cell lymphoma with a cytotoxic immunophenotype involving lymph node. Many of the neoplastic cells were TIA-1(+). (Right) PTCL with a cytotoxic immunophenotype involving lymph node. In situ hybridization showed that a subset of neoplastic cells was EBER(+).

ANGIOIMMUNOBLASTIC T-CELL LYMPHOMA

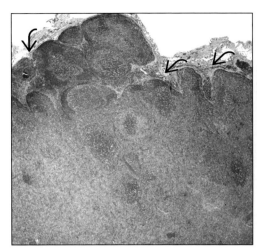

Lymph node involved by angioimmunoblastic T-cell lymphoma (AITL) shows residual follicles, expanded paracortical and interfollicular regions, and open subcapsular (peripheral) sinuses ⤷.

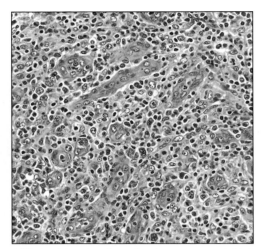

AITL involving lymph node shows increased high endothelial venules (HEV) and a mixed cellular infiltrate. Around the HEV are clusters of neoplastic clear cells.

TERMINOLOGY

Abbreviations
• Angioimmunoblastic T-cell lymphoma (AITL)

Synonyms
• Angioimmunoblastic lymphadenopathy with dysproteinemia (AILD)
  ○ AILD-like (type) T-cell lymphoma
• Immunoblastic lymphadenopathy

Definitions
• Peripheral T-cell lymphoma (PTCL) derived from CD4(+) follicular helper T cells characterized by
  ○ Lymphadenopathy, systemic disease, and, usually, immunodysregulation and immunodeficiency

ETIOLOGY/PATHOGENESIS

Immunodysregulation
• AITL is tumor of follicular helper T cells
  ○ Follicular helper T cells upregulate CXCR5 and CXCL13
    ▪ CXCL13 promotes B-cell recruitment through adherence of B cells on high endothelial venules (HEV)
    ▪ CD21(+) follicular dendritic cells expand from HEV
    ▪ Leads to B-cell expansion, plasmacytic differentiation, and hypergammaglobulinemia

Viral Infection
• EBV(+) B cells are detected in most cases of AITL
  ○ Most likely secondary event as result of host immunocompromise
• Human herpesvirus 6B (HHV6B) is also detected by PCR in almost 1/2 of AITL cases
• EBV and potentially HHV6B may

  ○ Modulate secretion of cytokines and chemokines or expression of membrane receptors
  ○ Influence development of tumor microenvironment, favoring disease progression

CLINICAL ISSUES

Epidemiology
• Incidence
  ○ Rate: 0.5 per 100,000 person years in USA
    ▪ More common in whites than in African-Americans or Asian-Americans
  ○ Represents 1.2% of all non-Hodgkin lymphomas and 18% of all PTCLs
  ○ AITL is more common in Europe than in North America or Asia
• Age
  ○ Median: 59-65 years in various studies
• Gender
  ○ Likely a slight male predominance (but varies in different studies)

Presentation
• Subacute or acute systemic illness
• Advanced stage with generalized lymphadenopathy, hepatomegaly, &/or splenomegaly
• B symptoms are common (fever, weight loss, night sweats)
• Skin rash in > 50% of patients
  ○ Generalized or predominantly truncal maculopapular eruption mimicking inflammatory dermatosis
  ○ Nodular lesions, plaques, purpura, and urticarial lesions also have been observed
  ○ Prior to, concurrent with, or following initial diagnosis of AITL
• Other systemic manifestations
  ○ Arthralgias or arthritis
  ○ Pleural effusions, ascites, &/or edema

ANGIOIMMUNOBLASTIC T-CELL LYMPHOMA

Key Facts

Terminology
- Peripheral T-cell lymphoma derived from CD4(+) follicular helper T cells characterized by
  - Lymphadenopathy, systemic disease, and, usually, immunodysregulation and immunodeficiency

Clinical Issues
- Advanced stage with generalized lymphadenopathy, hepatomegaly, &/or splenomegaly
- Aggressive, with median survival of < 3 years
- Anemia, hypereosinophilia, polyclonal hypergammaglobulinemia

Microscopic Pathology
- Lymph node
  - Partial or complete effacement of architecture
  - Neoplastic T cells with clear/pale cytoplasm
  - Proliferation of arborizing high endothelial venules
  - Proliferation of follicular dendritic cells

Ancillary Tests
- CD2(+), CD3(+), CD4(+) CD5(+), TCR-$\alpha\beta$(+)
- CD10(+/-), Bcl-6(+/-), CXCL13(+/-), PD-1(+/-)
- B immunoblasts(+) in variable numbers
- Monoclonal T-cell receptor rearrangements
- EBER(+) in ~ 80-90% of cases
- Neoplastic cells have gene expression profile of follicular helper T cells

Top Differential Diagnoses
- Viral lymphadenitis or drug reaction
- Classical Hodgkin lymphoma
- T-cell/histiocyte-rich large B-cell lymphoma
- Peripheral T-cell lymphoma, not otherwise specified

  - Lung, neurologic, or gastrointestinal involvement
- Cases of AITL have been reported after administration of antibiotics
  - Most likely, patients with undetected AITL predisposed to infection requiring antibiotic therapy

Laboratory Tests
- Complete blood cell count
  - Anemia
    - Cryoglobulins or cold agglutinins
    - Positive Coombs test in many patients
  - Hypereosinophilia
  - Lymphopenia (lymphocytosis is rare)
  - Thrombocytopenia
- Polyclonal hypergammaglobulinemia
  - Hypoalbuminemia
- ± autoantibodies
  - Rheumatoid factor, anti-nuclear factor, anti-smooth muscle
- Elevated erythrocyte sedimentation rate
- Elevated serum lactate dehydrogenase and β2-microglobulin levels

Treatment
- No consensus on optimal therapeutic regimen
- For medically eligible patients, combined chemotherapy followed by autologous hematopoietic cell transplantation after achieving remission
- For nontransplant candidates, combined chemotherapy
- Steroids have role for patients who are not candidates for chemotherapy
- Novel, investigational therapies are needed for patients with AITL

Prognosis
- Aggressive, with median survival of < 3 years
- ~ 30% of patients are long-term survivors
- Adverse prognostic factors
  - Male sex, mediastinal lymphadenopathy, and anemia adversely affect overall survival
  - Overall immune status also influences survival

- Histological features of AITL do not correlate with prognosis

IMAGE FINDINGS

Radiographic Findings
- Generalized lymphadenopathy, organ involvement, body effusions
  - Cannot distinguish AITL from other lymphoma types with disseminated disease

MICROSCOPIC PATHOLOGY

Histologic Features
- Lymph node
  - Partial or complete effacement of architecture; perinodal infiltration common
    - Paracortical distribution of neoplasm
    - Peripheral sinuses in lymph node cortex are often patent
  - Neoplastic cells are small- to medium-sized, with clear to pale cytoplasm, distinct cell membranes, and minimal atypia
    - Tumor cells often form small clusters around follicles and HEV
  - Background cells are polymorphous
    - Variable numbers of small reactive lymphocytes, eosinophils, plasma cells, and histiocytes
    - ± immunoblasts of B-cell lineage; number is variable and can be prominent
    - ± HRS-like cells of B-cell lineage; usually EBV(+)
  - Marked proliferation of arborizing high endothelial venules (HEV)
  - Increased proliferation of follicular dendritic cells (FDC), usually surrounding HEV
  - 3 patterns in lymph node have been described
    - I: Architecture is partially preserved and hyperplastic, or normal follicles are present
    - II: Architecture is mostly effaced with residual follicles present; ± follicles disrupted or irregular

ANGIOIMMUNOBLASTIC T-CELL LYMPHOMA

- III: Architecture is completely replaced; ± few regressed ("burned out") follicles
- Bone marrow
  - Nodular or interstitial aggregates in paratrabecular or nonparatrabecular distribution
    - Neoplastic cells are often small; ± clear cytoplasm; can be difficult to identify
    - Reactive cells include plasma cells, eosinophils, histiocytes, and B cells
    - Aggregates are associated with blood vessel proliferation
    - ± EBV(+) cells
  - Uninvolved bone marrow ± reactive changes associated with AITL
    - Erythroid hyperplasia, polyclonal plasmacytosis, eosinophilia, fibrosis, or hemophagocytosis
- Peripheral blood
  - Lymphocytosis is uncommon
  - ± atypical lymphocytes or activated lymphocytes (so-called immunocytes)
  - CD10(+) T cells have been shown in many patients by flow cytometric immunophenotyping
- Skin
  - Changes are variable, may not always result from direct tumor infiltration
    - Changes can range from nonspecific, mild perivascular dermal lymphocytic infiltrate to, more rarely, overt lymphoma
- Body effusions
  - Nonneoplastic in nature and their cause is poorly understood
  - Mixture of small lymphocytes, histiocytes, ± eosinophils
- **Morphological variants of AITL**
  - Epithelioid variant
    - High content of epithelioid histiocytes in small, poorly defined clusters (Lennert-like reaction)
  - Clear cell-rich variant
    - Overt lymphomatous proliferation with sheets of neoplastic cells with clear/pale cytoplasm
  - Plasma cell-rich variant
    - Plasma cells numerous; can resemble plasma cell neoplasm
    - Plasma cells lack cytologic atypia
    - Usually EBV(-)
  - B cell-rich variant
    - Background lymphocytes can be composed of numerous small B lymphocytes
    - EBV(+/-)
- **2nd lymphomas in patients with AITL**
  - Patients with AITL have increased risk of developing another lymphoma
  - Diffuse large B-cell lymphoma (DLBCL) is most common
    - Usually EBV(+)
    - EBV(+) DLBCL can precede diagnosis of AITL
  - Patients can develop classical Hodgkin lymphoma
    - Usually EBV(+)
  - Small B-cell lymphomas and plasmacytomas have been reported
    - Usually EBV(-)

Cytologic Features

- Diagnosis of AITL can be difficult to establish by fine needle aspiration because of polymorphous cell composition
  - Correlation with clinical features and ancillary studies to assess immunophenotype or clonality are necessary

ANCILLARY TESTS

Immunohistochemistry

- CD2(+), CD3(+), CD5(+), βF1/TCR-αβ(+)
- ± aberrant loss or reduced expression of CD7
- Usually CD4(+) and CD8(-)
- T cells have follicular helper T-cell immunophenotype in most cases
  - CD10(+), Bcl-6(+), CXCL13(+), &/or PD-1(+)
- FDC proliferation around HEV is highlighted by FDC-associated markers
  - CD21, CD23, CD35, clusterin, or other antibodies
- B-immunoblasts are present in variable number
  - CD19(+), CD20(+), pax-5(+), CD79a(+)
  - Commonly EBER(+); subset LMP1(+/-)

Flow Cytometry

- Normal CD4:CD8 ratio is common
  - Due to reactive T cells that outnumber neoplastic T cells
- ± decreased expression or loss of CD7 &/or CD26
- ± coexpression of CD10 by subset of T cells
- Monotypic B-cell population can be detected in ~ 15% of cases

Cytogenetics

- Most common recurrent abnormalities: Trisomies of chromosomes 3, 5, and 21, gain of X, and loss of 6q

In Situ Hybridization

- EBER(+) in ~ 80-90% of cases

Array CGH

- Gains of 22q, 19, and 11q13
- Loss of 13q

Molecular Genetics

- Monoclonal T-cell receptor (*TCR*) rearrangements in 75-90% of cases
- Monoclonal *Ig* rearrangements in ~ 25% of cases

Gene Expression Profiling

- These studies have shown 2 general components in biopsy specimens involved by AITL
  - Neoplastic T cells have the expression profile of follicular helper T cells
    - Express genes such as *CD10*, *BCL6*, and *CXCL13*
  - Other gene signature is consistent with reactive inflammatory and stromal cells

ANGIOIMMUNOBLASTIC T-CELL LYMPHOMA

DIFFERENTIAL DIAGNOSIS

Reactive Hyperplasia as Result of Viral Infection or Immunodysregulation
- These diseases can overlap with early involvement by AITL (pattern I)
- Absence of atypical clear T cells that are positive for CD10 or follicular T helper cell markers
- No FDC expansion
- Vasculature can be increased; often not HEV
- Often CD8(+) T cells are predominant (especially in viral infection)
- EBV(-) with exception of EBV(+) infectious mononucleosis
- Usually no evidence of monoclonal *TCR* rearrangements

Drug Reaction
- Patients with drug reaction can develop B symptoms, systemic lymphadenopathy, and effusions mimicking AITL
- Histologic findings in drug reaction also can mimic AITL
  o Paracortical expansion by polymorphous infiltrate
  o Proliferation of HEV
  o Oligoclonal or monoclonal *TCR* rearrangements
- Usually atypical clear cells are absent
- No immunophenotypic evidence of follicular T helper cell immunophenotype
- Clinical history is extremely helpful for establishing diagnosis

Classical Hodgkin Lymphoma, Mixed Cellularity Type
- In some cases of AITL, HRS-like cells can be present; EBV(+); B-cell antigens(+)
- Classical Hodgkin lymphoma lacks neoplastic T cells with clear cytoplasm; no increase in HEV or FDC
- No evidence of aberrant T-cell immunophenotype or monoclonal *TCR* rearrangements

T-cell/Histiocyte-rich Large B-cell Lymphoma (TCHRLBL)
- Features that support diagnosis of TCHRLBCL over AITL
  o B cells (tumor cells) are large; in AITL there are many small B cells as well as B immunoblasts
  o T cells lack atypia; no FDC proliferation; EBV(-)
  o Monoclonal *Ig* rearrangements

Peripheral T-cell Lymphoma (PTCL), Not Otherwise Specified (NOS)
- PTCL-NOS lacks features that allow diagnosis of AITL
  o No proliferation of FDC; ± increased HEV
  o Markedly reduced B cells; most cases are EBV(-)
- Gene expression profiling has shown that subset of PTCL-NOS has follicular helper T-cell profile
  o This suggests that some cases of early AITL are included within current PTCL-NOS category

EBV(+) DLBCL of the Elderly
- Polymorphous subtype can mimic AITL
- Features that support EBV(+) DLBCL of the elderly over AITL
  o No proliferation of FDC
  o EBV(+) large B cells, often markedly increased and forming sheets
  o No evidence of aberrant T-cell immunophenotype or monoclonal TCR rearrangements

Kimura Disease
- Subcutaneous mass of head and neck (including salivary glands), associated with regional lymphadenopathy
- Germinal center hyperplasia
  o With polykaryocytes, fibrosis, and proteinaceous material in germinal centers; also folliculolysis
- Interfollicular eosinophils and eosinophilic abscesses; increased paracortical plasma cells; variably hyalinized vessels

Angiolymphoid Hyperplasia with Eosinophilia (ALHE)/Epithelioid Hemangioma
- ALHE can be associated with marked polymorphous inflammatory infiltrate mimicking AITL
- ALHE is typically extranodal; no evidence of systemic symptoms or disease
- No evidence of aberrant T-cell immunophenotype or T-cell clonality

SELECTED REFERENCES

1. de Leval L et al: Advances in the understanding and management of angioimmunoblastic T-cell lymphoma. Br J Haematol. 148(5):673-89, 2010
2. Khokhar FA et al: Angioimmunoblastic T-cell lymphoma in bone marrow: a morphologic and immunophenotypic study. Hum Pathol. 41(1):79-87, 2010
3. Kyriakou C et al: Allogeneic stem cell transplantation is able to induce long-term remissions in angioimmunoblastic T-cell lymphoma: a retrospective study from the lymphoma working party of the European group for blood and marrow transplantation. J Clin Oncol. 27(24):3951-8, 2009
4. Rodriguez-Justo M et al: Angioimmunoblastic T-cell lymphoma with hyperplastic germinal centres: a neoplasia with origin in the outer zone of the germinal centre? Clinicopathological and immunohistochemical study of 10 cases with follicular T-cell markers. Mod Pathol. 22(6):753-61, 2009
5. Attygalle AD et al: Histologic evolution of angioimmunoblastic T-cell lymphoma in consecutive biopsies: clinical correlation and insights into natural history and disease progression. Am J Surg Pathol. 31(7):1077-88, 2007
6. Willenbrock K et al: Frequent occurrence of B-cell lymphomas in angioimmunoblastic T-cell lymphoma and proliferation of Epstein-Barr virus-infected cells in early cases. Br J Haematol. 138(6):733-9, 2007
7. Baseggio L et al: Identification of circulating CD10 positive T cells in angioimmunoblastic T-cell lymphoma. Leukemia. 20(2):296-303, 2006

ANGIOIMMUNOBLASTIC T-CELL LYMPHOMA

Microscopic and Immunohistochemical Features of AITL

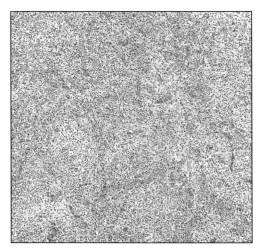 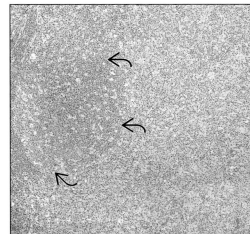

(Left) In a typical case of angioimmunoblastic T-cell lymphoma (AITL), the lymph node architecture is completely replaced by a polymorphous cellular infiltrate associated with arborizing vascular proliferation. (Right) In some cases of AITL, the lymph node is partially involved (so-called pattern I). A preserved follicle is present in the field. This follicle is hyperplastic but lacks a surrounding mantle zone ➡.

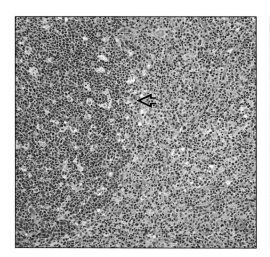 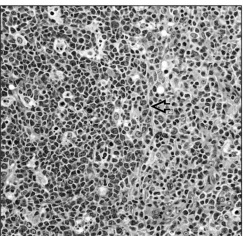

(Left) An "early" variant (so-called pattern I) of angioimmunoblastic T-cell lymphoma shows follicular hyperplasia ➡ and expanded paracortex. Histologic findings in AITL do not predict clinical stage or outcomes. (Right) High-power view of "early" variant of AITL shows a "naked" germinal center ➡ without a mantle zone. The follicle is surrounded by a polymorphous inflammatory infiltrate. Tumor cells are not discernible at this magnification.

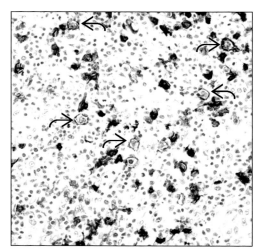 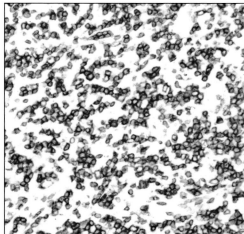

(Left) CD20 highlights B cells in angioimmunoblastic T-cell lymphoma, including small B cells as well as B immunoblasts ➡. The number of B cells in AITL is highly variable. (Right) In this case of AITL, CD3 highlights many small T cells. The T cells include reactive and neoplastic cells, and reactive cells are often predominant. Therefore, the CD4:CD8 ratio is often within the normal range.

9

ANGIOIMMUNOBLASTIC T-CELL LYMPHOMA

Microscopic and Immunohistochemical Features of AITL

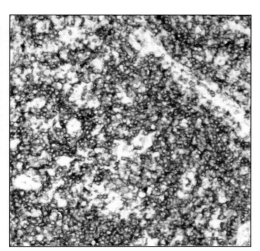

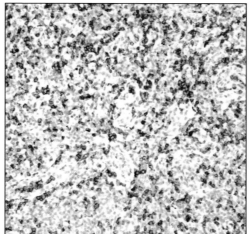

(Left) In angioimmunoblastic T-cell lymphoma, the CD4(+) cells appear to be abundant. The CD4(+) cells include reactive and tumor cells. The anti-CD4 antibody also reacts with histiocytes. (Right) In AITL, many CD8(+) T cells are also present. In contrast, either CD4 or CD8 is often predominant in peripheral T-cell lymphoma, not otherwise specified.

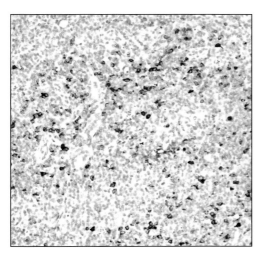

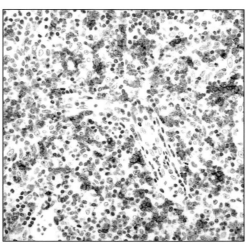

(Left) In angioimmunoblastic T-cell lymphoma, the neoplastic cells show a follicular T helper cell immunophenotype, expressing CD10, Bcl-6, CXCL13, &/or PD-1. This is a CD10 stain showing reactivity in a subset of tumor cells. (Right) The tumor cells in this case of AITL are PD-1(+). Also note that the neoplastic cells are mainly distributed around high endothelial venules.

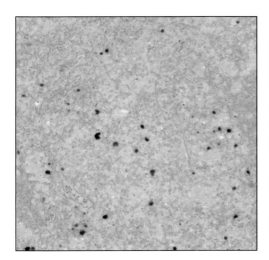

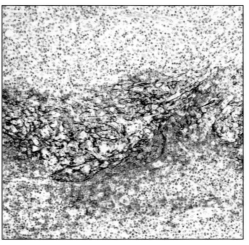

(Left) In many cases of angioimmunoblastic T-cell lymphoma, B immunoblasts are present that are EBV(+), shown here by in situ hybridization for EBER. (Right) In a typical case of AITL, follicular dendritic cells are expanded and form meshworks, often around high endothelial venules. This feature is highly characteristic of AITL and is uncommon in other types of T-cell lymphoma.

9

ANGIOIMMUNOBLASTIC T-CELL LYMPHOMA

Microscopic Features of AITL

(Left) Clear-cell variant of angioimmunoblastic T-cell lymphoma shows large aggregates of clear cells, a result of a marked proliferation of tumor cells. (Right) High-power magnification of a case of clear cell variant AITL shows that the tumor cells are small and lack significant atypia but have an abundance of clear cytoplasm. Many high endothelial venules are present in the field.

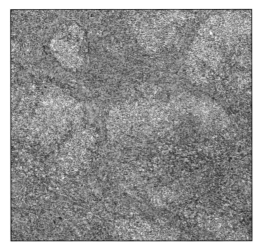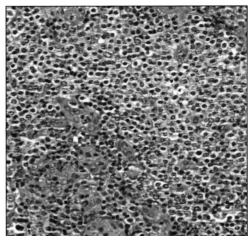

(Left) Approximately 20% of cases of angioimmunoblastic T-cell lymphoma contain a clonal B-cell population. In some cases, clonal B cells are markedly expanded and fulfill diagnostic criteria for the diagnosis of diffuse large B-cell lymphoma as seen in this case. (Right) CD20 highlights large, transformed B cells in this case of diffuse large B-cell lymphoma that coexisted with AITL.

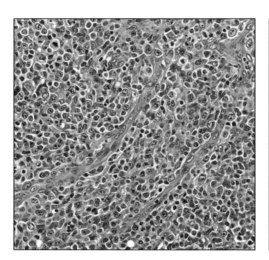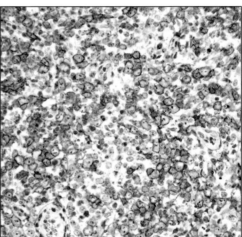

(Left) Angioimmunoblastic T-cell lymphoma involving bone marrow often presents as a nodular infiltrate, either paratrabecular or nonparatrabecular, or both patterns. (Right) The infiltrate of AITL in bone marrow is composed of polymorphous cells including small lymphocytes, eosinophils, and histiocytes. Tumor cells can be difficult to find. EBV(+) cells can be scant or absent in the bone marrow.

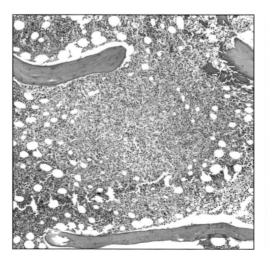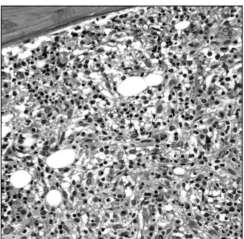

AITL and Differential Diagnosis

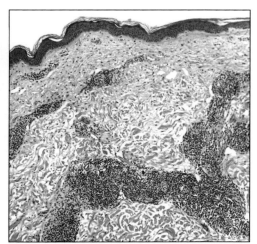

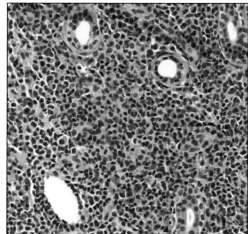

(Left) Skin involvement by angioimmunoblastic T-cell lymphoma shows a predominantly perivascular infiltrate. The histologic changes in skin lesions from AITL patients can be variable, ranging from subtle nonspecific perivascular lymphocytic infiltrates to, less often, overt lymphoma. (Right) High-power view of skin shows a perivascular infiltrate of AITL composed of a mixed cellular infiltrate of small lymphocytes, plasma cells, and rare eosinophils.

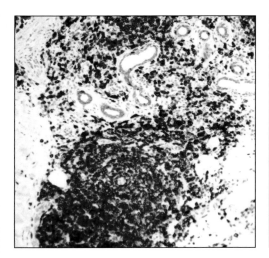

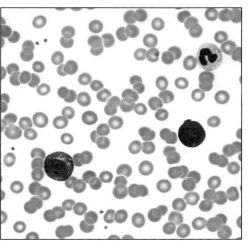

(Left) Angioimmunoblastic T-cell lymphoma involving skin shows many CD3(+) T cells. (Right) Peripheral blood smear obtained from a patient with AITL shows atypical/activated lymphocytes. By flow cytometric immunophenotyping, a subset of T cells in the blood of AITL patients has been shown to coexpress CD10, supporting the diagnosis of AITL.

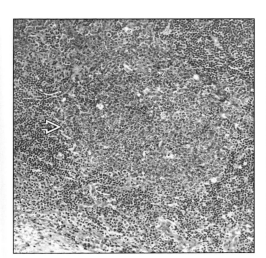

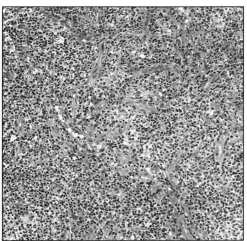

(Left) A reactive lymph node in a patient with a drug reaction shows marked follicular hyperplasia ➡. This degree of hyperplasia is unusual in angioimmunoblastic T-cell lymphoma. (Right) A reactive lymph node in a patient with a drug reaction shows expansion of the interfollicular region with vascular proliferation (not HEV) and a polymorphous cellular infiltrate including eosinophils. The changes can mimic "early" AITL.

ANGIOIMMUNOBLASTIC T-CELL LYMPHOMA

Differential Diagnosis

(Left) A case of mixed-cellularity Hodgkin lymphoma (MCHL) demonstrates a mixed cellular proliferation with scattered large atypical cells. *(Right)* A case of MCHL with atypical large cells that have features of HRS ➡ cells. Many eosinophils are present in the field.

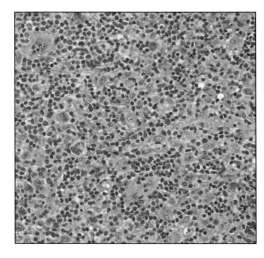
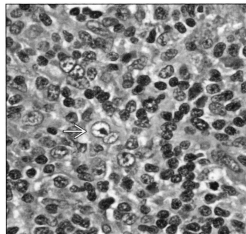

(Left) Paraffin section of a lymph node involved by Kimura disease shows hyperplastic lymphoid follicles and marked eosinophilia. The follicle contains a well-defined mantle zone ➘. *(Right)* Paraffin section of a lymph node involved by Kimura disease shows a hyperplastic lymphoid follicle (right field) ➡ and marked eosinophilia (left field). The follicle (follicle lysis) is also infiltrated by eosinophils with single-cell necrosis and karyorrhexis.

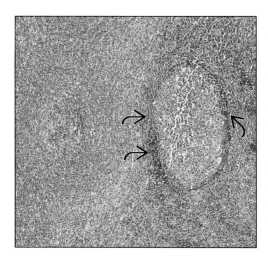
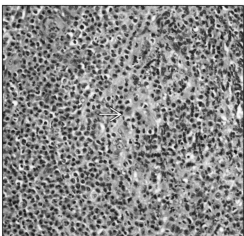

(Left) Paraffin section shows a case of angiolymphoid hyperplasia with eosinophilia (ALHE)/epithelioid hemangioma from the lip region of a 28-year-old man. This field shows soft tissue involved by a large reactive lymphoid follicle ➡ as well as increased blood vessels and eosinophils (top of field). *(Right)* ALHE/epithelioid hemangioma shows a marked proliferation of epithelioid endothelial cells in addition to eosinophils and lymphocytes.

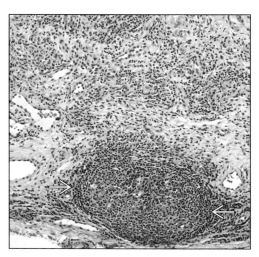
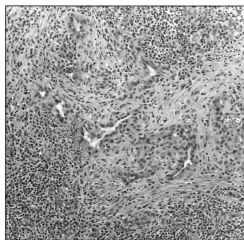

ANGIOIMMUNOBLASTIC T-CELL LYMPHOMA

Differential Diagnosis

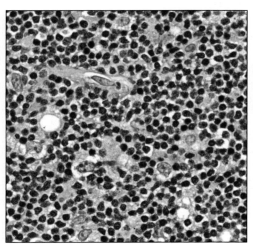

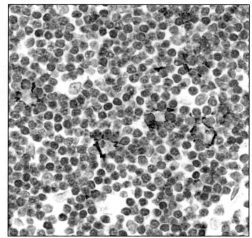

(Left) A case of T-cell/histiocyte-rich large B-cell lymphoma (TCHRLBCL) shows scattered large neoplastic cells in a background of small lymphocytes and histiocytes. *(Right)* CD20 highlights large neoplastic B cells in TCHRLBCL. The large B cells are usually EBV(-), unlike many cases of angioimmunoblastic T-cell lymphoma.

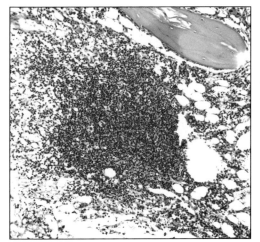

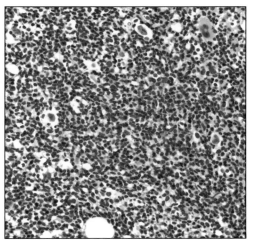

(Left) A case of peripheral T-cell lymphoma, not otherwise specified (PTCL-NOS), small-cell variant shows a nodular pattern of infiltration in the bone marrow. *(Right)* PTCL-NOS, small-cell variant in the bone marrow shows that the infiltrate is more monotonous than is seen in angioimmunoblastic T-cell lymphoma.

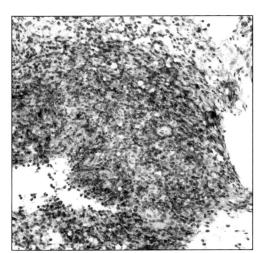

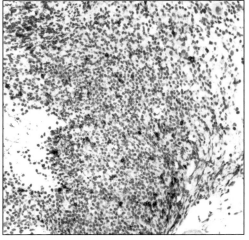

(Left) PTCL-NOS, small cell variant, in the bone marrow. The anti-CD4 antibody shows that the tumor cells are CD4(+). *(Right)* PTCL-NOS, small cell variant in the bone marrow. Very few CD8(+) T cells are present, unlike cases of angioimmunoblastic T-cell lymphoma in which there is usually a mixture of CD4(+) and CD8(+) T cells.

ADULT T-CELL LEUKEMIA/LYMPHOMA, HTLV-1+

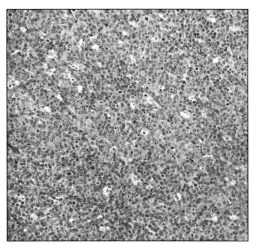

Adult T-cell leukemia/lymphoma (ATLL) diffusely involving lymph node. In this case a "starry sky" pattern can be appreciated, indicating a high cell turnover.

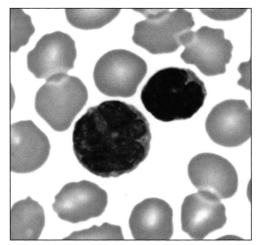

Peripheral blood smear of a patient with adult T-cell leukemia/lymphoma (ATLL). Note the markedly irregular, multilobulated nuclei ("flower cells") that are seen most frequently in the acute variant.

TERMINOLOGY

Abbreviations
- Adult T-cell leukemia/lymphoma (ATLL)

Synonyms
- HTLV-1-associated T-cell lymphoma
- T-cell lymphoma small cell type or pleomorphic medium and large cell type (HTLV-1[+])
- T-cell immunoblastic sarcoma

Definitions
- Peripheral T-cell leukemia/lymphoma caused by human T-cell lymphotropic virus type 1 (HTLV-1) infection
- 4 clinical variants are recognized
  - Acute, lymphomatous, chronic, smoldering
- 5th clinical variant has been proposed: Cutaneous

ETIOLOGY/PATHOGENESIS

Infectious Agents
- HTLV-1 is a type C retrovirus, delta retrovirus genus
- Single strand of RNA that, during infection is
  - Converted into double strand of DNA in host
  - Monoclonally integrated into host cell genome
    - All cells have same site of proviral integration

Pathogenesis
- HTLV-1 is spread in 4 general ways
  - Vertical transmission from mother to child via breast-feeding
  - Sexual intercourse with infected person
  - Transfusion of contaminated blood products
  - Sharing of contaminated needles and syringes among drug users
- HTLV-1 can infect immature thymocytes and mature CD4(+) T cells

- HTLV-1 infection occurs and spreads via cell-to-cell contact
- Genome of HTLV-1 is composed of
  - Long terminal repeat (LTR) regions at each end
  - Structural genes: *gag*, *pol*, and *env*
  - pX region that encodes for tax, rex, p12, p13, p21, and p30 proteins
- P40 tax viral protein is needed for HTLV-1 to transform cells in early stages of disease
  - Many cellular genes are transcriptionally activated by tax
    - Growth factor interleukin (IL)-2
    - Its high-affinity receptor α subunit (IL-2Rα; CD25) promotes autocrine stimulation
    - JAK/STAT pathway is constitutively activated in HTLV-1-infected cells
  - Tax can repress transcription of genes that
    - Negatively control cell cycle
    - Inhibit proteins involved in tumor suppression and DNA repair
- Host immunity is involved in control of HTLV-1 infection
  - Insults to host immune system in viral carrier can result in onset of ATLL
- Marked immunodeficiency that results from HTLV-1-infection can lead to opportunistic infections

Molecular Aberrations
- HTLV-1 infection alone is insufficient to cause ATLL
- Numerous cytogenetic and molecular abnormalities are present
- Molecular models suggest 6 or 7 "hits" involved in pathogenesis of full-blown ATLL

CLINICAL ISSUES

Epidemiology
- Incidence
  - HTLV-1 is endemic in

ADULT T-CELL LEUKEMIA/LYMPHOMA, HTLV-1+

Key Facts

Terminology
- Peripheral T-cell leukemia/lymphoma caused by human T-cell lymphotropic virus type 1 (HTLV-1)
- 4 clinical variants are recognized
  ○ Acute, lymphomatous, chronic, smoldering

Clinical Issues
- Lymphadenopathy that spares the mediastinum
- Hepatosplenomegaly, skin lesions
- Leukemic involvement, hypercalcemia, lytic lesions
- Seropositivity for HTLV-1 can be used as surrogate for HTLV-1 integration into tumor
  ○ Useful in areas with low prevalence of HTLV-1 infection

Microscopic Pathology
- Diffuse effacement of lymph node architecture

- Variable cytologic composition in tissues
- "Flower cells" in peripheral blood

Ancillary Tests
- Immunophenotype
  ○ CD2(+), CD3(+), CD5(+), TCR-α/β(+)
  ○ CD25(+), CCR4(+), FOXP3(+), CD62 (L-selectin)(+)
  ○ CD45RO(+); most cases CD4(+), CD8(-)
- Complex cytogenetic abnormalities
- Monoclonal integration of HTLV-1 into host genome
- Monoclonal *TCR* gene rearrangements

Top Differential Diagnoses
- Peripheral T-cell lymphoma, NOS
- Angioimmunoblastic T-cell lymphoma
- Anaplastic large cell lymphoma
- Mycosis fungoides/Sézary syndrome

- ■ Southwestern Japan, sub-Saharan Africa
- ■ Caribbean basin: Jamaica and Martinique
- ■ South America: Northern Brazil, Colombia, and French Guyana
- ○ Cumulative incidence of ATLL is estimated to be 2.5% among HTLV-1 carriers in Japan
  - ■ Over 1.2 million persons in Japan are infected with HTLV-1
- ○ Prevalence of HTLV-1 infection is very low in North America and Europe
- ○ Variable frequency of seroprevalence in various countries probably related to
  - ■ Genetic predisposition, cultural, and geographical factors
- ○ ~ 10% of patients have positive family history
- Age
  - ○ Range: 20-80 years; mean: 58 years
  - ○ Median age of onset of ATLL is younger in Central and South America, between 40-50 years of age
- Gender
  - ○ M:F ≈ 1.5:1

Site
- Lymph nodes
- Extranodal sites: Main sites are skin and peripheral blood
  - ○ Other sites: Spleen, lungs, liver, gastrointestinal (GI) tract, and central nervous system

Presentation
- Common widespread lymphadenopathy and peripheral blood involvement
- 4 clinical variants: Acute, lymphomatous, chronic, and smoldering
- Acute variant
  - ○ ~ 50% of cases in Japan
  - ○ Leukocytosis, skin rash, and lymphadenopathy
  - ○ Common peripheral blood involvement and hypercalcemia
- Lymphomatous variant
  - ○ ~ 20% of cases in Japan
  - ○ Lymphadenopathy and skin lesions

- Chronic variant
  - ○ ~ 20% of cases in Japan
  - ○ Lymphocytosis and mild organ involvement
- Smoldering variant
  - ○ ~ 5% of cases in Japan
  - ○ Skin or lung lesions
  - ○ Up to 5% of atypical lymphocytes in absence of leukocytosis
- Skin lesions
  - ○ Scaly and erythematous rash, cutaneous plaques, or nodules
  - ○ Acute and lymphomatous variants more frequently associated with skin lesions
- T-cell immunodeficiency is common
  - ○ Associated with *Pneumocystis jirovecii* pneumonia and strongyloidiasis

Endoscopic Findings
- Stomach, colon, and small intestine can be affected
  - ○ Edema, erosions, or polypoid lesions can be identified
- Upper GI tract endoscopy with biopsy is recommended for staging
  - ○ GI tract involvement is frequent in patients with aggressive ATLL

Laboratory Tests
- Seropositivity for HTLV-1 can be used as surrogate for monoclonal integration of virus
  - ○ Only useful in areas with low prevalence of HTLV-1 infection
- Complete blood count: Elevated leukocyte count and circulating neoplastic lymphocytes (leukemic phase)
- Elevated serum lactate dehydrogenase level reflects disease burden/activity
- Hypercalcemia is more common in patients with acute variant
  - ○ With or without associated lytic bone lesions
- Eosinophilia and neutrophilia are common
- Elevated soluble interleukin-2 receptor α-chain levels in patients with aggressive ATLL

ADULT T-CELL LEUKEMIA/LYMPHOMA, HTLV-1+

Natural History
- Patients with chronic or smoldering variant can progress to acute or lymphomatous picture

Treatment
- Options, risks, complications
  - Chronic and smoldering variants
    - Watchful waiting
  - Acute and lymphomatous variants
    - Antiviral agents; chemotherapy
    - Allogeneic hematopoietic stem-cell transplant
    - Novel targeted therapies
- Drugs
  - Zidovudine (AZT)/interferon (IFN) α therapy can achieve long-term response
    - Patients with wild-type p53 and low interferon regulatory factor 4 expression
  - No standard chemotherapy regimen
    - Usually transient response or no response

Prognosis
- Acute and lymphomatous variants
  - Median survival time is 13 months
- Chronic and smoldering variants have protracted clinical course

IMAGE FINDINGS

Radiographic Findings
- Extensive lytic lesions are present in some patients
  - Skull, pelvis, spine, and long bones can be affected
- "Punched-out" lesions similar to multiple myeloma can be found

CT Findings
- Computed tomography (CT) scans of body detect sites of nodal and extranodal disease

MICROSCOPIC PATHOLOGY

Cytologic Features
- ATLL cells show variable appearances
  - Irregular/polylobulated nuclei, homogeneous, condensed chromatin, small nucleoli
  - Agranular basophilic cytoplasm

Lymph Nodes
- ATLL initially involves paracortical T-cell zones, leaving B-cell regions unaffected
- Subsequently ATLL diffusely replaces lymph node
- Lymph nodes involved by ATLL have been subdivided according to cell type and pattern into
  - Pleomorphic small-cell (usually monotonous)
  - Pleomorphic medium- and large cell type/pattern; this is most common
  - Anaplastic large-cell (resembling anaplastic large cell lymphoma)
    - CD30(+), anaplastic lymphoma kinase(-)
  - Angioimmunoblastic T-cell lymphoma-like
    - Medium to large neoplastic cells with abundant clear cytoplasm

- Inflammatory cells and proliferation of high endothelial venules
- Neoplastic cells are CD3(+), CD10(-), PD-1(-), CXCL13(-)
- No proliferation of follicular dendritic cells
  - Hodgkin lymphoma-like; contains multinucleated HRS-like cells
    - Epstein-Barr virus positive B cells are interspersed within lesion
    - Smaller lymphocytes show marked atypia; distinguishing feature from Hodgkin lymphoma
- Mitotic and apoptotic rates are variable
  - Often very high in acute and lymphomatous variants
- Inflammatory background including eosinophils is sparse

Peripheral Blood and Bone Marrow
- ATLL cells are of intermediate or large size, up to 3x size of normal lymphocytes
  - Convoluted or multilobulated nuclei, coarse chromatin, and prominent nucleoli
  - Distinctive appearance of these cells has led to their designation as "flower cells"
  - Basophilic cytoplasm, with or without vacuoles
- In some ATLL patients, neoplastic cells are more uniform in size and shape
  - Nuclei are smaller and less pleomorphic
- Bone marrow involvement may be difficult to identify
  - Infiltrates of ATLL are usually patchy and interstitial
  - Diffuse replacement of the medullary space is rare
  - Increased bone resorption can be seen
    - Osteoclasts can be increased
  - Independent poor prognostic factor

Skin
- Skin lesions are common in ATLL patients: ~ 40-70%
- Erythematous rash, papules, or tumor nodules
- Erythematous lesions tend to be composed of smaller cells in perivascular pattern in dermis
- Papules and nodules tend to be composed of larger cells that replace dermis
- Epidermotropism, including well-formed Pautrier-like microabscesses, can occur

ANCILLARY TESTS

Immunohistochemistry
- Pan-T-cell antigens(+)
  - CD2, CD3, CD5, and T-cell receptor (TCR)-α/β
- CD25(+), CCR4(+), HLA-DR(+), CD62 (L-selectin)(+)
- FOXP3(+), which is a marker of regulatory T cells
- CD45RO(+); most cases CD4(+), CD8(-)
- IRF-4/MUM1(+/-), CD15(-/+), CD30(-/+), CD56(-/+)
- Ki-67/MIB-1 shows high proliferation index
- TdT(-), ALK1(-), TCL1(-), cytotoxic molecules(-)
- B-cell antigens(-), myeloid-associated antigens(-)

Flow Cytometry
- ATLL is neoplasm of mature T cells
  - CD2(+), CD3(+), CD5(+), CD45RO(+), TCR-αβ(+)
  - CD1a(-), CD2(+), CD7(-), CD10(-), PD-1(-)

ADULT T-CELL LEUKEMIA/LYMPHOMA, HTLV-1+

- ~ 90% of cases are CD4(+), CD8(-)
  - Rare cases can be CD4(-), CD8(+), or CD4(+), CD8(+)

Cytogenetics
- Complex abnormalities in acute and lymphomatous variants
- Numerical and structural abnormalities are common
- Higher number of chromosomal abnormalities
  - Acute > lymphomatous > chronic or smoldering

Array CGH
- Gains: 1q, 2p, 4q, 7p, 7q
- Losses: 10p, 13q, 16q, and 18p
- Acute variant: Gains of 3/3p

Molecular Genetics
- Monoclonal *TCR* gene rearrangements are present
- Monoclonal integration of HTLV-1 proviral DNA is found in all ATLL patients
- Integration of defective HTLV-1 into ATLL cells is observed in 1/3 of ATLL patients
  - Associated with clinical subtypes and prognosis
- Southern blot to identify presence of viral integration
- Polymerase chain reaction for HTLV-1 for quantitative purposes
- Mutations or deletions of tumor suppressor genes, such as *P53*, *P15*, or *P16*
  - Observed in ~ 50% of ATLL cases
- *NOTCH1* signaling is upregulated
- Functional impact of microRNAs induced by HTLV-1
  - Tax-driven overexpression: miR-146a, miR-130b
  - Probable tax protein independent mechanisms
    - miR-155, miR-93

Gene Expression Profiling
- Different variants of ATLL have differences in their gene expression signatures
- Therapy with AZT/IFNα induces upregulation of interferon response genes
  - Correlates with clinical response

Electron Microscopy
- Viral particles, 80-120 nm, are present in both cytoplasm and extracellular space

DIFFERENTIAL DIAGNOSIS

Peripheral T-cell Lymphoma (PTCL), Not Otherwise Specified (NOS)
- Complete effacement of architecture
- Spectrum of neoplastic cells, ranging from small cells to large pleomorphic
- Variable amounts of background inflammatory cells
- Features that favor PTCL, NOS over ATLL
  - Patient from Western hemisphere
  - Background of reactive cells including eosinophils, plasma cells, and histiocytes
  - Negative serologic or molecular evidence of HTLV-1

Angioimmunoblastic T-cell Lymphoma (AITL)
- Polymorphic infiltrate with proliferation of high endothelial venules
- Neoplastic cells with clear cytoplasm in small clusters

- Features that favor AITL over ATLL
  - CD10(+), PD-1(+), &/or CXCL13(+) lymphoma cells
  - Irregular proliferation of CD21(+) follicular dendritic cells
  - Hypergammaglobulinemia and eosinophilia
  - Significant B-cell infiltration including large B cells and monoclonal *Ig* gene rearrangements
- EBV infection can be detected in both AITL and ATLL

Anaplastic Large Cell Lymphoma (ALCL)
- Neoplastic cells usually large with abundant cytoplasm and pleomorphic, kidney-shaped nuclei
- Rare peripheral blood involvement
  - Small cell variant of ALK(+) ALCL can present as leukemia
- Downregulation of T-cell antigen expression is common
- Features that favor ALCL over ATLL
  - Sinusoidal distribution in partially involved lymph nodes
  - Lymphoma cells are strongly CD30(+)
  - Expression of cytotoxic granule-associated proteins
  - Translocations involving ALK gene and ALK(+)

Mycosis Fungoides/Sézary Syndrome (MF/SS)
- Long history of skin lesions with secondary lymph node involvement
- Features that favor MF/SS over ATLL
  - Sézary cells are cerebriform, small, hyperchromatic
  - CD25 is variably positive in MF/SS in contrast with strong positivity in ATLL
  - Smaller intraepidermal microabscesses and mild spongiosis

T-Lymphoblastic Leukemia/Lymphoma
- Small to intermediate cells, with fine chromatin and inconspicuous nucleoli
- Features that favor T-lymphoblastic leukemia/lymphoma over ATLL
  - Large mediastinal mass in adolescent or young adult
  - TdT(+), CD1a(+)

HTLV-1(+) Reactive Lymphadenitis
- Lymph node with preservation of architecture; no lymphocyte atypia
- Interfollicular and paracortical expansion of T-cell zones
- No evidence of aberrant immunophenotype or monoclonal T-cell population

DIAGNOSTIC CHECKLIST

Clinically Relevant Pathologic Features
- HTLV-1 is required for diagnosis
  - HTLV-1 is clonally integrated into tumor cell genome

Pathologic Interpretation Pearls
- Wide morphologic spectrum
- CD4(+) CD8(-), CD25(+), FOXP3(+), TCR-α/β(+)
- Monoclonal *TCR* gene rearrangements

ADULT T-CELL LEUKEMIA/LYMPHOMA, HTLV-1+

Differential Diagnosis of Adult T-cell Leukemia/Lymphoma (HTLV-1[+])

Features	ATLL	PTCL, NOS	AITL	ALCL	MF/SS
Clinical Features					
Male to female ratio	1.5 to 1	2 to 1	1 to 1	1.5 to 1	2 to 1
Presentation	From asymptomatic to disseminated node and organ involvement	Peripheral lymphadenopathy	Generalized lymphadenopathy; hepatosplenomegaly		Indolent skin disease with progression over many years
Skin lesions	Rash, papules, and nodules	Nodules	Rash or papules	Nodules in ALCL, ALK(-), or cutaneous CD30(+) lymphoproliferative disorder	Erythema, patch, papule, plaque, or tumor stage; erythroderma
Laboratory Findings					
	Hypercalcemia, HTLV-1(+)	± eosinophilia	Polytypic hypergammaglobulinemia	Nonspecific	Leukocytosis; circulating cerebriform cells
Pathologic Features					
Lymph node	Complete effacement of architecture; sparse reactive cells	Interfollicular to diffuse pattern with polymorphic background	Interfollicular to diffuse pattern with increased vascularity and polymorphic background including large B cells	Sinusoidal infiltration, large pleomorphic cells; kidney-shaped nuclei	Secondary involvement with progression from paracortical to complete replacement
Skin	Pautrier-like microabscesses are common	Nodules or tumor	Sparse perivascular infiltration	Nodule or tumor in cutaneous CD30(+) lymphoproliferative disorder	Lichenoid infiltrate; Pautrier microabscesses in up to 40% of cases
Cytologic Findings					
	Multilobulated, "flower cell"	Irregular, monomorphic or pleomorphic cells	Small to irregular with clear cytoplasm	Horseshoe- or kidney-shaped large nuclei	Cerebriform cell
Immunophenotype					
	CD4(+), CD25(+), FOXP3(+), CD7(-); cytotoxic molecules(-)	CD4(+), βF1(+); loss of CD7, CD5; variable expression of CD56, cytotoxic antigens, CD8	T cells(+) for CD10, Bcl-6, CCXL13, PD-1; increased B cells; EBV(+/-)	CD4(+); EMA(+/-), CD25(+), cytotoxic molecules(+); CD30(+), ALK(+) in ALCL, ALK(+)	Usually CD4(+), common loss of CD7, CD5, CD26
Cytogenetic or Molecular Features					
	Monoclonal integration of HTLV-1	Monoclonal *TCR* gene rearrangements; complex karyotype	Monoclonal *TCR* gene rearrangements common; monoclonal *IgH* gene rearrangements in ~ 20%	Translocations involving ALK at 2p23 in ALCL, ALK(+)	Monoclonal *TCR* gene rearrangements; complex karyotype

ATLL = adult T-cell leukemia/lymphoma; PTCL, NOS = peripheral T-cell lymphoma, not otherwise specified; AITL = angioimmunoblastic T-cell lymphoma; ALCL = anaplastic large cell lymphoma; MF/SS = mycosis fungoides/Sézary syndrome.

SELECTED REFERENCES

1. Alizadeh AA et al: Expression profiles of adult T-cell leukemia-lymphoma and associations with clinical responses to zidovudine and interferon alpha. Leuk Lymphoma. 51(7):1200-16, 2010
2. Gonçalves DU et al: Epidemiology, treatment, and prevention of human T-cell leukemia virus type 1-associated diseases. Clin Microbiol Rev. 23(3):577-89, 2010
3. Pancewicz J et al: Notch signaling contributes to proliferation and tumor formation of human T-cell leukemia virus type 1-associated adult T-cell leukemia. Proc Natl Acad Sci U S A. 107(38):16619-24, 2010
4. Ruggero K et al: Role of microRNAs in HTLV-1 infection and transformation. Mol Aspects Med. Epub ahead of print, 2010
5. Tanosaki R et al: Adult T-cell leukemia-lymphoma: current treatment strategies and novel immunological approaches. Expert Rev Hematol. 3(6):743-53, 2010
6. Tsukasaki K et al: Definition, prognostic factors, treatment, and response criteria of adult T-cell leukemia-lymphoma: a proposal from an international consensus meeting. J Clin Oncol. 27(3):453-9, 2009
7. Karube K et al: Adult T-cell lymphoma/leukemia with angioimmunoblastic T-cell lymphomalike features: Report of 11 cases. Am J Surg Pathol. 31(2):216-23, 2007
8. Shimizu K et al: Upregulation of CC chemokine ligand 18 and downregulation of CX3C chemokine receptor 1 expression in human T-cell leukemia virus type 1-associated lymph node lesions: Results of chemokine and chemokine receptor DNA chip analysis. Cancer Sci. 98(12):1875-80, 2007

ADULT T-CELL LEUKEMIA/LYMPHOMA, HTLV-1+

Imaging, Microscopic, and Immunohistochemical Features

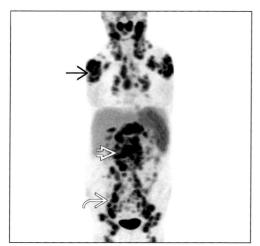

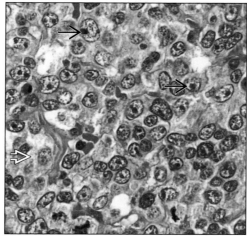

(Left) PET CT shows extensive FDG-avid disease above and below the diaphragm in a patient with adult T-cell leukemia/lymphoma (ATLL). Enlarged axillary ➔, mesenteric ⇒, and iliac-femoral ⇒ lymph nodes are noted. *(Right)* ATLL involving lymph node. In this case the neoplastic cells are large, and a subset has prominent nucleoli ➔ resembling immunoblasts. Note histiocytes ⇒ with ample, clear cytoplasm.

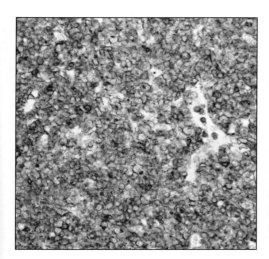

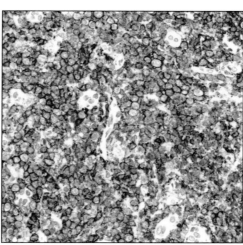

(Left) ATLL involving lymph node. Immunohistochemistry for CD3 shows that the neoplastic cells are CD3(+) T cells. Most cases of ATLL are positive for CD2, CD3, CD5, and TCR-αβ, and are commonly CD7(-). *(Right)* ATLL involving lymph node. CD4 immunohistochemistry highlights the neoplastic cells. Most cases of ATLL are CD4(+) and CD8(-).

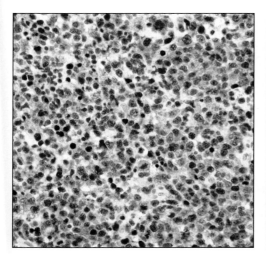

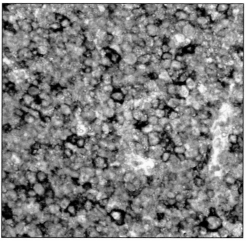

(Left) ATLL involving lymph node. The neoplastic cells are strongly positive for IRF-4/MUM1. Elevated expression of IRF-4/MUM1 has been observed in a large subset of ATLL. *(Right)* ATLL involving lymph node. Immunohistochemistry for CD25 highlights strong reactivity of neoplastic cells. The soluble form of IL-2 receptor α chain is elevated in patients with aggressive ATLL.

ADULT T-CELL LEUKEMIA/LYMPHOMA, HTLV-1+

Microscopic and Immunohistochemical Features

(Left) ATLL involving lymph node. A subset of lymphoma cells express CD30 ⊳. Note that reactivity is variable in contrast with diffuse, strong reactivity typically observed in anaplastic large cell lymphoma. *(Right)* ATLL, Hodgkin-like, involving lymph node. The large cells were CD15(+) and CD30(+). However the large cells were also CD3(+), and surrounding lymphocytes → exhibit cytologic atypia supporting ATLL over classical Hodgkin lymphoma.

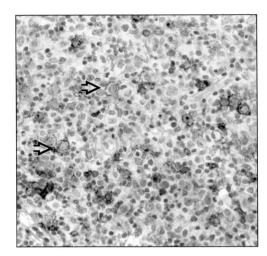
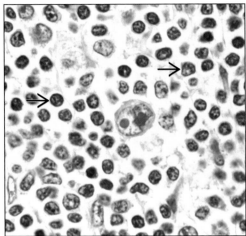

(Left) Fine needle aspirate of an axillary lymph node from a patient with adult T-cell leukemia/lymphoma (ATLL). There are large, atypical lymphocytes with irregular nuclear contours and basophilic, vacuolated cytoplasm ⊳. *(Right)* ATLL involving skin. A dense infiltrate involving the dermis is seen. This patient had cutaneous nodules.

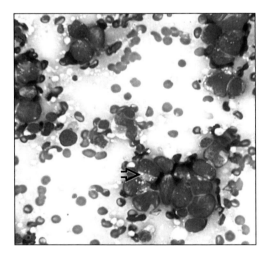
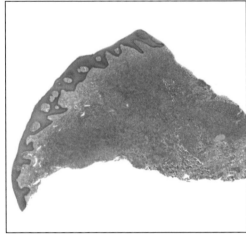

(Left) ATLL involving skin. In this case, abundant lymphoma cells in the epidermis form a well-circumscribed, Pautrier-like microabscess ⊳. Smaller and less-cellular aggregates are more characteristic of mycosis fungoides, although sometimes the distinction is not possible. *(Right)* ATLL involving the skin. Most of the neoplastic cells are pleomorphic and medium to large in size.

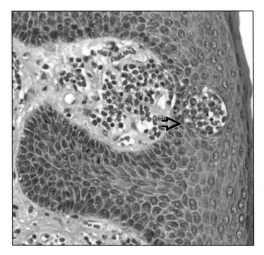
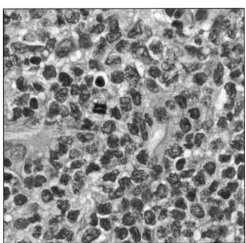

ADULT T-CELL LEUKEMIA/LYMPHOMA, HTLV-1+

Microscopic and Immunohistochemical Features

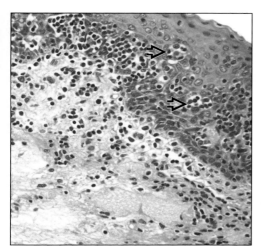

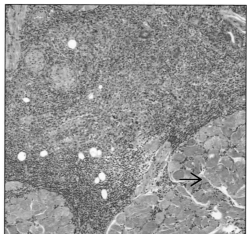

(Left) ATLL involving the tongue. Note the small lymphocytes with irregular, hyperchromatic nuclei infiltrating squamous mucosa, forming Pautrier-like microabscesses ⊅. *(Right)* ATLL involving the tongue. Note diffuse infiltration of the tongue by small to medium-sized lymphoma cells. Relatively uninvolved skeletal muscle is also present in this field ⊡.

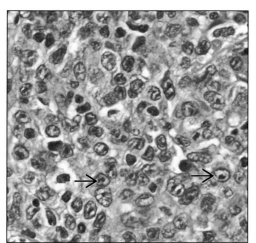

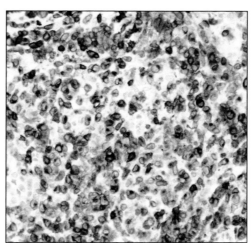

(Left) ATLL involving the tongue. The neoplasm is composed of a mixture of small and large lymphoma cells with irregular nuclei. Note large transformed cells with distinct nucleoli ⊡. *(Right)* ATLL involving the tongue. Immunohistochemistry for CD3 shows that the lymphoma cells are strongly positive, supporting T-cell lineage.

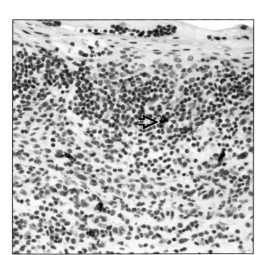

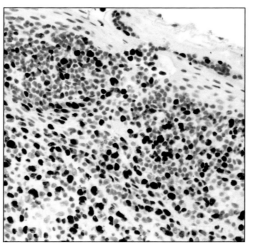

(Left) Adult T-cell leukemia/lymphoma (ATLL) involving the tongue. Immunohistochemistry for CD20 shows that the neoplastic cell are CD20(-). Scattered reactive B cells ⊅ are admixed within the neoplasm. *(Right)* ATLL involving the tongue. Immunohistochemistry for Ki-67 shows that ATLL cells have a proliferation rate of ~ 40% in this case.

ADULT T-CELL LEUKEMIA/LYMPHOMA, HTLV-1+

Microscopic and Flow Immunophenotypic Features

(Left) ATLL involving the femur in a 54-year-old African-American woman with osteolytic lesions; the woman did not have lymphadenopathy or hepatosplenomegaly. There is hypercellularity with a polymorphous proliferation of medium to large lymphoma cells ⮕. Numerous osteoclasts ⮕ cause resorption of bone trabeculae. *(Right)* ATLL involving the femur. Immunohistochemistry for CD3 highlights neoplastic cells, supporting T-cell lineage.

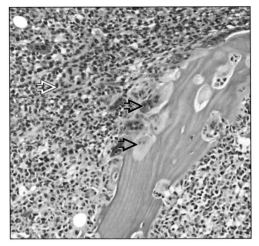
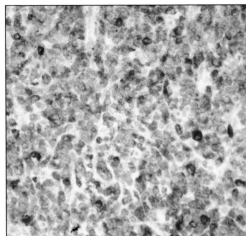

(Left) Adult T-cell leukemia/lymphoma (ATLL) involving bone marrow biopsy specimen. Note increased bone resorption and osteoclasts ⮕ on both sides of bone trabeculae, causing the appearance of an "apple core." Bone marrow involvement is an independent poor prognostic factor in patients with ATLL. *(Right)* ATLL in a bone marrow aspirate smear. The lymphoma cells are medium to large in size with basophilic, vacuolated cytoplasm and irregular nuclei ⮕.

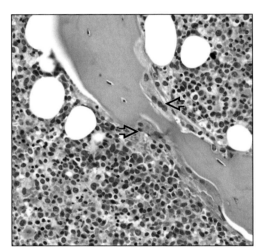
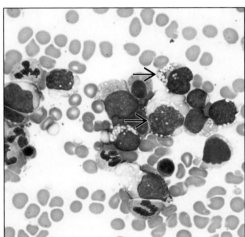

(Left) Adult T-cell leukemia/lymphoma (ATLL) in leukemic phase shows neoplastic lymphocytes with irregular nuclear contours ⮕. Note the intermediate to large size and the flower-like nuclei. *(Right)* ATLL assessed by flow cytometric immunophenotyping demonstrates a CD3(+), CD4(+), and CD25(+) cell population. The left histogram displays CD4 (y-axis) versus CD3; the right histogram displays CD25 (y-axis) versus CD19.

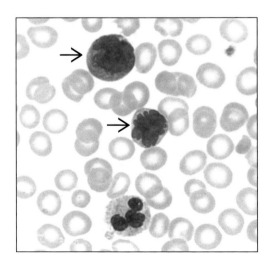
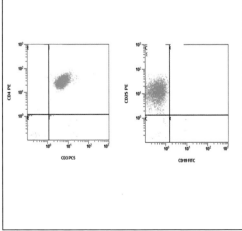

ALK+ ANAPLASTIC LARGE CELL LYMPHOMA

Microscopic Features

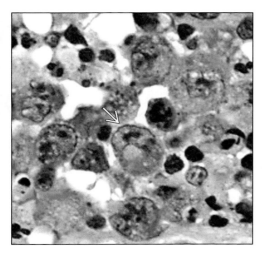
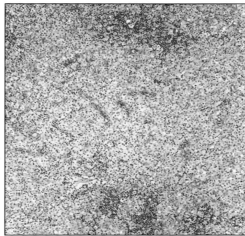

(Left) Hematoxylin & eosin shows neoplastic cells that are large and pleomorphic. Hallmark cells ➡ are usually present (cells with kidney-shaped nuclei and eosinophilic Golgi region). *(Right)* ALK(+) ALCL, lymphohistiocytic variant. Numerous histiocytes and clusters of small lymphocytes are noted at low power.

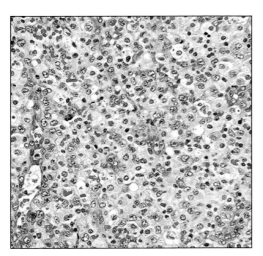
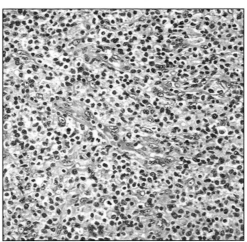

(Left) ALK(+) ALCL, lymphohistiocytic variant is composed of relatively few neoplastic cells associated with numerous reactive lymphocytes and histiocytes. CD30 or ALK immunostain help in recognizing this variant. *(Right)* ALCL, small cell variant characterized by numerous small neoplastic cells. Few large neoplastic cells are also seen but they are infrequent. CD30 or ALK immunostain helps in recognizing this variant.

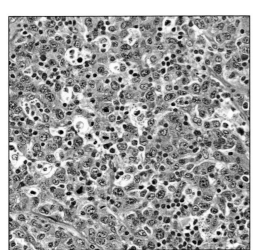
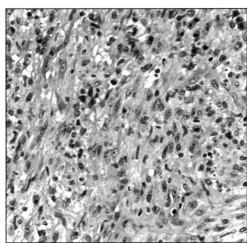

(Left) ALK(+) ALCL, monomorphic variant. The neoplastic cells are intermediate to large and have a monomorphic appearance. CD30 or ALK immunostain helps in recognizing this variant. *(Right)* ALK(+) ALCL, sarcomatoid variant. This variant is characterized by the presence of a subset of tumor cells with a spindle morphology.

ALK+ ANAPLASTIC LARGE CELL LYMPHOMA

Ancillary Techniques

(Left) ALK immunostain highlights prominent sinusoidal growth of the tumor cells in ALK(+) ALCL. This pattern is particularly seen in lymph nodes not involved extensively. *(Right)* CD30 is strongly expressed by the neoplastic cells in ALK(+) ALCL tumors. Note the characteristic membranous and paranuclear (Golgi) pattern (target-like appearance).

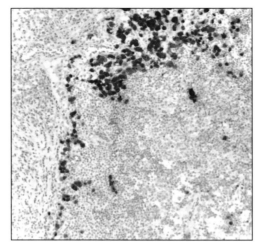 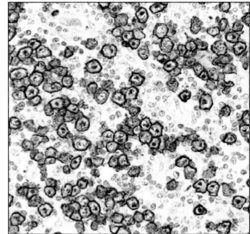

(Left) ALK(+) ALCL. ALK stain has a cytoplasmic and nuclear pattern indicating the presence of the t(2;5) (NPM-ALK). *(Right)* CD30 may help to identify ALCL in bone marrow. In some cases, very few tumor cells not seen by H&E can be highlighted using immunostains.

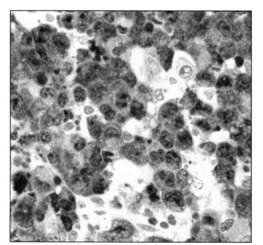 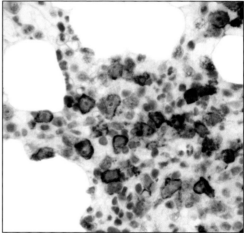

(Left) Frequently, the tumor cells in ALK(+) ALCL are CD3 negative. *(Right)* NPM-ALK encodes a fusion protein that contains the tyrosine kinase (TK) domain of ALK. The oligomerization domain (OD) of NPM allows the formation of homodimers between NPM-ALK proteins and heterodimers of NPM-ALK with wild type (WT) NPM. WT NPM has nuclear localization signals (NLS) that drive the heterodimers into the nucleus. Thus, in the presence of t(2;5), ALK immunostain is cytoplasmic and nuclear.

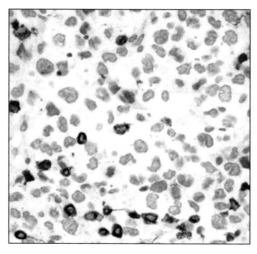 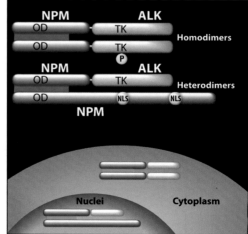

ALK+ ANAPLASTIC LARGE CELL LYMPHOMA

Differential Diagnosis

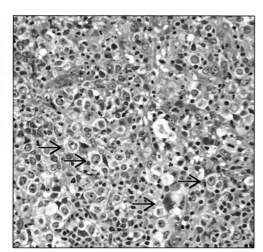

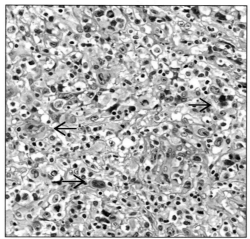

(Left) Classical Hodgkin lymphoma (CHL) may morphologically resemble ALCL. Note the presence of numerous large atypical cells ➡. However, tumor cells were positive for pax-5 & CD30 and negative for CD45 (LCA). This immunophenotype is characteristic of CHL. *(Right)* ALK(-) ALCL. Large anaplastic tumor cells ➡ are present in this case. They were positive for CD30, simulating ALK(+) ALCL, or CHL. However, tumor cells were negative for ALK and pax-5.

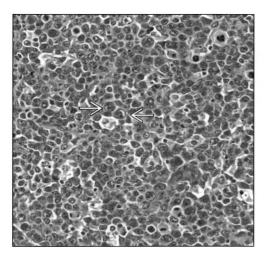

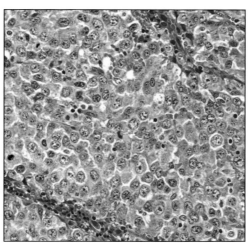

(Left) This case of ALK(-) ALCL is morphologically indistinguishable from ALK(+) ALCL. Note the presence of hallmark cells ➡. The tumor cells were positive for CD30, CD15 (subset), and CD3, and negative for ALK. *(Right)* The tumor cells in this case of DLBCL with t(2;17) have plasmablastic morphology and were positive for ALK (cytoplasmic, coarsely granular), CD79a (focally), and negative for CD30 and CD3.

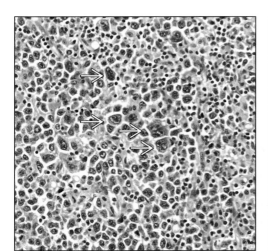

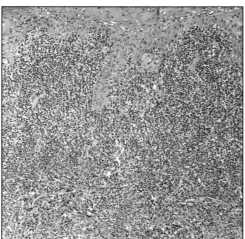

(Left) Diffuse large B-cell lymphoma (DLBCL). The tumor cells have anaplastic morphology ➡ and were strongly and uniformly positive for CD30 and negative for CD20. pax-5 immunostain confirmed the diagnosis of DLBCL instead of ALCL. *(Right)* ALK(-) ALCL involving skin. The dermis is extensively involved. The neoplasm has a diffuse pattern and is composed of large anaplastic cells strongly and uniformly CD30(+). The tumor cells were negative for ALK.

ALK- ANAPLASTIC LARGE CELL LYMPHOMA

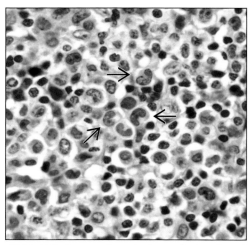

ALK(-) ALCL. Large and anaplastic neoplastic cells and occasional cells with horseshoe-shaped nuclei, so-called "hallmark" cells ⇨ are present.

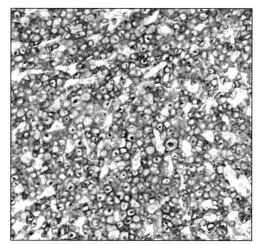

ALK(-) ALCL. The neoplastic cells are strongly positive for CD30 with the same pattern seen in ALK(+) ALCL (membranous and paranuclear; target-like pattern).

TERMINOLOGY

Abbreviations
- Anaplastic lymphoma kinase (ALK) negative, anaplastic large cell lymphoma (ALCL)

Definitions
- Lymphoma histologically resembling ALK(+) ALCL, with strong and uniform expression of CD30, but lacking ALK expression

CLINICAL ISSUES

Presentation
- No age preference
- No sex predilection or slight male predominance
- Extranodal involvement can be seen (skin, liver, and lungs)
- B-symptoms frequent

Treatment
- Doxorubicin-based chemotherapy regimens

Prognosis
- International prognosis index (IPI) often high
- Poorer prognosis than ALK(+) ALCL but better than peripheral T-cell lymphoma unspecified (PTCL-U)

MICROSCOPIC PATHOLOGY

Histologic Features
- Most common variant closely mimics classical ALK(+) ALCL
  - Large neoplastic cells including "hallmark" cells
  - Cohesive growth pattern
  - Extensive sinus involvement
- Hallmark cells less common than in classical variant of ALK(+) ALCL

- Anaplasia usually greater in ALK(-) ALCL than in ALK(+) ALCL

ANCILLARY TESTS

Immunohistochemistry
- Immunophenotype of ALK(-) ALCL shares many features with ALK(+) ALCL
- CD30 is uniformly and strongly positive
- ALK(-) ALCL expresses at least 1 T-cell antigen such as
  - CD2, CD3, CD4, CD5, CD7, CD43, CD45RO, and T-cell receptors
- Aberrant T-cell immunophenotype common
  - Loss of CD3, CD5, and T-cell receptors
- Expression of cytotoxic molecules (TIA-1, GZM-B, perforin) in 50%
- Clusterin usually positive
- CD15(-/+), Bcl-2(+/-)
- EBV LMP1(-)
- B-cell antigens are negative
- LCA/CD45 can be negative (more often by immunohistochemistry than by flow cytometry)

In Situ Hybridization
- EBER(-/+)

PCR
- Monoclonal T-cell receptor gene rearrangements

DIFFERENTIAL DIAGNOSIS

ALK(+) ALCL
- Histologically, ALK(+) ALCL and ALK(-) ALCL are indistinguishable
  - ALK(-) ALCL tumors are often more anaplastic
- Immunophenotypically ALK(+) ALCL shares many features with ALK(-) ALCL
  - Commonalities
    - Frequent aberrant T-cell immunophenotype

ALK- ANAPLASTIC LARGE CELL LYMPHOMA

Key Facts

Terminology
- Lymphoma histologically resembling spectrum of ALK(+) ALCL, with strong and uniform expression of CD30, but lacking ALK expression

Clinical Issues
- Poorer prognosis than ALK(+) ALCL
- Better prognosis than PTCL-U

Microscopic Pathology
- Most common variant closely mimics classical variant of ALK(+) ALCL
  - Hallmark cells less frequently seen in ALK(-) ALCL than ALK(+) ALCL
  - ALK(-) ALCL often more anaplastic than ALK(+) ALCL
  - Cohesive growth pattern
  - Sinus involvement

Ancillary Tests
- Immunophenotypic studies needed to confirm dx
  - CD30 strongly and uniformly positive
  - ALK negative
  - Frequent expression of cytotoxic molecules
  - Absence of B-cell markers
  - EBV positive in subset of cases
- Monoclonal T-cell receptor gene rearrangements

Top Differential Diagnoses
- ALK(+) ALCL
- PTCL-U
- Cutaneous ALCL
  - Staging studies needed to establish diagnosis of cutaneous ALCL

Immunohistochemistry

Antibody	Reactivity	Staining Pattern	Comment
CD30	Positive	Cell membrane & cytoplasm	Strong and uniformly positive
Clusterin	Positive	Golgi zone	Positive in 80-90% of cases
Bcl-2	Positive	Cytoplasmic	Positive in most cases
CD15	Positive	Cell membrane & cytoplasm	Positive in 50% of cases
EBV-LMP	Positive	Cell membrane & cytoplasm	Positive in subset of cases
ALK1	Negative	Not applicable	
CD3	Negative		Loss of CD3 expression is common

- CD30 positive (strong and uniform)
- Clusterin positive
- Cytotoxic molecules expressed in most cases
- Differences, ALK(+) ALCL is
  - ALK positive (in various patterns; most often nuclear and cytoplasmic)
  - Bcl-2 negative, CD15 usually negative
  - Epstein-Barr virus (EBER and LMP1) not expressed

Peripheral T-cell Lymphoma Unspecified (PTCL-U)
- ALK(-)ALCL has distinctive histologic and cytologic features unlike PTCL-U
  - Hallmark cells usually absent in PTCL-U
  - CD30 only focally positive in PTCL-U
  - PTCL-U usually express LCA (CD45), CD3, CD5, and T-cell receptors
  - Cytotoxic molecules infrequently expressed in PTCL-U (in western countries)
- ALK(-) ALCL appears to have better prognosis than PTCL-U

Cutaneous ALCL
- They are uniformly and strongly positive for CD30
- ALK absent (or very rare)
  - Up to 20% of patients with systemic ALCL can have skin disease
  - ALK expression useful for distinguishing systemic ALK(+) ALCL from cutaneous ALCL

- Cutaneous ALCL often negative for EMA and can express cutaneous lymphocyte antigen (CLA)
- Importantly, clinical and radiologic staging studies needed to establish diagnosis of cutaneous ALCL

SELECTED REFERENCES

1. Salaverria I et al: Genomic profiling reveals different genetic aberrations in systemic ALK-positive and ALK-negative anaplastic large cell lymphomas. Br J Haematol. 140(5):516-26, 2008
2. Savage KJ et al: ALK- anaplastic large-cell lymphoma is clinically and immunophenotypically different from both ALK+ ALCL and peripheral T-cell lymphoma, not otherwise specified: report from the International Peripheral T-Cell Lymphoma Project. Blood. 111(12):5496-504, 2008
3. Medeiros LJ et al: Anaplastic Large Cell Lymphoma. Am J Clin Pathol. 127(5):707-22, 2007
4. Kadin ME: Pathobiology of CD30+ cutaneous T-cell lymphomas. J Cutan Pathol. 33 Suppl 1:10-7, 2006
5. Bonzheim I et al: Anaplastic large cell lymphomas lack the expression of T-cell receptor molecules or molecules of proximal T-cell receptor signaling. Blood. 104(10):3358-60, 2004
6. Falini B et al: ALK+ lymphoma: clinico-pathological findings and outcome. Blood. 93(8):2697-706, 1999
7. Stein H et al: The expression of the Hodgkin's disease associated antigen Ki-1 in reactive and neoplastic lymphoid tissue: evidence that Reed-Sternberg cells and histiocytic malignancies are derived from activated lymphoid cells. Blood. 66(4):848-58, 1985

ALK- ANAPLASTIC LARGE CELL LYMPHOMA

Microscopic Features

(Left) A "starry sky" pattern is noted in this case of ALK(-) ALCL. Mitotic figures are easily seen. *(Right)* Hematoxylin & eosin shows occasional large cells with eccentric horseshoe-shaped nuclei and distinct paranuclear eosinophilic zone corresponding to the Golgi region ➡.

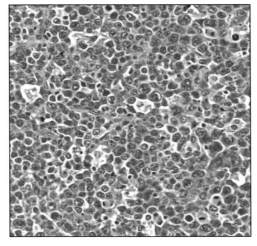
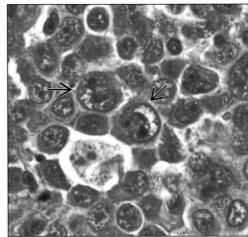

(Left) This ALK(-) ALCL tumor shows scattered large atypical tumor cells in an inflammatory background of small lymphocytes, neutrophils, and eosinophils simulating classical Hodgkin lymphoma. *(Right)* ALK(-) ALCL, sarcomatoid variant. Some neoplastic cells are spindled within a myxoid background. The tumor in this case was positive for CD2, CD4, CD30, and GZM-B, and negative for CD3, ALK, cytokeratin, S100, desmin, myogenin, CD21, and pax-5.

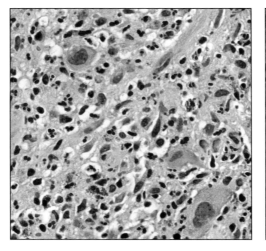
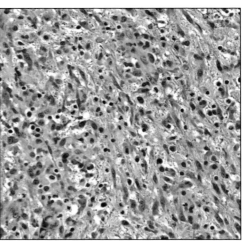

(Left) Lymph node involved by ALK(-) ALCL. Fine needle aspiration shows scattered large anaplastic cells are present with a background of numerous small, reactive lymphocytes. *(Right)* ALK(-) ALCL involving bone marrow. Note clusters of large atypical cells. The neoplastic cells were positive for CD3 and CD30 and negative for ALK. The patient had a history of ALK(-) ALCL involving lymph node.

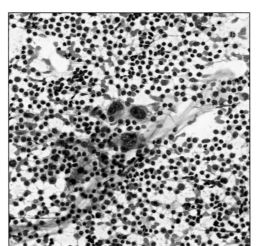
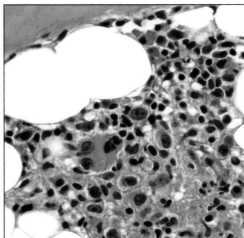

ALK- ANAPLASTIC LARGE CELL LYMPHOMA

Immunophenotypic Features

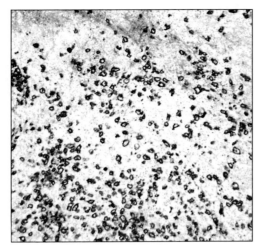
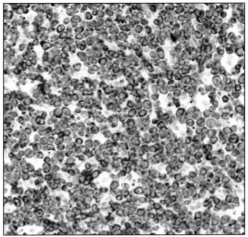

(Left) ALK(-) ALCL. The large neoplastic cells are strongly and uniformly positive for CD30. (Right) ALK(-) ALCL. The neoplastic cells are positive for CD3.

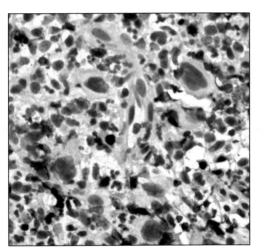
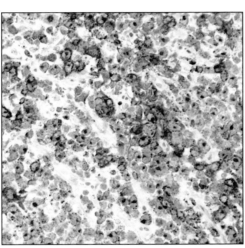

(Left) Not uncommonly, ALK(-) ALCL is negative for CD3 as shown in this case. (Right) ALK(-) ALCL. The neoplastic cells were positive for CD15. CD15 expression can be seen in approximately 50-60% of ALK(-) ALCL.

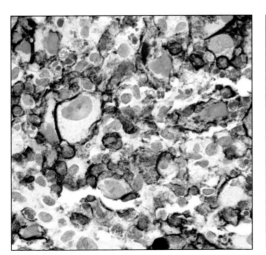
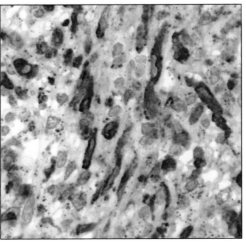

(Left) ALK(-) ALCL. The neoplastic cells are positive for CD43 and were negative for CD3 (not shown). (Right) ALK(-) ALCL (sarcomatoid variant). The neoplastic cells are spindled and strongly positive for GZM-B.

Extranodal T-/NK-cell Lymphomas

Non-Hodgkin Lymphoma Specimen Examination

BREAST IMPLANT-ASSOCIATED ANAPLASTIC LARGE CELL LYMPHOMA

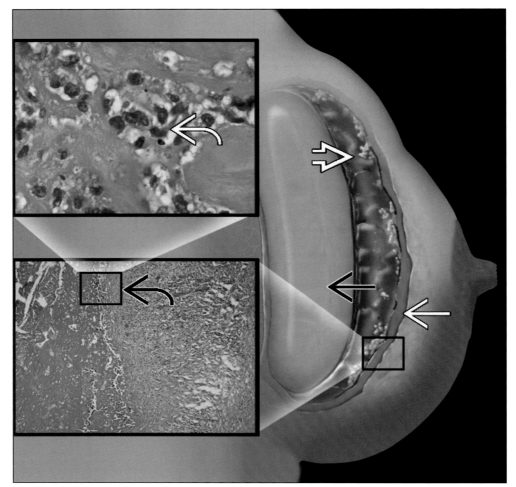

Artist reconstruction of anaplastic large cell lymphoma associated with breast implant shows fluid ⇒ accumulation around breast implant ⇒. Fibrous capsule ⇒ is displaced by fluid and is thickened where fibrinoid material and tumor cell clusters are identified ⇒ (sequence of rectangles). No distinct tumor is identified grossly. Areas where tumor cells ⇒ are found microscopically appear as slightly thickened capsule with fibrinoid deposition.

TERMINOLOGY

Abbreviations
- Breast implant-associated anaplastic large cell lymphoma (ALCL)

Synonyms
- Seroma-associated ALCL

Definitions
- ALCL of T-/null-cell lineage that arises around breast implant and is ALK(-)

ETIOLOGY/PATHOGENESIS

Etiology
- Unknown; occurs with saline and silicone breast implants
- Carcinogenic factors or mechanisms are not identified; suggested possibilities include
  - Implant contents or implant texture
  - Autoimmune-mediated cytokines
  - Genetic susceptibility

Pathogenesis
- Implant placed for purely cosmetic reasons or as part of reconstructive surgery for breast cancer
- Reactive fibrous capsule usually develops around implants
  - Microscopic leaking from implant may trigger surrounding reaction
- Almost all cases associated with implants and effusion are ALK(-) ALCL
  - Small subset of patients have history of primary cutaneous CD30(+) T-cell lymphoproliferative disorder

BREAST IMPLANT-ASSOCIATED ANAPLASTIC LARGE CELL LYMPHOMA

Key Facts

Terminology
- ALCL of T-/null-cell lineage that arises around breast implant and is ALK(-)

Etiology/Pathogenesis
- Unknown; occurs with saline and silicone implants

Clinical Issues
- ALK(-) ALCL accounts for > 90% of lymphomas associated with breast implants
- Tumor is usually detected a number of years after implant; median: 8 years

Microscopic Pathology
- Fibrinoid material on luminal side of capsule where individual cells or tumor cell clusters are contained
- Fibrinoid layer subtly merges with surrounding fibrous tissue to appear as thick capsule

- Cells are large, pleomorphic with abundant clear to eosinophilic cytoplasm
  - Occasional kidney-shaped nuclei identified

Ancillary Tests
- CD30(+) with uniform membranous or Golgi pattern
- T-cell antigens(+); aberrant immunophenotype(+/-)
- Cytotoxic antigens(+/-), EMA(+/-)
- Clusterin(+/-), CD45/LCA(+/-)
- Proliferation rate (Ki-67) is usually high
- Monoclonal T-cell receptor gene rearrangements(+)

Top Differential Diagnoses
- Primary cutaneous ALCL disseminated to breast
- ALK(-) ALCL
- ALK(+) ALCL
- Peripheral T-cell lymphoma, not otherwise specified

CLINICAL ISSUES

Epidemiology
- Incidence
  - Primary breast lymphomas are rare: 0.4 to 0.7% of all non-Hodgkin lymphomas
  - Most are B-cell lymphomas; most common types are
    - Diffuse large B-cell lymphoma (DLBCL)
    - Extranodal marginal zone B-cell lymphoma of mucosa-associated lymphoid tissue (MALT)
  - T-cell lymphomas represent < 10% of all breast lymphomas
    - Most common type is peripheral T-cell lymphoma, not otherwise specified
    - ALK(-) ALCL, by far, is most common lymphoma type associated with breast implants
  - Other lymphoma types rarely reported to be associated with breast implants
    - Follicular lymphoma
    - Lymphoplasmacytic lymphoma
  - Case control studies show association of ALK(-) ALCL with breast implants
    - However, risk of developing this lymphoma is minimal, estimated at 1 in 1,000,000 per year
    - Long-term follow-up of women with breast implants: No evidence for increased risk of carcinoma or lymphoma
- Age
  - Median: 52 years
- Gender
  - All reported patients are women

Site
- Around breast implant, contained within surrounding fibrous capsule

Presentation
- Tumor detected 3-19 years after implant; median: 8 years
  - Cases occurring in shorter interval after implant are very rarely reported

- Swelling around breast implant; all cases reported have been unilateral
- Disease is usually localized, stage IE; rare cases are stage IIE
- When present, effusion ranges from 80-720 mL
- Contractures or asymmetry of breasts can occur

Laboratory Tests
- Normal blood cell counts and serum chemistry results

Treatment
- Surgical approaches
  - Surgical removal (capsulectomy) has been most common therapeutic approach
- Adjuvant therapy
  - Variable, including adjuvant chemotherapy, radiation therapy, or none
    - CHOP (cyclophosphamide, doxorubicin, vincristine, and prednisone) regimen has been used most often

Prognosis
- Excellent, considering limited follow-up of reported cases
- Long-term follow-up not yet available for these patients
  - Median follow-up interval on published reports is 1 year; all patients alive, free of disease
  - No deaths attributable to disease to date

IMAGE FINDINGS

Radiographic Findings
- Various modalities can show breast effusion

MACROSCOPIC FEATURES

General Features
- Thickened capsule with luminal surface extensively covered by fibrinoid material
- Distinct tumor mass in small subset of cases

10

BREAST IMPLANT-ASSOCIATED ANAPLASTIC LARGE CELL LYMPHOMA

- Fibrinoid fluid may be identified within capsule
- Implant is usually intact; not disrupted
  - No gross evidence of implant leakage or retractions

MICROSCOPIC PATHOLOGY

Histologic Features
- Fibrinoid material on luminal side of capsule where individual tumor cells or clusters are present
- Fibrinoid layer subtly merges with surrounding fibrous tissue to appear as thick capsule
  - Neoplastic cells do not appear to grow through fibrous capsule
- Inflammatory cells are relatively few in background
- Foreign body giant cell reaction can develop as result of microscopic implant leakage
- Mitotic figures are numerous

Cytologic Features
- Cells are large and pleomorphic with hyperchromatic nuclei and abundant clear to eosinophilic cytoplasm
  - Occasional kidney-shaped nuclei identified

ANCILLARY TESTS

Cytology
- Neoplastic cells usually identified in aspirate specimens from effusions
- Cells are large with clear to eosinophilic cytoplasm; hyperchromatic and pleomorphic nuclei

Immunohistochemistry
- CD30(+), with uniform membranous or Golgi pattern
- T-cell antigens(+); aberrant immunophenotype common
  - Small subset of cases have "null-cell" immunophenotype in which no T-cell markers are detected
- Cytotoxic antigens(+/-): Granzyme B, perforin, and TIA-1
- EMA(+/-), clusterin(+/-), CD45/LCA(+/-)
- Proliferation rate (Ki-67) is usually high
- CD15(-/+), ALK(-), B-cell antigens(-), EBV-LMP1(-)

Cytogenetics
- Minimal data currently available

In Situ Hybridization
- Epstein-Barr virus encoded RNA(-) in few cases assessed

PCR
- Monoclonal T-cell receptor gamma chain gene rearrangements in all tested cases
  - Present in "null cell" cases
- No evidence of monoclonal *IgH* gene rearrangements
- No characteristic chromosomal translocations known
  - No evidence of abnormalities of *ALK* gene

DIFFERENTIAL DIAGNOSIS

Primary Cutaneous ALCL/CD30(+) T-cell Lymphoproliferative Disorder
- Primary cutaneous ALCL can disseminate to breast as ALK(-) ALCL
  - Cutaneous lesions usually do not involve breast skin initially
- Primary cutaneous ALCL can disseminate to breast in patients with implants
  - Initial skin ALCL has preceded breast implant-associated ALCL by 1-4 years
- Cytologic features of primary cutaneous ALCL in breast and breast implant-associated ALCL are similar
  - Primary cutaneous ALCL involving breast is usually **not** confined to serous fluid or fibrous capsule
  - Both tumors are
    - CD30(+)
    - T-cell markers(+)
    - Cytotoxic markers(+/-)
- In few cases described, primary cutaneous ALCL disseminated to breast had good prognosis

ALK(-) ALCL
- Disease usually stage IV when breast involvement
  - No history of primary cutaneous CD30(+) T-cell lymphoproliferative disorder
- ± palpable mass, not associated with breast implants
- Cytologic features of ALK(-) ALCL are similar to breast implant-associated ALCL
  - Both tumors are
    - CD30(+)
    - T-cell markers(+)
    - Cytotoxic markers(+/-)

ALK(+) ALCL
- Disease usually stage IV when breast involvement
- ± palpable mass, not associated with breast implants
- Cytologic features of ALK(+) ALCL are similar to breast implant-associated ALCL
  - ALK(+), t(2;5)(p23;q35) or other *ALK* gene abnormalities

Peripheral T-cell Lymphoma, Not Otherwise Specified
- Disease usually stage IV when breast involvement
- No cases associated with breast implants reported
- Variable cytologic appearance ranging from small to large, pleomorphic cells
- Immunophenotype
  - T-cell antigens(+)
  - CD30(-/+)
  - ALK(-)

Diffuse Large B-cell Lymphoma
- Can arise in breast or represent manifestation of disease dissemination (stage IV)
- No cases associated with breast implants reported
- Usually palpable mass histologically composed of sheets of large B cells

Differential Diagnosis of Breast Implant-associated Anaplastic Large Cell Lymphoma

	Implant-associated ALCL	Cutaneous ALCL	ALK(+) or ALK(-) ALCL
Clinical Features			
	Reconstructive surgery or cosmetic reasons	Recurrent cutaneous lesions in different body regions	Nodal or extranodal disease
Clinical stage	Stage I	Stage IV if disseminated to breast	Usually stage IV
Association with implant	Yes	Some cases	No
Association with effusion	Yes	No	No
Pathologic Features			
Gross appearance	Effusion around implant; usually after several years	Pain or mass effect; outside capsule when associated with breast implant	Infiltrative tumor mass
	Microgranular and fibrinoid deposits on luminal side of capsule	Single tumor mass; outside capsule when associated with implant	Single mass; not related with implant
Tumor size	Not grossly measurable; thickened capsule can be extensive	< 2 cm	> 3 cm
Low-magnification appearance	Small or large clusters of neoplastic cells contained within fibrinoid material	Confluent large cells within fibrous stroma on outer side of capsule or breast parenchyma	Sheets of large pleomorphic cells in breast parenchyma
High-magnification appearance	Large cells with abundant clear cytoplasm; pleomorphic vesicular nuclei; rare kidney-shaped cells	Large cells with pleomorphic, vesicular nuclei; frequent mitoses; occasional kidney-shaped nuclei	Large pleomorphic cells, hyperchromatic nuclei; frequent kidney-shaped nuclei
Special Studies			
Distinctive markers	CD30(+); ALK(-); T-cell markers(+)	CD30(+); ALK(-); T-cell markers(+)	If ALK(+), usually nuclear and cytoplasmic; T-cell markers(+)
Molecular genetics	Monoclonal T-cell receptor gamma chain gene rearrangements	Monoclonal T-cell receptor gamma chain gene rearrangements	ALK(+) cases carry t(2;5)(p23;q35); ALK(-) cases have no distinctive molecular changes

SELECTED REFERENCES

1. Lipworth L et al: Breast implants and lymphoma risk: a review of the epidemiologic evidence through 2008. Plast Reconstr Surg. 123(3):790-3, 2009
2. Miranda RN et al: Anaplastic large cell lymphoma involving the breast: a clinicopathologic study of 6 cases and review of the literature. Arch Pathol Lab Med. 133(9):1383-90, 2009
3. de Jong D et al: Anaplastic large-cell lymphoma in women with breast implants. JAMA. 300(17):2030-5, 2008
4. Newman MK et al: Primary breast lymphoma in a patient with silicone breast implants: a case report and review of the literature. J Plast Reconstr Aesthet Surg. 61(7):822-5, 2008
5. Roden AC et al: Seroma-associated primary anaplastic large-cell lymphoma adjacent to breast implants: an indolent T-cell lymphoproliferative disorder. Mod Pathol. 21(4):455-63, 2008
6. Talwalkar SS et al: Lymphomas involving the breast: a study of 106 cases comparing localized and disseminated neoplasms. Am J Surg Pathol. 32(9):1299-309, 2008
7. Wong AK et al: Anaplastic large cell lymphoma associated with a breast implant capsule: a case report and review of the literature. Am J Surg Pathol. 32(8):1265-8, 2008
8. Medeiros LJ et al: Anaplastic Large Cell Lymphoma. Am J Clin Pathol. 127(5):707-22, 2007
9. Olack B et al: Anaplastic large cell lymphoma arising in a saline breast implant capsule after tissue expander breast reconstruction. Ann Plast Surg. 59(1):56-7, 2007
10. Friis S et al: Cancer risk among Danish women with cosmetic breast implants. Int J Cancer. 118(4):998-1003, 2006
11. Fritzsche FR et al: Anaplastic large-cell non-Hodgkin's lymphoma of the breast in periprosthetic localisation 32 years after treatment for primary breast cancer--a case report. Virchows Arch. 449(5):561-4, 2006
12. Lin Y et al: Primary breast lymphoma: long-term treatment outcome and prognosis. Leuk Lymphoma. 47(10):2102-9, 2006
13. Kraemer DM et al: Lymphoplasmacytic lymphoma in a patient with leaking silicone implant. Haematologica. 89(4):ELT01, 2004
14. Sahoo S et al: Anaplastic large cell lymphoma arising in a silicone breast implant capsule: a case report and review of the literature. Arch Pathol Lab Med. 127(3):e115-8, 2003
15. Gaudet G et al: Breast lymphoma associated with breast implants: two case-reports and a review of the literature. Leuk Lymphoma. 43(1):115-9, 2002
16. Wong WW et al: Primary non-Hodgkin lymphoma of the breast: The Mayo Clinic Experience. J Surg Oncol. 80(1):19-25; discussion 26, 2002
17. Keech JA Jr et al: Anaplastic T-cell lymphoma in proximity to a saline-filled breast implant. Plast Reconstr Surg. 100(2):554-5, 1997
18. Cook PD et al: Follicular lymphoma adjacent to foreign body granulomatous inflammation and fibrosis surrounding silicone breast prosthesis. Am J Surg Pathol. 19(6):712-7, 1995

Imaging and Microscopic Features

(Left) Breast implant-associated anaplastic large cell lymphoma (ALCL). Asymmetry of implants on MR reflects displaced left breast implant ⇨. Effusion ➡ is noted under an enhanced fibrous capsule. No distinct tumor mass was identified. Note intact, nondisplaced right breast implant ➡. *(Courtesy N. Haideri, MD.)* *(Right)* Breast implant-associated ALCL. Hematoxylin & eosin highlights a sclerotic capsule ⇨. Luminal side of capsule shows fibrinoid exudate ➡, where neoplastic cells are contained.

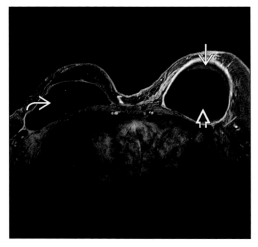
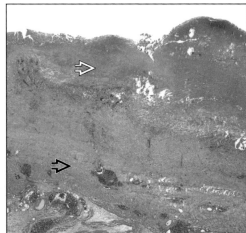

(Left) Breast implant-associated ALCL. Individual cells or clusters ⇨ of neoplastic cells are floating on the luminal side of the capsule, in the middle of fibrinoid exudate ➡. *(Right)* Breast implant-associated ALCL. Individual tumor and clusters of tumor cells ⇨ can be appreciated within the fibrinoid exudate on the luminal side of the capsule ➡.

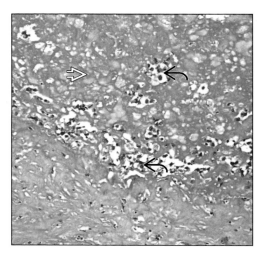
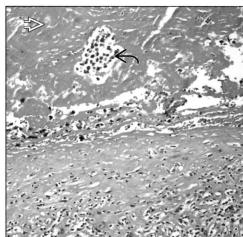

(Left) Breast implant-associated ALCL. High magnification of neoplastic cells ⇨ are seen within fibrinoid exudate ➡ on the luminal side of the capsule. *(Right)* Fibrous capsule surrounding a breast implant removed for cosmetic reasons. Microscopic leaking leads to sclerosis ➡ and an inflammatory reaction, including foamy histiocytes ⇨, lymphocytes ⇨, and plasma cells. No lymphoma or effusion were detected in this case.

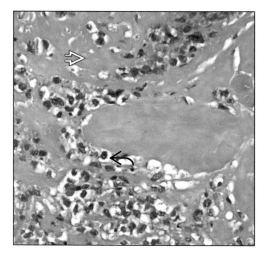
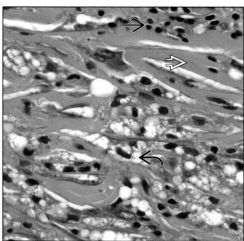

BREAST IMPLANT-ASSOCIATED ANAPLASTIC LARGE CELL LYMPHOMA

Microscopic Features

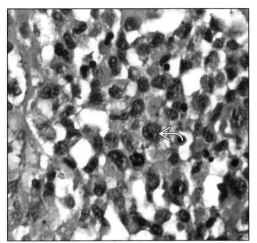
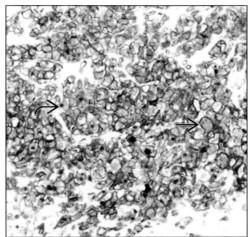

(Left) Breast implant-associated ALCL. This high magnification shows large neoplastic cells with clear or eosinophilic cytoplasm and hyperchromatic, pleomorphic nuclei ➡. (Right) Breast implant-associated ALCL. The neoplastic cells are strongly and uniformly CD30(+) in a membranous ➡ and Golgi-like ➡ pattern.

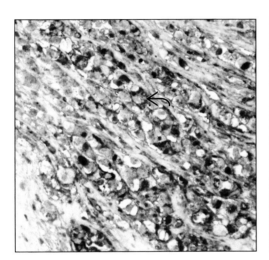
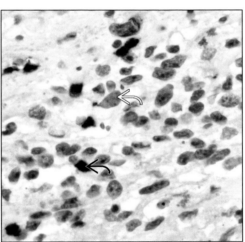

(Left) Breast implant-associated ALCL. Most of the neoplastic cells were reactive with the T-cell helper marker CD4 ➡, supporting the T-cell lineage. (Right) Breast implant-associated ALCL. Small reactive lymphocytes ➡ are positive for the T-cell marker CD7, whereas the large neoplastic cells ➡ are negative, consistent with aberrant loss of a T-cell marker. This tumor was positive for CD4.

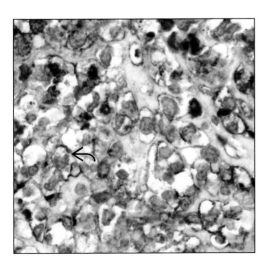
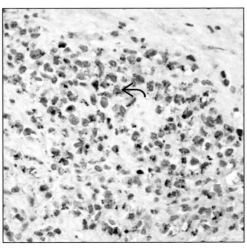

(Left) Breast implant-associated ALCL. The neoplastic cells are positive for epithelial membrane antigen (EMA) ➡. (Right) Breast implant-associated ALCL. The neoplastic cells are positive for T-cell intracellular antigen-1 (TIA-1) ➡, a marker that indicates the presence of cytotoxic granules. Most cases of ALCL associated with a breast implant exhibit a cytotoxic immunophenotype.

BREAST IMPLANT-ASSOCIATED ANAPLASTIC LARGE CELL LYMPHOMA

Differential Diagnosis

(Left) ALK(-) ALCL of breast in a patient with a breast implant, but not effusion. The patient had a distinct tumor mass within fibrous tissue ⇒, but not on the luminal side ⇒. This patient also had a history of primary cutaneous CD30(+) ALCL of non-breast skin, and this lesion may represent dissemination. *(Right)* ALK(-) ALCL of the breast associated with breast implant but not effusion shows large pleomorphic cells ⇒. Eosinophils ⇒ and fibrous stroma are noted.

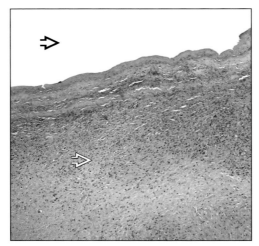
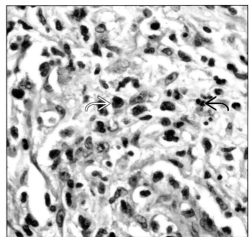

(Left) ALK(-) ALCL of the breast not associated with breast implant shows sheets of large, pleomorphic cells ⇒ and tingible body macrophages ⇒. *(Right)* ALK(-) ALCL of the breast in a patient with implants who had stage II disease and a 1.5 cm mass attached to the breast capsule of the implant. There was no effusion. These features differ from typical cases of breast implant-associated ALCL where tumor cells are present within the effusion.

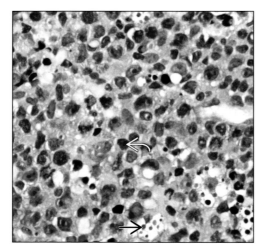
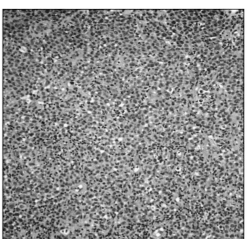

(Left) ALK(-) ALCL of the breast. A 1.5 cm mass attached to implant capsule was detected; no effusion was found. Tumor cells ⇒ admixed with inflammatory cells ⇒ are noted. This appearance differs from breast implant-associated ALCL in which there are usually few inflammatory cells. *(Right)* ALK(-) anaplastic large cell lymphoma of the breast. The tumor was stage II. Tumor cells are CD30(+) with a membranous ⇒ and Golgi ⇒ pattern.

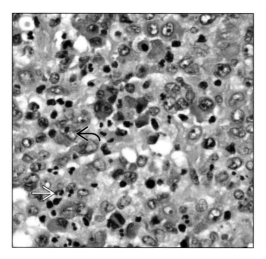
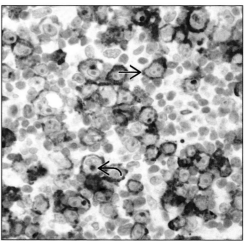

Differential Diagnosis

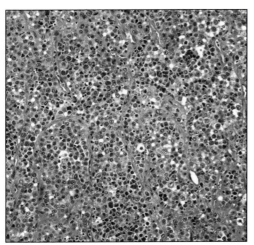

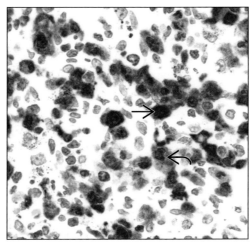

(Left) ALK(+) anaplastic large cell lymphoma (ALCL) of the breast. The patient had stage IV disease and a 4 cm tumor, not associated with a breast implant. This tumor is easily distinguished from implant-associated ALCL because of the presence of sheets of tumor cells and the ALK expression. *(Right)* ALK(+) ALCL involving the breast reveals reactivity of ALK in the nucleus ⤇ and cytoplasm ⤇, consistent with the t(2;5)(p23;q35).

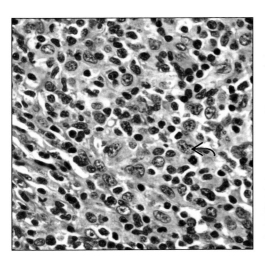

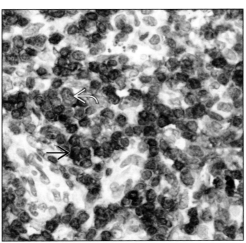

(Left) Peripheral T-cell lymphoma, not otherwise specified. The neoplastic cells can be large and pleomorphic ⤇, histologically similar to ALCL, but these tumors do not typically express CD30. If CD30 is (+), expression is often focal and dim. *(Right)* Peripheral T-cell lymphoma, not otherwise specified. Small ⤇ and large ⤇ neoplastic cells are reactive with the T-cell marker CD3.

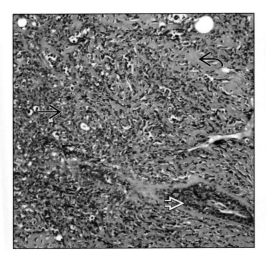

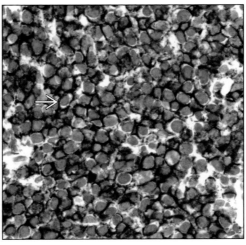

(Left) Diffuse large B-cell lymphoma. Note diffuse infiltrate ⤇ of large cells with reactive sclerosis ⤇. The infiltrate destroys breast architecture; a residual breast duct ⤇ remains surrounded by lymphoma. This tumor grows as an infiltrating and distinct mass and it is not associated with breast implants. *(Right)* Diffuse large B-cell lymphoma. The neoplastic cells show strong, membranous ⤇ reactivity with the B-cell marker CD20.

EXTRANODAL NK-/T-CELL LYMPHOMA, NASAL TYPE

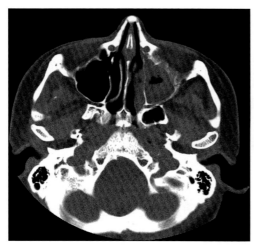

CT scan shows an almost completely opacified maxillary sinus and thickening of mucosa in the nasopharynx. This patient was shown to have extranodal NK/T-cell lymphoma, nasal type.

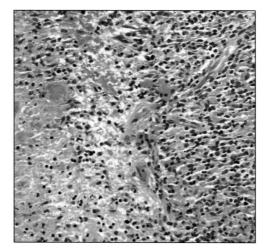

Extranodal NK/T-cell lymphoma, nasal type. Biopsy from the maxillary sinus shows extensive coagulative necrosis (left).

TERMINOLOGY

Synonyms
- Polymorphic reticulosis
- Malignant midline reticulosis
- Angiocentric T-cell lymphoma
- Angiocentric immunoproliferative lesion
  - Term is not completely synonymous but includes nasal-type extranodal NK/T-cell lymphoma

Definitions
- Predominantly extranodal lymphoma of either natural killer-cell (NK) or T-cell lineage
  - Characterized by necrosis, cytotoxic immunophenotype, and Epstein-Barr virus (EBV) infection
  - Vascular destruction is common

ETIOLOGY/PATHOGENESIS

Infectious Agents
- EBV is consistently present in these neoplasms, suggesting its involvement in pathogenesis
  - EBV is usually type A

Epidemiology
- Disease is common in Asia and in Native Americans of Central and South America
- Disease is rare in United States, but its incidence has risen since 1992

CLINICAL ISSUES

Presentation
- Mass that is nasal or extranasal
  - Nasal cases are usually defined as a neoplasm involving upper aerodigestive tract
    - Nasal cavity, nasopharynx, paranasal sinuses, palate
    - Patients suffer from obstruction, epistaxis, or midline destructive lesion
    - These neoplasms can disseminate
  - Extranasal cases are defined as neoplasm involving any site but without nasal involvement
    - Skin is most common extranasal site
    - Other sites: Testis, gastrointestinal tract, kidney, salivary glands
    - Primary involvement of lymph nodes is rare but has been reported
    - Bone marrow obtained as part of staging can be involved

Natural History
- Extranodal nasal-type NK/T-cell lymphoma can disseminate
  - Regional lymph node involvement is not uncommon
  - Bone marrow involvement and leukemic phase can occur
  - These neoplasms can disseminate to virtually any anatomic site

Treatment
- Options, risks, complications
  - Chemotherapy and radiation therapy are usually employed for nasal cases
  - Platelet-derived growth factor α overexpression shown by gene expression studies suggests role for imatinib

Prognosis
- Patients with nasal-type extranodal NK/T-cell lymphoma, in general, have poor prognosis
  - Patients with extranasal tumors have poorest prognosis
  - Factors associated with poorer prognosis for nasal cases include

EXTRANODAL NK-/T-CELL LYMPHOMA, NASAL TYPE

Key Facts

Etiology/Pathogenesis
- EBV is constant finding, present in clonal episomal form, and is likely involved in pathogenesis

Clinical Issues
- Nasal or extranasal

Microscopic Pathology
- Cytologic spectrum of nasal-type extranodal NK/T-cell lymphoma is wide
  - Small cell neoplasms can be misinterpreted as chronic inflammation
- Necrosis and superimposed acute and chronic inflammation can lead to incorrect diagnosis
- Angiocentricity and angiodestruction are helpful findings but are not constant
  - Most likely to be absent in small biopsy specimens

Ancillary Tests
- Approximately 2/3 of tumors are of NK cell lineage: CD2(+), cyt CD3-ϵ(+), CD56(+/-), CD5(-), CD8(-), *TCR* gene rearrangements(-)
- Approximately 1/3 of tumors are of cytotoxic T-cell lineage: CD2(+), CD3(+), CD5(+), CD8(+/-), TCR-β(+), *TCR* gene rearrangements(+)
- All tumors are positive for cytotoxic proteins and EBV (best shown by in situ hybridization for EBER)

Top Differential Diagnoses
- Cytotoxic EBV-peripheral T-cell lymphoma, not otherwise specified
- B-cell lymphomas involving upper aerodigestive tract (usually diffuse large B-cell lymphoma)
- Wegener granulomatosis

- High International Prognostic Index (IPI) or Korean NK/T-cell Prognostic Score
- Elevated C-reactive protein, anemia (< 11g/dL), or thrombocytopenia (< normal)
- Large cells > 40%
- Ki-67 (proliferation rate) > 50%
- Korean NK/T Prognostic Score is based on
  - B symptoms, stage, serum LDH, and regional lymph nodes

IMAGE FINDINGS

General Features
- Location
  - Nasal: Imaging studies show mass that can distort midline, displace adjacent organs, and destroy bone
  - Extranasal: Imaging studies usually show mass

MICROSCOPIC PATHOLOGY

Histologic Features
- Nasal-type NK/T lymphoma has diffuse pattern; commonly associated with coagulative necrosis
  - Cell size is variable, ranging from small to large
  - Mitotic figures are usually identified; common in large tumors
  - In touch imprints, neoplastic cells can have azurophilic cytoplasmic granules
  - Angiocentricity and angiodestruction are common but not invariable
    - Less common in small biopsy specimens
  - Ulcer and superimposed inflammation are common at mucosal sites
  - Overlying epithelium at mucosal sites can show pseudoepitheliomatous hyperplasia
  - Erythrophagocytosis can complicate clinical course; can be fatal
- Lymph node
  - Nasal-type NK/T preferentially involves paracortex ± medulla

- Bone marrow
  - Staging bone marrow is involved in ~ 10-20% of patients
    - Commonly an interstitial infiltrate without discrete aggregates
    - In situ hybridization for EBER helpful to detect disease

Cytologic Features
- Nasal-type NK/T-cell lymphoma is uncommonly assessed by fine needle aspiration
- Superimposed inflammation can make recognition of the disease challenging

ANCILLARY TESTS

Immunohistochemistry
- NK-cell lineage in ~ 65-75% of cases
  - CD2(+), cytoplasmic CD3-ϵ(+), CD56(+/-), CD94(+) cytotoxic markers (TIA, GZM-B, perforin)(+)
    - Both T and NK cells express epsilon chain of CD3 (CD3-ϵ)
  - CD4(-), CD5(-), CD8(-), TCR-β (BF1)(-)
- True T-cell lineage in approximately 25-35% of cases
  - CD2(+), CD3-ϵ(+), CD5(+), CD8(+/-), TCR-β (BF1)(+), CD56(-/+), cytotoxic markers(+)
- Both NK- and T-cell neoplasms are positive for Epstein-Barr virus
  - Can be shown by variety of molecular methods (Southern blotting, in situ hybridization)
    - In situ hybridization for EBV small-encoded RNA (EBER) is convenient and sensitive
  - Southern blot studies have shown that EBV is present in clonal episomal form
    - EBV is present prior to clonal expansion and implicates EBV in pathogenesis
  - EBV latent membrane protein is variably expressed (usually many less cells than EBER)

EXTRANODAL NK-/T-CELL LYMPHOMA, NASAL TYPE

PCR
- NK-cell tumors do not carry monoclonal T-cell receptor (*TCR*) rearrangements
- T-cell tumors carry monoclonal *TCR* rearrangements

Array CGH
- Comparative genomic hybridization studies have shown multiple gains and losses
  - Most common site of gain: 2q
  - Common sites of losses: 1p36, 6q16-q27, 4q12, 5q34-q35, 7q21-22, 11q22-q23, and 15q11-q14
- Nasal-type NK/T-cell lymphoma of skin
  - Gains of 1q, 7q, and 17p

Molecular Genetics
- Various gene deletions or mutations have been identified
  - *FAS*, *P53*, β-*catenin*, *KRAS*, *C-KIT*
  - More common in large cell tumors

Gene Expression Profiling
- Overexpression of genes related to angiogenesis and infection by EBV
- Activation of JAK-STAT, AKT, and NF-κB pathways
- Platelet-derived growth factor α is overexpressed

DIFFERENTIAL DIAGNOSIS

Lethal Midline Granuloma
- Term for clinical syndrome that includes nasal-type extranodal NK/T-cell lymphoma as well as
  - Aggressive variants of Wegener granulomatosis
  - Infections
  - Cocaine abuse (usually marked inflammation but without vasculitis)

Wegener Granulomatosis
- Typically patients also have lung and kidney disease
- Classic histologic triad is uncommon (< 25% of cases)
  - Vasculitis, granulomatous inflammation, and geographic necrosis
- Epithelial ulceration is common
- Inflammatory infiltrate is mixed
  - Granulocytes (including eosinophils), lymphocytes, histiocytes, and plasma cells are present
  - Wegener granulomatosis is not lymphocyte-rich

B-cell Lymphomas Involving Upper Aerodigestive Tract
- Most often diffuse large B-cell lymphoma
- These tumors are usually monotonous; large cells
- Blood vessel involvement is less common than in nasal-type extranodal NK/T-cell lymphoma
- Superimposed inflammation is also less common
- Immunophenotype: CD19(+), CD20(+), CD79a(+), pax-5(+), CD3(-)
- Molecular studies show monoclonal *IgH* gene rearrangements; EBV(-)

Peripheral T-cell Lymphoma, Not Otherwise Specified, Involving Upper Aerodigestive Tract
- Histologic features can mimic nasal-type extranodal NK/T-cell lymphoma
  - Necrosis and involvement of vessels
  - These tumors usually lack CD56 and are negative for EBV

Infections
- A number of infectious organisms can involve nasal region
- Mixed inflammatory infiltrate with granulocytes
- No evidence of monoclonal gene rearrangements
- EBV(-)

STAGING

Staging
- Ann Arbor staging is not ideal for nasal-type extranodal NK/T-cell lymphoma
  - 3-tier system for staging has been suggested in Korea
    - Limited stage upper aerodigestive tract disease without local invasion
    - Advanced stage upper aerodigestive tract disease or limited stage with extensive local invasion
    - Involvement of non-nasal sites

SELECTED REFERENCES

1. Berti E et al: Cutaneous extranodal NK/T-cell lymphoma: a clinicopathologic study of 5 patients with array-based comparative genomic hybridization. Blood. 116(2):165-70, 2010
2. Huang Y et al: Gene expression profiling identifies emerging oncogenic pathways operating in extranodal NK/T-cell lymphoma, nasal type. Blood. 115(6):1226-37, 2010
3. Au WY et al: Clinical differences between nasal and extranasal natural killer/T-cell lymphoma: a study of 136 cases from the International Peripheral T-Cell Lymphoma Project. Blood. 113(17):3931-7, 2009
4. Coppo P et al: STAT3 transcription factor is constitutively activated and is oncogenic in nasal-type NK/T-cell lymphoma. Leukemia. 23(9):1667-78, 2009
5. Kim TM et al: Extranodal NK / T-cell lymphoma, nasal type: new staging system and treatment strategies. Cancer Sci. 100(12):2242-8, 2009
6. Abouyabis AN et al: Incidence and outcomes of the peripheral T-cell lymphoma subtypes in the United States. Leuk Lymphoma. 49(11):2099-107, 2008
7. Kim TM et al: Clinical heterogeneity of extranodal NK/T-cell lymphoma, nasal type: a national survey of the Korean Cancer Study Group. Ann Oncol. 19(8):1477-84, 2008
8. Takahashi E et al: Nodal T/NK-cell lymphoma of nasal type: a clinicopathological study of six cases. Histopathology. 52(5):585-96, 2008
9. Lee J et al: Extranodal natural killer T-cell lymphoma, nasal-type: a prognostic model from a retrospective multicenter study. J Clin Oncol. 24(4):612-8, 2006

Microscopic and Immunohistochemical Features

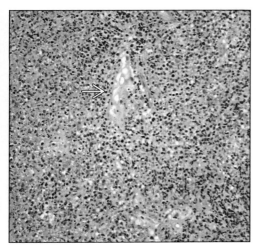

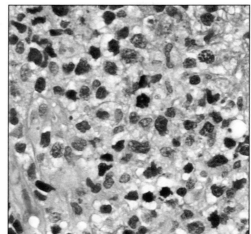

(Left) Extranodal NK/T-cell lymphoma, nasal type, of NK cell lineage. The neoplastic cells are predominantly medium-sized cells. Necrosis (left) and a blood vessel ➡ are present. *(Right)* High magnification of cells in extranodal NK/T-cell lymphoma, nasal type, of NK cell lineage. The neoplastic cells are medium-sized with irregular nuclear contours & pale cytoplasm. Mitotic figures are present in this field.

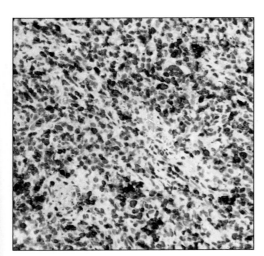

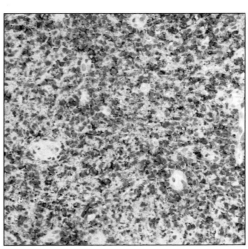

(Left) CD3 IHC stain shows that the neoplastic cells are positive. This antibody detects the epsilon chain of CD3 within the cell cytoplasm. Expression of CD3-ε chain is (+) in both T cells & NK cells. *(Right)* CD56 immunohistochemical stain shows many positive neoplastic cells. CD56 is commonly (but not invariably) expressed in extranodal NK/T-cell lymphoma, nasal type. CD56 is highly suggestive of, but not specific for, NK cell lineage.

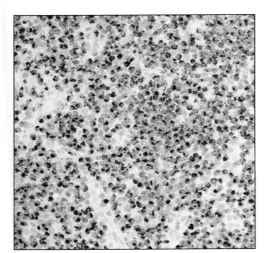

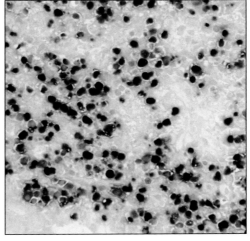

(Left) TIA-1 immunohistochemical stain shows that all of the neoplastic cells are strongly (+). TIA, as well as GZM-B and perforin, are cytotoxic markers that are usually expressed in extranodal NK/T-cell lymphoma, nasal type. *(Right)* Positive in situ hybridization for Epstein-Barr virus small-encoded RNA (EBER). EBV infection is an invariable feature of extranodal NK/T-cell lymphoma, nasal type, as defined in the 2008 WHO classification of lymphoid tumors.

ENTEROPATHY-ASSOCIATED T-CELL LYMPHOMA

Comparison of Types 1 and 2 Enteropathy-associated T-cell Lymphoma (EATL)

Feature	Type 1	Type 2
Frequency	80-90%	10-20%
Geographic distribution	More common in northern Europe	Worldwide
History of celiac disease	Usually present	Often absent
Histology	Variable; can be large and highly pleomorphic	Monomorphous; medium-sized cells
Immunophenotype	CD3(+), CD4(-), CD5(-), CD7(+), CD8(-/+), CD30(+/-), CD103(+), TCR-β(+)	CD3(+), CD4(-), CD5(-), CD8(+), CD56(+), TCR-β(+)
Comparative genomic hybridization		
Gains of 9q31.3-qter	Common	Common
Losses of 16q.12.1	Common	Common
Gains of 5q34-q36.2	Common	Uncommon
Gains of 8q24/MYC	Uncommon	Common

- o Most common extranodal sites are bone, skin, and soft tissue
- Morphologic features overlap with some EATL, type 1
- No enteropathy-associated changes
- CD30 strong and uniformly (+)

ALK(+) ALCL
- Uncommonly involves small intestine
- Morphologic features overlap with some EATL, type 1
- No enteropathy-associated changes
- CD30 strong and uniform (+); ALK(+); *ALK* gene abnormalities

Extranodal NK-/T-cell Lymphoma, Nasal Type
- Morphologic features overlap with EATL
- No enteropathy-associated changes
- Often show angiocentric and angiodestructive growth pattern
- Surface CD3(-), cytoplasmic CD3-ε(+)
- CD2(+), CD4(-), CD8(-), CD5(-), CD56(+)
- Cytotoxic proteins(+)
- EBV-encoded RNA (EBER)(+) in virtually all cases

T-Lymphoblastic Lymphoma
- Small to medium-sized blasts with high nuclear to cytoplasmic ratio
- No enteropathy-associated changes
- Immature T-cell immunophenotype; TdT(+), CD1a(+/-), CD34(+/-)

Adult T-cell Leukemia/Lymphoma (ATLL)
- Can present as small intestine mass
- Morphologic features overlap with EATL
  - o No enteropathy-associated changes
- Most cases are CD4(+), CD8(-)
  - o CD25 is strongly (+) in virtually all cases
  - o Few cases are CD4(-), CD8(+) or CD4(+), CD8(+)
- Associated with HTLV-1 infection

DIAGNOSTIC CHECKLIST

Pathologic Interpretation Pearls
- Clinicopathologic and genetic data suggest that EATL can be divided into types 1 and type 2

- Enteropathy-associated changes are almost always present in both types
- Association with celiac disease is proven for type 1

SELECTED REFERENCES

1. Ferreri AJ et al: Enteropathy-associated T-cell lymphoma. Crit Rev Oncol Hematol. Epub ahead of print, 2010
2. Ko YH et al: Enteropathy-associated T-cell lymphoma-- a clinicopathologic and array comparative genomic hybridization study. Hum Pathol. 41(9):1231-7, 2010
3. Rubio-Tapia A et al: Clinical staging and survival in refractory celiac disease: a single center experience. Gastroenterology. 136(1):99-107; quiz 352-3, 2009
4. Chuang SS et al: The phenotype of intraepithelial lymphocytes in Taiwanese enteropathy-associated T-cell lymphoma is distinct from that of the West. Histopathology. 53(2):234-6, 2008
5. de Mascarel A et al: Mucosal intraepithelial T-lymphocytes in refractory celiac disease: a neoplastic population with a variable CD8 phenotype. Am J Surg Pathol. 32(5):744-51, 2008
6. Laird J et al: The value of small bowel magnetic resonance imaging in the management of enteropathy associated T-cell lymphoma. Br J Haematol. 2008 Jul;142(1):136-7. Epub 2008 May 8. Erratum in: Br J Haematol. 143(2):304, 2008
7. Verbeek WH et al: Incidence of enteropathy--associated T-cell lymphoma: a nation-wide study of a population-based registry in The Netherlands. Scand J Gastroenterol. 43(11):1322-8, 2008
8. Deleeuw RJ et al: Whole-genome analysis and HLA genotyping of enteropathy-type T-cell lymphoma reveals 2 distinct lymphoma subtypes. Gastroenterology. 132(5):1902-11, 2007
9. Zettl A et al: Enteropathy-type T-cell lymphoma. Am J Clin Pathol. 127(5):701-6, 2007
10. Hoffmann M et al: 18F-fluoro-deoxy-glucose positron emission tomography (18F-FDG-PET) for assessment of enteropathy-type T cell lymphoma. Gut. 52(3):347-51, 2003
11. Carey MJ et al: Primary anaplastic large cell lymphoma of the small intestine. Am J Clin Pathol. 112(5):696-701, 1999

Microscopic Features

(Left) Enteropathy-associated T-cell lymphoma, type 1. The lymphoma cells are pleomorphic. Many intraepithelial lymphoma cells ⊞ are present in crypts. *(Right)* Enteropathy-associated T-cell lymphoma, type 1. The lymphoma infiltrate is associated with ulcer, marked inflammation, and granulation tissue, as illustrated here. The tumor infiltrate can be obscured by the background inflammation, especially in a small biopsy specimen.

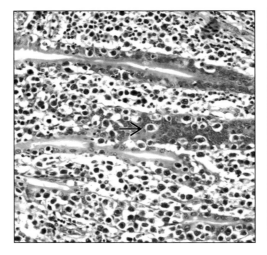 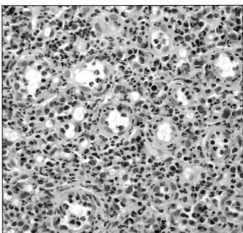

(Left) Enteropathy-associated T-cell lymphoma, type 2, involving jejunum. The neoplasm is composed of small, monomorphic lymphoma cells. The history of this patient was negative for celiac disease. *(Right)* Enteropathy-associated T-cell lymphoma, type 2, involving jejunum. The neoplasm is strongly CD56(+).

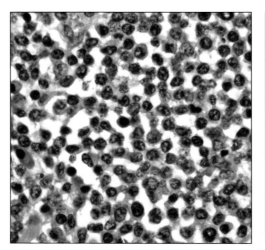 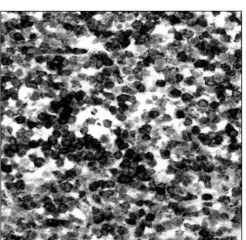

(Left) Mesenteric lymph node involved by type 2 enteropathy associated T-cell lymphoma. Reactive follicles ⊞ are present. The lymphoma infiltrate partially replaces lymph node architecture ⊡. *(Right)* Histologic section of mucosa adjacent to a tumor mass in small intestine involved by enteropathy-associated T-cell lymphoma. A small focus of lymphoma ⊟ within the mucosa can be seen. Also noted are increased numbers of intraepithelial lymphocytes.

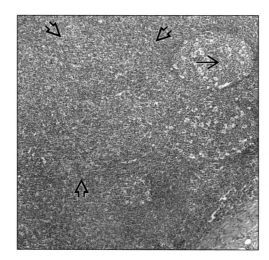 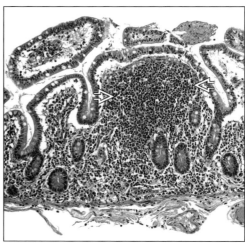

ENTEROPATHY-ASSOCIATED T-CELL LYMPHOMA

Microscopic Features

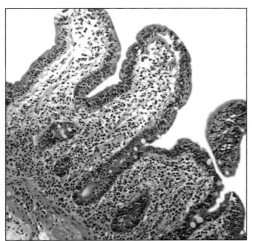
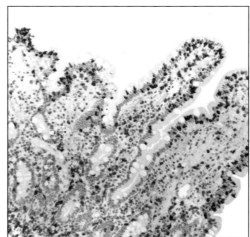

(Left) Adjacent uninvolved small intestinal mucosa in a patient with enteropathy-associated T-cell lymphoma shows increased numbers of intraepithelial lymphocytes and mild flattening of the villi. *(Right)* Adjacent uninvolved small intestinal mucosa in a patient with enteropathy-associated T-cell lymphoma. The intraepithelial lymphocytes are CD3(+).

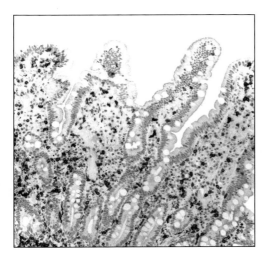
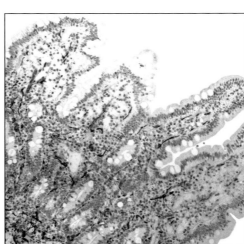

(Left) Adjacent uninvolved small intestinal mucosa in a patient with enteropathy-associated T-cell lymphoma. The intraepithelial lymphocytes are CD8(-). *(Right)* Adjacent uninvolved small intestinal mucosa in a patient with enteropathy-associated T-cell lymphoma. The intraepithelial lymphocytes are CD56(-).

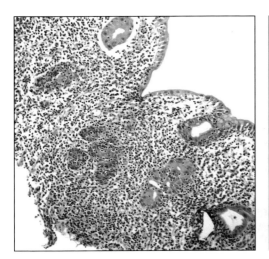
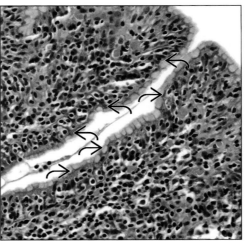

(Left) A gastric biopsy specimen shows severe celiac disease-related changes in a patient with enteropathy-associated T-cell lymphoma. *(Right)* A gastric biopsy specimen shows mucosa with numerous intraepithelial lymphocytes ➢ in a patient with suspected enteropathy-associated T-cell lymphoma.

SUBCUTANEOUS PANNICULITIS-LIKE T-CELL LYMPHOMA

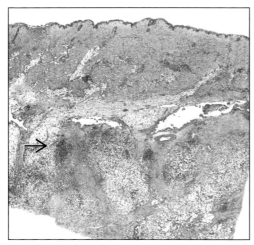

Low-magnification view of skin shows lymphoid infiltration ➡ of subcutaneous tissue involved by subcutaneous panniculitis-like T-cell lymphoma (SPTCL). The dermis and epidermis are not involved.

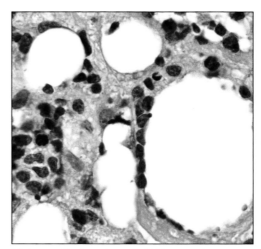

High-magnification view of SPTCL in subcutaneous adipose tissue. The neoplastic cells are cytologically atypical and "rim" adipocytes.

TERMINOLOGY

Abbreviations
- Subcutaneous panniculitis-like T-cell lymphoma (SPTCL)

Synonyms
- T-cell lymphoma involving subcutaneous tissue

Definitions
- T-cell lymphoma that preferentially involves subcutaneous tissue and expresses T-cell receptor α/β and cytotoxic proteins
- Definition of SPTCL was revised in World Health Organization (WHO) 2008 classification
  - Cases that express T-cell receptor γ/δ are now excluded
    - Instead, classified as primary cutaneous γ/δ T-cell lymphoma
  - In effect, SPTCL has become a more indolent disease by excluding patients with aggressive disease

ETIOLOGY/PATHOGENESIS

Infectious Agents
- Rare cases of SPTCL are associated with Epstein-Barr virus infection
  - Usually in setting of immune suppression or dysregulation
    - e.g., methotrexate therapy for arthritis

Possible Role of Autoimmunity
- Autoimmune diseases occur in ~ 20% of patients
  - Systemic lupus erythematosus most common
  - Rheumatoid, juvenile rheumatoid, or psoriatic arthritis
  - Sjögren syndrome
  - Immune thrombocytopenic purpura

CLINICAL ISSUES

Epidemiology
- Incidence
  - < 1% of non-Hodgkin lymphomas
- Age
  - Median: ~ 35 years (range: 9–79 years)
- Gender
  - Female predominance (male:female ratio is 1:2)
- Ethnicity
  - No ethnic predisposition

Site
- Legs > arms > trunk (in frequency of involvement)
- Lymph nodes are not involved at initial diagnosis
- SPTCL can disseminate, though uncommon
  - Lymphadenopathy and leukemic phase of disease have been reported

Presentation
- Patients present with solitary or multiple subcutaneous nodules or plaques
  - Size can range from 0.5-20 cm
  - Lesions often painless
  - Ulceration rare
  - Local symptoms related to ulceration or mass effect can occur
- Skin lesions can regress, in part, and show a range in stages of "healing"
- Systemic symptoms: ~ 60% of patients
  - Fever most common; weight loss and night sweats can occur
  - Symptoms related to hemophagocytosis
- Full-blown hemophagocytic syndrome (HPS) develops in ~ 15-20% of patients
- Hepatomegaly can occur; often associated with HPS
- Substantial delay can occur between onset of symptoms and specific diagnosis of SPTCL

SUBCUTANEOUS PANNICULITIS-LIKE T-CELL LYMPHOMA

Key Facts

Terminology

- Cytotoxic T-cell lymphoma that preferentially involves subcutaneous tissue and expresses TCR-αβ
- Definition of SPTCL substantially revised in WHO 2008 classification
  - Cases that express TCR-γδ are excluded

Clinical Issues

- Patients present with solitary or multiple subcutaneous nodules or plaques
- Legs > arms > trunk
- Full-blown HPS arises in ~ 15-20% of patients
- SPTCL is clinically indolent
  - Recent trend toward using single immunosuppressive agents, at least initially
  - Multi-agent chemotherapy reserved for patients with progressive disease

Microscopic Pathology

- SPTCL primarily involves subcutaneous adipose tissue
- Predominantly involves lobules and spares septa
- Neoplastic cells often rim individual adipocytes
- Lymphoma cells small to intermediate in size
- Apoptotic cells, karyorrhectic debris, fat necrosis

Ancillary Tests

- βF1/TCR-αβ(+); pan-T-cell antigens(+)
- CD8(+), CD4(-); cytotoxic proteins(+)
- Monoclonal *TCR* gene rearrangements

Top Differential Diagnoses

- Lupus erythematosus panniculitis
- Primary cutaneous γ/δ T-cell lymphoma
- Primary cutaneous CD30(+) lymphoproliferative disorders

Laboratory Tests

- Elevated erythrocyte sedimentation rate &/or C-reactive protein
- Abnormalities often associated with onset of HPS
  - Anemia, leukopenia, thrombocytopenia
  - Elevated liver function tests

Natural History

- SPTCL is clinically indolent
  - Disease can wax and wane
- Prolonged remissions with therapy are common

Treatment

- Surgical approaches
  - Rare patients with solitary lesion have undergone excision with no new lesions during follow-up
- Drugs
  - Many patients have received conventional chemotherapy
    - Cyclophosphamide, doxorubicin, vincristine, and prednisone (CHOP)
    - May be combined with alemtuzumab (anti-CD52)
  - Recent trend is toward using single immunosuppressive agents, at least initially
    - Corticosteroids, cyclosporine, chlorambucil
    - Long-term complete remission has been reported in subset of patients
    - Multi-agent chemotherapy reserved for patients with progressive disease
- Radiation
  - May have role in localized disease
    - Can lead to long-term remissions
    - May have role in palliation
- Stem cell transplantation appears to have role in patients with primary refractory, recurrent, or disseminated disease
  - Complete remission rate reported in subset of patients
    - Did these patients truly have SPTCL or primary cutaneous γ/δ T-cell lymphoma?

- Reevaluation of earlier published case series is needed, as disease was redefined in WHO 2008 classification

Prognosis

- Clinically indolent disease
  - ~ 80% 5-year overall survival (OS)
  - > 90% in patients who never develop HPS
- Prolonged remission with therapy
- Dissemination is rare

IMAGE FINDINGS

Ultrasonographic Findings

- Diffuse, hyperechoic areas with linear vascular markings

CT Findings

- Enhancing nodules with infiltrative pattern in subcutaneous tissue

F18 FDG PET Scan

- SPTCL can be moderately avid

MICROSCOPIC PATHOLOGY

Histologic Features

- SPTCL primarily involves subcutaneous adipose tissue
  - Overlying dermis and epidermis are not involved
    - Minimal involvement of deep dermis can be present
- Dense pattern of lymphoid infiltration
  - Neoplastic cells predominantly involve lobules and spare septa
  - Neoplastic cells often rim individual adipocytes
    - Characteristic feature but not specific for SPTCL
- Lymphoma cells
  - Size varies from case to case
    - Usually small to intermediate in size
    - Subset of cases have large cells
  - Pleomorphic

SUBCUTANEOUS PANNICULITIS-LIKE T-CELL LYMPHOMA

- o Hyperchromatic, irregular nuclear contours
- o Pale or clear cytoplasm
- o Mitotic figures present and can be numerous
- o Tumor cell apoptosis with karyorrhectic debris common
- Angioinvasion occurs in subset of cases
  - o Associated with poorer prognosis
  - o SPTCL lesions are not angiocentric
- Reactive cells are common in SPTCL lesions
  - o Numerous histiocytes admixed
    - ▪ Vacuolated due to ingested lipid
    - ▪ Loose granuloma formation can occur
    - ▪ Multinucleated giant cells in occasional cases
  - o Plasma cells can be present in ~ 10% of cases
  - o Neutrophils and eosinophils are uncommon
- Fat necrosis is very common
- Hemophagocytosis is common in skin lesions
- Bone marrow
  - o May demonstrate hemophagocytosis

Cytologic Features

- SPTCL lesions studied by fine needle aspiration are rarely reported
  - o Granulomas and mixed inflammatory infiltrate can make diagnosis challenging to establish

ANCILLARY TESTS

Immunohistochemistry

- Mature T-cell lineage
  - o βF1/TCR-αβ(+); pan-T-cell antigens(+)
  - o Aberrant loss of CD5, CD7, and CD2 in decreasing order
- CD8(+), CD4(-) in > 95% of cases
  - o Rare cases are CD4(-), CD8(-) or CD4(+), CD8(-)
- CD43(+), CD45RO(+)
- Cytotoxic proteins(+): TIA-1, perforin, and granzyme B
- Ki-67 (MIB-1 proliferation index) variable, ranging from low to high
- BAX(+), p53(+) in cases with large cells
- CD30(-), CD56(-), Bcl-2(-)
- CD45RA(-), CD56(-), TCR-δ-1(-), TCR-γ(-)
- B-cell antigens (-), EBV-LMP1(-)

Cytogenetics

- Relatively few cases analyzed by conventional cytogenetics
- No consistent abnormalities identified

In Situ Hybridization

- EBER(-) in almost all cases
  - o Rare cases reported to be EBER(+), more often in
    - ▪ Asian patients
    - ▪ Immunocompromised patients

PCR

- Monoclonal rearrangements of TCR β, γ, and δ genes
- No evidence of monoclonal IgH gene rearrangements

Array CGH

- Single cell CGH has shown many DNA copy number changes

- o Losses of chromosomes
  - ▪ 1p, 2p, 2q, 5p, 7p, 9q, 10q, 11q, 12q, 16, 17q, 19, 20, and 22
- o Gains of chromosomes
  - ▪ 2q, 4q, 5q, 6q, and 13q
  - ▪ 5q and 13q may be characteristic of SPTCL

Molecular Genetics

- NAV3 aberrations identified in ~ 50% of cases
  - o Shown by loss of heterozygosity or FISH methods

Terminal Deoxynucleotidyl Transferase-Mediated dUTP Nick End Labeling (TUNEL)

- Apoptosis rate is usually high

DIFFERENTIAL DIAGNOSIS

Systemic Lupus Erythematosus Panniculitis

- SPTCL can be misdiagnosed as benign panniculitis in early stages of disease
  - o Lesions resolve spontaneously; often respond to steroids
  - o Mixed infiltrate of lymphocytes and histiocytes
  - o Lymphoid atypia can be minimal in early disease
- Unlike SPTCL, in benign panniculitis
  - o Germinal center formation may be present
  - o B-cell aggregates and T cells present; latter are a mixture of CD4(+) and CD8(+) cells
  - o No rimming of individual fat cells by CD8(+) T cells
  - o T cells are negative for cytotoxic proteins

Cytophagocytic Histiocytic Panniculitis (CHP)

- Many cases of SPTCL were once designated as CHP
- Small subset of true CHP lesions remains
- Histiocyte rich; no evidence of lymphoid atypia
- No evidence of monoclonal TCR gene rearrangements

Atypical Lymphocytic Lobular Panniculitis

- Defined as clonal lymphoid-rich infiltrate that does not meet histopathologic criteria for lymphoma
- Chronic condition often with spontaneous resolution
  - o T-cell clone may increase progressively
  - o Unequivocal SPTCL may develop in some cases
- Lobular infiltrate
  - o Small to intermediate-sized lymphocytes
  - o Minimal nuclear atypia
- Interstitial plump histiocytes also present
- In contrast to SPTCL
  - o Infiltrate is less dense; rimming around adipocytes is less prominent
  - o Hemorrhage, karyorrhexis absent
  - o CD4(+) T cells present; can be decreased

Primary Cutaneous Gamma-Delta T-cell Lymphoma

- Median age at diagnosis: ~ 60 years
- Generalized lesions on legs, arms, trunk
- Lymphadenopathy, hepatosplenomegaly common
- Hemophagocytic syndrome develops in ~ 50% of patients; often fatal
- 5-year overall survival: ~ 10%

SUBCUTANEOUS PANNICULITIS-LIKE T-CELL LYMPHOMA

- Lesions can show 3 patterns: Epidermotropic, dermal, and subcutaneous
  - Subcutaneous involvement can closely mimic SPTCL
    - Rimming around adipocytes is less prominent
- Necrosis and ulceration common
- Angioinvasion and angiodestruction common
- Immunophenotype
  - CD4(-), CD8(-), CD56(+) in 60% of cases
    - Subset of cases are CD8(+)
  - TCR-δ(+), βF1/TCR-αβ(-)
  - Strongly (+) for cytotoxic proteins: TIA-1, granzyme B, perforin
- Monoclonal *TCR* gene rearrangements

Primary Cutaneous CD30(+) Lymphoproliferative Disorders
- Primary cutaneous anaplastic large cell lymphoma
  - Usually single large nodule or localized nodules
    - Ulceration common
  - Diffuse cohesive sheets of anaplastic large cells in dermis
    - Tumor can involve subcutaneous adipose tissue
    - No rimming of fat cells by CD8(+) T cells
- Lymphomatoid papulosis
  - Multifocal skin lesions that spontaneously regress
  - Ulceration with healing typical
- Immunophenotype
  - CD30(+), bright and uniform; often CD4(+)
  - TCRs often negative

T- and B-cell Lymphomas and Myeloid Leukemias
- Virtually any hematopoietic neoplasm can infiltrate subcutaneous adipose tissue
  - Neoplastic cells can rim adipocytes, morphologically can mimic SPTCL
- Immunophenotypic analysis essential to distinguish these entities from SPTCL

Blastic Plasmacytoid Dendritic Cell Neoplasm (BPDCN)
- Patients present with solitary or multiple skin lesions
- Regional lymphadenopathy: 20% of cases
- Bone marrow and peripheral blood involved commonly
  - Disease progresses to acute or chronic myelomonocytic leukemia in subset of patients
- In skin, BPDCN is diffuse infiltrate that involves
  - Dermis and subcutaneous tissue; epidermis spared
- Neoplastic cells
  - Monomorphic, intermediate-sized cells with scant cytoplasm
  - Irregular nuclear contours, blastic chromatin
- Immunophenotype
  - CD4(+), CD56(+), CD123(+), CD303(+)
  - Tcl-1(+), CD43(+), CD45RA(+)
  - CD7(+/-), CD33(-/+), CD68(-/+)
  - TdT(+) in 30-50% of cases
  - Cytotoxic proteins(-)

DIAGNOSTIC CHECKLIST

Clinically Relevant Pathologic Features
- In WHO 2008 classification, criteria for SPTCL were revised
  - TCR-γδ(+) cases were reclassified as primary cutaneous γ/δ T-cell lymphoma
  - In effect, worst prognostic subset of what had been designated as SPTCL is now excluded
- SPTCL, therefore, has relatively good prognosis
  - Conservative therapy (e.g., immunosuppressive agents) recommended currently
  - Multi-agent chemotherapy reserved for patients with progressive disease

Pathologic Interpretation Pearls
- In its early stages, SPTCL can closely mimic benign forms of panniculitis
  - Clues to early diagnosis
    - Lymphoid atypia
    - Cytotoxic immunophenotype
- Rimming of adipocytes by atypical cells is not specific for SPTCL; also seen in
  - Primary and secondary cutaneous lymphomas
    - T- and B-cell lineage
  - Myeloid leukemias

SELECTED REFERENCES
1. Parveen Z et al: Subcutaneous panniculitis-like T-cell lymphoma: redefinition of diagnostic criteria in the recent World Health Organization-European Organization for Research and Treatment of Cancer classification for cutaneous lymphomas. Arch Pathol Lab Med. 133(2):303-8, 2009
2. Hahtola S et al: Clinicopathological characterization and genomic aberrations in subcutaneous panniculitis-like T-cell lymphoma. J Invest Dermatol. 128(9):2304-9, 2008
3. Kong YY et al: Subcutaneous panniculitis-like T-cell lymphoma: a clinicopathologic, immunophenotypic, and molecular study of 22 Asian cases according to WHO-EORTC classification. Am J Surg Pathol. 32(10):1495-502, 2008
4. Willemze R et al: Subcutaneous panniculitis-like T-cell lymphoma: definition, classification, and prognostic factors: an EORTC Cutaneous Lymphoma Group Study of 83 cases. Blood. 111(2):838-45, 2008
5. Kang BS et al: Subcutaneous panniculitis-like T-cell lymphoma: US and CT findings in three patients. Skeletal Radiol. 36 Suppl 1:S67-71, 2007
6. Ghobrial IM et al: Clinical outcome of patients with subcutaneous panniculitis-like T-cell lymphoma. Leuk Lymphoma. 46(5):703-8, 2005
7. Massone C et al: Lupus erythematosus panniculitis (lupus profundus): clinical, histopathological, and molecular analysis of nine cases. J Cutan Pathol. 32(6):396-404, 2005
8. Magro CM et al: Atypical lymphocytic lobular panniculitis. J Cutan Pathol. 31(4):300-6, 2004
9. Sen F et al: Apoptosis and proliferation in subcutaneous panniculitis-like T-cell lymphoma. Mod Pathol. 15(6):625-31, 2002
10. Gonzalez CL et al: T-cell lymphoma involving subcutaneous tissue. A clinicopathologic entity commonly associated with hemophagocytic syndrome. Am J Surg Pathol. 15(1):17-27, 1991

SUBCUTANEOUS PANNICULITIS-LIKE T-CELL LYMPHOMA

Microscopic and Immunohistochemical Features

(Left) Subcutaneous tissue involved by subcutaneous panniculitis-like T-cell lymphoma (SPTCL). Atypical lymphoid cells infiltrate between adipocytes. *(Right)* The neoplastic cells of SPTCL are often medium-sized and hyperchromatic with irregular nuclear contours. Numerous apoptotic cells and karyorrhectic debris ➡ are often present. Rimming of individual adipocytes by lymphoma cells ⇒ is well shown in this field.

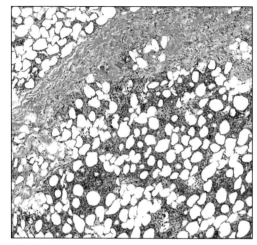 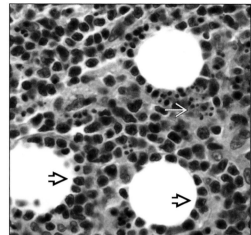

(Left) Subcutaneous panniculitis-like T-cell lymphoma (SPTCL) often shows a mixture of lymphoma cells ➡ and reactive histiocytes ⮕. Histiocytes often have lipid-laden or "foamy" cytoplasm and can be vacuolated as shown in this field. *(Right)* Subcutaneous tissue involved by SPTCL. Neoplastic cells are strongly CD3(+); the immunostaining highlights rimming of adipocytes by neoplastic T cells.

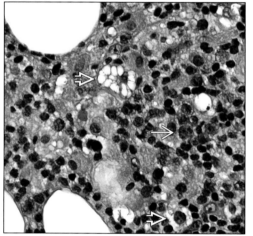 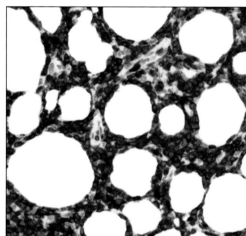

(Left) Subcutaneous tissue involved by subcutaneous panniculitis-like T-cell lymphoma (SPTCL). Neoplastic cells are strongly βF1(+). This antibody reacts with an epitope of the framework of the α/β T-cell receptor. *(Right)* Subcutaneous tissue involved by SPTCL. The lymphoma cells ➡ are strongly CD8(+). The lymphoma cells also expressed cytotoxic proteins and were CD4(-) (not shown), as is typical of SPTCL.

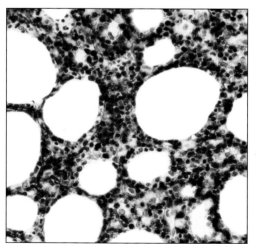 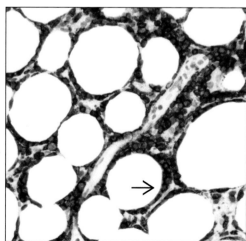

SUBCUTANEOUS PANNICULITIS-LIKE T-CELL LYMPHOMA

Differential Diagnosis

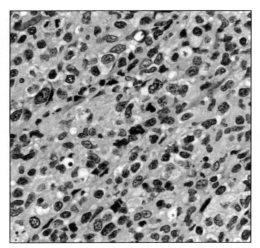

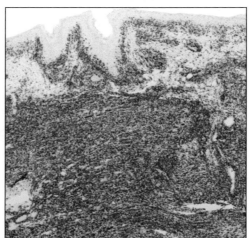

(Left) Primary cutaneous γ/δ T-cell lymphoma. The neoplastic cells in this case show marked cytologic atypia. *(Right)* Primary cutaneous γ/δ T-cell lymphoma CD7(+) neoplastic cells. This image also shows that the neoplasm primarily involves the dermis and subcutaneous tissue.

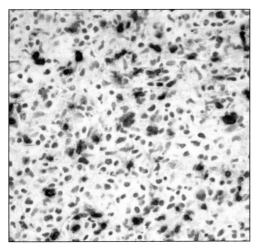

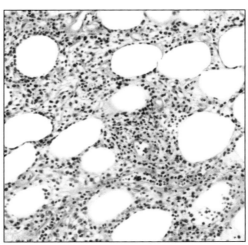

(Left) Primary cutaneous γ/δ T-cell lymphoma. The neoplastic cells are βF1(-). The absence of βF1 immunoreactivity implies that the neoplastic cells may express the γ/δ T-cell receptor. *(Right)* Systemic ALK(-) anaplastic large cell lymphoma involving subcutaneous tissue. Many types of T- and B-cell lymphoma as well as myeloid leukemia can involve subcutaneous adipose tissue and morphologically mimic SPTCL.

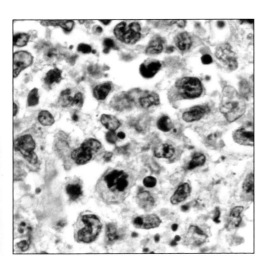

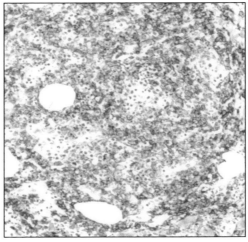

(Left) Systemic ALK(-) anaplastic large cell lymphoma involving subcutaneous tissue. The neoplastic cells are large and anaplastic, to a degree that would be highly unusual in cases of SPTCL. *(Right)* Systemic ALK(-) anaplastic large cell lymphoma involving subcutaneous tissue. The neoplastic cells are strongly CD30(+) and are negative for anaplastic lymphoma kinase (ALK) (not shown).

PRIMARY CUTANEOUS GAMMA-DELTA T-CELL LYMPHOMA

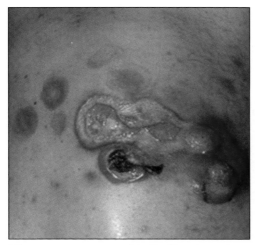

Primary cutaneous gamma-delta T-cell lymphoma shows a large raised lesion with ulcer and satellite lesions. (Courtesy C. Sander, MD.)

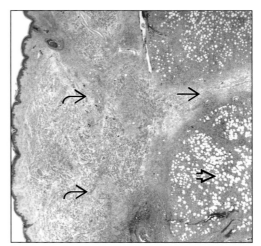

PCGDTCL involving skin. The neoplasm predominantly involves the subcutaneous adipose tissue ➢ in a lobular pattern sparing septae ➾. Foci of dermal involvement are also present ➚.

TERMINOLOGY

Abbreviations
- Primary cutaneous γ/δ T-cell lymphoma (PCGDTCL)

Definitions
- Neoplasm arising in skin composed of cytotoxic T-cells that express γ/δ T-cell receptor

ETIOLOGY/PATHOGENESIS

Possible Role of Antigen Drive
- Chronic antigenic stimulation is suggested as being involved in pathogenesis
- Involves cutaneous T-cells expressing γ/δ T-cell receptor
  - Increased frequency of expression of Vδ2

Immunosuppression &/or Immunodysregulation Involvement
- Case reported in patient with rheumatoid arthritis treated with tumor necrosis factor inhibitor

CLINICAL ISSUES

Epidemiology
- Incidence
  - Rare; < 1% of cutaneous T-cell lymphomas
- Age
  - Adults
- Gender
  - No sex preference

Presentation
- B-type symptoms are common
- Patients present with skin lesions, often multiple
  - Most common on extremities

- Neoplasm can involve epidermis, dermis, &/or subcutaneous tissue
  - Epidermal disease can appear as patches or plaques
  - Dermal or subcutaneous disease appears as nodules
- Epidermal ulcer and necrosis in subset of patients
- PCGDTCL can disseminate
  - Other extranodal or mucosal sites
  - Lymph nodes, liver, spleen, and bone marrow are involved uncommonly
- Hemophagocytic syndrome can occur in subset of patients
  - More common in patients with subcutaneous tumors
- Rare patients had prolonged indolent course before developing aggressive behavior

Laboratory Tests
- High serum LDH in subset of patients
- No serologic evidence of HHV8, EBV, HTLV-1

Treatment
- Drugs
  - Combination chemotherapy ± radiation therapy
    - Tumors are often resistant

Prognosis
- Poor
  - Median overall survival: ~ 15 months
  - Patients with subcutaneous tumors have worst overall survival
    - In part, related to higher frequency of hemophagocytic syndrome

MICROSCOPIC PATHOLOGY

Histologic Features
- 3 histologic patterns that are not mutually exclusive
  - Epidermotropic pattern represents wide spectrum
    - Minimal to marked epidermotropism

PRIMARY CUTANEOUS GAMMA-DELTA T-CELL LYMPHOMA

Key Facts

Terminology
- Neoplasm arising in skin composed of cytotoxic T-cells that express γ/δ T-cell receptor

Clinical Issues
- Adults who present with skin lesions; often multiple
  ○ Epidermal disease appears as patches or plaques
  ○ Dermal or subcutaneous disease appears as nodules
- B-type symptoms are common
- PCGDTCL can disseminate to other extranodal or mucosal sites
  ○ Lymph nodes, liver, spleen, and bone marrow are rarely involved
- Hemophagocytic syndrome in subset of patients
- Poor prognosis despite multiagent chemotherapy ± irradiation

Microscopic Pathology
- 3 histologic patterns of involvement
  ○ Epidermotropic, dermal, &/or subcutaneous
- Apoptosis and necrosis are common
- Cytologic spectrum of neoplastic cells is wide

Ancillary Tests
- TCR-δ(+), TCR-γ(+), βF1/TCR-αβ(-)
- CD2(+), CD3(+), cytotoxic proteins(+), CD56(+)
- CD4(-), CD8(-) in most cases; CD5(-)
- Monoclonal rearrangements of TCRγ and TCRδ genes

Top Differential Diagnoses
- Subcutaneous panniculitis-like T-cell lymphoma
- Primary cutaneous anaplastic large cell lymphoma
- Pagetoid reticulosis
- Peripheral T-cell lymphoma, NOS

  ○ Dermal; reticular dermis commonly involved
  ○ Subcutaneous; often associated with dermal involvement
    ■ Neoplastic cells often rim adipocytes
- Apoptosis and necrosis are very common; ± angioinvasion

Cytologic Features
- Neoplastic cells show spectrum of cell size (small to large) with cytologic atypia

ANCILLARY TESTS

Immunohistochemistry
- PCGDTCL has mature but aberrant T-cell immunophenotype
  ○ TCR-δ(+), TCR-γ(+), βF1/TCR-αβ(-)
  ○ CD2(+), CD3(+), CD56(+), cytotoxic proteins(+)
  ○ Vδ2(+) in subcutaneous tumors; CD7(+/-)
  ○ CD4(-), CD8(-); subset of tumors can be CD8(+)
  ○ CD5(-), CD1a(-), TdT(-), B-cell antigens(-)

In Situ Hybridization
- EBER(-)

Molecular Genetics
- Monoclonal rearrangements of TCRγ and TCRδ genes
- ± monoclonal rearrangement of TCRβ gene
- No monoclonal rearrangements of Ig genes

DIFFERENTIAL DIAGNOSIS

Subcutaneous Panniculitis-like T-cell Lymphoma (SPTCL)
- SPTCL is confined to subcutaneous tissue
- SPTCL has indolent clinical course with ~ 80-90% 5-year survival rate
- Subset of cases of PCGDTCL were previously designated as "γ/δ TCR(+) SPTCL"
- Immunophenotype

  ○ CD3(+), CD8(+), βF1/TCR-αβ(+)
  ○ Cytotoxic proteins(+), TCR-δ(-), TCR-γ(-), CD56(-)

Primary Cutaneous Anaplastic Large Cell Lymphoma
- Neoplasm of large and anaplastic cells usually situated in dermis
- CD30(+) strong and uniform; CD4(+/-), cytotoxic proteins(+)

Pagetoid Reticulosis
- In some case of PCGDTCL, marked epidermotropism can mimic pagetoid reticulosis
- Pagetoid reticulosis (PR) differs from PCGDTCL
  ○ PR is restricted to foot or ankle; usually CD8(+)

Peripheral T-cell Lymphoma, NOS
- Often involves dermis ± involvement of subcutaneous tissue
- Usually cytologic atypia is prominent
- Neoplasms can be CD4(+) or CD8(+); usually βF1/TCR-αβ(+)

Benign Causes of Panniculitis
- Lupus profundus panniculitis
  ○ Often clinical or laboratory evidence of autoimmune disease
- Other types of lobular panniculitis
- Minimal or absent cytologic atypia
- T cells are mixture of CD4(+) and CD8(+) cells
- No evidence of monoclonal TCR gene rearrangements

SELECTED REFERENCES

1. Koens L et al: Cutaneous gamma/delta T-cell lymphoma during treatment with etanercept for rheumatoid arthritis. Acta Derm Venereol. 89(6):653-4, 2009
2. Tripodo C et al: Gamma-delta T-cell lymphomas. Nat Rev Clin Oncol. 6(12):707-17, 2009
3. Hosler GA et al: Transformation of cutaneous gamma/delta T-cell lymphoma following 15 years of indolent behavior. J Cutan Pathol. 35(11):1063-7, 2008

PRIMARY CUTANEOUS GAMMA-DELTA T-CELL LYMPHOMA

Microscopic and Immunohistochemical Features

(Left) Primary cutaneous γ/δ T-cell lymphoma involving subcutaneous adipose tissue. In this case the neoplasm exhibited extensive involvement of the subcutaneous adipose tissue. Both atypical lymphoid cells and histiocytes are interspersed among adipocytes. (Right) PCGDTCL involving subcutaneous adipose tissue. The neoplastic cells exhibit cytologic atypia and rim the adipocyte in this field. Mitotic figures are present ➡.

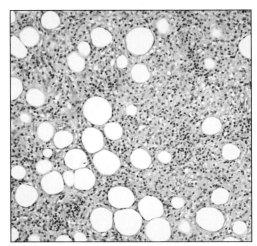
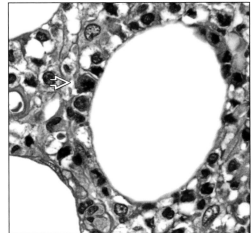

(Left) PCGDTCL involving subcutaneous adipose tissue. The neoplastic T cells are strongly CD3(+) and rim adipocytes. (Right) PCGDTCL involving subcutaneous adipose tissue. The neoplastic T cells are negative for βF1. βF1 is reactive with an epitope of the α/β T-cell receptor (TCR). Absence of βF1 expression is presumptive evidence that the neoplastic cells express the γ/δ TCR. Scattered reactive T cells are positive.

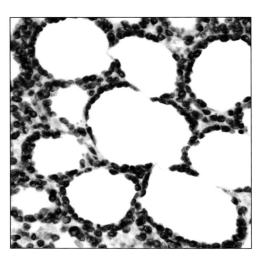
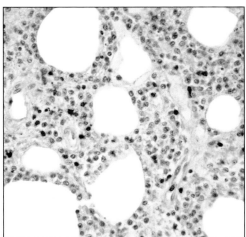

(Left) Primary cutaneous γ/δ T-cell lymphoma involving subcutaneous adipose tissue. The neoplastic cells express granzyme B and have a cytotoxic T-cell immunophenotype. (Right) PCGDTCL involving skin biopsy specimen shows neoplastic cells primarily involving the epidermis in this field. This neoplasm also involved the deep dermis and subcutaneous tissue (not shown).

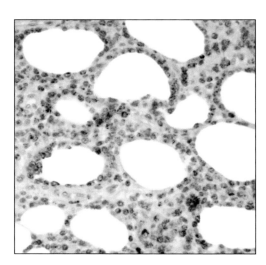
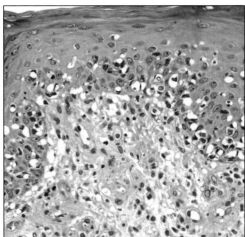

PRIMARY CUTANEOUS GAMMA-DELTA T-CELL LYMPHOMA

Microscopic and Immunohistochemical Features

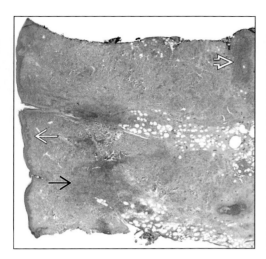

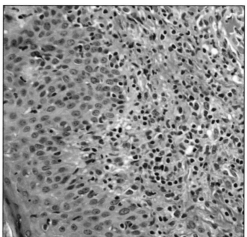

(Left) Primary cutaneous γ/δ T-cell lymphoma involving skin. The neoplasm involves the epidermis ➡, dermis ⇨, and subcutaneous tissue ⇢, with the most extensive disease in the dermis and subcutis. (Right) PCGDTCL involving skin. Neoplastic cells involve the papillary dermis with a lesser degree of epidermotropism. In this case most of the neoplastic cells are small and highly irregular.

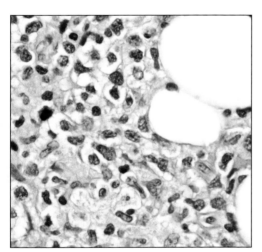

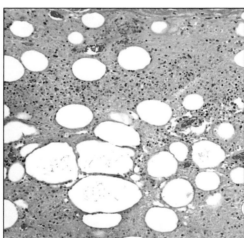

(Left) Primary cutaneous γ/δ T-cell lymphoma involving subcutaneous adipose tissue of skin. The neoplastic cells exhibit cytologic atypia and are admixed with histiocytes in this field. (Right) PCGDTCL involving subcutaneous adipose tissue of skin. This area of the neoplasm showed extensive fat necrosis.

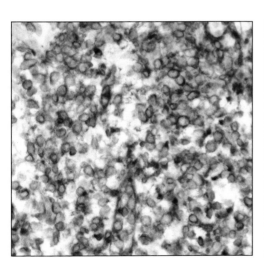

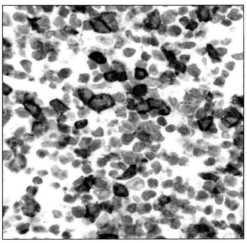

(Left) Primary cutaneous γ/δ T-cell lymphoma involving a skin biopsy specimen. The neoplastic cells are strongly CD3(+). (Right) PCGDTCL involving a skin biopsy specimen. A subset of the neoplastic cells in this neoplasm are CD8(+). Most cases of PCGDTCL are CD4(-) and CD8(-), but a subset of neoplasms can show partial or total CD8 expression.

PRIMARY CUTANEOUS GAMMA-DELTA T-CELL LYMPHOMA

Microscopic and Immunohistochemical Features

(Left) Primary cutaneous γ/δ T-cell lymphoma involving a biopsy of the eyelid. The neoplasm involved the dermis and skeletal muscle ⊅ underlying the skin. *(Right)* PCGDTCL involving an eyelid biopsy specimen shows an area of necrosis with karyorrhexis within the neoplasm. Both atypical neoplastic lymphoid cells and histiocytes ⊅ are present in this field.

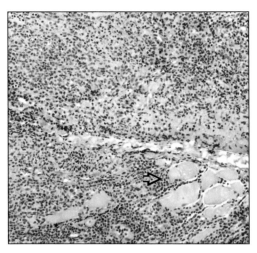
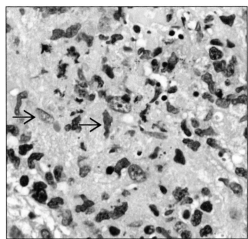

(Left) Primary cutaneous γ/δ T-cell lymphoma involving a biopsy of the eyelid. The neoplastic lymphocytes show cytologic atypia, and a mitotic figure is present at the upper left of the field ⊅. Reactive histiocytes ⊅ are also admixed within the neoplasm. *(Right)* PCGDTCL involving an eyelid biopsy specimen. Epithelium overlies the lesion. The neoplastic cells are strongly CD7(+).

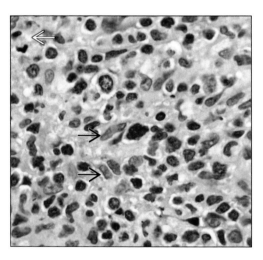
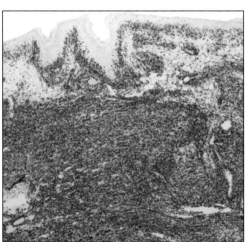

(Left) Primary cutaneous γ/δ T-cell lymphoma involving a biopsy of the eyelid. The neoplastic cells are βF1(-). Reactive T cells in the field are βF1(+). *(Right)* High-power magnification of PCGDTCL involving an eyelid biopsy specimen. The neoplastic cells are βF1(-). This result suggests that the neoplastic cells express the γ/δ TCR. Reactive T cells in the field are βF1(+).

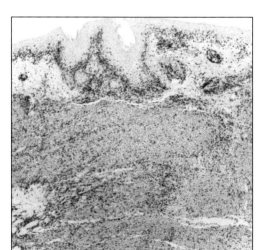
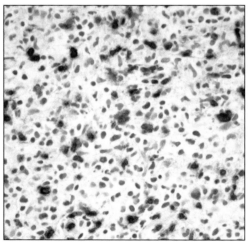

PRIMARY CUTANEOUS GAMMA-DELTA T-CELL LYMPHOMA

Differential Diagnosis

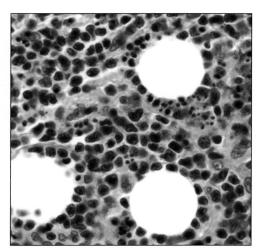

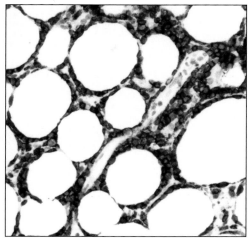

(Left) Skin biopsy specimen involved by subcutaneous panniculitis-like T-cell lymphoma (SPTCL). Neoplastic cells infiltrate between and surround adipocytes. Apoptosis and karyorrhexis are present. *(Right)* SPTCL involving subcutaneous adipose tissue. The neoplastic cells are strongly CD8(+). Unlike SPTCL, most cases of PCGDTCL are CD8(-), although ~ 20% of cases can show partial or dim CD8 expression.

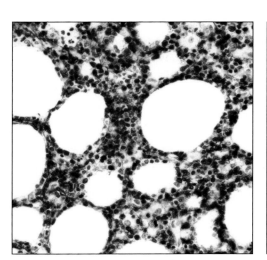

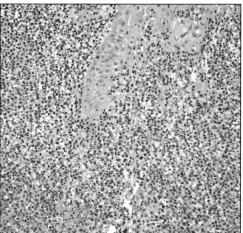

(Left) Subcutaneous panniculitis-like T-cell lymphoma involving subcutaneous adipose tissue. The neoplastic cells are strongly βF1(+). This result indicates that the neoplastic cells express the α/β T-cell receptor. Primary cutaneous gamma-delta T-cell lymphoma is βF1(-) *(Right)* Primary cutaneous anaplastic large cell lymphoma (C-ALCL) involving skin. Most cases of C-ALCL are based in the dermis. Epidermal &/or subcutaneous adipose tissue also can be involved.

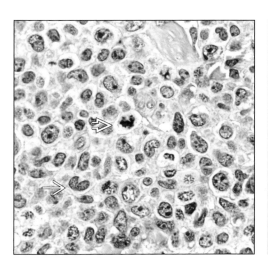

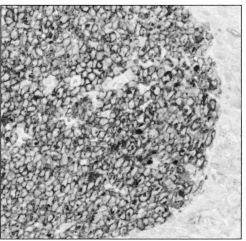

(Left) Primary cutaneous anaplastic large cell lymphoma. The neoplastic cells are large and anaplastic. Hallmark cells ⇒ and a mitotic figure ⇒ are present in this field. *(Right)* Primary cutaneous anaplastic large cell lymphoma involving skin. The neoplastic cells are strongly CD30(+). CD30 is typically absent or expressed only focally in primary cutaneous gamma-delta T-cell lymphoma.

MYCOSIS FUNGOIDES

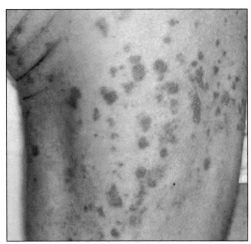

The plaque stage of mycosis fungoides shows the presence of multiple red plaques on much of the body surface of this patient.

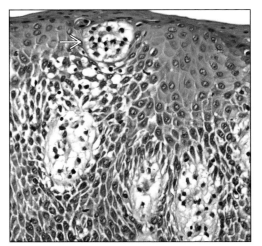

The plaque stage of mycosis fungoides shows the presence of a Pautrier microabscess ➡ containing small atypical tumor cells.

TERMINOLOGY

Abbreviations
- Mycosis fungoides (MF)

Definitions
- Primary cutaneous T-cell lymphoma characterized by
  o Epidermotropism
  o Clinical course showing stepwise evolution of patches, plaques, and tumors

ETIOLOGY/PATHOGENESIS

Unknown
- Chronic antigenic stimulation, possibly due to infectious agent, may play role
- Genetic abnormalities are likely to be involved

CLINICAL ISSUES

Epidemiology
- Incidence
  o 0.6/100,000 people per year
  o 50% of all cases of primary cutaneous lymphoma
- Age
  o Adults, 5th-6th decade
  o Can be seen in patients < 35 years
- Gender
  o M:F = 2:1
- Ethnicity
  o Incidence is 1.7x higher in African-Americans than in whites

Presentation
- Premycotic period
  o Nonspecific skin lesions; often slight scaling, pruritus

- Lesions can wax and wane for years; may never progress to MF
- Skin biopsy findings are nondiagnostic
- Stepwise evolution of disease with appearance of patches, plaques, and tumors
  o Patches
    - Mostly on trunk but can arise anywhere on body including palms and toes
    - Can be associated with alopecia
  o Plaques
    - Palpable lesions raised above skin surface
    - Can be associated with patch lesions
  o Tumors
    - Usually manifest as skin nodule(s)
    - Can coexist with patches and plaques
- MF variants
  o Pagetoid reticulosis
    - Also referred to as Woringer-Kolopp disease
    - Solitary, slow-growing, psoriasiform, crusty or hyperkeratotic patches or plaques
    - Often arises on distal limb
  o Folliculotropic (pilotropic) MF
    - Often involves head and neck area
    - Follicular papules (often grouped), alopecia, and acneiform lesions
    - Clinically more aggressive than other MF types; responds less well to skin-directed therapy
  o Syringotropic MF
    - Solitary, well-circumscribed, red-brown plaque, often associated with alopecia
    - Skin-directed therapy may be inadequate (similar to folliculotropic MF)
  o Granulomatous slack skin
    - Circumscribed areas of pendulous folds of lax skin in major folds (axillae, groin)
    - May coexist with classical MF lesions or classical Hodgkin lymphoma

MYCOSIS FUNGOIDES

Key Facts

Terminology
- Primary cutaneous T-cell lymphoma characterized by
  - Epidermotropism
  - Clinical course showing stepwise evolution of patches, plaques, and tumors

Clinical Issues
- Overall indolent clinical course
- Clinical stage is most important predictor of prognosis

Microscopic Pathology
- Skin biopsy findings are nondiagnostic in premycotic and some early patch stage lesions
- Superficial band-like or lichenoid infiltrate in patch and thin plaque stage

- Dense, subepidermal band-like infiltrate in thick plaque stage
- Prominent dermal infiltrate in tumor stage
- Large cell transformation: Large tumor cells are > 25%

Ancillary Tests
- Immunophenotype
  - CD3(+), CD5(+), TCR-αβ/βF1(+)
  - CD4(+), CD8(-), CD7(-), CD26(-)

Top Differential Diagnoses
- Drug reaction, inflammatory dermatoses
- Primary cutaneous CD30(+) T-cell lymphoproliferative disorders
- Primary cutaneous γ/δ T-cell lymphoma
- Rare variants of T-cell lymphoma involving skin

Laboratory Tests
- Morphologic assessment of peripheral blood for Sézary cells
  - Insensitive
- Flow cytometry immunophenotypic analysis
  - Aberrant T-cell immunophenotypes support involvement by MF
- Assessment of T-cell clonality by PCR
- Serum lactate dehydrogenase &/or β-2-microglobulin
  - High levels associated with poorer prognosis

Natural History
- Over time, some patients develop visceral involvement by MF
- Most common sites: Lungs, liver, spleen

Treatment
- Early-stage disease (stages I and IIA) requires direct skin therapy
  - Topical chemotherapy with nitrogen mustard or carmustine
  - Topical corticosteroids and retinoids
  - Phototherapy; local radiation (x-ray or electron beam)
- Advanced-stage disease (stages IIB-IV)
  - Extracorporeal photopheresis
  - Single-agent chemotherapy
    - Methotrexate, pegylated liposomal doxorubicin (Doxil), purine analogs (fludarabine, 2-deoxycoformycin), others
  - Combination chemotherapy: Many regimens have been used
    - Cyclophosphamide, doxorubicin, vincristine, and prednisone (CHOP)
    - Cyclophosphamide, vincristine, and prednisone (CVP)
    - CVP with methotrexate (COMP)
  - Hematopoietic cell transplantation

Prognosis
- Indolent clinical course overall
- Disease prognosis depends on clinical stage

- Clinical significance of T-cell receptor (TCR) gene rearrangements in MF staging is controversial
  - Monoclonal TCR gene rearrangement in blood is extremely common in early-stage disease
    - Not synonymous with blood involvement by MF in absence of morphologic or immunophenotypic evidence of disease
  - Monoclonal TCR gene rearrangement in lymph nodes is common finding
    - Not prognostically significant in multivariate analysis

MACROSCOPIC FEATURES

General Features
- Patches
  - Circumscribed lesions with discoloration of variable size, color, and shape
  - Little scaling, not palpable
- Plaques
  - Palpable infiltrate of variable stage (thin and thick)
- Tumors
  - Often exophytic and ulcerated (hence term "fungoides")

MICROSCOPIC PATHOLOGY

Histologic Features of Skin
- Premycotic stage (parapsoriasis)
  - Skin biopsy findings are nondiagnostic
  - Lymphocytic infiltrate
    - Mainly in upper dermis, not in subepidermal zone
    - No epidermotropism
- Patch and early (thin) plaque stage
  - Superficial band-like or lichenoid infiltrate by lymphocytes and histiocytes
    - Atypical lymphocytes infiltrate basal layer, especially tips of rete ridges
    - Epidermotropism with single-cell infiltrate

MYCOSIS FUNGOIDES

- Neoplastic lymphocytes are small, slightly cerebriform, some with halos
  - Other changes
    - Mild acanthosis, hyperkeratosis; basal layer damage
    - Edema and fibrosis, increased postcapillary venules
  - In some early lesions, skin biopsy findings are nondiagnostic
- Thick plaque stage
  - Dense, subepidermal, band-like infiltrate with many cerebriform lymphocytes
  - Epidermotropism is more prominent with
    - Intraepidermal clusters and Pautrier microabscesses
    - Confluent Pautrier microabscesses that can result in subcorneal and subepidermal bullae
- Tumor stage
  - Dermal infiltrate becomes more diffuse and prominent
    - Tumor cells range in size from small to large
  - Epidermotropism may be lost
  - Large cell transformation
    - Often occurs in tumor stage
    - Large tumor cells ≥ 25%
    - CD30 can be (+); high proliferation rate (Ki-67)
- MF variants
  - Pagetoid reticulosis
    - Intraepidermal proliferation of neoplastic T cells
    - Sponge-like disaggregation of epidermis
    - Atypical cells have medium-sized or large, sometimes hyperchromatic and cerebriform nuclei
    - CD4(+), CD8(-), or CD4(-), CD8(+)
    - Often CD30(+); Ki-67 > 30%
  - Folliculotropic MF (pilotropic MF)
    - Atypical lymphocyte infiltrating epithelium of hair follicles
    - Infiltrate spares epidermis
    - Often associated with mucinosis (mucinous degeneration)
  - Syringotropic MF
    - Hyperplastic eccrine ducts and glands infiltrated by atypical lymphocytes
    - Often abundant eosinophils present
  - Granulomatous slack skin
    - Dense granulomatous dermal infiltrate containing atypical T cells, macrophages, and often many multinucleated giant cells
    - Infiltrate often shows destruction of elastic tissue; ± epidermotropism
    - CD4(+), CD8(-)

Histologic Features of Lymph Nodes

- Best to biopsy lymph nodes draining area of involved skin or lymph node with highest standardized uptake value on FDG PET scan
- Early involvement by MF (N1 and N2)
  - Lymph node architecture is well maintained
  - Dermatopathic changes common
  - Cerebriform lymphocytes are either absent, singly scattered, or in small clusters or aggregates
    - Often difficult to identify morphologically

- Ancillary testing is important to demonstrate involvement by MF
  - Flow cytometric immunophenotyping
  - Assessment for *TCR* gene rearrangement
- Extensive involvement by MF (N3)
  - Overt involvement or complete effacement of architecture
  - May show large cell transformation

Cytologic Features

- Small- to medium-sized lymphocytes
- Cerebriform nuclear contours and hyperchromatic nuclei

ANCILLARY TESTS

Immunohistochemistry

- CD2(+), CD3(+), CD5(+), βF1(+)
- Often shows CD7 loss (all disease stages)
- CD4(+), CD8(-)
  - Rare cases can be CD4(-), CD8(+)
- CD45/LCA(+), CLA(+), CD52(+), CD25(-/+)
- CD30(+/-), usually expressed by large cells
- Ig(-), B-cell antigens(-)

Flow Cytometry

- Can be performed on skin, peripheral blood, lymph nodes, and other tissue specimens
- Flow panel should include
  - CD2, CD3, CD4, CD5, CD7
  - CD8, CD25, CD26, TCR-αβ, TCR-γδ
- CD4:CD8 ratio is often increased
- Typical immunophenotype: CD3(+), CD4(+), CD8(-), CD5(+), TCR-αβ(+)
- Frequent immunophenotypic aberrancies
  - CD26(-), loss of/decreased CD7
  - Dim expression of CD2, CD3, CD4, or CD5
- Clonality assessment by Vβ analysis
  - Can identify clonality and quantify clonal T cells
  - Can be used to follow treatment response

Cytogenetics

- Complex karyotypes occur in subset of patients
  - Most common in patients with advanced-stage disease

Molecular Genetics

- Monoclonal *TCR* gene rearrangements
- No evidence of monoclonal *Ig* gene rearrangements
- Inactivation of *P16/CDKN2A* or *PTEN* in subsets of cases

Gene Expression Profiling

- Deregulation of genes involved in tumor necrosis factor (TNF) signaling pathway

DIFFERENTIAL DIAGNOSIS

Drug Reaction, Inflammatory Dermatoses

- Epidermotropism of lymphocytes (exocytosis) can simulate MF
- Perivascular lymphocytic infiltrate

MYCOSIS FUNGOIDES

- Increased eosinophils and plasma cells in dermis
- Dyskeratotic keratinocytes, parakeratosis (+/-)

Lymphomatoid Papulosis, Type B

- Recurrent, self-healing, waxing and waning skin lesions
  - Papular, papulonecrotic, &/or nodular skin lesions at different stages of development
- Morphological features
  - Often wedge-shaped lesions
  - Epidermotropic infiltrate of small atypical cells with cerebriform nuclei similar to MF
- Immunophenotype: T-cell antigens(+), TCR-αβ(+), TCL1(+)
- Differential diagnosis in some cases can only be made by obtaining complete clinical information

Cutaneous Anaplastic Large Cell Lymphoma (C-ALCL)

- Cases of MF with large cell transformation can be uniformly CD30(+) mimicking C-ALCL
- Clinical history or histologic evidence of MF elsewhere is helpful

Primary Cutaneous γ/δ T-cell Lymphoma

- Clinical presentation
  - Patients often present with generalized skin lesions, preferentially affecting extremities
  - Disease may be predominantly epidermotropic and present with patches/plaques that simulate MF
  - Patients can present with deep dermal or subcutaneous tumor, ± epidermal necrosis and ulceration
  - B-symptoms are common
- Morphologic features
  - Can be epidermotropic, dermal, or subcutaneous infiltrate
  - Medium to large lymphoid cells with coarse chromatin
  - Apoptosis and necrosis are common
- Immunophenotype
  - CD2(+), CD3(+), CD7(+/-), CD56(+), TCR-γδ(+)
  - Cytotoxic proteins (+), CD30(-/+), TCR-αβ/βF1(-)
  - CD4(-), CD5(-), CD8(-)

Primary Cutaneous Aggressive Epidermotropic CD8(+) Cytotoxic T-cell Lymphoma

- Clinical presentation
  - Generalized skin lesions
  - Eruptive papules, nodules, and tumors with central ulceration and necrosis
  - May disseminate to other visceral sites but often spares lymph nodes
  - Aggressive clinical course; median survival 32 months
- Morphological features
  - Variable, ranging from lichenoid pattern to marked, pagetoid epidermotropism and subepidermal to deeper nodular infiltrates
  - Epidermis may show necrosis, ulceration, and blister formation

- Tumor cells are small to medium in size
- Angiocentricity and angioinvasion may be present, and tissue destruction is often present
- Immunophenotype
  - βF1(+), CD3(+), CD8(+)
  - Cytotoxic proteins(+), CD45RA(+/-), CD2(-/+), CD7(+/-)
  - CD4(-), CD5(-), CD45RO(-)

Primary Cutaneous Small/Medium CD4(+) T-cell Lymphoma

- Clinically indolent
  - Most cases present with solitary skin lesion, no evidence of patches and plaques typical of MF
    - Commonly on face, neck, or upper trunk
- Morphological features
  - Dense, diffuse, or nodular infiltrates within dermis with tendency to infiltrate subcutis
  - Epidermotropism may be present focally, but if conspicuous, consideration should be given to diagnosis of MF
  - Small/medium-sized pleomorphic T-cells
- Immunophenotype
  - CD3(+), CD4(+), CD8(-), βF1(+)

T-cell Prolymphocytic Leukemia (T-PLL) Involving Skin

- T-PLL can involve skin, usually with dermal involvement, but epidermotropism can be seen
- Clinical history is helpful as patients usually have history of T-PLL with
  - High peripheral blood leukocyte count; bone marrow involvement
- Immunophenotype: T-cell antigens(+), TCR-αβ(+), TCL1(+)

STAGING

Advanced Stage Predicts Poor Prognosis

- Erythematous skin (T4)
- Blood involvement with high tumor volume (blood stage B2)
- Histologic evidence of lymph node involvement (N3)
- Visceral organ involvement (M1)

SELECTED REFERENCES

1. Feng B et al: Flow cytometric detection of peripheral blood involvement by mycosis fungoides and Sézary syndrome using T-cell receptor Vbeta chain antibodies and its application in blood staging. Mod Pathol. 23(2):284-95, 2010
2. Olsen E et al: Revisions to the staging and classification of mycosis fungoides and Sezary syndrome: a proposal of the International Society for Cutaneous Lymphomas (ISCL) and the cutaneous lymphoma task force of the European Organization of Research and Treatment of Cancer (EORTC). Blood. 2007 Sep 15;110(6):1713-22. Epub 2007 May 31. Review. Erratum in: Blood. 111(9):4830, 2008

MYCOSIS FUNGOIDES

TMNB Staging of Mycosis Fungoides

TMNB Stage

Tumor Stage (T)

T1: Limited patches, papules, &/or plaques covering < 10% of skin surface; may further stratify into T1a (patch only) vs. T1b (plaque ± patch)

T2: Patches, papules, or plaques covering 10% or more of skin surface; may further stratify into T2a (patch only) vs. T2b (plaque ± patch)

T3: 1 or more tumors (1 cm diameter)

T4: Confluence of erythema covering 80% of body surface area

Extracutaneous Disease (visceral involvement) (M)

M0: No visceral organ involvement

M1: Visceral involvement (must have pathologic confirmation)

Splenomegaly as visceral disease, even without biopsy confirmation

Bone marrow involvement has not been considered as visceral involvement by ISCL/EORTC

Lymph Node Stage* (lymph nodes > 1.5 cm in greatest dimension) (N)

N0: No clinically abnormal peripheral lymph nodes; biopsy not required

N1: Dermatopathic lymphadenopathy; no or a few scattered atypical cerebriform mononuclear cells with nuclei > 7.5 μm

N2: Dermatopathic lymphadenopathy; aggregates or clusters of atypical cerebriform mononuclear cells with nuclei > 7.5 μm; architecture is preserved

N3: Partial or complete effacement of architecture with many atypical lymphocytes

Blood Stage** (B)

B0: Absence of significant blood involvement: 5% of peripheral blood lymphocytes are atypical (Sézary) cells

B1: Low blood tumor burden: > 5% of peripheral blood lymphocytes are atypical (Sézary) cells but < 1,000/μL or > 1,000/μL atypical cells; no clonality

B3: High blood tumor burden: 1,000/μL Sézary cells with positive clonality studies

*Central adenopathy may be secondary to a 2nd malignancy (especially a 2nd lymphoma), infection, or a reactive process. The ISCL/EORTC recommends that central enlarged nodes be excluded from the determination of "N" status except in cases where an excisional biopsy of a central node has proven lymphomatous (N3) involvement with MF. **Morphological assessment of Sézary cells is insensitive to identify tumor cells. Flow cytometry immunophenotyping with proven clonality either by TCR gene rearrangement or Vβ flow cytometric analysis can better assess tumor cell burden.

Clinical Staging of Patients with Mycosis Fungoides (ISCL/EORTC)*

Clinical Stage	TMNB Classification	Description of Clinical Presentation
Stage I		
Stage IA	T1 N0 M0 B0 or B1	Disease confined to skin with patches/papules/plaques < 10% of skin surface; no clinically abnormal lymph nodes
Stage IB	T2 N0 M0 B0 or B1	Disease confined to skin with patches/papules/plaques > 10% of skin surface; no clinically abnormal lymph nodes
Stage II		
Stage IIA	T1 or T2 N1 or N2 M0 B0 or B1	Skin involvement with patches/papules/plaques associated with no or early lymph node involvement
Stage IIB	T3 N0 to N2 M0 B0 or B1	Skin involvement with patches/papules/plaques and with 1 or more tumors (> 1 cm) associated with no or early lymph node involvement
Stage III		
Stage IIIA	T4 N0 to N2 M0 B0	Skin involvement with erythroderma, no or early lymph node involvement, and absent blood tumor burden (< 5% Sézary cells)
Stage IIIB	T4 N0 to N2 M0 B0	Skin involvement with erythroderma, no or early (N1-N2) lymph node involvement, and low blood tumor burden (> 5% but < 1,000/μL circulating Sézary cells)
Stage IV		
Stage IVA1	T1 to T4 N0 to N2 M0 B2	High blood tumor burden (> 1,000/μL circulating Sézary cells) with no or early lymph node involvement and no visceral involvement
Stage IVA2	T1 to T4 N3 M0 B0 to B2	High blood tumor burden (> 1,000/μL circulating Sézary cells) with extensive lymph node involvement and no visceral involvement
Stage IVB	T1 to T4 N0 to N3 M1 B0 to B2	High blood tumor burden (> 1,000/μL circulating Sézary cells) with or without extensive lymph node involvement and positive for visceral involvement

*International Society for Cutaneous Lymphomas (ISCL) and the Cutaneous Lymphoma Task Force of the European Organization of Research and Treatment of Cancer (EORTC).

Mycosis Fungoides, Different Stages of Disease

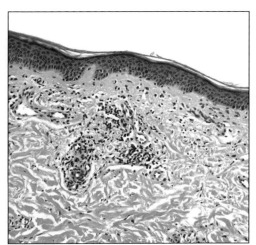
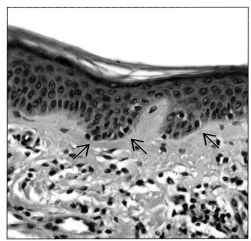

(Left) This biopsy specimen shows the patch stage of mycosis fungoides of the skin. Changes in the early patch stage are often very subtle. The biopsy specimen shows a perivascular lymphocytic infiltrate consisting of small lymphocytes and minimal epidermal infiltrate. *(Right)* Patch stage of mycosis fungoides of the skin. This higher power view reveals an epidermal basal layer infiltrate ➡. The tumor cells are small but have irregular nuclear contours.

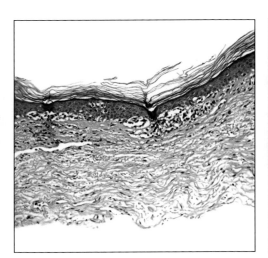
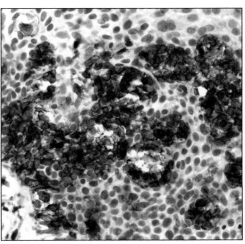

(Left) Later patch stage and early plaque stage of mycosis fungoides shows intraepidermal clusters of atypical lymphocytes. There is minimal subepidermal infiltrate. *(Right)* Plaque stage of mycosis fungoides. The intraepidermal atypical cerebriform lymphocytes within Pautrier microabscesses are CD4(+).

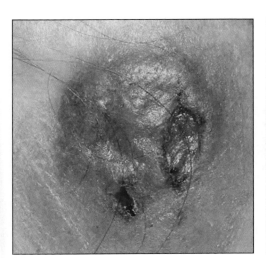
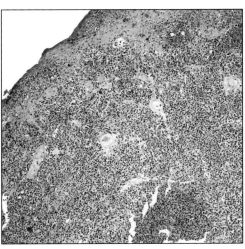

(Left) The tumor stage is shown in a patient with mycosis fungoides. *(Right)* The tumor stage of mycosis fungoides shows a diffuse and prominent dermal infiltrate. Also present is epidermal hemorrhage with focal ulceration.

Mycosis Fungoides with Large Cell Transformation

(Left) High-power view of the tumor stage of mycosis fungoides shows no significant epidermotropism and tumor cells growing in sheets. *(Right)* A case of mycosis fungoides with large cell transformation shows a diffuse dermal infiltrate with increased large cells. There is no significant epidermotropism.

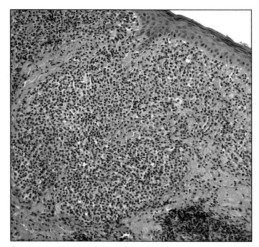 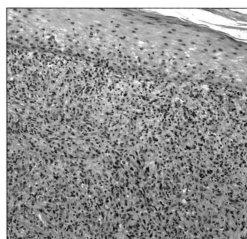

(Left) Mycosis fungoides with large cell transformation involving skin. The tumor cells are large and pleomorphic with angulated nuclei and nuclear hyperchromasia. *(Right)* Mycosis fungoides with large cell transformation involving skin. The large tumor cells are CD3(+).

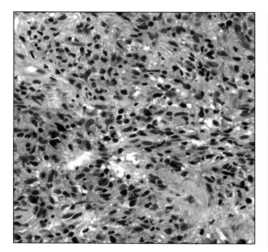 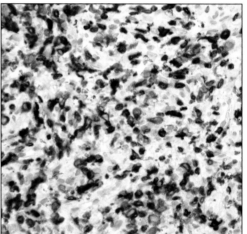

(Left) Mycosis fungoides with large cell transformation involving skin. The large tumor cells are CD7(-). *(Right)* Mycosis fungoides with large cell transformation involving skin. The large tumor cells are CD30(+). Large cell transformation may or may not show CD30 expression.

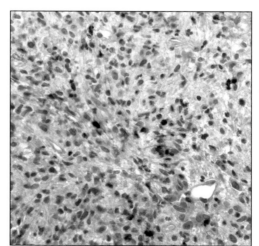 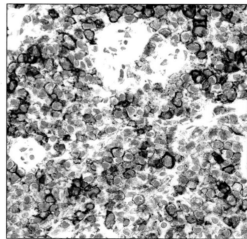

MYCOSIS FUNGOIDES

Variants of Mycosis Fungoides

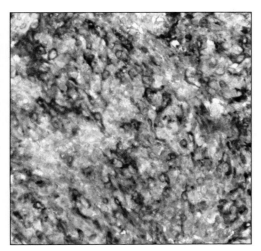

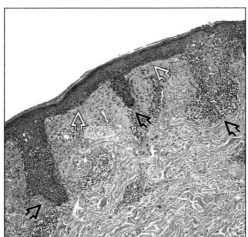

(Left) Mycosis fungoides with large cell transformation involving skin. The large tumor cells are CD25(+). *(Right)* A case of folliculotropic variant mycosis fungoides (pilotropic mycosis fungoides) shows a lymphocytic infiltrate in and around the hair follicles ⧫ with sparing of the interfollicular skin ⧫.

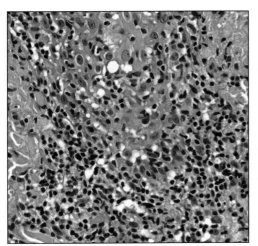

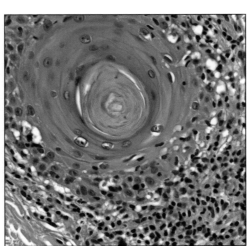

(Left) Folliculotropic mycosis fungoides shows atypical lymphocytes within and surrounding the hair follicle epithelium. *(Right)* A cornified hair follicle is infiltrated by atypical lymphocytes in folliculotropic mycosis fungoides.

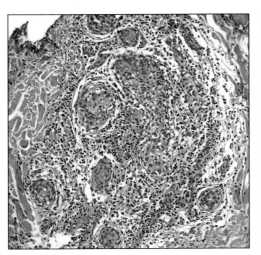

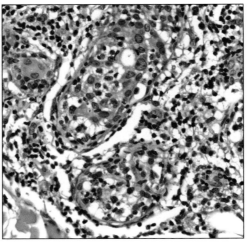

(Left) A case of syringotropic variant mycosis fungoides shows a lymphocytic infiltrate predominantly involving eccrine sweat glands. *(Right)* A case of syringotropic variant mycosis fungoides shows atypical small cerebriform lymphocytes inside and around eccrine glands.

MYCOSIS FUNGOIDES

Variants of Mycosis Fungoides

(Left) Granulomatous slack skin disease is a variant of mycosis fungoides. This is an advanced-stage lesion and shows a dense lymphohistiocytic infiltrate in the dermis. (Right) Granulomatous slack skin disease. The dense, lymphohistiocytic infiltrate extends to the deep dermis with many giant cells.

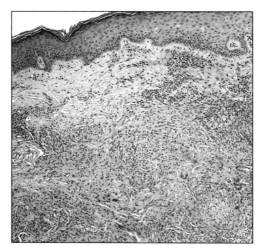
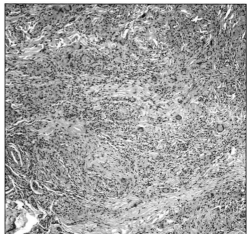

(Left) Granulomatous slack skin disease with giant cells containing 20-30 nuclei. Some of the giant cells have nuclei localized in the periphery of the cytoplasm. Focal elastophagocytosis is present ➔. The lymphocytes between the giant cells are small with less pronounced cytological atypia. (Right) Granulomatous slack skin disease. The infiltrating lymphocytes are CD3(+).

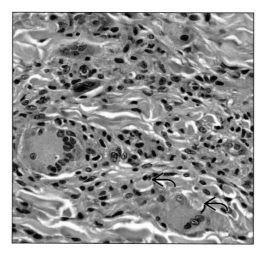
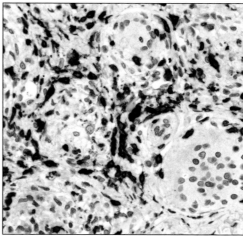

(Left) Pagetoid reticulosis is a slow-growing, psoriasiform crusty patch or plaque typically found in the distal limb. Note the hyperkeratotic, crusty epithelium with a lymphocytic infiltrate that shows vacuolized changes. (Right) Pagetoid reticulosis of the distal limb. The infiltrating lymphocytes are atypical and small to medium in size with perinuclear halos.

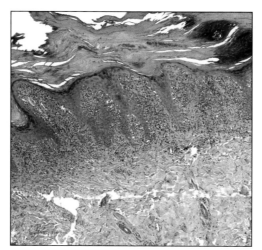
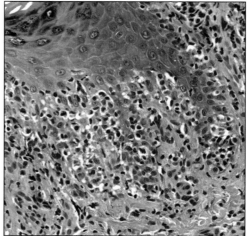

MYCOSIS FUNGOIDES

Variants of Mycosis Fungoides and Lymph Node

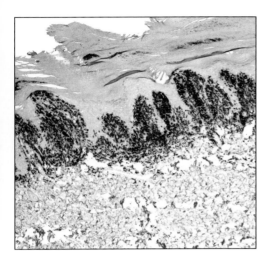
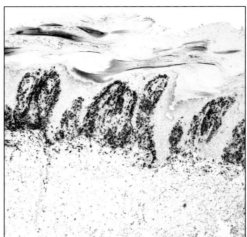

(Left) Biopsy specimen of pagetoid reticulosis. The lymphocytes are CD3(+) and CD8(+) (not shown). CD8(+) pagetoid reticulosis is not uncommon. (Right) Pagetoid reticulosis. The lymphocytes are CD8(+).

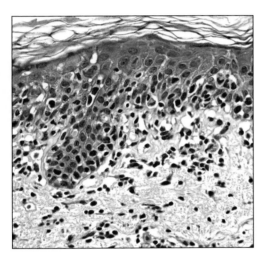
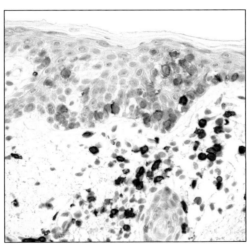

(Left) This case of typical mycosis fungoides is CD8(+). The histologic features are very similar to conventional CD4(+) mycosis fungoides and differ from pagetoid reticulosis and primary cutaneous aggressive epidermotropic CD8(+) cytotoxic T-cell lymphoma. (Right) This case of typical mycosis fungoides is CD8(+). The CD8 immunostain highlights the neoplastic intraepidermal T cells that express CD8 more dimly than reactive CD8(+) T cells in this field.

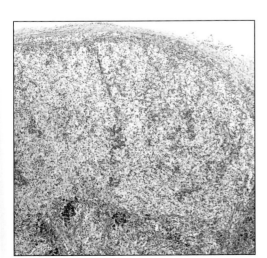
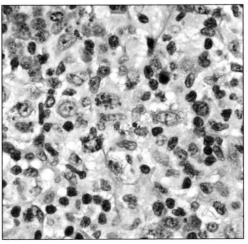

(Left) Lymph node biopsy specimen from a patient with mycosis fungoides shows marked dermatopathic changes and maintained nodal architecture. (Right) Lymph node biopsy specimen from a patient with mycosis fungoides shows many interdigitating dendritic cells, Langerhans cells, and melanin-containing macrophages. The lymphocytes are not atypical. This would be interpreted as no histologic evidence of mycosis fungoides (N1).

MYCOSIS FUNGOIDES

Lymph Node and Flow Cytometry

(**Left**) Lymph node biopsy specimen from a patient with mycosis fungoides shows scattered, larger, atypical cells ➡; the histological grading of this involvement is still N1. (**Right**) Lymph node biopsy specimen from a patient with mycosis fungoides shows sheets of tumor cells present (N3). Macrophages containing melanin pigment are also present.

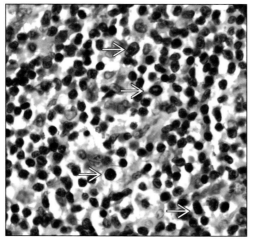
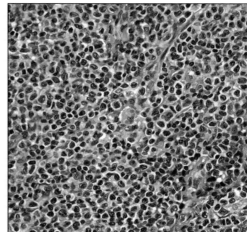

(**Left**) Flow cytometric immunophenotyping of lymph node tissue reveals an immunophenotypically aberrant T-cell population ⇨ (CD3[dim +], CD4[dim +]). (Courtesy J. Jorgenson, MD.) (**Right**) Flow cytometric immunophenotyping of lymph node reveals an aberrant T-cell population ⇨ (CD3[dim +], CD4[bright+]). Both cases indicate lymph node involvement. Also noted are many immunophenotypically normal T cells in both cases. (Courtesy J. Jorgenson, MD.)

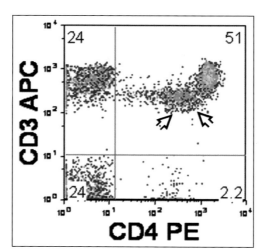
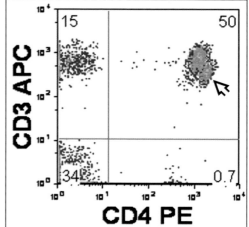

(**Left**) Peripheral blood smear shows many large cerebriform (Sézary) cells consistent with mycosis fungoides in the leukemic phase (so-called secondary Sézary syndrome). (**Right**) Mycosis fungoides. The peripheral blood smear shows lymphocytosis. The lymphocytes are small with round nuclei and lack typical Sézary cell morphology. However, flow cytometry and molecular studies confirmed the lymphocytes to be neoplastic T cells.

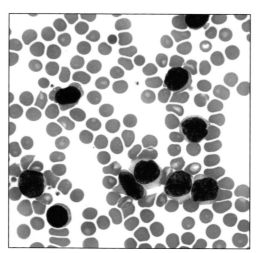
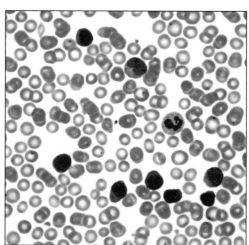

MYCOSIS FUNGOIDES

Blood, Bone Marrow, and Flow Cytometry

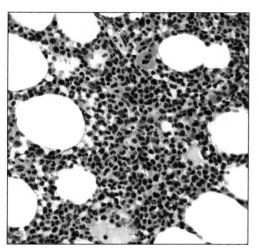

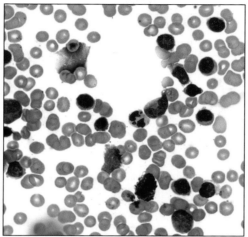

(Left) Bone marrow involvement by mycosis fungoides is uncommon. When bone marrow is involved, the neoplasm often has an interstitial pattern of infiltration. (Right) Bone marrow aspirate smear reveals many atypical small- to medium-sized lymphocytes, consistent with bone marrow involvement by mycosis fungoides.

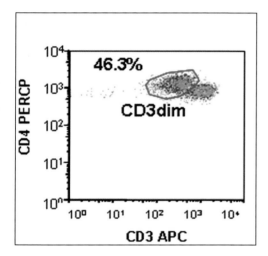

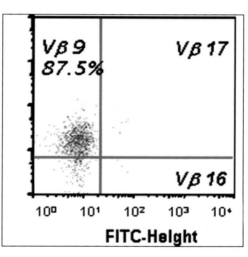

(Left) Flow cytometric immunophenotyping identifies an immunophenotypically aberrant T-cell population (CD3[dim], circled). (Courtesy J. Jorgensen, MD.) (Right) These immunophenotypically aberrant T-cells are Vβ 9-restricted by flow cytometric Vβ analysis, which confirms T-cell clonality. (Courtesy J. Jorgensen, MD.)

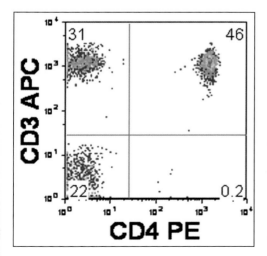

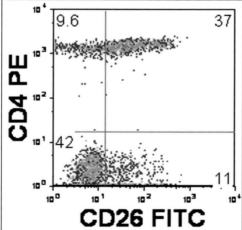

(Left) A normal peripheral blood sample shows a normal CD4:CD8 ratio. (Courtesy J. Jorgensen, MD.) (Right) A normal peripheral blood sample shows a normal expression pattern of CD26 on CD4(+) T cells. (Courtesy J. Jorgensen, MD.)

MYCOSIS FUNGOIDES

Flow Cytometry and Differential Diagnosis

(Left) A peripheral blood sample obtained from a mycosis fungoides patient reveals a markedly increased CD4:CD8 ratio as well as an immunophenotypically aberrant T-cell population (CD3[dim], CD4[dim]). (Courtesy J. Jorgensen, MD.) (Right) The aberrant T cells (CD3[dim]) are CD26(-). (Courtesy J. Jorgensen, MD.)

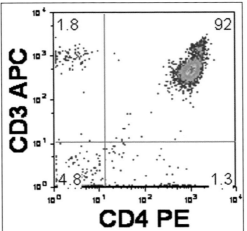
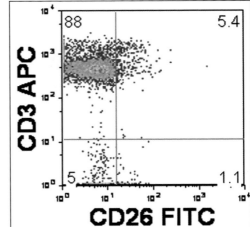

(Left) A peripheral blood sample obtained from a mycosis fungoides patient reveals a slightly increased CD4:CD8 ratio as well as an immunophenotypically aberrant T-cell population (CD3[dim], CD4[dim]) ⮞. (Courtesy J. Jorgensen, MD.) (Right) The aberrant T cells (CD3[dim]) are CD26(-) ⮞. (Courtesy J. Jorgensen, MD.)

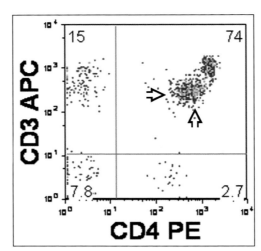
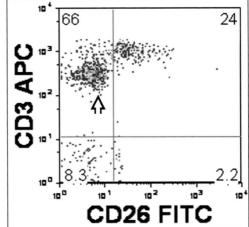

(Left) Primary cutaneous aggressive epidermotropic CD8(+) cytotoxic T-cell lymphoma shows a pronounced epidermal and dermal infiltrate. (Right) Primary cutaneous aggressive epidermotropic CD8(+) cytotoxic T-cell lymphoma. The lymphoma cells are CD8(+).

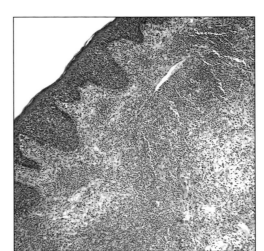
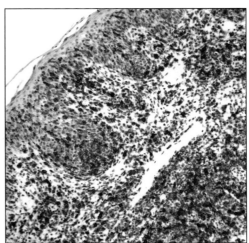

MYCOSIS FUNGOIDES

Differential Diagnosis

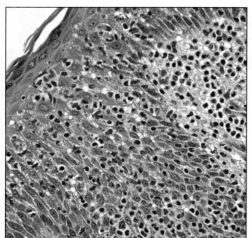

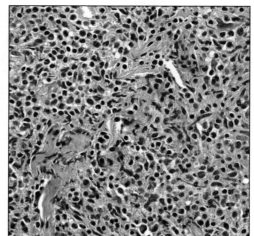

(Left) Primary cutaneous aggressive epidermotropic CD8(+) cytotoxic T-cell lymphoma. The lymphoma cells are small- to medium-sized with irregular nuclear contours and infiltrate the epidermis. *(Right)* Primary cutaneous aggressive epidermotropic CD8(+) cytotoxic T-cell lymphoma. The lymphoma cells infiltrate the dermis. Morphologically, the cells are medium-sized, angulated, and infiltrative.

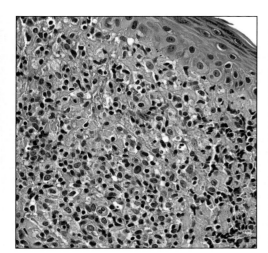

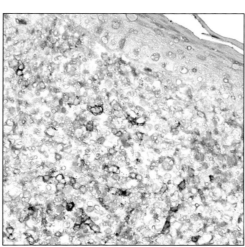

(Left) Primary cutaneous CD30(+) T-cell lymphoproliferative disorder consistent with lymphomatoid papulosis, type A. A dermal infiltrate consisting of a mixture of small lymphocytes, histiocytes, and scattered large cells is present. *(Right)* Primary cutaneous CD30(+) T-cell lymphoproliferative disorder consistent with lymphomatoid papulosis, type A. Anti-CD30 highlights scattered large cells.

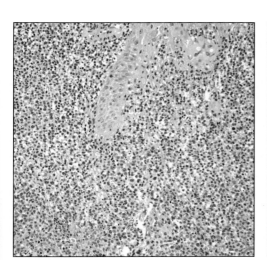

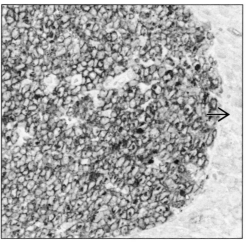

(Left) Cutaneous anaplastic large cell lymphoma (C-ALCL). Some cases of mycosis fungoides (MF) in large cell transformation can be uniformly CD30(+) and mimic C-ALCL. A history of MF or evidence of MF elsewhere on the patient, or at the margins of the lesion in the biopsy specimen, is helpful in differential diagnosis. *(Right)* C-ALCL. The neoplastic cells are uniformly CD30(+). Epidermis is present at the right ⇒.

SEZARY SYNDROME

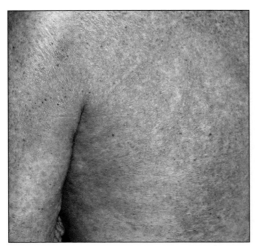

Skin of patient with Sézary syndrome shows erythroderma. The patient's back and left arm are shown in this field.

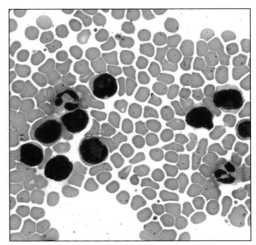

Peripheral blood smear from a patient with Sézary syndrome shows many large Sézary cells with folded cerebriform nuclei and scant to moderate cytoplasm; they are larger than neutrophils.

TERMINOLOGY

Abbreviations
- Sézary syndrome (SS)

Synonyms
- Erythrodermic cutaneous T-cell lymphoma (E-CTCL)

Definitions
- SS defined by triad of
  - Pruritic erythroderma
  - High number of Sézary cells in peripheral blood (> 1,000/μL) with
    - Confirmed T-cell clonality **or**
    - Increased CD4:CD8 ratio > 10 **or**
    - T-cell immunophenotypic aberrancies demonstrated by flow cytometric immunophenotyping
  - Lymphadenopathy, usually generalized

ETIOLOGY/PATHOGENESIS

Unknown
- Genetics, infectious agents, or environmental exposures may play a role

CLINICAL ISSUES

Epidemiology
- Incidence
  - 5% of all cutaneous T-cell lymphomas
- Age
  - Adults; median: 60 years (range: 45-70 years)
- Gender
  - M:F = 1.5:1
- Ethnicity
  - Incidence in blacks 2x as high as in whites

Presentation
- SS occurs de novo in most patients
- Can be preceded by prodromal phase
  - Pruritus or nonspecific dermatitis
- Can be preceded by mycosis fungoides (MF)
  - Patients must fulfill blood criteria for SS (T4B2)
  - These cases should be designated as "SS preceded by MF"
    - Recommendation of International Society for Cutaneous Lymphomas (ISCL)
- Skin: Intractable pruritus and generalized erythroderma with edema (≥ 80% of skin surface)
  - Associated with alopecia, ectropion, leonine facies
  - Nail dystrophy, plantar hyperkeratoses with extremely painful fissuring
  - Secondary bacterial infection
  - Some cases show marked photosensitivity
    - Mimic chronic actinic dermatitis
- Extracutaneous involvement
  - Lymph nodes
  - Liver, lung, spleen, central nervous system, and any other organs
  - Bone marrow is relatively spared
- Increased prevalence of secondary malignancies, especially lymphoma
  - May be attributable to decreased normal CD4(+) T cells
- Hypereosinophilic syndrome has been reported to be associated with SS
  - Can cause end organ dysfunction

Laboratory Tests
- Work-up should include
  - Complete blood count with differential
  - Serum chemistry tests of liver and renal function, electrolytes, and lactate dehydrogenase (LDH)
  - Serologic tests for viruses
    - HTLV-1, HIV, hepatitis B

SEZARY SYNDROME

Key Facts

Terminology
- Sézary syndrome (SS) is defined by triad of
  - Pruritic erythroderma
  - High number of Sézary cells in blood (> 1,000/μL)
  - Lymphadenopathy, usually generalized

Clinical Issues
- SS presents de novo in most patients
- Can be preceded by mycosis fungoides (MF)
  - Cases should be designated as "SS preceded by MF"
- Skin: Intractable pruritus and generalized erythroderma with edema (≥ 80% of skin surface)
- Extracutaneous sites of involvement
  - Lymph nodes, lung, liver
  - Spleen, central nervous system, other organs
  - Bone marrow is relatively spared
- Most treatments are palliative, not curative

- Total skin electron beam radiation with nonmyeloablative allogeneic SCT may be curative
- Poor survival: Median < 2.5 years

Microscopic Pathology
- Sézary cells (cells with cerebriform nuclei) in peripheral blood
- Skin changes are very similar to mycosis fungoides
- Lymph nodes show partial or total effacement of normal architecture

Top Differential Diagnoses
- Nonneoplastic causes of erythroderma
- Adult T-cell leukemia/lymphoma (ATLL)
- T-cell prolymphocytic leukemia
- Leukemia cutis (especially monocytic leukemia)
- Peripheral T-cell lymphoma, not otherwise specified

- Flow cytometric immunophenotyping of peripheral blood useful for
  - Confirming clonality
  - Detecting immunophenotypic aberrancies
- Molecular analysis of T-cell receptor (*TCR*) genes for assessment of clonality
  - T-cell clone can be seen in up to 20% of reactive skin conditions

Treatment
- Most therapies are palliative and not curative
  - Extracorporeal photoimmunotherapy
  - Bexarotene (retinoid)
  - Methotrexate
  - Vorinostat (histone deacetylase inhibitor)
  - Alemtuzumab (anti-CD52)
  - Denileukin diftitox (anti-CD25 IL-2 diphtheria fusion protein)
  - High-dose chemotherapy
    - Etoposide, vincristine, doxorubicin, bolus cyclophosphamide, oral prednisone (EPOCH)
  - Autologous hematopoietic stem-cell transplantation following high-dose chemotherapy
    - Can produce remissions, but early relapses are common
- Total skin electron beam radiation with nonmyeloablative allogeneic stem cell transplantation (SCT)
  - Possibly curative approach

Prognosis
- Poor; median survival < 2.5 years
  - Predictors of poor prognosis
    - Advanced age
    - Elevated serum LDH

MICROSCOPIC PATHOLOGY

Histologic Features
- Peripheral blood
  - Cells with cerebriform nuclei (Sézary cells)

- Can range in size from small to large
  - Small Sézary cells (< 12 μm in diameter)
  - Large Sézary cells (> 14 μm in diameter)
  - Sézary cells are not completely specific
    - Especially small forms can be seen in reactive conditions
    - Most large cells are neoplastic
- Skin
  - Changes are very similar to MF
  - In ~ 2/3 patients with SS, skin biopsy shows diagnostic findings
  - Epidermotropism is variable
    - Can be absent in some biopsy specimens
    - Atypical cells are present only in dermis; often perivascular
  - Tumor cell size can be variable
    - Cell population is often monotonous (more so than MF)
  - In ~ 1/3 of patients, only nonspecific changes without abnormal lymphocytes
    - Cannot distinguish from nonneoplastic erythroderma using histologic criteria
- Bone marrow
  - Often not involved or only minimal involvement
  - When involved, Sézary cell infiltrate is often sparse
    - Mainly interstitial pattern; often patchy

Cytologic Features
- Cerebriform cells; can be small, medium, or large

Lymph Nodes
- Involved lymph nodes show partial or total effacement of normal architecture by Sézary cells
  - Dense, monotonous infiltrate of Sézary cells
  - Capsular invasion or extranodal invasion is often present
  - B-cell follicles may be reduced in number or small
- Changes of dermatopathic lymphadenopathy are often present with
  - Increased interdigitating dendritic and Langerhans cells

o Increased epithelioid venules and scattered melanophages

ANCILLARY TESTS

Immunohistochemistry
- Pan-T-cell antigens(+), TCR-αβ(+)
  o Loss or dim expression of T-cell antigens(+/-)
- CD4(+), CD8(-)
- CD25(-/+), CD30(-/+), CD52(+)
- B-cell antigens(-)
- Ki-67 moderate to high

Flow Cytometry
- CD2(+), CD3(+), CD5(+), CD7(+), TCR-αβ(+)
- CD4(+), CD8(-)
- TdT(-), CD1a(-), CD10(-), B-cell antigens(-)
- Immunophenotypic aberrancies are common; best detected by flow cytometry
  o Increased CD4:CD8 ratio
  o Loss of CD7, CD26, or other antigens
  o Altered expression levels of CD2, CD3, CD4, or CD5
- Vβ analysis is useful to confirm clonality and for quantifying neoplastic cells
  o Can be used for initial diagnosis and monitoring treatment response

Cytogenetics
- No specific chromosomal abnormalities
  o Complex karyotypes are common
  o Both numeric and structural abnormalities are observed
    ▪ High frequency of unbalanced translocations
    ▪ Deletions of chromosomes 1p, 6q, 10q, 17p, and 19
- Abnormal clone is independent hematologic criterion of SS

Molecular Genetics
- Monoclonal *TCR* gene rearrangements
  o Blood, skin, or lymph node
- No evidence of monoclonal *Ig* gene rearrangements
- T-cell clonality is not specific for SS
  o T-cell clone can be seen in up to 20% of reactive skin conditions
  o However, presence of identical T-cell clone in blood and skin/lymph node is specific
- *P53* or *CDKN2A* gene mutations are common; *JUNB* amplification in subset

DNA Ploidy Analysis
- DNA ploidy assessed by flow cytometry can identify cells with abnormal DNA content
- Indicative of numerical chromosomal abnormality

DIFFERENTIAL DIAGNOSIS

Nonneoplastic Erythroderma (Pseudo-E-CTCL)
- Common causes: Drug reaction, erythrodermic psoriasis, and erythrodermic eczema

o Variety of drugs can cause pseudo-E-CTCL
  ▪ Anticonvulsants (hydantoin, phenobarbital, carbamazepine, and sodium valproate)
  ▪ Angiotensin-converting enzyme inhibitors
  ▪ β-blockers
  ▪ Antidepressants, phenothiazine
  ▪ H1/2 histamine-receptor antagonists
- Chronic actinic dermatitis (actinic reticuloid)
  o Some are HIV-associated cutaneous lymphoproliferative disease
  o Infiltrate lymphocytes are mainly CD8(+) T cells
- Circulating Sézary cells can be present
  o Usually small in size
  o Except for decreased CD7 expression, often no other immunophenotypic aberrancies
  o Sézary cells often negative for clonality by flow cytometric Vβ analysis
  o Small monoclonal *TCR* gene rearrangement can be present
  o If absolute number of Sézary cells ≥ 1,000/µL or CD4/CD8 ratio ≥ 10
    ▪ Such cases can be designated as pseudo-SS

Adult T-cell Leukemia/Lymphoma (ATLL)
- HTLV-1(+); endemic in Southwestern Japan, Caribbean basin, and parts of Central Africa
- Acute variant is most common and is characterized by
  o Leukemic phase, often with markedly elevated white blood cell count
  o Skin rash and generalized lymphadenopathy
  o Hypercalcemia
  o Frequent opportunistic infections
    ▪ *Pneumocystis jirovecii* pneumonia
    ▪ *Strongyloides stercoralis*
    ▪ *Cryptococcus neoformans* meningitis
    ▪ Disseminated herpes zoster
- Skin is involved in up to 50% of patients with ATLL
  o Nodules or tumors are most common
  o Erythematous plaques and macules are 2nd most common
  o Erythroderma occurs in 3-5% of patients
  o Cutaneous type of ATLL has skin-limited lesions without lymph node involvement or leukemic presentation
    ▪ Belongs to group of smoldering ATLL
  o Skin biopsy findings can be indistinguishable from MF or SS
    ▪ Epidermotropism is often present
    ▪ ± Pautrier microabscesses
  o ATLL often infiltrates dermis and subcutaneous fat
  o Tumor cells are often medium to large in size, pleomorphic
- Peripheral blood smear shows polylobated (flower) cells with basophilic cytoplasm
  o CD3(+), CD4(+), CD5(+), CD7(-), CD25(+), FOXP3(+)
    ▪ Suggests derivation from CD4(+), CD25(+), FOXP3(+) regulatory T cells
- Bone marrow (BM) infiltrate is usually patchy, ranging from sparse to moderate
  o Osteoclastic activity may be prominent, even if tumor absent in BM

T-cell Prolymphocytic Leukemia
- Involves peripheral blood, bone marrow, lymph nodes, spleen, liver
  - Cells are predominantly small to medium-sized
    - Nongranular basophilic cytoplasm; round, oval, or markedly irregular nuclei
    - Nucleolus usually prominent; can be absent in "small cell variant"
  - In some cases, nuclear outline is very irregular and can be cerebriform
- Skin infiltrate occurs in 20% of patients
  - Perivascular or more diffuse dermal infiltrates without epidermotropism
- In lymph nodes
  - Involvement is diffuse and preferentially involves paracortical areas
- Immunophenotype
  - CD4(+), CD8(-): ~ 60%; CD4(+), CD8(+): ~ 25%
  - CD4(-), CD8(+): ~ 15%; TCL1(+)

Leukemia Cutis
- Especially monocytic leukemia
- Skin involvement occurs in ~ 10% of patients
- Superficial and deep perivascular or dermal infiltrate; no epidermotropism
- Cells are large with high nuclear to cytoplasmic ratio
- CD3(-), CD4(+), CD68(+), lysozyme(+), MPO (focal +)

Peripheral T-cell Lymphoma, Not Otherwise Specified
- Predominantly lymph node-based disease
- Peripheral blood is sometimes involved, but leukemic presentation is uncommon
- Skin is occasionally involved, but erythroderma is uncommon

DIAGNOSTIC CHECKLIST

Pathologic Interpretation Pearls
- Sézary cells can be seen in reactive conditions, especially small forms; not necessarily indicative of neoplastic cells
  - ISCL requires the following to establish diagnosis of SS
    - Confirmation of clonality **or**
    - Immunophenotypical aberrancies **or**
    - CD4:CD8 ratio > 10
- Erythroderma can develop during course of disease in MF, but patients often lack blood findings
  - Not classified as SS; is erythrodermic MF (stage T4)
- Cases that fail to fulfill diagnostic criteria for either erythrodermic MF or SS
  - This category was previously designated as "pre-SS"; now designated as E-CTCL

SELECTED REFERENCES

1. Duvic M et al: Total skin electron beam and non-myeloablative allogeneic hematopoietic stem-cell transplantation in advanced mycosis fungoides and Sezary syndrome. J Clin Oncol. 28(14):2365-72, 2010
2. Feng B et al: Flow cytometric detection of peripheral blood involvement by mycosis fungoides and Sézary syndrome using T-cell receptor Vbeta chain antibodies and its application in blood staging. Mod Pathol. 23(2):284-95, 2010
3. Agar N et al: Case report of four patients with erythrodermic cutaneous T-cell lymphoma and severe photosensitivity mimicking chronic actinic dermatitis. Br J Dermatol. 160(3):698-703, 2009
4. Vidulich KA et al: Overall survival in erythrodermic cutaneous T-cell lymphoma: an analysis of prognostic factors in a cohort of patients with erythrodermic cutaneous T-cell lymphoma. Int J Dermatol. 48(3):243-52, 2009
5. Duarte RF et al: Haematopoietic stem cell transplantation for patients with primary cutaneous T-cell lymphoma. Bone Marrow Transplant. 41(7):597-604, 2008
6. Olsen E et al: Revisions to the staging and classification of mycosis fungoides and Sezary syndrome: a proposal of the International Society for Cutaneous Lymphomas (ISCL) and the cutaneous lymphoma task force of the European Organization of Research and Treatment of Cancer (EORTC). Blood. 2007 Sep 15;110(6):1713-22. Epub 2007 May 31. Review. Erratum in: Blood. 111(9):4830, 2008
7. Huang KP et al: Second lymphomas and other malignant neoplasms in patients with mycosis fungoides and Sezary syndrome: evidence from population-based and clinical cohorts. Arch Dermatol. 143(1):45-50, 2007
8. Lee CH et al: Erythrodermic cutaneous T cell lymphoma with hypereosinophilic syndrome: Treatment with interferon alfa and extracorporeal photopheresis. Int J Dermatol. 46(11):1198-204, 2007
9. Vonderheid EC et al: Sézary cell counts in erythrodermic cutaneous T-cell lymphoma: implications for prognosis and staging. Leuk Lymphoma. 47(9):1841-56, 2006
10. Vonderheid EC: On the diagnosis of erythrodermic cutaneous T-cell lymphoma. J Cutan Pathol. 33 Suppl 1:27-42, 2006
11. Ponti R et al: T-cell receptor gamma gene rearrangement by multiplex polymerase chain reaction/heteroduplex analysis in patients with cutaneous T-cell lymphoma (mycosis fungoides/Sézary syndrome) and benign inflammatory disease: correlation with clinical, histological and immunophenotypical findings. Br J Dermatol. 153(3):565-73, 2005
12. Russell-Jones R: Diagnosing erythrodermic cutaneous T-cell lymphoma. Br J Dermatol. 153(1):1-5, 2005
13. Wang S et al: Flow cytometric DNA ploidy analysis of peripheral blood from patients with Sezary syndrome: detection of aneuploid neoplastic T cells in the blood is associated with large cell transformation in tissue. Am J Clin Pathol. 122(5):774-82, 2004
14. Vonderheid EC et al: Update on erythrodermic cutaneous T-cell lymphoma: report of the International Society for Cutaneous Lymphomas. J Am Acad Dermatol. 46(1):95-106, 2002
15. Trotter MJ et al: Cutaneous histopathology of Sézary syndrome: a study of 41 cases with a proven circulating T-cell clone. J Cutan Pathol. 24(5):286-91, 1997
16. Scheffer E et al: A histologic study of lymph nodes from patients with the Sézary syndrome. Cancer. 57(12):2375-80, 1986

SEZARY SYNDROME

Skin of Patients with SS

(Left) Skin biopsy specimen from a patient with Sézary syndrome shows a band-like dermal infiltrate of small, atypical lymphoid cells. There was minimal epidermotropism in this case. *(Right)* High-power view from a skin biopsy specimen from a patient with Sézary syndrome. Note a few scattered intraepidermal atypical lymphocytes ➡.

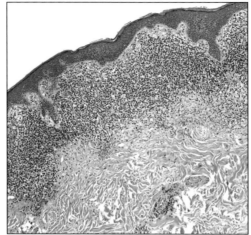 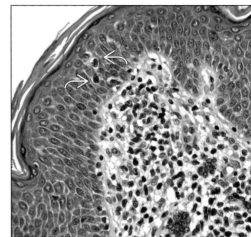

(Left) Skin biopsy specimen from a patient with Sézary syndrome. CD4 highlights the tumor cells predominantly in the dermis. Epidermotropism is minimal in this field. *(Right)* Skin biopsy specimen from a patient with Sézary syndrome that evolved from mycosis fungoides shows epidermotropism with many Pautrier microabscesses ➡. There is a prominent dermal and perivascular infiltrate.

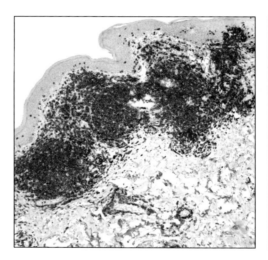 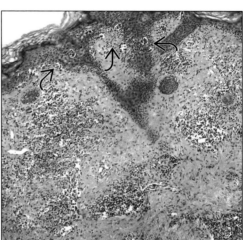

(Left) Skin biopsy specimen from a patient with Sézary syndrome (SS) that evolved from mycosis fungoides. The perivascular lymphocytic infiltrate is composed of medium- to large-sized lymphocytes with hyperchromatic and irregular nuclei. *(Right)* Skin biopsy specimen from a patient with SS that evolved from mycosis fungoides. Some of the larger forms are CD30(+).

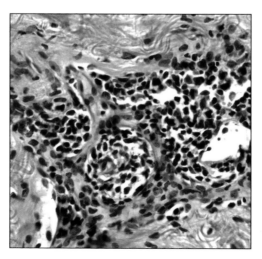 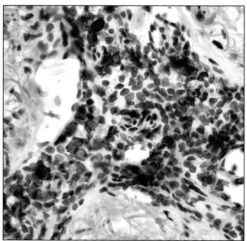

Bone Marrow and Peripheral Blood of Patients with SS

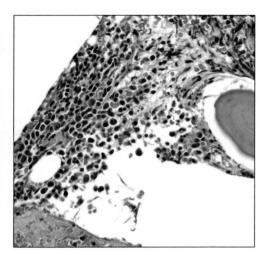

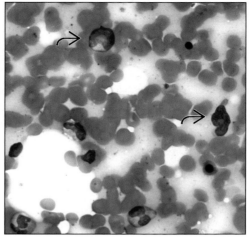

(Left) Bone marrow biopsy specimen of a patient with Sézary syndrome shows a focal and interstitial lymphocytic infiltrate present in this case. *(Right)* Bone marrow touch imprint of a patient with Sézary syndrome reveals large atypical Sézary cells ➡.

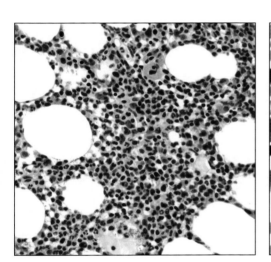

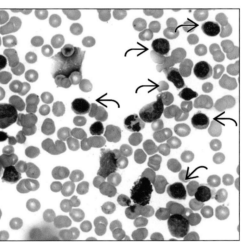

(Left) Bone marrow biopsy specimen of a patient with Sézary syndrome. The field shows a patchy lymphocytic infiltrate. *(Right)* Bone marrow aspirate smear of a patient with Sézary syndrome. Many small lymphocytes with irregular nuclear contours are seen, consistent with small forms of Sézary cells ➡.

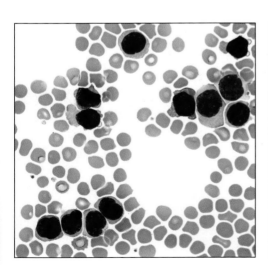

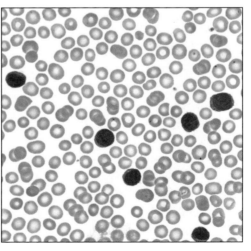

(Left) Peripheral blood smear of a patient with Sézary syndrome. Note many large forms of Sézary cells. *(Right)* Peripheral blood smear of a patient with Sézary syndrome shows smaller forms of Sézary cells.

Lymph Node of Patients with SS

(Left) Lymph node biopsy specimen of a patient with Sézary syndrome. Infiltration of the capsule by medium-sized lymphocytes is shown. **(Right)** Lymph node biopsy specimen of a patient with Sézary syndrome (SS). Lymph nodes obtained from SS patients often show complete or partial architectural effacement, as illustrated in this figure. The tumor cells are of medium size with irregular nuclei.

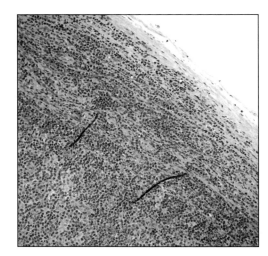 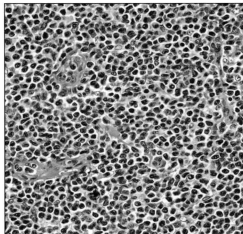

(Left) Lymph node biopsy specimen of a patient with Sézary syndrome (SS). In some areas, the lymph node showed pale areas consistent with dermatopathic lymphadenopathy ⊡, common in lymph nodes from SS patients. **(Right)** High-power view of a lymph node biopsy specimen of a patient with SS shows dermatopathic changes with many pigment-containing macrophages, admixed with small to medium-sized lymphocytes.

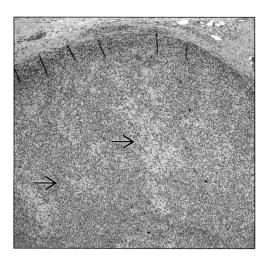 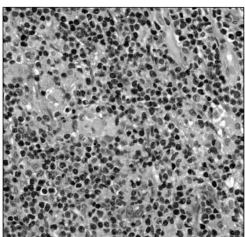

(Left) Lymph node biopsy specimen of a patient with Sézary syndrome (SS). This field shows Langerhans cells, interdigitating cells, and pigmented macrophages, consistent with dermatopathic changes. Sézary cells are also present. **(Right)** Touch imprint of lymph node biopsy specimen involved by SS shows many Sézary cells, mainly medium-sized. Also present are cells consistent with either Langerhans or interdigitating dendritic cells ⊡.

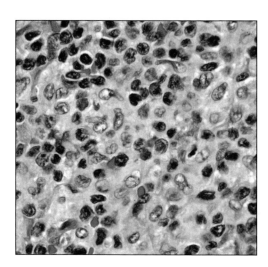 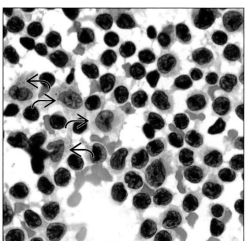

10

SEZARY SYNDROME

Differential Diagnosis

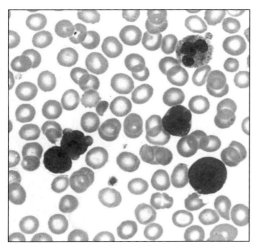

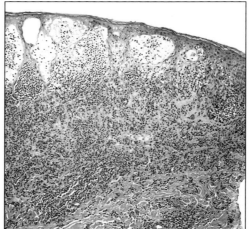

(Left) Peripheral blood smear shows neoplastic flower-like cells typical of HTLV-1-associated adult T-cell leukemia/lymphoma. *(Right)* Skin biopsy specimen involved by adult T-cell leukemia/lymphoma (ATLL). Skin involvement is seen in approximately 50% of patients with ATLL. This field shows an epidermal and dermal lymphocytic infiltrate, with bullae in the epidermis.

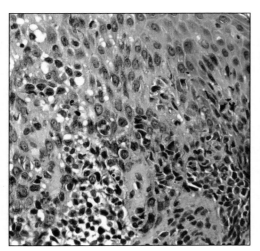

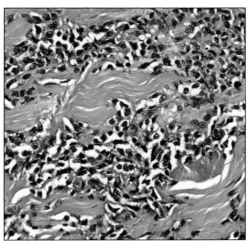

(Left) Skin biopsy specimen involved by adult T-cell leukemia/lymphoma (ATLL). The lymphocytes are of medium to large size and exhibit epidermotropism. *(Right)* Skin biopsy specimen involved by adult T-cell leukemia/lymphoma (ATLL). The lymphocytes infiltrate the collagen of the dermis, are of medium to large size, and have angulated nuclear contours.

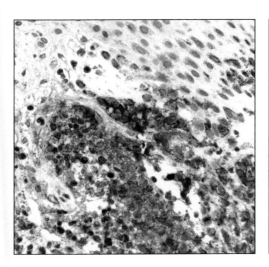

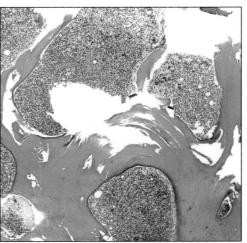

(Left) Skin biopsy specimen involved by adult T-cell leukemia/lymphoma (ATLL). The ATLL cells are strongly CD25(+). The tumor cells of ATLL have an immunophenotype of regulatory T cells: CD4(+), CD25(+), FOXP3(+). *(Right)* Bone marrow biopsy specimen of a patient with T-prolymphocytic leukemia shows an extensive lymphocytic infiltrate in a diffuse pattern.

Differential Diagnosis

(Left) Bone marrow biopsy specimen of a patient with T-prolymphocytic leukemia. The tumor cells are predominantly small and are present in an interstitial and diffuse pattern. *(Right)* Peripheral blood smear involved by T-cell prolymphocytic leukemia shows small neoplastic lymphocytes, each with a prominent nucleolus.

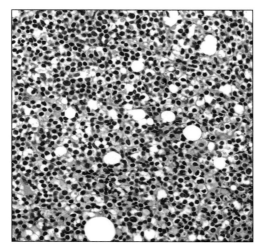
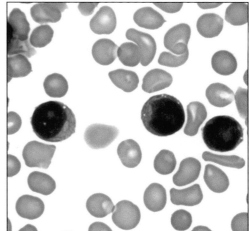

(Left) Skin biopsy specimen involved by acute monocytic leukemia (leukemia cutis). The neoplasm diffusely involves the deep dermis and has a perivascular pattern in the upper dermis. The patient had a history of acute monocytic leukemia. *(Right)* Skin biopsy specimen involved by acute monocytic leukemia (leukemia cutis). High-power view shows that the cellular infiltrate consists of intermediate to large cells with irregular nuclear contours.

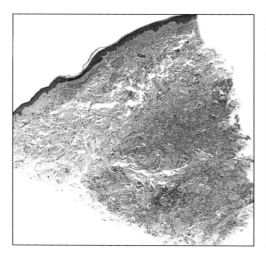
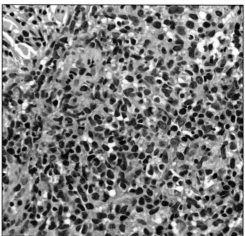

(Left) Skin biopsy specimen involved by acute monocytic leukemia (leukemia cutis). The tumor cells are CD4(+), supporting monocytic lineage. *(Right)* Skin biopsy specimen involved by acute monocytic leukemia (leukemia cutis). The tumor cells are strongly CD68(+), supporting monocytic lineage.

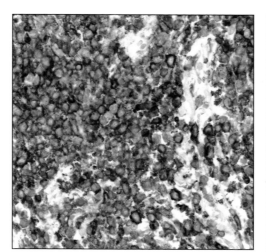
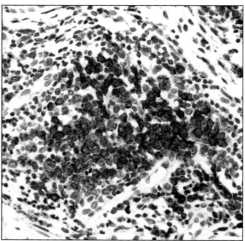

SEZARY SYNDROME

Flow Cytometric Immunophenotyping and Vβ Analysis

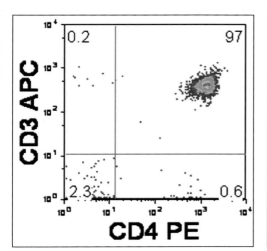
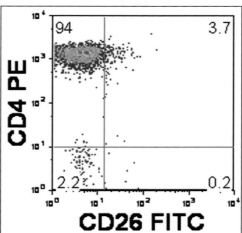

(*Left*) *Peripheral blood specimen involved by Sézary syndrome (SS). Almost all events are CD3(+), CD4(+) T cells. A markedly increased CD4:CD8 ratio supports the diagnosis of SS.* (*Right*) *Peripheral blood specimen involved by Sézary syndrome. CD4(+) T cells are CD26(-), which is aberrant. Normal CD4(+) T cells are mostly CD26(+).*

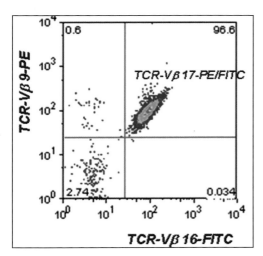
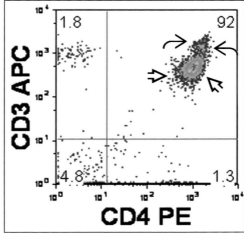

(*Left*) *Peripheral blood specimen involved by Sézary syndrome. The CD4(+) Sézary cells are Vβ 17-restricted, confirming clonality.* (*Right*) *Another case of SS shows a large population of CD3 (dimmer +), CD4 (dimmer+) ⊵ cells as well as a small number of CD4(+) T cells with normal expression of CD3 and CD4 ⊳.*

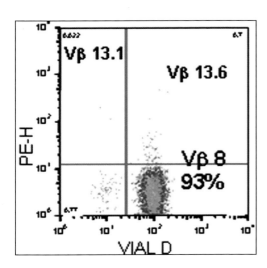
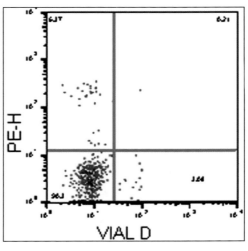

(*Left*) *Peripheral blood specimen involved by Sézary syndrome. A large population of CD3 (dimmer +), CD4 (dimmer +) T cells is Vβ 8-restricted, confirming clonality of immunophenotypically aberrant T cells.* (*Right*) *Peripheral blood specimen involved by Sézary syndrome. The small population of CD3(+), CD4(+) T cells shows no Vβ restriction, confirming that they are normal CD4(+) T cells (a total of 24 Vβ repertoires tested).*

PRIMARY CUTANEOUS ANAPLASTIC LARGE CELL LYMPHOMA

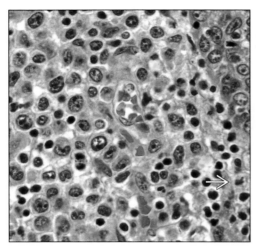

Excisional skin biopsy specimen shows cutaneous anaplastic large cell lymphoma (C-ALCL) composed of sheets of intermediate and large anaplastic lymphoid cells with frequent mitoses ➔.

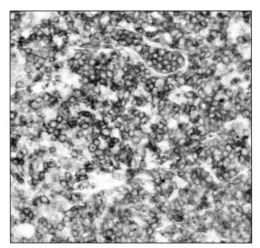

Skin biopsy specimen of C-ALCL. Immunohistochemistry showed that the neoplastic cells are uniformly and strongly CD30(+).

TERMINOLOGY

Abbreviations
- Primary cutaneous anaplastic large cell lymphoma (C-ALCL)

Synonyms
- Primary cutaneous CD30(+) T-cell lymphoproliferative disorder
  - This term also includes lymphomatoid papulosis

Definitions
- Cutaneous lymphoma composed of large T cells that express CD30 (> 75%)

ETIOLOGY/PATHOGENESIS

Unknown
- CD30/TRAF1/IRF-4 activation induced upregulation of NF-κB is implicated
- Other suggested factors
  - Viral infection, reduced immunosurveillance
  - Chronic antigenic stimulation, direct oncogenic effect of immunosuppressive drugs
- Gene expression profiling has failed to show genes that clearly distinguish C-ALCL from ALK(-) systemic ALCL
  - Increased expression of skin-homing chemokine receptors may play a role in confining C-ALCL to skin

CLINICAL ISSUES

Epidemiology
- Age
  - Median: 60 years
- Gender
  - M:F = 2-3:1

Site
- Common sites: Face, trunk, and extremities

Presentation
- Solitary nodule or localized nodules or papules; ± ulceration
- Multifocal lesions occur in ~ 20% of patients
- Extracutaneous dissemination in ~ 10% of patients
  - Regional lymph nodes; rarely viscera
- Partial or complete spontaneous regression can occur; relapse is common

Treatment
- Irradiation for localized nodules
- Low-dose methotrexate for multifocal lesions
- Extracutaneous tumors require systemic chemotherapy

Prognosis
- Favorable, with 10-year survival of ~ 90%
- Similar prognosis for patients with localized vs. multifocal skin lesions

MICROSCOPIC PATHOLOGY

Histologic Features
- Diffuse infiltrates of large neoplastic cells mainly located in dermis; can extend into subcutaneous tissue
  - Epidermal involvement ± ulcer
- Variable degree of inflammatory infiltrate consisting of reactive T-cells, histiocytes, eosinophils, and neutrophils
  - Biopsy lesions can be eosinophil-rich or neutrophil-rich (pyogenic)

Cytologic Features
- Anaplastic cells with round to irregular nuclei, prominent eosinophilic nucleoli, and abundant cytoplasm

PRIMARY CUTANEOUS ANAPLASTIC LARGE CELL LYMPHOMA

Key Facts

Terminology
- Cutaneous lymphoma composed of large T cells that express CD30 (> 75%)

Clinical Issues
- Common sites: Face, trunk, and extremities
- Solitary nodule or localized nodules/papules; ± ulceration
- Multifocal lesions occur in ~ 20% of patients
- Extracutaneous dissemination in ~ 10% of patients
- Spontaneous regression can occur; relapse is common
- Favorable prognosis with 10-year survival of ~ 90%

Microscopic Pathology
- Diffuse infiltrates of large neoplastic cells mainly located in dermis; can extend into subcutaneous tissue

- Variable inflammatory cell infiltrate in background
- Anaplastic cells in most cases; ~ 20% nonanaplastic

Ancillary Tests
- > 75% of neoplastic large cells CD30(+)
- CD4(+), cytotoxic proteins(+), cutaneous lymphocyte antigen (+/-)
- CD56(-/+), EMA(-), CD15(-), ALK(-)
- No specific cytogenetic abnormalities identified
- Monoclonal T-cell receptor rearrangements

Top Differential Diagnoses
- Systemic ALK(-) ALCL with cutaneous involvement
- Large cell transformation of mycosis fungoides
- Lymphomatoid papulosis, type C
- Peripheral T-cell lymphoma, NOS

- ~ 20% of cases appear nonanaplastic (pleomorphic or immunoblastic)

ANCILLARY TESTS

Immunohistochemistry
- > 75% of neoplastic large cells are CD30(+)
- Activated CD4(+) T-cell phenotype
- Rarely show CD8(+) T cell or null CD4(-)/CD8(-) immunophenotype
- Variable loss of pan-T-cell antigens: CD2, CD3, CD5, T-cell receptor (βF1)
- Cytotoxic proteins(+), cutaneous lymphocyte antigen (+/-)
- CD56(-/+), EMA(-), CD15(-), ALK(-)

Cytogenetics
- No specific cytogenetic abnormalities identified
- No translocations involving ALK gene at chromosome 2p23
- Array-based comparative genomic hybridization has revealed chromosomal imbalances
  - Gains in 7q, 17q, 21; losses in 3p, 6q, 8p, 13q

Molecular Genetics
- Most cases show monoclonal T-cell receptor rearrangements

DIFFERENTIAL DIAGNOSIS

Systemic ALK(+) ALCL with Cutaneous Involvement
- Children and young adults
- Peripheral lymph nodes and extranodal sites (+)
- CD30(+), ALK(+)
- Translocations involving ALK

Systemic ALK(-) ALCL with Cutaneous Involvement
- Any age; no sex predominance

- Peripheral lymph nodes and extranodal sites
- Poorer prognosis
- CD30(+), ALK(-)

Large Cell Transformation of Mycosis Fungoides (MF)
- Defined in some studies as > 25% large lymphoid cells in infiltrate
  - Cells can be anaplastic and morphologically mimic C-ALCL
  - Epidermotropism may be lost in anaplastic lesions
  - CD30(+), ALK(-)
- Usually adults (often elderly)
- Characteristic clinical course of MF: Patches, plaques, tumors
- At margins of anaplastic lesion look for typical features of MF
- CD4(+) CD8(-) (> 95% of cases)
- Pan-T-cell antigens (+) but CD7 often (-)
- Unfavorable prognosis similar to other cases of tumor phase MF

Lymphomatoid Papulosis (LyP) Type C
- Lesions closely mimic C-ALCL morphologically and are CD30(+)
- Individual skin lesions spontaneously regress within 3-12 weeks
  - May persist in waxing and waning manner
- In some patients, only clinical findings at follow-up can distinguish LyP from C-ALCL

Peripheral T-cell Lymphoma, NOS, with Cutaneous Involvement
- Sheets of medium to large pleomorphic cells involving dermis ± subcutaneous tissue
- Usually spares epidermis
- CD30(-), cutaneous lymphocyte antigen (-)

Subcutaneous Panniculitis-like T-cell Lymphoma
- Median age: 35 years; females > males

T-CELL PROLYMPHOCYTIC LEUKEMIA INVOLVING LYMPH NODE AND OTHER TISSUES

Microscopic Features

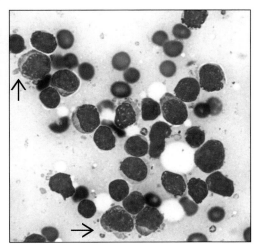

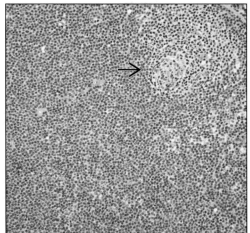

(Left) Fine needle aspirate of cervical lymph node in a patient with T-cell prolymphocytic leukemia (T-PLL). The neoplastic cells have cytoplasmic blebs ➡; nucleoli can be appreciated in a subset of cells. *(Right)* Lymph node involved by T-PLL. The neoplastic cells fill the paracortical region and spare a lymphoid follicle ➡.

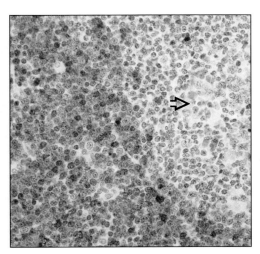

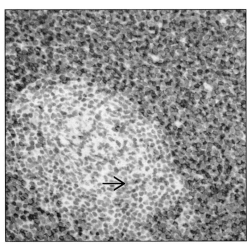

(Left) Lymph node involved by T-cell prolymphocytic leukemia (T-PLL). Tcl-1 immunohistochemical stain shows that the neoplastic cells express Tcl-1 in a nuclear and cytoplasmic pattern. A reactive lymphoid follicle ➡ in the field is negative. *(Right)* Immunohistochemical stain of a lymph node involved by T-PLL shows that the neoplastic cells are CD3(+). A reactive lymphoid follicle is negative except for admixed reactive T cells ➡.

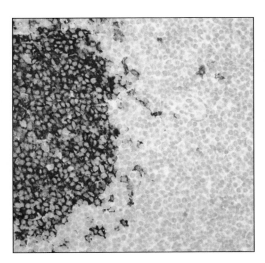

(Left) Immunohistochemical stain of a lymph node involved by T-cell prolymphocytic leukemia (T-PLL) shows that the neoplastic cells are CD20(-). A reactive lymphoid follicle (left of field) is positive for CD20. *(Right)* Spleen involved by T-cell prolymphocytic leukemia (T-PLL). The red and white pulp are infiltrated by neoplastic cells. The spleen of this patient was 832 grams and was removed after chemotherapy and relapse.

T-CELL PROLYMPHOCYTIC LEUKEMIA INVOLVING LYMPH NODE AND OTHER TISSUES

Microscopic Features

(Left) High-power magnification of a spleen involved by T-cell prolymphocytic leukemia (T-PLL) shows red and white pulp with extensive infiltration by neoplastic cells. (Right) High-power magnification of a spleen involved by T-PLL shows neoplastic cells in splenic red pulp.

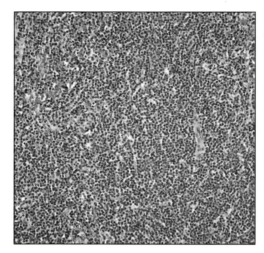 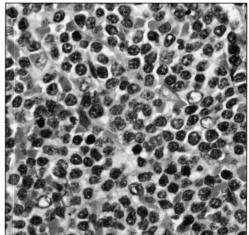

(Left) Immunohistochemical stain of a spleen involved by T-cell prolymphocytic leukemia (T-PLL) shows that the neoplastic cells are CD3(+). Residual B cells in the white pulp are CD3(-) ➡. (Right) Liver involved by T-PLL. Neoplastic cells fill and distend sinuses within a portal tract.

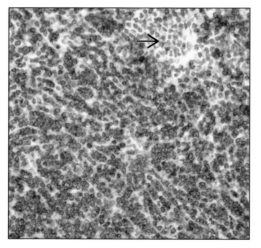 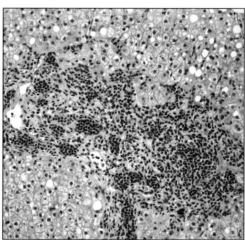

(Left) High-power magnification shows neoplastic cells within a portal tract in this liver involved by T-cell prolymphocytic leukemia (T-PLL). (Right) T-PLL involving peripheral blood. The smear shows that the neoplastic cells have round or irregular nuclear contours and distinctly visible or prominent nucleoli.

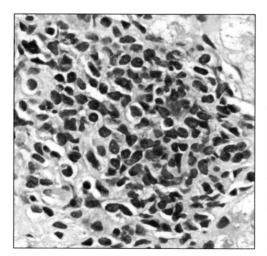 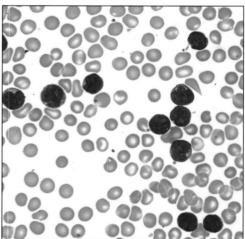

T-CELL PROLYMPHOCYTIC LEUKEMIA INVOLVING LYMPH NODE AND OTHER TISSUES

Microscopic and Clinical Features

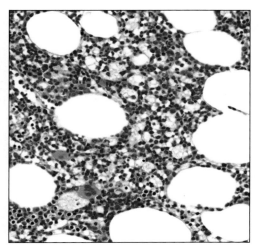

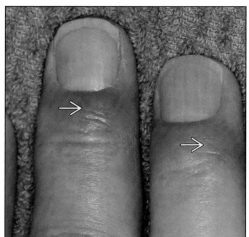

(Left) Bone marrow biopsy specimen involved by T-cell prolymphocytic leukemia (T-PLL). The neoplastic cells are present in an intersitial pattern. (Right) Red skin lesions ➡ are seen on the fingers of a patient with T-PLL. Skin biopsy showed T-PLL in skin.

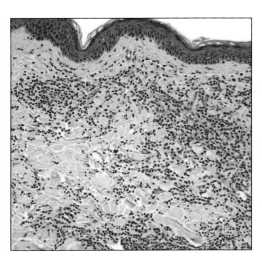

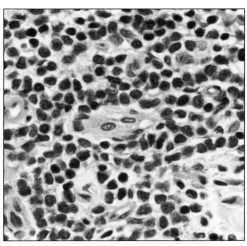

(Left) Skin involved by T-cell prolymphocytic leukemia (T-PLL). Neoplastic lymphocytes involve the dermis in a perivascular pattern. These skin lesions were detected at the time of relapse. (Right) Skin involved by T-PLL. Neoplastic lymphocytes surround a blood vessel in the dermis. These skin lesions were detected at the time of relapse.

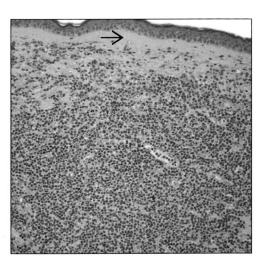

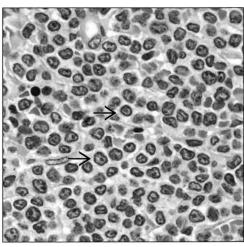

(Left) Skin involved by T-cell prolymphocytic leukemia (T-PLL). Neoplastic lymphocytes fill the dermis. Note the Grenz zone ➡ between the infiltrate and the uninvolved epidermis. (Right) High-power magnification of involved skin in this case of T-PLL shows the neoplastic cells in dermis. The cells have either round or irregular nuclear contours and a subset of cells has prominent nucleoli ➡.

Non-Hodgkin Lymphoma/Lymphoid Neoplasms: Biopsy, Resection

Surgical Pathology Cancer Case Summary (Checklist)

Specimen (select all that apply)

____ Lymph node(s)

____ Other (specify): _____

____ Not specified

Procedure

____ Biopsy

____ Resection

____ Other (specify): _____

____ Not specified

Tumor Site (select all that apply)

____ Lymph node(s), site not specified

____ Lymph node(s)

    Specify site(s): _____

____ Other tissue(s) or organ(s): _____

____ Not specified

Histologic Type

____ Histologic type cannot be assessed

Precursor lymphoid neoplasms

____ B lymphoblastic leukemia/lymphoma, not otherwise specified (NOS)#

____ B lymphoblastic leukemia/lymphoma with t(9;22)(q34;q11.2); *BCR-ABL1*

____ B lymphoblastic leukemia/lymphoma with t(v;11q23); *MLL* rearranged

____ B lymphoblastic leukemia/lymphoma with t(12;21)(p13;q22); *TEL-AML1 (ETV6-RUNX1)*

____ B lymphoblastic leukemia/lymphoma with hyperdiploidy

____ B lymphoblastic leukemia/lymphoma with hypodiploidy (hypodiploid acute lymphoblastic leukemia/lymphoma [ALL])

____ B lymphoblastic leukemia/lymphoma with t(5;14)(q31;q32); *IL3-IGH*

____ B lymphoblastic leukemia/lymphoma with t(1;19)(q23;p13.3); *E2A-PBX1 (TCF3-PBX1)*

____ T lymphoblastic leukemia/lymphoma

Mature B-cell neoplasms

____ B-cell lymphoma, subtype cannot be determined (Note: Not a category within the WHO classification)

____ Chronic lymphocytic leukemia/small lymphocytic lymphoma

____ B-cell prolymphocytic leukemia

____ Splenic B-cell marginal zone lymphoma

____ Hairy cell leukemia

____ Splenic B-cell lymphoma/leukemia, unclassifiable†

____ Splenic diffuse red pulp small B-cell lymphoma†

____ Hairy cell leukemia-variant†

____ Lymphoplasmacytic lymphoma

____ Gamma heavy chain disease

____ Alpha heavy chain disease

____ Plasma cell myeloma

____ Solitary plasmacytoma of bone

____ Extraosseous plasmacytoma

____ Extranodal marginal zone lymphoma of mucosa-associated lymphoid tissue (MALT lymphoma)

____ Nodal marginal zone lymphoma

____ Pediatric nodal marginal zone lymphoma†

____ Follicular lymphoma

____ Pediatric follicular lymphoma†

____ Primary intestinal follicular lymphoma†

____ Primary cutaneous follicle center lymphoma

____ Primary cutaneous follicle center lymphoma

_____ Mantle cell lymphoma

_____ Diffuse large B-cell lymphoma (DLBCL), NOS

_____ T-cell/histiocyte-rich large B-cell lymphoma

_____ Primary DLBCL of central nervous system (CNS)

_____ Primary cutaneous DLBCL, leg type

_____ Epstein-Barr virus (EBV) positive DLBCL of the elderly†

_____ DLBCL associated with chronic inflammation

_____ Lymphomatoid granulomatosis

_____ Primary mediastinal (thymic) large B-cell lymphoma

_____ Intravascular large B-cell lymphoma

_____ Anaplastic lymphoma kinase (ALK) positive large B-cell lymphoma

_____ Plasmablastic lymphoma

_____ Large B-cell lymphoma arising in HHV8-associated multicentric Castleman disease

_____ Primary effusion lymphoma

_____ Burkitt lymphoma

_____ B-cell lymphoma, unclassifiable, with features intermediate between diffuse large B-cell lymphoma and Burkitt lymphoma

_____ Other (specify): _____

Mature T- and NK-cell neoplasms

_____ T-cell lymphoma, subtype cannot be determined (Note: Not a category within the WHO classification)

_____ T-cell prolymphocytic leukemia

_____ T-cell large granular lymphocytic leukemia

_____ Chronic lymphoproliferative disorder of NK cells†

_____ Aggressive NK-cell leukemia

_____ Systemic EBV positive T-cell lymphoproliferative disease of childhood

_____ Hydroa vacciniforme-like lymphoma

_____ Adult T-cell leukemia/lymphoma

_____ Extranodal NK/T-cell lymphoma, nasal type

_____ Enteropathy-associated T-cell lymphoma

_____ Hepatosplenic T-cell lymphoma

_____ Subcutaneous panniculitis-like T-cell lymphoma

_____ Primary cutaneous anaplastic large cell lymphoma

_____ Lymphomatoid papulosis

_____ Primary cutaneous gamma-delta T-cell lymphoma

_____ Primary cutaneous CD8 positive aggressive epidermotropic cytotoxic T-cell lymphoma†

_____ Peripheral T-cell lymphoma, NOS

_____ Angioimmunoblastic T-cell lymphoma

_____ Anaplastic large cell lymphoma, ALK positive

_____ Anaplastic large cell lymphoma, ALK negative†

_____ Other (specify): _____

Histiocytic and dendritic cell neoplasms

_____ Histiocytic sarcoma

_____ Langerhans cell histiocytosis

_____ Langerhans cell sarcoma

_____ Interdigitating dendritic cell sarcoma

_____ Fibroblastic reticular cell tumor†

_____ Indeterminate dendritic cell tumor†

_____ Disseminated juvenile xanthogranuloma

Post-transplant lymphoproliferative disorders (PTLD)##

Early lesions

_____ Plasmacytic hyperplasia

_____ Infectious mononucleosis-like PTLD

_____ Polymorphic PTLD

_____ Monomorphic PTLD (B- and T/NK cell types)

Specify subtype: _____

PROTOCOL FOR EXAMINATION OF NON-HODGKIN LYMPHOMA SPECIMENS

____ Classical Hodgkin lymphoma type PTLD###

Pathologic Extent of Tumor (select all that apply)

*____ Involvement of a single lymph node region

    *Specify site: _____

*____ Involvement of ≥ 2 lymph node regions on same side of diaphragm

    *Specify site: _____

*____ Spleen involvement

*____ Liver involvement

*____ Bone marrow involvement

*____ Other site involvement

    *Specify site(s): _____

Additional Pathologic Findings

    *Specify: _____

Immunophenotyping (Flow Cytometry &/or Immunohistochemistry)

____ Performed, see separate report: _____

____ Performed

    *Specify method(s) and results: _____

*____ Not performed

Cytogenetic Studies

____ Performed, see separate report: _____

____ Performed

    *Specify method(s) and results: _____

*____ Not performed

Molecular Genetic Studies

____ Performed, see separate report: _____

____ Performed

    *Specify method(s) and results: _____

*____ Not performed

Clinical Prognostic Factors and Indices (select all that apply)

*____ International Prognostic Index (IPI) (specify): _____

*____ Follicular Lymphoma International Prognostic Index (FLIPI) (specify): _____

*____ B symptoms present

*____ Other (specify): _____

†Denotes provisional entities in the 2008 WHO classification. #An initial diagnosis of "B lymphoblastic leukemia/lymphoma, NOS" may need to be given before the cytogenetic results are available. ##These disorders are listed for completeness, but not all of them represent frank lymphomas. ###Classical Hodgkin lymphoma type PTLD can be reported using either this protocol or the separate College of American Pathologists protocol for Hodgkin lymphoma. Adapted with permission from College of American Pathologists, "Protocol for the Examination of Specimens from Patients with Non-Hodgkin Lymphoma/Lymphoid Neoplasms." Web posting date June 2010, www.cap.org.

Immunodeficiency-associated Lymphoproliferations

OVERVIEW OF LYMPHOPROLIFERATIVE DISORDERS ASSOCIATED WITH PRIMARY IMMUNE DEFICIENCY DISORDERS

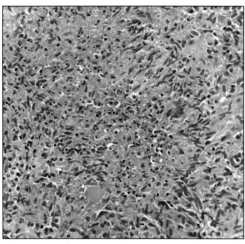

Chronic granulomatous inflammation involving lymph node in a patient with common variable immunodeficiency (CVID).

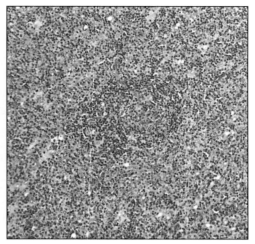

B-cell lymphoma with polymorphous features in a patient with ataxia-telangiectasia (AT).

TERMINOLOGY

Definitions
- Lymphomas and lymphoma-like lesions arising in clinical setting of primary immunodeficiency
  - Primary immunodeficiency disorders are a heterogeneous group of genetic diseases that result in an immunocompromised state

Abbreviations
- Primary immunodeficiency disorders (PID)

Synonyms
- Primary immune disorders
- Congenital immunodeficiency diseases (disorders)

EPIDEMIOLOGY

Incidence
- Variable incidence of clinically evident PID in USA
  - Cumulative incidence: 1 in 10,000
  - Incidence likely higher but some diseases are not evident clinically
- Lymphoproliferative disorders (LPDs) associated with PID
  - LPDs are most common neoplasms in patients with PID
    - Up to 75% of all neoplasms in a given PID
  - Risk of developing LPD varies by type of PID, ranging 0.7-15% (accurate estimation is difficult due to low incidence)

Age Range
- PIDs are more common in pediatric age group
  - Exception: Common variable immunodeficiency disease (CVID) occurs in adults
- Median age of LPD onset: 7.1 years (per Immunodeficiency-Cancer Registry)
- Recent increase in LPDs at older ages due to better survival of PID patients

Gender
- More common in males; true for X-linked as well as for autosomal recessive disorders

ETIOLOGY/PATHOGENESIS

Etiology
- Gene mutations account for many PIDs
  - X-linked hyper-IgM syndrome (XHIGM): *CD40* or *CD40 ligand (CD40LG)*
  - Autoimmune lymphoproliferative syndrome (ALPS): *FAS* or *FAS ligand (FASLG)*
  - Ataxia-telangiectasia (AT): *ATM*
  - Nijmegen breakage syndrome (NBS): *NBS1 (nibrin)*
- Complex abnormalities account for other PIDs
  - Wiskott-Aldrich syndrome exhibits defective function of T cells, B cells, neutrophils, and macrophages

Pathogenesis
- Basis for increased risk of hematologic neoplasms is poorly understood; likely multifactorial
  - Epstein-Barr virus infection drives subset of LPDs in PID settings
  - Defective DNA mismatch repair involved in AT and NBS
  - Possible underlying immune defect against cancer cells

CLINICAL IMPLICATIONS

Clinical Presentation
- Patients with PID often present with recurrent infection
  - Fever, fatigue, infectious-mononucleosis-like syndrome

OVERVIEW OF LYMPHOPROLIFERATIVE DISORDERS
ASSOCIATED WITH PRIMARY IMMUNE DEFICIENCY DISORDERS

- Lymphadenopathy &/or hepatosplenomegaly occur in ALPS and X-linked lymphoproliferative syndrome (XLP)
  - In XLP, fulminant infectious mononucleosis (FIM) can occur, which is marked by fever, rash, generalized lymphadenopathy, and hepatomegaly

Site
- LPDs in PID often present in extranodal sites

Treatment
- Reduced risk of LPD after allogeneic stem cell transplant in PIDs
- Limited data due to rarity of PIDs and lack of randomized trials
- Recommendation is to treat with histologic subtype-specific protocol
- Possible role for immunoregulatory therapy (e.g., interferon-α 2b)

Prognosis
- Related to both underlying PID and type of LPD
  - Most LPDs in PID patients are clinically aggressive
  - Self limited, ALPS; clinically indolent, common variable immunodeficiency (CVID)
- Newer antimicrobial therapies that allow more aggressive treatments have improved prognosis
- Fatal hemophagocytic syndrome can occur in EBV-driven infectious mononucleosis
  - Occurs in XLP and severe combined immunodeficiency (SCID)

MICROSCOPIC FINDINGS

Nonneoplastic Lesions in Lymph Nodes
- Spectrum of morphologic abnormalities
- Subtle alterations may require immunophenotyping
- Common findings
  - Lymphoid depletion
  - Atrophic follicles with progressive depletion of germinal centers
  - Depletion of small lymphocytes in paracortical region with increase in histiocytes and plasma cells
  - Similar findings observed in spleen and tonsils at autopsy
- Secondary changes
  - Chronic granulomatous inflammation secondary to infections
  - Florid reactive hyperplasia
  - Atypical hyperplasia
- Fatal infectious mononucleosis (FIM) resulting from EBV infection (XLP, SCID)
  - Extreme atypical hyperplasia
  - Polymorphous lymphoid cells with plasmacytoid and immunoblastic differentiation
  - Systemic uncontrolled proliferation of abnormal B cells
  - Frequent hemophagocytic syndrome, most readily identified on bone marrow aspirates
- Waxing and waning lymphoproliferations (CVID)
  - Variable morphology showing follicular hyperplasia and paracortical expansion with many EBV(+) cells

- Characteristic nodular lymphoid hyperplasia in gastrointestinal tract
- Autoimmune lymphoproliferative syndrome
  - Expansion of CD4(-), CD8(-) T cells (so-called double negative cells)
  - Increased CD5(+) polyclonal B cells
  - Prominent follicular hyperplasia
- X-linked hyper-IgM syndrome
  - Extensive accumulation of IgM-producing plasma cells in extranodal sites without malignant transformation
  - Peripheral blood B-cells express only IgM and IgD

Precursor Lesions
- Broad morphologic spectrum
- Increasingly dominant clonal population, from polyclonal, to oligoclonal, to monoclonal
- Monoclonal expansions may or may not progress to major persistent lesions

Neoplastic Lesions
- Increased risk of developing leukemias, lymphomas and nonhematopoietic tumors (lymphoma > leukemia)
- In general, morphology and immunophenotype similar to lymphomas in immunocompetent hosts
- Polymorphous cytologic features commonly seen
- Non-Hodgkin lymphoma
  - Overall, B-cell more common than T-cell lymphomas
    - Exception: In ataxia-telangiectasia, T-cell lymphoma/leukemia is common
  - Diffuse large B-cell lymphoma (DLBCL) is most common NHL in PID patients
    - Immunophenotype similar to DLBCLs in immunocompetent patients
    - If EBV(+): Focal expression or absence of CD20 and CD79a; aberrant CD30(+)
  - Many cases are polymorphous with plasmacytoid differentiation
  - Frequently EBV(+)
  - Burkitt lymphoma is more common in XLP than in other PIDs
- Hodgkin lymphoma (HL)
  - 2nd most common LPD per Immunodeficiency Cancer Registry
    - ~ 10% of all lymphomas in PID patients
  - Classical HL most common in PID patients
    - Lymphocyte depleted and mixed cellularity types more common due to feeble immune response
    - HRS cells: CD15(+/-), CD30(+), pax-5(+, dim), CD45/LCA(-)
  - NLPHL relatively uncommon except in patients with ALPS

CLASSIFICATION

Immunodeficiencies
- Combined T- and B-cell immunodeficiencies
  - Severe combined immunodeficiency (SCID)
  - X-linked hyper-IgM syndrome
- Predominantly antibody deficiencies

11

OVERVIEW OF LYMPHOPROLIFERATIVE DISORDERS ASSOCIATED WITH PRIMARY IMMUNE DEFICIENCY DISORDERS

- ○ Common variable immunodeficiency (CVID)
- Other well-defined immunodeficiency syndromes
  - ○ Ataxia-telangiectasia (AT)
  - ○ Nijmegen breakage syndrome (NBS)
  - ○ Wiskott-Aldrich syndrome (WAS)
- Diseases of immune dysregulation
  - ○ Autoimmune lymphoproliferative syndrome (ALPS)
  - ○ X-linked lymphoproliferative disorder (XLP)
- Congenital defects of phagocyte number, function, or both
- Defects in innate immunity
- Autoinflammatory disorders
- Complement deficiencies

DIAGNOSTIC TESTS

Laboratory Tests to Diagnose PID
- Multiple tests may be required to establish diagnosis of PID; however, testing for LPD in PID is same as in immunocompetent hosts
- Complete blood count
- Immunophenotyping of T and B cells
- Serum protein electrophoresis and immunofixation
- Measurement of serum levels of vitamins, cytokines, ligands, and immunoglobulins
- In vitro functional assays
- Testing for autoantibodies
- Molecular genetic testing for gene mutations

Molecular Genetic Testing to Diagnose LPD
- Antigen receptor gene rearrangement
  - ○ Gene clonality useful for establishing diagnosis of LPD; may not predict clinical behavior
    - Polyclonal LPD can be fatal, such as in fatal infectious mononucleosis; monoclonal LPD can be indolent
  - ○ Monoclonal immunoglobulin heavy and light chain gene rearrangements present in overt B-cell lymphomas, limited information on T-cell clonality
- EBV DNA
  - ○ EBV infection common in many LPDs in PID
  - ○ Demonstration of EBV possible at molecular level using specific probes
  - ○ EBV terminal repeat analysis may be helpful in establishing monoclonality
- Oncogenes
  - ○ Defects related to primary immune defect: *FAS* mutation in ALPS, mutations in gene encoding *SAP/SLAM* in XLP
  - ○ Defects occurring during course of LPDs: Inversions &/or translocations of *T-cell receptor (TCR)* genes in AT
- Chromosomal translocations
  - ○ Limited information available
  - ○ AT: In normal state, ~ 10% of lymphocytes have aberrations corresponding to *TCR* genes and *TCL-1*

DIFFERENTIAL DIAGNOSIS FOR NONNEOPLASTIC LESIONS

Neoplastic Hematologic Lesions in PID
- Critical to determine whether LPD is benign or malignant since benign lesions can histologically mimic lymphoma
- Immunophenotyping and molecular studies are useful for this purpose

Benign Lymphoid Tissue in Neonates
- Morphologic spectrum in normal newborns may be difficult to distinguish from PID-related changes
- Lymph nodes at birth are primarily composed of small primary B-follicles in cortex and poorly developed paracortex

Lymphoid Depletion in Longstanding Infections
- Lymphoid depletion in non-PID babies with longstanding infections can be difficult to distinguish from lymphoid depletion in PID

Angioimmunoblastic T-cell Lymphoma
- Overlapping features: Lymphoid depletion, paracortical expansion, polymorphous cell population
- Distinguishing features: AITL occurs mainly in elderly, T cells in PID do not express CD10, Bcl-6, or CXCL13

Castleman Disease, Hyaline Vascular Type
- Overlapping features: Atrophic follicles with lymphocyte depletion and hypervascularity
- Distinguishing features: Clinical history; lymph nodes are not enlarged in PID and lack features such as twinning and "onion skin" appearance

DIFFERENTIAL DIAGNOSIS FOR NEOPLASTIC LESIONS

PID-associated LPDs
- In general, LPDs in PID are histologically and immunophenotypically indistinguishable from lesions arising in immunocompetent hosts
- Differential diagnosis is same as for lesions in immunocompetent hosts
- Clinical history is critical for establishing PID setting

DIAGNOSTIC CHECKLIST

Clinically Relevant Pathologic Features
- Presentation of LPD usually early in life
- Propensity to involve extranodal sites; high frequency of EBV infection
- Broad morphologic and biologic spectrum of lymphoproliferations
- Knowledge of preexisting PID is critical

OVERVIEW OF LYMPHOPROLIFERATIVE DISORDERS ASSOCIATED WITH PRIMARY IMMUNE DEFICIENCY DISORDERS

Epidemiology and Clinical Features of PID

Category	Disease	Inheritance	Population Frequency	Frequency of PID (%)	Clinical Features
T- and B-cell immunodeficiencies	SCID	AR, X	1 in 100,000 live births	1-5	Severe recurrent infections
	XHIGM	X	1 in 20,000,000 live male births	1-2	Pancytopenia, hepatobiliary tract disease, *Pneumocystis jiroveci* infections, diarrhea
Antibody deficiencies	CVID	AD, S	1 in 10-50,000 live births	21-31	Variable phenotype, recurrent bacterial infections
	IgA deficiency	AD, S	1 in 700 individuals of European origin	> 50 (most common)	Prone to bacterial infections
Immune dysregulation	XLP	X	400 documented cases	< 1	EBV infections trigger clinical and immunologic abnormalities
	ALPS	AD, AR	Unknown	< 1	Present in infancy with autoimmune cytopenias, autoimmune diseases
Other syndromes	WAS	X	1 in 250,000 live male births	1-3	Thrombocytopenia with small platelets, eczema
	AT	AR	1 in 40-100,000 live births	2-8	Cerebellar degeneration with progressive ataxia, oculocutaneous telangiectasia
	NBS	AR	1 in 100,000 live births	1-2	Microcephaly, café au lait spots, hypersensitivity to ionizing radiation

SCID = severe combined immunodeficiency; XHIGM = X-linked hyper-IgM syndrome; CVID = common variable immunodeficiency; XLP = X-linked lymphoproliferative syndrome; ALPS = autoimmune lymphoproliferative syndrome; WAS = Wiskott-Aldrich syndrome; AT = ataxia-telangiectasia; NBS = Nijmegen breakage syndrome (NBS); AD = autosomal dominant; AR = autosomal recessive; X = X-linked; S = sporadic.

Malignancies in PID*

Category	Disease	Malignancy Rate (%)	Median Age (years)	Gender (M to F)	Hematologic	Nonhematologic
T- and B-cell immunodeficiencies	SCID	1.5	1.6	3.3 to 1	EBV-associated, FIM, NHL, HL, leukemias	Renal and pulmonary leiomyomata
	XHIGM	7.8	7.2		EBV-associated (DLBCL, HL), LGL leukemia	NA
Antibody deficiencies	CVID	2.5 (onset < 16 years), 8.5 (onset > 16 years)	23	1.3 to 1	NHL (50%); EBV-associated (DLBCL, HL), SLL, MALT lymphoma, LPL, PTCL (2-7%)	Epithelial tumors (39%; stomach, breast, bladder, cervix, vulva)
	IgA deficiency	Rare	NA	NA	HL, leukemia or lymphoma (25%)	NA
Immune dysregulation	XLP	30	NA	NA	EBV-associated (FIM, DLBCL, Burkitt), aplastic anemia	NA
	ALPS	10-20	< 1	NA	Increased risk of NHL (50x) and HL (10x); NLPHL, classical HL, DLBCL, Burkitt, PTCL (3-10%)	NA
Other syndromes	WAS	13	6.2	M only	EBV associated (DLBCL, HL)	Cerebellar astrocytoma, Kaposi sarcoma, muscle tumors
	AT	33	8.5	1.7 to 1	Non-leukemic clonal T-cell proliferations, DLBCL, Burkitt, T-PLL (young adults), T-ALL/LBL (age: 1-5 years), HL (10-30%)	Epithelial tumors
	NBS	Rare	NA	NA	DLBCL, PTCL, T-ALL/LBL, HL (28-36%)	Brain tumors

*Data based on Immunodeficiency Cancer Registry; FIM = fatal infectious mononucleosis; NHL = non-Hodgkin lymphoma; HL = Hodgkin lymphoma; NA = information not available; LGL = large granular lymphocyte; SLL = small lymphocytic lymphoma; MALT = mucosa-associated lymphoid tissue; LPL = lymphoplasmacytic lymphoma; PTCL = peripheral T-cell lymphoma; NLPHL = nodular lymphocyte predominant HL; ALL/LBL = acute lymphoblastic leukemia/lymphoblastic lymphoma.

SELECTED REFERENCES

1. International Union of Immunological Societies Expert Committee on Primary Immunodeficiencies et al: Primary immunodeficiencies: 2009 update. J Allergy Clin Immunol. 2009 Dec;124(6):1161-78. Erratum in: J Allergy Clin Immunol. 125(3):771-3, 2010
2. Ioachim HL et al: Ioachim's Lymph Node Pathology. 4th ed. Philadelphia: Lippincott Williams & Wilkins. 2009
3. Van Krieken JH et al: Lymphoproliferative disorders associated with primary immune disorders. In Swerdlow SH et al: WHO Classification of Tumours of Haematopoietic and Lymphoid Tissues. Lyon: IARC. 336-9, 2008

OVERVIEW OF LYMPHOPROLIFERATIVE DISORDERS ASSOCIATED WITH PRIMARY IMMUNE DEFICIENCY DISORDERS

Microscopic and Immunohistochemical Features

(Left) Lymph node biopsy specimen shows atypical paracortical hyperplasia in a CVID patient. The overall nodal architecture is distorted but not effaced. The paracortical regions are expanded, vascular proliferation is present, and sinuses are patent. *(Right)* Lymph node shows atypical paracortical hyperplasia in a CVID patient. Higher magnification of paracortical region shows a heterogeneous cell population. There was no evidence of T- or B-cell clonality by PCR analysis.

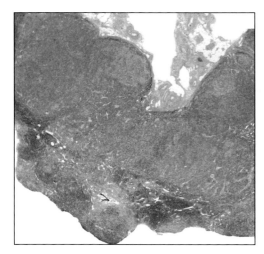
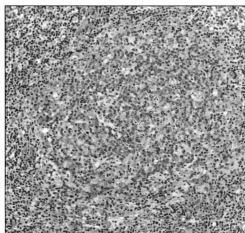

(Left) Lymph node involved by polymorphous B-cell lymphoproliferative disorder (LPD) in a patient with AT. Note the effacement of the interfollicular region. Monoclonal immunoglobulin heavy chain gene rearrangement was detected by PCR. *(Right)* Lymph node involved by polymorphous B-cell LPD in an AT patient. The interfollicular region shows a polymorphic lymphoid infiltrate of predominantly medium-sized lymphocytes ⇨ admixed with large transformed cells ⇨.

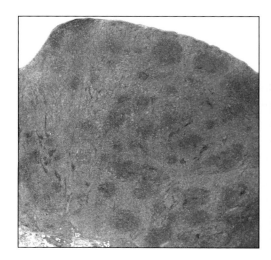
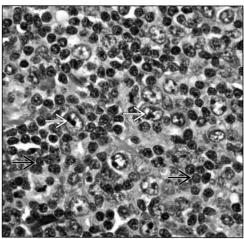

(Left) Lymph node involved by polymorphous B-cell LPD in an AT patient is shown. Most lymphocytes are CD20(+) and show primarily interfollicular staining pattern. By flow cytometry, B cells were CD19(+), CD20(+), and dim monotypic immunoglobulin kappa(+). *(Right)* Lymph node involved by polymorphous B-cell LPD in an AT patient. The atypical cells are CD3(-). There is a marked increase of CD3(+) T-lymphocytes in a dystrophic follicle ⇨.

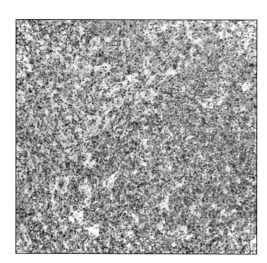
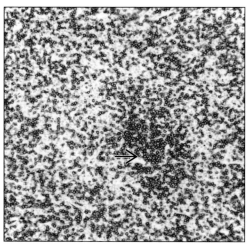

OVERVIEW OF LYMPHOPROLIFERATIVE DISORDERS ASSOCIATED WITH PRIMARY IMMUNE DEFICIENCY DISORDERS

Microscopic and Immunohistochemical Features

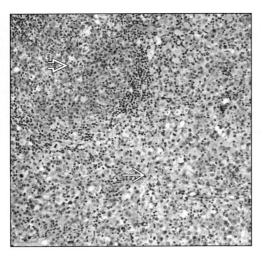
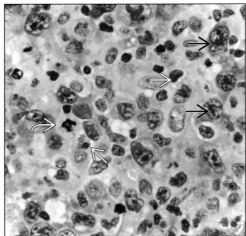

(Left) Lymph node involved by diffuse large B-cell lymphoma (DLBCL) with an interfollicular pattern ➡ in a patient with Wiskott-Aldrich syndrome (WAS). A reactive follicle is also present ➡. (Right) Lymph node involved by DLBCL in a WAS patient. The neoplastic cells ➡ are predominantly intermediate to large sized with irregular nuclear contours, prominent nucleoli, and abundant cytoplasm. There are scattered interspersed eosinophils ➡, and a mitotic figure ➡ is present.

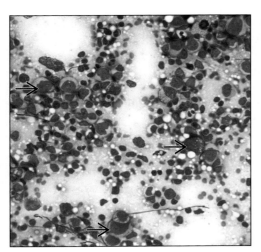
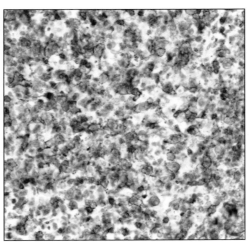

(Left) Touch imprint of lymph node involved by DLBCL in a WAS patient. Note the many large cells ➡. A mixed inflammatory cell infiltrate is also present in the background. (Right) Lymph node involved by DLBCL in a WAS patient. Anti-CD20 antibody highlights large atypical B cells. Flow cytometric immunophenotyping showed that the B cells were CD19(+), CD20(+), and monotypic immunoglobulin κ light chain(+).

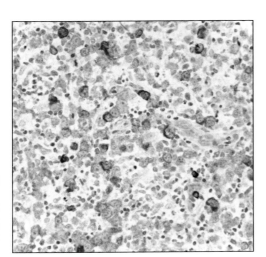
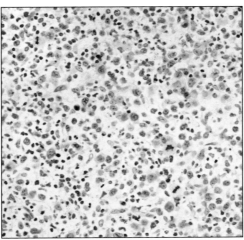

(Left) Lymph node involved by DLBCL in a WAS patient. The large neoplastic cells are immunoglobulin κ light chain(+), shown by immunohistochemistry. (Right) Lymph node involved by DLBCL in a WAS patient. The large neoplastic cells are immunoglobulin λ light chain(-) by immunohistochemistry.

11

AUTOIMMUNE LYMPHOPROLIFERATIVE SYNDROME

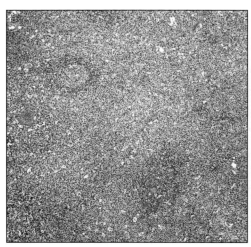

Autoimmune lymphoproliferative syndrome (ALPS) involving lymph node. The paracortex of the lymph node is markedly expanded. Small lymphoid follicles are also present.

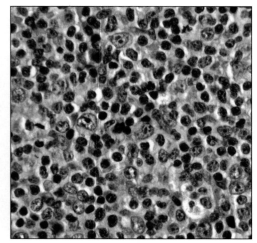

ALPS involving lymph node. The paracortex is populated by small lymphocytes and many large immunoblasts with prominent nucleoli.

TERMINOLOGY

Abbreviations
- Autoimmune lymphoproliferative syndrome (ALPS)

Definitions
- Disease of disrupted lymphocyte homeostasis as result of defective Fas-mediated apoptosis

ETIOLOGY/PATHOGENESIS

Genetic Mutations in FAS Pathway
- FAS pathway mutations cause ALPS
- FAS mutations are usually heterozygous
- Multiple types have been described
- **Type I**: Accounts for approximately 65% of all ALPS cases
  - 3 type I subtypes
    - Ia: Germline mutations in FAS (TNFRSF6, CD95, APO1) gene
    - Ib: Germline mutations in FAS ligand gene
    - Is: Somatic mutations in FAS gene
- **Type II**: Germline mutations in gene encoding caspase 10
- **Type III**: No identifiable genetic mutations in FAS pathway
  - Accounts for approximately 20-30% of all ALPS cases
- **Type IV**: Very rare
  - Gain-of-function mutation in NRAS
  - Patients have ALPS phenotype but normal Fas-mediated apoptosis
- ALPS is multistep process requiring more than a single genetic hit for clinical expression
- In most cases, mutations are inherited in autosomal dominant fashion
  - Therefore, penetrance is 100% at cellular level
  - Penetrance for clinical phenotype of ALPS is variable
- Significant proportion of family members can have mutation without phenotype of ALPS
- Additional factors must contribute to expression of disease

CASPASE 8 Mutations
- Once considered part of ALPS
- Present with lymphadenopathy and defective Fas-mediated apoptosis
- Profound apoptotic defects in B, T, and NK cells
- Patients often have mucocutaneous herpes virus infections
- Therefore, CASP8 mutations are now considered to represent a distinct disease

CLINICAL ISSUES

Presentation
- Chronic nonmalignant lymphoproliferation, often appearing in 1st year of life
  - Chronic &/or recurrent lymphadenopathy in ~ 80% of patients
  - Splenomegaly with/without hypersplenism in ~ 85% of patients
  - Hepatomegaly in ~ 45% of patients
  - Lymphocytic interstitial pneumonia
- Autoimmune diseases in ~ 70% of patients
  - Cytopenias are most frequent
    - Autoimmune hemolytic anemia
    - Immune thrombocytopenia
    - Autoimmune neutropenia
    - More than 1 lineage is often affected
  - Evans syndrome
    - Originally described in 1951
    - Autoimmune destruction of erythrocytes and platelets
    - Subset of these patients has ALPS
  - Other less common autoimmune phenomena in ALPS include

11

AUTOIMMUNE LYMPHOPROLIFERATIVE SYNDROME

Key Facts

Etiology/Pathogenesis

- Disease of disrupted lymphocyte homeostasis as result of defective Fas-mediated apoptosis
- Many mutations have been identified in ALPS
- Type I: Accounts for approximately 65% of all ALPS cases; 3 subtypes
  - Ia: Germline mutations in *FAS* gene
  - Ib: Germline mutations in *FAS ligand* gene
  - Is: Somatic mutations in *FAS* gene
- Type II: Germline mutations in gene encoding caspase 10
- Type III: Accounts for approximately 20-30% of all ALPS cases
  - No identifiable genetic mutations in *FAS* pathway
- Type IV: Very rare; gain-of-function mutation in *NRAS*

Clinical Issues

- Chronic nonmalignant lymphoproliferation
  - Lymph nodes, spleen, liver
- Autoimmune disease
- Increased risk for lymphoma

Microscopic Pathology

- Marked paracortical expansion with increased DNT cells

Ancillary Tests

- Flow cytometry
  - Increased DNT cells: TCR-α/β(+), CD3(+), CD4(-), CD8(-)
- Apoptosis assay: Defective FAS-induced apoptosis in ALPS types Ia and Ib

---

- Skin rash: Often of urticarial nature
- Autoimmune hepatitis
- Autoimmune glomerulonephritis
- Autoimmune thyroiditis
- Uveitis and Guillain-Barré syndrome
- Vasculitis and panniculitis
- Autoimmune colitis
- Autoimmune cerebellar syndrome
- Patients followed into adulthood have increased risk of pulmonary fibrosis
- ALPS patients have increased risk of malignancies of various types
  - Increased risk of Hodgkin lymphoma and non-Hodgkin lymphoma
    - 51x increased risk of Hodgkin lymphoma
    - 14x increased risk of non-Hodgkin lymphoma
    - Usually not related to Epstein-Barr virus infection
  - Increased risk of carcinomas
    - Thyroid, breast, liver, tongue, skin
  - Increased risk of leukemias
  - Some ALPS patients present with multiple neoplasms (thyroid/breast adenomas, gliomas)
- Presentation related to type of genetic mutation
  - Homozygous or compound heterozygous *FAS* mutations lead to
    - Severe lymphoproliferation before, at, or shortly after birth
    - Patients typically succumb to lymphoproliferation &/or autoimmunity at early age
  - Mutations in any domain of Fas lead to same clinical phenotype of ALPS
    - Lymphoma is most often associated with mutations affecting intracellular domains of Fas

Laboratory Tests

- Peripheral blood lymphocytosis
- Serum
  - Elevated concentrations of IgG, IgA, and IgE; normal or decreased concentration of IgM
  - Increased levels of interleukin (IL)-10
  - Increased levels of vitamin B12
- Autoimmune antibodies

- Autoantibodies to red cells, platelets, and neutrophils are often found
- Anti-smooth muscle and anti-phospholipid antibodies can be positive
- Anti-nuclear antibodies and rheumatoid factor can be positive
- Flow cytometric immunophenotyping of peripheral blood shows increased double negative T cells
  - Double negative T cells (DNT) = TCR-α/β(+), CD3(+), CD4(-), CD8(-)
    - Normal range: DNT cells have been expressed as percentage of total lymphocytes; total T cells and TCR-α/β(+) T cells in various studies
    - Normal range may differ according to patient age and flow cytometry gating strategy
    - DNT cells are increased if > 1% of total T cells (peripheral blood)
    - Markedly increased (3-60%) DNTs in peripheral blood is very specific for ALPS
    - Present in all subtypes of ALPS
    - Found in peripheral blood, lymph nodes, spleen, and other tissues
    - Role of DNT cells in ALPS, and whether these cells are pathogenic or merely a marker of disease, remains to be determined
  - Other flow cytometry findings
    - Increased TCR-γ/δ(+) DNT cells
    - Increased CD8(+), CD57(+) T cells
    - Increased CD5(+) B cells
    - Increased HLA-DR(+) T cells
    - Decreased CD27(+) B cells
    - Decreased CD4(+), CD25(+) regulatory T cells
  - DNT can be increased in other autoimmune diseases
    - Usually low-level increase of DNT in these diseases
    - Systemic lupus erythematosus
    - Immune thrombocytopenic purpura
  - *FAS* mutations in 100% of DNT population in somatic ALPS patients suggests that these cells contribute to disease pathogenesis
- In vitro Fas-mediated apoptosis assays are helpful for diagnosis of ALPS

AUTOIMMUNE LYMPHOPROLIFERATIVE SYNDROME

- ○ Isolate peripheral blood mononuclear cells from ALPS patient
- ○ Activate T cells with mitogen and expand with IL-2 in culture for 28 days
- ○ Expose T cells to anti-Fas IgM antibody
  - ■ Normal T cells: Rapid cell death and apoptosis
  - ■ ALPS T cells: No or impaired cell death
- ○ Type of ALPS mutation yields different results for in vitro Fas-mediated apoptosis
  - ■ Type I: Often exhibit defective FAS-induced apoptosis
  - ■ Types II and III: No defective FAS-induced apoptosis
- Molecular genetic assays
  - ○ FAS
    - ■ FAS germline mutations identified throughout entire coding region and exons/introns of FAS
    - ■ Sequencing of entire coding region and intron/exon boundaries of FAS gene detects ~ 90% of mutations
    - ■ FAS somatic mutation detection often performed on sorted DNT cells
  - ○ FASLG
    - ■ Sequence analysis of entire coding region of FASLG gene is available clinically
  - ○ CASP10
    - ■ Sequence analysis of entire coding region of CASP10 gene is available clinically

Natural History
- Nonmalignant lymphoproliferative manifestations in ALPS often regress or improve over time
- Autoimmunity shows no permanent remission with advancing age
- Risk for development of lymphoma appears to be lifelong

Treatment
- Some patients with ALPS require no treatment
- Hemolytic anemia and thrombocytopenia
  - ○ Prednisone
  - ○ Immunosuppressant
    - ■ Mycophenolate mofetil (Cellcept)
    - ■ Sirolimus (rapamycin)
  - ○ Only a few patients respond to intravenous immunoglobulin
  - ○ Rituximab: Anti-CD20 monoclonal chimeric antibody
    - ■ Percentage of ALPS patients are predisposed to develop common variable immunodeficiency disease (CVID) upon rituximab treatment
    - ■ Reserved for patients who fail all other therapies
  - ○ Splenectomy to control autoimmune cytopenias is discouraged
    - ■ ALPS patients have increased risk of developing post-splenectomy sepsis despite vaccination and antibiotic prophylaxis
    - ■ No long-term effect to control cytopenia(s)
- Bone marrow (hematopoietic stem cell) transplantation carries risks
  - ○ Reduced-intensity transplant can reduce transplant-associated risks

Prognosis
- Refer to natural history

Recently Proposed Diagnostic Criteria for ALPS
- Major
  - ○ 1: Chronic nonmalignant lymphoproliferation
    - ■ > 6 months
    - ■ Splenomegaly &/or lymphadenopathy of at least 2 nodal groups
  - ○ 2: Marked elevation of peripheral blood DNTs of at least 5%
  - ○ 3: Defective in vitro Fas-mediated apoptosis
  - ○ 4: Identifiable genetic mutation, germline or somatic
    - ■ FAS, FASL, CASP10, NRAS
- Minor
  - ○ 1: Autoimmune cytopenias
    - ■ Thrombocytopenia, neutropenia, &/or hemolytic anemia
    - ■ Proven to be immune-mediated by autoantibody detection or response to immunosuppressive agent
  - ○ 2: Moderate elevation in DNTs
  - ○ 3: Elevated serum IgG
  - ○ 4: Elevated serum IL-10
  - ○ 5: Elevated serum vitamin B12
  - ○ 6: Elevated plasma Fas ligand level
- Diagnosis established if
  - ○ 3 major criteria present or
  - ○ 2 major + 2 minor criteria present

IMAGE FINDINGS

Radiographic Findings
- Imaging studies detect lymphadenopathy or hepatosplenomegaly
- Lymphoproliferations in ALPS are FDG PET avid
- Cannot distinguish benign from malignant; therefore, biopsy needed

MICROSCOPIC PATHOLOGY

Lymph Nodes
- Marked expansion of paracortical (T-cell) zones
  - ○ Lymphocytes show various stages of immunoblastic transformation
    - ■ Small, intermediate, and large lymphocytes; often with clear cytoplasm
    - ■ Increased immunoblasts
    - ■ Mitotic figures increased
  - ○ Small plasma cells without atypia are common
  - ○ Eosinophils or neutrophils are typically absent
  - ○ Reduced or absent tingible body macrophages
  - ○ Some cases may show prominent postcapillary venules
- Germinal centers show a spectrum of reactive changes ranging from
  - ○ Florid follicular hyperplasia
    - ■ Tingible body macrophages can be prominent

AUTOIMMUNE LYMPHOPROLIFERATIVE SYNDROME

Immunodeficiency-associated Lymphoproliferations

o Progressive transformation of germinal centers (PTGC)
o Atrophic follicles with regressive changes (Castleman-like)
• Changes resembling Rosai-Dorfman disease can occur

Spleen
• Expanded white pulp
  o Reactive follicular hyperplasia
  o Reactive marginal zone hyperplasia
• Expanded red pulp
  o Increased DNT cells
  o Immunoblasts
  o Polytypic plasma cells

Bone Marrow
• ± interstitial lymphoid aggregates
  o Large lymphoid cells

Liver
• Portal tract triaditis
• DNT cells can be increased

ANCILLARY TESTS

Immunohistochemistry
• Immunohistochemistry of lymph node or other tissue site
  o Increased DNT cells
    ▪ TCR-α/β(+), CD3(+), CD4(-), CD8(-)
    ▪ CD45RO(-), CD45RA(+), CD25(-)
  o Large subset of T cells are CD57(+), TIA-1(+), and perforin(+)
  o Small subset of T cells are CD4(+)
  o Small subset of T cells are CD8(+)
  o CD16(-), CD56(-) assessed in frozen tissue
• Follicles express polytypic Ig light chains
  o B-cell antigens(+), Bcl-6(+), Bcl-2(-)
• Plasma cells express polytypic Ig light chains
• Tests for Epstein-Barr virus (EBV) are usually negative
  o EBV-LMP1(-)
  o EBER(-) by in situ hybridization

Flow Cytometry
• Flow cytometry can be performed on cell suspension of lymph node or other tissue site
  o Increased DNT cells

Molecular Genetics
• No evidence of monoclonal *TCR* gene rearrangements
• No evidence of monoclonal *Ig* gene rearrangements
• No distinctive chromosomal translocations
• *FAS* gene mutations

DIFFERENTIAL DIAGNOSIS

Common Variable Immunodeficiency Disease (CVID)
• Specific genetic mutations are unknown, but CVID is likely to be heterogeneous

• Cases with low/absent B cells and low serum concentrations of immunoglobulin (Ig) are usually not confused with ALPS
  o ALPS patients often have normal or increased number of B cells
• Cases with presence of B cells can cause difficulty in differential diagnosis
  o Lymph node
    ▪ Reactive follicular hyperplasia
    ▪ Paracortical expansion without increased DNT cells
    ▪ Often many EBV(+) cells in paracortical areas
    ▪ Frequently associated with granulomatous inflammation of infectious causes
    ▪ Some cases can show atypical lymphoid hyperplasia with markedly expanded B- and T-cell populations
  o Gastrointestinal tract
    ▪ Nodular lymphoid hyperplasia, some with monoclonal Ig rearrangement
  o Nodular lymphoid hyperplasia and granulomas can be seen in many organs
    ▪ Lung, spleen, skin, liver, bone marrow, endocrine organs, brain, etc.

X-linked Lymphoproliferative Syndrome (XLP)
• Mutations in *SH2D1A* gene
• Patients do not manifest significant immune defects until exposure to EBV
• 75% of patients develop fulminant infectious mononucleosis
  o Lymph node shows changes of fulminant infectious mononucleosis
    ▪ Increased immunoblasts and plasma cells
    ▪ Significant necrosis
  o Often associated with hemophagocytic lymphohistiocytosis
  o Most patients succumb to hepatic necrosis &/or bone marrow failure
  o Survivors are at risk for subsequent hypogammaglobulinemia, lymphoma, hemophagocytic syndrome, and aplastic anemia
• Laboratory findings
  o Serologic tests for EBV IgM antibodies(+)
  o Quantitative EBV-specific polymerase chain reaction(+)

Wiskott-Aldrich Syndrome (WAS)
• X-linked; *WASP* mutations
  o WASP is key regulator of signaling and cytoskeletal reorganization in hematopoietic cells
• Clinical presentation
  o Thrombocytopenia
  o Immunodeficiency, eczema
  o Autoimmune manifestations
    ▪ Autoimmune hemolytic anemia, cutaneous vasculitis, arthritis, and nephropathy
  o High susceptibility to developing tumors
• Histologic features of lymph node
  o In early phase of disease, often shows follicular hyperplasia

○ Later stage of disease often shows progressive depletion of germinal centers
○ Paracortical lymphocyte depletion with the following
  ▪ Increased immunoblasts (transformed cells)
  ▪ Increased eosinophils and atypical plasma cells
  ▪ Extramedullary hematopoiesis

Evans Syndrome
• Originally described as patient with 2 autoimmune cytopenias
  ○ Platelets and erythrocytes
• Now clear that some patients with this syndrome have ALPS
• All patients with Evans syndrome should be tested for defects in Fas-mediated apoptosis

Autoimmune Diseases
• Low-level increases in DNTs in blood occur in autoimmune diseases
  ○ Can lead to misdiagnosis as ALPS
• Full autoimmune work-up will show evidence that suggests specific autoimmune disease
• No defects in Fas-mediated apoptosis

Peripheral T-cell Lymphoma (PTCL)
• In most cases, lymph node is completely replaced by PTCL
• Neoplastic cells in PTCL are often associated with eosinophils
• Immunophenotype: PTCL cells are commonly CD4(+), CD8(-) or CD4(-), CD8(+)
• EBV(+) in some types of PTCL
• Monoclonal *TCR* gene rearrangements

DIAGNOSTIC CHECKLIST

Clinically Relevant Pathologic Features
• Lymphadenopathy and hepatosplenomegaly
• Autoimmune diseases
  ○ Cytopenias are most common
  ○ Various organs can be involved
• Defective apoptosis leading to expansion of antigen-specific lymphocyte populations
  ○ Defects are related to gene mutations (mainly of FAS pathway)
• Most mutations are congenital, with germline mutations in *FAS*, *FASL*, and *CASP10*
  ○ Somatic mutations of *FAS* also occur
  ○ In some patients, known mutations have not been found

Pathologic Interpretation Pearls
• Lymph nodes show marked paracortical expansion
  ○ Lymphocytes show various stages of immunoblastic transformation
    ▪ Mitotic figures can be numerous
  ○ Varying degrees of follicular hyperplasia or regressive changes
  ○ Immunophenotyping shows increased DNT cells in paracortex

○ Changes resembling Rosai-Dorfman disease can occur
○ Increased risk of Hodgkin and non-Hodgkin lymphoma
• Immunophenotyping of peripheral blood is helpful
  ○ Increased DNT cells (> 1%)
    ▪ DNT cells = TCR-α/β(+), CD3(+), CD4(-), CD8(-), CD45RA(+); CD45RO(-)
  ○ Increased TCR-γ/δ(+) DNT cells
  ○ Increased CD8(+) and CD57(+) T cells
  ○ Increased CD5(+) B cells and HLA-DR(+) T cells
  ○ Decreased CD27(+) B cells
  ○ Decreased CD4(+), CD25(+) regulatory T cells

SELECTED REFERENCES

1. Dowdell KC et al: Somatic FAS mutations are common in patients with genetically undefined autoimmune lymphoproliferative syndrome. Blood. 115(25):5164-9, 2010
2. Seif AE et al: Identifying autoimmune lymphoproliferative syndrome in children with Evans syndrome: a multi-institutional study. Blood. 115(11):2142-5, 2010
3. Teachey DT et al: Advances in the management and understanding of autoimmune lymphoproliferative syndrome (ALPS). Br J Haematol. 148(2):205-16, 2010
4. Bosticardo M et al: Recent advances in understanding the pathophysiology of Wiskott-Aldrich syndrome. Blood. 113(25):6288-95, 2009
5. Bristeau-Leprince A et al: Human TCR alpha/beta+ CD4-CD8- double-negative T cells in patients with autoimmune lymphoproliferative syndrome express restricted Vbeta TCR diversity and are clonally related to CD8+ T cells. J Immunol. 181(1):440-8, 2008
6. Seif A et al: Testing patients with Evans syndrome for the autoimmune lymphoproliferative syndrome (ALPS): results of a large multi-institutional clinical trial (ASPHO supplement). Pediatric Blood & Cancer. 50: S22-S23, 2008
7. Maric I et al: Histologic features of sinus histiocytosis with massive lymphadenopathy in patients with autoimmune lymphoproliferative syndrome. Am J Surg Pathol. 29(7):903-11, 2005
8. Straus SE et al: The development of lymphomas in families with autoimmune lymphoproliferative syndrome with germline Fas mutations and defective lymphocyte apoptosis. Blood. 98(1):194-200, 2001
9. Jackson CE et al: Autoimmune lymphoproliferative syndrome with defective Fas: genotype influences penetrance. Am J Hum Genet. 64(4):1002-14, 1999
10. Jackson CE et al: Autoimmune lymphoproliferative syndrome, a disorder of apoptosis. Curr Opin Pediatr. 11(6):521-7, 1999
11. Lim MS et al: Pathological findings in human autoimmune lymphoproliferative syndrome. Am J Pathol. 153(5):1541-50, 1998
12. Elenitoba-Johnson KS et al: Lymphoproliferative disorders associated with congenital immunodeficiencies. Semin Diagn Pathol. 14(1):35-47, 1997
13. Sander CA et al: Lymphoproliferative lesions in patients with common variable immunodeficiency syndrome. Am J Surg Pathol. 16(12):1170-82, 1992
14. Snover DC et al: Wiskott-Aldrich syndrome: histopathologic findings in the lymph nodes and spleens of 15 patients. Hum Pathol. 12(9):821-31, 1981

11

AUTOIMMUNE LYMPHOPROLIFERATIVE SYNDROME

Microscopic Features

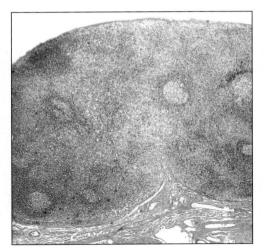

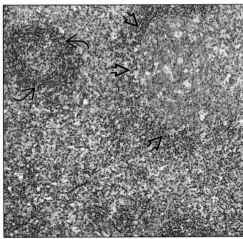

(Left) ALPS involving lymph node. This lymph node is relatively small, and the overall architecture is maintained. The paracortical regions are expanded, and follicular hyperplasia is also present. (Right) ALPS involving lymph node. This image shows a hyperplastic follicle ⊟ and an adjacent small follicle with regressive changes ⊟. The follicles in ALPS lymph nodes often exhibit a spectrum of changes, ranging from hyperplastic to regressive (Castleman-like).

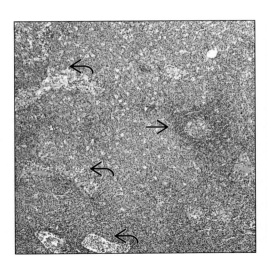

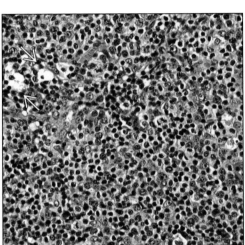

(Left) ALPS involving lymph node. The lymph node shows marked hyperplasia and expansion in the paracortex. Lymph node sinuses are patent ⊟, and a small but hyperplastic follicle is also shown ⊟. (Right) ALPS involving lymph node. Lymphocytes in the paracortex often show reduced apoptosis manifested histologically by rare tingible body macrophages being present ⊟.

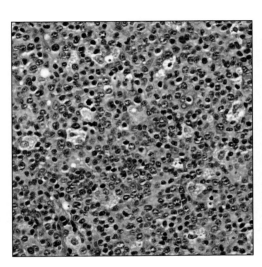

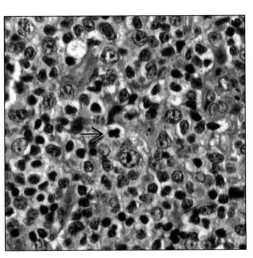

(Left) ALPS involving lymph node. High-power magnification of a reactive germinal center in a non-ALPS case shows normal apoptosis, including many tingible body macrophages. (Right) ALPS involving lymph node. High-magnification view shows immunoblasts and mitotic figures in the paracortex. Mitotic figures ⊟ can be conspicuous in ALPS, and a high proliferation rate shown by Ki-67 immunostaining also can be high (not shown).

AUTOIMMUNE LYMPHOPROLIFERATIVE SYNDROME

Microscopic Features

(Left) ALPS involving lymph node. The overall architecture of the lymph node is preserved. At this low-power magnification, marked follicular hyperplasia is easily appreciated. Paracortical hyperplasia is also present, better seen at higher power magnification. *(Right)* ALPS involving lymph node. This image shows paracortical expansion and small reactive follicles ➡.

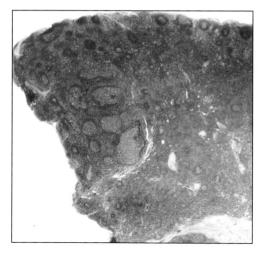
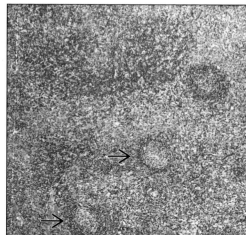

(Left) ALPS involving lymph node. This high magnification of the paracortical region of lymph node shows a mixture of cell types, including small lymphocytes, histiocytes, and immunoblasts with prominent nucleoli. Mitotic figures are present ➡. *(Right)* ALPS involving lymph node. Most T cells in the paracortical region of an ALPS case are CD3(+) and negative for CD4 and CD8 (not shown). A CD3(-) reactive follicle ➡ is also present.

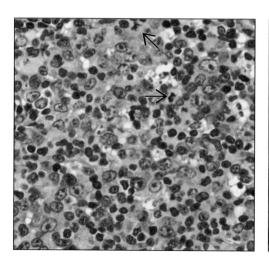
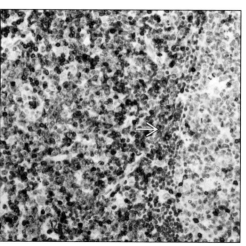

(Left) ALPS involving lymph node. Some T cells and histiocytes in the paracortex of this field are dimly CD4(+), but most of the T cells are CD4(-). A reactive follicle ➡ is also present. *(Right)* ALPS involving lymph node. Most T cells in the paracortical region are also CD8(-). A reactive follicle ➡ is present.

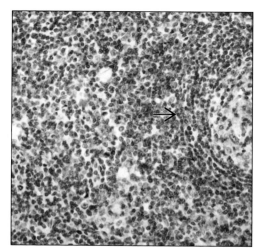
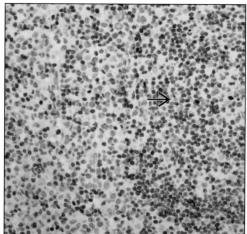

AUTOIMMUNE LYMPHOPROLIFERATIVE SYNDROME

Microscopic Features

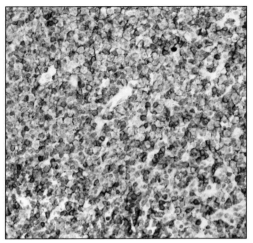
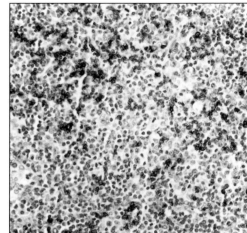

(Left) ALPS involving lymph node. Most T cells in the paracortical region are CD45RA(+). Increased T cells that are CD45RA(+) and CD45RO(-) are typically present in lymph nodes of ALPS patients. (Right) ALPS involving lymph node. Most T cells in the paracortical region are CD45RO(-).

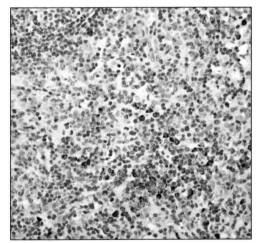
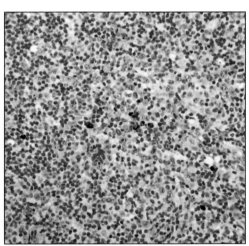

(Left) ALPS involving lymph node. Small plasma cells without atypia are commonly present in the paracortical region and express polytypic immunoglobulin light chains. Kappa is shown here. (Right) ALPS involving lymph node. Small plasma cells without atypia are commonly present in the paracortical region and express polytypic immunoglobulin light chains. Lambda is shown here.

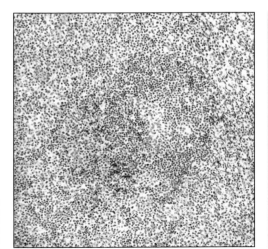
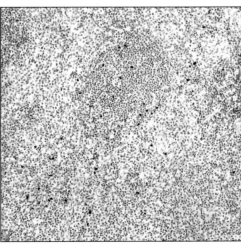

(Left) ALPS involving lymph node. In situ hybridization is usually negative for Epstein-Barr virus encoded RNA (EBER), as shown in this image. (Right) ALPS involving lymph node. Scattered TdT(+) lymphoid cells can be present in the paracortical regions of ALPS lymph nodes, especially in patients of a very young age.

AUTOIMMUNE LYMPHOPROLIFERATIVE SYNDROME

Microscopic Features

(Left) ALPS involving lymph node. In some cases, such as the one shown here, the paracortical areas are markedly expanded and confluent, demonstrating a diffuse proliferation pattern. These cases can raise the differential diagnosis with peripheral T-cell lymphoma. (Right) ALPS involving lymph node. Increased postcapillary high endothelial venues are often observed in the paracortical regions of lymph nodes from patients with ALPS.

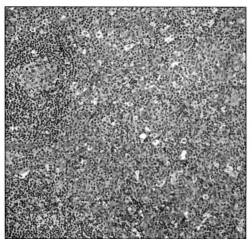

(Left) ALPS involving lymph node. CD3 highlights many T cells in the expanded paracortex and, in this field, the T cells surround a regressed follicle ➡. (Right) ALPS involving lymph node. CD20 highlights small follicles, and most B cells are confined to the follicles in ALPS lymph nodes.

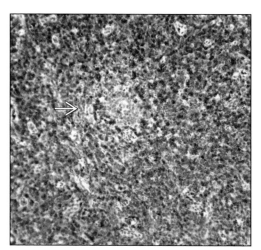
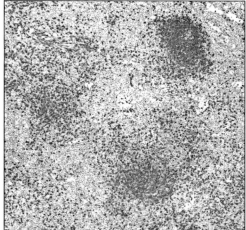

(Left) ALPS involving lymph node. CD4 highlights scattered T cells and some histiocytes. Most of the T cells are CD4(-) and CD8(-) (not shown). (Right) ALPS involving lymph node. CD8 highlights very few T cells. Most of the T cells are CD8(-) and CD4(-) (not shown).

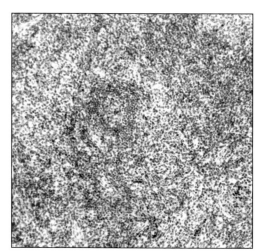
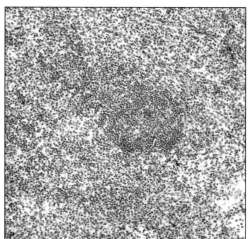

11

Flow Cytometric Immunophenotyping

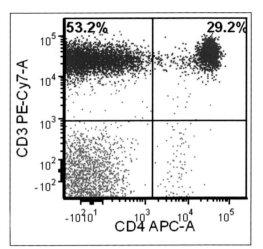

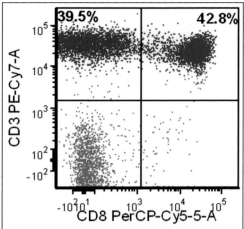

(Left) Peripheral blood of ALPS patient. Flow cytometry shows 29.2% CD4(+) T cells. *(Right)* Peripheral blood of ALPS patient. Flow cytometric immunophenotypic analysis shows 42.8% CD8(+) T cells. These percentages do not add up to 100%, indicative of the presence of double-negative T cells.

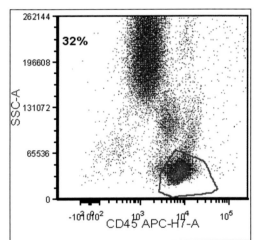

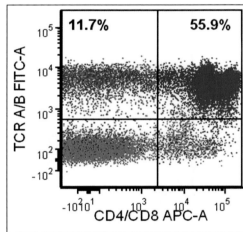

(Left) Peripheral blood of ALPS patient. Flow cytometric immunophenotyping panels designed for regular blood testing are often gated on total lymphocytes, based on side scatter/CD45. This approach is not optimal for ALPS analysis. *(Right)* PB of ALPS patient. Gating based on the lymphocyte gate, DNT cells represent 11.7% of total lymphocytes. DNT cells are TCR-α/β(+), CD4(-), CD8(-). CD4 and CD8 antibodies are labeled with same fluorochrome to detect CD4(-) CD8(-) cells.

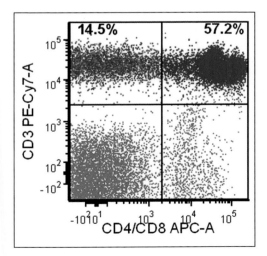

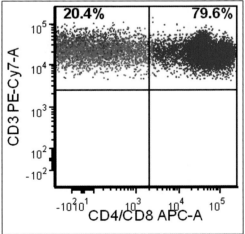

(Left) Peripheral blood of ALPS patient. Gating based on lymphocyte gate, the DNT cells are CD3(+), TCR-α/β(+), CD4(-), and CD8(-) (in fuchsia color). Note that not all the CD3(+), CD4(-), CD8(-) cells are TCR-α/β(+) DNT; some are γ/δ(+) DNT cells. *(Right)* Peripheral blood of ALPS patient. CD3(+) T cells are gated. The percentage of cells that are CD3(+), CD4(-), CD8(-) is different from that obtained by gating on total lymphocytes (20.4% vs. 14.5%).

11

Immunodeficiency-associated Lymphoproliferations

Flow Cytometric Immunophenotyping

(Left) Peripheral blood of ALPS patient. Double-negative T (DNT) cells (highlighted in fuchsia color) are CD45RA(+). *(Right)* Peripheral blood of ALPS patient. The DNT cells (highlighted in fuchsia color) are CD45RO(-).

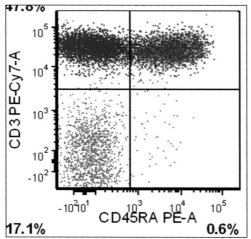

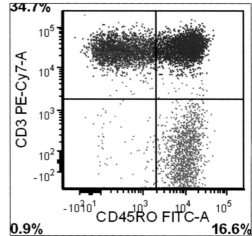

(Left) Peripheral blood of ALPS patient. TCR-γ/δ(+), CD4(-), CD8(-) T cells, a component of CD3(+), CD4(-), CD8(-) cells, are also increased in ALPS (4.1% of total T cells in this case). *(Right)* Peripheral blood of ALPS patient. DNT cells normally express CD2 and CD5 (not shown).

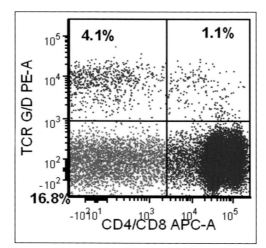

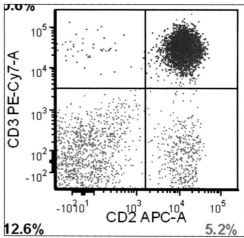

(Left) Peripheral blood of ALPS patient. DNT cells show heterogeneous and decreased expression of CD7. CD7 expression on T cells also can be down-regulated in inflammatory conditions. *(Right)* Peripheral blood of ALPS patient. There are very few CD4(+), CD25(+) regulatory T cells. DNT cells are typically CD25(-), another feature of ALPS.

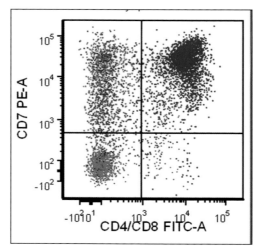

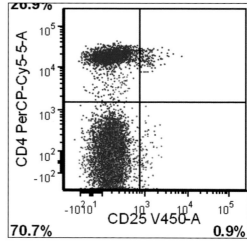

11

Flow Cytometric Immunophenotyping

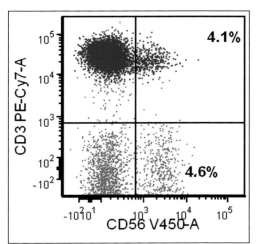 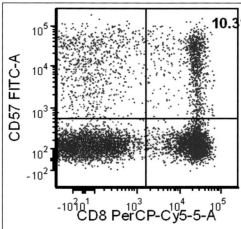

(Left) Peripheral blood of ALPS patient. NK cells that are CD3(-) and CD56(+) are often normal in number (4.6% of total lymphocytes in this case). *(Right)* Peripheral blood of ALPS patient. Large granular lymphocytes that are CD3(+), CD8(+), and CD57(+) are often increased in ALPS (10.3% of T cells in this case).

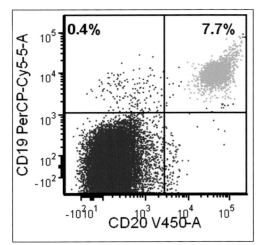 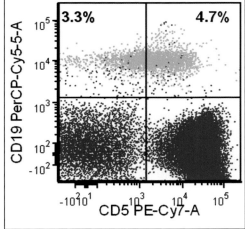

(Left) Peripheral blood of an ALPS patient who had a normal or increased absolute number of B cells. This differs from common variable immunodeficiency patients who have reduced B cells. *(Right)* Peripheral blood of ALPS patient. CD5(+) B cells are often increased in ALPS patients. In this case, CD5(+) B cells represented > 50% of total B cells.

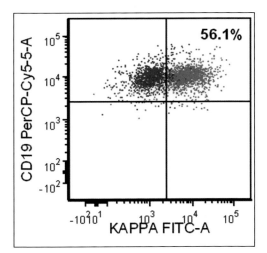 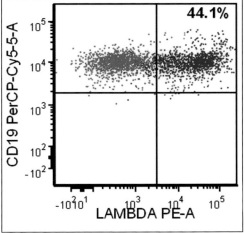

(Left) Peripheral blood of ALPS patient. B cells are polytypic as assessed by light chain expression. Kappa B cells are highlighted in red and lambda is highlighted in blue. *(Right)* Peripheral blood of ALPS patient. B cells are polytypic as assessed by light chain expression. Kappa B cells are highlighted in red with lambda highlighted in blue.

IMMUNOMODULATING AGENT-ASSOCIATED LYMPHOPROLIFERATIVE DISORDERS

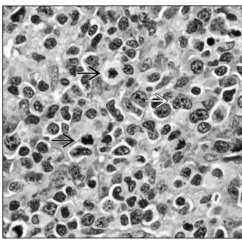

Lymph node from a patient treated with methotrexate (MTX) for rheumatoid arthritis shows diffuse large B-cell lymphoma. There are many centroblasts ⮞ and mitotic figures ⇥.

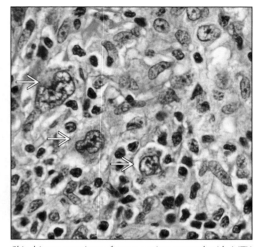

Skin biopsy specimen from a patient treated with MTX for dermatomyositis shows a Hodgkin-like LPD. The HRS cells ⮞ were CD15(+), CD20(+), and CD30(+) (not shown).

TERMINOLOGY

Abbreviations
- Immunomodulating agent-associated lymphoproliferative disorders (IA-LPD)

Definitions
- LPDs in patients treated with immunosuppressive drugs, usually for autoimmune diseases
  - LPDs arising in setting of transplantation are excluded

ETIOLOGY/PATHOGENESIS

Risk Factors for IA-LPD
- Type of immunosuppressive drug
  - Methotrexate (MTX), tumor necrosis factor (TNF)-α antagonists, etc.
- Duration of drug therapy
- Underlying disease type and disease activity
  - Rheumatoid arthritis (RA) appears to have highest risk
- Patient genetic background
- Difficult to tease out relative contributions of these factors
  - Risk factors point to potential pathogenesis

Immunosenescence and Lymphomagenesis in RA
- RA patients with lymphoma have mean age of 70 years (range 32–91)
  - Increased age is correlated with immunosenescence
- B-cell immune dysregulation in RA could drive B cell expansion
  - B-cell autoimmune activity increased due to
    - Rheumatoid factor, anti-cyclic citrullinated peptide antibodies, and free light chains
  - Systemic inflammation

- Elevated erythrocyte sedimentation rate, C-reactive protein
- Elevated B-cell survival factors: B-cell activating factor (BAFF) and APRIL (a proliferation-inducing ligand)
- Increased B cells infected by Epstein-Barr virus (EBV) in circulation
- T-cell immune dysregulation in RA could lead to loss of tolerance
  - T cells have marked contraction in diversity and premature telomere shortening
- Leads to permissive conditions for EBV(+) B-cell proliferation

Epstein-Barr Virus and Lymphomagenesis in Autoimmune Disease
- Virus is often present in lymphomas arising in patients with immune dysregulation
- Virus transforms primary B cells in vitro
- EBV(+) B-cell proliferation could be due to
  - Immunosenescence in autoimmune disease
  - MTX activated lytic EBV infection in host cells
- However, EBV can account for only fraction of increased risk
- MTX withdrawal can lead to spontaneous regression of EBV(+) diffuse large B-cell lymphoma (DLBCL)

Lymphomas in RA Patients: General Considerations
- RA is a multisystemic disease with increased risk of lymphoma
  - Risk correlates with cumulative inflammatory activity
  - Risk may be reduced with aggressive treatment by decreasing cumulative inflammation
  - DLBCL is most common type of lymphoma
    - Risk of DLBCL increased 100x from 1st to 3rd tertile of cumulative inflammation
- Long duration of RA before diagnosis of lymphoma; mean: 20 years (range: 4–50 years)

Key Facts

Etiology/Pathogenesis
- Risk factors for IA-LPDs
  - Type of immunosuppressive drug
  - Duration of drug therapy
  - Underlying disease type and disease activity
  - Patient genetic background
- EBV plays role in subset of cases

Clinical Issues
- Presentation and therapy similar to corresponding LPDs in immunocompetent patients
- Methotrexate-associated LPD
  - Partial regression after drug withdrawal in subset of cases, especially if EBV(+)
- TNF-α inhibitors
  - Regression after drug withdrawal is uncommon
- HSTCL in Crohn disease

- Fatal in most patients

Microscopic Pathology
- Many lymphoma types described in patients on immunomodulator therapy
- Analogous to other immunodeficiency states; most common are
  - Diffuse large B-cell lymphoma
  - Classical Hodgkin lymphoma; Hodgkin-like LPD
  - Polymorphic/lymphoplasmacytic LPD
  - Hepatosplenic T-cell lymphoma

Ancillary Tests
- Immunophenotype similar to corresponding LPDs in immunocompetent patients

Diagnostic Checklist
- Knowledge of drug therapy essential for diagnosis

RA Patients Treated with Methotrexate
- Methotrexate is a potent immunosuppressive agent
  - Activates lytic EBV infection in host cells
  - Appears to cause IA-LPD in at least some patients in whom drug cessation leads to regression
    - Regression is more common in EBV(+) IA-LPDs
    - Complete or partial remission usually occurs within 4 weeks of cessation; remission sustained
- However, no increase in risk of lymphoma attributable to MTX demonstrated in large, population-based studies
- Risk associated with MTX therapy may appear falsely elevated due to selection bias
  - Patients on immunomodulating therapy are more likely to have active disease
- Types of lymphomas described in patients treated with MTX
  - DLBCL (~ 50% of cases)
  - Classical Hodgkin lymphoma (CHL) (20% of cases)
  - Polymorphic/lymphoplasmacytic LPD (15% of cases)
  - Follicular lymphoma (~ 10% of cases)
  - Peripheral T-cell lymphoma (rare)
- Risk of DLBCL correlates with prolonged duration of RA, therapy, and dose of MTX
  - Duration of RA: Median 96 months
  - Duration of MTX treatment: Median 56 months
  - Cumulative MTX dose: Median ~ 900 mg

RA Patients Treated with Azathioprine
- Risk of lymphoma increased
  - Lower risk than patients treated with MTX

RA Patients Treated with TNF-α Antagonists
- Drugs include
  - Infliximab, Adalimumab, Etanercept
- Current data indicate that treatment up to 4 years does not increase risk
- DLBCL and CHL have been reported
- Risk of lymphoma is difficult to estimate because
  - TNF-α antagonists are administered to RA patients with most severe disease

  - Underlying risk for lymphoma is very high in these patients
  - These drugs are often combined with MTX or used in patients who previously received MTX
- Polymorphous LPDs that do not meet criteria for lymphoma can regress with drug cessation

RA Patients Treated with Other Drugs
- Risk of lymphoma does not appear to be increased in patients treated with intramuscular gold or sulfasalazine
- Risk decreased with oral steroids (odds ratio of 0.6); and intraarticular steroids
- Risk of lymphoma not yet clear for rituximab, Abatacept, Anakinra

Crohn Disease and Lymphoma
- Risk of LPD in inflammatory bowel disease increased
  - ~ 2x increase independent of therapy
  - DLBCL (most common); T-cell lymphomas, CHL reported
- Risk increased further by therapy with azathioprine and 6-mercaptopurine (6-MP)
  - DLBCL, MALT lymphoma, CHL, and plasmacytoma
  - ~ 40% of these are EBV(+)
- Risk with infliximab
  - Incidence of LPDs in patients receiving infliximab for Crohn disease is 0.2-1.4%
    - Small subset of cases have regressed following drug cessation
  - T-cell lymphomas have been reported
    - HSTCL (n=8), Sézary syndrome (n=2)
    - Systemic anaplastic large cell lymphoma (n=1), cutaneous CD30(+) T-cell lymphoma (n=1)
  - Infliximab may predispose to or cause lymphomagenesis due to
    - Impaired T-cell apoptosis leading to decreased activated T cells in peripheral blood
    - Impaired T-cell immune surveillance
- Crohn disease and HSTCL
  - 100% of patients were treated with azathioprine or 6-MP in past

11

IMMUNOMODULATING AGENT-ASSOCIATED LYMPHOPROLIFERATIVE DISORDERS

- 4-year gap between thiopurine therapy and development of HSTCL
- ~ 80% of patients had prior treatment with infliximab
  - Interval between 1st dose and development of HSTCL: Median 33 months
- No reported cases of HSTCL in patients treated only with TNF-α inhibitor
- Causal role of infliximab remains unproven

CLINICAL ISSUES

Epidemiology
- Incidence
  - Not well characterized
    - Overall risk of LPDs increased 2x in RA
    - Severe disease activity associated with higher risk
    - Concurrent treatment with ≥ 2 immunomodulator agents confounds risk assessment for specific drug
- Age
  - DLBCL
    - Median: 62 years
  - HSTCL in Crohn disease
    - Median at diagnosis: 22 years (range: 12-40 years)
- Gender
  - Sex ratio related to underlying disease in most instances
  - HSTCL in Crohn disease: ~ 90% of patients are male

Site
- Methotrexate-associated LPD
  - ~ 50% are extranodal
  - Gastrointestinal (GI) tract, liver, spleen, lung, kidney
  - Skin, soft tissue, thyroid gland, bone marrow
- Classical Hodgkin lymphoma
  - Usually involves lymph nodes
- HSTCL
  - Spleen, liver, and bone marrow
- EBV(+) mucocutaneous ulcer
  - Recently described entity that can occur in patients treated with IAs
    - Azathioprine, MTX, or cyclosporin A
  - Circumscribed ulcer of oropharyngeal mucosa, skin, or GI tract

Presentation
- Similar to counterparts in patients not treated with IAs
- DLBCL
  - ± rapidly enlarging lymph nodes or extranodal mass
  - B-type symptoms in subset
- HSTCL
  - Splenomegaly in 100%, hepatomegaly in ~ 80% of patients

Laboratory Tests
- DLBCL: Lactate dehydrogenase elevated in almost all patients
- HSTCL: Hepatic transaminases elevated in ~ 75% of patients

Natural History
- Methotrexate-associated LPD
  - Complete or partial regression after drug withdrawal in subset of cases
    - Especially true for polymorphous &/or EBV(+) lesions
  - Disease may recur subsequently mandating chemotherapy
- TNF-α inhibitors
  - Regression after drug withdrawal uncommon
- HSTCL in Crohn disease
  - Fatal course; death within 12 months in most patients

Treatment
- Options, risks, complications
  - Treatment similar to corresponding LPDs in patients not treated with IAs
- Drugs
  - DLBCL
    - Cyclophosphamide, doxorubicin (Adriamycin), vincristine, prednisone (CHOP)
    - Role of rituximab under evaluation
  - CHL
    - Doxorubicin, bleomycin, vincristine, dacarbazine (ABVD)
    - Role of rituximab under evaluation

Prognosis
- RA patients on immunomodulating drugs with DLBCL
  - Overall survival: ~ 50%
  - ~ 80% of patients have intermediate or high International Prognostic Index
  - Independent risk factors for outcome
    - Ann Arbor lymphoma stage
    - Age at diagnosis
  - Non-germinal center type of DLBCL more likely to have
    - Disseminated disease (Ann Arbor stage IV)
    - Worse 5-year overall survival
- EBV(+) mucocutaneous ulcer
  - Usually regresses if drug therapy discontinued

IMAGE FINDINGS

General Features
- Radiographic findings according to underlying autoimmune disease

MICROSCOPIC PATHOLOGY

Histologic Features
- Diffuse large B-cell lymphoma
  - Sheets of centroblasts or immunoblasts
  - ± plasmacytoid differentiation
  - ± geographic necrosis
- Classical Hodgkin lymphoma
  - Mixed cellularity common; nodular sclerosis can occur
  - Extranodal location in some cases
  - Typical HRS cells in inflammatory background

IMMUNOMODULATING AGENT-ASSOCIATED LYMPHOPROLIFERATIVE DISORDERS

- Hodgkin-like LPDs
  - These lesions resemble CHL, in part, but do not fulfill criteria for Hodgkin lymphoma
  - Contain HRS-like cells
- Polymorphic/lymphoplasmacytic LPD
  - Partial effacement of architecture due to polymorphic infiltrate in interfollicular distribution
    - Small lymphocytes, plasmacytoid lymphocytes
    - Immunoblasts, HRS-like cells, histiocytes
  - Recent description of so-called EBV(+) mucocutaneous ulcer
    - Polymorphous infiltrate; ± HRS cells; and usually EBV(+)
- Low-grade B-cell lymphomas
  - Uncommon; a number of tumors described
    - MALT lymphoma, Waldenström macroglobulinemia
    - Follicular lymphoma, chronic lymphocytic leukemia/small lymphocytic lymphoma
- T-cell lymphomas
  - ~ 5% of cases of IA-LPDs; tumors described include
    - Peripheral T-cell lymphoma, NOS
    - Extranodal NK/T-cell lymphoma, nasal type
  - Hepatosplenic T-cell lymphoma
    - Resembles HSTCL as occurs in patients without infliximab therapy
    - Effacement of splenic red pulp
    - Infiltration of liver and bone marrow sinusoids
    - Intermediate-sized cells with irregular nuclear contours, indistinct nucleoli, and pale cytoplasm
    - Brisk mitotic rate and karyorrhectic debris present

ANCILLARY TESTS

Immunohistochemistry

- DLBCL
  - Most information available is from RA patients on MTX
  - CD20(+), CD79a(+), pax-5(+)
  - Bcl-6(+) ~ 70%, IRF-4/MUM1(+) in ~ 50%
  - CD10(+) ~ 30%, Bcl-2(+) ~ 20%
  - Can be divided into germinal center (GC) and non-GC phenotypes
    - GC: ~ 40% of cases; CD10(+), Bcl-6(+), IRF-4/MUM1(-)
    - Non-GC: ~ 60% of cases; more likely to be EBV(+)
    - EBV(+) shows latency type II pattern: LMP-1(+) and EBNA2(-)
  - Both GC and non-GC DLBCLs
    - Associated with RA disease activity
    - Similar drug history
  - MIB-1 (Ki-67) index high; T-cell antigens(-)
- Classical Hodgkin lymphoma
  - HRS cells
    - CD30(+), CD15(+/-), pax-5(+ dim)
    - EBV(+/-), CD45/LCA(-), T-cell antigens(-)
- EBV(+) mucocutaneous ulcer
  - HRS-like cells: CD30(+), CD20(+), EBV(+), CD15(+/-)
- HSTCL
  - CD3(+), CD4(-), CD8(-/+), CD5(-), CD56(+/-)

- TIA(+), granzyme M(+), granzyme B(-/+), perforin(-), EBV(-)
- TCR-γ/δ subtype in ~ 75% of cases
- TCR-α/β subtype in ~ 25% cases

Flow Cytometry

- Immunophenotype similar to corresponding LPDs in patients not treated with IAs

Cytogenetics

- Methotrexate-associated DLBCL in RA
  - t(14;18)(q32;q21) in subset of cases
    - IgH-BCL2 fusion gene rearrangement positive by fluorescence in situ hybridization (FISH)
  - t(3;14)(q27;q32) or der(3)(q27) in subset of cases
- Hepatosplenic T-cell lymphoma
  - Isochromosome 7 in most cases
  - Trisomy 8, rarely trisomy 13

In Situ Hybridization

- EBV small encoded RNA (EBER) positive in EBV(+) cases

PCR

- Monoclonal IgH rearrangements in B-cell lymphomas
- Monoclonal TCR rearrangements in T-cell lymphomas

DIFFERENTIAL DIAGNOSIS

Classical Hodgkin Lymphoma vs. Hodgkin-like LPD

- Classical Hodgkin lymphoma
  - HRS cells in reactive inflammatory milieu
    - HRS are CD30(+), CD15(+), CD45/LCA(-)
- Hodgkin-like LPD has HRS-like cells
  - Large cells are: CD20(+), CD30(+), CD45/LCA(+), CD15(-)
- This differential diagnosis includes EBV(+) mucocutaneous ulcer
  - A lesion that fits within broader group of Hodgkin-like LPD

SELECTED REFERENCES

1. Dojcinov SD et al: EBV positive mucocutaneous ulcer-- a study of 26 cases associated with various sources of immunosuppression. Am J Surg Pathol. 34(3):405-17, 2010
2. Niitsu N et al: Clinicopathologic correlations of diffuse large B-cell lymphoma in rheumatoid arthritis patients treated with methotrexate. Cancer Sci. 101(5):1309-13, 2010
3. Ochenrider MG et al: Hepatosplenic T-cell lymphoma in a young man with Crohn's disease: case report and literature review. Clin Lymphoma Myeloma Leuk. 10(2):144-8, 2010
4. Goldin LR et al: Autoimmunity and lymphomagenesis. Int J Cancer. 124(7):1497-502, 2009
5. Hasserjian RP et al: Immunomodulator agent-related lymphoproliferative disorders. Mod Pathol. 22(12):1532-40, 2009
6. Rizzi R et al: Spontaneous remission of "methotrexate-associated lymphoproliferative disorders" after discontinuation of immunosuppressive treatment for autoimmune disease. Review of the literature. Med Oncol. 26(1):1-9, 2009

IMMUNOMODULATING AGENT-ASSOCIATED LYMPHOPROLIFERATIVE DISORDERS

Lymphomas Associated with Autoimmune Diseases

Autoimmune Disease	Relative Risk	Lymphoma Types
Sjögren syndrome	9-18	DLBCL, MALT lymphoma, WM
Dermatomyositis	5-15	DLBCL, CHL
Dermatitis herpetiformis	2-10	Enteropathy-type T-cell lymphoma
Systemic lupus erythematosus	3-6	DLBCL, MALT lymphoma, HL, T-cell lymphoma
Hashimoto thyroiditis	3-6	MALT lymphoma, DLBCL
Celiac disease	3-6	Enteropathy-type T-cell lymphoma, MALT lymphoma
Rheumatoid arthritis	2-3	DLBCL, FL (modest increase), T-cell lymphoma, WM, CHL

DLBCL = diffuse large B-cell lymphoma; FL = follicular lymphoma; MALT lymphoma = extranodal marginal zone lymphoma of mucosa-associated lymphoid tissue; CHL = classical Hodgkin lymphoma; WM = Waldenström macroglobulinemia.

Biologic Drugs Used in Autoimmune Diseases

Drugs	mAB Type
TNF-α Inhibitors	
Etanercept	Fusion protein
Infliximab	Chimeric
Adalimumab	Fully human
IL-1 Inhibitors	
Anakinra	Fully human
Rilonacet	Fusion protein
IL-1β Inhibitor	
Canakinumab	Fully human
IL-2 Receptor α Subunit (CD25) Inhibitors	
Daclizumab	Humanized
Basiliximab	Chimeric
IL-6 Inhibitors	
Tocilizumab	Humanized
CTLA4 Ig	
Abatacept	Fusion protein
B-lymphocyte Stimulator (BLyS) Inhibitor	
Belimumab	Fully human
CD20 Antagonist	
Rituximab	Chimeric
CD-22 Inhibitor	
Epratuzumab	Humanized

mAB = monoclonal antibody; CTLA4 = cytotoxic T-lymphocyte-associated antigen 4; IL = interleukin.

7. Sokol H et al: Inflammatory bowel disease and lymphoproliferative disorders: the dust is starting to settle. Gut. 58(10):1427-36, 2009
8. Baecklund E et al: Expression of the human germinal-centre-associated lymphoma protein in diffuse large B-cell lymphomas in patients with rheumatoid arthritis. Br J Haematol. 141(1):69-72, 2008
9. Kleinschmidt-DeMasters BK et al: Epstein Barr virus-associated primary CNS lymphomas in elderly patients on immunosuppressive medications. J Neuropathol Exp Neurol. 67(11):1103-11, 2008
10. Baecklund E et al: Characteristics of diffuse large B cell lymphomas in rheumatoid arthritis. Arthritis Rheum. 54(12):3774-81, 2006
11. Kamel OW et al: Lymphoid neoplasms in patients with rheumatoid arthritis and dermatomyositis: frequency of Epstein-Barr virus and other features associated with immunosuppression. Hum Pathol. 25(7):638-43, 1994

Microscopic and Immunohistochemical Features

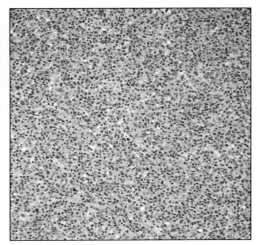
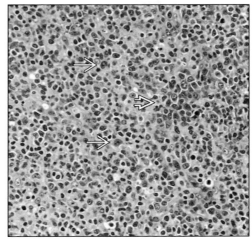

(Left) Lymph node from a patient treated with methotrexate (MTX) for rheumatoid arthritis (RA) involved by polymorphous B-cell lymphoproliferative disorder (LPD) shows effaced architecture. Lymphoid cells of varying size including many large B cells and scattered plasmacytoid cells are present. *(Right)* Lymph node from a patient treated with MTX for RA involved by polymorphous B-cell LPD shows numerous centroblasts ➡ intermixed with plasmacytoid cells ➡.

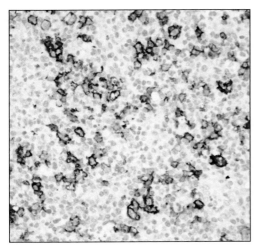
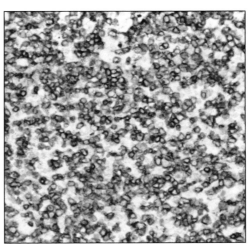

(Left) Lymph node in a patient treated with methotrexate (MTX) for rheumatoid arthritis (RA) shows involvement by a polymorphous B-cell lymphoproliferative disorder (LPD). This field demonstrates clusters of large atypical cells that are CD20(+). *(Right)* Lymph node in a patient treated with MTX for RA shows involvement by polymorphous B-cell LPD. Numerous small T cells in the background are CD3(+).

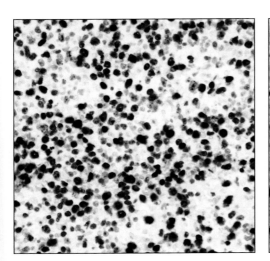
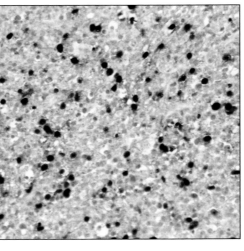

(Left) Lymph node in a patient treated with methotrexate (MTX) for rheumatoid arthritis (RA) shows involvement by polymorphous B-cell lymphoproliferative disorder (LPD). This lesion has a high proliferation (Ki-67) index of 60-70% (nuclear stain). *(Right)* Lymph node in a patient treated with MTX for RA shows involvement by polymorphous B-cell LPD. In situ hybridization studies demonstrate that numerous cells are positive for Epstein-Barr virus (EBV) small encoded RNA (EBER).

IMMUNOMODULATING AGENT-ASSOCIATED LYMPHOPROLIFERATIVE DISORDERS

Microscopic and Immunohistochemical Features

(Left) Hodgkin-like LPD is seen in a patient treated with methotrexate (MTX). *(Right)* Biopsy specimen of forehead skin of a patient with dermatomyositis treated with MTX. The dermis is extensively replaced by a Hodgkin-like lymphoproliferative disorder. Numerous Hodgkin and Reed-Sternberg (HRS)-like cells are present ➡. A reactive lymphocytic infiltrate ➡ and numerous eosinophils ➡ are present in the background.

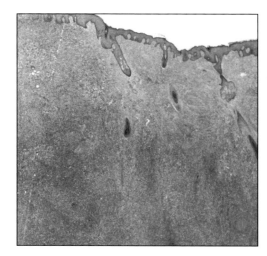
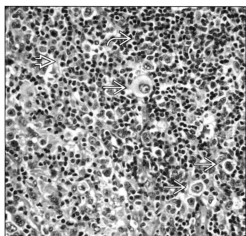

(Left) Biopsy specimen of forehead skin of a patient with dermatomyositis treated with methotrexate (MTX). The HRS-like cells are CD20(+). *(Right)* Biopsy specimen of forehead skin of a patient with dermatomyositis treated with MTX. The HRS-like cells are CD15(+) with a membranous and Golgi zone pattern ➡.

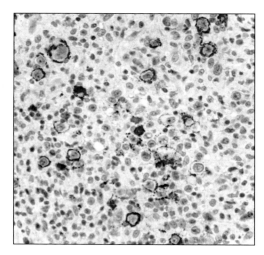
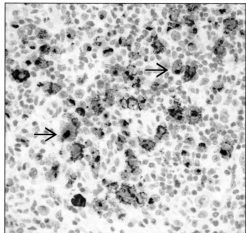

(Left) Biopsy specimen of forehead skin from a patient with dermatomyositis treated with methotrexate (MTX). The Reed-Sternberg and Hodgkin-like cells are EBV-LMP1(+). *(Right)* Biopsy specimen of forehead skin from a patient with dermatomyositis treated with MTX. The HRS-like cells are negative for CD45/LCA ➡.

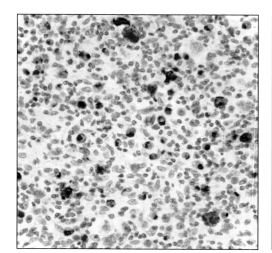
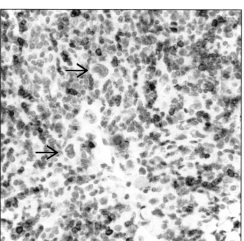

Microscopic and Immunohistochemical Features

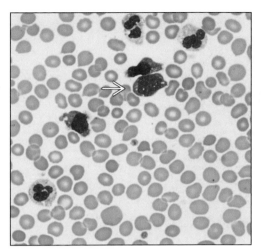

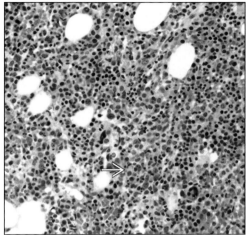

(Left) Peripheral blood smear of a patient treated with methotrexate (MTX) and anti-TNF-α for rheumatoid arthritis (RA) shows a T-cell lymphoproliferative disorder (LPD) characterized by large atypical lymphoid cells ➡. *(Right)* Bone marrow of a patient treated with MTX and anti-TNF-α for RA shows T-cell LPD. The bone marrow shows an interstitial infiltrate of atypical lymphoid cells ➡ of predominantly intermediate size, with variably dispersed chromatin and inconspicuous nucleoli.

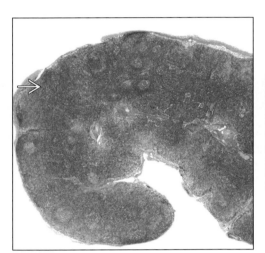

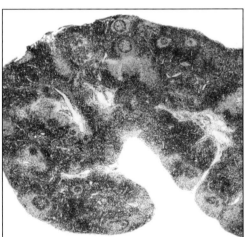

(Left) Lymph node of a patient treated with methotrexate (MTX) for rheumatoid arthritis (RA) shows a T-cell lymphoproliferative disorder (LPD). The lymph node demonstrates focal paracortical expansion ➡. The architecture is otherwise relatively preserved. *(Right)* Lymph node of a patient treated with MTX for RA shows a T-cell LPD. The anti-CD3 antibody highlights expansion of the paracortical zones by T-cells.

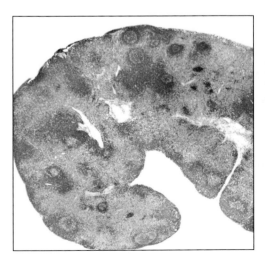

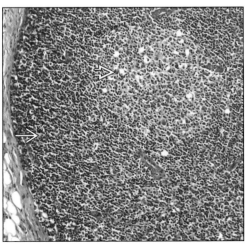

(Left) Lymph node of a patient treated with methotrexate (MTX) for rheumatoid arthritis (RA) shows a T-cell lymphoproliferative disorder (LPD). The anti-CD20 antibody demonstrates residual follicles composed of B cells expressing CD20. *(Right)* Lymph node of a patient treated with MTX for RA shows a T-cell LPD. High-power view of a reactive germinal center ➡ with tingible-body macrophages. The surrounding cells are neoplastic T-cells ➡.

POST-TRANSPLANT LYMPHOPROLIFERATIVE DISORDER, EARLY LESIONS AND POLYMORPHIC

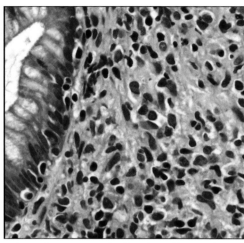

Polymorphic post-transplant lymphoproliferative disorder (PTLD) involving the rectum. Note the mixture of cell types present.

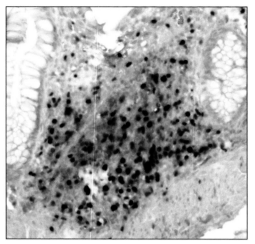

Polymorphic PTLD involving the rectum. In situ hybridization for Epstein-Barr virus (EBV) encoded small RNA (EBER) is positive in many cells.

TERMINOLOGY

Abbreviations
• Post-transplant lymphoproliferative disorder (PTLD)

Definitions
• Plasmacytic or lymphoid proliferations occurring as result of immunosuppression following solid organ or bone marrow transplantation
  ○ Early lesions are PTLDs characterized by architectural preservation of involved site
  ○ Polymorphic lesions are PTLDs that efface architecture but are morphologically heterogeneous and do not fulfill criteria for any known lymphoma type

ETIOLOGY/PATHOGENESIS

Infectious Agents
• Epstein-Barr virus plays a central role
  ○ 80% of all PTLDs are EBV(+)
    ▪ Usually type A
  ○ Serum EBV antibody titers and blood EBV DNA load increase prior to onset of PTLD
  ○ Number of EBV(+) cytotoxic T cells drops prior to onset of PTLD
  ○ Treatment with EBV-specific T cells induces remission or responses in some patients
  ○ Analysis of EBV terminal repeat regions by Southern blot analysis has shown monoclonal form of virus
    ▪ Indicates presence of EBV before monoclonal expansion began
  ○ EBV can transform germinal center (GC) B cells
    ▪ Extended half-life of EBV-infected B cells increases likelihood of acquiring additional molecular aberrations that confer a growth advantage

Pathogenesis
• Arise from GC or post-GC B cells

○ In solid organ allograft recipients, most PTLDs are of host origin
○ In bone marrow or stem cell allograft recipients, most PTLDs are of donor origin
• Iatrogenically decreased host immunosurveillance
• Risk factors for PTLD in general
  ○ EBV seronegativity before transplant
  ○ Degree of overall immunosuppression
  ○ Type of immunosuppression
    ▪ Higher risk with tacrolimus, OKT3 monoclonal antibody, or antithymocyte globulin
  ○ Type of organs transplanted
    ▪ Most common in intestinal and multiorgan transplant recipients
    ▪ Lowest in renal transplant recipients
    ▪ May be attributable to differences in immunosuppressive regimens used
  ○ Age
    ▪ Pediatric patients have a higher incidence of PTLD
    ▪ Most likely related to more frequent EBV seronegativity prior to transplant
  ○ Additional risk factors for patients who receive autologous bone marrow or stem cell transplants
    ▪ HLA-mismatched allograft
    ▪ T-cell-depleted allograft
    ▪ Immunosuppressive therapy for graft vs. host disease

CLINICAL ISSUES

Epidemiology
• Incidence
  ○ Frequency of PTLD is related to type of transplant and associated immunosuppression
    ▪ Kidney: 1-3% of all transplant patients
    ▪ Liver: 1-3% of all transplant patients
    ▪ Heart: 1-6% of all transplant patients
    ▪ Heart-lung: 2-6% of all transplant patients
    ▪ Lung: 4-10% of all transplant patients

POST-TRANSPLANT LYMPHOPROLIFERATIVE DISORDER, EARLY LESIONS AND POLYMORPHIC

Key Facts

Etiology/Pathogenesis
- Epstein-Barr virus infection and impaired host immunosurveillance important
  - 80% of all PTLDs are EBV(+)
- Risk factors for developing PTLD
  - EBV seronegativity before transplant; age
  - Degree of overall immunosuppression
  - Types of immunosuppression or transplanted organ

Clinical Issues
- Early lesions: Involve lymph nodes or Waldeyer ring
  - Reduction of immunosuppression often adequate
- Polymorphic PTLDs: Involve lymph nodes &/or extranodal sites
  - Reduction of immunosuppression ± effective
  - Subset of patients require cytotoxic chemotherapy

Microscopic Pathology
- Plasmacytic hyperplasia
  - Preserved architecture; plasma cells, lymphocytes, and scattered immunoblasts
- IM-like PTLD
  - Paracortical expansion by lymphocytes, plasma cells, and immunoblasts
- Polymorphic PTLD
  - Effacement of architecture by plasma cells, lymphocytes, and immunoblasts; ± necrosis

Ancillary Tests
- Early lesions
  - Polytypic plasma cells and B cells; EBV(+/-)
- Polymorphic PTLD
  - ~ 50% monotypic &/or monoclonal; EBV(+/-)

- Small intestine: ~ 20% of all transplant patients
- Age
  - Predicted by age of patient population undergoing transplant
    - Younger patients are at increased risk of developing PTLD

Site
- Early lesions
  - Primarily involving lymph nodes
  - Tonsils, adenoids
- Polymorphic
  - Lymph nodes
  - Extranodal masses can occur

Presentation
- Highly variable
  - ± nonspecific findings: Weight loss, fever, lethargy or malaise
- Early lesions
  - Lymphadenopathy, enlarged tonsils or adenoids
    - ± obstructive symptoms
  - Patients can present with infectious mononucleosis-like syndrome
- Polymorphic lesions
  - Lymphadenopathy or extranodal mass
    - ± organ-specific compromise

Natural History
- Early lesions
  - Usually regress; either spontaneously or after reduction of immunosuppression
  - Small subset of patients subsequently develop polymorphous or monomorphous PTLD
  - Rare patients with infectious mononucleosis (IM)-like lesions have aggressive course
- Polymorphic
  - A subset of cases regresses after reduction of immunosuppression
  - Other patients have progressive disease and require chemotherapy

Treatment
- No established treatment recommendations for PTLDs due to
  - Clinical & pathologic heterogeneity of these lesions
  - General lack of prospective, randomized studies
- 3-step approach is often taken in treating patients with PTLDs
  - Reduction of immunosuppression
  - Single agent rituximab (anti-CD20)
  - Cytotoxic chemotherapy
- Early lesions often only require first step in management
- Other therapeutic approaches
  - Infusion of EBV-specific cytotoxic T lymphocytes
  - Radiation therapy has potential role for localized and bulky disease

Prognosis
- In general, pediatric patients or patients with localized disease have best prognosis
- Early lesions
  - Prognosis usually excellent
  - Can regress spontaneously and most cases regress following reduction in immunosuppression
- Polymorphic lesions
  - Patients have variable prognosis
  - Subset of polymorphous PTLD regress with reduction of immunosuppression
  - Many polymorphous PTLD persist and require chemotherapy
    - Subset of these patients do poorly

MICROSCOPIC PATHOLOGY

Histologic Features
- 2 types of early lesions: Plasmacytic hyperplasia and IM-like PTLD
- Plasmacytic hyperplasia
  - Preserved architecture
  - Sheets or aggregates of plasma cells, small lymphocytes, and scattered immunoblasts

- IM-like PTLD
  - Prominent paracortical expansion
  - Proliferation of mixed population of EBV(+) B cells and reactive T cells
  - Numerous immunoblasts
  - Germinal center can be hyperplastic or small
- Polymorphic PTLD
  - These lesions exhibit some degree of effacement of normal architecture of involved organ
  - ± focal or confluent areas of necrosis
  - Mixed population of plasma cells, variably sized lymphoid cells, and immunoblasts
    - ± HRS-like cells
  - Mitotic figures can be common
  - Sheets of large cells should not be seen; indicate presence of monomorphic PTLD

ANCILLARY TESTS

Immunohistochemistry
- Early lesions
  - Polytypic plasma cells and B cells
  - Plasmacytoid lymphocytes and plasma cells: CD38(+), CD138(+), and often CD20(+)
  - Immunoblasts are CD30(+)
  - EBV-LMP1(+/-), HHV8(-)
- Polymorphic PTLD
  - ~ 50% of cases express monotypic Ig in plasmacytoid cells
  - Plasmacytoid lymphocytes and plasma cells: CD38(+), CD138(+), and often CD20(+)
  - MIB-1/Ki-67 can be high
  - EBV-LMP1(+/-), HHV8(-)
  - EBV-LMP2(+/-), EBV-LMP3(+/-)

Flow Cytometry
- B-lymphocyte clonality in ~ 50% of polymorphic PTLD
- T cells show no immunophenotypic aberrancies

In Situ Hybridization
- EBER usually positive in both early & polymorphic PTLDs
- Some cases can be EBER negative

Molecular Genetics
- Early lesions
  - Plasmacytic hyperplasia
    - No evidence of monoclonal *Ig* or T-cell receptor *(TCR)* gene rearrangements
  - IM-like PTLD
    - Small monoclonal or oligoclonal *Ig* or *TCR* gene rearrangements
    - EBV terminal repeat analysis: Polyclonal or oligoclonal patterns
- Polymorphic PTLD
  - ~ 50% monoclonal *IgH* rearrangements
  - EBV terminal repeat analysis: Usually monoclonal pattern; less commonly oligoclonal or polyclonal
  - *BCL6* gene mutations or aberrant methylation in subset of cases

DIFFERENTIAL DIAGNOSIS

Plasma Cell Neoplasm
- Plasmacytic hyperplasia can have some resemblance to plasma cell neoplasm
- Features that support plasma cell neoplasm
  - No history of transplantation
  - Effacement of architecture; EBV(-)

EBV(+) Diffuse Large B-cell Lymphoma (DLBCL)
- IM-like PTLD or polymorphic PTLD can resemble, in part, EBV(+) DLBCL
  - High mitotic rate and focal necrosis
- Features that support EBV(+) DLBCL over IM-like PTLD
  - No history of transplantation
  - Effacement of architecture by sheets of large centroblasts/immunoblasts
  - Large cells are of B-cell lineage and monoclonal
- Features supporting EBV(+) DLBCL over polymorphic PTLD
  - No history of transplantation
  - Sheets of large centroblasts/immunoblasts
  - Subsets of polymorphic PTLD are EBV(-) or polyclonal

Classical Hodgkin Lymphoma (CHL)
- Cases of polymorphic PTLD can resemble CHL
- Features that distinguish polymorphic PTLD from CHL
  - Hodgkin and Reed-Sternberg cells in
    - Polymorphic PTLD: CD30(+), CD20(+), CD15(-)
    - CHL: CD15(+), CD30(+), CD20(-/+)
  - History of transplantation is helpful
  - ~ 50% of polymorphic PTLD is monoclonal

Reactive Follicular Hyperplasia
- Florid reactive follicular hyperplasia can occur in PTLD patients
- No effacement of architecture; no evidence of clonality; EBV(+/-)
- Not considered an early lesion by some authors; can be lumped with early lesions

SELECTED REFERENCES
1. Parker A et al: Diagnosis of post-transplant lymphoproliferative disorder in solid organ transplant recipients - BCSH and BTS Guidelines. Br J Haematol. 149(5):675-92, 2010
2. Parker A et al: Management of post-transplant lymphoproliferative disorder in adult solid organ transplant recipients - BCSH and BTS Guidelines. Br J Haematol. 149(5):693-705, 2010
3. Styczynski J et al: Outcome of treatment of Epstein-Barr virus-related post-transplant lymphoproliferative disorder in hematopoietic stem cell recipients: a comprehensive review of reported cases. Transpl Infect Dis. 11(5):383-92, 2009
4. Bakker NA et al: Post-transplant lymphoproliferative disorders: from treatment to early detection and prevention? Haematologica. 92(11):1447-50, 2007

POST-TRANSPLANT LYMPHOPROLIFERATIVE DISORDER, EARLY LESIONS AND POLYMORPHIC

Microscopic and Immunohistochemical Features

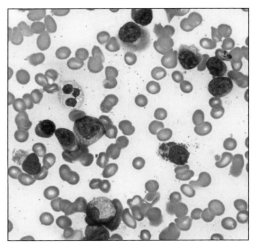

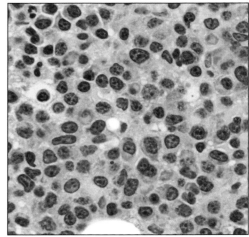

(Left) Post-transplant lymphoproliferative disorder (PTLD), early lesion, plasmacytic hyperplasia, involving bone marrow. Numerous bland plasma cells were present in the bone marrow aspirate smear. This case arose in a patient who previously underwent allogeneic stem cell transplantation. *(Right)* PTLD, early lesion, plasmacytic hyperplasia, involving bone marrow. Numerous plasma cells were present in the bone marrow aspirate clot specimen.

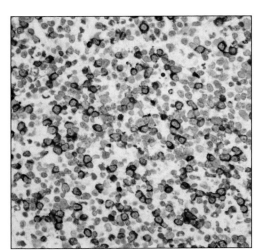

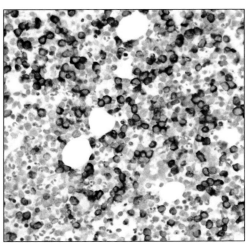

(Left) PTLD, early lesion, plasmacytic hyperplasia, involving bone marrow. Immunohistochemistry of the aspirate clot specimen showed that the plasma cells were polytypic, kappa(+) in this field. *(Right)* PTLD, early lesion, plasmacytic hyperplasia, involving bone marrow. Immunohistochemistry of the aspirate clot specimen showed that the plasma cells were polytypic, lambda(+) in this field.

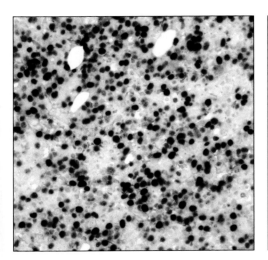

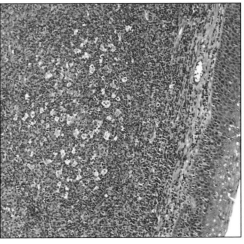

(Left) PTLD, plasmacytic hyperplasia, involving bone marrow. In situ hybridization showed many EBER(+) plasma cells. *(Right)* Reactive follicular hyperplasia involving oropharynx of a patient who underwent kidney transplantation within the past year. In situ hybridization showed that the lesion was EBER(+). Some authors consider this lesion to be an early lesion PTLD, whereas other authors separately designate these cases as reactive lymphoid hyperplasia.

POST-TRANSPLANT LYMPHOPROLIFERATIVE DISORDER, EARLY LESIONS AND POLYMORPHIC

Microscopic and Immunohistochemical Features

(Left) Polymorphic post-transplant lymphoproliferative disorder (PTLD) involving skin. This field shows the lesion in the dermis surrounding blood vessels. *(Right)* Polymorphic PTLD involving skin. This field shows a spectrum of cell types.

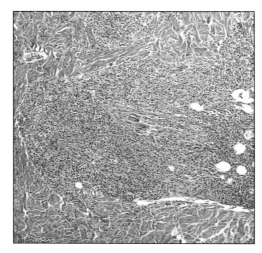 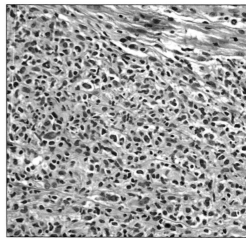

(Left) Polymorphic post-transplant lymphoproliferative disorder (PTLD) involving skin. Immunohistochemical stain for CD20 shows that many lymphoid cells are CD20(+). *(Right)* Polymorphic PTLD involving skin. Immunohistochemical stain for CD3 highlights reactive T cells in the background.

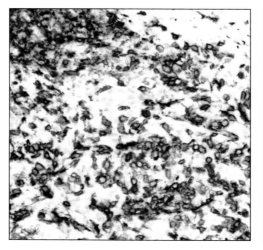 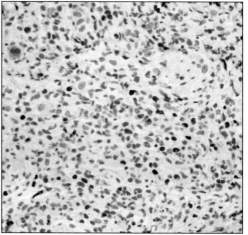

(Left) Polymorphic post-transplant lymphoproliferative disorder (PTLD) involving skin. Immunohistochemical stain for CD30 highlights scattered CD30(+) immunoblasts. *(Right)* Polymorphic PTLD involving skin. In situ hybridization for EBV encoded small RNA (EBER) shows many EBER(+) cells.

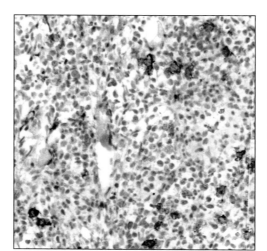 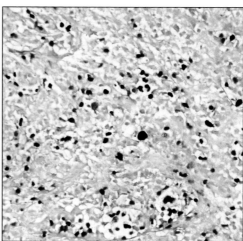

POST-TRANSPLANT LYMPHOPROLIFERATIVE DISORDER, EARLY LESIONS AND POLYMORPHIC

Microscopic and Immunohistochemical Features

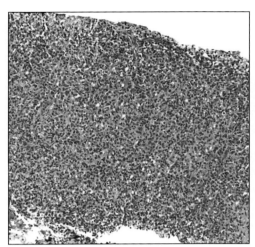
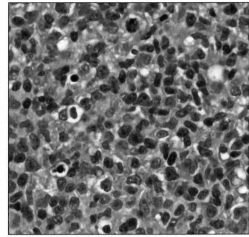

(Left) Needle biopsy shows a cervical lymph node involved by polymorphic post-transplant lymphoproliferative disorder (PTLD). *(Right)* Needle biopsy of a cervical lymph node involved by polymorphic PTLD. A mixture of small and large lymphocytes and histiocytes is shown in this field.

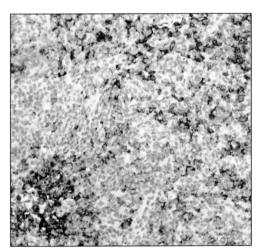
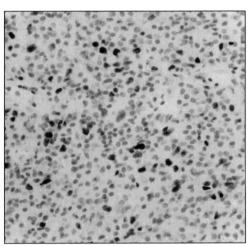

(Left) Needle biopsy shows a cervical lymph node involved by polymorphic post-transplant lymphoproliferative disorder (PTLD). Immunohistochemical stain for CD20 shows that many lymphocytes are CD20(+). *(Right)* Needle biopsy of a cervical lymph node involved by polymorphic PTLD. Immunohistochemical stain for pax-5 shows that many cells are B cells that are pax-5(+).

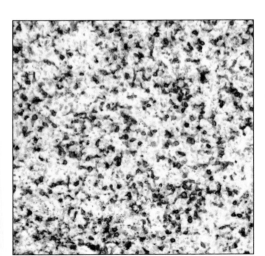
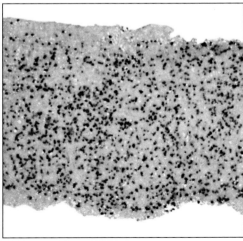

(Left) Needle biopsy shows a cervical lymph node involved by polymorphic post-transplant lymphoproliferative disorder (PTLD). Immunohistochemical stain for CD3 highlights reactive T cells. *(Right)* Needle biopsy of a cervical lymph node involved by polymorphic PTLD. In situ hybridization for EBV encoded small RNA (EBER) is positive.

POST-TRANSPLANT LYMPHOPROLIFERATIVE DISORDER, MONOMORPHIC

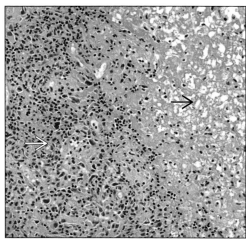

Monomorphic post-transplant lymphoproliferative disorder (PTLD), consistent with diffuse large B-cell lymphoma, involving brain shows atypical lymphoid infiltrate ➡ and necrosis ➡.

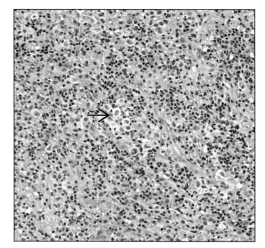

Monomorphic PTLD, consistent with diffuse large B-cell lymphoma, involving brain. Numerous large atypical lymphoid cells ➡ are present in a background of reactive T cells.

TERMINOLOGY

Abbreviations
- Post-transplant lymphoproliferative disorder (PTLD)

Synonyms
- Post-transplantation lymphoproliferative disease (PTLD)

Definitions
- PTLDs are plasmacytic or lymphoid proliferations that occur as a result of immunosuppressive therapy following solid organ or bone marrow transplantation
- Monomorphic PTLDs fulfill criteria for lymphomas as observed in immunocompetent patients
  - All cells appear to be transformed but lesions are not completely monotonous
    - Plasmacytoid/plasmacytic differentiation &/or pleomorphism of neoplastic cells are common

ETIOLOGY/PATHOGENESIS

Infectious Agents
- Epstein-Barr virus (EBV) infection plays important role in pathogenesis
  - ~ 80% of all PTLDs are EBV(+); usually type A
  - Prior to onset of PTLDs
    - Serum EBV antibody titers and EBV DNA levels in blood increase
    - Numbers of EBV(+) cytotoxic T cells decrease prior to onset of PTLD
  - Therapy with EBV-specific T cells effective in subset of patients
  - EBV genomes are monoclonal shown by EBV terminal repeat analysis
    - Virus is present prior to monoclonal expansion
- EBV can transform germinal center B cells
  - Extends lifespan of B cells

  - Increases likelihood of additional genetic abnormalities that confer growth advantage
  - EBV latent membrane protein (LMP)1 and LMP2A proteins activate B-cell receptor and intracellular signaling pathways

Decreased Host Immunosurveillance Resulting from Therapeutic Immunosuppression
- Underlying immune deficiency can be involved (e.g., cystic fibrosis, hepatitis C infection)
- Cumulative amount of immunosuppression
  - Cyclosporin A, antithymocyte globin (ATG) or OKT3 monoclonal antibodies
- Type of organ transplanted
  - Multiorgan > lung > liver > heart > pancreas > kidney > bone marrow and stem cell transplantation
  - Kidney transplant patients are more susceptible to NK/T-cell lymphoma and EBV(-)
  - Stem cell transplant patients are more susceptible to Hodgkin lymphoma
    - T-cell depletion in donor allograft increases risk

Cell of Origin
- B-cell PTLDs arise from germinal center (GC) or post-GC B-cells
- Cell of origin of T-cell PTLDs is unknown
- 90% of PTLD in recipients of solid organ transplants are of host origin
- Most PTLD in recipients of bone marrow/stem cell transplant are of donor origin

Risk Factors for PTLDs in General
- EBV seronegativity before transplant
- Degree of overall immunosuppression
  - Higher risk if multiple regimens are used or if patients receive multiple transplants
- Type of immunosuppression
  - Higher risk with

POST-TRANSPLANT LYMPHOPROLIFERATIVE DISORDER, MONOMORPHIC

Key Facts

Terminology
- Monomorphic PTLDs fulfill criteria for lymphomas as observed in immunocompetent patients

Etiology/Pathogenesis
- Epstein-Barr virus (EBV) infection plays important role in pathogenesis
- ~ 80% of all PTLDs are EBV(+); usually type A
- Risk factors for developing PTLDs
  - EBV seronegativity before transplant; young age
  - Degree of overall immunosuppression
  - Types of immunosuppression or organs transplanted

Clinical Issues
- Lymphadenopathy &/or extranodal sites
- EBV(+) PTLDs usually occur < 5 years after transplant

- EBV(-) PTLDs develop later (median: 50 months)
- 3-step approach is taken for treating PTLD patients
  - Reduction of immunosuppression
  - Single agent rituximab (anti-CD20 antibody)
  - Cytotoxic chemotherapy

Microscopic Pathology
- ~ 80% monomorphic PTLDs are of B-cell origin
  - Diffuse large B-cell lymphoma is most common
- ~ 15% are NK/T-cell
- ~ 5% plasma cell neoplasms and Hodgkin lymphoma

Ancillary Tests
- Karyotypic aberrations are detectable in most cases
- Monomorphic B-cell PTLD: Monoclonal *Ig* rearrangements
- NK/T-cell PTLDs: Monoclonal *TCR* rearrangements

- Tacrolimus
- Monoclonal antibody OKT3
- Antithymocyte globulin
- Type of organs transplanted
  - Highest risk in patients receiving intestinal or multi-organ transplants
  - Lowest risk in patients who receive kidney allograft
  - Likely attributable, in part, to immunosuppressive regimens used
- Age
  - Children who receive allografts have higher frequency of PTLD
  - Likely related to higher frequency of EBV seronegativity at time of transplant
- Patients who receive bone marrow/stem cell transplants have additional risk factors
  - HLA-mismatched allograft
  - Allograft that has been T cell depleted
  - Immunosuppressive therapy for graft vs. host disease

CLINICAL ISSUES

Epidemiology
- Incidence
  - PTLD occurs in < 2-3% of all patients who receive organ allografts
    - Kidney: 1-3% of transplant patients
    - Liver: 1-3% of transplant patients
    - Heart: 1-6% of transplant patients
    - Heart-lung: 2-6% of transplant patients
    - Lung: 4-10% of transplant patients
    - Small intestine: ~ 20% of transplant patients
  - Younger patients have higher incidence
- Age
  - Predicted by age of population undergoing transplant
- Gender
  - Predicted, in part, by underlying diseases of population undergoing transplant

Presentation
- Highly variable; depends on
  - Organ(s) involved by PTLD
  - Histology of PTLD
  - Status of EBV infection
- EBV(+) PTLDs usually occur within 5 years of transplant
  - Commonly arise within 1st year after transplant
- EBV(-) cases occur a median of 50 months after transplantation
- Constitutional symptoms are common
- Lymphadenopathy; can be localized or systemic
- Extranodal sites are commonly involved (up to 75% of cases)
  - Often involve gastrointestinal (GI) tract or brain
  - PTLD commonly involves allograft, but can be generalized
    - Associated with allograft failure
  - Most NK/T-cell PTLDs involve extranodal sites
    - Skin, blood, bone marrow, spleen, lung, GI tract
- Bone marrow transplant recipients can develop generalized PTLD that mimics graft vs. host disease
  - ± pancytopenia
- Classical Hodgkin lymphoma type of PTLD is more common in patients with kidney or bone marrow/stem cell transplants

Natural History
- Some monomorphic PTLDs may regress after discontinuation of immunosuppression
  - Relapse is common
  - Regression less likely if PTLD is EBV(-)
- Most patients with monomorphic PTLDs require aggressive therapy

Treatment
- No established therapeutic recommendations for PTLDs because of
  - Clinical and pathologic heterogeneity
  - General lack of prospective, randomized studies
- 3-step approach is often taken in treating PTLD patients

EPITHELIAL INCLUSIONS IN LYMPH NODE

Epithelial Inclusions in Axilla and Pelvis

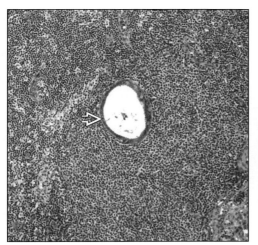
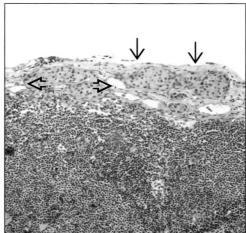

(Left) Axillary lymph node with marginal zone lymphoma displays an incidentally detected glandular epithelial inclusion ⮞. Benign epithelial inclusions are usually subcapsular but can also be found deep in the lymph node parenchyma. *(Right)* Lymph node with subcapsular metastasis of breast carcinoma. Nests are round to oval and contained within subcapsular sinus ⮞. The overlying capsule is thin ➡.

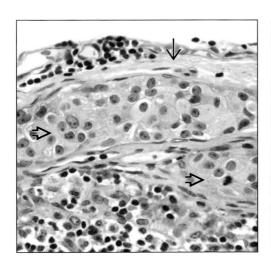
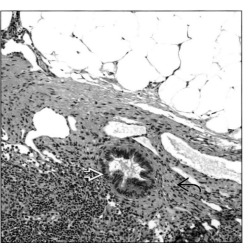

(Left) High magnification of breast cancer metastasis. A metastatic nest fills the subcapsular sinus ⮞. The overlying capsule is thin and poorly cellular ➡. *(Right)* Pelvic lymph node with endosalpingiosis. There is an isolated gland ⮞ contained within capsular fibrous stroma ➡. There is no associated hemorrhage or hemosiderin-laden histiocytes that could suggest endometriosis.

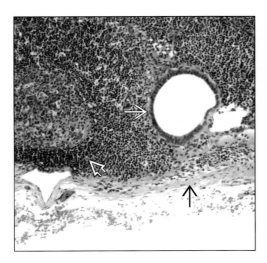
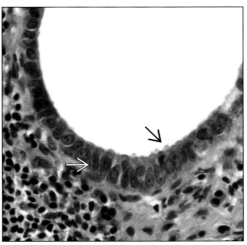

(Left) Endosalpingiosis in an iliac lymph node. There is a distinct dilated gland ⮞ near the capsule ➡. A lymphoid follicle is also noted ⮞. *(Right)* Endosalpingiosis in an iliac lymph node. Epithelial lining is low columnar ➡ with bland nuclear features and occasional luminal blebs ➡. Although cilia are common in endosalpingiosis, they are not always detected.

NEVUS CELL INCLUSIONS IN LYMPH NODE

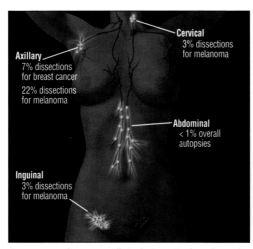

Frequency of nevus cell inclusions in lymph nodes according to anatomical site. Frequency varies according to case selection and with the use of immunohistochemistry for S100 protein.

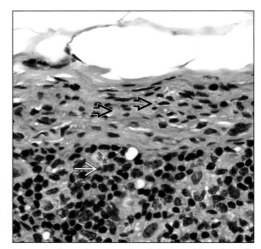

Hematoxylin and eosin stain of thickened lymph node capsule displays spindle cells with pale cytoplasm ⊳, corresponding to nevus cells. Reactive lymphocytes are noted in subcapsular sinus ➡.

TERMINOLOGY

Abbreviations
- Nevus cell inclusions (NCI)

Synonyms
- Nevus cell aggregates (NCA)
- Blue nevus of lymph node

Definitions
- Conventional definition for aggregates of melanocytes in lymph node capsule or trabeculae
- Recent literature also includes (benign) nevus cells within sinuses or lymph node (LN) parenchyma

ETIOLOGY/PATHOGENESIS

Possible Theories
- May explain presence of melanocytic cells in lymph nodes
- 2 distinct patterns of NCI in LNs support 2 theories
  - Suggests that these mechanisms represent independent processes
- Theory #1: Nevus cells result from abnormal (arrested) migration and trapping of neural crest cells in LN capsule
  - Applies better for spindled, usually heavily pigmented lesions in LN capsule or trabeculae
  - Occurs during embryonic development
    - Concurrent timing of neural crest cell migration and lymphatic development
  - Theory supported by coincidental presence of congenital nevi in skin
  - Similar mechanisms may explain blue nevus in prostate, cervix, and vagina
  - NCI in LN capsule share spindle cell morphology with congenital nevus
- Theory #2: Nevus cells embolize from skin nevus, representing "benign metastasis"

- Applies better for small clusters of embolic nevus cells
- Also designated as "mechanical transport"
  - Displacement may result from biopsy procedure or tumor pushing nevus cells into lymphatics
- Theory supported by occasional presence of nevus cells within LN sinuses or parenchyma
  - Nevus cell clusters may also be found within cutaneous lymphatics as well as in afferent lymphatics of LNs
  - These nevus cell clusters are emphasized in recent literature
  - NCI in LN sinuses share oval or cuboidal morphology of conventional (not congenital) cutaneous nevus cells
  - In addition, nevus cells are rare in LNs draining noncutaneous sites
  - Oncogene *BRAF* point mutations found in concurrent skin nevus and in LN nevus cells

CLINICAL ISSUES

Site
- Can be found in superficial skin-draining axillary, inguinal, or cervical LNs
  - Usually affects single LN (even in specimens with many LNs)
  - Overall, NCI are more frequent in axillary region than in cervical or inguinal regions
    - NCI are rare in visceral LNs
- Using routine histologic examination, frequency of NCI in LNs is relatively low
  - ~ 3-4% of inguinal LN dissections for malignant melanoma
  - < 1% of axillary LN dissections for breast cancer
- Using immunohistochemistry, reported frequency of NCI is higher
  - 22% of cases of LN dissections for melanoma

NEVUS CELL INCLUSIONS IN LYMPH NODE

Key Facts

Terminology
- Aggregates of melanocytes or nevus cells in lymph node (LN) capsule or trabeculae
  - Presence of nevus cells within LN sinuses or parenchyma is unusual

Etiology/Pathogenesis
- Nevus cells may represent arrested migration and trapping of neural crest cells in LN capsule
- Alternatively, nevus cells may embolize from skin nevus, representing "benign metastasis"

Clinical Issues
- Nevus cells can be found in superficial skin-draining axillary, inguinal, or cervical LNs

Microscopic Pathology
- Benign nevus cells can coexist with malignancy in sentinel LNs

Ancillary Tests
- Nevus cell aggregates are usually surrounded by reticulin meshwork
- Nevus cell inclusions are S100 protein(+), tyrosinase(+), Melan-A(+)
- RT-PCR for tyrosinase mRNA on sentinel LNs is not specific; can be positive in
  - Benign nevus cell inclusions
  - Metastatic melanoma

Top Differential Diagnoses
- Nevus cell inclusions in LN sinuses or parenchyma raises suspicion for metastasis

---

- Apparent higher incidence of LN NCI when melanoma Breslow thickness is > 2.5 mm
- ~ 7% of axillary LN dissections for breast cancer using immunohistochemistry

Presentation
- Usually found incidentally
  - Sentinel LN biopsy or dissection may be performed for diagnosis or for staging of carcinomas or melanoma
- Nevus cell aggregates in LNs can be associated with malignant or benign processes
  - Malignant melanoma
  - Breast carcinoma
  - Adnexal skin carcinoma
  - Congenital cutaneous nevi
  - Blue nevus and cellular blue nevus
  - Plexiform spindle cell nevus and atypical spitzoid tumors
  - Neurofibromatosis

Treatment
- Therapy is not needed for benign melanocytic or nevus cell inclusions
  - However, these lesions are found incidentally in procedures performed for underlying malignancies
  - Positive sentinel LN biopsy followed by lymphadenectomy improves survival of patients with melanoma
  - Positive cases identify patients who may benefit from adjuvant therapy
- Sentinel LN biopsy is considered efficient approach for early detection of metastasis of melanoma to LNs

Prognosis
- Nevus cells in lymph nodes
  - Excellent prognosis when nevus cells are only lesion in LN
    - Nevus cells may not be capable of completing multistep process of conventional metastasis
    - Nevus cells are not capable of proliferation and colonization

- Variable prognosis when associated with malignancy that prompted LN dissection
- Rare cases of melanoma in LN are thought to arise from benign nevus aggregates
  - Variable prognosis for melanoma found only in LN without primary site

MICROSCOPIC PATHOLOGY

Histologic Features
- Nevus cell inclusions in lymph nodes
  - Usually extend over small fraction of LN capsule; mean size ~ 3 mm
    - NCI may grow under influence of cytokines in cases associated with melanoma
  - Typically, nevus cells distributed as band within LN capsule
    - Small, slender, uniform, bipolar, cytologically bland cells
    - Indistinct cell membranes; usually with finely granular pigmented cytoplasm
    - Histologically reminiscent of blue nevus
    - Pigment may be dispersed along collagen fibers, inside endothelial cells, or within macrophages
    - Nevus cell aggregates may extend along fibrous trabeculae of LN in larger lesions
  - Subcapsular NCI may be nodular and composed of solid clusters of oval cells with empty clefts
    - Usually display clear cytoplasm; pigmentation is dusty and focal
    - No multinucleation
    - No mitotic figures
  - Occasionally found adjacent to small blood vessels
  - NCI are usually surrounded by reticulin meshwork
- Cellular blue nevus in LNs is usually in peripheral sinuses or parenchyma
  - Rarely found within lymphatics around lymph nodes
  - This pattern is distinct from usual capsular NCI
  - Therefore, intrasinusoidal nevus cell aggregates are not necessarily malignant melanoma

NEVUS CELL INCLUSIONS IN LYMPH NODE

ANCILLARY TESTS

Immunohistochemistry
- Immunohistochemical evaluation of sentinel LNs of patients with melanoma is standard procedure
- S100 protein(+), tyrosinase(+), and Melan-A(+) in melanocytic inclusions
- HMB-45(+/-), Ki-67(-), IMP3(-), keratin(-)

PCR
- RT-PCR for tyrosinase mRNA performed on sentinel LNs can be positive in NCI and melanoma-bearing cases
  - Sensitivity ~ 70%
  - Positive test in ~ 11% of control cases
    - Therefore, poor specificity
    - Some of these (+) cases probably due to nevus cell inclusions
- RT-PCR of sentinel LNs of melanoma patients has been recommended to increase sensitivity provided by immunohistochemistry
  - Positive molecular result should trigger review of original biopsy, including immunohistochemistry

Molecular Genetics
- *BRAF* oncogene point mutation V600E is considered most common genetic alteration in melanoma (~ 80%)
  - Thymine to adenine missense mutation at nucleotide 1799 of *BRAF* gene
    - Substitutes glutamic acid for valine at codon 600 (V600E)
  - However, *BRAF* oncogene point mutation is detected in ~ 50% of NCI in LNs

DIFFERENTIAL DIAGNOSIS

Lymph Node Dissections for Melanoma
- Location of cells beyond capsule into subcapsular sinus or LN parenchyma favors metastasis
  - Skin nevus can rarely be associated with floating nevus cells within sinuses ("benign metastasis")
- Cellular atypia, including prominent nucleoli and mitotic activity
  - Melanoma cells are usually positive for HMB-45, IMP3, and Ki-67
  - Melanoma cells are not usually surrounded by reticulin meshwork as noted with reticulin stain

Lymph Node Dissections for Carcinoma
- Carcinoma cells usually present as large aggregates within sinuses
- Cellular atypia, including prominent nucleoli and mitotic activity
- Immunohistochemistry for cytokeratin or EMA supports metastatic carcinoma
- Fibroblastic reticular cells can be positive for low molecular weight cytokeratin

Atypical Spitzoid Melanocytic Tumors in Children
- Skin tumor of children, adolescents, and young adults

  - Skin lesions show benign architecture with large melanocytes with "glassy" cytoplasm and frequent mitoses
- Positive sentinel LNs occur in ~ 50% of cases and do not adversely affect prognosis

Glomus Tumor
- Glomus cells may simulate nevus cell aggregates
- Immunohistochemistry: Smooth muscle actin (+), S100 protein (-), and CD34(-)

DIAGNOSTIC CHECKLIST

Pathologic Interpretation Pearls
- Typically, nevus cells are distributed as band within LN capsule
  - Occasional nevus cells within sinuses or LN parenchyma
- Lesions with high proliferation index favor metastasis
  - Ki-67 helpful

SELECTED REFERENCES

1. Busam KJ et al: Atypical spitzoid melanocytic tumors with positive sentinel lymph nodes in children and teenagers, and comparison with histologically unambiguous and lethal melanomas. Am J Surg Pathol. 33(9):1386-95, 2009
2. Taube JM et al: Benign nodal nevi frequently harbor the activating V600E BRAF mutation. Am J Surg Pathol. 33(4):568-71, 2009
3. Dadzie OE et al: Incidental microscopic foci of nevic aggregates in skin. Am J Dermatopathol. 30(1):45-50, 2008
4. Holt JB et al: Nodal melanocytic nevi in sentinel lymph nodes. Correlation with melanoma-associated cutaneous nevi. Am J Clin Pathol. 121(1):58-63, 2004
5. Patterson JW: Nevus cell aggregates in lymph nodes. Am J Clin Pathol. 121(1):13-5, 2004
6. Biddle DA et al: Intraparenchymal nevus cell aggregates in lymph nodes: a possible diagnostic pitfall with malignant melanoma and carcinoma. Am J Surg Pathol. 27(5):673-81, 2003
7. Starz H et al: Tyrosinase RT-PCR as a supplement to histology for detecting melanoma and nevus cells in paraffin sections of sentinel lymph nodes. Mod Pathol. 16(9):920-9, 2003
8. Bautista NC et al: Benign melanocytic nevus cells in axillary lymph nodes. A prospective incidence and immunohistochemical study with literature review. Am J Clin Pathol. 102(1):102-8, 1994
9. Lamovec J: Blue nevus of the lymph node capsule. Report of a new case with review of the literature. Am J Clin Pathol. 81(3):367-72, 1984
10. Ridolfi RL et al: Nevus cell aggregates associated with lymph nodes: estimated frequency and clinical significance. Cancer. 39(1):164-71, 1977

Microscopic and Diagrammatic Features

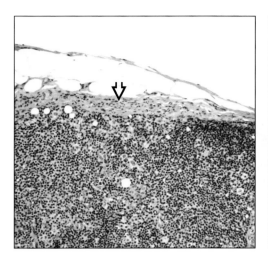

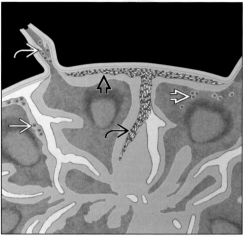

(Left) Lymph node with spindle nevus cells in the capsule ⮞. The remainder of the lymph node shows reactive changes. (Courtesy C. Torres-Cabala, MD.) *(Right)* Distribution of melanocytic and nevus cell inclusions in lymph nodes. Melanocytes are spindled and pigmented and usually distributed within the capsule ⮞ and trabeculum ⮞. Occasionally, nevus cells can be found in afferent lymphatics ⮞, sinuses ⮞, or, rarely, within nodal parenchyma ⮞.

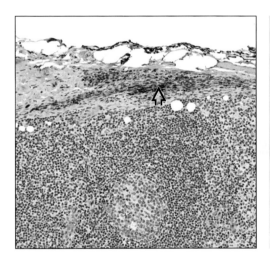

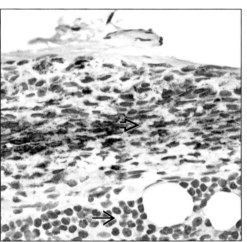

(Left) Melan-A103 immunohistochemistry of a lymph node highlights the distribution of nevus cell inclusions along the lymph node capsule ⮞. Benign nevus cells are not seen within sinuses. *(Right)* Melan-A103 immunohistochemistry highlights nevus cells within lymph node capsule. Nevus cells are small and spindled ⮞. Benign nevus cells do not infiltrate the subcapsular sinus ⮞. (Courtesy C. Torres-Cabala, MD.)

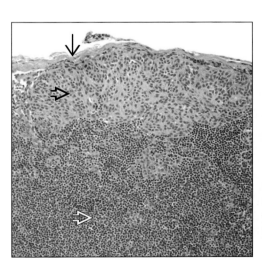

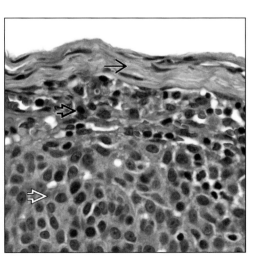

(Left) Metastatic melanoma fills a subcapsular sinus ⮞. Overlying capsule is thin ⮞. Underlying lymph node shows preserved architecture ⮞. *(Right)* Metastatic melanoma in subcapsular sinus ⮞ admixed with small lymphocytes ⮞. Overlying capsule is thin and contains scattered spindled fibroblasts ⮞.

VASCULAR TRANSFORMATION OF LYMPH NODE SINUSES

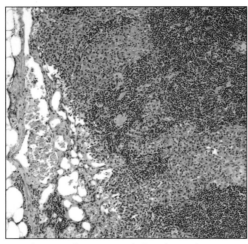

Vascular transformation of lymph node sinuses. Hematoxylin and eosin stain shows expansion and fibrosis of the subcapsular sinuses by a vasoproliferative process.

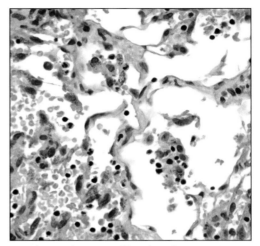

Vascular transformation of lymph node sinuses. Sinuses are distended by blood-filled, anastomosing, endothelial-lined vascular channels, fibrosis, and hemosiderosis.

TERMINOLOGY

Abbreviations
• Vascular transformation of lymph node sinuses (VTS)

Synonyms
• Nodal angiomatosis, stasis lymphadenopathy

Definitions
• Conversion of nodal sinuses into complex, anastomosing, endothelial-lined channels
• Vasoproliferative process
• Fibrosis is frequent

ETIOLOGY/PATHOGENESIS

VTS Associations
• Occlusion of efferent lymphatics, with or without venous obstruction
  ○ Factors contributing to lymphovascular obstruction
    ▪ Vascular thrombosis, severe heart failure, and previous surgery
    ▪ Possible secretion of pro-angiogenesis factors

CLINICAL ISSUES

Epidemiology
• Age
  ○ Adults; often patients with cancer

Site
• Lymph nodes
  ○ Typically, regional lymph nodes excised for cancer operations
  ○ Intraabdominal > axillary, inguinal > cervical, supraclavicular > mediastinal

Presentation
• Usually asymptomatic

• No laboratory abnormalities
• In some patients, no apparent cause or associated disease

Treatment
• Excision is curative

Prognosis
• Excellent; VTS is innocuous

MICROSCOPIC PATHOLOGY

Histologic Features
• Lymph node
  ○ Architecture intact and normal capsule
  ○ Sinuses: Distended by blood-filled, anastomosing, endothelial-lined vascular channels
    ▪ Fibrosis and hemosiderosis; fibrin deposits
    ▪ Subcapsular sinus is most often involved
    ▪ Intermediate or medullary sinuses also commonly involved
  ○ Follicles: Normal or depleted
  ○ Interfollicular areas: Normal
  ○ Blood vessels in perinodal tissue are prominent, with thickened muscle coat
    ▪ No evidence of vasculitis; thrombi rare

Cytologic Features
• No cellular atypia
• Well-formed capillary-sized vessels occur in sinus with fibrosis
• 4 patterns of vascular proliferation are described
  ○ Cleft-like spaces; most common pattern (71%)
  ○ Rounded vascular channels, most often in subcapsular sinus (60%)
  ○ Solid spindle cell foci interspersed with collagen (41%)
    ▪ Solid spindle cell foci merge and "mature" into better-formed blood vessels near capsule

VASCULAR TRANSFORMATION OF LYMPH NODE SINUSES

Key Facts

Clinical Issues
- Any age group
- No sex preference
- Usually incidental finding
- Involves lymph nodes
  ○ Either single or multiple
  ○ Commonly involves regional lymph nodes draining cancer

Macroscopic Features
- 4 patterns of vascular proliferation involving diffuse or segmental pattern
  ○ Cleft-like spaces
  ○ Rounded vascular channels, most often found in subcapsular sinus
  ○ Solid foci of spindled cells interspersed with collagen
  ○ Plexiform pattern

Microscopic Pathology
- Benign vasoproliferative process in which lymph node sinuses are converted into vascular channels
- Confined to sinuses; sclerosis common and can be prominent
- Vascular slits are complex and branching
- Pericytes are present
- VTS does not
  ○ Involve lymph node capsule
  ○ Have cellular atypia
  ○ Have PAS-positive hyaline globules (except rarely)

Ancillary Tests
- Immunostaining for smooth muscle highlights pericytes

○ Plexiform pattern (12%)
  ▪ Intraabdominal lymph nodes
  ▪ Complex intercommunicating channels lined by attenuated endothelium
- Nodular spindle cell variant
  ○ Most frequent in retroperitoneal lymph nodes removed because of renal cell carcinoma
  ○ Nodules comprise interlacing fascicles of spindle cells with interspersed vascular clefts
  ○ Most spindle cells are pericytes or smooth myocytes
  ○ Pushing, lobulated borders
- Coexistence of 2 or more patterns is common

ANCILLARY TESTS

Immunohistochemistry
- Spindle cells: Smooth muscle actin(+), vimentin(+)
  ○ Keratin(-), S100(-), desmin(-), and FVIIIRAg(-)
- Endothelial cells lining vascular channels: FVIIIRAg(+) and CD34(+)

DIFFERENTIAL DIAGNOSIS

Kaposi Sarcoma
- Occurs most frequently in immunocompromised hosts
- Histologic features
  ○ Lymph node capsule and trabeculae are involved
  ○ Vascular slits short and nonbranching
  ○ Spindle cell fascicles are seen
  ○ PAS-positive hyaline globules common
- Unlike VTS, Kaposi sarcoma typically lacks
  ○ Rounded vascular spaces in subcapsular sinuses
  ○ Sinusoidal sclerosis or pericytic component

Nodal Hemangioma
- Nodular growth centered on lymph node hilum or medulla
- Discrete mass lesion of vascular channels
- Closely packed blood vessels with barely visible lumina creates cellular, spindle cell pattern

- Immunostaining for smooth muscle actin highlights pericytes
- Sinuses not involved; no dominant solid smooth muscle component

Bacillary Angiomatosis
- Immunocompromised subjects
- Haphazard, coalescent nodules in nodal parenchyma
- Deeply eosinophilic interstitial material
- Warthin-Starry stain shows clusters of bacilli in macrophages and extracellular areas

Inflammatory Pseudotumor of Lymph Node
- Vascular and myofibroblastic proliferation
- Involves capsule and trabeculae of lymph node
- Prominent inflammatory infiltrate rich in plasma cells
- Vasculitis is common

DIAGNOSTIC CHECKLIST

Pathologic Interpretation Pearls
- Vascular slits in VTS are complex and branching
- Pericytic component is present
- Confined to sinuses; capsule is spared
- Sclerosis is common and can be prominent
- No cellular atypia

SELECTED REFERENCES

1. Cook PD et al: Nodular spindle-cell vascular transformation of lymph nodes. A benign process occurring predominantly in retroperitoneal lymph nodes draining carcinomas that can simulate Kaposi's sarcoma or metastatic tumor. Am J Surg Pathol. 19(9):1010-20, 1995
2. Chan JK et al: Vascular transformation of sinuses in lymph nodes. A study of its morphological spectrum and distinction from Kaposi's sarcoma. Am J Surg Pathol. 15(8):732-43, 1991
3. Haferkamp O et al: Vascular transformation of lymph node sinuses due to venous obstruction. Arch Pathol. 92(2):81-3, 1971

VASCULAR TRANSFORMATION OF LYMPH NODE SINUSES

Microscopic Features

(Left) Vascular transformation of lymph node sinuses. Immunohistochemical stain for CD34 shows strong positivity of blood vessels in sinuses in this case. Note the absence of staining of spindle cells forming cuffs around blood vessels. (Right) Vascular transformation of lymph node sinuses. Immunohistochemical stain for smooth muscle actin accentuates the cuff-like arrangement for spindle cells around vascular channels in this case.

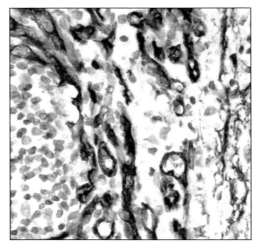
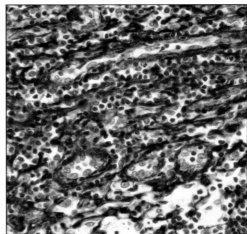

(Left) Vascular transformation of lymph node sinuses. Hematoxylin and eosin stain shows lymph node with prominent vascular transformation associated with lymphocyte depletion in the parenchyma. Note the rounded vascular channels in the subcapsular sinus ⊇. (Right) Vascular transformation of lymph node sinuses. Hematoxylin and eosin stain shows both a solid, nodular pattern ⊅ and more "mature," better-formed vessels underneath the lymph node capsule ⊅.

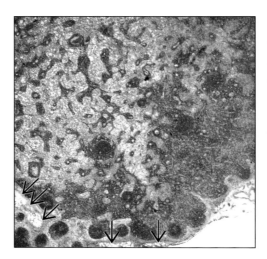
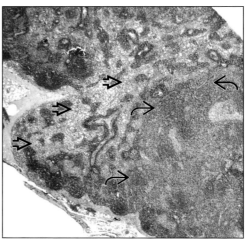

(Left) Vascular transformation of lymph node sinuses. Hematoxylin and eosin stain of an intraabdominal lymph node shows a plexiform pattern of VTS. Note the complex intercommunicating channels lined by attenuated endothelium. (Right) Vascular transformation of lymph node sinuses. Hematoxylin & eosin stain shows vascular transformation with both solid foci composed of sclerosis ⊇ and well-formed vessels ⊅ distending sinuses.

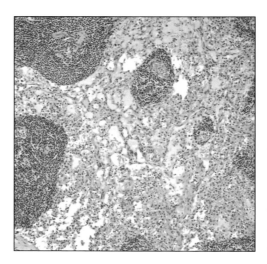
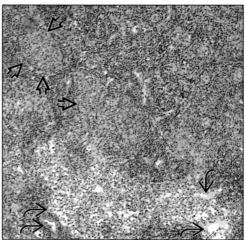

VASCULAR TRANSFORMATION OF LYMPH NODE SINUSES

Microscopic Features and Differential Diagnosis

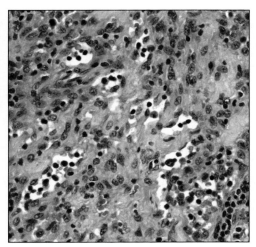

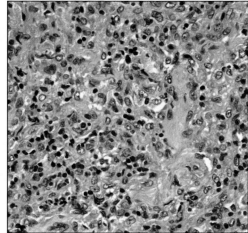

(Left) Vascular transformation of lymph node sinuses. Hematoxylin and eosin stain shows an area of vascular transformation with a solid pattern composed of plump cells and poorly formed vascular channels. *(Right)* Vascular transformation of lymph node sinuses. Hematoxylin and eosin stain shows an area of vascular transformation composed of solid foci of spindle cells interspersed with collagen.

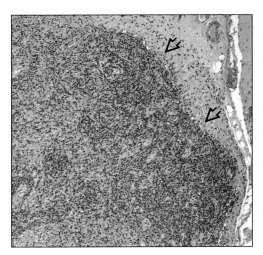

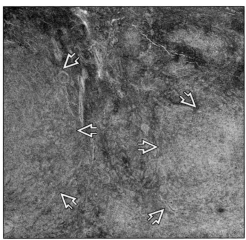

(Left) Nodular variant of vascular transformation of lymph sinuses. This was a retroperitoneal lymph node removed as part of a nephrectomy for renal cell carcinoma. Nodules are composed of interlacing fascicles of spindle cells with interspersed vascular clefts. Note the pushing, lobulated borders ⊳. *(Right)* Lymph node involved by bacillary angiomatosis. Note haphazard, coalescent nodules ⊳ in the parenchyma without a sinusoidal distribution.

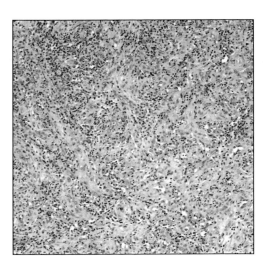

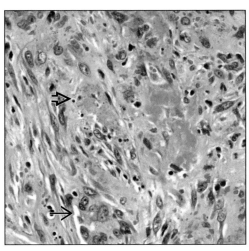

(Left) Lymph node involved by bacillary angiomatosis. Hematoxylin and eosin shows a low-power pale or pink appearance as a result of abundant eosinophilic, amorphous interstitial material. *(Right)* Lymph node involved by bacillary angiomatosis. Hematoxylin and eosin stain shows deeply eosinophilic interstitial material (bacillary aggregates) ⊳ and scattered neutrophils. Plump endothelial cells ⊳ are present. Mitotic figures in spindle cells are also seen.

ANGIOMYOMATOUS HAMARTOMA

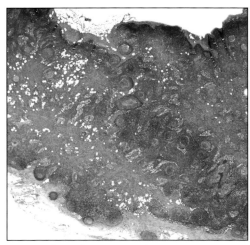

Hematoxylin and eosin stain shows angiomyomatous hamartoma extensively replacing the lymph node parenchyma.

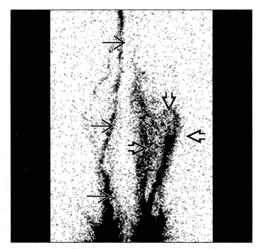

Anterior view from a lymphangioscintigram of the lower extremities shows normal lymphatic drainage ➡ of the right leg but dermal backflow ⮥ on the left. The left leg was edematous on exam.

TERMINOLOGY

Abbreviations
- Angiomyomatous hamartoma (AH)

Definitions
- Benign smooth muscle proliferation that begins in hilum and extends into medulla and cortex of lymph node
  - Involves inguinal lymph nodes almost exclusively

ETIOLOGY/PATHOGENESIS

Unknown
- Unknown but may represent
  - Acquired hamartomatous lesion
  - Unusual reparative reaction to previous lymph node inflammation
  - Result of interference with normal lymphatic drainage

CLINICAL ISSUES

Epidemiology
- Age
  - Mean: 42 years
  - Range: 3-80 years
- Gender
  - M:F ratio = 5:1

Site
- Edema or swelling of ipsilateral limb sometimes accompanies lymphadenopathy
- Lesion is clinically innocuous but may recur after excision

Presentation
- Patients present with enlarged inguinal lymph nodes
  - Lymph nodes can be matted

- Lymphadenopathy is often of long duration
- Pain and swelling
- Occurrence
  - 13 of 17 cases developed in inguinal lymph nodes
  - 2 cases in femoral lymph nodes
  - 1 case each in popliteal and cervical lymph nodes, respectively

Treatment
- Surgical approaches
  - Excision

Prognosis
- Excellent

IMAGE FINDINGS

General Features
- Ultrasonography
  - Poorly circumscribed mass with heterogeneous echo levels
  - Relatively well circumscribed; low echoic areas

Lymphoscintigraphy Findings
- Extensive lymph node abnormalities
- Anarchic lymphatic vessel drainage
- Dermal backflow
- Absence of superficial lymphatic vessels and deep lymphatic drainage
- Absence of visualization of iliac lymph nodes

MACROSCOPIC FEATURES

Size
- 1-3.5 cm

Lymph Node
- Lymph node is replaced by firm white tissue
  - Preferential involvement of hilum and medulla

ANGIOMYOMATOUS HAMARTOMA

Key Facts

Terminology
- Benign smooth muscle proliferation that begins in hilum and extends into medulla and cortex of lymph node
  - Involves inguinal lymph nodes almost exclusively

Clinical Issues
- Wide age range; male predominance
- Lymph node enlargement is often of long duration
- Pain, edema, or swelling of ipsilateral limb may be present
- Lesion clinically innocuous

Image Findings
- Poorly circumscribed mass with heterogeneous echo levels

- Extensive lymph node abnormalities by lymphoscintigraphy studies

Microscopic Pathology
- Characterized by extensive lymph node parenchymal replacement by
  - Smooth muscle with absence of cellular fascicles
  - Blood vessels
  - Fibrous tissue
- No mitoses

Ancillary Tests
- Immunohistochemistry
  - Smooth muscle cells: H-caldesmon(+), muscle specific actin(+), desmin(+), CD34(-)
  - Endothelial cells: CD31(+), CD34(+)

MICROSCOPIC PATHOLOGY

Histologic Features
- Lymph Node
  - Hilum
    - Smooth muscle proliferation closely related to narrow or ectatic vascular spaces
    - Haphazardly and sparsely dispersed bland-looking smooth muscle cells in sclerotic stroma
    - Increased in fibrous tissue; sclerosis
    - Process extends into and replaces nodal parenchyma
    - Congested, proliferated, thin-walled blood vessels interspersed within lesion
  - Medulla and cortex
    - Process extends into medulla and cortex

Cytologic Features
- Smooth muscle cells are spindled with eosinophilic cytoplasm but do not form fascicles
  - No mitoses

ANCILLARY TESTS

Immunohistochemistry
- Smooth muscle cells are
  - H-caldesmon(+), muscle specific actin(+), desmin(+)
  - CD31(-), CD34(-)
- Endothelial cells are
  - CD31(+), CD34(+)

DIFFERENTIAL DIAGNOSIS

Primary Nodal Leiomyomatosis (Vascular Leiomyomatosis)
- Benign; usually intraabdominal lymph nodes
- Proliferation of compact bundles of smooth muscle
- Mitotically inactive

Lymphangiomyomatosis
- Female predominance
- Thoracic and abdominal lymph nodes or as part of more widespread disease
- Fascicles of smooth muscle cells surround anastomosing ectatic vascular spaces
- Endothelium-lined anastomosing vascular channels
- HMB-45(+)

Lymphangioma
- Cystic endothelium-lined spaces
  - Filled with lymph fluid and lymphocytes

Palisaded Myofibroblastoma
- More cellular tumor with amianthoid fibers
- Spindle cells form fascicles; no vascular proliferation
- Smooth muscle actin(+), vimentin(+)

DIAGNOSTIC CHECKLIST

Angiomyomatous Hamartoma
- Male predominance
- Inguinal lymph nodes
- Involves lymph node hilum, medulla, and portions of cortex
- Spindled cells with eosinophilic cytoplasm haphazardly arranged
- Proliferation of thick-walled blood vessels
- H-caldesmon(+), muscle specific actin(+), HMB-45(-)

SELECTED REFERENCES

1. Bourgeois P et al: Lymphoscintigraphy in angiomyomatous hamartomas and primary lower limb lymphedema. Clin Nucl Med. 34(7):405-9, 2009
2. Mauro CS et al: Angiomyomatous hamartoma of a popliteal lymph node: an unusual cause of posterior knee pain. Ann Diagn Pathol. 12(5):372-4, 2008
3. Chan JK et al: Primary vascular tumors of lymph nodes other than Kaposi's sarcoma. Analysis of 39 cases and delineation of two new entities. Am J Surg Pathol. 16(4):335-50, 1992

12

Microscopic and Imaging Features

(Left) Angiomyomatous hamartoma involving lymph node. This image shows smooth muscle cells sparsely and haphazardly dispersed in collagenous stroma. Note thick ➡ and thin ➡ blood vessels, respectively. *(Right)* Angiomyomatous hamartoma involving a lymph node. Immunohistochemical stain for muscle specific actin shows abundant smooth muscle in the muscle wall of the blood vessels ➡ and intervening spaces.

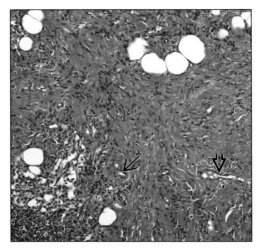
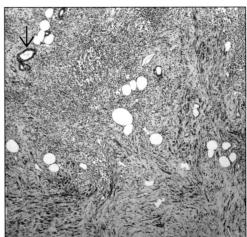

(Left) Angiomyomatous hamartoma involving a lymph node. Immunohistochemical stain for muscle specific actin at high magnification shows smooth muscle cells that are positive for actin spraying into the sclerotic stroma. *(Right)* Angiomyomatous hamartoma involving a lymph node. Immunohistochemical staining for caldesmon shows the abnormal and haphazard thick-walled blood vessels in the hilum.

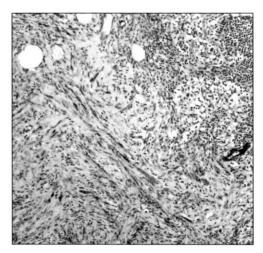
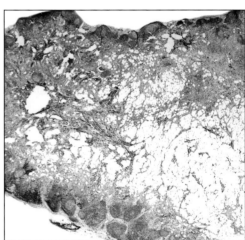

(Left) Angiomyomatous hamartoma involving lymph node. This is an immunohistochemical stain for caldesmon at high magnification. *(Right)* CT image of the right leg shows an enlarged inguinal lymph node ➡. Surgical clips ➡ are seen from a prior lymph node biopsy, which confirmed the diagnosis of angiomatous hamartoma.

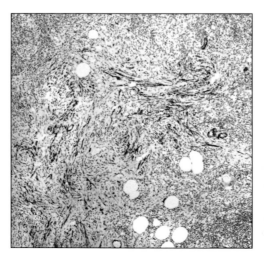
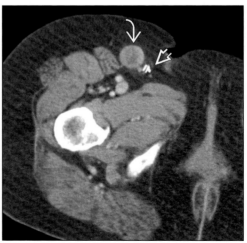

Differential Diagnosis

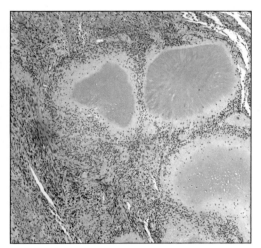

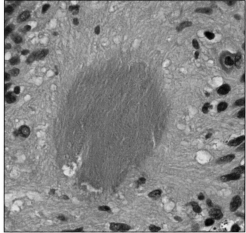

(Left) Palisaded myofibroblastoma with amianthoid bodies composed of fine collagen fibers. Note the hemorrhagic rim and hemosiderin deposits. (Right) Palisaded myofibroblastoma (PM) shows stellate-shaped areas containing thick collagen fibers (so-called amianthoid bodies). PM is a rare benign mesenchymal tumor of lymph node with myofibroblastic/smooth muscle differentiation.

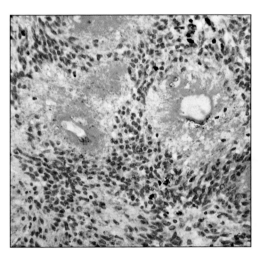

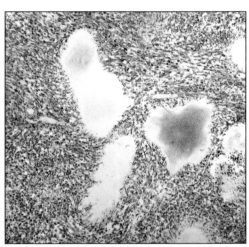

(Left) Palisaded myofibroblastoma shows positivity for smooth muscle actin. (Right) Palisaded myofibroblastoma shows immunopositivity for vimentin. The spindled cells were also immunoreactive for myosin but not for desmin, S100 protein, or factor VIII-related antigen (not shown).

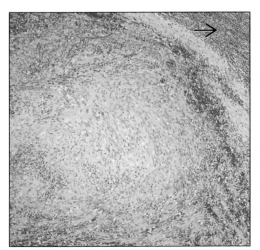

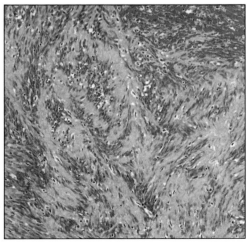

(Left) Palisaded myofibroblastoma in an inguinal lymph node from a 40-year-old man. Low-power view shows an attenuated rim of lymph node tissue on top ⇒. Note the prominent interstitial hemorrhagic rim. Spindle cells are evident. (Right) PM. Parallel and criss-cross fascicles of spindle cells are separated by degenerated collagen. PM is benign and does not need any further therapy except total surgical resection of the mass.

PALISADED MYOFIBROBLASTOMA

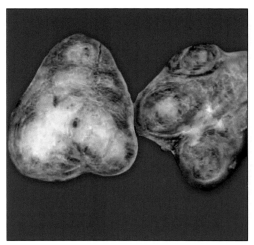

A fixed excisional lymph node biopsy specimen shows replacement by palisaded myofibroblastoma. Note the central gray-white areas and subcapsular hemorrhage ("milk freshly poured into tea").

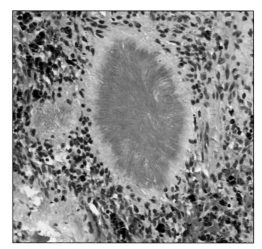

Amianthoid fibers were prominent in this case of palisaded myofibroblastoma. Amianthoid fibers are composed of eosinophilic mats of degenerated collagen fibers with a starburst quality in this field.

TERMINOLOGY

Abbreviations
- Palisaded myofibroblastoma (PM)

Synonyms
- Intranodal palisaded myofibroblastoma
- Intranodal hemorrhagic spindle cell tumor with amianthoid fibers
- Myofibroblastoma

Definitions
- Benign tumor of probable myofibroblastic origin that almost always arises in inguinal lymph nodes
  - Minority view suggests smooth muscle origin (from vessels or capsule)

ETIOLOGY/PATHOGENESIS

Acquired Abnormality
- Inguinal lymph nodes have increased numbers of myofibroblasts compared with other lymph nodes
- May be related to increased lymphatic drainage at this site
  - Predisposes to benign proliferation of myofibroblastic cells

CLINICAL ISSUES

Epidemiology
- Incidence
  - Rare tumor; approximately 50 cases reported in literature
- Age
  - Wide age range: 19-71 years
    - Median: 6th decade
- Gender
  - Slight male predominance (M:F = 4:1)

- Ethnicity
  - No ethnic preference reported

Presentation
- Painful mass
- Unilateral; no side preference
- Unicentric; rare multicentric cases reported
- Almost all cases arise in inguinal lymph nodes
  - Located deeply; under inguinal ligament
  - Overlying skin is not involved
- Rare cases reported in submandibular or cervical lymph nodes

Treatment
- Surgical approaches
  - Excision is curative
  - No additional therapy required

Prognosis
- Excellent
  - Benign lesion
  - Only 2 cases have recurred locally and needed reexcision
    - Recurrence at 6 years and 9 years

MACROSCOPIC FEATURES

General Features
- Size: Range 0.6-5.0 cm in greatest dimension
- Well encapsulated
- Cut surface is gray-white and nodular with subcapsular hemorrhage
  - Likened to "milk freshly poured into tea"

MICROSCOPIC PATHOLOGY

Histologic Features
- Often nodular pattern at low power
- Surrounded by pseudocapsule

PALISADED MYOFIBROBLASTOMA

Key Facts

Terminology
- Intranodal palisaded myofibroblastoma
- Synonyms
  - Intranodal hemorrhagic spindle-cell tumor with amianthoid fibers
  - Myofibroblastoma

Clinical Issues
- Rare benign tumor of probable myofibroblastic origin
- Almost always involves inguinal lymph nodes
- Excision is curative

Macroscopic Features
- Well encapsulated

Microscopic Pathology
- Crisscrossed fascicles of parallel, slender, spindled cells

- Often display palisading pattern
- Can resemble Antoni type A areas of schwannoma
- Mats of eosinophilic material (amianthoid fibers)
  - Stellate or circular shapes depending on plane of section
  - Homogeneous, deeply eosinophilic

Ancillary Tests
- Immunohistochemistry
  - Actin-sm(+), myosin(+)
  - Vimentin(+), Cyclin-D1(+/-)
  - Desmin(-), S100(-), HMB-45(-), CD34(-), CD117(-)

Top Differential Diagnoses
- Schwannoma
- Angiomyomatous hamartoma

- Uninvolved lymph node parenchyma often compressed
- Crisscrossed fascicles of parallel, slender, spindled cells
  - Often display palisading pattern
    - Can resemble Antoni type A areas of schwannoma
  - Spindle cells have eosinophilic cytoplasm and nuclei with tapered ends
    - No nuclear atypia
    - Mitotic figures rare or absent
- Extravasated erythrocytes between spindle cells common
  - Hemosiderin can be abundant
- Amianthoid fibers are present
  - Mats of eosinophilic material
    - Stellate or circular shapes depending on plane of section
    - Homogeneous, deeply eosinophilic
    - Trichrome stain very positive (collagen)
    - Small vessels lined by flattened endothelial cells can be at center
- Metaplastic bone has been reported in PM rarely

Cytologic Features
- Few case reports of PM assessed by fine needle aspiration
- Touch imprint findings
  - Cellular with bland spindled cells
  - Arranged in vague palisades
  - Amianthoid fibers can be seen on imprints

ANCILLARY TESTS

Immunohistochemistry
- Actin-sm(+), muscle specific actin(+), myosin(+)
  - Actin-sm expression accentuated around amianthoid fibers
- Vimentin(+), Cyclin-D1(+/-)
- Extracellular material
  - Collagen types I(+), III(+), IV(+)
  - Fibronectin(+), laminin(+)
- Desmin(-), S100(-), HMB-45(-)

- FVIIIRAg(-), CD34(-), CD117/KIT(-)
- Keratins(-), CEA(-), synaptophysin(-)
- EBV-latent membrane protein type 1(-)
- Herpes simplex(-), human papilloma virus(-)

In Situ Hybridization
- EBV-encoded RNA (EBER)(-)

Electron Microscopy
- Intracytoplasmic inclusions support myofibroblastic origin
- Amianthoid fibers represent loosely parallel collagen fibers
- No Weibel-Palade bodies, secretory granules, or desmosomes

DNA Content Analysis
- Diploid

DIFFERENTIAL DIAGNOSIS

Schwannoma (Neurilemmoma)
- No preference for inguinal lymph nodes
- Benign tumor of Schwann cells
  - Commonly Antoni type A and B areas are present
  - Hemorrhage can occur but uncommon
  - No amianthoid fibers
- Immunohistochemistry
  - S100(+), actin-sm(-), desmin(-)
- PM was initially considered to be intranodal schwannoma

Angiomyomatous Hamartoma
- Occurs in inguinal lymph nodes
- Predominantly affects men; wide age range
- Benign lesion; excision is curative
- Smooth muscle proliferation associated with medium-to-large blood vessels
- Arises in hilum but often extends into medulla and cortex
- No amianthoid fibers
- Immunohistochemistry

PALISADED MYOFIBROBLASTOMA

○ Desmin(+), actin-sm(+)

Leiomyoma
- No preference for inguinal lymph nodes
- Benign tumor of smooth muscle cells
  ○ Whorls of smooth muscle cells
  ○ Hemorrhage rare
  ○ No amianthoid fibers
- Immunohistochemistry
  ○ Desmin(+), caldesmon(+), EMA(+/-), LMWK(+/-)

Inflammatory Pseudotumor
- Any lymph node group can be involved
- Lesion is centered in capsule and trabeculae of lymph node
- Mixed inflammatory cell infiltrate

Kaposi Sarcoma
- Common history of HIV infection and associated skin lesions
- No preference for inguinal lymph nodes
- Malignant tumor of endothelial cells
  ○ Cell fascicles are thinner (than PM) and lined by endothelial cells
  ○ Often abundant hemorrhage
  ○ High mitotic activity and nuclear atypia
- Immunohistochemistry
  ○ Vascular markers(+), HHV8(+)
  ○ Actin(-), myosin(-)

Leiomyosarcoma
- No preference for inguinal lymph nodes
- Malignant tumor of smooth muscle cells
  ○ Hemorrhage and necrosis common
  ○ Nuclear atypia and high mitotic activity
- Immunohistochemistry
  ○ Desmin(+), caldesmon(+), EMA(+/-), LMWK (+/-)

Follicular Dendritic Cell Sarcoma
- Lymph nodes of head and neck and thorax
- Malignant tumor of follicular dendritic cells
  ○ Whorls of plump cells: Spindled or epithelioid
  ○ Nuclear atypia and mitotic figures (variable)
  ○ Small lymphocytes often admixed with tumor cells
    ■ Can be CD23(+)
- Immunohistochemistry
  ○ CD21(+), CD23(+), CD35(+)
  ○ Clusterin(+), EGFR(+/-), vimentin(+)
  ○ Actin-sm(-), actin(-), myosin(-)

Interdigitating Dendritic Cell Sarcoma
- Malignant tumor of interdigitating dendritic cells
  ○ Epithelioid or spindled neoplastic cells
  ○ Nuclear atypia and mitotic figures (often high)
- Immunohistochemistry
  ○ S100(+), histiocyte markers(+/-)
  ○ Actin-sm(-), muscle specific actin(-), myosin(-)

Metastatic Spindle Cell Melanoma
- Any lymph node group can be involved
- Nuclear atypia and mitotic figures (often high)
- Melanosomes often present by EM
- Immunohistochemistry

○ S100(+), HMB-45(-)
○ Actin-sm(-), muscle specific actin(-), myosin(-)

Metastatic Spindle Cell Carcinoma
- Any lymph node group can be involved
- Nuclear atypia and mitotic figures (often high)
- Desmosomes often present by EM
- Immunohistochemistry
  ○ Keratins(+), actin(-), myosin(-)

Inflammatory Myofibroblastic Tumor
- No preference of inguinal lymph nodes
- Can metastasize
- Nuclear atypia and mitoses are variable
- Immunohistochemistry
  ○ S100(+), ALK(+/-)

DIAGNOSTIC CHECKLIST

Clinically Relevant Pathologic Features
- Organ distribution
  ○ Almost always involves inguinal lymph nodes
- Benign lesion but can rarely recur locally

Pathologic Interpretation Pearls
- Spindle cells and amianthoid fibers are distinctive
  ○ No nuclear atypia and only rare mitoses

SELECTED REFERENCES

1. Koseoglu RD et al: Intranodal palisaded myofibroblastoma; a case report and review of the literature. Pathol Oncol Res. 15(2):297-300, 2009
2. Skagias L et al: Imprint cytology of intranodal palisaded myofibroblastoma. Diagn Cytopathol. Epub ahead of print, 2009
3. Kleist B et al: Intranodal palisaded myofibroblastoma with overexpression of cyclin D1. Arch Pathol Lab Med. 127(8):1040-3, 2003
4. Creager AJ et al: Recurrent intranodal palisaded myofibroblastoma with metaplastic bone formation. Arch Pathol Lab Med. 123(5):433-6, 1999
5. Hisaoka M et al: Intranodal palisaded myofibroblastoma with so-called amianthoid fibers: a report of two cases with a review of the literature. Pathol Int. 48(4):307-12, 1998
6. Michal M et al: Intranodal "amianthoid" myofibroblastoma. Report of six cases immunohistochemical and electron microscopical study. Pathol Res Pract. 188(1-2):199-204, 1992
7. Bigotti G et al: Selective location of palisaded myofibroblastoma with amianthoid fibres. J Clin Pathol. 44(9):761-4, 1991
8. Suster S et al: Intranodal hemorrhagic spindle-cell tumor with "amianthoid" fibers. Report of six cases of a distinctive mesenchymal neoplasm of the inguinal region that simulates Kaposi's sarcoma. Am J Surg Pathol. 13(5):347-57, 1989
9. Weiss SW et al: Palisaded myofibroblastoma. A benign mesenchymal tumor of lymph node. Am J Surg Pathol. 13(5):341-6, 1989
10. Deligdish L et al: Malignant neurilemmoma (Schwannoma) in the lymph nodes. Int Surg. 49(3):226-30, 1968

Microscopic Features

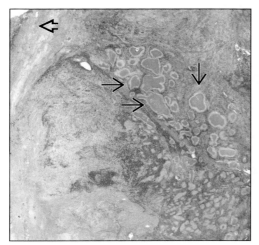

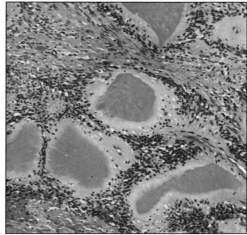

(Left) Low magnification shows a case of palisaded myofibroblastoma involving inguinal lymph node. The lymph node is completely replaced. Pseudocapsule is present ⊵. Numerous amianthoid fibers ⊠ and hemorrhage and fibrosis are also present. **(Right)** Amianthoid fibers in a case of palisaded myofibroblastoma involving an inguinal lymph node. The amianthoid fibers are surrounded by basophilic spindle cells.

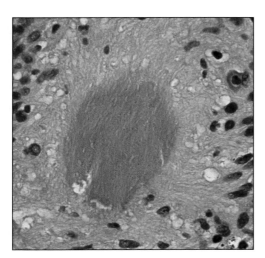

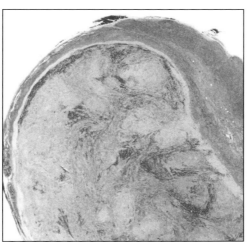

(Left) High-power magnification (oil immersion) of amianthoid fibers in a case of palisaded myofibroblastoma involving lymph node. Spindle cells are present at the periphery. **(Right)** Low-power magnification shows a palisaded myofibroblastoma that involved lymph node. Normal lymph node tissue is compressed and displaced. The lesion is cellular with many spindle cells and foci of hemorrhage.

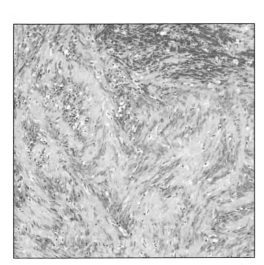

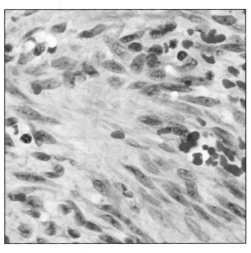

(Left) In this field of palisaded myofibroblastoma, the spindle cells are palisading and mimic Antoni type A structures as can be seen in schwannoma (neurilemmoma). Foci of hemorrhage are present in this field. **(Right)** High-power magnification (oil immersion) shows a palisaded myofibroblastoma that involved inguinal lymph node. Note the bland-appearing spindle cells and the absence of nuclear atypia or mitotic figures.

METASTATIC KAPOSI SARCOMA

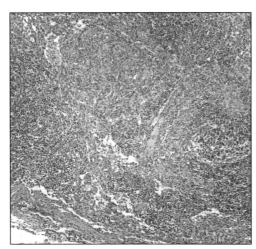

Kaposi sarcoma (KS) associated with multicentric Castleman disease. In the center of the field, focal KS is present among hyaline-vascular follicles. KS is predominantly sinusoidal.

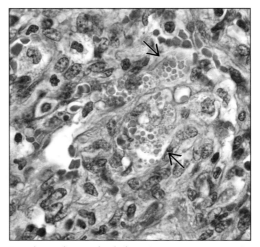

Lymph node involved by Kaposi sarcoma (KS). Note spindle cells and histiocytes with cytoplasmic, eosinophilic hyaline globules ➡. The globules stain a lighter color than erythrocytes.

TERMINOLOGY

Abbreviations
- Kaposi sarcoma (KS)
- Human herpes virus type 8 (HHV8)

Definitions
- Kaposi sarcoma (KS): Distinctive type of vascular neoplasm that can involve any body site
  - Almost always associated with HHV8 infection
  - Occurs sporadically at low frequency but is much more frequent in setting of immunosuppression

ETIOLOGY/PATHOGENESIS

Infectious Agents
- HHV-8, a *Gammaherpesviridae*, is uniformly expressed in KS
  - a.k.a. Kaposi sarcoma-associated herpes virus (KSHV)
- HHV8 establishes latent infection in most infected KS cells; lytic replication occurs in small subset of KS cells
- Transmission via sexual and nonsexual routes
  - Saliva contains shed epithelial cells infected by HHV-8

Pathogenesis
- KS may be multicentric neoplasm at time of conception
- HHV8 interacts with other factors in pathogenesis
  - e.g., HIV TAT protein has mitogenic and modulating effects on KS cells
- Angiogenic factors and cytokines are likely to be involved
- Viral proteins expressed during both latent and lytic phases of viral life cycle contribute to KS pathogenesis

Cell of Origin
- KS involves progenitor cell from either blood vessel or lymphatic endothelia

  - CD34(+) suggests progenitor endothelial cells

CLINICAL ISSUES

Epidemiology
- Incidence
  - Varies greatly depending on presentation
- Age
  - Varies depending on presentation
- Gender
  - Male predominance in all types of KS
- Ethnicity
  - Sporadic cases more common around Mediterranean sea

Site
- Skin, mucosal surfaces, lymph nodes, and all internal organs
  - Skin most common site
  - Oral mucosa and gastrointestinal tract are frequent sites
  - Lymph node involvement usually associated with skin disease
    - Rare patients reported with only lymph node disease

Presentation
- Presentation of KS can be divided into 4 clinical subsets
  - Sporadic (classic)
    - Involves distal extremities of elderly patients
    - Common in men of Mediterranean and Jewish Ashkenazi origin
    - Clinically indolent
    - Subset of cases can be clinically aggressive; associated with coexistent non-Hodgkin lymphoma
    - In USA, 0.2 per 100,000 tumors
  - African (endemic)

METASTATIC KAPOSI SARCOMA

Key Facts

Etiology/Pathogenesis
- HHV8 infection plays critical role in most cases
  - Interacts with other factors

Clinical Issues
- Multiple presentations of KS
  - Sporadic (Mediterranean countries)
  - Endemic (equatorial Africa)
  - Iatrogenic (e.g., post transplantation)
  - Epidemic (HIV-associated)
- Common sites: Skin, lymph nodes, gastrointestinal tract
  - Often multifocal

Microscopic Pathology
- Wide histologic spectrum
  - Lacework of thin-walled capillaries
  - Ectatic vessels without pericytes
  - Cleft-like vascular spaces, nonbranching
  - Well-formed bundles and whorls of spindle cells
- Extravasated erythrocytes
- Intracytoplasmic eosinophilic hyaline globules
- Plasma cells and small lymphocytes common
- Hemosiderin-laden macrophages common

Ancillary Tests
- Immunohistochemistry
  - HHV8(+), CD31(+), CD34(+)
  - FVIIIRAg(+) in well-differentiated tumors

Top Differential Diagnoses
- Bacillary angiomatosis
- Vascular transformation of lymph node sinuses
- Angiosarcoma

- Sub-Saharan central Africa
- 9% of malignant neoplasms in Uganda
- Children often have generalized lymphadenopathy and aggressive clinical course
- Subset of aggressive cases likely related to HIV infection
- Middle-aged adults have KS on extremities; more indolent
- Iatrogenic immunosuppression
  - KS arises more frequently after organ transplantation or steroid therapy
  - 128x increased incidence after kidney transplantation
  - Usually clinically indolent; can be aggressive
- AIDS-associated (epidemic)
  - 451x increased incidence in setting of AIDS infection
  - More common in homosexuals; less frequent in IV drug users and hemophiliacs

Natural History
- In patients who die, KS can be widespread at autopsy
  - Organs: Virtually any organ can be involved
    - Lungs common

Treatment
- Drugs
  - Highly active antiretroviral therapy (HAART)

Prognosis
- Depends, in large part, on clinical presentation and associated illness
- HAART therapy has reduced frequency and improved prognosis for epidemic KS

MACROSCOPIC FEATURES

Lymph Nodes
- Enlarged and matted

Skin
- Size range: 0.1 cm up to 3 cm
- Pink-red or purple lesions
- Patches, plaques, or nodules

MICROSCOPIC PATHOLOGY

Histologic Features
- Lymph node
  - Early lesions usually involve capsule
  - KS cells proliferate along trabeculae or infiltrate in wedge-shaped pattern
  - KS eventually replaces most or all of lymph node
  - Uninvolved lymph node shows preserved architecture
    - Reactive follicles with prominent germinal centers
    - Plasmacytosis of medullary cords
- Histologic patterns of KS (in any site)
  - Ectatic or thick-walled blood vessels (well differentiated)
    - Blood lakes can be present
  - Anastomosing vascular channels
  - Glomeruloid aggregates of vessels
  - Spindle cells with vascular cleft-like spaces that contain erythrocytes
  - Pure spindle cell pattern; often with whorls of cells (sarcoma-like)
- KS is commonly associated with
  - Hemorrhage
  - Small lymphocytes &/or plasma cells
  - Hemosiderin-laden macrophages
    - Highlighted by iron stain
  - Cytoplasmic hyaline globules
    - Periodic acid-Schiff (PAS)(+), with and without diastase digestion
    - Probably represent degenerated, phagocytosed erythrocytes
- Nuclei are large, slightly pleomorphic
- Mitoses are usually present
- Early lesions can be difficult to recognize
  - Appear as lacework of irregularly shaped, thin-walled capillary vessels

METASTATIC KAPOSI SARCOMA

ANCILLARY TESTS

Immunohistochemistry
- HHV8(+), strong and diffuse
  - Antibody specific for latent nuclear antigen-1 (LANA-1)
- CD31(+), CD34(+), vimentin(+)
- FVIIIRAg(+/-), *Ulex europaeus*(+/-)
  - Positive in tumors with well-differentiated blood vessels

PCR
- HHV8 present in most (if not all) KS
  - Shown by PCR or Southern blot methods
  - Nuclear localization by in situ hybridization

Electron Microscopy
- Mixture of endothelial cells, pericytes, fibroblasts, and myofibroblasts
- Weibel-Palade bodies infrequent
- Phagocytosis of erythrocytes present

DIFFERENTIAL DIAGNOSIS

Bacillary Angiomatosis
- Prevalent in HIV-infected patients; forms cutaneous vascular lesions
- Bacillary angiomatosis usually causes skin lesions
- Capillaries are lined by typical endothelial cells
  - No nuclear atypia
- Bacilli stain with Warthin-Starry stain

Vascular Transformation of Lymph Node Sinuses
- Confined predominantly to lymph node sinuses
- Capsule involvement is not present (unlike KS)
- No atypia or mitotic figures; no cytoplasmic hyaline globules

Vascular Hyperplasia of HIV Lymphadenitis
- In late stages of HIV lymphadenitis, vascular proliferation can be abundant
- Blood vessels are not cleft-like but well formed
- Bundles or whorls of spindle-shaped cells are not present
- No nuclear atypia and rare or absent mitoses

Angiosarcoma
- Usually no history of immunosuppression or HIV infection
- Angiosarcomas exhibit endothelial multilayering, nuclear atypia, and mitoses

Follicular Dendritic Cell Sarcoma
- Highly spindled but without vascular clefts
- Can have marked atypia and many mitoses
- CD21(+), CD23(+), CD35(+), clusterin(+)
- CD31(-), CD34(-)
- Usually no history of immunosuppression or HIV infection

Angioimmunoblastic T-cell Lymphoma (AITL)
- Branching vascular pattern located in paracortex
- AITL is thought to arise in or around follicles
  - In contrast, KS arises in capsule and grows in along trabeculae
- Atypical T-cell population, often with clear cytoplasm
- ± aberrant T-cell immunophenotype
- Monoclonal T-cell receptor gene rearrangements

Metastatic Spindle Cell Carcinoma or Melanoma
- Evidence of primary neoplasm elsewhere
- Nuclear atypia and mitoses more prominent
- Immunohistochemistry helpful
  - Carcinoma: Keratin(+); melanomas: S100(+), HMB-45(+)

DIAGNOSTIC CHECKLIST

Clinically Relevant Pathologic Features
- 4 clinical forms of disease with similar histologic findings

Pathologic Interpretation Pearls
- In lymph nodes, KS preferentially involves capsule, trabeculae, and medulla
- HHV8(+)

SELECTED REFERENCES
1. Arkin LM et al: Kaposi's sarcoma in the pediatric population: the critical need for a tissue diagnosis. Pediatr Infect Dis J. 28(5):426-8, 2009
2. Koreishi A et al: Synchronous Follicular Lymphoma, Kaposi Sarcoma, and Castleman's Disease in a HIV-Negative Patient With EBV and HHV-8 Coinfection. Int J Surg Pathol. Epub ahead of print, 2009
3. Naresh KN et al: Lymph nodes involved by multicentric Castleman disease among HIV-positive individuals are often involved by Kaposi sarcoma. Am J Surg Pathol. 32(7):1006-12, 2008
4. Schulz TF: The pleiotropic effects of Kaposi's sarcoma herpesvirus. J Pathol. 208(2):187-98, 2006
5. Courville P et al: [Detection of HHV8 latent nuclear antigen by immunohistochemistry. A new tool for differentiating Kaposi's sarcoma from its mimics.] Ann Pathol. 22(4):267-76, 2002
6. Ioachim HL et al: Kaposi's sarcoma of internal organs. A multiparameter study of 86 cases. Cancer. 75(6):1376-85, 1995
7. Templeton AC: Kaposi's sarcoma. Pathol Annu. 16(Pt 2):315-36, 1981

Microscopic Findings

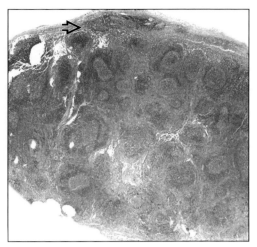

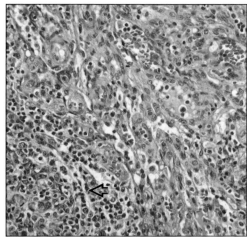

(Left) Lymph node involved by Kaposi sarcoma (KS) and multicentric Castleman disease. Note the capsular and subcapsular proliferation of KS with wedge-shaped penetration into the cortex ➡. (Right) Well-developed Kaposi sarcoma (KS) characterized by curved fascicles of spindle cells with intertwined short slits contains extravasated erythrocytes. A lymphoid follicle is present ➡.

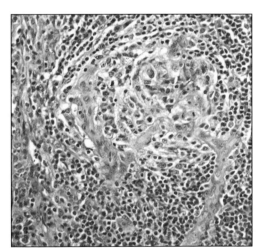

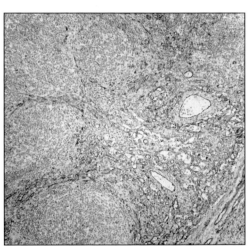

(Left) Lymph node involved by Kaposi sarcoma (KS) and multicentric Castleman disease. A hyalinized, regressed follicle (hyaline-vascular lesion) is shown in this field. Lymphadenopathy, hepatosplenomegaly, and pancytopenia were present in this patient. (Right) KS is composed of well-differentiated vascular spaces that strongly stain with anti-CD34 antibody in this field.

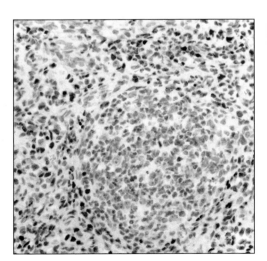

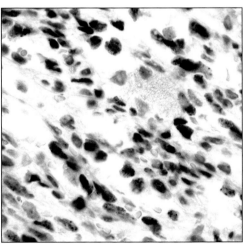

(Left) Lymph node involved by Kaposi sarcoma (KS). In this field, the nuclei of KS surround a reactive lymphoid follicle. The nuclei of the KS cells express human herpes virus type 8 (HHV8). The lymphoid cells are negative for HHV8. (Right) High magnification view shows Kaposi sarcoma (KS) cells in a lymph node. The nuclei of the KS cells are strongly positive for HHV8 using an antibody specific for latent nuclear antigen (LANA-1).

MYELOID/MONOCYTIC SARCOMA

Microscopic and Immunohistochemical Features

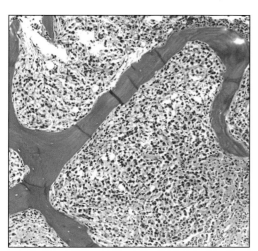

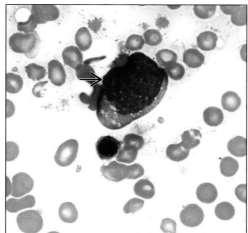

(Left) Acute myeloid leukemia extensively involving bone marrow is shown in this patient with monocytic sarcoma involving skin. *(Right)* An aspirate smear shows a large monoblast ➡. Flow cytometric analysis showed that the blasts had monocytic differentiation, being positive for CD13, CD14, CD15, CD33, CD45, and CD56. Conventional cytogenetics showed a complex hyperdiploid karyotype.

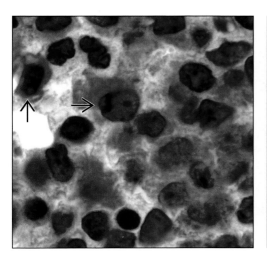

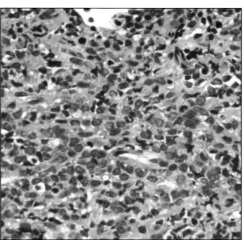

(Left) Myeloid sarcoma. Blasts show cytoplasmic positivity for nucleophosmin (NPM) (mAb 376) ➡. Cytoplasmic NPM correlates with NPM1 gene mutation, the most frequent molecular lesion in myeloid sarcoma (~ 15% of cases). *(Right)* Myeloid sarcoma involving soft tissue. The neoplasm is composed of medium to large cells with irregular nuclear contours. This lesion, in part, mimics diffuse large B-cell lymphoma. Immunohistochemistry is needed for diagnosis of myeloid sarcoma.

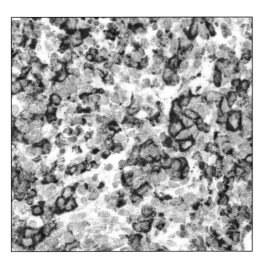

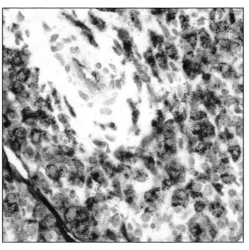

(Left) Myeloid sarcoma involving soft tissue. The neoplastic cells are MPO(+). Myeloid sarcoma should be considered as synonymous with AML. Evaluation of morphologic, immunophenotypic, genetic, and molecular features is needed to classify the neoplasm into AML subgroups or myeloid blast phase of an MPN. *(Right)* Myeloid sarcoma involving soft tissue. The neoplastic cells in this case were CD34(+). CD34 is expressed by ~ 50% of cases of MS.

BLASTIC PLASMACYTOID DENDRITIC CELL NEOPLASM

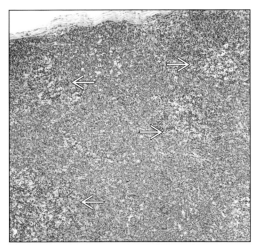

Blastic plasmacytoid dendritic cell neoplasm (BPDCN) involving lymph node. The neoplasm incompletely replaces the lymph node in a paracortical pattern. Uninvolved areas ➡ can be appreciated.

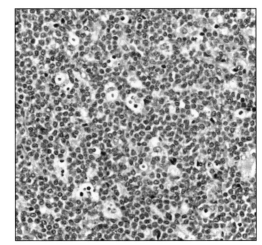

BPDCN involving lymph node. The neoplasm has a "starry sky" pattern in this field, indicating a high cell turnover rate. The neoplastic cells are blast-like.

TERMINOLOGY

Abbreviations
- Blastic plasmacytoid dendritic cell neoplasm (BPDCN)
  - Current term in 4th edition of World Health Organization (WHO) classification

Synonyms
- CD4(+), CD56(+) hematodermic neoplasm/tumor
- CD4(+), CD56(+) blastic tumor of skin
- Blastic NK-cell lymphoma (3rd edition of WHO classification)

Definitions
- Highly aggressive neoplasm derived from precursors of plasmacytoid dendritic cells

ETIOLOGY/PATHOGENESIS

Normal Plasmacytoid Dendritic Cells (PDCs)
- Other terms used for PDCs
  - Type 2 dendritic cells (DC2)
  - Plasmacytoid monocytes (obsolete)
  - Plasmacytoid T cells (obsolete)
- Mostly located in T-zones of lymphoid tissues
- Also present in bone marrow and blood
- PDCs are characterized by
  - High expression of IL-3α chain receptor
  - Production of interferon-γ
  - Differentiate into dendritic cells in culture after treatment with IL3 and CD40 ligand
- PDCs are increased in a number of diseases including
  - Lymph nodes
    - Chronic granulomatous inflammation
    - Kikuchi-Fujimoto disease, Castleman disease
    - Classical Hodgkin lymphoma
  - Skin
    - Psoriasis
    - Lupus erythematosus

- Immunophenotype of normal PDCs
  - CD4(+), CD123(+), HLA-DR(+)
  - CD303/BDCA-2(+), CLA(+), TCL1(+)
  - GZM-B(+), CD43(+, dim), CD68(+, dim)
  - CD11c(-), CD56(-), TIA1(-), perforin(-)

Etiology & Pathogenesis of BPDCN Unknown
- Associated with myelomonocytic leukemia in ~ 10-20% of cases
  - With or without underlying myelodysplasia

CLINICAL ISSUES

Epidemiology
- Incidence
  - Rare
    - < 1% of all lymphomas that involve skin
- Age
  - Median age: ~ 65 years
  - Wide age range: 8-96 years
- Gender
  - Male to female ratio: ~ 2-3:1
- Ethnicity
  - No known ethnic predilection

Site
- Skin is most common initial site of disease
- Other common sites of disease at time of initial diagnosis
  - Lymph nodes
  - Bone marrow and blood
    - Usually low-level involvement
- Staging studies can show involvement of
  - Spleen, liver, other viscera
- Other rare sites of disease
  - Tonsils, nasopharynx, gums
  - Lacrimal gland, conjunctiva
  - Kidneys, gynecologic tract

BLASTIC PLASMACYTOID DENDRITIC CELL NEOPLASM

Key Facts

Clinical Issues
- Median age: ~ 65 years
  - Wide age range: 8-96 years
- Male to female ratio: ~ 2-3:1
- Skin is most common initial site of disease
- Other common sites of disease at initial diagnosis
  - Lymph nodes
  - Bone marrow and blood
- No established standard therapy
- Very aggressive clinical course; median survival 12-14 months

Microscopic Pathology
- Skin: Diffuse dermal infiltrate
- Lymph nodes: Paracortical or diffuse replacement
- Bone marrow: Interstitial pattern
- Neoplastic cells can exhibit spectrum of findings
  - Small/intermediate size resembling lymphoblasts
  - Intermediate size and resembling myeloblasts

Ancillary Tests
- Characteristic immunophenotype
  - CD123(+), TCL1(+), CD303(+), bcl-11A(+)
  - CD4(+), CD56(+)
- TdT expressed in ~ 50% of cases
- CD45/LCA(+), CD99(+/-)
- Conventional cytogenetics
  - Complex karyotype common

Top Differential Diagnoses
- Myeloid/monocytic sarcoma or leukemia
- T lymphoblastic leukemia/lymphoma
- PDC proliferations associated with myeloid neoplasms

- Central nervous system involvement is rare at diagnosis
  - Involved in ~ 33% of patients at time of relapse
- Mediastinum is rarely involved

Presentation
- Solitary or multiple skin lesions
  - Nodules, patch-like, or plaques
  - ± erythema, ± purpura
  - Can be asymptomatic
  - Disease restricted to skin in ~ 50% of patients
- Regional lymph nodes positive in ~ 50% of patients
- Low-level blood and bone marrow involvement
- Systemic B symptoms are uncommon

Laboratory Tests
- Complete blood count
  - ± cytopenias
  - ± monocytosis
- BPDCN can progress to full-blown leukemic phase
  - Neoplastic cells may be either BPDCN or myelomonocytic leukemia

Treatment
- No established standard therapy; options usually employed
  - Combination chemotherapy
  - Allogeneic stem cell transplantation at first relapse
- Localized radiotherapy has limited utility

Prognosis
- Very aggressive clinical course
- Median survival: 12-14 months
  - Patients often have good initial response to chemotherapy
  - Relapse and disease progression very common
- Skin lesions respond to radiotherapy, but this modality has limited utility
- Few patients enter long-term remission after stem cell transplantation
- Prognosis is relatively better for patients < 40 years
  - Median survival: ~ 3 years

IMAGE FINDINGS

Radiographic Findings
- Increased uptake by [18F] fluorodeoxyglucose positron emission tomography

MACROSCOPIC FEATURES

General Features
- Nodules, plaques, or bruise-like lesions of skin
  - ± ulcer

MICROSCOPIC PATHOLOGY

Histologic Features
- Skin
  - Monomorphous infiltrate predominantly involving dermis
    - Perivascular and periadnexal pattern in lesions with minimal involvement
    - Diffuse pattern with extensive involvement
    - Grenz zone usually present between infiltrate and epidermis
    - No or minimal epidermotropism
  - Erythrocyte extravasation is common
  - Modest inflammatory infiltrate associated with neoplasm
    - Small number of T cells
    - Usually no plasma cells or eosinophils
- Lymph node
  - Diffuse effacement of lymph node architecture
  - In cases with partial involvement
    - Preferential paracortical replacement
    - Sinuses can be involved
- Bone marrow
  - Mild to marked interstitial infiltration
  - Dysplasia in residual hematopoietic cells
    - Can be prominent in megakaryocytes

13

BLASTIC PLASMACYTOID DENDRITIC CELL NEOPLASM

Cytologic Features

- Neoplastic cells can exhibit spectrum of findings
  - Small to intermediate size and resembling lymphoblasts
    - Small amount of cytoplasm
    - Fine (blast-like) chromatin with indistinct nucleoli
  - Intermediate size and resembling myeloblasts
    - Moderate, pale to eosinophilic cytoplasm
    - 1 to several nucleoli
- Mitotic figures are numerous
- Bone marrow and peripheral blood smears
  - Agranular cytoplasm (Wright-Giemsa stain)
  - Neoplastic cells often resemble monoblasts with
    - Submembranous ("pearl necklace") cytoplasmic vacuoles
    - Pseudopodia

ANCILLARY TESTS

Immunohistochemistry

- Characteristic profile
  - CD4(+), CD56(+)
    - CD4 and CD56 can show weak/dim expression
  - CD123/IL-3α chain receptor(+)
  - CD303/BDCA2(+), TCL1(+)
  - bcl-11A(+), CD2AP(+)
  - MxA(+)
    - MxA is a surrogate for interferon-γ
- TdT(+/-); expressed in ~ 50% of all cases
  - Subset of cells positive with variable intensity
- CLA(+), CD45RA(+), CD101(+)
- CD45/LCA(+), CD99(+/-)
- Cytotoxic proteins(-), EBV-LMP(-), CD57(-)
- CD23(-), CD30(-), CD138(-)
- T-cell markers
  - CD43(+), CD7(+/-)
  - CD3(-), CD5(-), CD8(-), T-cell receptors(-)
- Myelomonocytic markers
  - CD33(-/+), CD36(+/-), CD68(+/-)
  - CD13(-), CD15(-), CD117(-)
  - Lysozyme(-), MPO(-), CD163(-)
- B-cell markers
  - Surface Ig(-), B-cell antigens(-)

Flow Cytometry

- As above for immunohistochemistry except
  - More sensitive and can detect dim expression more readily
  - Some antigens better assessed by flow cytometry
- CD36(+/-), CD14(-), CD16(-)
- CD57(-), HLA-DR(-)
- BDCA4(+)

Cytogenetics

- Complex karyotypes found in ~ 60-70% of cases
  - 6-8 abnormalities common
  - Gross genomic imbalances predominate
    - Usually hypodiploid
  - 6 major recurrent chromosomal targets have been identified
    - 5q, 12p, 13q, 6q, 15q, and 9

In Situ Hybridization

- EBER(-)

Molecular Genetics

- Few cases have shown monoclonal *TCR* gene rearrangement
- No monoclonal *IgH* gene rearrangements
- *P16* and *P27* abnormalities are common

Cytochemistry

- Naphthol-butyrate esterase(-)
- MPO(-)

DIFFERENTIAL DIAGNOSIS

Myeloid/Monocytic Sarcoma or Leukemia

- Clinical presentation of BPDCN and myelomonocytic sarcoma/leukemia overlap
  - Skin and bone marrow disease, ± lymphadenopathy
- In leukemia, the blasts of myelomonocytic leukemia may have granules (Giemsa stain)
- Cytochemistry
  - MPO or naphthol-butyrate esterase(+) supports myelomonocytic leukemia
- Immunophenotype
  - Unequivocal evidence of granulocytic or monocytic differentiation
  - Best shown by using a panel of markers
    - MPO(+), CD11c(+), CD13(+)
    - CD14(+), CD15(+), CD33(+)
    - CD34(+/-), CD56(+), CD68(+)
  - CD303/BDCA-2, TCL1, bcl-11A , CD2AP are usually negative

T-Lymphoblastic Leukemia/Lymphoma (T-LBL)

- Lymphoblasts and cells of BPDCN show morphologic overlap
  - TdT(+) in both entities can further lead to misdiagnosis
- T-LBL differs from BPDCN as follows
  - Most patients with T-LBL are adolescents or young adults
  - A mediastinal mass is common
  - TdT(+) is usually uniform and bright
  - T-cell antigens are positive in T-LBL dependent on maturational stage
    - Cytoplasmic CD3(+), surface CD3(+/-),
    - CD2(+/-), CD5(+/-), CD7(+), T-cell receptors(+/-)
  - CD123, CD303/BDCA-2, bcl-11A usually (-)
  - CD10(+/-), CD1a(+/-)
- Monoclonal *TCR* rearrangements in T-LBL
  - Reported in small subset of BPDCN

PDC Proliferations Associated with Myeloid Neoplasms

- Previously designated as plasmacytoid T-cell lymphoma
- PDC proliferation most common in lymph nodes
  - Also reported in bone marrow or skin (dermis)
- Patients present with underlying myeloid neoplasm

BLASTIC PLASMACYTOID DENDRITIC CELL NEOPLASM

- Immunohistochemical profile is similar to that of benign PDCs
  - CD4(+), CD56(+), CD123(+)
  - Granzyme B(+), perforin(-), TIA-1(-)
- PDCs can show cytogenetic abnormalities identical to underlying myeloid neoplasm
  - FISH has shown shared abnormalities in chromosomes 7 and 17
  - Therefore, PDC nodules likely to be part of myeloid neoplasm

B-Lymphoblastic Leukemia/Lymphoma (B-LBL)

- Lymphoblasts and BPDCN show morphologic overlap
- B-LBL can rarely present as skin nodules
- B-LBL differs from BPDCN as follows
  - TdT(+) is usually uniform and bright
  - B-cell antigens are positive
    - pax-5(+), CD19(+), CD20(+/-), CD22(+/-)
  - CD10(+/-), CD1a(+/-)
  - Monoclonal *Ig* rearrangements in B-LBL(+)

Extranodal NK-/T-cell Leukemia/Lymphoma, Nasal Type, Involving Skin

- Angiocentric/angiodestructive infiltrate with necrosis
- Variable cytologic features
  - Small to large cells; atypia can be marked
    - Chromatin is usually not blast-like
  - ± azurophilic cytoplasmic granules
- Typical immunophenotype
  - CD2(+), CD56(+)
  - Surface CD3(-), cytoplasmic CD3-ε(+)
  - Cytotoxic molecules(+), CD30(-/+)
  - CD4(-), CD5(-), CD8(-), T-cell receptors(-)
  - CD16(-), CD57(-)
- EBER(+) in all cases
- No evidence of monoclonal *TCR* rearrangements
- ~ 10% of cases are of T-cell lineage
  - T-cell antigens(+)
  - Monoclonal *TCR* rearrangements

T-cell Prolymphocytic Leukemia (T-PLL)

- Patients with T-PLL can develop skin lesions and lymphadenopathy
- Neoplastic cells are TCL1(+) and often CD4(+)
- Most patients present with high leukocyte count and extensive bone marrow disease
- Neoplasm is of true T-cell lineage
  - CD3(+), CD5(+), CD123(-), CD303(-)
  - Monoclonal *TCR* rearrangements

Peripheral T-cell Lymphoma

- Neoplasms showing spectrum of cytologic findings
  - Small, medium-sized, or large neoplastic cells with irregular nuclei
- Certain subtypes show prominent epidermotropism
- Immunophenotype
  - T-cell markers(+)
  - CD4(+) or CD8(+) or negative for both
  - Aberrant immunophenotypes are common
  - CD303(-), CD123(-), CD56(-/+)

- Monoclonal *TCR* rearrangements(+)

DIAGNOSTIC CHECKLIST

Clinically Relevant Pathologic Features

- Skin disease is almost invariable
  - Localized or generalized macules, plaques, or nodules
  - Regional lymph nodes positive in ~ 50% of patients
- Occasionally associated with
  - Acute myeloid or myelomonocytic leukemia
  - Myelodysplastic/myeloproliferative neoplasm (e.g., CMML)
- Very poor prognosis

Pathologic Interpretation Pearls

- Skin
  - Dermal involvement is characteristic
- Lymph node
  - Paracortical/interfollicular or diffuse pattern
- Bone marrow
  - Often shows focal involvement at initial presentation
    - IHC or flow cytometry are essential to identify involvement
  - Can progress to myelomonocytic leukemia
- Neoplastic cells show cytologic spectrum
  - Small to medium-sized cells with blast-like chromatin resembling lymphoblasts
  - Medium-sized cells with more abundant cytoplasm and nuclei with nucleoli
- Immunophenotype
  - CD123(+), CD303(+), TCL1(+)
  - CD4(+), CD56(+), TdT(+/-)
  - CD3(-), MPO(-)

SELECTED REFERENCES

1. Cota C et al: Cutaneous manifestations of blastic plasmacytoid dendritic cell neoplasm-morphologic and phenotypic variability in a series of 33 patients. Am J Surg Pathol. 34(1):75-87, 2010
2. Wiesner T et al: Alterations of the cell-cycle inhibitors p27(KIP1) and p16(INK4a) are frequent in blastic plasmacytoid dendritic cell neoplasms. J Invest Dermatol. 130(4):1152-7, 2010
3. Pilichowska ME et al: CD4+/CD56+ hematodermic neoplasm ("blastic natural killer cell lymphoma"): neoplastic cells express the immature dendritic cell marker BDCA-2 and produce interferon. Am J Clin Pathol. 128(3):445-53, 2007
4. Petrella T et al: Blastic NK-cell lymphomas (agranular CD4+CD56+ hematodermic neoplasms): a review. Am J Clin Pathol. 123(5):662-75, 2005
5. Petrella T et al: TCL1 and CLA expression in agranular CD4/CD56 hematodermic neoplasms (blastic NK-cell lymphomas) and leukemia cutis. Am J Clin Pathol. 122(2):307-13, 2004

BLASTIC PLASMACYTOID DENDRITIC CELL NEOPLASM

Microscopic and Immunohistochemical Features

(Left) Blastic plasmacytoid dendritic cell neoplasm (BPDCN) involving lymph node. The neoplasm completely replaces lymph node and has a diffuse pattern. *(Right)* BPDCN involving lymph node. In this case, the neoplastic cells are small and have immature chromatin resembling, in part, lymphoblasts.

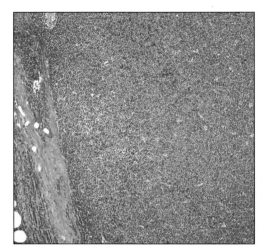
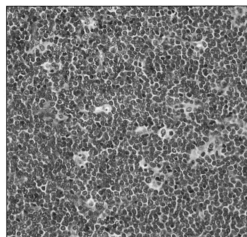

(Left) Blastic plasmacytoid dendritic cell neoplasm involving lymph node. The neoplastic cells in this case expressed CD4 with dim intensity. *(Right)* BPDCN involving lymph node. The neoplastic cells are CD56(+). A residual follicle ➡ is CD56(-).

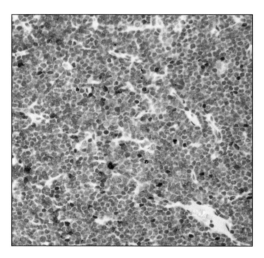
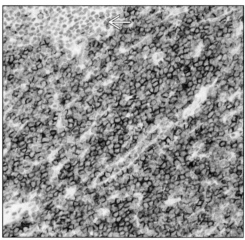

(Left) Blastic plasmacytoid dendritic cell neoplasm involving lymph node. The neoplastic cells are strongly TCL1(+) with a nuclear pattern of expression. TCL1 expression is present in these neoplasms and helpful in the differential diagnosis. *(Right)* BPDCN involving lymph node. The neoplastic cells are strongly CD123(+). Expression of CD123 is characteristic of this neoplasm and very helpful in the differential diagnosis.

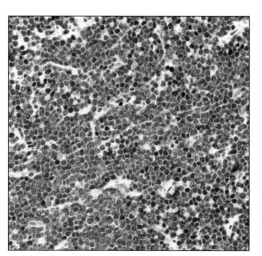
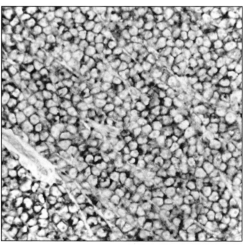

BLASTIC PLASMACYTOID DENDRITIC CELL NEOPLASM

Immunohistochemical and Cytologic Features

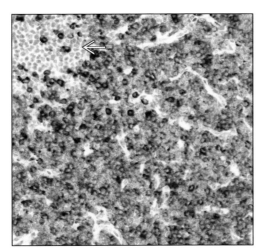
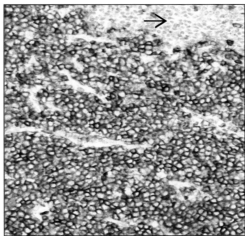

(Left) Blastic plasmacytoid dendritic cell neoplasm involving lymph node. The neoplastic cells are CD7(+). A residual follicle is CD7(-) ➡. *(Right)* BPDCN involving lymph node. The neoplastic cells are CD43(+). A residual follicle is CD43(-) ➡.

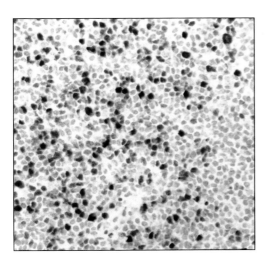
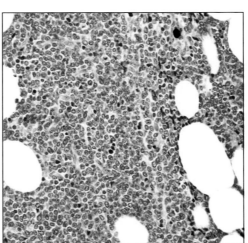

(Left) Blastic plasmacytoid dendritic cell neoplasm involving lymph node. TdT is expressed with variable intensity by a subset of neoplastic cells. *(Right)* BPDCN involving lymph node and perinodal adipose tissue. The neoplastic cells are lysozyme(-).

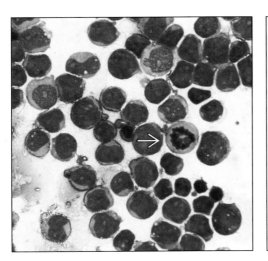
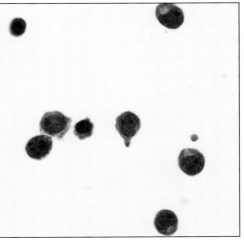

(Left) Fine needle aspiration of cervical lymph node involved by blastic plasmacytoid dendritic cell neoplasm. The neoplastic cells show a range of cell sizes. A mitotic figure ➡ is present in this field. *(Right)* Cerebrospinal fluid is involved by BPDCN.

BLASTIC PLASMACYTOID DENDRITIC CELL NEOPLASM

Microscopic and Immunohistochemical Features

(Left) Blastic plasmacytoid dendritic cell neoplasm involving lymph node. The neoplasm incompletely replaces the lymph node in this field. Residual lymph node tissue ➡ is seen at left of the field. *(Right)* BPDCN involving lymph node. The neoplastic cells have moderately pale cytoplasm and nuclei with small nucleoli. A mitotic figure ➡ is present.

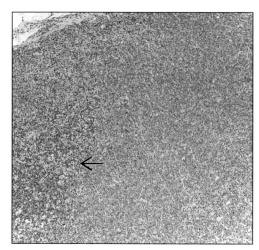
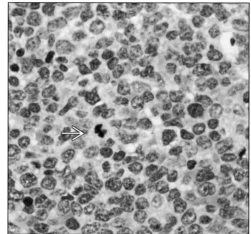

(Left) Blastic plasmacytoid dendritic cell neoplasm involving lymph node. The neoplastic cells are CD56(+). A residual follicle ➡ is CD56(-). *(Right)* BPDCN involving lymph node. The neoplastic cells are CD3(-), which is true in almost all cases of BPDCN. Reactive T cells in this field are CD3(+).

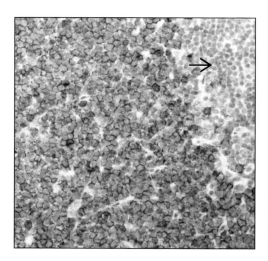
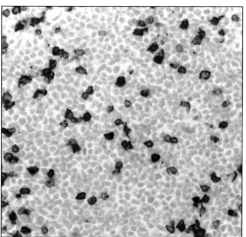

(Left) Blastic plasmacytoid dendritic cell neoplasm involving skin. The neoplastic cells fill the dermis but spare the epidermis. A grenz zone ➡ is present. *(Right)* BPDCN involving skin. The neoplastic cells are strongly TCL1(+).

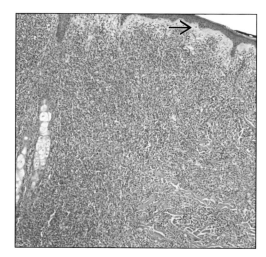
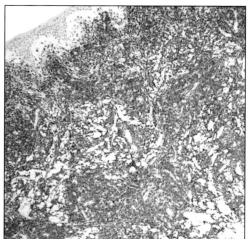

BLASTIC PLASMACYTOID DENDRITIC CELL NEOPLASM

Microscopic and Immunohistochemical Features

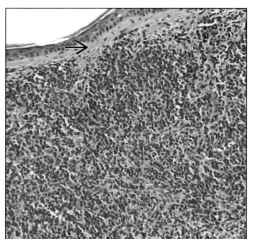

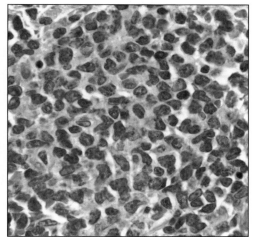

(Left) Blastic plasmacytoid dendritic cell neoplasm involving skin. The dermis is replaced by the neoplasm. The epidermis is not involved, and a grenz zone ⇒ can be appreciated. *(Right)* BPDCN involving skin. The neoplastic cells are small to intermediate in size. These cytologic features suggest a differential diagnosis with lymphoblastic lymphoma and small cell T-cell lymphomas.

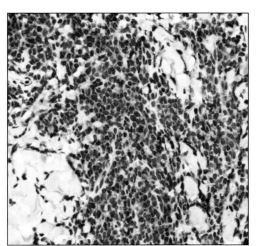

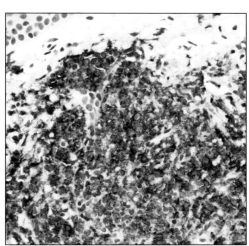

(Left) Blastic plasmacytoid dendritic cell neoplasm involving dermis of skin. The neoplastic cells are CD4(+). *(Right)* BPDCN involving dermis of skin. The neoplastic cells are CD56(+).

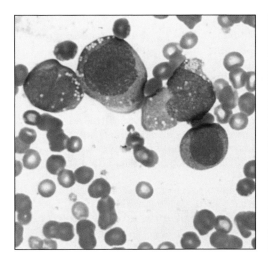

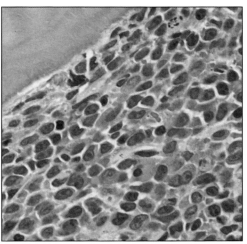

(Left) Wright-Giemsa stain shows acute myelomonocytic leukemia involving bone marrow in a patient with blastic plasmacytoid dendritic cell neoplasm involving skin and lymph node diagnosed 6 months previously. The blasts were MPO(+). *(Right)* Acute myelomonocytic leukemia involving bone marrow. This patient had a BPDCN involving skin and lymph node diagnosed 6 months previously. The medullary space was 100% cellular with numerous blasts.

HISTIOCYTIC SARCOMA

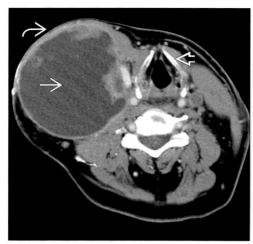

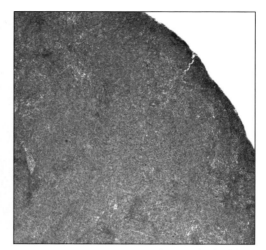

CT of neck shows a 10 cm histiocytic sarcoma of soft tissue ⟹, displaying extensive necrosis ⟹. Calcified thyroid cartilage ⟹ is noted as a reference. (Courtesy P. Bhosale, MD.)

Histiocytic sarcoma. Low magnification shows diffuse effacement of the nodal architecture.

TERMINOLOGY

Abbreviations
- Histiocytic sarcoma (HS)

Synonyms
- True histiocytic lymphoma
- Extramedullary monocytic tumor
- Malignant histiocytosis is historical term
  - Not a true synonym as this term encompassed a number of entities

Definitions
- Malignant neoplasm composed of mature histiocytes
  - Diagnosis mainly based on morphology and immunophenotype
    - Tumor cells are positive for histiocyte-associated markers, such as CD68, CD163, and lysozyme
    - Tumor cells are negative or show minor reactivity for dendritic or follicular dendritic cell markers
- Monocytic/histiocytic neoplasms associated with acute myeloid leukemia, myeloproliferative neoplasms, or myelodysplastic syndromes are excluded
  - Better considered as monocytic sarcoma

ETIOLOGY/PATHOGENESIS

Postulated Normal Cell Counterpart
- Phagocytic histiocyte or macrophage derived from bone marrow monocytes

Etiology
- Unknown

Pathogenesis
- Histiocytic and monocytic tumors are closely related
- Some cases arise as 2nd malignancy after chemotherapy

Concept of "Transdifferentiation"
- Patient has both lymphoid and histiocytic tumors that are clonally related
  - In most patients, histiocytic tumors follow or are synchronous with lymphoid neoplasms
    - Rare histiocytic tumors precede lymphoid neoplasms
  - This occurrence suggests that mature lymphoid cells can switch phenotypes to histiocytic lineage
    - Process may require initial de-differentiation &/or subsequent re-differentiation
- Examples in literature include
  - HS and follicular lymphoma
  - HS and splenic marginal zone lymphoma
  - HS and B-lymphoblastic leukemia/lymphoma
  - Interdigitating dendritic cell sarcoma (IDCS) and follicular lymphoma
  - IDCS and chronic lymphocytic leukemia/small lymphocytic lymphoma
- Histiocytic neoplasms associated with follicular lymphoma share
  - t(14;18)(q32;q21)/IgH-BCL2 and IgH rearrangements
  - Suggests common clonal origin of follicular lymphoma and histiocytic neoplasms
  - Supports that lymphoid neoplasms can transform into histiocytic neoplasms
    - An example of lineage plasticity
  - This concept also may encompass subset of sporadic histiocytic or dendritic cell sarcomas that
    - Bear monotypic IgH gene rearrangements
    - Show IgH/BCL2 translocation also identified in histiocytes
    - Express B-cell transcription factor Oct-2 but are negative for CD20, CD79a, and PAX-5
- Possible mechanisms explaining monoclonal IgH gene rearrangements in HS
  - Lineage infidelity of primitive cells, supported by association with germ cell tumors

HISTIOCYTIC SARCOMA

Microscopic Features

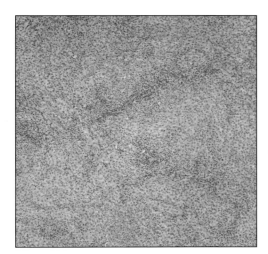

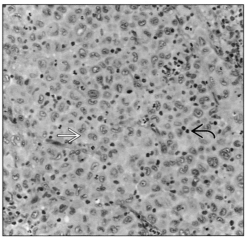

(Left) Histiocytic sarcoma shows diffuse effacement of the lymph node architecture. (Right) Histiocytic sarcoma shows sheets of large cells ⇒ admixed with scattered lymphocytes ⇒.

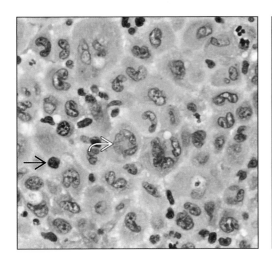

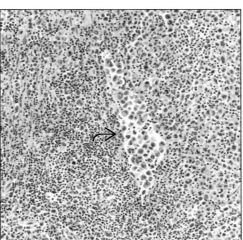

(Left) Histiocytic sarcoma. Large histiocytes ⇒ display abundant cytoplasm and folded nuclei with pleomorphic shapes. There are scattered lymphocytes ⇒ admixed with the neoplastic cells. (Right) Histiocytic sarcoma is seen displaying a sinusoidal pattern ⇒. Histiocytic sarcoma most characteristically is paracortical rather than sinusoidal when there is partial nodal involvement.

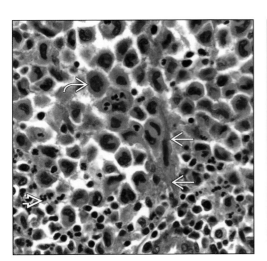

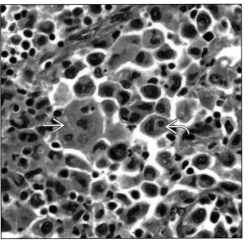

(Left) Histiocytic sarcoma. Large noncohesive histiocytes ⇒ appear contained in a dilated sinusoid ⇒. There are abundant reactive neutrophils ⇒ admixed with the neoplastic cells. (Right) Histiocytic sarcoma. There are pleomorphic neoplastic cells ⇒ as well as reactive histiocytes ⇒ with hemophagocytosis. Hemophagocytosis is more characteristic of lymphohistiocytic hemophagocytic syndromes rather than histiocytic sarcoma.

HISTIOCYTIC SARCOMA

Microscopic and Immunohistochemical Features

(Left) Histiocytic sarcoma. CD68 immunohistochemistry highlights dim reactivity in large neoplastic cells ➜ and strong reactivity in small nonneoplastic histiocytes ➔. *(Right)* Histiocytic sarcoma. CD4 immunohistochemistry highlights membrane reactivity in the large neoplastic cells ➔.

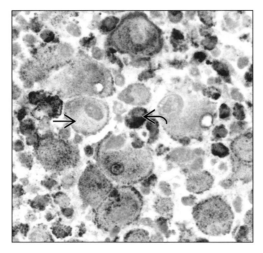
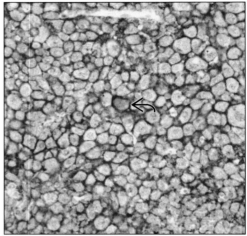

(Left) Histiocytic sarcoma. A neoplastic cell is positive for S100 protein ➔ by immunohistochemistry. Reactivity occurs in the nucleus and in the cytoplasm. In certain cases of histiocytic sarcoma, a subset (< 25%) of neoplastic cells may express S100 protein. *(Right)* Histiocytic sarcoma. Numerous reactive neutrophils are positive for myeloperoxidase ➔ by immunohistochemistry. Neoplastic histiocytes are negative ➔.

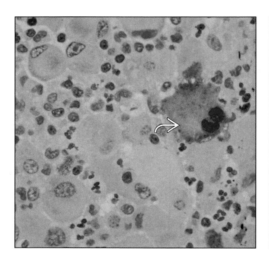
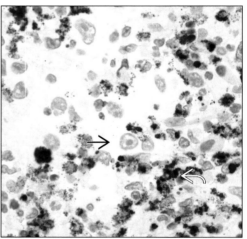

(Left) Histiocytic sarcoma. Touch imprint of lymph node shows large neoplastic cells with abundant cytoplasm and irregular nuclei ➔. *(Right)* Positron emission tomography (PET) of large lateral neck histiocytic sarcoma shows high ➔ standardized uptake value (SUV). Other structures of the neck are negative or very faint ➔. (Courtesy P. Bhosale, MD.)

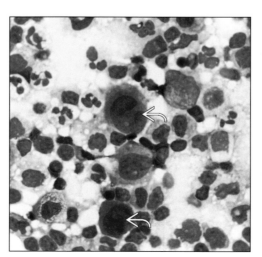
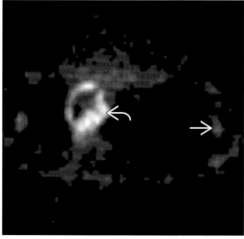

Bone Marrow HS and Monocytic Sarcoma

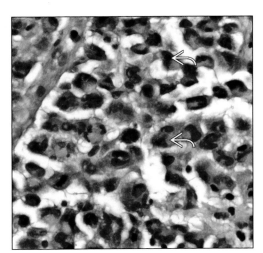
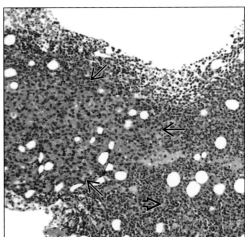

(Left) Histiocytic sarcoma involving lymph node. Large pleomorphic cells ⇨ involve a sinus. In the older literature, cases like this were classified as malignant histiocytosis, but only a small subset of these tumors were truly histiocytic like this tumor. *(Right)* Histiocytic sarcoma (HS) vs. acute monocytic leukemia involving bone marrow (BM). A compact cluster of pleomorphic cells ⇨ is surrounded by uninvolved BM ⇨, suggestive of HS.

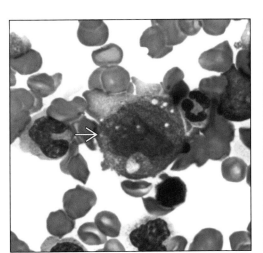
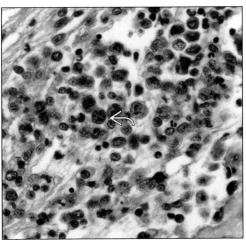

(Left) Histiocytic sarcoma (HS) vs. acute monocytic leukemia (AMoL) in bone marrow (BM) aspirate shows a large cell ⇨ with irregular nucleus and abundant cytoplasm. The WHO recommends classifying this case as AMoL, but a diagnosis of HS can be suggested if these cells are few or < 25% of cellularity. *(Right)* Acute monocytic leukemia in bone marrow. The neoplastic cells ⇨ are similar to histiocytic sarcoma cells and represent ≥ 25% of BM cellularity.

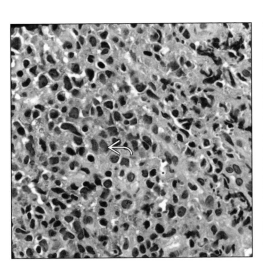
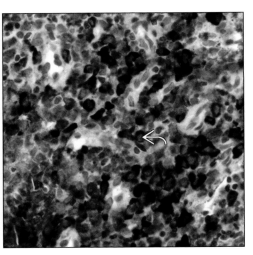

(Left) Monocytic sarcoma in a lymph node. Neoplastic cells show a moderate amount of cytoplasm and central, irregular nuclei ⇨. These cells appear more monocytic than histiocytic. Bone marrow showed refractory anemia with excess blasts. *(Right)* Monocytic sarcoma in a lymph node. Neoplastic cells show strong reactivity with lysozyme ⇨.

Differential Diagnoses: LCH, SHML, and ALCL

(Left) Langerhans cell histiocytosis (LCH). Histiocytes have twisted ➡ or grooved ➡ nuclei with bland fine chromatin. *(Right)* Langerhans cell histiocytosis (LCH). Histiocytes have grooved nuclei ➡ with bland fine chromatin and are associated with frequent eosinophils ➡.

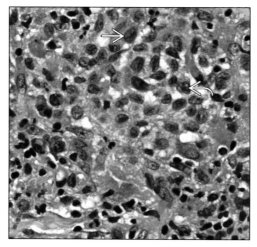 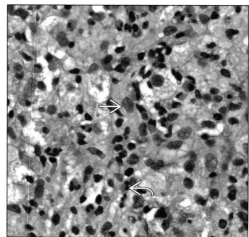

(Left) Rosai-Dorfman disease (RDD). There are scattered histiocytes with abundant cytoplasm, some of which contain intact lymphocytes or plasma cells ➡, a process known as emperipolesis. Histiocytes display vesicular nuclei ➡ with distinct nucleoli. Small lymphocytes and plasma cells ➡ are common in the background. *(Right)* RDD. A large histiocyte containing intact lymphocytes ➡ is S100 protein(+) ➡.

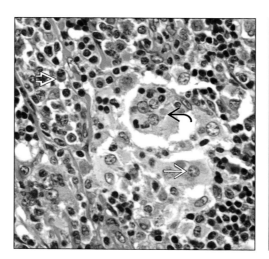 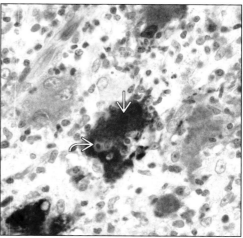

(Left) Anaplastic large cell lymphoma (ALCL). There are large cells ➡ with irregular and pleomorphic nuclei and abundant cytoplasm, similar to histiocytic sarcoma. Scattered small histiocytes ➡ and small lymphocytes are noted in the background. *(Right)* Anaplastic large cell lymphoma. The large neoplastic cells are positive for CD30 ➡, contrary to what occurs in histiocytic sarcoma.

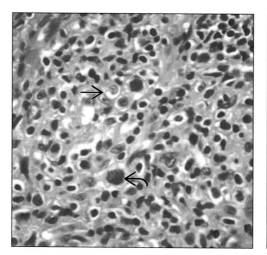 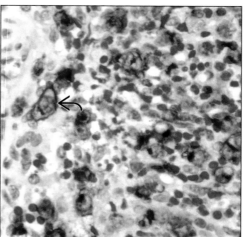

HISTIOCYTIC SARCOMA

"Transdifferentiation" of Histiocytic Neoplasms

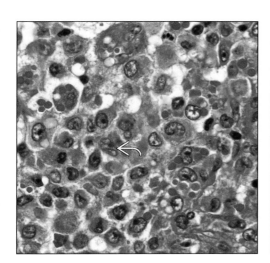
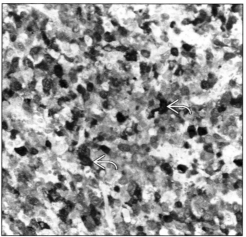

(Left) Interdigitating dendritic cell sarcoma shows neoplastic cells with abundant eosinophilic cytoplasm and folded nuclei ➜. The patient developed follicular lymphoma a few months later, a phenomenon known as transdifferentiation, in which both neoplasms are clonally related as determined by similar IgH gene rearrangements. *(Right)* Interdigitating dendritic cell sarcoma of soft tissue. The neoplastic cells are strongly positive for S100 protein ➜.

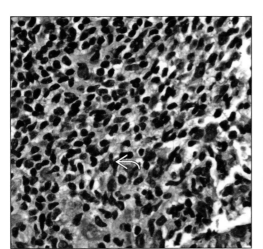
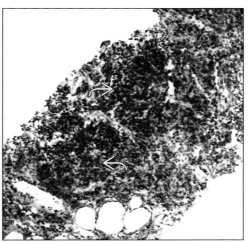

(Left) Follicular lymphoma grade 1 in lymph node. Neoplastic cells are small centrocytes ➜. This lymphoma developed a few months after the patient was diagnosed with interdigitating dendritic cell sarcoma, a process known as transdifferentiation. *(Right)* Follicular lymphoma grade 1 in lymph node. Two neoplastic follicles are highlighted with Bcl-2 ➜. This tumor developed a few months after the patient was diagnosed with interdigitating dendritic cell sarcoma.

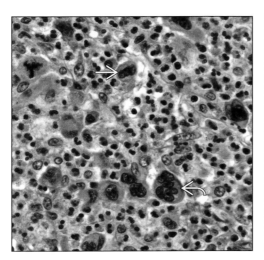
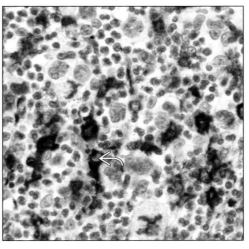

(Left) Malignant histiocytic tumor, unclassifiable. Large pleomorphic cells ➜, some of which are multinucleated ➜ are shown. All histiocytic markers were negative. Approximately 10% of histiocytic malignancies may fall into this category. *(Right)* Malignant histiocytic tumor, unclassifiable. Neoplastic cells are (-) for histiocytic markers, including CD163. Reactive histiocytes are CD163(+) ➜. Histiocytic nature was implied from morphology, CD45/LCA(+), and ultrastructure.

FOLLICULAR DENDRITIC CELL SARCOMA

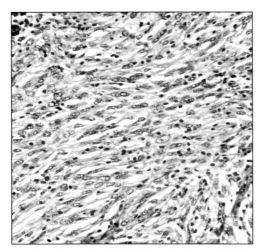

Lymph node involved by follicular dendritic cell (FDC) sarcoma. The neoplastic cells have indistinct cell borders, a moderate amount of eosinophilic cytoplasm, and oval or elongated bland nuclei.

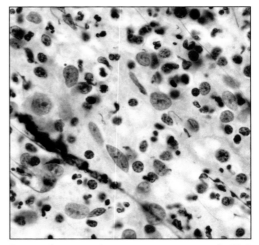

Papanicolaou-stained scrape preparation of FDC sarcoma. The neoplastic cells are large and oval or spindle-shaped, with inflammatory cells in the background.

TERMINOLOGY

Abbreviations
- Follicular dendritic cell (FDC) sarcoma

Synonyms
- FDC tumor
- Dendritic reticulum cell sarcoma

Definitions
- Neoplastic proliferation of follicular dendritic cells
  - Immunophenotype supports FDC lineage

ETIOLOGY/PATHOGENESIS

Normal FDCs
- Localized to B-cell areas in primary and secondary lymphoid follicles
  - Form a meshwork via cell to cell attachments and desmosomes
  - Do not migrate
- Trap and present antigens to B cells that are involved in B-cell proliferation and differentiation
  - Store antigen on cell surface as immune complexes
- Closely related to bone marrow stromal progenitors
  - Have features of myofibroblasts

Etiology of FDC Sarcoma
- Unknown in most cases
- Small subset of cases of FDC sarcoma are associated with Castleman disease (CD)
  - Hyaline-vascular variant
  - FDC "dysplasia" has been reported in hyaline-vascular CD
- Inflammatory pseudotumor-like variant of FDC sarcoma
  - Consistently associated with Epstein-Barr virus (EBV)
  - EBV is present in monoclonal form

CLINICAL ISSUES

Epidemiology
- Incidence
  - Rare
- Age
  - Adults; median age: 40-50 years
- Gender
  - Overall, no gender preference
    - Inflammatory pseudotumor-like variant shows female predominance
- Ethnicity
  - No known predisposition

Presentation
- Often presents as slow-growing, painless mass
  - Lymph nodes
    - Cervical lymphadenopathy is most common
    - Other lymph node groups: Axillary, mediastinal, mesenteric, and retroperitoneal may or may not present
  - Extranodal sites
    - Waldeyer ring is most common, such as tonsil, oral cavity
    - Gastrointestinal tract
    - Soft tissue, skin
    - Thyroid, breast, mediastinum
    - Liver and spleen
  - Inflammatory pseudotumor-like variant FDC sarcoma
    - Often arises in intraabdominal sites: Liver, spleen, and peripancreatic area
- Systemic symptoms
  - Uncommon in most patients with FDC sarcoma
  - Systemic symptoms are common in patients with inflammatory pseudotumor-like variant
    - Weight loss and fever
  - Paraneoplastic pemphigus can occur rarely

FOLLICULAR DENDRITIC CELL SARCOMA

Key Facts

Terminology
- Neoplastic proliferation of follicular dendritic cells

Clinical Issues
- Presents as slow-growing, painless mass
  ○ Lymph nodes
  ○ Extranodal sites; Waldeyer ring common
- Most cases behave like low- to intermediate-grade soft tissue sarcoma
  ○ Local excision, frequent recurrence
  ○ Insensitive to chemotherapy
- Subset of cases are clinically aggressive

Microscopic Pathology
- Spindled to ovoid cells forming fascicles, storiform arrays, whorls, diffuse sheets, or vague nodules
- Morphologic variants
  ○ Spindled/typical, epithelioid
  ○ Inflammatory pseudotumor-like variant
- High-grade features correlate with aggressive clinical course

Ancillary Tests
- Immunophenotype
  ○ Variable expression of CD21, CD23, CD35, CXCL13, clusterin, or EGFR
- Electron microscopy
  ○ Well-formed desmosomes

Top Differential Diagnoses
- Interdigitating dendritic cell sarcoma
- Langerhans cell histiocytosis/sarcoma
- Inflammatory myofibroblastic tumor
- Diffuse large B-cell lymphoma

Treatment
- Most patients are treated by complete surgical excision
  ○ With or without adjuvant radiotherapy or chemotherapy
    ▪ Various chemotherapy regimens have been used with limited success
    ▪ Adjuvant radiotherapy may prolong disease-free survival

Prognosis
- Most cases behave like low- to intermediate-grade soft tissue sarcoma
  ○ Local recurrences occur in > 50% of patients
  ○ Metastases occur in ~ 25% of patients
    ▪ Lymph nodes, lung, liver
  ○ 10-20% of patients ultimately die of the disease after many years
- Poor prognostic indicators
  ○ Large tumor size (> 6 cm)
  ○ Intraabdominal location
    ▪ Often in liver, spleen, or peripancreatic or retroperitoneal lymph nodes
    ▪ Inflammatory pseudotumor-like variant of FDC sarcoma is more indolent
  ○ High-grade histologic features

IMAGE FINDINGS

General Features
- FDC sarcoma cannot be distinguished from other malignant processes by imaging
- CT and MR
  ○ Mass lesion, expansile
  ○ ± invasion of surrounding structures
- Positron emission tomography (PET) shows abnormal radiotracer uptake

MACROSCOPIC FEATURES

Size
- Mean: 5 cm; range: 1-21 cm

MICROSCOPIC PATHOLOGY

Histologic Features
- Typical histologic features
  ○ Spindled to ovoid cells forming fascicles, storiform arrays, whorls, diffuse sheets, or nodules
  ○ Often admixed with small lymphocytes
    ▪ Lymphocytes often aggregate around blood vessels
  ○ Many cases have low-grade cytologic features
- Epithelioid variant
  ○ Oval or round nuclei and moderate amount of cytoplasm
  ○ Myxoid stroma often present
  ○ Neoplastic cells can show clear or eosinophilic (oncocytic) changes
- Histologic features of high-grade FDC sarcoma
  ○ Significant cytologic atypia
  ○ Mitotic figures numerous; up to > 30/10 high-power fields
  ○ Coagulative necrosis(+)
- **Inflammatory pseudotumor-like variant of FDC sarcoma**
  ○ Well demarcated from surrounding parenchyma
  ○ Admixture of lymphocytes, plasma cells, and histiocytes
    ▪ Striking histologic resemblance to inflammatory pseudotumor or inflammatory myofibroblastic tumor
    ▪ Some cases can resemble classical Hodgkin lymphoma with HRS-like cells
  ○ Center of tumor often shows hemorrhage and necrosis
    ▪ Blood vessels frequently show fibrinoid deposits in walls

13

FOLLICULAR DENDRITIC CELL SARCOMA

- **FDC sarcoma associated with hyaline-vascular variant of Castleman disease (CD)**
  - Often see coexistent changes of hyaline-vascular CD
    - ± regressed (involuted) germinal centers with hyalinization
    - Thick and hyalinized blood vessel walls
    - Vascular proliferation in interfollicular areas
    - Effaced lymph node sinuses
  - Proliferation of FDC
    - In large sheets, nodular or confluent
    - Often CXCL13(+)
  - Not associated with HHV8 infection

Cytologic Features

- Neoplastic cells have indistinct cell borders and a moderate amount of cytoplasm
- Nuclei are often bland
  - Oval or elongated with vesicular or granular, finely dispersed chromatin
  - Small but distinct nucleoli
  - Delicate nuclear membranes
  - Nuclear pseudoinclusions are common
  - Binucleated and multinucleated forms often present
- High-grade FDC sarcoma
  - Marked nuclear pleomorphism, cytologic atypia, prominent nucleoli
  - Many mitotic figures

ANCILLARY TESTS

Immunohistochemistry

- FDC sarcoma is positive for 1 or more FDC-associated markers
  - CD21, CD35, CD23, KiM4p, and CNA.42
  - Reactivity can be patchy and focal
    - Especially in high-grade tumors, epithelioid variant, or inflammatory pseudotumor-like variant
- Epidermal growth factor receptor (EGFR)(+)
- CXCL13(+), clusterin(+)
- Desmoplakin, vimentin, fascin are usually positive
- EMA(+/-), CD68(+/-), S100 protein(+/-)
- Rare cases can be CD45/LCA(+), CD20(+), or keratin(+)
- Inflammatory pseudotumor-like variant
  - LMP1(+) in subset of tumor cells
  - CD30(-), ALK-1(-)

In Situ Hybridization

- EBER(-) in most cases of FDC sarcoma
- EBER(+) in inflammatory pseudotumor-like variant

Molecular Genetics

- Limited molecular or cytogenetic data available

Electron Microscopy

- Transmission
  - Numerous interwoven long villous processes that are connected by desmosomes
  - Abundant organelles, including mitochondria and endoplasmic reticulum
  - Birbeck granules(-)

DIFFERENTIAL DIAGNOSIS

Interdigitating Dendritic Cell Sarcoma

- Tumor cells usually form fascicles, storiform pattern, and whorls of spindled to ovoid cells
- Tumor cells usually have bland cytology; low number of mitoses
- Admixed with small lymphocytes and, less commonly, with plasma cells
- In lymph nodes, ± paracortical distribution
- Immunohistochemistry
  - S100 protein(+), vimentin(+)
  - Fascin(+), CD68(+/-), lysozyme(+/-)
  - FDC-associated markers(-)
    - CD21, CD23, and CD35
  - HMB-45(-), CD1a(-), langerin(-)
  - CD30(-), B- and T-cell antigens(-)
- Ultrastructure
  - Complex interdigitating cell processes but no well-formed desmosomes
  - No Birbeck granules

Langerhans Cell Histiocytosis/Sarcoma

- In lymph nodes: Mainly in sinus pattern with secondary infiltration of paracortex
- Langerhans cells are oval with grooved, folded, indented, or lobulated nuclei
- Admixed with variable number of eosinophils, histiocytes, neutrophils, and small lymphocytes
- Immunohistochemistry
  - CD1a(+), langerin(+), S100 protein(+)
  - Vimentin(+), CD68(+)
  - FDC-associated markers(-)
- Electron microscopy
  - Birbeck granules(+)
  - No desmosomes/junctional specializations

Inflammatory Myofibroblastic Tumor

- Morphologically resembles inflammatory pseudotumor-like variant of FDC sarcoma
- Spindle cells are myofibroblasts
  - Vimentin(+), actin(+), desmin(+)
  - ALK-1(+) in ~ 60% of cases
  - FDC-associated markers(-), EBER(-)

Inflammatory Pseudotumor of Lymph Node

- Process tends to involve lymph node capsule and trabeculae
- Spindle cells and inflammatory cells ± many plasma cells
- Spindle cells do not exhibit cytologic atypica
- Spindle cells are negative for FDC-associated markers

Diffuse Large B-cell Lymphoma (DLBCL)

- Small subset of DLBCLs shows spindled cell morphology and resemble FDC sarcoma
  - CD21(+) or CD23(+) in some cases
- Panel of immunophenotypic markers will show B-cell lineage
- Molecular studies show monoclonal *Ig* gene rearrangements

FOLLICULAR DENDRITIC CELL SARCOMA

- Chromosomal translocations in subset: t(14;18) (q32;q21) or bcl-6/3q27 translocations

Metastatic Carcinoma in Lymph Node
- Spindle cell carcinoma can resemble FDC sarcoma
- Lymphoepithelioma-like carcinoma can resemble epithelioid variant of FDC sarcoma
- History of primary site of neoplasm is helpful
- Immunohistochemistry
  - Keratin(+), EMA(+), FDC-associated markers(-)

Metastatic Melanoma in Lymph Node
- Melanoma can resemble epithelioid variant of FDC sarcoma
- Melanin pigment can be present in melanoma
- S100 protein(+), HMB-45(+), Melan-A(+), FDC-associated markers(-)

Mycobacterial Spindle Cell Pseudotumor
- Partial/complete effacement of lymph node architecture by storiform pattern of bland spindle cells
- Spindle cells are macrophages distended by large amounts of mycobacteria
  - Ziehl-Neelsen(+) with numerous bacteria identified
- Spindle cells are CD68(+), FDC-associated markers(-)

Kaposi Sarcoma
- History of HIV is common
- Spindle cells form slits containing red blood cells
- HHV8(+), CD31(+)
- CD34(+), factor-VIII-related antigen(+)
- FDC-associated markers(-)

Sarcoma Involving Extranodal Sites
- FDC sarcoma can closely mimic other types of sarcoma
- Immunohistochemistry is usually needed
  - FDC-associated markers(+), other lineage markers(-)

Classical Hodgkin Lymphoma (CHL)
- Rare cases of FDC sarcoma can have HRS-like cells
  - Referred to as Hodgkin lymphoma-like variant
- In CHL
  - Usually more granulocytes in background than in FDC sarcoma
  - Fewer neoplastic cells in CHL than in FDC sarcoma
  - Hodgkin and Reed-Sternberg cells are
    - CD15(+), CD30(+), pax-5(+ dim), FDC-associated markers(-)

DIAGNOSTIC CHECKLIST

Clinically Relevant Pathologic Features
- FDC sarcoma is not a hematolymphoid neoplasm
  - Most FDC sarcomas
    - Behave as low- to intermediate-grade neoplasms
    - Present as localized mass lesion involving lymph nodes or extranodal sites
- Complete excision is treatment of choice
  - Local recurrences are common; dissemination can occur
  - High-grade morphology and intraabdominal location correlates with aggressive clinical course

- Patients with disseminated disease respond poorly to chemotherapy

Pathologic Interpretation Pearls
- FDC sarcoma has several morphologic variants
  - Spindled/typical
  - Epithelioid
  - Inflammatory pseudotumor-like
  - Hodgkin lymphoma-like
- FDC sarcoma can be associated with hyaline-vascular variant of Castleman disease
- Immunohistochemistry
  - FDC sarcoma is positive for 1 or more FDC-associated markers
    - Often expressed variably
- Electron microscopy
  - Long cellular processes connected by well-formed desmosomes

SELECTED REFERENCES

1. Li L et al: Clinicopathological features and prognosis assessment of extranodal follicular dendritic cell sarcoma. World J Gastroenterol. 16(20):2504-19, 2010
2. Orii T et al: Differential immunophenotypic analysis of dendritic cell tumours. J Clin Pathol. 63(6):497-503, 2010
3. Vermi W et al: Identification of CXCL13 as a new marker for follicular dendritic cell sarcoma. J Pathol. 216(3):356-64, 2008
4. Youens KE et al: Extranodal follicular dendritic cell sarcoma. Arch Pathol Lab Med. 132(10):1683-7, 2008
5. Kairouz S et al: Dendritic cell neoplasms: an overview. Am J Hematol. 82(10):924-8, 2007
6. Soriano AO et al: Follicular dendritic cell sarcoma: a report of 14 cases and a review of the literature. Am J Hematol. 82(8):725-8, 2007
7. Shia J et al: Extranodal follicular dendritic cell sarcoma: clinical, pathologic, and histogenetic characteristics of an underrecognized disease entity. Virchows Arch. 449(2):148-58, 2006
8. Cossu A et al: Classic follicular dendritic reticulum cell tumor of the lymph node developing in a patient with a previous inflammatory pseudotumor-like proliferation. Hum Pathol. 36(2):207-11, 2005
9. Cokelaere K et al: Hyaline vascular Castleman's disease with HMGIC rearrangement in follicular dendritic cells: molecular evidence of mesenchymal tumorigenesis. Am J Surg Pathol. 26(5):662-9, 2002
10. Cheuk W et al: Inflammatory pseudotumor-like follicular dendritic cell tumor: a distinctive low-grade malignant intra-abdominal neoplasm with consistent Epstein-Barr virus association. Am J Surg Pathol. 25(6):721-31, 2001
11. Fonseca R et al: Follicular dendritic cell sarcoma and interdigitating reticulum cell sarcoma: a review. Am J Hematol. 59(2):161-7, 1998
12. Perez-Ordoñez B et al: Follicular dendritic cell tumor: review of the entity. Semin Diagn Pathol. 15(2):144-54, 1998
13. Chan JK et al: Follicular dendritic cell sarcoma. Clinicopathologic analysis of 17 cases suggesting a malignant potential higher than currently recognized. Cancer. 79(2):294-313, 1997

FOLLICULAR DENDRITIC CELL SARCOMA

Microscopic Features

(Left) FDC sarcoma involving lymph node. The lymph node architecture is effaced by a nodular proliferation of spindle cells. **(Right)** FDC sarcoma involving lymph node. The neoplastic cells are admixed with small lymphocytes, and the lymphocytes are often aggregated around the blood vessels ➡.

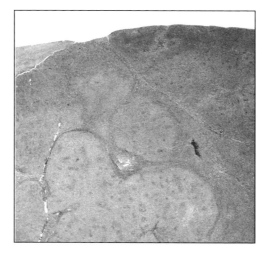 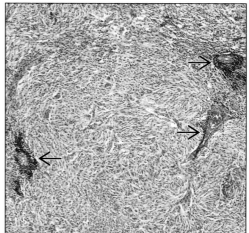

(Left) FDC sarcoma involving spleen. In this field, an infiltrate of spindle cells replaces the red pulp. **(Right)** FDC sarcoma involving spleen. The neoplasm infiltrates the red pulp along the sinuses. The pattern resembles, in part, Kaposi sarcoma with slit-like vasculature. The neoplastic cells are admixed with many small lymphocytes.

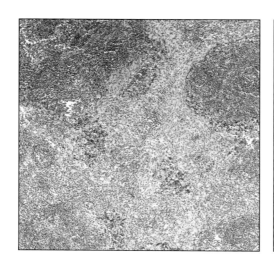 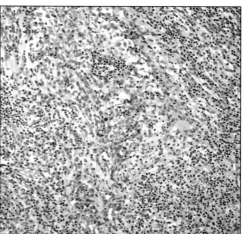

(Left) FDC sarcoma involving lymph node. The neoplastic cells often have low-grade histologic features with very few mitoses. The background inflammatory cells can include small lymphocytes, plasma cells, and histiocytes. **(Right)** In this case of FDC sarcoma, the nuclei are oval or elongated with vesicular or granular, finely dispersed chromatin, indistinct nucleoli, and delicate nuclear membranes. Note plasma cell ➡ and small lymphocytes ➡ in the background.

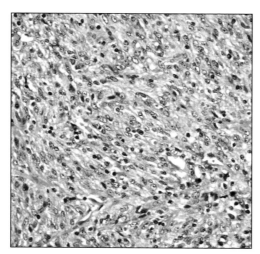 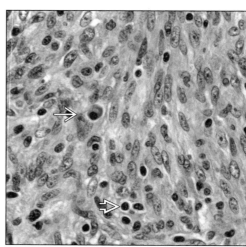

FOLLICULAR DENDRITIC CELL SARCOMA

Immunohistochemical Features

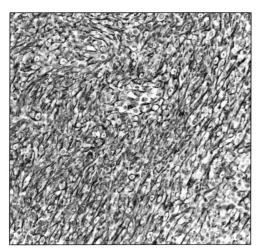

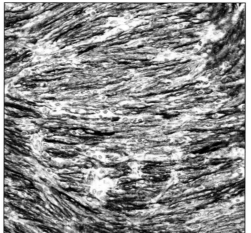

(Left) FDC sarcoma involving lymph node. The neoplastic cells are strongly vimentin positive. *(Right)* FDC sarcoma involving lymph node. The neoplastic cells are strongly CD21 positive.

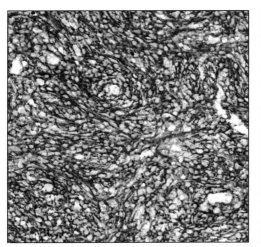

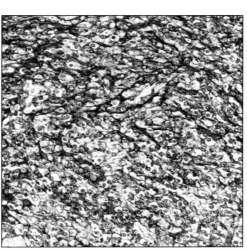

(Left) FDC sarcoma involving lymph node. The neoplastic cells are strongly CD35 positive. *(Right)* FDC sarcoma involving lymph node. The neoplastic cells are strongly CD23 positive.

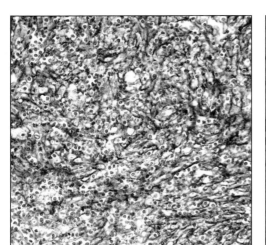

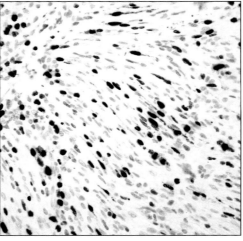

(Left) FDC sarcoma involving lymph node. The neoplastic cells are positive for epidermal growth factor receptor (EGFR). *(Right)* FDC sarcoma involving lymph node. MIB-1 (Ki-67) shows a proliferation fraction of approximately 20% in this case.

FOLLICULAR DENDRITIC CELL SARCOMA

Variant Microscopic Features

(Left) FDC sarcoma, epithelioid variant, involving a lymph node. The neoplastic cells with round nuclei have open chromatin, distinct nucleoli, and eosinophilic cytoplasm. Many admixed small lymphocytes are present. *(Right)* FDC sarcoma, epithelioid variant, involving lymph node. As illustrated with the anti-CD21 antibody in this case, it is common for FDC-associated markers to be expressed variably.

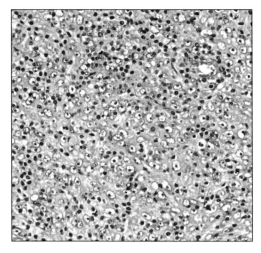
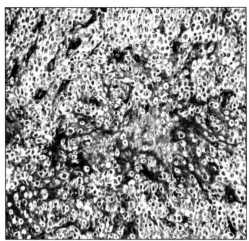

(Left) Positron emission tomography (PET) of a patient with high-grade FDC sarcoma shows increased radiotracer uptake in the liver and paraaortic lymph nodes. *(Right)* FDC sarcoma with high-grade histologic features. The neoplastic cells show marked nuclear pleomorphism and cytologic atypia. In such cases, it is difficult to differentiate FDC sarcoma from other types of high-grade sarcoma without immunohistochemistry.

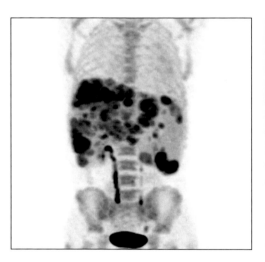
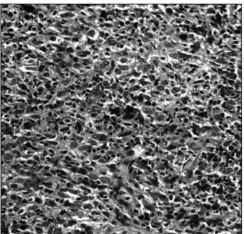

(Left) FDC sarcoma with high-grade histologic features and Hodgkin-like giant cells. The neoplastic cells are large with prominent nucleoli. Mitoses are easily seen ⇗. Focal necrosis is present ⇨. *(Right)* FDC sarcoma with high-grade histologic features. CD21 is expressed by a small subset of the neoplastic cells, in a staining pattern typical of FDCs.

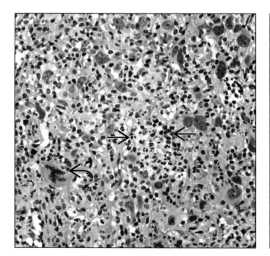
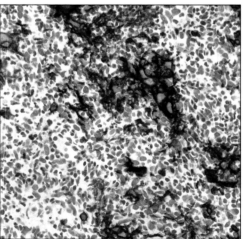

FOLLICULAR DENDRITIC CELL SARCOMA

Variant Microscopic Features

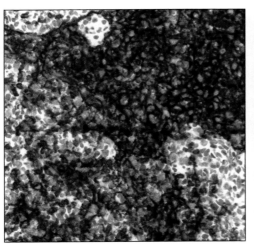

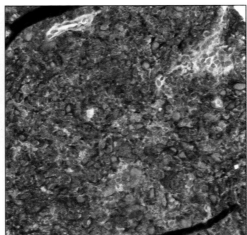

(Left) FDC sarcoma with high-grade histologic features. CD23 is expressed by most of the neoplastic cells in this case, unlike CD21, which was focally expressed. FDC sarcoma often shows different reactivity patterns with different FDC-associated markers, and therefore, a panel of markers should be performed in cases with a suspected diagnosis of FDC sarcoma. *(Right)* FDC sarcoma, high grade. The tumor cells are strongly and diffusely positive for clusterin.

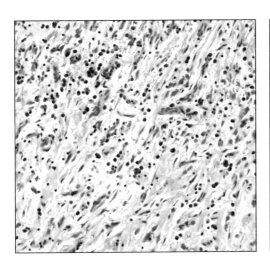

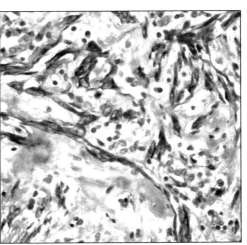

(Left) Inflammatory myofibroblastic tumor can closely resemble the inflammatory pseudotumor-like variant FDC sarcoma. The spindle cells in inflammatory myofibroblastic tumor are myofibroblasts. *(Right)* Inflammatory myofibroblastic tumor with spindle cells expressing anaplastic lymphoma kinase (ALK). ALK is expressed in approximately 60% of cases of inflammatory myofibroblastic tumor.

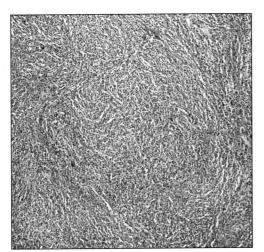

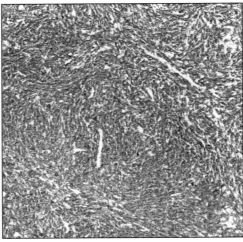

(Left) Diffuse large B-cell lymphoma is seen with many lymphoma cells that have spindle cell morphology resembling FDC sarcoma. *(Right)* Diffuse large B-cell lymphoma (DLBCL) with spindled lymphoma cells. The lymphoma cells are diffusely CD20(+). Rare cases of FDC sarcoma can exhibit weak and focal CD20 expression, but strong and uniform CD20(+), as seen here, supports DLBCL.

INTERDIGITATING DENDRITIC CELL SARCOMA

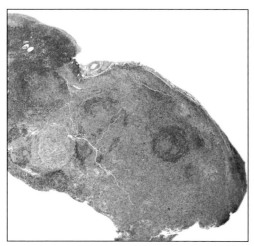

Interdigitating dendritic cell sarcoma subtotally replacing lymph node. The neoplasm tends to spare lymphoid follicles. The neoplasm was S100 protein(+).

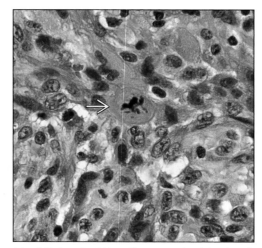

Interdigitating dendritic cell sarcoma involving lymph node. The neoplastic cells are spindled and epithelioid with abundant eosinophilic cytoplasm. A mitotic figure is present ➡.

TERMINOLOGY

Abbreviations
- Interdigitating dendritic cell (IDC) sarcoma

Synonyms
- Interdigitating cell dendritic cell tumor
- Interdigitating dendritic reticulum cell sarcoma

Definitions
- Neoplastic proliferation of cells with immunophenotypic profile that is similar to normal IDCs

ETIOLOGY/PATHOGENESIS

Postulated Normal Cell Counterpart is IDC
- Antigen-presenting cell that is involved in T-cell immunity
- Derived from CD34(+) lymphoid/myeloid progenitor cell in bone marrow that homes to lymph node
- Normally found in
  - T-cell regions of lymph node
  - Periarteriolar lymphoid sheaths
  - Interfollicular areas of extranodal lymphoid tissue

Concept of "Transdifferentiation"
- Rare patients with histiocytic neoplasms also have clonally related B-cell lymphoma
  - Usually B-cell lymphoma precedes histiocytic neoplasm
  - Examples in literature include
    - IDC sarcoma and follicular lymphoma
    - Histiocytic sarcoma and follicular lymphoma
    - IDC sarcoma and chronic lymphocytic leukemia/ small lymphocytic lymphoma
    - Histiocytic sarcoma and splenic marginal zone lymphoma
  - Histiocytic neoplasms associated with follicular lymphoma share
    - t(14;18)(q32;q21)/*BCL2-IgH* &/or identical *IgH* gene rearrangements
  - Histiocytic tumors and nonfollicular B-cell lymphomas share identical *IgH* gene rearrangements
- These results suggest that B-cell lymphoma can transform to histiocytic phenotype via "transdifferentiation"
  - Possibly as result of loss of key components of B-cell differentiation

CLINICAL ISSUES

Epidemiology
- Incidence
  - Very rare
- Age
  - Wide age range
    - Most patients are adults with median age in 6th or 7th decades
    - Youngest patient reported was 2 years of age
- Gender
  - Male to female ratio: 1.2 to 1

Site
- Lymph node
  - Most commonly a single lymph node is involved
  - Cervical, axillary, or inguinal lymph node groups most often affected
- Extranodal sites can be involved
  - Wide variety of extranodal sites
    - Skin and soft tissue most common
    - Liver and spleen
    - Gastrointestinal tract, lung, kidney
  - Bone marrow is involved in < 20% of patients

Presentation
- Slow-growing, asymptomatic mass is most common

INTERDIGITATING DENDRITIC CELL SARCOMA

Key Facts

Clinical Issues
- Wide age range
- Single lymph nodes most commonly involved
  - Cervical, axillary, or inguinal groups
  - Slow-growing, asymptomatic mass
- Rare cases associated with B- or T-cell lymphomas or leukemias

Microscopic Pathology
- Partial or complete replacement of lymph node architecture
- Sheets, whorls, nests, or fascicles
- Spindle-shaped or epithelioid cells
- Cytologic atypia can be mild or prominent

Ancillary Tests
- Immunohistochemistry

- S100 strongly positive
- CD68(+/-), often variable
- Vimentin(+), fascin(+), CD45/LCA(+/-), lysozyme(+/-)
- Molecular genetics
  - HUMARA has shown clonality in small subset of cases tested
  - Antigen receptor genes are usually in germline configuration
  - No chromosomal translocations
  - IDC sarcoma in patients with follicular lymphoma carry *IgH* rearrangements and t(14;18)/*IgH-BCL2*

Top Differential Diagnoses
- Langerhans cell sarcoma
- Follicular dendritic cell sarcoma
- Histiocytic sarcoma

- Systemic symptoms occur in subset of patients
  - Fever, night sweats, fatigue
- Small subset of patients have IDC sarcoma and another hematopoietic neoplasm including
  - Chronic lymphocytic leukemia/small lymphocytic lymphoma
  - Mycosis fungoides
  - Acute lymphoblastic leukemia (mostly of T-cell lineage)
- Small subset of patients with IDC sarcoma also have carcinoma
  - Most common types: Breast, stomach, liver, colon

Treatment
- Surgical resection and radiation therapy for patients with localized disease
- Currently, there is no established chemotherapy regimen
  - ABVD (doxorubicin, bleomycin, vincristine, and dacarbazine) and other regimens have been used
    - Many patients initially respond but relapse, and death is common in this patient subset

Prognosis
- Variable clinical course
  - 40-50% of patients develop disseminated disease with poor outcome

IMAGE FINDINGS

Radiographic Findings
- Lymphadenopathy
- Positron emission tomography (PET) often shows increased fluorodeoxyglucose (FDG) uptake

MACROSCOPIC FEATURES

General Features
- Hemorrhage and necrosis can be present

Size
- Variable; ranging from 1.0-6.0 cm in most studies
- Lobulated mass with firm cut surface

MICROSCOPIC PATHOLOGY

Histologic Features
- Partial or complete replacement of lymph node architecture
  - Paracortical pattern in cases of partial involvement
    - Spares lymphoid follicles
  - Sinusoidal pattern of involvement can be prominent
- Sheets, whorls, nests, or fascicles
- Spindle-shaped or epithelioid cells
  - Vesicular nuclei; nucleoli can be small or prominent
  - Abundant eosinophilic cytoplasm with indistinct cell borders
- Cytologic atypia can be mild or prominent
  - Mitotic rate is variable; usually high in cases with marked atypia
- Inflammatory cells are common in background
  - Small lymphocytes present; usually T cells
  - ± eosinophils and plasma cells
- Hemophagocytosis is uncommon but has been reported

Cytologic Features
- Difficult diagnosis to establish by fine needle aspiration (FNA)
- Neoplastic cells in FNA smears are cytologically similar to those observed in tissue sections

ANCILLARY TESTS

Immunohistochemistry
- All cases are strongly positive for S100 protein
- CD11c(+), HLA-DR(+), vimentin(+), and fascin(+) in most cases
- CD68(+/-) but can be variable
- CD45/LCA(+/-), CD68(+/-), CD4(+/-), lysozyme(+/-)

INTERDIGITATING DENDRITIC CELL SARCOMA

- P53(+), but only a few cases have been assessed and reported
- CD14(-/+), CD15(-/+), CD33(-/+), CD43(-/+), CD45RO(-/+)
- Pan-B-cell and pan-T-cell antigens(-)
  - pax-5 reported as weakly (+) in IDC sarcoma associated with B-cell lymphomas
- CD1a(-); rare cases reported as focally and variably positive
- Negative markers
  - CD21(-), CD23(-), CD35(-)
  - Langerin(-), CD163(-)
  - CD30(-), CD34(-), myeloperoxidase(-)

Cytogenetics
- No recurrent cytogenetic abnormalities have been reported

In Situ Hybridization
- Epstein-Barr virus encoded RNA (EBER) is negative

Molecular Genetics
- Human androgen receptor assay (HUMARA) has shown clonality in small subset of cases tested
- In accord with origin from IDC
  - Antigen receptor genes are usually in germline configuration
  - No chromosomal translocations
- IDC sarcoma in patients with follicular lymphoma share
  - Monoclonal *IgH* rearrangements and t(14;18) (q32;q21)/*IgH-BCL2*

Electron Microscopy
- Transmission
  - Long, complex interdigitating cell processes and irregularly shaped nuclei
  - No Birbeck granules, well-formed desmosomes, or melanosomes

Cytochemistry
- Generally has a limited role in diagnosis
  - Adenosine triphosphatase activity (strongly +)
  - Myeloperoxidase usually negative
  - Chloroacetate esterase(-)

DIFFERENTIAL DIAGNOSIS

Langerhans Cell Sarcoma
- Most commonly occurs in extranodal sites (e.g., skin, bone)
  - ~ 20% of patients present with lymph node disease
- Sinusoidal pattern can be present in Langerhans cell sarcoma
- Neoplastic IDC and Langerhans cells are cytologically similar
- Mitotic rate is usually high in Langerhans cell sarcoma
  - Often 50 per 10 HPFs (400x)
- Immunohistochemistry
  - S100(+), CD1a(+), langerin(+)
    - Expression of CD1a and langerin can be focal
- Birbeck granules by EM(+/-)

Follicular Dendritic Cell Sarcoma
- Commonly FDC sarcoma is more spindled than IDC sarcoma, but they can be indistinguishable
- Features suggestive of FDC sarcoma, if present
  - Nuclear pseudoinclusions
  - Binucleated, squared off, FDCs
  - Reactive small lymphocytes of B-cell lineage
- Immunohistochemistry
  - CD21(+/-), CD23(+/-), CD35(+/-)
  - Clusterin(+), EGFR(+)
  - S100(-), CD68(-/+)
- Electron microscopy shows desmosomes

Histiocytic Sarcoma
- Tumor cells typically have epithelioid appearance without spindling
- Immunohistochemistry
  - CD68(+), CD163(+), lysozyme(+/-), S100(-/+)

Metastatic Melanoma
- Usually more pleomorphic with more necrosis than IDC sarcoma
- History of primary neoplasm or melanoma elsewhere is helpful
- Immunohistochemistry
  - S100(+), HMB-45(+), tyrosinase(+), Mart-1(+)
  - CD45/LCA(-), fascin(-)

Metastatic Carcinoma
- Usually more pleomorphic with more necrosis than IDC sarcoma
  - Cells are obviously cohesive
- History of primary neoplasm or carcinoma elsewhere is helpful
- Immunohistochemistry
  - Keratins(+), EMA(+)
  - CD45/LCA(-), S100(-)

SELECTED REFERENCES

1. Orii T et al: Differential immunophenotypic analysis of dendritic cell tumours. J Clin Pathol. 63(6):497-503, 2010
2. Wang E et al: Histiocytic sarcoma arising in indolent small B-cell lymphoma: report of two cases with molecular/genetic evidence suggestive of a 'transdifferentiation' during the clonal evolution. Leuk Lymphoma. 51(5):802-12, 2010
3. Zhang D: Histiocytic sarcoma arising from lymphomas via transdifferentiation pathway during clonal evolution. Leuk Lymphoma. 51(5):739-40, 2010
4. Fraser CR et al: Transformation of chronic lymphocytic leukemia/small lymphocytic lymphoma to interdigitating dendritic cell sarcoma: evidence for transdifferentiation of the lymphoma clone. Am J Clin Pathol. 132(6):928-39, 2009
5. Feldman AL et al: Clonally related follicular lymphomas and histiocytic/dendritic cell sarcomas: evidence for transdifferentiation of the follicular lymphoma clone. Blood. 111(12):5433-9, 2008

INTERDIGITATING DENDRITIC CELL SARCOMA

Microscopic Features

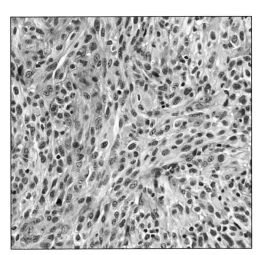

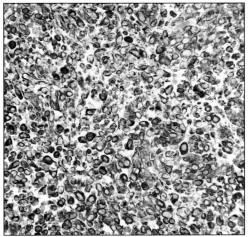

(Left) Interdigitating dendritic cell (IDC) sarcoma replacing lymph node. The neoplastic cells have abundant eosinophilic cytoplasm, are spindle-shaped, and form a storiform pattern in this field. This case of IDC sarcoma showed mild to moderate atypia and had a relatively low mitotic rate. *(Right)* Interdigitating dendritic cell sarcoma replacing lymph node. This field shows strong expression of vimentin. The neoplastic cells were also positive for S100 protein (not shown).

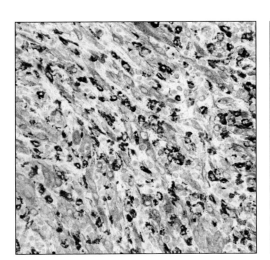

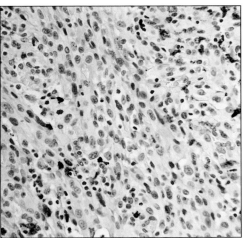

(Left) Interdigitating dendritic cell sarcoma replacing lymph node. This field shows moderate and variable expression of the lysosomal antigen CD68. The neoplastic cells were also positive for S100 protein (not shown). *(Right)* Interdigitating dendritic cell sarcoma replacing lymph node. This field shows that whereas the neoplastic cells are negative for CD45/LCA, small reactive lymphocytes in the background are positive. This neoplasm was positive for S100 protein (not shown).

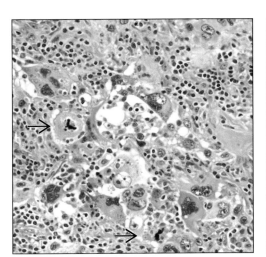

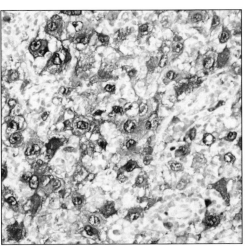

(Left) IDC sarcoma involving lymph node. The neoplastic cells in this case show marked nuclear atypia and abundant eosinophilic cytoplasm and are oval to round in shape. This case of IDC sarcoma showed marked atypia and had a high mitotic rate, with 2 mitotic figures ⇒ being present in this field. *(Right)* Interdigitating dendritic cell sarcoma involving lymph node. The neoplastic cells strongly express S100 protein.

13

MAST CELL DISEASE

Key Facts

Clinical Issues
- Multiple clinical variants; common variants are
  - Cutaneous mastocytosis
  - Indolent systemic mastocytosis
  - Systemic mastocytosis with associated clonal hematological non-mast cell lineage disease
  - Aggressive systemic mastocytosis
- Cutaneous mastocytosis is localized to skin
- Systemic mastocytosis usually involves bone marrow
  - Less often: Spleen, lymph nodes, and liver ± skin

Microscopic Pathology
- Lymph node
  - Mast cells usually present in interfollicular or diffuse pattern
  - Mast cells have clear/pale cytoplasm with abundant fine granules
  - Delicate sclerosis; eosinophils are common

Ancillary Tests
- Mast cells have metachromatic granules: Giemsa(+), toluidine blue(+), chloroacetate esterase(+)
- Immunophenotype: Tryptase(+), CD117/KIT(+), aberrant CD2(-/+), CD25(+/-)
- ± activating KIT point mutation D816V

Top Differential Diagnoses
- Mast cell hyperplasia
- Acute myeloid leukemia with tryptase(+) blasts
- Myeloid and lymphoid neoplasms with PDGFRA rearrangements
- Nodal marginal zone B-cell lymphoma

Natural History
- CM is usually self-limited
- Indolent SM is characterized by
  - Limited lesions, mild symptoms, prolonged course
- Aggressive SM is characterized by
  - BM or multiorgan dysfunction ("C" findings)

Treatment
- Osteoporosis often responds to bisphosphonates
- Patients with SM usually have slowly progressive disease
  - Interferon-α, 2-chlorodeoxyadenosine
- Patients with SM and rapidly progressive disease &/or mast cell leukemia
  - Polychemotherapy
  - Hematopoietic stem cell transplant
- SM with associated clonal hematological non-mast cell lineage disease (SM-AHNMD)
  - Therapy mainly directed to AHNMD component

Prognosis
- Excellent prognosis for patients with CM and indolent SM
- Patients with aggressive SM have poor prognosis
- Poor prognosis when associated with BM or organ dysfunction

Cutaneous Mastocytosis: Diagnostic Criteria
- Skin lesions associated with typical clinical findings of UP
  - Less frequent diffuse CM or solitary mastocytoma
- Typical histological infiltrates of mast cells in multifocal or diffuse pattern
- Absence of features/criteria that establish diagnosis of SM

Systemic Mastocytosis: Diagnostic Criteria
- Diagnosis requires 1 major criterion and 1 minor criterion, or at least 3 minor criteria
- Tissue diagnosis based on examination of BM or extracutaneous organs
- Major criterion
  - Multifocal, dense infiltrates of mast cells (≥ 15 mast cells per aggregate)
- Minor criteria
  - > 25% of mast cells in infiltrate are spindle-shaped or have atypical morphology or
  - > 25% of mast cells in BM aspirate smears are immature or atypical
  - Detection of an activating point mutation at codon 816 of KIT (usually D816V) in BM, blood, or another extracutaneous organ
  - Mast cells in BM, blood, or other extracutaneous organs express CD2 &/or CD25
  - Serum total tryptase persistently exceeds 20 ng/mL
    - Except when there is associated clonal myeloid neoplasm

Criteria for Variants of Systemic Mastocytosis
- All variants meet criteria for SM; in addition, distinctive features and subgroups are described
- Extracutaneous mastocytoma
  - Unifocal mast cell tumor with low-grade cytology and without destructive growth pattern
  - No evidence of SM; no skin lesions
- Indolent SM
  - No "C" findings; no evidence of SM-AHNMD
  - Subtype: BM mastocytosis
    - Absence of skin lesions
  - Subtype: Smoldering SM
    - ≥ 2 "B" findings and no "C" findings
- SM with associated clonal hematological non-mast cell lineage disease (SM-AHNMD)
  - Meets criteria for AHNMD, which include
    - Myelodysplastic syndrome, myeloproliferative neoplasm, acute myeloid leukemia, lymphomas, or other hematological neoplasm
    - Associated neoplasm meets criteria for distinct entity as defined in WHO classification
    - Poor prognosis
- Aggressive SM

MAST CELL DISEASE

- 1 or more "C" findings; no evidence of mast cell leukemia; usually without skin lesions
- Subtype: Lymphadenopathic mastocytosis with eosinophilia
  - Progressive lymphadenopathy with peripheral blood eosinophilia
  - Often with extensive bone involvement and hepatosplenomegaly; usually without skin lesions
- Mast cell leukemia
  - BM biopsy specimen showing diffuse, compact infiltration by atypical, immature mast cells
  - BM aspirate smears show 20% or more mast cells
  - Mast cells usually account for ≥ 10% of peripheral blood white cells
  - Usually without skin lesions
- Mast cell sarcoma
  - Unifocal mast cell tumor with destructive growth pattern and high-grade cytology
  - No evidence of SM

"B" Findings

- BM biopsy specimen showing > 30% infiltration by mast cells (focal, dense aggregates) &/or serum total tryptase level > 200 ng/mL
- Signs of dysplasia or myeloproliferation in non-mast cell lineage(s)
  - But insufficient criteria for diagnosis of clonal hematopoietic non-mast cell neoplasm (AHNMD)
    - Normal or only slightly abnormal blood counts
- Hepatomegaly without liver dysfunction &/or
  - Splenomegaly without hypersplenism &/or
  - Lymphadenopathy on palpation or imaging

"C" Findings

- BM dysfunction manifested by 1 or more cytopenias (ANC < 1.0 x 10⁹/L, Hb < 10 g/dL, or platelet count < 100 x 10⁹/L)
  - But no obvious clonal hematological non-mast cell hematopoietic disorder
- Palpable hepatomegaly with impairment of liver function, ascites, &/or portal hypertension
- Skeletal involvement with large osteolytic lesions &/or pathological fracture(s)
- Palpable splenomegaly with hypersplenism
- Malabsorption with weight loss due to mast cell infiltrates in gastrointestinal tract

IMAGE FINDINGS

Radiographic Findings

- Radiograph of bone and bone mineral density assessment show
  - Osteosclerosis in ~ 80% of patients
  - Osteoporosis in ~ 30% of patients; mixed osteolytic and osteosclerotic lesions
  - Rare vertebral fracture, osteolytic lesions
  - No skeletal alterations in ~ 20% of patients

CT Findings

- Loss of corticomedullary differentiation in bones of axial skeleton
- Thickening of cortical bone in appendicular skeleton

- Can mimic myelofibrosis and osteosclerosis
- Increased fluorodeoxyglucose (FDG) uptake in cortical bone by FDG-PET/CT scan

MACROSCOPIC FEATURES

General Features

- Cut surface of spleen reveals micronodules and fibrous streaks
- Lymph nodes are firm

MICROSCOPIC PATHOLOGY

Cytologic Features

- Medium-sized round, oval, or spindled cells
- Abundant pale/clear cytoplasm and indented nuclei

Cutaneous Mastocytosis

- Spindle-shaped mast cells in papillary dermis that may extend to reticular dermis
  - Usually perivascular or periadnexal
  - Lesions in adults reveal relatively fewer mast cells than lesions in children
- Diffuse CM
  - Sheets of mast cells filling papillary and upper reticular dermis
- Solitary mastocytoma of skin
  - Large aggregates or sheets of mast cells that may extend into subcutaneous tissue
  - Mast cells with abundant granular cytoplasm

Bone Marrow

- Multifocal, compact infiltrates of ≥ 15 mast cells in BM biopsy or clot specimen
  - Major diagnostic criterion for SM
- Monomorphic, spindle-shaped mast cells that affect or stream along bone trabeculae
- Mast cells appear as oval to spindle cells with faintly visible granules filling cytoplasm
  - Oval, round, elongated, or bilobed nuclei
    - Clumped chromatin with indistinct nucleoli
- Predominantly paratrabecular or perivascular
- Reticulin fibrosis within mast cell clusters and thickening of adjacent bone
- Variable mixture of lymphocytes, eosinophils, histiocytes, and fibroblasts
- Rarely, compact infiltrates composed of round, hypergranular MC
  - Tryptase(+) round cell infiltration of BM (TROCI-BM)
- BM aspirate smears
  - Mast cells are found within fair distance from particles
  - ≥ 20% mast cells in BM aspirate smears indicate mast cell leukemia
- BM not affected by SM
  - Normal distribution of fat and hematopoietic precursors
  - If abnormal, hypercellularity requires exclusion of MPN, MDS, or MDS/MPN

- Also exclude lymphoproliferative disorders, plasma cell myeloma, lymphoma

Spleen
- Splenomegaly in 25-40% of patients
- "C" finding, if associated with hypersplenism
- Clusters of mast cells with sclerosis around Malpighian follicles
  - Often associated with fibrosis or eosinophils
- Less frequently, diffuse infiltration of parenchyma with minimal sclerosis

Liver
- "C" finding, if associated with liver dysfunction
- Small mast cell clusters in periportal tracts or in sinusoids
- Mast cell clusters associated with fibrosis or eosinophils

Lymph Node
- Eosinophils are commonly associated with mast cells; may be numerous
- Mast cell infiltrate can be centered on arterioles
- Mast cell infiltrate may be accompanied by
  - Prominent vascular proliferation
  - Follicular lymphoid hyperplasia
- Lymphadenopathic mastocytosis with eosinophilia is rare subtype (~ 10%)
  - Prominent, rapid development of lymphadenopathy with mast cell infiltrate
  - Peripheral blood eosinophilia
  - Features may be similar to cases with rearrangements of *PDGFR*α

Bone
- Osteosclerotic or osteolytic lesions can be found
- "C" finding, when large osteolytic lesions or pathologic fractures present
- Irregular remodeling of bone trabeculae

Gastrointestinal Tract Mucosa
- Mast cells can infiltrate mucosa; a "C" finding when associated with malabsorption and weight loss
  - Diffuse or multifocal mucosal lesions throughout intestines
- Gastric rugal hypertrophy or flattening of folds

Histochemical Stains Helpful for Diagnosis
- Naphthol AS-D chloroacetate esterase
- Giemsa and toluidine blue highlight metachromatic cytoplasmic granules

ANCILLARY TESTS

Histochemistry
- Wright-Giemsa stain
  - Reactivity: Positive
  - Staining pattern
    - Cytoplasmic
- Toluidine blue
  - Reactivity: Positive
  - Staining pattern
    - Cytoplasmic

Immunohistochemistry
- Tryptase(+), CD117/CKIT(+)
  - Highly sensitive for detecting mast cells
  - Tryptase helpful for identifying multifocal, compact infiltrates of atypical mast cells
- CD25(+/-), CD2(-/+)
  - Aberrantly expressed by neoplastic mast cells
- CD43(+), CD68(+/-), chymase(+/-)
- B-cell antigens(-), CD3(-), CD5(-), CD7(-), MPO(-)
- CD15(-), CD21(-), CD30(-), CD34(-)
- MIB1/Ki-67 usually low

Flow Cytometry
- Normal mast cells
  - High side scatter
  - CD9(+), CD32(+), CD33(+), CD45(+), CD117(+)
  - CD59(+), CD63(+), CD69(+), CD203c(+), CD23(+)
  - HLA-I cytoplasmic carboxypeptidase(+/-), cytoplasmic total tryptase(+/-)
  - CD2(-), CD14(-), CD15(-), CD16(-)
  - CD25(-), CD34(-), CD123(-)
- Neoplastic mast cells
  - CD25(+) in 88% of cases, CD2(+) in 39% of cases
    - CD2 is often dim or negative compared with CD25
    - Stain with CD2 should be conjugated with bright fluorochrome, such as phycoerythrin
- Abnormal mast cells in SM
  - Higher side scatter
  - Aberrant expression of CD25 (high), CD2, and CD123
  - Abnormally high reactivity for
    - CD59 complement regulatory protein
    - CD63, CD69, CD203c activation markers
    - Fc γ R11 (CD32)
    - CD45
- Maturation-related immunophenotypic profiles
  - Immature with clonal involvement of all myeloid lineages
    - CD25(+), CD2(-), CD63(+), CD69(+)
    - Aberrantly low side scatter
    - Detected in aggressive SM, mast cell leukemia
  - Mature activated immunophenotype in indolent SM
    - Aberrantly increased side scatter
    - Uniform and high CD25 expression

Molecular Genetics
- Clonally expanded mast cells usually carry D816V *KIT* mutation
- Less frequently, other activating *KIT* mutations are present

Electron Microscopy
- Mast cell granules, which are bound by unit membrane and filled with electron-dense material

Cytochemistry
- Mast cells show enzyme cytochemical activity
  - Naphthol AS-D chloroacetate esterase and elastase; strong
  - Tartrate-resistant acid phosphatase; moderate

13

MAST CELL DISEASE

- Mast cell tryptase is detectable in early stages of mast cell development
- Mast cells do not show reactivity with
  - Myeloperoxidase
  - α-naphthyl acetate and butyrate esterases

DIFFERENTIAL DIAGNOSIS

Mast Cell Hyperplasia
- Occasionally, increase of mast cells in BM
  - Associated with primary or secondary neoplasms or reactive processes
- Extreme cases show abundant mast cells interspersed with hematopoietic cells
- Features that favor SM over mast cell hyperplasia
  - Compact clusters with ≥ 15 mast cells
  - Aberrant immunophenotype: CD2(+), CD25(+)
  - Abnormal morphology including spindle shapes and degranulation
- Mast cell hyperplasia may show overlapping features with UP in adults

Acute Myeloid Leukemia with Tryptase(+) Blasts
- Occasionally, blasts of AML show reactivity with tryptase ± *KIT* mutation
  - Usually no morphologic evidence of SM
  - If blasts show metachromatic granules, neoplasm may represent distinct subgroup
    - Constitute part of leukemic clone
    - Designation of myelomastocytic leukemia has been suggested
- Complete remission leads to disappearance of blasts
  - No residual tryptase(+) cells
  - Distinct from SM with associated clonal hematological non-mast cell lineage disease

Myeloid and Lymphoid Neoplasms with PDGFRα Rearrangements
- Neoplasms usually associated with eosinophilia
  - Less frequently present as acute myeloid leukemia or T-lymphoblastic leukemia/lymphoma
- Bone marrow mast cells increased, arranged in loose rather than compact clusters of SM
- Diagnosis requires FISH to detect a 4q12 microdeletion
  - Results in a *FIP1L1-PDGFRA* fusion
  - Other fusion partners may be detected with conventional cytogenetics
- Responsive to imatinib

Hairy Cell Leukemia (HCL)
- Infiltrate is diffuse with massive involvement of splenic red pulp or BM
- B-cell antigens(+), CD11c(+), CD25(+), CD103(+), annexin-A1(+)
- Tartrate-resistant acid phosphatase (+, strong)
- Features that favor SM over HCL
  - SM is often nodular and associated with sclerosis and eosinophils

Nodal Marginal Zone B-cell Lymphoma (NMZL)
- Mast cells in lymph node can have abundant pale cytoplasm and mimic NMZL
- Features that favor NMZL over SM
  - More heterogeneous cell population; ± plasmacytoid differentiation
  - B-cell antigens(+), tryptase(-)

Peripheral T-cell Lymphoma
- Clear cells in parafollicular distribution may mimic SM
- Polymorphic lymphoid population
- T-cell phenotype and T-cell receptor gene rearrangements

Langerhans Cell Histiocytosis (LCH)
- Bone lesions can be single with sclerotic margin
- Eosinophilic microabscesses
- Grooved nuclei and abundant cytoplasm
- S100 protein(+), CD1a(+), langerin/CD207(+)

DIAGNOSTIC CHECKLIST

Pathologic Interpretation Pearls
- Major diagnostic criterion of SM is presence of compact clusters of mast cells
  - In bone marrow or extracutaneous sites
- Mast cells contain metachromatic granules
  - Giemsa(+), toluidine blue(+), naphthol AS-D chloroacetate esterase(+)
- Immunophenotype: Tryptase(+), CD117(+), aberrant CD25(+/-), CD2(-/+)
- Common association with other clonal hematologic disorders
- Activating *KIT* point mutation D816V is a minor criterion for diagnosis of SM

SELECTED REFERENCES

1. Brockow K et al: Mastocytosis. Chem Immunol Allergy. 95:110-24, 2010
2. Johnson MR et al: Utility of the World Heath Organization classification criteria for the diagnosis of systemic mastocytosis in bone marrow. Mod Pathol. 22(1):50-7, 2009
3. Pullarkat VA et al: Systemic mastocytosis with associated clonal hematological non-mast-cell lineage disease: analysis of clinicopathologic features and activating c-kit mutations. Am J Hematol. 73(1):12-7, 2003
4. Valent P et al: Myelomastocytic overlap syndromes: biology, criteria, and relationship to mastocytosis. Leuk Res. 25(7):595-602, 2001
5. Allpress SM et al: Diagnosis of mastocytosis by fine-needle aspiration cytology. Diagn Cytopathol. 18(5):368-70, 1998
6. Miranda RN et al: Systemic mast cell disease presenting with peripheral blood eosinophilia. Hum Pathol. 25(7):727-30, 1994
7. Horny HP et al: Lymph node findings in generalized mastocytosis. Histopathology. 21(5):439-46, 1992
8. Metcalfe DD: The liver, spleen, and lymph nodes in mastocytosis. J Invest Dermatol. 96(3 Suppl):45S-46S; discussion 46S, 60S-65S, 1991

MAST CELL DISEASE

Skin

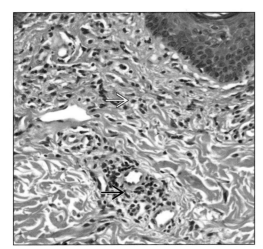 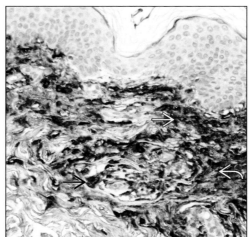

(Left) Skin biopsy of an adult with cutaneous mastocytosis (CM). The infiltrate is perivascular ⇒ and interstitial ➡ in superficial dermis. Mast cells are oval to spindle-shaped with pale cytoplasm with fine granularity. *(Right)* Skin biopsy of an adult with CM. Immunohistochemistry for tryptase highlights numerous perivascular ⇒ and interstitial ➡ mast cells. Extracellular reactivity ⇗ is consistent with mast cell degranulation.

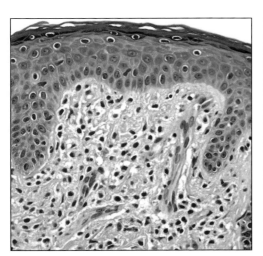 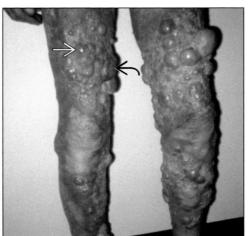

(Left) Skin biopsy of cutaneous mastocytosis (CM) in a child with maculopapular lesions. Mast cells are oval and relatively more abundant in lesions of children as compared with adults. CM in children is usually self-limiting and eventually disappears. (Courtesy N. Quintanilla, MD.) *(Right)* Multiple cutaneous mastocytomas in a patient with systemic mastocytosis (SM). In this patient, the skin tumors are confluent ⇗ with blisters ➡.

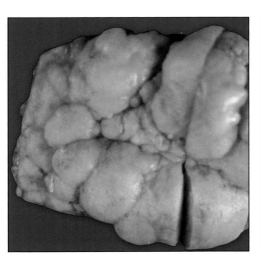 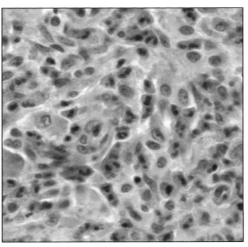

(Left) Gross photograph shows excision of skin and subcutaneous tissue involved by mastocytomas in a patient with SM. Note fibrosis creating a nodular, tan appearance. *(Right)* Mastocytoma of skin. The mast cells have oval and spindle-shaped nuclei and are associated with many eosinophils.

13

MAST CELL DISEASE

Lymph Node

(Left) Touch imprint preparation of a lymph node involved by systemic mastocytosis (SM). Note that the mast cells ⇥ are round to oval with abundant cytoplasm filled with faintly visible granules. *(Right)* SM involving lymph node. The mast cells have round or bilobed nuclei and clear cytoplasm. Note increased vascularity ⇛ and eosinophils.

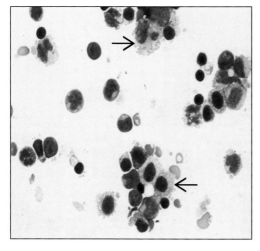
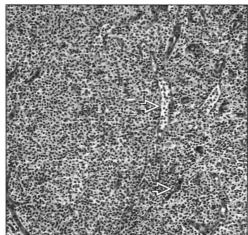

(Left) Systemic mastocytosis (SM) involving lymph node. There is a tendency for the mast cell infiltrate to exhibit a perifollicular distribution of growth ⇥. *(Right)* SM involving lymph node. Mast cells have abundant clear cytoplasm and reniform nuclei ⇥. Note increased eosinophils and delicate collagenous fibers ⇛.

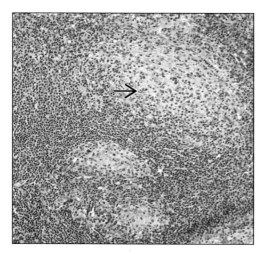
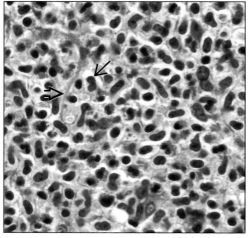

(Left) Systemic mastocytosis (SM) involving lymph node. Mast cells have strong enzyme cytochemical activity with naphthol AS-D chloroacetate esterase. *(Right)* SM involving lymph node. Immunohistochemistry for KIT/CD117 highlights many neoplastic mast cells.

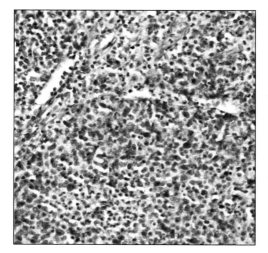
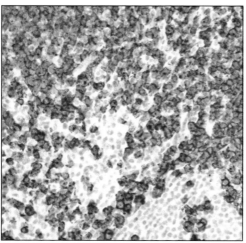

MAST CELL DISEASE

Spleen, Liver, and Gastrointestinal Tract

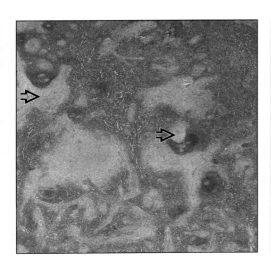

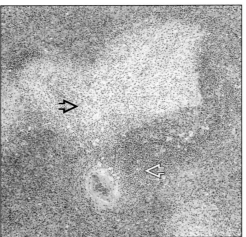

(Left) Spleen in a patient with systemic mastocytosis (SM). Note perifollicular mast cell aggregates ⊳. Characteristically patchy fibrosis is associated with and can obscure mast cells. *(Right)* Spleen in a patient with SM. A large mast cell aggregate ⊳ partially destroys a Malpighian follicle ⇒. This is a common pattern of SM in the spleen.

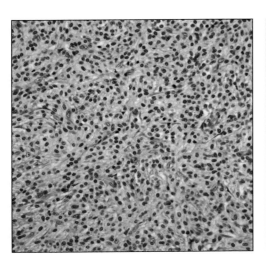

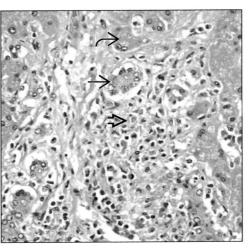

(Left) This micrograph depicts a diffuse mast cell infiltrate in the spleen of a patient with systemic mastocytosis (SM). This pattern occurs less frequently than the presence of aggregates of mast cells. *(Right)* SM in the liver. This mast cell aggregate ⊳ is associated with eosinophilia and is adjacent to a portal space, which is where this tumor usually localizes. Bile ducts ⇒ and hepatocytes ⇗ are also noted.

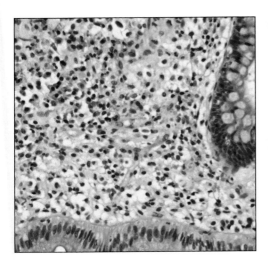

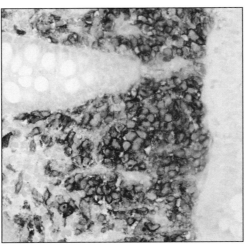

(Left) Systemic mastocytosis (SM) involving the mucosa of the left colon. The mucosa is expanded by mast cells with pale cytoplasm associated with eosinophils. This patient had symptoms of malabsorption and had many lesions involving the small and large intestines. *(Right)* SM involving the mucosa of the left colon. Mast cells in the mucosa are CD117(+).

MAST CELL DISEASE

Bones

(Left) Radiograph of vertebrae removed at autopsy shows diffuse osteosclerosis ⇨ in a patient with systemic mastocytosis (SM). Osteosclerosis is the most frequent alteration of the bone in patients with SM. A control radiograph is shown for comparison ➡. *(Right)* Cross section of vertebrae removed at autopsy shows osteosclerosis and osteolytic lesions ➡ in a patient with SM. The skull, spine, ribs, and pelvis are the most commonly involved sites in SM.

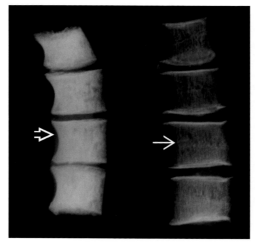
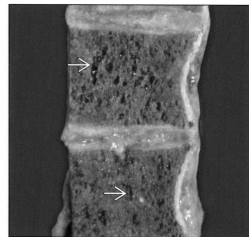

(Left) Bone lesions in systemic mastocytosis (SM) are variable. In this case there is prominent osteosclerosis ⇨. Trapped bone marrow space is filled with clusters of mast cells ⇨. *(Right)* Bone lesion in SM reveals irregular remodeling with mosaic lines ➡ that mimics Paget disease. Clusters of mast cells ⇨ are noted in the bone marrow space.

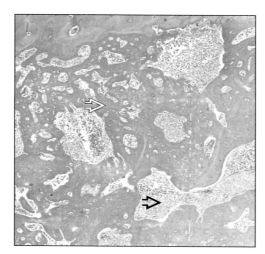
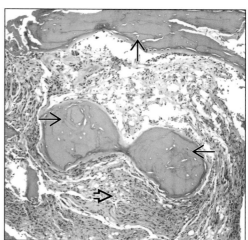

(Left) In this case of systemic mastocytosis (SM), the bone marrow is infiltrated by large aggregates of mast cells in a paratrabecular ⇨ distribution. Bone trabeculae may be thin/osteoporotic ⇨ or focally osteosclerotic ➡. *(Right)* In this case of SM, the bone marrow is infiltrated by oval to fusiform mast cells in a paratrabecular ⇨ distribution. Normal hematopoiesis ⇨ is noted in unaffected areas.

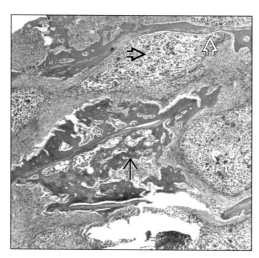
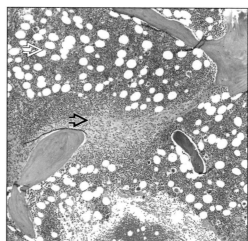

MAST CELL DISEASE

Bone Marrow

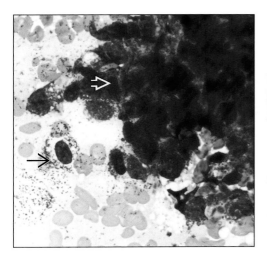

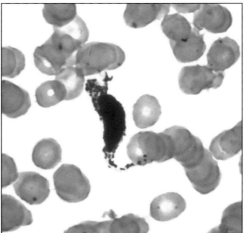

(Left) Bone marrow aspirate smear of a patient with systemic mastocytosis (SM) shows mast cells ⇒ that contain abundant cytoplasmic granules ➡. Low-power examination of aspirate smears is useful to detect these clusters. *(Right)* Bone marrow aspirate smear in a patient with SM shows an atypical spindle-shaped mast cell with cytoplasmic granules. A minor criterion for SM is fulfilled if > 25% of mast cells on the smear display an atypical morphology.

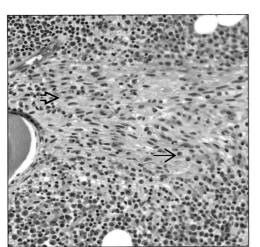

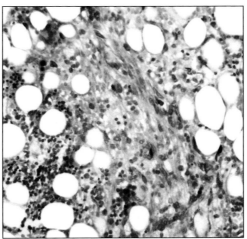

(Left) In this case of systemic mastocytosis (SM) in a 40-year-old man, the bone marrow shows paratrabecular ⇒ mast cell aggregates with associated fibrosis and an admixture of small lymphocytes and eosinophils ➡. *(Right)* Bone marrow biopsy specimen of a patient with SM. Giemsa stain highlights metachromatic granules in mast cell cytoplasm.

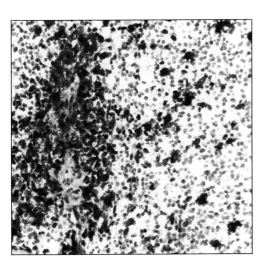

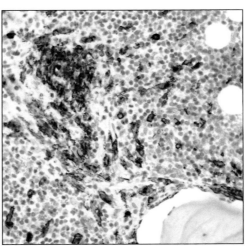

(Left) Antitryptase antibody highlights a compact cluster of mast cells in this bone marrow biopsy specimen of a patient with systemic mastocytosis (SM). This cluster fulfills the major diagnostic criterion for the diagnosis of SM. *(Right)* Anti-CD117 highlights a compact cluster of mast cells in this bone marrow involved by systemic mastocytosis (SM). In addition, this patient had follicular lymphoma, grade 1, involving a retroperitoneal lymph node.

MAST CELL DISEASE

Extracutaneous Mastocytoma

(Left) Extracutaneous mastocytoma involving soft tissue of the shoulder displays a diffuse and multinodular pattern. This was the only lesion in an adult patient who underwent excision and has not had evidence of recurrence after 9 years of follow-up. *(Right)* High-power magnification shows extracutaneous mastocytoma involving soft tissue of the shoulder. Note the cytoplasmic granularity and associated eosinophils.

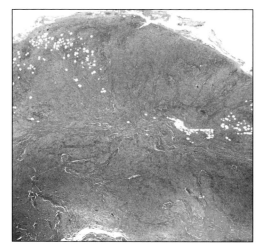
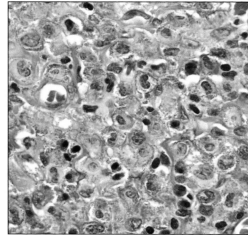

(Left) Extracutaneous mastocytoma involving soft tissue of the shoulder. Giemsa stain shows abundant metachromatic granules in the cytoplasm of the mast cells. *(Right)* Extracutaneous mastocytoma involving soft tissue of the shoulder. Immunohistochemistry for tryptase highlights abundant cytoplasmic granularity of the mast cells.

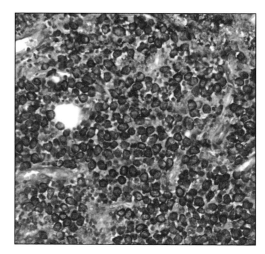
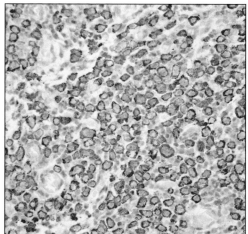

(Left) Extracutaneous mastocytoma involving soft tissue of the shoulder. Immunohistochemistry for CD2 highlights the mast cells. CD2 expression by mast cells is aberrant and supports mast cell neoplasia. *(Right)* Extracutaneous mastocytoma involving soft tissue of the shoulder. Immunohistochemistry for Ki-67 shows that the lesion has a low mitotic rate.

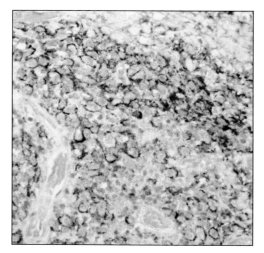
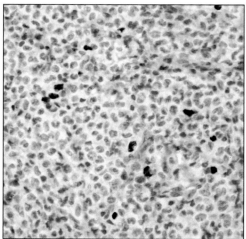

13

MAST CELL DISEASE

Mast Cell Leukemia and SM-AHNMD

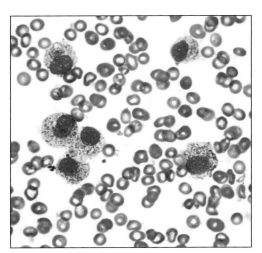
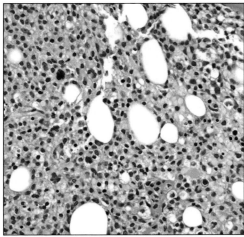

(Left) Peripheral blood smear involved by mast cell leukemia (MCL). Most cases of MCL show > 10% of mast cells in peripheral blood. In this patient, longstanding systemic mastocytosis preceded the onset of leukemia. *(Right)* MCL extensively involving bone marrow. MCL is characterized by a diffuse, compact mast cell infiltrate of the medullary space.

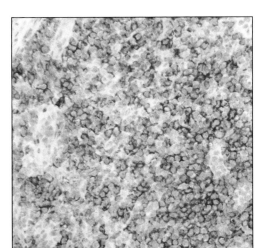
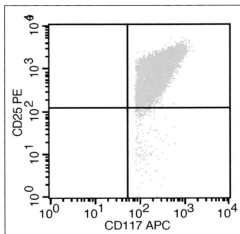

(Left) Immunohistochemistry for CD25 highlights a compact cluster of mast cells in this bone marrow biopsy specimen. Reactivity of mast cells with CD25 fulfills a minor diagnostic criterion for the diagnosis of systemic mastocytosis (SM). *(Right)* Flow cytometric immunophenotype of bone marrow aspirate material demonstrates CD25(+) and CD117(+) mast cells. Reactivity of mast cells with CD25 is aberrant and fulfills a minor diagnostic criterion for the diagnosis of SM.

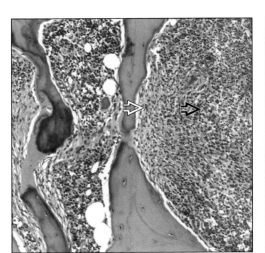
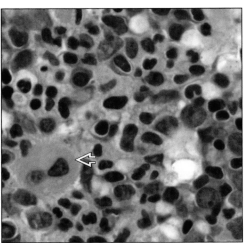

(Left) Systemic mastocytosis (SM) with associated clonal hematological non-mast cell lineage disease (AHNMD). In this case, there is a diagnostic lesion of SM ⇒ associated with bone marrow hypercellularity due to chronic myelomonocytic leukemia ⇒. *(Right)* SM with AHNMD. In this field, chronic myelomonocytic leukemia replaces normal bone marrow. A dysplastic megakaryocyte ⇒ is shown.

MAST CELL DISEASE

SM-AHNMD

(Left) Systemic mastocytosis with associated clonal hematological non-mast cell lineage disease (SM-AHNMD). SM and chronic myelomonocytic leukemia (CMML) involving an axillary lymph node of a patient with previously diagnosed CMML is shown. (Right) SM-AHMD. SM with chronic myelomonocytic leukemia involving an axillary lymph node. The neoplastic mast cells are tryptase(+).

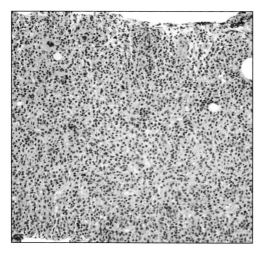
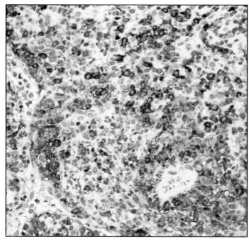

(Left) SM-AHMD. The bone marrow shows a mast cell cluster ⮞ adjacent to acute myeloid leukemia (AML) with t(8;21)(q22;q22). (Courtesy K. Reichard, MD.) (Right) SM-AHNMD. In this bone marrow aspirate smear, there are mast cells ⮞ and blasts ➡ of AML with t(8;21)(q22;q22). Therapy succeeded in removing the acute leukemia but not the mast cells. (Courtesy Kaaren Reichard, MD.)

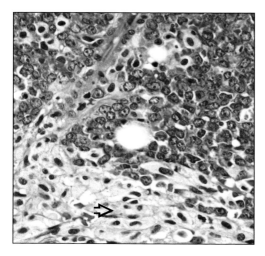
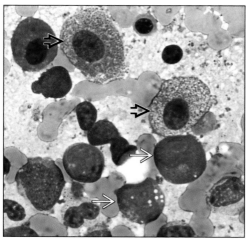

(Left) Systemic mastocytosis with associated clonal hematological non-mast cell lineage disease (SM-AHNMD) in bone marrow shows a compact mast cell aggregate ➡ and chronic lymphocytic leukemia ⮞. Immunophenotyping showed a monotypic B-cell population, CD5(+), CD19(+), CD20(+), CD23(+), and immunoglobulin κ light chain(+). (Right) Bone marrow aspirate smear in a case of SM-AHNMD shows spindle mast cells ➡ of SM associated with chronic lymphocytic leukemia ⮞.

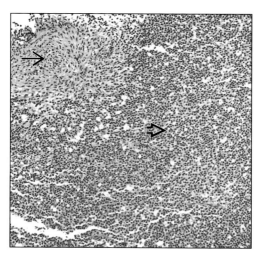
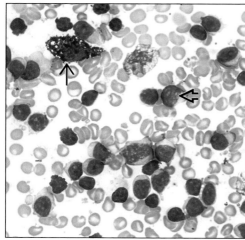

13

MAST CELL DISEASE

SM-AHNMD and Differential Diagnosis

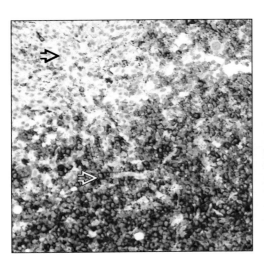

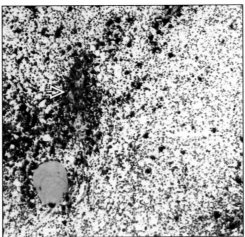

(Left) Systemic mastocytosis with associated clonal hematological non-mast cell lineage disease (SM-AHNMD). In this case, SM is associated with chronic lymphocytic leukemia. The lymphoid infiltrate shows reactivity with CD20 ➡. The mast cells are negative for CD20 ➡. *(Right)* SM-AHNMD. In this case, SM is associated with chronic lymphocytic leukemia involving bone marrow. The neoplastic mast cells strongly express tryptase ➡.

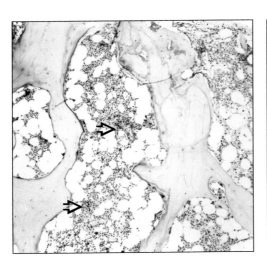

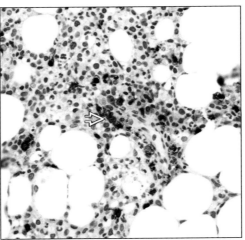

(Left) Acute myeloid leukemia involving bone marrow associated with tryptase(+) hyperplastic mast cells ➡ appearing in an interstitial pattern. The mast cells do not form compact clusters as occurs in systemic mastocytosis (SM). *(Right)* Acute myeloid leukemia involving bone marrow associated with tryptase(+) hyperplastic mast cells ➡ present in a perivascular and interstitial pattern. These mast cells do not form compact clusters as it occurs in SM.

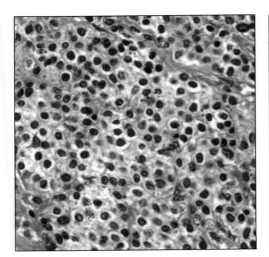

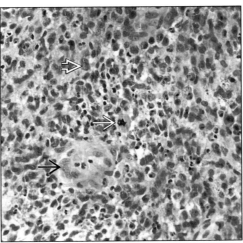

(Left) Hairy cell leukemia (HCL) in the spleen shows oval cells with clear cytoplasm that can mimic sheets of mast cells. However, this infiltrate is diffuse and is not associated with eosinophils. *(Right)* Langerhans cell histiocytosis (LCH) in involving bone shows numerous Langerhans cells ➡, eosinophils, and a multinucleated giant cell ➡. A mitotic figure ➡ is noted; LCH lesions often show rare to occasional mitotic figures.

Spleen

SPLENIC INFLAMMATORY PSEUDOTUMOR

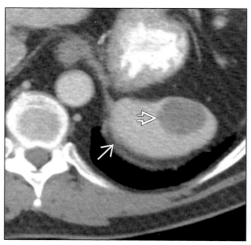

CT of abdomen shows a normal-sized spleen ➡ with a 2.5 cm in diameter inflammatory pseudotumor ➡. Lesion was 1 cm 16 months before, when it was found during staging for renal cell carcinoma.

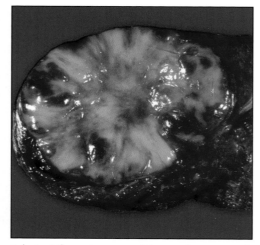

Splenic inflammatory pseudotumor shows a well-circumscribed fleshy mass with focal hemorrhage surrounded by congested splenic parenchyma.

TERMINOLOGY

Abbreviations
- Splenic inflammatory pseudotumor (IPT)

Definitions
- Reactive lesion of spleen composed of inflammatory cells and spindled cells with or without sclerosis
- Etiology of splenic IPT is unknown
- Classification is controversial since other entities have been classified as IPT; in particular
  - Inflammatory pseudotumor-like follicular dendritic cell tumor (IPT-FDCT)
    - True neoplasm that involves mainly liver and spleen
  - ALK(+) inflammatory myofibroblastic tumor (IMT)
    - Most often involves soft tissues of children and young adults
  - IPT-FDCT and ALK(+) IMT are now excluded from the category of IPT

ETIOLOGY/PATHOGENESIS

Infectious Agents
- Etiology of splenic IPT is unknown
- Most likely a number of causes may ultimately result in splenic IPT
  - Infectious causes are likely
    - Variable association reported with *Streptococcus*, *Legionella*, and Epstein-Barr virus
  - Vascular events may be involved
  - Autoimmunity has been hypothesized to play a role
- Regardless of initiating event, exuberant tissue repair is probably involved in pathogenesis
- Splenic IPT appears to be pathobiologically similar to IPT of lymph nodes

CLINICAL ISSUES

Epidemiology
- Incidence
  - Uncommon; ~ 3% of splenic masses
  - Rare when compared with IPT at other sites of body
- Age
  - Range: 19-87 years; median: 53 years
  - Rare in children
- Gender
  - Slight female predominance; M:F ratio = 1:1.3

Site
- Typically involves spleen as single lesion
  - Rare cases can be multicentric

Presentation
- Affected patients are immunocompetent
- Fever and weight loss in about half of patients
- Asymptomatic in 50% of cases
- Epigastric or left flank pain, usually associated with larger lesions
  - Splenomegaly may be noted in some cases
- Occasional IPT are associated with malignancies, e.g., colon or renal cell carcinoma

Laboratory Tests
- Usually unremarkable
  - Occasionally patients have mild leukocytosis, (< 15 x 10^9/L), anemia, and hypergammaglobulinemia

Treatment
- Due to rarity and nonspecific CT or MR imaging, these lesions are not diagnosed preoperatively
  - Diagnosis first established after splenectomy
    - Splenectomy is effective treatment
- Symptoms and laboratory abnormalities disappear after splenectomy

SPLENIC INFLAMMATORY PSEUDOTUMOR

Key Facts

Terminology
- Splenic inflammatory pseudotumor (IPT)

Clinical Issues
- Age: 19-87 years (median: 53 years)
  - Rare in children
- Slight female predominance
- Excision is curative

Macroscopic Features
- Well-circumscribed mass
  - Median: 10 cm (range: 1.5-22 cm)

Microscopic Pathology
- Cellular spindle cells of short fascicles with bland nuclear features
- Mixed infiltrate of plasma cells, lymphocytes, and histiocytes

Ancillary Tests
- Spindle cells
  - Vimentin(+) and CD68([+], focal)
  - ~ 70% of cases (+) for smooth muscle actin (focal)
  - CD8(-), CD21(-), CD23(-), CD30(-), desmin(-)
- Lymphocytes and plasma cells
  - Polytypic
- Molecular genetic studies
  - No evidence of monoclonal Ig or T-cell receptor gene rearrangements

Top Differential Diagnoses
- Inflammatory pseudotumor-like follicular dendritic cell tumor
- Inflammatory myofibroblastic tumor
- Follicular dendritic cell sarcoma

Prognosis
- Excellent prognosis; no deaths attributable to splenic IPT
- Tumors are cured by splenectomy, and there are no reported recurrences of similar lesions elsewhere

IMAGE FINDINGS

CT Findings
- Discrete, single splenic mass
- Associated with splenomegaly when tumors are larger
- Lymphadenopathy is unusual

MACROSCOPIC FEATURES

General Features
- Spleen weight
  - Mean: 331 g (range: 140-1,030 g)
    - Splenomegaly > 250 g in 50% of cases
- Well-circumscribed, nonencapsulated single mass
  - Cut surface is white-tan, gray, or yellow; soft to firm lesions
  - Rarely multinodular
  - Mean size: 10 cm (range: 1-22 cm)

MICROSCOPIC PATHOLOGY

Histologic Features
- Lesions are usually well circumscribed
  - Lesions may be partially encapsulated
  - Islands of white or red pulp may be trapped at periphery of lesion
- 3 growth patterns are recognized; may occur simultaneously
  - Cellular spindle cell, composed of short fascicles
    - Most common
    - Can be focally storiform; rare mitoses identified
    - Bland spindle cells with oval vesicular nuclei and small nucleoli
  - Hypocellular fibrous pattern, similar to scar tissue
  - Myxoid and vascularized, similar to granulation tissue
- Abundant mixed inflammatory infiltrate of plasma cells, lymphocytes, and histiocytes
  - Variable proportions of inflammatory cells in different areas of same lesions
    - Marked variability from case to case
  - Lymphocytes are usually small with occasional immunoblasts
  - Mature plasma cells, with occasional Russell bodies
- Other features
  - Focal, central necrosis usually associated with neutrophilic infiltrate
    - Histiocytes and eosinophils are less frequent
  - Hemorrhage and hemosiderin deposition
- Compressed and congested splenic parenchyma around tumor; otherwise unremarkable spleen

ANCILLARY TESTS

Immunohistochemistry
- Spindle cells
  - Vimentin(+) and CD68([+], focal)
  - ~ 70% of cases are positive for smooth muscle actin (focal) and desmin(-)
    - Smooth muscle actin(+) cells are considered myofibroblasts
  - Occasionally positive for S100 protein (focal) and Factor XIII
  - CD8(-), CD21(-), CD23(-), and CD30(-)
  - HMB-45(-), ALK-1(-), HHV8(-), and cytokeratin(-)
  - Epstein-Barr virus(+) in small subset of cases
    - Infected cells are spindle cells, some of which can focally express smooth muscle actin
- Lymphocytes and plasma cells
  - Mixture of T and B cells; usually with predominance of CD3(+) cells
  - B cells and plasma cells are polytypic

SPLENIC INFLAMMATORY PSEUDOTUMOR

Cytogenetics
- Normal karyotype

Molecular Genetics
- No evidence of monoclonal immunoglobulin (Ig) or T-cell receptor gene rearrangements
- No known oncogene abnormalities

DIFFERENTIAL DIAGNOSIS

Inflammatory Pseudotumor-like Follicular Dendritic Cell Tumor (IPT-FDCT)
- Female predominance
- Considered variant of follicular dendritic cell sarcoma
- More aggressive clinically, contrary to splenic IPT
  - Recurrences are common
  - Recurrent tumors show pleomorphic large cells usually not detected in primary tumors
- Immunohistochemistry helpful as FDC can be
  - CD21(+), CD23(+), Factor XIII(+)
- Commonly EBV(+)
  - Monoclonal EBV when assessing EBV DNA terminal repeat regions
- IPT-FDCT of spleen is pathobiologically similar to liver IPT

Inflammatory Myofibroblastic Tumor (IMT)
- Affects soft tissues of children and young adults
- Ill-defined mass grossly
- Myofibroblasts positive for smooth muscle actin (100%) and cytokeratin (15-30%)
  - Negative for follicular dendritic cell markers and H-caldesmon
- Scattered large atypical cells, sometimes ganglion-like cells with prominent nucleoli
- Harbors balanced translocations involving anaplastic lymphoma kinase (ALK) gene at 2p23
  - Anaplastic lymphoma kinase (ALK) is expressed in ~ 50% of cases
  - ALK is not expressed in splenic IPT
- Has locally aggressive clinical behavior with recurrences
- Rare reports of IMT in spleen, but those reported have been ALK(-)

Follicular Dendritic Cell Sarcoma (FDCS)
- Formerly designated as follicular dendritic cell tumor
- Affects primarily lymph nodes but can involve spleen and other sites
  - Intraabdominal cases are often clinically aggressive
- More aggressive than IPT-FDCT, with recurrences and distal metastasis
- No gender predilection, except in splenic or hepatic forms where there is female predominance
- FDCS can show range of histologic features
  - Composed of spindled or epithelioid cells
  - Bland or pleomorphic cytologic features
  - May display scattered inflammatory cells
- Immunohistochemistry helpful as FDCS can be
  - CD21(+), CD23(+), CD35(+), CNA.42(+)
  - Clusterin(+), fascin(+), and EGFR(+)

- Rare or no association with EBV

Inflammatory Pseudotumor (IPT) Involving Other Sites
- Usually present with systemic findings; sometimes asymptomatic
- IPT has been diagnosed in various anatomic sites
  - Respiratory tract, lungs, orbit, spinal meninges, digestive tract, heart, and lymph nodes
- Encompasses lesions where myofibroblasts are detected but are not main component
  - Variable mix of small and activated lymphocytes
  - Polytypic plasma cells, histiocytes, and sclerosis
- Fibrotic process in lymph node extends along capsule or trabeculae and then throughout parenchyma
- EBV small encoded RNA (EBER)(+) in 20% of nodal IPT; in scattered lymphocytes
  - Spindle cells are negative for EBER

Sclerosing Angiomatoid Nodular Transformation (SANT)
- Involves splenic red pulp
- Recently described entity with overlapping features with splenic IPT
  - Some researchers consider that SANT is subset or end stage of splenic IPT
- Single mass composed of multiple small nodules
- Nodules display dense network of capillaries as well as remnants of sinuses
  - Endothelial cells positive for CD34 and CD31; usually negative for CD8
  - EBER(-); EBV latent membrane protein type 1(-)
  - Negative for follicular dendritic cell markers CD21, CD35, and CNA.42
- Collagenous fibrosis with scattered spindle cells may occur around and in center of lesion
  - Spindle cells around nodules react as myofibroblasts and are smooth muscle actin(+)
- Angiomatoid nodules occasionally show dense inflammatory infiltration
  - Polytypic plasma cells, small lymphocytes, and histiocytes are not unusual
- Hyalinization of arterial walls and organizing thrombosis in veins

Splenic Hamartoma
- No gender predilection
- Usually found incidentally after splenectomy for other medical or surgical conditions
  - Sometimes found at autopsy
- Involves splenic red pulp
  - Considered to be malformation
- Usually single lesion, less commonly presents as multiple lesions
- Disorganized red pulp displacing normal white and red pulp
  - Indistinct interface with white and red pulp
- Sinus or cord-like spaces are characteristic of splenic hamartoma and not seen in splenic IPT
  - Inflammatory cells, including plasma cells and histiocytes, are unusual but occur
  - Occasional sclerosis

- Sometimes anemia and thrombocytopenia due to hamartoma sequestration
  - These cases most frequently show extramedullary hematopoiesis
- Cells lining sinuses are CD8(+)

Littoral Cell Angioma
- Rare, benign splenic tumor that arises in red pulp
- Composed of splenic sinus lining cells
- Grossly presents as solitary or multiple bloody nodules
- Anastomosing vascular channels merge with surrounding cords and sinuses
- Vascular channels are lined by tall or large cells with abundant clear or faintly granular cytoplasm
  - Cell nuclei are vesicular, nonatypical
  - Absent or rare mitoses are noted
- Lining cells are Factor VIII-related antigen(+)

Diffuse Large B-cell Lymphoma (DLBCL)
- DLBCL often presents as large solitary mass
  - Cases presenting as solitary mass with central necrosis may be similar to IPT by imaging studies
  - Less frequently it presents with diffuse pattern
  - Involves red or white pulp; usually both are involved
- Histologically DLBCL of spleen is characterized by
  - Sheets of large lymphoid cells
    - Centroblastic, immunoblastic, or highly pleomorphic cytologic features
  - Necrosis and mitotic figures are common
  - Can show admixture of inflammatory cells and sclerosis
- Immunophenotype: Monotypic immunoglobulin expression or aberrant B-cell population
- Monoclonal immunoglobulin gene rearrangements are present

Classical Hodgkin Lymphoma (CHL)
- Usually involves white pulp in incipient lesions
  - Commonly involves both white and red pulp
- Reed-Sternberg and Hodgkin cells are large with vesicular nuclei and prominent nucleoli
  - Immunohistochemically react with CD15, CD30, and pax-5
- Inflammatory component is prominent and includes
  - Eosinophils, plasma cells, histiocytes, and small lymphocytes
- Variable association with EBV, as detected both by LMP1 and EBER
  - ~ 75% in mixed cellularity CHL
  - 10-40% in nodular sclerosis CHL

Mycobacterial Spindle Cell Pseudotumor
- HIV(+) patients
- Most often affects lymph nodes, but spleen can be involved
  - In spleen, presents as mass mimicking splenic IPT
- Multinodular, granulomatous reaction with spindle cells
- Stains for acid-fast bacilli reveal *Mycobacterium* organisms

Smooth Muscle Tumors
- Leiomyomas and leiomyosarcomas arising in immunosuppressed patients can be EBV(+)
- Usually affect children and young adults with acquired immunodeficiency syndrome
- EBV is monoclonal and infects smooth muscle cells

DIAGNOSTIC CHECKLIST

Clinically Relevant Pathologic Features
- Usually single mass in spleen
- Commonly incidental finding detected by imaging studies or splenectomy
- Surgical excision is curative

Pathologic Interpretation Pearls
- Mixture of inflammatory cells and histologically bland spindled cells
  - Spindle cells distributed loosely or as short fascicles
  - Inflammatory cells are mainly lymphocytes, plasma cells, and histiocytes
- Secondary changes include sclerosis and necrosis

SELECTED REFERENCES

1. Rosenbaum L et al: Epstein-Barr virus-associated inflammatory pseudotumor of the spleen: report of two cases and review of the literature. J Hematop. Epub ahead of print, 2009
2. Yamamoto H et al: Inflammatory myofibroblastic tumor versus IgG4-related sclerosing disease and inflammatory pseudotumor: a comparative clinicopathologic study. Am J Surg Pathol. 33(9):1330-40, 2009
3. Diebold J et al: Is sclerosing angiomatoid nodular transformation (SANT) of the splenic red pulp identical to inflammatory pseudotumour? Report of 16 cases. Histopathology. 53(3):299-310, 2008
4. Horiguchi H et al: Inflammatory pseudotumor-like follicular dendritic cell tumor of the spleen. Pathol Int. 54(2):124-31, 2004
5. Lewis JT et al: Inflammatory pseudotumor of the spleen associated with a clonal Epstein-Barr virus genome. Case report and review of the literature. Am J Clin Pathol. 120(1):56-61, 2003
6. Cheuk W et al: Inflammatory pseudotumor-like follicular dendritic cell tumor: a distinctive low-grade malignant intra-abdominal neoplasm with consistent Epstein-Barr virus association. Am J Surg Pathol. 25(6):721-31, 2001
7. Selves J et al: Inflammatory pseudotumor of the liver. Evidence for follicular dendritic reticulum cell proliferation associated with clonal Epstein-Barr virus. Am J Surg Pathol. 20(6):747-53, 1996
8. Arber DA et al: Frequent presence of the Epstein-Barr virus in inflammatory pseudotumor. Hum Pathol. 26(10):1093-8, 1995
9. Suster S et al: Mycobacterial spindle-cell pseudotumor of the spleen. Am J Clin Pathol. 101(4):539-42, 1994
10. Thomas RM et al: Inflammatory pseudotumor of the spleen. A clinicopathologic and immunophenotypic study of eight cases. Arch Pathol Lab Med. 117(9):921-6, 1993
11. Cotelingam JD et al: Inflammatory pseudotumor of the spleen. Am J Surg Pathol. 8(5):375-80, 1984

SPLENIC INFLAMMATORY PSEUDOTUMOR

Differential Diagnosis of Splenic Inflammatory Pseudotumor

Features	Splenic IPT	Hepatic or Splenic IPT-FDCT	IMT	FDCS	IPT in Other Sites	SANT
Male to Female Ratio						
	1:1.3	1:3-1:6	1:1.3	1:1	1:1.6	1:2
Age Range (Median)						
	19-87 y (53 y)	1-87 y (44 y)	< 1-46 y (9 y)	25-69 y (44 y)	1-68 y (24 y)	22-82 y (44 y)
Preferential Geographic Distribution						
	Worldwide	Asian	Worldwide	Worldwide	Worldwide	Not established
Gross Appearance						
	Well-circumscribed single mass; focal necrosis	Single or multiple masses in liver; single mass in spleen	Poorly circumscribed	Poorly circumscribed	Poorly circumscribed	Multinodular
Size Range (Median)						
	1.5-22 cm (10 cm)	3-22 cm (11 cm)	1-17 cm (6 cm)	1-19 cm (5 cm)	1-12 cm (3 cm)	1.0-12 cm (6 cm)
Histopathologic Features						
Pattern	Spindle cells or storiform	Spindle cells or storiform	Spindle cell fascicles	Cellular fascicles	Spindle cells or storiform	Multiple nodules
Main cell component	Spindle cells; not atypical	Follicular dendritic cell; significant atypia, more in recurrences	Myofibroblast, usually bland cytology; occasionally pleomorphic	Follicular dendritic cell with bland to aggressive features	Myofibroblasts and histiocytes	Benign endothelial cells
Inflammatory cells	Small lymphocytes, polytypic plasma cells, histiocytes	Small lymphocytes, polytypic plasma cells, histiocytes	Small lymphocytes and polytypic plasma cells	Scattered small lymphocytes, polytypic plasma cells, histiocytes	Small lymphocytes, polytypic plasma cells, histiocytes	Small lymphocytes and polytypic plasma cells around nodules
Ancillary Studies						
Markers	CD21(-), CD35(-), CNA.42(-)	CD21(+), CD35(+), CNA.42(+)	Smooth muscle actin, ALK(+), cytokeratin (~ 15-30%)	CD21(+), CD35(+), or CNA.42(+)	CD68(+); CD21(-), ALK(-), smooth muscle actin(-)	CD31(+), CD34(+), CD8(-/+)
EBV status	Negative	Positive in spindle cells in 40-70% of cases	Negative	0-4% EBER(+)	Negative; if EBV(+), infected cells are lymphocytes	Negative
Prognosis After Surgical Resection						
	Excellent; no recurrence	Good; some recurrence (~ 40% in hepatic cases; no recurrence in splenic cases); rare metastasis in hepatic cases (< 10%)	Recurrence; metastasis (~ 10%)	Recurrence and metastasis	Excellent	Excellent

IPT = inflammatory pseudotumor; IPT-FDCT = IPT-like follicular dendritic cell tumor; IMT = inflammatory myofibroblastic tumor; FDCS = follicular dendritic cell sarcoma; SANT = sclerosing angiomatoid nodular transformation of spleen.

SPLENIC INFLAMMATORY PSEUDOTUMOR

Microscopic Features

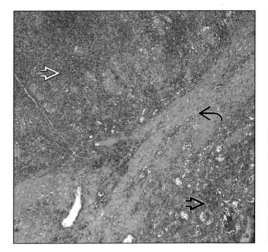

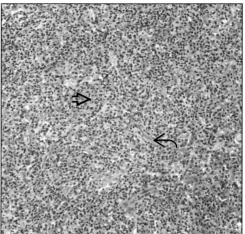

(Left) Splenic inflammatory pseudotumor ⮆ surrounded by a capsule ➡. Capsule is usually incomplete in inflammatory pseudotumor. Other parts of spleen display red pulp congestion ⮆. *(Right)* Splenic inflammatory pseudotumor is characterized by a mixed inflammatory infiltrate ⮆ and scattered spindle cells ➡.

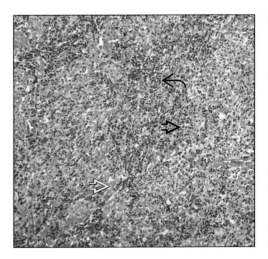

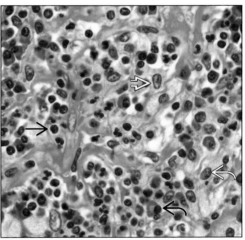

(Left) Low magnification of splenic inflammatory pseudotumor displays a subtle cellular spindle cell component ⮆, inflammatory cells ➡, and mild sclerosis ⮆. *(Right)* High magnification of splenic inflammatory pseudotumor displays the characteristic cell mixture of small lymphocytes ➡, plasma cells ➡, histiocytes ⮆, and plump spindle cells ⮆. Atypia of spindle cells is not a feature of splenic inflammatory pseudotumor.

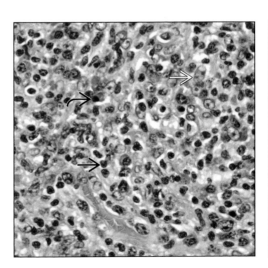

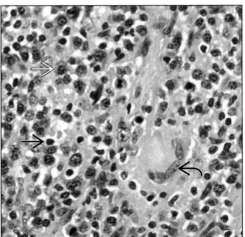

(Left) Splenic inflammatory pseudotumor displays a mixed inflammatory infiltrate composed of small lymphocytes ➡ and plasma cells ➡. There are also scattered bland, plump, uniform spindle cells ⮆. *(Right)* Splenic inflammatory pseudotumor displays abundant inflammatory cells, including small lymphocytes ➡, plasma cells ⮆, and a multinucleated giant cell ➡. Rarely, well-formed granulomas can occur.

SPLENIC INFLAMMATORY PSEUDOTUMOR

Microscopic Features and Differential Diagnosis: IPT-FDCT

(Left) Splenic inflammatory pseudotumor with necrosis appearing as granular debris ⭲. Necrosis is focal, usually in the middle of the lesion. *(Right)* Splenic inflammatory pseudotumor with extensive sclerosis ⭲ leaving only few remaining inflammatory cells ⭲. This pattern can be focal and sometimes may mimic amyloid or a scar.

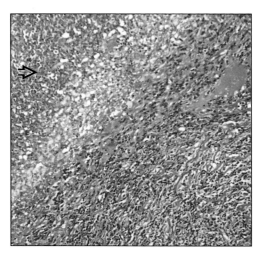
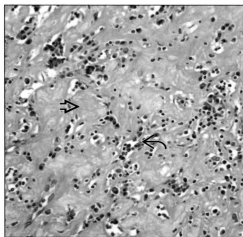

(Left) Splenic inflammatory pseudotumor-like follicular dendritic cell tumor (IPT-FDCT) shows a mixture of spindle cells and abundant inflammatory cells. *(Courtesy M. Vasef, MD.)* *(Right)* Immunohistochemistry for CD35 in IPT-FDCT shows reactivity in follicular dendritic cell processes ⭲. *(Courtesy M. Vasef, MD.)*

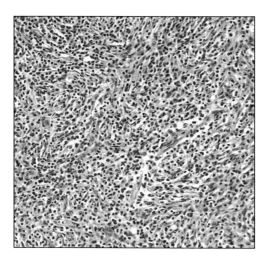
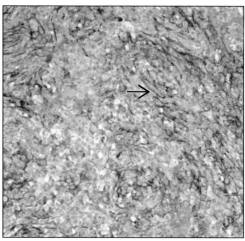

(Left) In situ hybridization for EBV-encoded RNA (EBER) in a case of IPT-FDCT shows reactivity in spindle cells ⭲. Approximately 40% of these tumors are positive for EBER. *(Courtesy M. Vasef, MD.)* *(Right)* Follicular dendritic cell sarcoma (FDCS) displays a spindle cell proliferation ⭲. The spindle cells form compact fascicles. This tumor involved spleen, liver, and intraabdominal lymph nodes.

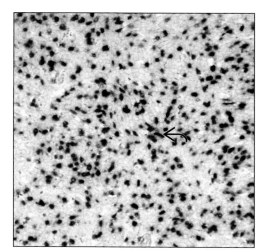
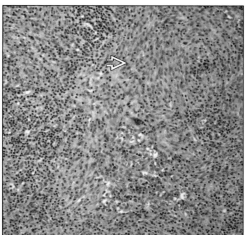

Differential Diagnosis: FDCS and SANT

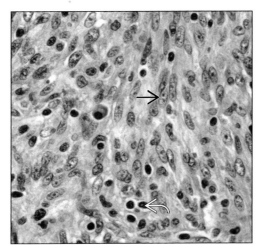

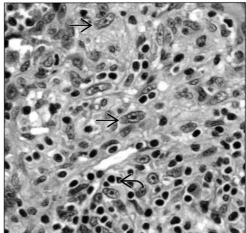

(Left) High magnification of follicular dendritic cell sarcoma displays a uniform spindle cell proliferation with indistinct cytoplasm, and oval vesicular nuclei ➡ with small, distinctive nucleoli. Tumor is admixed with rare inflammatory cells ➡. This pattern is the usual FDCS pattern. *(Right)* FDCS displays scattered neoplastic cells with pleomorphic nuclei ➡ admixed with many inflammatory cells ➡ that are focally similar to splenic inflammatory pseudotumor.

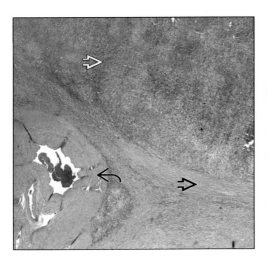

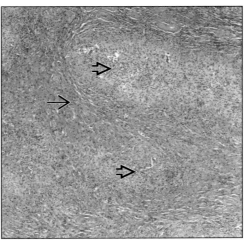

(Left) Sclerosing angiomatoid nodular transformation (SANT) ➡ of splenic red pulp appears as a large nodule surrounded by a thick collagenous capsule ➡ and well demarcated from surrounding spleen. A large hyalinized vessel is also noted ➡. Hyalinized vessels or organizing thrombosis of veins can also be found around this tumor. *(Right)* SANT is composed of multiple vascular nodules ➡ surrounded by collagen ➡.

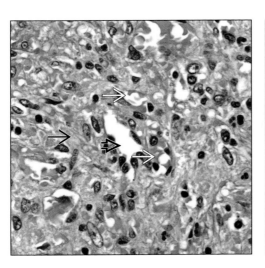

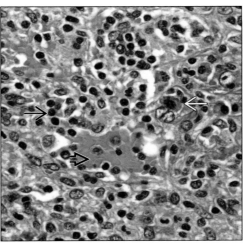

(Left) Center of a nodule in SANT displays a blood vessel ➡ with small endothelial cells, surrounded by collagenous stroma ➡ and satellite small vessels ➡. *(Right)* Center of SANT displays blood vessel ➡. This area shows, in addition, small lymphocytes ➡ and plasma cells ➡ that focally are similar to splenic inflammatory pseudotumor. Inflammatory cells are more frequently found around vascular nodules.

POST-CHEMOTHERAPY HISTIOCYTE-RICH PSEUDOTUMOR OF SPLEEN

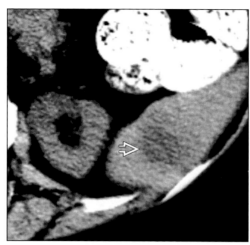

Post-chemotherapy histiocyte-rich pseudotumor of spleen shows an ill-defined nodular lesion ⇗ that did not change size after 3 months following chemotherapy for metastatic ovarian carcinoma.

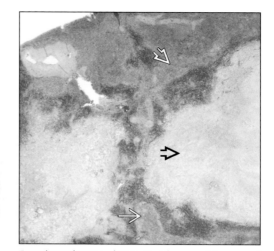

Post-chemotherapy histiocyte-rich pseudotumor of spleen ⇗ at the interface with normal spleen ⇗. There are large nodular, ill-defined masses with trapped splenic parenchyma ⇗.

TERMINOLOGY

Synonyms
- Xanthomatous pseudotumor
- Benign histiocytic proliferation with xanthomatous changes

Definitions
- Residual splenic mass after chemotherapy composed of viable nonneoplastic cells and necrotic neoplastic cells
  - Similar masses can occur in other sites

ETIOLOGY/PATHOGENESIS

Chemotherapy-induced Tumor Necrosis
- Sensitive tumors usually resolve after effective chemotherapy
- However, large or bulky masses may persist after chemotherapy; more frequent with
  - Hodgkin lymphoma
  - Aggressive non-Hodgkin lymphomas
  - Metastatic carcinomas
  - Pediatric malignancies of primitive cells

Pathogenesis
- Presumably, toxic effects of therapy kill neoplastic cells, which then elicits tissue reaction
  - Toxic effects of normal tissue stroma also may occur
- Tumor necrosis releases chemotactic substances
- Circulating monocytes are attracted and recruited to site of necrosis and become histiocytes
- Role of lipid-accumulating macrophages in the pathogenic process is complex
  - There is transcription of genes associated with M2 activation
    - Mannose receptor/CD206
    - Scavenger receptor/CD163
    - Chemokine CCL18

- Anti-inflammatory cytokine IL-10

CLINICAL ISSUES

Site
- Spleen is focus of this chapter
  - Involved by tumor before therapy
    - Occasionally splenic mass is detected after chemotherapy
  - Rare site of post-chemotherapy histiocyte-rich pseudotumor
    - Other anatomic sites also can be involved: Mediastinum, lymph nodes, gastrointestinal tract

Presentation
- Wide age range, in accordance with type of lymphoma and carcinoma
- Variable time of follow-up depending on clinical assessment
  - Usually 1-6 months after completion of therapy
- Splenic mass can be asymptomatic or associated with pain
- Persistent mass after chemotherapy usually prompts suspicion of recurrent malignancy
  - Clinical or radiologic evidence of residual mass used to prompt "2nd look" surgery
    - Highly sensitive CT scans can detect smaller lesions of unknown clinical significance
    - PET scans can show high uptake
  - Post-therapy, splenic mass can be of similar size or larger than viable tumor mass before therapy
- In general, the larger the size of residual mass, the higher the likelihood of residual viable cancer
  - Residual masses > 3 cm have greater chance of harboring viable tumor
- Post-chemotherapy evaluation has clinical relevance
  - Hodgkin lymphoma
    - Assessment of response to chemotherapy may lead to further chemotherapy or radiation therapy

POST-CHEMOTHERAPY HISTIOCYTE-RICH PSEUDOTUMOR OF SPLEEN

Key Facts

Terminology
- Residual splenic mass after chemotherapy composed of viable nonneoplastic cells and necrotic neoplastic cells

Etiology/Pathogenesis
- Chemotherapy is toxic to neoplastic cells in spleen
  - Tumor necrosis releases chemotactic substances
  - Circulating monocytes are attracted and recruited to site of necrosis and become histiocytes

Clinical Issues
- Residual masses after successful chemotherapy are rarely diagnosed in spleen
- More common in patients with bulky tumors
- In lymphoma patients, post-chemotherapy histiocyte-rich pseudotumors can

- Revert to normal upon follow-up for > 1 year in ~ 50%
- Relapse in about 20% of those with residual masses

Image Findings
- FDG-PET is considered one of the most helpful noninvasive imaging techniques

Microscopic Pathology
- Nonviable tumor cells usually appear as cell ghosts
- Many lipid-laden histiocytes; other inflammatory cells common

Top Differential Diagnoses
- Residual viable tumor associated with necrosis
- Storage diseases
- Splenic inflammatory pseudotumor

- Nonseminomatous germ cell tumors with persistent lymphadenopathy (> 1 cm)
  - Revealed 2% residual viable cancer, 62% teratoma, and 36% necrosis; 4% had recurrence elsewhere
  - Resection is needed for better outcome in cases of teratoma or residual cancer
- Wilms tumor
  - Post-chemotherapy complete tumor necrosis is considered as "low risk" in Wilms tumor
  - If tumor is stage I, may not require further chemotherapy
- Residual masses can occur in ~ 60% of patients after chemotherapy for lymphomas
  - More common in patients with bulky tumors
  - Symptoms are variable depending on site of involvement
  - Smaller, asymptomatic lesions may go undetected

Natural History
- Related to underlying malignant neoplasm, including recurrences
- Post-chemotherapy masses in lymphoma patients can
  - Revert to normal upon follow-up for > 1 year (~ 50%)
  - Lead to sclerosis, fibrous scars, or calcification after longer periods of follow-up
  - Relapse in about 20% of those with residual masses
- Mass is smaller or remains stable after chemotherapy has been completed
- Occasionally splenic masses are 1st detected following chemotherapy for disease elsewhere
  - Splenic mass inapparent prior to therapy and resultant development of pseudotumor

Treatment
- Observation or follow-up only
  - If imaging studies show evidence of progression, then resection, further chemotherapy, or radiotherapy may be indicated
- Overdiagnosis of malignancy may lead to unnecessary additional therapy

Prognosis
- Long-term prognosis related to underlying malignancy
- Discovery of residual mass in mediastinum of Hodgkin lymphoma patients after chemotherapy correlates with higher 5-year relapse rate
- 2nd-line regimens (salvage therapy) are becoming more successful when residual disease is detected

IMAGE FINDINGS

MR Findings
- Considered poorly sensitive for staging and follow-up of lymphoma patients

CT Findings
- Sensitive technique to diagnose and monitor therapy
  - Advantage of being noninvasive and accurately determines extent of disease
    - Eliminates need for lymphangiography and staging laparotomy for Hodgkin lymphoma
  - In untreated lymphoma patients, any mass or lymph nodes > 1.5 cm is considered active disease
    - CT diagnosis of residual disease may lead to further chemotherapy, change of drug regimens, or radiotherapy
    - CT is considered nonspecific to assess tumor viability in patients who received chemotherapy

F18 Fluorodeoxyglucose (FDG) Positron Emission Tomography (PET)
- Considered one of the most helpful noninvasive imaging techniques
- Based on increased glucose metabolism of tumor cells
- FDG is taken up by cell, but not metabolized, and it is retained intracellularly
- Hodgkin lymphoma and aggressive non-Hodgkin lymphomas are generally FDG avid
  - Suggested that FDG PET is more sensitive for B-cell rather than T-cell lymphoma
  - Indolent non-Hodgkin lymphomas show variable FDG avidity

- Advantageous over CT scan in assessing stage and detection of residual disease or early tumor relapse
- Assessment of metabolic activity of cells in mass can predict tumor viability (high standardized uptake value [SUV])
  - Nonmetabolically active pseudotumors predict nonviable tumor and may prevent splenectomy
  - Approximately 10-30% false-positive rate as determined by concomitant biopsies
    - Refining may be required for cases with higher SUV values
    - Current recommendation is to obtain histological confirmation in these lesions
  - Metabolically active necrotic masses may indicate presence of inflammatory or histiocytic reaction
    - This pattern is more significant in 1st few months after completion of therapy
- Necrotic tumor is usually not metabolically active (low SUV)
- Gallium-scintigraphy was formerly considered valuable to evaluate metabolic activity
  - This approach has been largely abandoned

MACROSCOPIC FEATURES

General Features
- Single or multiple tan-white firm nodules
  - Variable size, 3.5 cm mean diameter
  - Yellow appearance when foamy histiocytes are predominant
- Larger tumor masses usually have central necrosis

MICROSCOPIC PATHOLOGY

Histologic Features
- Nonviable tumor cells usually appear as eosinophilic cell ghosts
- Associated inflammation or sclerosis at periphery of lesion
  - Most histiocytes are oval or polygonal and display pale foamy (xanthomatous) cytoplasm
- Cholesterol clefts, multinucleated giant cells, and ill-defined granulomas can be present
  - Dystrophic calcification can be present
- Longstanding lesions (> 8 months) may be predominantly sclerotic

ANCILLARY TESTS

Immunohistochemistry
- In B-cell lymphomas, ghosts of neoplastic cells can be CD20(+)
  - Nuclear-associated antigens usually lost in cell ghosts
- Foamy histiocytes are CD68(+), CD163(+), lysozyme(+)
- Reactive T cells are often present: CD3(+)

DIFFERENTIAL DIAGNOSIS

Post-Chemotherapy Residual Viable Tumor
- Imaging studies demonstrate evidence of viability
  - Growth over time or metabolic activity
- Microscopically, there is extensive necrosis with focal areas of viable tumor

Storage Diseases
- Usually history of systemic disease
- Diffuse enlargement of spleen
- Glycolipid-laden macrophages infiltrate red pulp
  - Histiocytes are highlighted by periodic acid-Schiff (PAS) reaction

Ceroid Histiocytosis
- Histiocytes accumulate ceroid: Product of oxidation and polymerization of unsaturated lipids
- Patients often present with splenomegaly and hepatomegaly
- Primary processes are called "sea-blue" histiocyte syndrome
  - May be familial, such as in Hermansky-Pudlak syndrome
- Many causes for secondary ceroid histiocytosis
  - Lipidoses and chronic myelogenous leukemia
  - Immune thrombocytopenic purpura and sickle cell anemia
- Histiocytes are prominent in cords and display granular cytoplasm ("ceroid" histiocytes)
  - Sinuses may also have increased histiocytes
  - Histiocytes appear blue-green with Romanowsky stains, hence the name "sea-blue" histiocytes
  - Foamy histiocytes may also occur
- Occasionally, scattered ceroid histiocytes may occur in spleen as isolated feature

Splenic Inflammatory Pseudotumor
- Partially circumscribed single tumor mass
- Spindle cell proliferation admixed with lymphocytes, neutrophils, plasma cells, and histiocytes
  - Histiocytes display pink, uniform, but not vacuolated cytoplasm
- Spindle cells are myofibroblasts: S100(+), smooth muscle actin(+)

Langerhans Cell Histiocytosis
- Large histiocytes with twisted and grooved nuclei
  - Frequent necrosis and eosinophilic infiltrate
- Immunohistochemistry is very helpful
  - Langerhans cells: S100(+), langerin/CD207(+), CD1a(+)
- Xanthomatous histiocytes can be prominent in regressing lesions

Histiocytic Sarcoma
- Rarely involves spleen; most commonly affected sites are soft tissues, skin, and lymph nodes
- Causes mass effect and shows frequent necrosis
- Neoplastic cells are histiocytes that show nuclear atypia and frequent mitoses
- Histiocytic sarcoma is often clinically aggressive

POST-CHEMOTHERAPY HISTIOCYTE-RICH PSEUDOTUMOR OF SPLEEN

Differential Diagnosis of Post-Chemotherapy Histiocyte-rich Pseudotumor of Spleen

	Post-Chemotherapy Histiocyte-rich Pseudotumor	Storage Diseases	Splenic Inflammatory Pseudotumor	Langerhans Cell Histiocytosis	Post-Chemotherapy Residual Viable Tumor
Clinical features	History of splenic malignancy treated with chemotherapy	Systemic disease	Recently discovered mass	Single or multiple masses	History of splenic malignancy and chemotherapy
Imaging studies	Mass with central necrosis, inactive metabolically	Enlargement of spleen, liver, or lymph nodes	Uniform mass; low metabolic activity	Uniform mass; low metabolic activity	Necrotic mass; metabolically active
Macroscopic features	Single or multiple masses	Diffuse splenic enlargement	Single mass	Diffusely enlarged or single mass	Single or multiple masses
Microscopic features	Tumor necrosis and xanthomatous histiocytes	Red pulp expansion by benign histiocytes with foamy cytoplasm	Mixture of inflammatory cells and histiocytes	Large histiocytes with grooved or twisted nuclei	Tumor necrosis and viable tumor
Ancillary studies	Histiocytes are CD68(+), lysozyme(+)	CD68(+), lysozyme(+), PAS with diastase(+)	Spindle cells (+) for smooth muscle actin; occasionally EBV(+)	S100(+), CD1a(+), langerin(+)	Immunohistochemical markers positive in viable tumor
	Immunohistochemical markers for lymphoma may be positive in necrotic tumor cell ghosts				Positive for markers of previously diagnosed malignancy

Follicular Dendritic Cell (FDC) Sarcoma
- Neoplastic proliferation of bland or atypical, spindle or epithelioid FDCs
  - Sheets of tumor cells or admixed with inflammatory cells
- Immunohistochemistry is helpful
  - FDCs: CD21(+), CD23(+), CD35(+), CNA.42(+), clusterin(+), EGFR(+)
- FDC sarcoma commonly recurs and can metastasize
  - Intraabdominal FDC sarcoma can be particularly aggressive

Metastatic Carcinoma
- Patients may have underlying malignancy, such as breast or prostate carcinoma
- Persistent mass may raise suspicion of 2nd neoplasm
- Microscopic features may include epithelial cells with clear cytoplasm
  - Foamy cytoplasm can be seen in some cases of prostatic carcinoma
    - Immunohistochemistry shows reactivity for cytokeratin and prostate-specific antigen
  - Clear cytoplasm is characteristic of most renal cell carcinomas; atypia may be noted
    - Immunohistochemistry shows reactivity for cytokeratin, epithelial membrane antigen, or WT1

DIAGNOSTIC CHECKLIST

Clinically Relevant Pathologic Features
- Often splenic histiocyte-rich pseudotumor is detected by imaging studies
  - Performed for staging after chemotherapy

Pathologic Interpretation Pearls
- Nonviable tumor cells usually appear as eosinophilic cell ghosts
  - Can retain cytoplasmic antigens detectable by immunohistochemistry
- Lipid-laden (foamy) histiocytes: CD68(+), CD163(+), lysozyme(+), etc.

SELECTED REFERENCES
1. Ehrlich Y et al: Long-term follow-up of Cisplatin combination chemotherapy in patients with disseminated nonseminomatous germ cell tumors: is a postchemotherapy retroperitoneal lymph node dissection needed after complete remission? J Clin Oncol. 28(4):531-6, 2010
2. Nakamura L et al: Current management of wilms' tumor. Curr Urol Rep. 11(1):58-65, 2010
3. van Eijk M et al: Differential expression of the EGF-TM7 family members CD97 and EMR2 in lipid-laden macrophages in atherosclerosis, multiple sclerosis and Gaucher disease. Immunol Lett. 129(2):64-71, 2010
4. Chandra P et al: Postchemotherapy histiocyte-rich pseudotumor involving the spleen. Am J Clin Pathol. 132(3):342-8, 2009
5. Zinzani PL et al: Histological verification of positive positron emission tomography findings in the follow-up of patients with mediastinal lymphoma. Haematologica. 92(6):771-7, 2007
6. Ford CD et al: False-positive restaging PET scans involving the spleen in two patients with aggressive non-Hodgkin lymphoma. Clin Nucl Med. 31(7):391-3, 2006
7. Ashfaq R et al: Xanthomatous pseudotumor of the small intestine following treatment for Burkitt's lymphoma. Arch Pathol Lab Med. 116(3):299-301, 1992
8. Durkin W et al: Benign mass lesions after therapy for Hodgkin's disease. Arch Intern Med. 139(3):333-6, 1979

POST-CHEMOTHERAPY HISTIOCYTE-RICH PSEUDOTUMOR OF SPLEEN

Microscopic Features

(Left) Post-chemotherapy histiocyte-rich pseudotumor of spleen. There is a fibrous scar ⇨ that partially surrounds the lesion. *(Right)* Post-chemotherapy histiocyte-rich pseudotumor of spleen. Pink necrosis ⇨ and cholesterol crystals ⇨, which appear as negative images of needles, are noted.

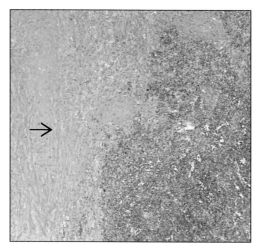
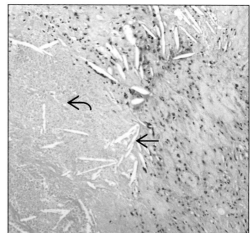

(Left) Post-chemotherapy histiocyte-rich pseudotumor of spleen. There are confluent histiocytes with abundant vacuolated cytoplasm ⇨, lymphocytes ⇨, and sclerosis. *(Right)* Post-chemotherapy histiocyte-rich pseudotumor of spleen. There are confluent histiocytes with abundant vacuolated cytoplasm ⇨ and central, bland nuclei ⇨.

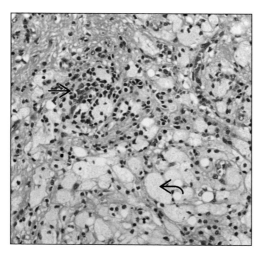
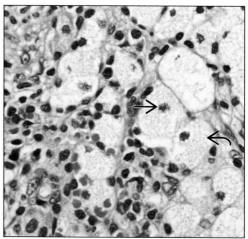

(Left) Post-chemotherapy histiocyte-rich pseudotumor of spleen. More cellular areas can display a spindle or epithelioid appearance of histiocytes with only focal cytoplasmic vacuolation ⇨. *(Right)* Post-chemotherapy histiocyte-rich pseudotumor of spleen. There is pink granular necrotic material ⇨ admixed with dystrophic calcification that appears as basophilic granules ⇨.

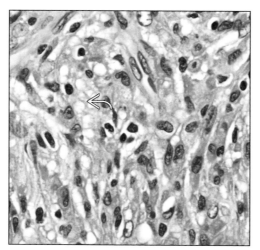
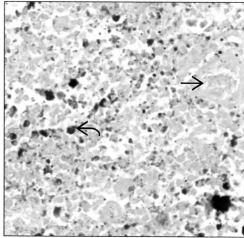

Differential Diagnosis

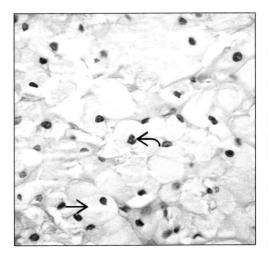
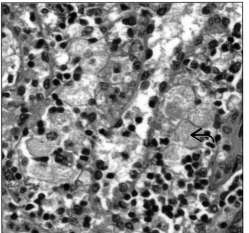

(Left) Histiocytes in storage disease disorders, such as in Tangier disease, show ample clear cytoplasm ➡ with central and small bland nuclei ➡. *(Right)* Ceroid histiocytosis. Red pulp cords contain numerous histiocytes with granular (ceroid) cytoplasm ➡. In this case, the accumulation of ceroid was likely attributable to phagocytosis of structurally abnormal platelets in a child with splenomegaly and mutation of the GATA-1 gene.

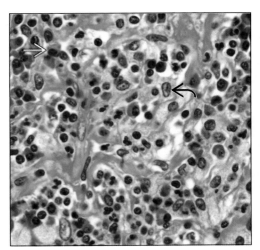
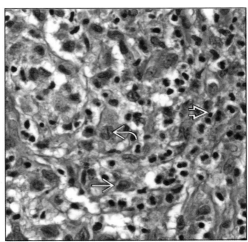

(Left) Inflammatory pseudotumor of the spleen. There are scattered histiocytes ➡ that are admixed with lymphocytes, plasma cells ➡, and vascular proliferation. *(Right)* Langerhans cell histiocytosis. Histiocytes are large with finely granular cytoplasm ➡ and central twisted ➡ or grooved ➡ nuclei. Scattered or clustered eosinophils ➡ are usually prominent.

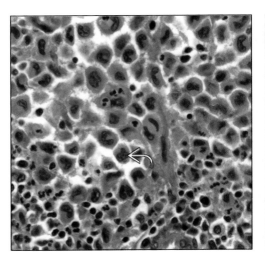
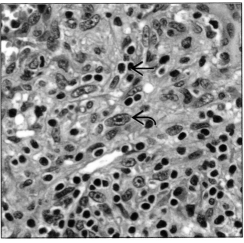

(Left) Histiocytic sarcoma. Histiocytes are large with irregular, atypical nuclei ➡. Cytoplasm is dense, uniform, and rarely vacuolated. *(Right)* Follicular dendritic cell sarcoma. Histiocytes are arranged in variable patterns and usually show mild atypia ➡. In this case, histiocytes are admixed with numerous lymphocytes ➡.

INFLAMMATORY PSEUDOTUMOR-LIKE FOLLICULAR DENDRITIC CELL TUMOR

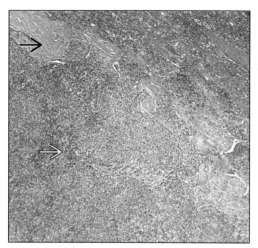

Inflammatory pseudotumor-like follicular dendritic cell tumor displays cellular ➡ and sclerotic ➡ areas. (Courtesy M. Vasef, MD.)

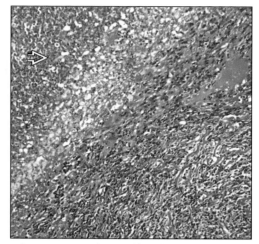

Inflammatory pseudotumor-like follicular dendritic cell tumor shows extensive necrosis ➡, which is a feature that may mislead to a diagnosis of malignancy when detected by imaging studies.

TERMINOLOGY

Abbreviations
- Inflammatory pseudotumor-like follicular dendritic cell tumor (IPT-FDCT)

Synonyms
- Terms inflammatory pseudotumor and inflammatory myofibroblastic tumor have been used as synonyms in the literature
  - This is confusing and may be incorrect
  - In this chapter these entities are distinguished

Definitions
- IPT-FDCT is considered a variant of follicular dendritic cell sarcoma
- Classification is controversial since several entities were previously lumped into category of splenic IPT
  - IPT-FDCT
    - True neoplasm of low malignant potential
    - Frequent association with Epstein-Barr virus (EBV)
    - Tends to involve spleen &/or liver
    - May overlap with EBV(+) cases without follicular dendritic cell markers
  - ALK(+) inflammatory myofibroblastic tumor (IMT)
    - Most often involves soft tissues of children and young adults
    - ~ 50% of tumors have rearrangements at 2p23 involving anaplastic lymphoma kinase (ALK)
  - Splenic inflammatory pseudotumor (IPT)
    - Reactive process composed of admixed bland spindle cells and inflammatory cells
    - Probably results from multiple etiologies, including infections and repair
    - Benign lesions that do not recur after surgical excision

ETIOLOGY/PATHOGENESIS

Infectious Agents
- Etiology is unknown
- Strong association with Epstein-Barr virus
  - Epstein-Barr virus is monoclonal when assessed by EBV DNA terminal repeat regions

Cell of Origin
- Spindled cells express 1 or more follicular dendritic cell markers
- Spindled cells also can express focally smooth muscle actin or S100 protein
- Cell of origin may be mesenchymal cell with differentiation along fibroblastic, myofibroblastic, or follicular dendritic cell lineages

CLINICAL ISSUES

Epidemiology
- Incidence
  - Uncommon; ~ 1% of splenic tumors
  - Rare when compared with IPT at other sites of body
- Age
  - Median: 44 years (range: 19-87 years)
    - Rare in children
- Gender
  - Female predominance

Site
- Appears in spleen as single lesion

Presentation
- Affected patients are immunocompetent
- Fever and weight loss in approximately 1/2 of patients
- Epigastric or left flank pain in subset of patients
  - Splenomegaly may be noted in some cases
- Can be incidental finding in asymptomatic patients

INFLAMMATORY PSEUDOTUMOR-LIKE FOLLICULAR DENDRITIC CELL TUMOR

Key Facts

Terminology
- Inflammatory pseudotumor-like follicular dendritic cell tumor (IPT-FDCT)
- Considered variant of follicular dendritic cell sarcoma
- Classification is controversial

Clinical Issues
- Marked female predominance
- Good prognosis; no deaths attributable to IPT-FDCT of spleen
- IPT-FDCT affecting liver can be recurrent and metastatic in rare cases

Microscopic Pathology
- Well-demarcated single mass with occasional incomplete fibrous capsule

- Loosely aggregated or dispersed oval or spindle cells admixed with abundant inflammatory cells

Ancillary Tests
- Usual reactivity with follicular dendritic cell markers
- Epstein-Barr virus encoded RNA (EBER)(+) in spindle cells in 40% of cases
- Cases that are EBV(+) show that viral genome is monoclonal

Top Differential Diagnoses
- Splenic inflammatory pseudotumor
- Follicular dendritic cell sarcoma
- Inflammatory myofibroblastic tumor
- Sclerosing angiomatoid nodular transformation of red pulp

- o Lesion in spleen detected by radiologic imaging performed for other diseases
- o Imaging studies can demonstrate significant tumor growth in patients followed with less than 1 year intervals

Laboratory Tests
- Usually unremarkable when not associated with other disease

Natural History
- Cases of splenic IPT-FDCT appear to be closely related to liver IPT-FDCT
  - o Histologically similar
  - o Share association with EBV
- More clinical information and follow-up are available for liver IPT-FDCT
  - o Recurrences and metastases have been reported
  - o Rare transformation of IPT-FDCT into overt follicular dendritic cell sarcoma

Treatment
- Patients usually are diagnosed/treated with splenectomy
  - o Due to rarity and nonspecific CT or MR imaging, these tumors are not diagnosed preoperatively
- Symptoms and any laboratory abnormalities disappear after tumor resection

Prognosis
- Good; no deaths attributable to IPT-FDCT of spleen

IMAGE FINDINGS

CT Findings
- Discrete, single splenic mass and occasional splenomegaly
- Lymphadenopathy is unusual

MACROSCOPIC FEATURES

General Features
- Spleen weight: Ranges from 140-1,030 g
- Well-circumscribed single mass
  - o Cut surface is tan, gray, and firm; bulges in cross section
    - May have focal necrosis
  - o Size: Ranges from 3-22 cm

MICROSCOPIC PATHOLOGY

Histologic Features
- Well-demarcated tumor with occasional incomplete fibrous capsule
- Loosely aggregated or dispersed oval or spindle cells admixed with abundant inflammatory cells
  - o Spindled cells with moderate amount of pale to faintly eosinophilic cytoplasm
    - Oval vesicular nuclei with minimal atypia and distinct small nucleoli
  - o Occasional small fascicles or focal storiform pattern
  - o Rare mitotic figures
  - o Occasional large cells with abundant cytoplasm and pleomorphic nuclei
- Mixed inflammatory infiltrate of plasma cells, lymphocytes, and histiocytes
  - o Lymphocytes are usually small admixed with occasional immunoblasts
  - o Mature plasma cells with occasional Russell bodies
- Other microscopic features
  - o Focal necrosis with neutrophilic infiltrate
  - o Histiocytes &/or eosinophils can be numerous

ANCILLARY TESTS

Immunohistochemistry
- Spindled cells
  - o Usually focal and weak reactivity with 1 or more follicular dendritic cell markers

Microscopic Features: Lymph Node and Bone Marrow

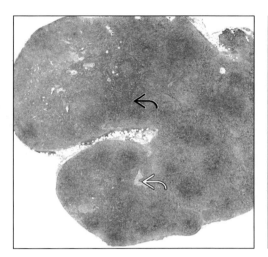

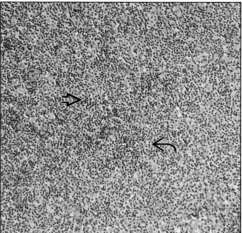

(Left) Hilar lymph node removed together with spleen in a case of SMZL shows a vague nodularity with residual lymphoid follicles ➡ and dilated sinuses ➡. (Right) Splenic hilar lymph node infiltrated by SMZL. An ill-circumscribed germinal center ➡ is almost completely replaced, and it appears as a mixture of small residual lymphocytes and intermediate-sized cells with clear cytoplasm ➡.

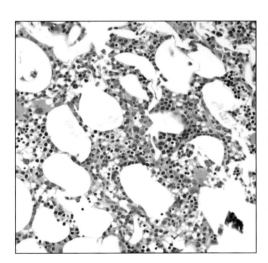

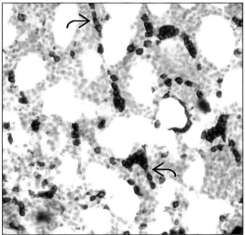

(Left) Bone marrow biopsy infiltrated by SMZL shows an apparent normocellularity with trilineage hematopoiesis and no apparent lymphoid infiltration. (Right) CD20 immunostain highlights sinusoidal pattern ➡ of SMZL in the bone marrow, characterized as a linear pattern of infiltration. This pattern can be seen in about 30% of cases of SMZL, but it is also seen in other lymphomas.

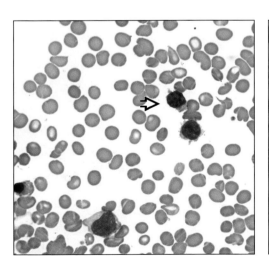

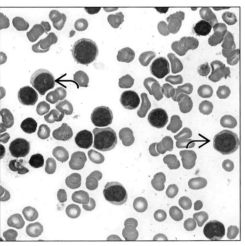

(Left) Wright-Giemsa stain of peripheral blood smear shows 3 lymphocytes. Two lymphocytes show cytoplasmic projections, one of which shows the characteristic "polar" villi ➡. Cytoplasmic villi may disappear if blood specimen has been sitting for more than a few hours. (Right) Wright-Giemsa stain of bone marrow smear shows numerous lymphocytes of SMZL. This is a case of transformation of SMZL and shows nucleolated cells ➡.

SPLENIC MARGINAL ZONE LYMPHOMA

Differential Diagnosis: SMZH and CLL

(Left) Splenic marginal zone hyperplasia. White pulp ⊳ and red pulp ⇒ are displayed. *(Right)* Splenic marginal zone hyperplasia at the interface between white pulp and red pulp. Follicular center ⊳, mantle zone ⇒, marginal zone ⇒, and red pulp ⇒ are identified. There is a sharp demarcation between marginal zone and red pulp.

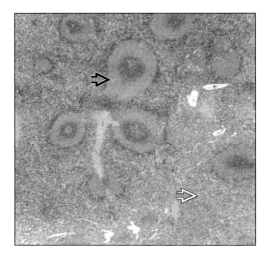
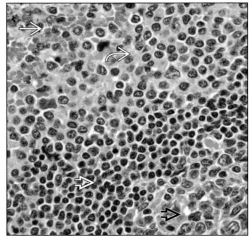

(Left) Red pulp in a case of splenic marginal zone hyperplasia. Sinuses contain blood ⊳, and splenic cord contains scattered small lymphocytes ⇒. *(Right)* Positive Bcl-6 immunostain shows a preserved germinal center (GC) ⇒ in splenic marginal zone hyperplasia. No Bcl-6 positive cells are noted outside GC, in the marginal zone ⇒, or in the red pulp ⊳ (unlike follicular lymphoma). An eccentric arteriole ⇒ is noted at the marginal zone.

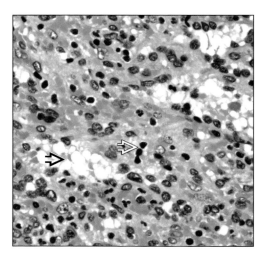
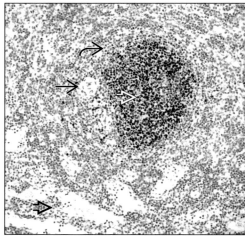

(Left) CLL/SLL replacing a preexisting germinal center. Lymphocytes are uniform throughout. Red pulp is seen at the periphery ⊳. *(Right)* CLL/SLL in a preexisting germinal center. Neoplastic lymphocytes are uniform, round, and show distinct chromocenters ⇒.

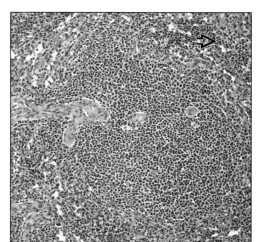
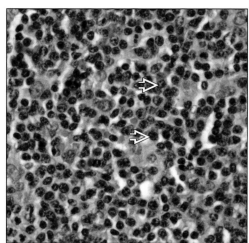

SPLENIC MARGINAL ZONE LYMPHOMA

Differential Diagnosis: MCL, HCL, and FL

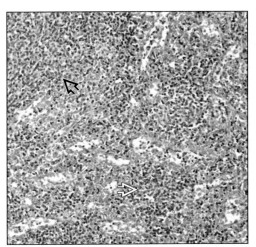

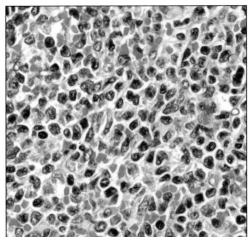

(Left) Mantle cell lymphoma replacing the white pulp ⊟ and infiltrating the red pulp ⊟. There is no evidence of a "biphasic" pattern unlike SMZL. Small lymphocytic aggregates can be seen in the red pulp. *(Right)* Cellular features of mantle cell lymphoma. Lymphocytes are intermediate in size with irregular nuclear contours (centrocyte-like). Diagnosis was confirmed by cyclin-D1 immunohistochemistry.

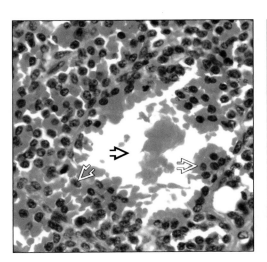

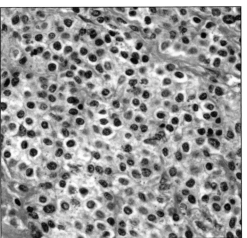

(Left) Hematoxylin and eosin shows a "blood lake" ⊟ in a case of hairy cell leukemia. A large space containing red cells is surrounded by HCL cells ⊟ and not by endothelial cells and may occur in normal or in dilated sinuses. *(Right)* Hematoxylin and eosin shows hairy cell leukemia with a sheet-like distribution of cells displaying central oval to indented hyperchromatic nuclei surrounded by abundant clear cytoplasm ("fried egg" appearance). Cell membranes can be seen.

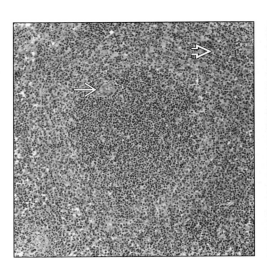

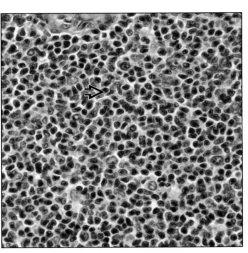

(Left) Hematoxylin and eosin shows follicular lymphoma on a preexisting germinal center identified as such by the presence of eccentric arteriole ⊟. Red pulp is at the periphery ⊟. *(Right)* Follicular lymphoma grade I in a preexisting germinal center. More than 95% of cells are small, and many show irregular nuclear outlines (centrocytes or cleaved cells) ⊟. Scattered round hyperchromatic lymphocytes represent reactive T cells.

HAIRY CELL LEUKEMIA

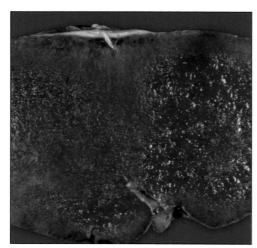

Hairy cell leukemia (HCL). Gross photograph shows a diffuse effacement of the splenic surface, without white pulp nodularity.

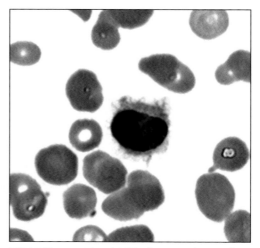

Wright-Giemsa stain of HCL shows an intermediate-sized lymphocyte with oval nucleus and abundant cytoplasm. The depicted cytoplasmic projections are best appreciated in peripheral blood smears.

TERMINOLOGY

Abbreviations
- Hairy cell leukemia (HCL)

Synonyms
- Leukemic reticuloendotheliosis (no longer used)

Definitions
- B-cell neoplasm composed of small lymphocytes with oval nuclei and abundant cytoplasm with "hairy" projections
- Primarily involves blood, bone marrow, and spleen

ETIOLOGY/PATHOGENESIS

Etiology
- Unknown; risk associated with genetic features and exposure to agricultural pesticides

Cell of Origin
- Mature memory B cell arising at post-germinal center cell stage of maturation

Pathogenesis
- Mitogen activated protein kinases (MAPKs) regulate tumor growth
- Hairy cells overexpress an isoform of β-actin that support "hairy" cytoplasmic projections
- TNF-α has anti-apoptotic effect
- Leukemic cells overexpress integrins that bind to splenic red pulp and sinusoids

CLINICAL ISSUES

Epidemiology
- Incidence
  - HCL is rare (~ 2% of lymphoid leukemias)
  - Middle-aged or elderly adults (median age: 52 years)
    - Uncommon in young adults and exceptionally rare in children
  - M:F = 5:1

Presentation
- Weakness and fatigue
- Left abdominal pain due to splenomegaly
- Fever secondary to neutropenia and recurrent opportunistic infections
  - More common in advanced disease
- Bleeding secondary to thrombocytopenia
- Massive splenomegaly used to be common; currently less frequent
  - Smaller spleen size is related to earlier detection of disease
- Hepatomegaly
- Lymph node involvement is uncommon and often minimal
  - More common 20-30 years ago (due to late disease detection)

Laboratory Tests
- Pancytopenia is typical
  - Monocytopenia is characteristic of HCL
  - Circulating hairy cells are identified; usually in small numbers
- Hairy cells are small to intermediate in size, with moderately abundant pale cytoplasm
  - Cytoplasmic projections or "hairs" are typically circumferential
  - Central oval to bean-shaped nucleus with uniform chromatin; no nucleolus
  - ± cytoplasmic vacuoles or inclusions
    - Represent ribosome-lamellar complexes
- Bone marrow
  - HCL involves bone marrow in interstitial or diffuse pattern
    - Reticulin fibrosis common
  - Aspiration often "dry tap" due to reticulin fibrosis

HAIRY CELL LEUKEMIA

Key Facts

Terminology
- Hairy cell leukemia (HCL)

Clinical Issues
- Weakness, fatigue, and left abdominal pain
- Pancytopenia with monocytopenia; few HCL cells in blood smear
- HCL is now often detected at early stage
  - Splenomegaly not massive
  - Lymphadenopathy uncommon
- Excellent prognosis

Microscopic Pathology
- Blood and bone marrow smears
  - Central nuclei without nucleoli
  - Pale blue cytoplasm with circumferential "hairs"
- Spleen
  - Extensive and diffuse red pulp involvement with atrophic or effaced white pulp
  - Central nuclei and pale cytoplasm ("fried egg")

Ancillary Tests
- Characteristic immunophenotype by flow cytometry
  - Bright surface Ig, pan-B, CD11c, and CD22
  - CD25(+), CD103(+), CD123(+), CD5(-), CD10(-)
- Immunohistochemistry: DBA.44/CD76(+), annexin-A1(+), T-bet(+)

Top Differential Diagnoses
- Hairy cell leukemia-variant
- Splenic marginal zone lymphoma/splenic lymphoma with villous lymphocytes

Treatment
- Current therapy: Cladribine or pentostatin (purine analogs) administered as single agents
  - > 80% of patients achieve complete remission
  - Relapse rate at 10 years: ~ 40%
- Rituximab may be useful for patients with refractory or recurrent disease
  - Anti-CD22 and anti-CD25 monoclonal antibodies are experimental
- Splenectomy or IFN-α was used in the past; relapse occurred in up to 1/3 of patients

Prognosis
- Excellent prognosis with overall survival rate ~ 90% at 10 years; median survival > 12 years
- High risk of 2nd malignant neoplasm
  - Up to 30% of long-term survivors
  - Hodgkin lymphoma, non-Hodgkin lymphoma
  - Many different types of solid tumors

MACROSCOPIC FEATURES

General Features
- Enlarged spleen with grossly dark red, homogeneous, and firm surface
  - White pulp nodules absent or inconspicuous
  - Necrosis is unusual (unless secondary infarct)

MICROSCOPIC PATHOLOGY

Histologic Features
- Diffuse effacement of red pulp (cords and sinuses)
- Red cell "lakes" and "pseudosinuses"; range from microscopic to grossly visible
  - Consequence of disruption of normal blood flow to red pulp
- White pulp is absent or atrophic
- Cytologic features
  - Hairy cells have oval to bean-shaped nuclei and abundant clear cytoplasm
  - Nonoverlapping, widely spaced nuclei and pale cytoplasm ("fried egg" appearance)
  - Mitotic figures are rare or absent
- Rare cases of blastic HCL are reported
  - Cells are intermediate to large in size with cytologic atypia and numerous mitotic figures present
  - Necrosis can be present
  - Typical immunophenotype (see below)
  - Some patients have history of typical HCL

Lymph Nodes
- HCL typically involves paracortical regions of lymph node
  - Follicles spared; sinuses usually patent

Predominant Pattern/Injury Type
- Lymphoid, diffuse

Predominant Cell/Compartment Type
- Hematopoietic, lymphoid

ANCILLARY TESTS

Cytology
- Tartrate-resistant acid phosphatase (TRAP) cytochemistry shows cytoplasmic granules in HCL cells
  - Acid phosphatase often appears brighter after tartrate in HCL cells
  - Technique is challenging and therefore not performed in some laboratories

Immunohistochemistry
- Positive for pan-B-cell antigens; negative for pan-T-cell antigens
- DBA.44/CD76(+), CD25(+), CD123(+), T-bet(+)
- Annexin-A1 is specific for HCL among B-cell lymphoid neoplasms
  - Annexin-A1 is positive in granulocytes and T cells; not very useful in bone marrow
- Bcl-2(+), CD45/LCA(+); CD10(-), Bcl-6(-)
- Cyclin-D1 weakly positive in subset of neoplasms

HAIRY CELL LEUKEMIA

- Associated T-lymphocytes are cytotoxic: CD3(+), CD8(+), CD57(+)

Flow Cytometry
- Immunophenotype of HCL is characteristic
- Bright surface Ig light chain (λ > κ), CD19, CD20 and bright expression of CD11c and CD22
- CD25(+), CD103(+), CD123(+), CD200/OX2(+), and FMC7(+)
- HCL can express surface IgM, IgD, IgG, or all at once
- Negative for CD5, CD10, and CD23
  - Exceptional cases reported positive for CD5 or CD10

Cytogenetics
- No recurrent structural or numerical cytogenetic abnormalities

Molecular Genetics
- Monoclonal *Ig* gene rearrangements
- Most cases show somatic hypermutation in the *IgH* variable (V) region genes
  - Consistent with post-germinal center cell stage of maturation
  - Unmutated *IgH* V genes correlate with aggressive course
- Gene expression profiling shows up-regulation of cytokines and adhesion molecules
- Array comparative genomic hybridization: HCL has stable genome
- Associated T-lymphocytes can show monoclonal or oligoclonal T-cell receptor gene rearrangements

Electron Microscopy
- Ribosome-lamellar bodies are characteristic, but not specific

DIFFERENTIAL DIAGNOSIS

Hairy Cell Leukemia Variant (HCL-v)
- Uncommon frequency compared with HCL
- Diffuse splenic red pulp involvement similar to HCL
- Peripheral blood shows lymphocytosis (often high WBC) and normal monocyte count
  - By contrast, in HCL pancytopenia with monocytopenia is common
- HCL-v cells have different cytologic features compared with HCL
  - Nuclei have distinct (but not large) nucleoli
  - Cytoplasm is clear to basophilic and often has fewer cytoplasmic projections ("hairs")
- TRAP cytochemistry is typically negative (or weak [+])
- Immunophenotype: Bright sIg(+), CD11c(+), DBA.44/CD76(+), CD103(+/-)
  - Annexin-A1(-), CD25(-); CD123(-)
- Currently considered provisional entity in 2008 WHO classification

Splenic Diffuse Red Pulp Small B-cell Lymphoma (SDRP SBCL)
- Predominant red pulp involvement with effacement of white pulp, similar to HCL
- Peripheral blood may show villous lymphocytes

- Bone marrow involvement commonly has sinusoidal pattern
- Immunophenotype: IgM(+), IgD(-), CD5(-), CD11c(+), CD25(-), CD103(-/+), CD123(-)
- Relationship of this entity to HCL-v is unclear since both frequently overlap
- Currently considered provisional entity in 2008 WHO classification

Chronic Lymphocytic Leukemia/Small Lymphocytic Lymphoma (CLL/SLL)
- Expansion of white pulp forming uniform nodules without marginal zone
  - Proliferation centers can be observed with extensive involvement
- Red pulp also commonly involved
- Lymphocytes are round to oval with clumped chromatin and scant cytoplasm
- Immunophenotype is distinctive
  - Dim surface Ig light chain (κ > λ), IgD(+/-), CD19, CD20(dim)
  - CD5(+), CD23(+), CD11c(+/-), CD22(-), CD25(-), CD103(-)
  - Annexin-A1(-), T-bet(+)
- Del(13q14), del(11q23), trisomy 12, del(17p) common

Splenic Marginal Zone Lymphoma/Splenic Lymphoma with Villous Lymphocytes (SMZL/SLVL)
- Marked expansion of white pulp with "biphasic" pattern
  - Centers composed of small lymphocytes (darker) surrounded by larger marginal zone cells with pale cytoplasm
- Secondary involvement of red pulp by nodules
- TRAP cytochemistry often weakly positive
- Immunophenotype: Bright sIg(+), pan-B-cell antigens(+)
  - Dim CD5(-/+), dim CD23(-/+), CD10(-)
- Conventional cytogenetics: Del(7q) in ~ 40-50%

Mantle Cell Lymphoma (MCL)
- Expansion of white pulp forming large nodules with frequent coalescence of nodules
  - Mantle zone pattern rare
- Red pulp involvement as lymphoid aggregates
- Lymphocytes are intermediate in size with round to irregular nuclear contours
  - Large lymphoid cells rare or absent (unless blastoid variant)
- Immunophenotype: sIg(+), pan-B-cell antigens(+), CD5(+), CD10(-), CD23(-)
  - Cyclin-D1 is strongly positive by immunohistochemistry (HCL is dim)
  - ~ 10% of MCL can be dim CD23(+); < 5% of MCL can be CD5(-)
- Conventional cytogenetics/FISH: t(11;14) (q13;q32)/*IgH-CCND1*

Systemic Mastocytosis (SM)
- Mast cells with pale cytoplasm can mimic HCL or MZL cells

HAIRY CELL LEUKEMIA

Differential Diagnosis of Small Lymphocytic Infiltrates in Spleen

	HCL	HCL-v	SDRP SBCL	CLL/SLL	SMZL/SLVL	MCL
Histopathologic Features						
Pattern	Diffuse red pulp with obliteration of white pulp	Diffuse red pulp with obliteration of white pulp	Diffuse red pulp with obliteration of white pulp	Nodular white pulp and secondary red pulp involvement	Nodular white pulp; biphasic pattern; secondary red pulp involvement	Nodular white pulp and secondary red pulp involvement
Cytologic features in tissue sections	Small round to oval hyperchromatic lymphocytes with clear cytoplasm and thick membranes	Small to intermediate size lymphocytes with nucleoli and clear cytoplasm	Small to intermediate size lymphocytes with nucleoli and clear to pink cytoplasm	Small round lymphocytes with small chromocenters admixed with prolymphocytes	Small lymphocytes in center of white pulp surrounded by marginal zone lymphocytes	Uniform small round to irregular lymphocytes; pink histiocytes
Cytologic features in touch imprint or blood smear	Oval or bean-shaped lymphocytes with long cytoplasmic projections	Round lymphocytes; distinct nucleolus; abundant bluish cytoplasm; small villi	Round lymphocytes with small nucleolus and occasional small villi	Small round lymphocytes with clumped chromatin and scant cytoplasm	Round to oval lymphocytes with polar cytoplasmic projections	Round to irregular lymphocytes; scant cytoplasm
Flow Cytometry Immunophenotype						
Positive (all CD19[+] and CD20[+])	CD11c, CD22, CD25, CD103, CD123, CD200, FMC7	CD11c, CD22, CD103, IgG(+/-), FMC7	CD11c, CD103 (-/+), IgG, IgD(+/-), FMC7	CD5, CD11c(-/+), CD23	CD5(-/+), CD11c, CD25, IgM	CD5, CD79b, FMC7
Negative	CD5, CD10 (up to 20% [+])	CD5, CD10, CD25, CD123	CD5, CD10, CD25, CD123	CD10, CD22, CD79b, CD103, FMC7	CD5 (10% dim [+]), CD10, CD103, CD123	CD23 (10% dim [+]), CD10
Immunohistochemistry						
DBA.44/CD76 & TRAP* combined	100%	Rare	Negative	8%	5%	5%
Annexin-A1	Positive	Rare	Negative	Negative	Negative	Negative

TRAP by immunohistochemistry is less specific than TRAP by enzyme cytochemistry.

- Aggregates often associated with eosinophils or granulomas
- Perivascular involvement is typical
- Disease can involve white pulp, red pulp, or both
- Air-dried touch preps stained for Giemsa helpful
- Immunophenotype: CD2(+/-), CD25(+/-), CD43(+), CD68(+), CD117(+), tryptase(+)
- *C-KIT* mutation (D816V) in subset of cases

Acute Myeloid Leukemia (AML)/Myeloid Sarcoma

- AML can involve red pulp (alone or preferentially)
- Myeloid sarcoma forms mass that often replaces red and white pulp
- Cytologic features helpful: Eosinophilic myelocytes, cytoplasmic granules
- Air-dried touch preps stained for myeloperoxidase (MPO) helpful
- Immunophenotype: MPO(+), CD13(+), CD33(+), CD34(+), CD117(+)

DIAGNOSTIC CHECKLIST

Pathologic Interpretation Pearls

- Pancytopenia with monocytopenia
- Relatively few HCL cells in peripheral blood smear
- Interstitial or diffuse pattern in bone marrow biopsy
- Diffuse involvement of red pulp of spleen with effacement of white pulp nodularity

o "Fried egg" appearance at low power

SELECTED REFERENCES

1. Nordgren A et al: Characterisation of hairy cell leukaemia by tiling resolution array-based comparative genome hybridisation: a series of 13 cases and review of the literature. Eur J Haematol. 84(1):17-25, 2010
2. Forconi F et al: Hairy cell leukemias with unmutated IGHV genes define the minor subset refractory to single-agent cladribine and with more aggressive behavior. Blood. 114(21):4696-702, 2009
3. Cannon T et al: Hairy cell leukemia: current concepts. Cancer Invest. 26(8):860-5, 2008
4. Hisada M et al: Second cancer incidence and cause-specific mortality among 3104 patients with hairy cell leukemia: a population-based study. J Natl Cancer Inst. 99(3):215-22, 2007
5. Tiacci E et al: Evolving concepts in the pathogenesis of hairy-cell leukaemia. Nat Rev Cancer. 6(6):437-48, 2006
6. Else M et al: Long remissions in hairy cell leukemia with purine analogs: a report of 219 patients with a median follow-up of 12.5 years. Cancer. 104(11):2442-8, 2005
7. Went PT et al: High specificity of combined TRAP and DBA.44 expression for hairy cell leukemia. Am J Surg Pathol. 29(4):474-8, 2005
8. Miranda RN et al: Immunohistochemical detection of cyclin D1 using optimized conditions is highly specific for mantle cell lymphoma and hairy cell leukemia. Mod Pathol. 13(12):1308-14, 2000

HAIRY CELL LEUKEMIA

Microscopic Features

(Left) Hairy cell leukemia (HCL). Hematoxylin and eosin shows a diffuse infiltrate of small to intermediate size lymphocytes with round to oval nuclei and moderately abundant pale cytoplasm (400x). *(Right)* Hematoxylin and eosin of HCL shows a "blood lake" containing red cells ⇨ and hairy cells ➡. The "lake" is delimited by hairy cells ⇨ and not by an endothelial lining (400x).

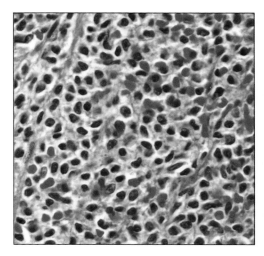
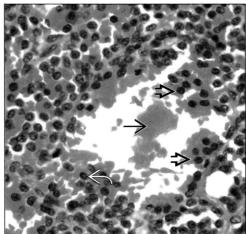

(Left) CD20 of HCL highlights distinct cell membranes ⇨ of hairy cells. Abundant clear cytoplasm also is noted ➡. *(Right)* Annexin-A1 is a granulocytic protein that also reacts with HCL cells. Annexin-A1 is difficult to interpret when leukemic cells are scant or when admixed with granulocytes, as in bone marrow specimens. Erythroid precursors ⇨ and megakaryocytes ⇨ are negative for Annexin-A1.

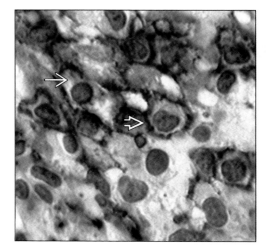
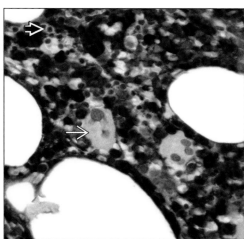

(Left) Cyclin-D1 reactivity in HCL shows that only a fraction of hairy cells are positive ⇨, usually with weak intensity. *(Right)* Tartrate-resistant acid phosphatase (TRAP) cytochemistry of HCL shows typical reactivity pattern characterized by abundant small cytoplasmic granules (red) that almost obscure the nucleus (counterstain with hematoxylin).

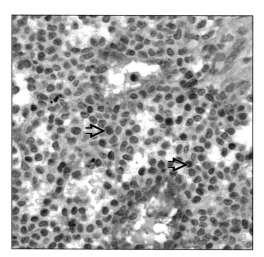
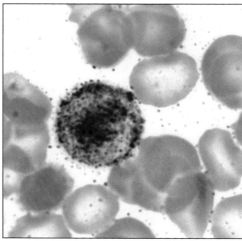

HAIRY CELL LEUKEMIA

Differential Diagnosis: HCL-v and SDRP SBCL

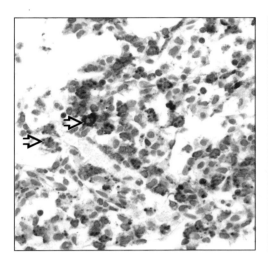

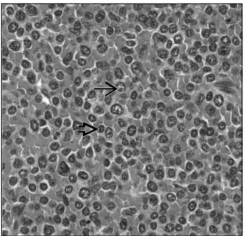

(Left) DBA.44/CD76 in a case of HCL shows granular reactivity ⮞ in most tumor cells. DBA.44/CD76 is also sometimes positive in other lymphoid neoplasms, including HCL-v. *(Right)* Hairy cell leukemia variant (HCL-v) diffusely infiltrates red pulp and sinuses, similar to HCL. Neoplastic cells may display a moderate amount of cytoplasm and nuclei may appear vesicular ➔ with distinctive nucleoli ⮞.

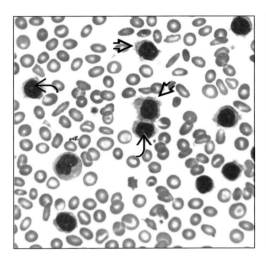

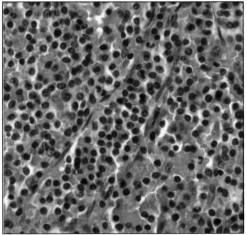

(Left) Wright-Giemsa stain in a case of HCL-v shows characteristic, intermediately sized lymphocytes with moderately abundant light basophilic cytoplasm with focal membrane projections ⮞ and oval nuclei with dispersed chromatin. A distinct but not prominent nucleolus is noted ➔. *(Right)* Splenic diffuse red pulp small B-cell lymphoma (SDRP SBCL). There is diffuse infiltration of spleen by intermediately sized lymphocytes, with distinct cytoplasm and round nuclei without nucleoli.

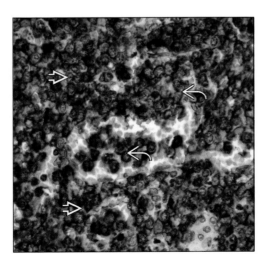

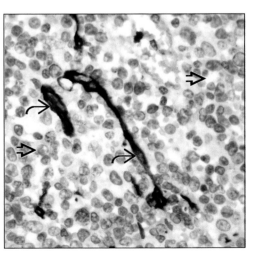

(Left) SDRP SBCL. CD20 immunostain shows diffuse reactivity of neoplastic cells with expansion of cords ⮞. Sinuses also contain neoplastic B cells ⮭. *(Right)* SDRP SBCL. CD34 immunostain displays obliteration of sinuses ➔ secondary to marked expansion of splenic cords by neoplastic cells ⮞. (Courtesy J. Cok, MD.)

HAIRY CELL LEUKEMIA

Differential Diagnosis: CLL and SMZL/SLVL

(Left) Chronic lymphocytic leukemia/small lymphocytic lymphoma (CLL/SLL). Tumor is distributed mainly in the white pulp ⊡ with secondary involvement of red pulp ⊡. From this low magnification it is apparent that the tumor cell population is uniform. *(Right)* CLL/SLL in white pulp of spleen. The tumor cells are small, round to oval, hyperchromatic lymphocytes with clumped chromatin and occasionally distinct chromocenters ➡. Proliferation centers are unusual in the spleen.

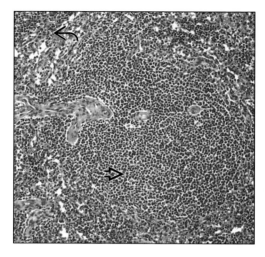
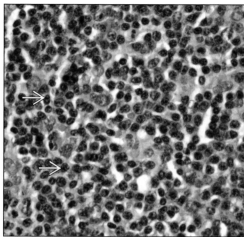

(Left) CLL/SLL involving the splenic red pulp can occasionally disrupt the stromal framework and form "blood lakes" characterized by red blood cell accumulation ⊡ amidst sheets of neoplastic cells ➡, similar to what occurs in HCL. *(Right)* CLL/SLL cells usually show scant cytoplasm with round to oval nuclei and clumped chromatin ⊡. Sometimes lymphocytes show moderately abundant basophilic cytoplasm ⊡ and irregular nuclei ⊡. No cytoplasmic projections are noted.

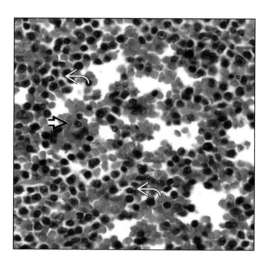
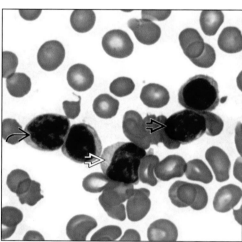

(Left) Splenic marginal zone lymphoma (SMZL) shows predominant white pulp involvement with a biphasic pattern characterized by a darker center ⊡ with many small lymphocytes, surrounded by a paler marginal zone ⊡. Tumor secondarily involves the red pulp ⊡. *(Right)* SMZL/ splenic lymphoma with villous lymphocytes (SLVL) in blood smear shows a lymphocyte with round to oval nuclei with polar cytoplasmic projections ⊡, a feature seen in approximately 50% of cases of SMZL/SLVL.

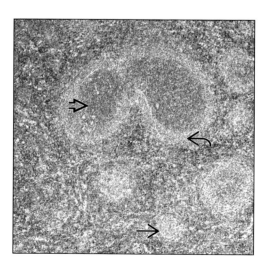
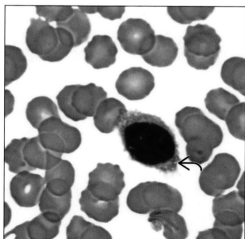

HAIRY CELL LEUKEMIA

Differential Diagnosis: MCL, SM and AML

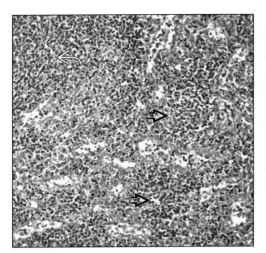
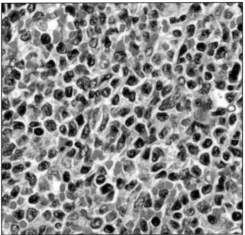

(Left) Mantle cell lymphoma (MCL) involving predominantly white pulp ➤ with secondary aggregates ➤ in red pulp cords is represented in this field. *(Right)* MCL infiltrate is characterized by a homogeneous population of small to intermediate size lymphocytes with clumped chromatin and irregular nuclear contours.

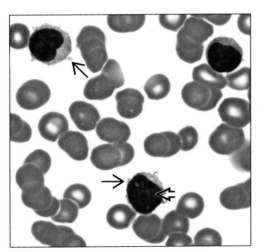
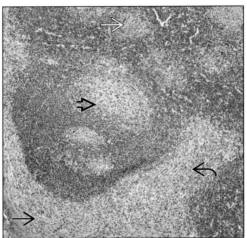

(Left) Wright-Giemsa stain of peripheral blood smear in a case of MCL shows small to intermediate size lymphocytes with round to oval nuclei, with occasional distinct eccentric nucleolus ➤. Cytoplasm may be scant with or without small cytoplasmic projections ➤. *(Right)* Hematoxylin and eosin of systemic mastocytosis (SM) shows tumor nodules in the white pulp ➤ and red pulp ➤. There is a fibrous capsule ➤ and thickened fibrous trabeculae ➤.

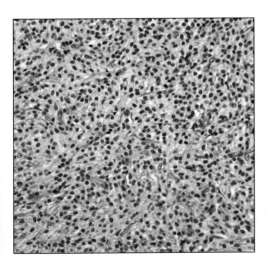
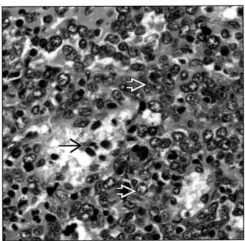

(Left) Hematoxylin and eosin shows a high magnification of SM with a diffuse pattern. The neoplastic cells show oval, hyperchromatic nuclei and clear cytoplasm that may mimic the "fried egg" appearance of hairy cell leukemia. Neoplastic cells were positive for CD117 and tryptase. *(Right)* Hematoxylin and eosin shows acute myeloid leukemia blasts within cords ➤. Cells are intermediate in size with oval nuclei and vesicular chromatin. Sinuses contain neutrophils ➤.

HAIRY CELL LEUKEMIA VARIANT

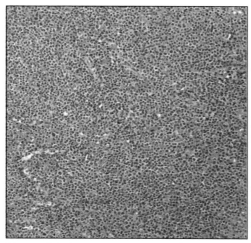

Hairy cell leukemia variant (HCL-v) shows a diffuse infiltrate throughout splenic red pulp cords and sinuses, with complete obliteration of white pulp nodules.

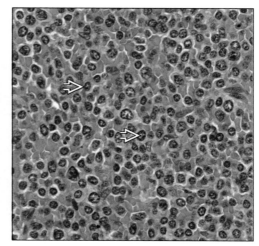

HCL-v shows a diffuse red pulp infiltrate of small to intermediately sized lymphocytes with small nucleoli ⇨ and indistinct cytoplasm. Cords and sinuses are inapparent due to lymphocyte density.

TERMINOLOGY

Abbreviations
- Hairy cell leukemia variant (HCL-v)

Synonyms
- Splenic B-cell lymphoma with villous lymphocytes
  - Also used for splenic marginal zone lymphoma (SMZL)
- Prolymphocytic variant of hairy cell leukemia (HCL); term is obsolete

Definitions
- Mature small B-cell neoplasm that primarily involves peripheral blood, bone marrow, and spleen
- Resembles classical HCL but has atypical laboratory, morphologic, or immunophenotypic features
- Provisional entity in 2008 WHO classification

ETIOLOGY/PATHOGENESIS

Environmental Exposure
- No known association with exposure to carcinogens, viral infections, or radiation

Cell of Origin
- Activated mature memory B cell

CLINICAL ISSUES

Epidemiology
- Incidence
  - HCL-v is less frequent than classical HCL, < 0.4% of all lymphoid leukemias
  - HCL-v may be more frequent in Asian countries (Japanese form of HCL-v)
- Age
  - Predominantly affects elderly people
    - Median: 71 years

- Gender
  - M:F = 1.6:1

Presentation
- Splenomegaly (85%)
- Hepatomegaly (20%)
- Lymphadenopathy (15%)

Laboratory Tests
- Leukocytosis (> 10 x 10⁹/L) in 90%, with lymphocytosis and normal monocyte count
  - Median leukocyte count: 34 x 10⁹/L
- Thrombocytopenia (< 100 x 10⁹/L) in 40%
- Anemia (Hgb < 10 g/L) in 30%

Treatment
- Partial response with purine analogues in 50% of patients
  - Pentostatin or cladribine
- Interferon-α is not effective
- Splenectomy is good palliative alternative for symptomatic anemia, thrombocytopenia, or abdominal pain
  - Usually partial response; median duration of 4 years

Prognosis
- Indolent clinical course; median survival: 9 years
- Morbidity related to splenomegaly, hypersplenism, and cytopenias
- Histologic transformation of disease in 6%
  - B-symptoms, marked lymphocytosis, or lymphadenopathy may indicate transformation
  - Poor prognosis

MACROSCOPIC FEATURES

General Features
- Splenomegaly with diffuse effacement

HAIRY CELL LEUKEMIA VARIANT

Key Facts

Terminology

- Hairy cell leukemia variant (HCL-v)
- Mature B-cell neoplasm involving peripheral blood, bone marrow, and spleen
- Resembles classical HCL but has atypical hematologic, morphologic, &/or immunophenotypic features

Clinical Issues

- Splenomegaly (85%), hepatomegaly (20%), and lymphadenopathy (15%)
- Leukocytosis in 90%, with lymphocytosis and normal monocytes
- Splenectomy is palliative for symptomatic anemia, thrombocytopenia, and abdominal pain
- Partial response with purine analogues in 50% of patients

Microscopic Pathology

- Diffuse infiltration of red pulp cords and sinusoids with effacement of white pulp
- Small cells with round to oval nuclei and nucleoli
- Histologic transformation to large cell or blastic lymphoma can occur

Ancillary Tests

- SIg([+] bright), usually IgG(+), CD11c(+), CD22(+), CD103(+/-), FMC7(+)
- CD5(-), CD10(-), CD23(-), CD25(-)

Top Differential Diagnoses

- Classical HCL
- Splenic diffuse red pulp small B-cell lymphoma
- Splenic marginal zone lymphoma/SLVL

MICROSCOPIC PATHOLOGY

Histologic Features

- Spleen
  - Diffuse infiltration of red pulp cords and sinusoids
    - Dilated sinusoids with abundant lymphocytes
    - Red blood cell lakes may be noted
  - Atrophy or complete effacement of white pulp
- Liver
  - Infiltration in portal tracts and within sinusoids
- Bone marrow
  - Interstitial and nodular lymphocytic distribution; occasional intrasinusoidal pattern

Cytologic Features

- Peripheral blood smear
  - Circulating HCL-v cells easily identified
    - Some authors require 20-30% of villous lymphocytes for diagnosis
  - Cytoplasm is abundant, bluish to basophilic
    - Cytoplasmic projections around part of cell circumference
  - Round to oval nuclei with distinct nucleoli
- Spleen and other tissue sites
  - Intermediate size lymphocytes with scant to moderately abundant indistinct cytoplasm
  - Variation in nuclear features; most commonly round with distinct, eccentric nucleoli
  - "Fried egg" or "honeycomb" appearance uncommon
- Histologic transformation is characterized by large cells or cells with blastic chromatin
  - High mitotic rate

Predominant Pattern/Injury Type

- Lymphoid, diffuse

Predominant Cell/Compartment Type

- Lymphocytosis

ANCILLARY TESTS

Immunohistochemistry

- B-cell antigens(+), DBA.44/CD76(+)
- Tartrate-resistant acid phosphatase (TRAP)
  - Immunohistochemistry can be positive
  - Cytochemistry usually negative or weakly positive
- CD123(-), annexin-A1(-), HC2(-), CD10(-), Bcl-6(-)

Flow Cytometry

- Mature B cells with strong surface immunoglobulin (Ig)
  - Usually IgG, sometimes IgM and IgD are coexpressed
- CD11c(+), CD22(+), CD79b([+] ~ 20%), CD103([+] ~ 70%), FMC7(+)
- CD5(-), CD10(-), CD23(-), CD25(-), CD27(-/+)

Cytogenetics

- No specific changes
- Some cases show complex karyotypes
  - Involving 8q24/*MYC*, 14q32/*IgH*, and del(17p)/*p53*

Molecular Genetics

- Monoclonal *IgH* and *Ig* light chain gene rearrangements
- HCL-v cells carry *MYC* transcripts; associated with resistance to interferon-α therapy
- *P53* gene deleted in subset of cases is common
  - Higher risk of histologic transformation

DIFFERENTIAL DIAGNOSIS

Hairy Cell Leukemia (HCL), Classical

- Patients present with pancytopenia and monocytopenia
- Few leukemic HCL cells in blood smear
- "Fried egg" appearance in tissue sections
- CD25(+), CD123(+), annexin-A1(+), HC2(+)
- T-bet(+), c-MAF(+)

Splenic Diffuse Red Pulp Small B-cell Lymphoma (SDRP SBCL)

- Provisional entity in 2008 WHO Classification
- Mature B-cell small lymphocytes with diffuse pattern involving red pulp and sinuses
- Cytologically display central round nuclei with indistinct nucleoli; occasional cytoplasmic projections
- Less degree of lymphocytosis; more IgM/IgD expression than HCL-v
- Appears to have substantial overlap with HCL-v

Splenic Marginal Zone Lymphoma (SMZL)/ Splenic Lymphoma with Villous Lymphocytes (SLVL)

- Prominent nodular involvement of white pulp with secondary red pulp involvement
  - White pulp has biphasic histologic appearance
- Neoplastic lymphocytes of intermediate size with moderately abundant cytoplasm
- In blood smear: Cells have polar cytoplasmic projections (villous lymphocytes)
- IgM(+), IgD(+/-), CD11c(+), CD79b(+)
- CD5(-/+), CD10(-), CD23(-/+), CD43(-), CD103(-), annexin-A1(-)

B-cell Prolymphocytic Leukemia (B-PLL)

- Aggressive disease with marked peripheral blood lymphocytosis
  - Intermediate size lymphocytes with prominent central nucleoli
  - Cells lack cytoplasmic villous projections
- Marked splenomegaly
  - Prominent nodular white pulp with secondary red pulp involvement
  - Nucleoli are difficult to appreciate in tissue sections without 1,000x (oil) magnification
- IgM(+), IgD(+/-), B-cell antigens(+), CD5(+/-), CD79b(+), CD10(-)

Chronic Lymphocytic Leukemia/Small Lymphocytic Lymphoma (CLL/SLL)

- Prominent nodular involvement of white pulp with secondary red pulp involvement
  - White pulp has monophasic appearance
- Small, round lymphocytes, prolymphocytes, and paraimmunoblasts
- IgM(+), IgD(+/-), CD5(+), CD23(+), CD10(-), CD22(-), CD79b(-/+)

Mantle Cell Lymphoma (MCL)

- Prominent nodular involvement of white pulp with secondary red pulp involvement
  - White pulp has monophasic appearance
- Monotonous tumor cell population; no large cells (in typical cases)
- IgM(+), IgD(+), CD5(+); Cyclin-D1(+, bright), CD23(-/+), CD10(-), DBA.44/CD76(-)

DIAGNOSTIC CHECKLIST

Clinically Relevant Pathologic Features
- Leukocytosis and lymphocytosis common

Pathologic Interpretation Pearls
- Spleen: Diffuse expansion of red pulp cords and sinuses with effacement of white pulp
- Blood: Small cells with distinct nucleoli and cytoplasmic projections
- CD11c(+), CD22(+), CD103(+/-), CD25(-), and TRAP cytochemistry(-)

SELECTED REFERENCES

1. Dong HY et al: Immunophenotypic analysis of CD103+ B-lymphoproliferative disorders: hairy cell leukemia and its mimics. Am J Clin Pathol. 131(4):586-95, 2009
2. Hashimoto Y et al: Hairy Cell Leukemia-Related Disorders Consistently Show Low CD27 Expression. Pathol Oncol Res. Epub ahead of print, 2009
3. Petit B et al: Among 157 marginal zone lymphomas, DBA.44(CD76) expression is restricted to tumour cells infiltrating the red pulp of the spleen with a diffuse architectural pattern. Histopathology. 54(5):626-31, 2009
4. Cannon T et al: Hairy cell leukemia: current concepts. Cancer Invest. 26(8):860-5, 2008
5. Matutes E et al: Splenic marginal zone lymphoma proposals for a revision of diagnostic, staging and therapeutic criteria. Leukemia. 22(3):487-95, 2008
6. Traverse-Glehen A et al: Splenic red pulp lymphoma with numerous basophilic villous lymphocytes: a distinct clinicopathologic and molecular entity? Blood. 111(4):2253-60, 2008
7. Razaq M et al: Hairy cell leukemia variant transforming into aggressive lymphoma with prostatic involvement in a patient with polycythemia vera. Leuk Lymphoma. 47(4):754-7, 2006
8. Cessna MH et al: Hairy cell leukemia variant: fact or fiction. Am J Clin Pathol. 123(1):132-8, 2005
9. Del Giudice I et al: The diagnostic value of CD123 in B-cell disorders with hairy or villous lymphocytes. Haematologica. 89(3):303-8, 2004
10. Kansal R et al: Histopathologic features of splenic small B-cell lymphomas. A study of 42 cases with a definitive diagnosis by the World Health Organization classification. Am J Clin Pathol. 120(3):335-47, 2003
11. Matutes E et al: The variant form of hairy-cell leukaemia. Best Pract Res Clin Haematol. 16(1):41-56, 2003
12. Mollejo M et al: Splenic small B-cell lymphoma with predominant red pulp involvement: a diffuse variant of splenic marginal zone lymphoma? Histopathology. 40(1):22-30, 2002
13. Matutes E et al: The natural history and clinico-pathological features of the variant form of hairy cell leukemia. Leukemia. 15(1):184-6, 2001
14. Sun T et al: Relationship between hairy cell leukemia variant and splenic lymphoma with villous lymphocytes: presentation of a new concept. Am J Hematol. 51(4):282-8, 1996
15. Wu CD et al: Splenic marginal zone cell lymphoma. An immunophenotypic and molecular study of five cases. Am J Clin Pathol. 105(3):277-85, 1996

HAIRY CELL LEUKEMIA VARIANT

Differential Diagnosis of Hairy Cell Leukemia-Variant in Spleen

	HCL	HCL-v*	SDRP SBCL*	SMZL/SLVL	B-PLL
Clinical Findings					
Median age	50 y	71 y	77 y	66 y	70 y
Splenomegaly	Yes	Yes (85%)	Yes	Yes	Yes
Lymphadenopathy	Uncommon	10-30%	NA	10-30%	10-30%
Laboratory Findings					
	Pancytopenia with lymphopenia and monocytopenia	Leukocytosis with lymphocytosis and normal monocyte count	Lymphocytes are normal or mildly elevated; normal monocyte count	Normal or elevated leukocyte count with lymphocytosis	Marked leukocytosis with lymphocytosis
Histopathologic Features					
Predominant distribution	Red pulp	Red pulp	Red pulp	White pulp	White and red pulp
Pattern	Effacement of white pulp; blood lakes frequent	Effacement of white pulp; occasional blood lakes	Effacement of white pulp; no blood lakes	Prominent white pulp with secondary extension into red pulp	Prominent white pulp
Cellular features	"Fried egg" appearance	Uniform intermediate size cells; round nucleus; distinct nucleolus	Uniform intermediate size cells; round nucleus; indistinct nucleolus	Biphasic pattern with small cells and some large cells	Intermediate size cells; oil immersion usually needed to detect nucleoli
Bone marrow features	Diffuse infiltration; depletion of normal hematopoietic cells; reticulin fibrosis	Interstitial or nodular pattern; no reticulin fibrosis	Intrasinusoidal pattern	Intrasinusoidal, interstitial, or nodular	Interstitial or nodular intertrabecular
Cytologic Features in Blood and Bone Marrow Smears or Touch Imprints					
Cytoplasm	Abundant, clear with projections around entire cell	Abundant, pale to basophilic, with partial small projections	Moderate to abundant; occasional polar villous projections	Short villi or polar cytoplasmic projections	Scant to moderate without projections
Nucleus	Oval or bean-shaped with dispersed chromatin; no nucleolus	Round with condensed chromatin and distinct to prominent nucleolus	Round without or with small distinct nucleolus	Small, round to oval with occasional small nucleolus	Large, round to oval with prominent nucleolus
Flow Cytometric Immunophenotypic Markers					
CD25 (IL2-R)	96%	0-6%	Negative	10%	10-30%
CD103	100%	36-60%	0-38%	0-25%	Negative
CD11c	100%	87-100%	97%	20-40%	10-30%
HC2 or CD123 (IL3-R)	95%	7%	16%	3%	Negative
HCL score**	3-4	0-2	0-2	0-2	NA
Heavy chain isotype	IgG; uncommon IgD and IgM; multiple isotypes at once	IgG; IgD or IgM (uncommon)	IgM, IgM/IgD, or IgG (uncommon)	IgM, IgD, or both; IgG or IgA (uncommon)	IgM and IgD
Other markers	CD22(+), Cyclin-D1(+), FMC7(+), CD79b(+/-), CD5(-), CD10(-), CD43(-)	CD22(+), FMC7(+), CD5(-), CD10(-), CD23(-), CD79a(-), CD79b(+/-)	IgD(-/+), CD5(-), CD10(-), CD23(-)	FMC7(+), CD22(+), CD79b(+), CD5([+] ~ 10%), CD10(-), CD23(-)	CD22(+), CD79b(+), CD5([+] 30%), CD23([+] 20%), ZAP-70([+] 60%)
Immunohistochemical Markers					
Annexin-A1	Positive	Negative	Negative	Negative	Negative
DBA.44/CD76	100%	Positive	Positive (25%)	40-85%	NA
Other markers	MNDA(+), T-bet(+), c-MAF(+)		P53(+/-), Cyclin-D1(-)	MNDA(+)	
TRAP cytochemistry	Positive (bright)	Negative or weak positive	Negative	Negative or weak positive	Negative
Therapy					
	Purine analogs; rituximab in recurrent or resistant cases	Partial response to purine analogs in 50% of cases	Good response to splenectomy	Splenectomy may be better than chemotherapy	Splenectomy and R-CHOP chemotherapy achieve partial response

*Provisional entities in the 2008 WHO Classification of Tumors of Hematopoietic Tissues; these are closely related. **1 point for each positive marker: CD25, CD11c, CD103, or HC2/CD123.

HAIRY CELL LEUKEMIA VARIANT

Microscopic Features

(Left) HCL-v as seen in peripheral blood smear shows characteristic appearance of cells that have lightly basophilic cytoplasm with small villous projections ⇨, oval nuclei with dispersed chromatin, and small nucleoli ⇨. *(Right)* HCL-v highlighted by an immunohistochemical stain for the B-cell marker CD79a. Neoplastic cells infiltrate red pulp cords ⇨ and sinuses ⇨.

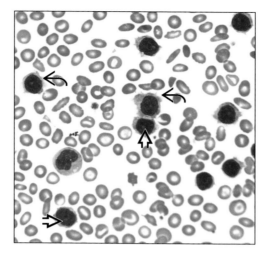
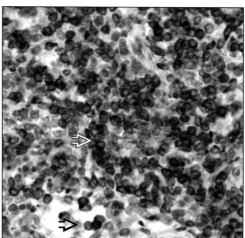

(Left) Immunohistochemical stain for annexin-A1 shows that HCL-v cells within cords ⇨ and sinuses ⇨ are negative. The cells that are positive for annexin-A1 are granulocytes ⇨. *(Right)* HCL-v with blastoid morphology. Histologic transformation can occur in a subset of patients with HCL-v. In this case the neoplastic cells are large with immature chromatin and abundant cytoplasm ⇨. The clinical course of transformed HCL-v is usually aggressive.

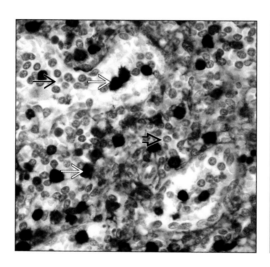
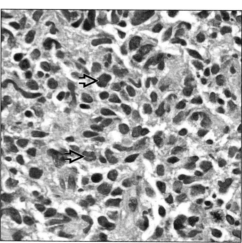

(Left) HCL-v involving liver sinusoids. Numerous small to intermediate size lymphocytes can be observed circulating within sinusoids ⇨. Hepatocyte cords ⇨ are well preserved. *(Right)* HCL-v involving liver sinusoids. Granulocytes ⇨ are positive for annexin-A1, while HCL-v lymphocytes ⇨ are negative. Hepatocytes ⇨ surround sinusoids.

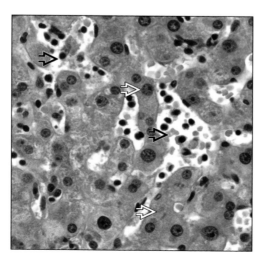
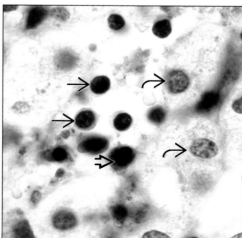

HAIRY CELL LEUKEMIA VARIANT

Differential Diagnosis: HCL and SDRP SBCL

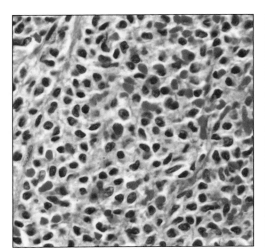

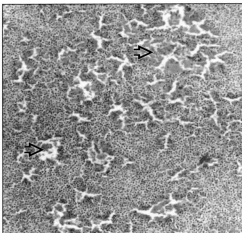

(Left) Classical hairy cell leukemia (HCL) diffusely infiltrating the red pulp of the spleen. The HCL cells have abundant clear cytoplasm imparting a "fried egg" appearance. HCL-v may display a "fried egg" appearance, but in HCL-v this is usually focal. (Right) Classical HCL shows "blood lakes" ⊟➤ surrounded by neoplastic lymphocytes. "Blood lakes" are infrequent in HCL-v.

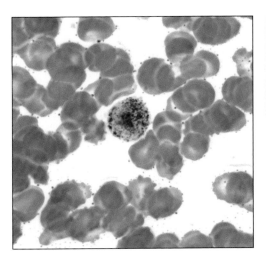

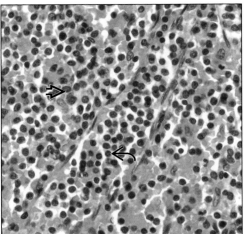

(Left) Classical HCL cell assessed by cytochemistry shows abundant cytoplasmic granules of tartrate-resistant acid phosphatase (TRAP). TRAP is absent or sparse in HCL-v. (Right) Splenic diffuse red pulp small B-cell lymphoma/leukemia (SDRP SBCL) replacing red pulp cords ⊟➤ and sinuses ➔ shows the neoplastic cells are small to intermediate in size with round nuclei and absent nucleoli. (Courtesy J. Cok, MD.)

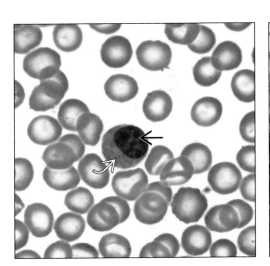

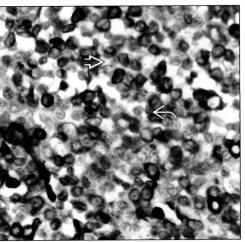

(Left) Wright-Giemsa stain of peripheral blood smear in a case of splenic diffuse red pulp B-cell lymphoma (SDRP SBCL) shows a neoplastic lymphocyte with an oval nucleus, vesicular chromatin ➔, and moderate cytoplasm ➔. A lower degree of lymphocytosis favors SDRP SBCL over HCL-v. (Right) SDRP SBCL. IgM immunohistochemical stain highlights neoplastic cells within cords ⊟➤ and sinusoids ➔ of spleen. IgM is more characteristic of SDRP SBCL, whereas IgG is more common in HCL-v.

HAIRY CELL LEUKEMIA VARIANT

Differential Diagnosis: SMZL/SLVL and B-PLL

(Left) Hematoxylin and eosin stain of splenic marginal zone lymphoma (SMZL)/splenic lymphoma with villous lymphocytes (SLVL) displays a biphasic pattern of white pulp involvement, with central darker small lymphocytes ⇨ surrounded by peripheral, paler zones ⇨. *(Right)* Bcl-6 immunohistochemical stain in SMZL shows Bcl-6 reacts with cells in a partially preserved, reactive germinal center ⇨. The neoplasm in the surrounding white pulp ⇨ or red pulp ⇗ is negative for Bcl-6.

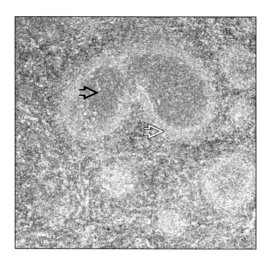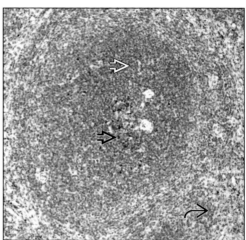

(Left) High-power magnification of SMZL involving the central region of a white pulp nodule shows a population of predominantly small cells with minimal cytoplasm imparting a darker appearance. *(Right)* Hematoxylin and eosin stain of spleen involved by B-cell prolymphocytic leukemia (B-PLL). There is extensive infiltration of the white ⇨ and red pulp ⇗ in this field.

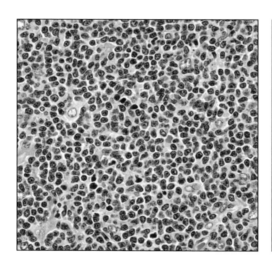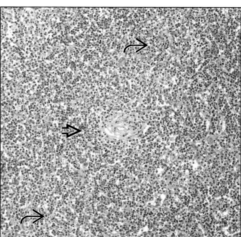

(Left) Hematoxylin and eosin of B-PLL involving the spleen shows infiltration of splenic cords ⇨ and sinuses ⇗ by intermediate to large lymphocytes, many with nucleoli ⇨. Some cells show a scant to moderate amount of cytoplasm ⇗. *(Right)* Wright-Giemsa stain of a peripheral blood smear shows involvement by B-PLL. The neoplastic cells are intermediate to large in size with oval to irregular nuclei and prominent nucleoli ⇨.

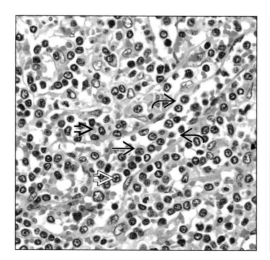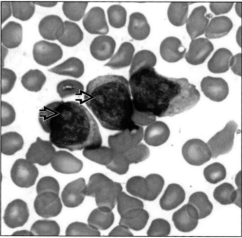

HAIRY CELL LEUKEMIA VARIANT

Differential Diagnosis: CLL and MCL

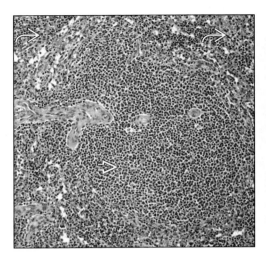

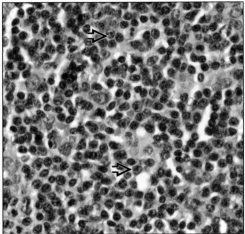

(Left) Chronic lymphocytic leukemia/small lymphocytic lymphoma (CLL/SLL) shows homogeneous, "monophasic" replacement of the splenic white pulp ⇒ with lesser, secondary red pulp involvement ⇉. (Right) High-power magnification of CLL/SLL involving spleen. The neoplastic cells are small, round to oval lymphocytes with clumped chromatin and scant cytoplasm; occasional lymphocytes show chromocenters ⇒. Scattered larger cells are also present.

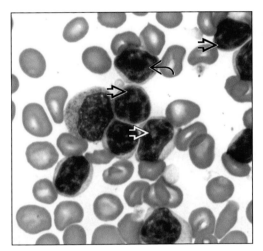

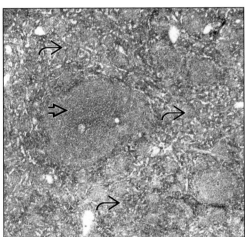

(Left) Wright-Giemsa stain of bone marrow smear of a CLL/SLL case displays usual morphology, with clumped chromatin ⇒ interspersed by clear spaces ⇉ (so-called "soccer ball" appearance). Small distinct, eccentric nucleoli ⇒ may be seen. (Right) Hematoxylin and eosin stain of spleen involved by mantle cell lymphoma (MCL). This field shows uniform expansion of white pulp nodules ⇒ with secondary involvement of red pulp ⇉.

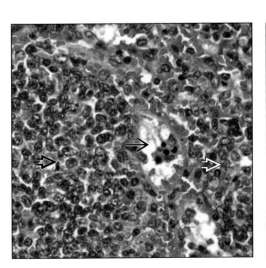

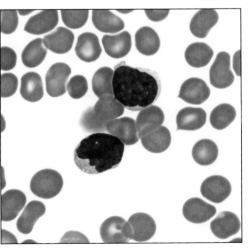

(Left) Hematoxylin and eosin stain of MCL in white pulp ⇒ and a cord ⇒ of the red pulp. An open sinus ⇒ divides white from red pulp. (Right) Wright-Giemsa stain of peripheral blood smear shows MCL. The neoplastic cells are of small to intermediate size with irregular nuclear outlines and clumped chromatin.

SPLENIC DIFFUSE RED PULP SMALL B-CELL LYMPHOMA

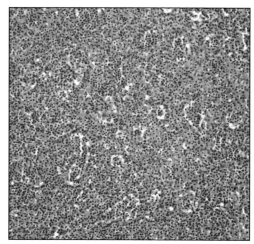

Hematoxylin and eosin stain of small diffuse red pulp small B-cell lymphoma (SDRP SBCL) shows a diffuse effacement of the splenic architecture. No residual white pulp nodularity is noted.

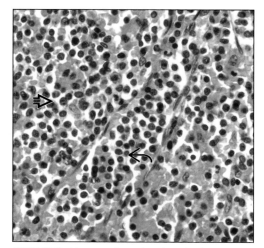

SDRP SBCL. Hematoxylin and eosin stain shows tumor cells in cords ⇨ and sinuses ➾ of spleen. Lymphocytes are small and round with compact chromatin and inconspicuous or absent nucleoli.

TERMINOLOGY

Abbreviations
- Splenic diffuse red pulp small B-cell lymphoma (SDRP SBCL)

Synonyms
- Splenic marginal zone lymphoma, diffuse variant
- Splenic B-cell lymphoma with villous lymphocytes
- Splenic red pulp lymphoma with numerous basophilic villous lymphocytes
- Lymphocytic lymphoma simulating hairy cell leukemia (obsolete term)

Definitions
- Mature B-cell neoplasm that involves peripheral blood, bone marrow, and spleen
- Overlap with hairy cell leukemia variant
- Provisional entity in 2008 WHO classification

ETIOLOGY/PATHOGENESIS

Etiology
- Unknown
- Cell of origin is a peripheral blood B cell of unknown stage and function

CLINICAL ISSUES

Epidemiology
- Incidence
  - Rare type of lymphoma; < 1% of all non-Hodgkin lymphomas
  - ~ 10% of B-cell lymphomas diagnosed by splenectomy
    - ~ 1% of chronic lymphoid leukemias
- Age
  - Most patients are > 40 years

- Median: 77 years
- Gender
  - No obvious gender bias; may be slight male predominance

Presentation
- Clinically indolent
  - B symptoms rare
- Splenomegaly; usually massive
- Usually presents as stage IV with bone marrow involvement
- Erythematous and pruritic skin papules in subset
- Lymphadenopathy rare

Laboratory Tests
- Low-level lymphocytosis in 76% of patients
  - Median lymphocyte count: 15.8×10^9/L
- Thrombocytopenia ($< 100 \times 10^9$/L) in 22%
- Anemia (Hgb < 10 g/L) in 8%
- Serum paraproteinemia is rare

Treatment
- Surgical approaches
  - Good clinical response following splenectomy

Prognosis
- Clinically indolent but incurable disease
  - 63% of patients alive with median follow-up of 48 months in 1 study
  - Rare transformation to diffuse large B-cell lymphoma occurs

MACROSCOPIC FEATURES

General Features
- Marked splenomegaly with diffuse congested pattern
  - Median weight: 1,820 g

SPLENIC DIFFUSE RED PULP SMALL B-CELL LYMPHOMA

Key Facts

Terminology
- Abbreviation: SDRP SBCL
- Provisional entity in 2008 WHO classification

Clinical Issues
- Low level of lymphocytosis
- Splenomegaly; usually massive
- Bone marrow involvement very common
- Clinically indolent B-cell lymphoma presenting at clinical stage IV
- Patients have good response after splenectomy

Microscopic Pathology
- Diffuse infiltration of red pulp cords and sinuses with effacement of white pulp
- Monomorphic round, small to intermediate-sized lymphocytes
- Vesicular nuclei; subset has small, distinct nucleolus
- Bone marrow: Intrasinusoidal pattern with or without interstitial or nodular pattern
- Blood and bone marrow smears
  - Lymphocytes show small cytoplasmic projections (villi) that are broad based
  - Villi are unevenly distributed around cell

Ancillary Tests
- IgM(+), IgD(-/+), pan-B cell(+), CD11c(+), CD25(-), CD103(+/-), CD123(-)
- Complex cytogenetic abnormalities in ~ 33%

Top Differential Diagnoses
- Hairy cell leukemia (HCL)
- Hairy cell leukemia-variant (HCL-v)

MICROSCOPIC PATHOLOGY

Histologic Features
- Spleen
  - Diffuse infiltration of red pulp cords and sinuses with effacement of white pulp
- Bone marrow
  - Intrasinusoidal pattern with or without interstitial or nodular pattern

Cytologic Features
- Monomorphic population of round, small to intermediate-sized lymphocytes
  - Vesicular nuclei and occasional distinct nucleoli
  - Scant to moderate pale or eosinophilic cytoplasm; occasionally cells show plasmacytoid features
- Peripheral blood and bone marrow smears
  - Lymphocytes show small, broad-based cytoplasmic projections (villi)
  - Villi are unevenly distributed around cell circumference

ANCILLARY TESTS

Immunohistochemistry
- Pan-B-cell antigens(+), DBA.44/CD76(+)
- p53(+) in subset
- CD5(-), CD10(-), CD25(-), annexin-A1(-)
- TRAP(-) by enzyme cytochemistry

Flow Cytometry
- Characteristic immunophenotype
  - IgG(+), CD20(+), DBA.44/CD76(+), CD5(-), CD10(-), CD11c(-), CD25(-)
- Subset of cases can be IgM(+), IgD(+), CD103(+)
- Rare cases CD5(+) or CD123(+)

Cytogenetics
- Complex cytogenetic abnormalities in ~ 33% of cases
  - Del(7q), trisomy 3q, &/or trisomy 18 reported

- Cytogenetic abnormalities are less frequent than in SMZL
- t(9;14)(p13;q32)/PAX5-IgH reported in subset of cases

Molecular Genetics
- Low frequency of somatic mutations in IgH variable region genes
- IgH variable region use similar to classical HCL
  - Overrepresentation of VH3-23 and VH4-34
  - No bias of VH1.2 usage of genes (similar to SMZL)
- P53 gene mutations in subset

DIFFERENTIAL DIAGNOSIS

Hairy Cell Leukemia
- Diffuse splenic red pulp involvement
- Diffuse replacement of bone marrow
  - "Fried egg" cytologic appearance
- Blood and bone marrow smears
  - Lymphocytes evenly surrounded by "hairy" cytoplasmic projections
- Blood: Pancytopenia with monocytopenia
- Immunophenotype: CD11c(+), CD25(+), CD103(+), CD123(+)

Hairy Cell Leukemia Variant
- Many similarities and overlap with SDRP SBCL
- Polar cytoplasmic projections and central nuclei, each with distinct nucleolus
- Anemia and thrombocytopenia more common than in SDRP SBCL
- Higher degree of lymphocytosis than in SDRP SBCL

Splenic Marginal Zone Lymphoma (SMZL), Diffuse Variant
- Synonymous with SDRP SBCL
- Considered a morphologic variant of SMZL/SLVL

SPLENIC DIFFUSE RED PULP SMALL B-CELL LYMPHOMA

Differential Diagnosis of Splenic Diffuse Red Pulp Small B-Cell Lymphoma

	HCL	HCL-v	SDRP SBCL
Clinical Findings			
	Splenomegaly	Splenomegaly	Splenomegaly
Lymphadenopathy	Rare	10-30%	Not available
Laboratory Findings			
	Pancytopenia with lymphopenia and monocytopenia	Leukocytosis with lymphocytosis and normal monocyte count	Low degree of lymphocytosis
Histopathologic Features			
Distribution	Red pulp; blood lakes common	Red pulp; uncommon blood lakes	Red pulp; rare blood lakes
White pulp	Effaced	Effaced	Effaced
Cellular features	"Fried egg" appearance	Intermediated-size round cells; distinct eccentric nucleoli	Intermediate-sized cells with round or irregular nuclei; vesicular chromatin; no nucleoli
Cytologic Features in Peripheral Blood or Bone Marrow Smears or Touch Imprints			
Cell size	Intermediate	Small to intermediate	Intermediate
Cytoplasm	Abundant, clear with long projections	Abundant, pale to bluish with some small villi	Moderate to abundant; occasional small villi
Nucleus	Oval to bean-shaped with dispersed chromatin	Round to oval with distinct nucleoli	Round to oval without nucleoli
Flow Cytometry Immunophenotypic Markers			
CD25	95%	0%	0%
CD103	100%	36%	38%
CD11c	100%	100%	97%
HCL score*	3-4	0-2	0-2
Immunohistochemical Markers			
Annexin-A1	Positive	Negative	Negative
TRAP (enzyme cytochemistry)	Positive	Negative	Not available
DBA.44/CD76	100%	Positive	86%
HC2/CD123	95%	9%	16%
Heavy chain isotype	IgG or multiple isotypes at once	IgG most cases	IgM, IgM/IgD, or IgG
Other markers	FMC7(+), CD79b(+/-), Cyclin-D1 (weak [+])	FMC7(+), CD5([+] 10%), CD23(-), CD79b(+/-)	CD5(14%), CD43(13%)
Therapy			
	Purine analogs; rituximab for recurrences or cases resistant to chemotherapy	Partial response to purine analogs in 50% of cases	Not available

*HCL score = 1 point for each positive marker (CD25, CD11c, CD103, HC2/CD123).

DIAGNOSTIC CHECKLIST

Pathologic Interpretation Pearls
- Diffuse involvement of splenic red pulp due to homogeneous small cell infiltrate
- Intrasinusoidal/interstitial or nodular patterns in bone marrow
- In smears, lymphocytes show small cytoplasmic projections that partially surround cell

SELECTED REFERENCES

1. Dong HY et al: Immunophenotypic analysis of CD103+ B-lymphoproliferative disorders: hairy cell leukemia and its mimics. Am J Clin Pathol. 131(4):586-95, 2009
2. Matutes E et al: Splenic marginal zone lymphoma proposals for a revision of diagnostic, staging and therapeutic criteria. Leukemia. 22(3):487-95, 2008
3. Traverse-Glehen A et al: Splenic red pulp lymphoma with numerous basophilic villous lymphocytes: a distinct clinicopathologic and molecular entity? Blood. 111(4):2253-60, 2008
4. Matutes E: Immunophenotyping and differential diagnosis of hairy cell leukemia. Hematol Oncol Clin North Am. 20(5):1051-63, 2006
5. Matutes E et al: The variant form of hairy-cell leukaemia. Best Pract Res Clin Haematol. 16(1):41-56, 2003
6. Mollejo M et al: Splenic small B-cell lymphoma with predominant red pulp involvement: a diffuse variant of splenic marginal zone lymphoma? Histopathology. 40(1):22-30, 2002

Microscopic Features

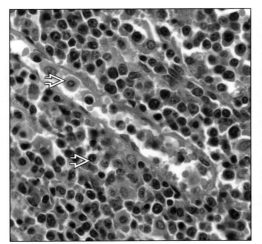

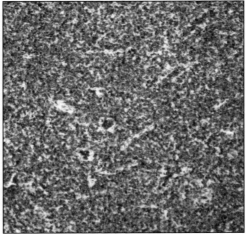

(Left) Hematoxylin and eosin stain of SDRP SBCL displays an infrequent appearance of the neoplastic lymphocytes. In this case, the lymphocytes show a distinct pink cytoplasm ➡. *(Courtesy J. Cok, MD.)* *(Right)* CD20 immunostain of SDRP SBCL shows a diffuse replacement by CD20(+) lymphocytes at this low-power magnification. No residual white pulp nodularity is present.

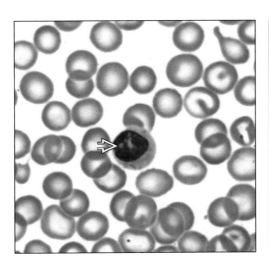

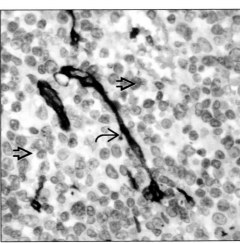

(Left) Wright-Giemsa stain of SDRP SBCL in peripheral blood smear shows a low level of lymphocytosis. This lymphocyte has a small nucleolus ➡ and moderately abundant cytoplasm; no villi are seen in this field. *(Courtesy J. Cok, MD.)* *(Right)* CD34 immunostain highlights endothelium of sinusoids in a case of SDRP SBCL. The neoplastic lymphocytes, negative for CD34, expand cords ➡ and obliterate sinuses ➡ in this field.

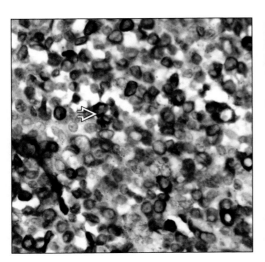

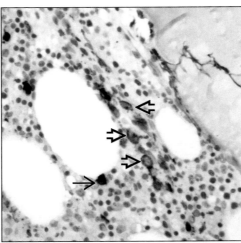

(Left) SDRP SBCL expressing IgM ➡. Cases of SDRP SBCL also can be positive for IgD, both IgM and IgD, or IgG. *(Right)* CD20 immunostain of bone marrow biopsy specimen in a case of SDRP SBCL shows a characteristic sinusoidal distribution of neoplastic B lymphocytes ➡. Reactive small B lymphocytes are also seen in the interstitium ➡. *(Courtesy J. Cok, MD.)*

SPLENIC DIFFUSE RED PULP SMALL B-CELL LYMPHOMA

Differential Diagnosis: HCL

(Left) Hematoxylin and eosin of classical hairy cell leukemia (HCL) shows diffuse red pulp infiltration by small to intermediate-sized lymphocytes with round to oval or bean-shaped nuclei. The nuclear chromatin is uniform and the cells have abundant pale to clear cytoplasm ⮕. (Right) Wright-Giemsa stain of a case of HCL shows an intermediate-sized lymphocyte with an oval nucleus and "hairy" membrane projections all over the cell circumference.

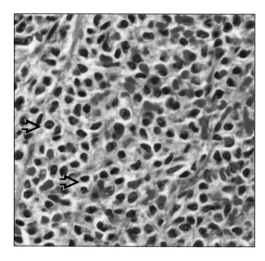
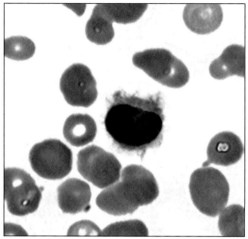

(Left) Cyclin-D1 immunostain in a case of classical HCL shows weak nuclear reactivity ⮕ in a fraction of neoplastic lymphocytes. (Right) CD20 immunostain in a case of classical HCL shows distinct membranous reactivity ⮕ of neoplastic cells, leaving a clear cytoplasm with a "fried egg" appearance ⮕.

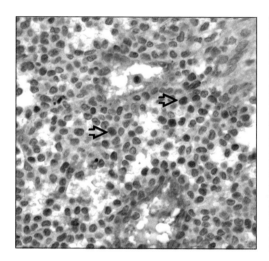
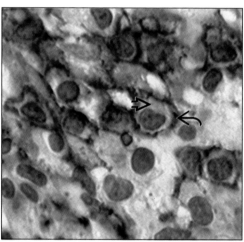

(Left) Hematoxylin and eosin stain of a case of classical HCL displays a characteristic "blood lake" ⮕, a feature that is only rarely seen in SDRP SBCL. (Right) Tartrate-resistant acid phosphatase (TRAP) in a case of classical HCL shows a fine diffuse reactivity throughout the cytoplasm. TRAP is usually negative in cases of SDRP SBCL.

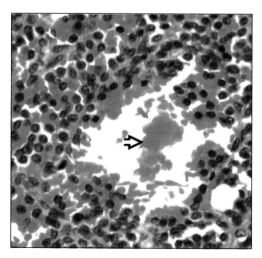
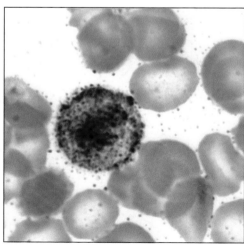

SPLENIC DIFFUSE RED PULP SMALL B-CELL LYMPHOMA

Differential Diagnosis: HCL-v

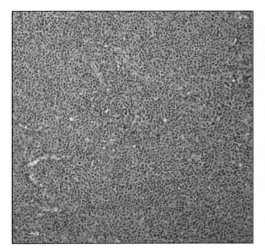

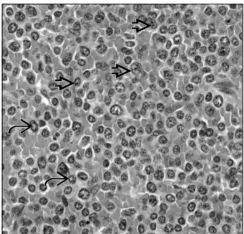

(Left) Hematoxylin and eosin stain of hairy cell leukemia variant (HCL-v) shows diffuse effacement of the architecture without remnants of white pulp nodularity. *(Right)* Hematoxylin and eosin stain of HCL-v shows a diffuse infiltrate of small to intermediate-sized lymphocytes with vesicular chromatin ➡. Lymphocytes show distinctive central nucleoli ➡.

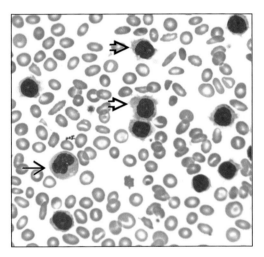

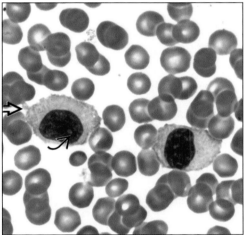

(Left) Wright-Giemsa stain of peripheral blood smear of HCL-v shows numerous neoplastic lymphocytes. Short villi are noted in some lymphocytes ➡. A monocyte is present in this field ➡. *(Right)* Wright-Giemsa stain of peripheral blood smear of HCL-v displays small to intermediately sized lymphocytes with abundant cytoplasm with projections ➡ around only part of the cell circumference. Nuclei are oval and 1 nucleus has a small nucleolus ➡.

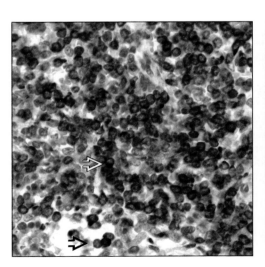

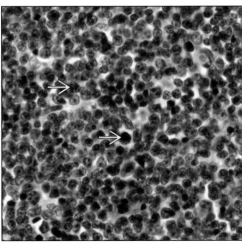

(Left) CD79a immunostain of HCL-v highlights neoplastic B lymphocytes in the red pulp cords ➡ and within sinusoids ➡. *(Right)* p53 immunostain of HCL-v shows overexpression ➡ in a subset of cells. Overexpression of p53 may be due to gene mutations or deletions.

DIFFUSE LARGE B-CELL LYMPHOMA ARISING IN THE SPLEEN

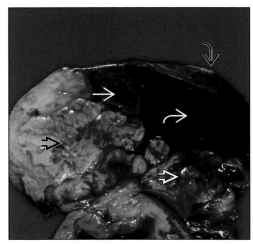

Gross photograph shows a multinodular tumor ⇨. Tumor extends into hilar fat ⇨ and shows focal infarction ➡. Well-preserved spleen is dark brown ⇘. Spleen capsule is noted ➘.

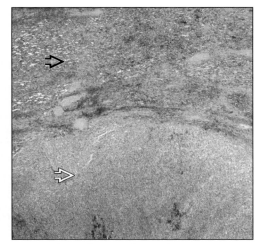

Hematoxylin and eosin shows the most common presentation of DLBCL characterized by a well-circumscribed tumor mass ⇨ surrounded by nonneoplastic spleen ➘.

TERMINOLOGY

Abbreviations
- Diffuse large B-cell lymphoma (DLBCL)

Synonyms
- Large cell lymphoma

Definitions
- Diffuse large B-cell lymphoma that arises in spleen
- Involvement of splenic hilar lymph nodes and bone marrow (usually focal) can occur in primary DLBCL
  - Liver involvement may be part of definition of splenic DLBCL with micronodular or diffuse patterns
- Primary DLBCL of spleen can be associated with splenic marginal zone B-cell lymphoma
- Primary DLBCL of spleen is rare, but represents up to 40% of splenectomy specimens involved by DLBCL
- Patients with history of lymphoma or evidence of disseminated DLBCL at diagnosis are excluded (secondary DLBCL)

ETIOLOGY/PATHOGENESIS

Infectious Agents
- No known etiology
- Primary DLBCL of spleen is rarely associated with hepatitis C or Epstein-Barr virus infection

CLINICAL ISSUES

Epidemiology
- Age
  - Adults are mainly affected; median age: 64 years
    - M:F ratio approximately 1:1

Presentation
- Abdominal pain
- Pain is often left-sided
- Systemic symptoms such as fever, malaise, and weight loss often occur
- Fine needle aspiration may yield necrosis only and be wrongly diagnosed as splenic abscess
- Diagnosis can be suspected in presence of splenomegaly and abdominal or retroperitoneal adenopathy
- Most patients are immunocompetent
  - Occasionally reported in HIV(+) patients

Treatment
- Chemotherapy similar to systemic cases of DLBCL
  - R-CHOP is most common chemotherapy used
- Splenectomy usually performed for diagnostic purposes

Prognosis
- 80% 5-year survival for patients with primary DLBCL presenting as mass
- Poor survival for DLBCL with T-cell-rich pattern or neoplasms that diffusely replace spleen
  - These cases often have disseminated disease shown by staging (probably not primary)

MACROSCOPIC FEATURES

General Features
- Most cases show solitary or multiple distinct nodular masses surrounded by nonneoplastic spleen
  - Neoplasms that diffusely replace red pulp can be subtle grossly
- Splenic weight can range from normal to > 3,000 g (average: 1,000 g)
- Tumor size usually ranges from 5-18 cm
- Multinodular tumor can replace up to 90% of spleen
- Extensive necrosis is usual
- Tumor may extend through capsule into adjacent diaphragm, stomach, pancreas, or abdominal wall

DIFFUSE LARGE B-CELL LYMPHOMA ARISING IN THE SPLEEN

Key Facts

Terminology
- Primary DLBCL of spleen is rare
- Involvement of splenic hilar lymph nodes and bone marrow (usually focal) can occur in primary DLBCL
- Liver involvement may be part of definition of primary DLBCL of spleen with micronodular or diffuse patterns
- Patients with history of DLBCL or dissemination at diagnosis are excluded (secondary DLBCL)

Clinical Issues
- Adults are mainly affected; median age: 64 years
- 80% 5-year survival for primary DLBCL presenting as distinct mass

Macroscopic Features
- Solitary or multiple distinct nodular masses surrounded by nonneoplastic spleen

Microscopic Pathology
- Sheets of large cells with variable cytomorphology
- B-cell lineage and surface immunoglobulin light chain restriction

Top Differential Diagnoses
- Diffuse large B-cell lymphoma, systemic
- Peripheral T-cell lymphoma
- T-cell/histiocyte-rich large B-cell lymphoma
- Classical Hodgkin lymphoma

Diagnostic Checklist
- Single or multiple masses composed of large B cells

MICROSCOPIC PATHOLOGY

Histologic Features
- Primary splenic DLBCL usually presents as large nodule or mass
  - Nodule/mass typically destroys white and red pulp
  - Approximately 1/3 of cases involve white pulp exclusively or predominantly
  - Approximately 20% of cases involve red pulp predominantly and diffusely
  - Adjacent Malpighian corpuscles may be focally involved
- Variable cell morphology (centroblastic, immunoblastic, anaplastic, etc.)
  - Relative increased frequency of immunoblastic cases
- Necrosis within neoplasm is common; sclerosis within or around neoplasm can be observed
- Surrounding uninvolved spleen is distinctly separated from tumor, sometimes by fibrous bands

Predominant Pattern/Injury Type
- Lymphoid, diffuse

Predominant Cell/Compartment Type
- Hematopoietic, lymphoid

Immunophenotype
- Neoplasms are of B-cell lineage: CD19(+), CD20(+), CD22(+), and pax-5(+)
- Surface immunoglobulin light chain restriction is detected by flow cytometry in most cases
- Most cases express Bcl-6 and about 1/3 express CD10
- CD43 is positive in 20-30% of cases
- CD3(-), CD5(-), CD23(-/+)
- Absence of follicular dendritic cells (CD21, CD23) in tumor nodules

Cytogenetic and Molecular Findings
- Monoclonal *IgH* rearrangements; *TCR* genes are usually germline
- No distinctive cytogenetic or molecular findings

DIFFERENTIAL DIAGNOSIS

Diffuse Large B-cell Lymphoma (DLBCL), Systemic
- Gross, microscopic, immunophenotypic, and molecular features can be identical to DLBCL arising in spleen
- Distinction can be made after complete staging
- Most DLBCL of spleen represent systemic or secondary involvement

T-cell/Histiocyte-rich Large B-cell Lymphoma (TCRLBCL)
- Subtype of DLBCL that if identified in spleen, is suggestive of disseminated disease
- Similar to any DLBCL both grossly and microscopically
- Predominance of small T lymphocytes; large neoplastic B cells represent < 10% of cell infiltrate
- Recently described micronodular variant (MTCRBL) does not produce large discrete mass but micronodules
- MTCRBL distributed mainly in white pulp leaving no residual normal white pulp

DLBCL Primarily Involving Red Pulp
- Unusual variant, clinically aggressive; median age: 69 years
- Diffuse splenic involvement, predominantly in splenic cords
- Frequent bone marrow and liver sinusoids infiltration; rare lymph node involvement
- Mature B cells that usually coexpress CD5; Cyclin-D1 and CD23 negative

Peripheral T-cell Lymphoma (PTCL)
- May involve white or red pulp
- Cell composition is more polymorphic than DLBCL with mixture of eosinophils and plasma cells
  - Vascularity is often increased
- Some cases may have increased histiocytes as well as erythrophagocytosis

CHRONIC LYMPHOCYTIC LEUKEMIA/SMALL LYMPHOCYTIC LYMPHOMA

Differential Diagnosis: MCL

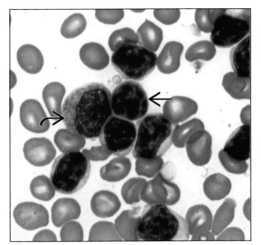

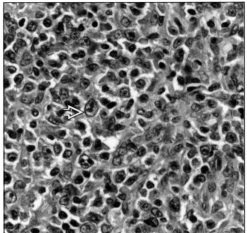

(Left) Bone marrow aspirate of a case of chronic lymphocytic leukemia/small lymphocytic lymphoma (CLL/SLL) shows small mature lymphocytes with clumped ("soccer ball") chromatin ➡. A myelocyte is also noted ➡. (Right) Richter transformation in CLL/SLL involving spleen demonstrates a predominance of large cells ➡, histologically similar to diffuse large B-cell lymphoma.

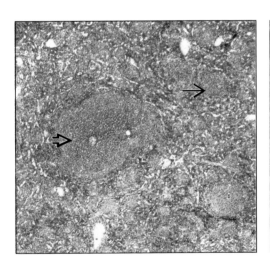

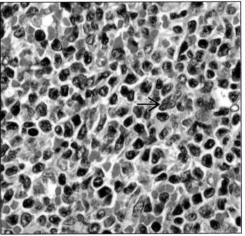

(Left) Mantle cell lymphoma (MCL) shows expansion of the white pulp ➡ and involvement of the red pulp presenting as small lymphoid aggregates ➡. (Right) Mantle cell lymphoma involving white pulp shows a uniform population of intermediate-sized lymphocytes with irregular nuclear outlines ➡.

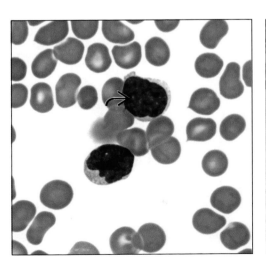

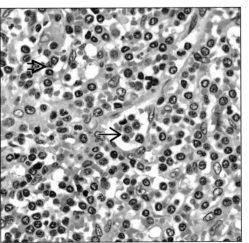

(Left) Mantle cell lymphoma in peripheral blood smear. This image shows 2 intermediate-sized lymphocytes with irregular nuclear outlines, small distinct nucleoli ➡, and scant cytoplasm. (Right) Prolymphocytoid variant of mantle cell lymphoma involving splenic red pulp shows expansion of cords ➡ and sinuses containing neoplastic lymphocytes ➡.

CHRONIC LYMPHOCYTIC LEUKEMIA/SMALL LYMPHOCYTIC LYMPHOMA

Differential Diagnosis: MCL, LPL, SMZL

(Left) Prolymphocytoid variant of MCL involving peripheral blood. The lymphocytes are of intermediate size, and many cells have a single prominent nucleolus ⇗ with perinuclear accentuation of chromatin. Occasional typical MCL cells are also present ⇗. *(Right)* Prolymphocytoid variant of MCL involving bone marrow biopsy. Many neoplastic cells have a single prominent nucleolus, but nucleoli are often more difficult to appreciate in hematoxylin & eosin stained sections.

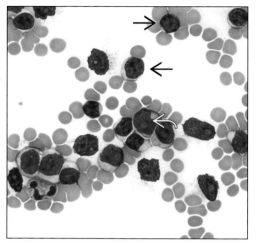
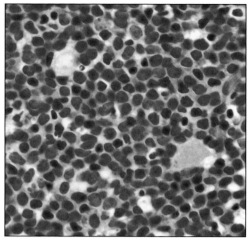

(Left) This is a high magnification of white pulp in a case of lymphoplasmacytic lymphoma in spleen that shows a mixture of small lymphocytes ⇗, intermediate-sized lymphocytes ⇗, plasmacytoid lymphocytes, and plasma cells ⇗, including some cells with intranuclear inclusions (Dutcher bodies) ⇗. *(Right)* Lymphoplasmacytic lymphoma in peripheral blood shows a plasmacytoid lymphocyte ⇗ and a plasma cell ⇗. The patient had > 3 g of IgM paraprotein.

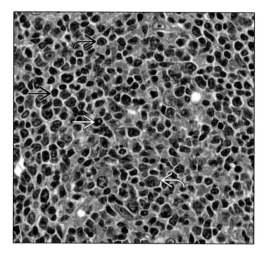
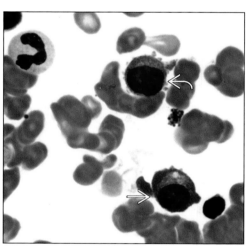

(Left) Splenic marginal zone lymphoma (SMZL) displays a "biphasic pattern" in which lymphocytes in the marginal zone ⇗ become larger and acquire more abundant cytoplasm. *(Right)* Peripheral blood of patient with SMZL displays small lymphocytes with cytoplasmic projections on part ("polar") of the cells ⇗.

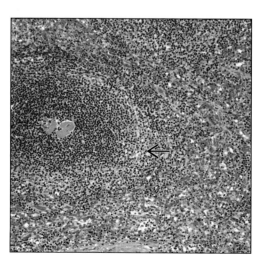
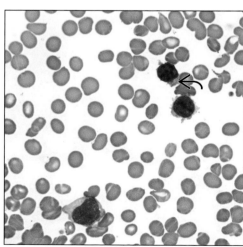

CHRONIC LYMPHOCYTIC LEUKEMIA/SMALL LYMPHOCYTIC LYMPHOMA

Differential Diagnosis: HCL and HCL-V

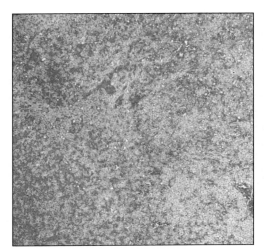
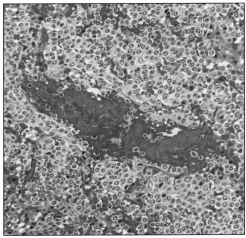

(Left) Hairy cell leukemia (HCL) involving the spleen. The red pulp is diffusely replaced by lymphocytes with abundant pale cytoplasm imparting a pale or clear appearance at low-power magnification. *(Right)* HCL involving the spleen. A blood lake, composed of pooled blood surrounded by hairy cells, is present within the red pulp.

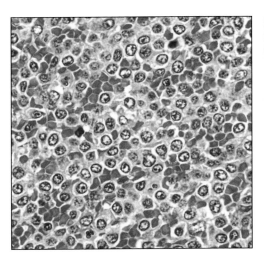
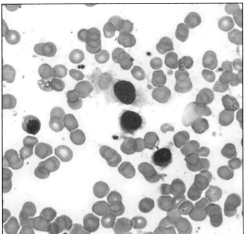

(Left) Hairy cell leukemia involving the spleen. Oil immersion lens magnification shows a homogeneous population of small cells with abundant cytoplasm. Small indistinct nucleoli in a subset of hairy cells can be appreciated in H&E stained tissue sections. *(Right)* Peripheral blood smear of hairy cell leukemia. The neoplastic cells have central nuclei with homogeneous chromatin, indistinct nucleoli, & abundant cytoplasm with villous ("hairy") cytoplasmic projections.

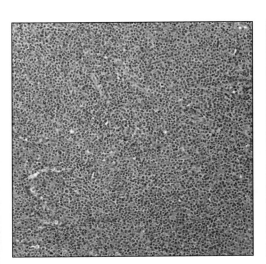
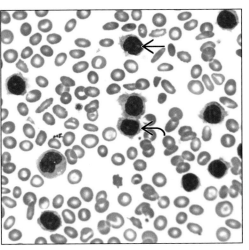

(Left) Hairy cell leukemia-variant (HCL-v) shows a diffuse infiltration of splenic red pulp with total obliteration of white pulp. *(Right)* Peripheral blood smear of HCL-v shows lymphocytosis. Lymphocytes are intermediate in size with moderately abundant cytoplasm and partial cytoplasmic projections ➚. Lymphocytes display round to oval nuclei with distinct nucleoli ➔.

FOLLICULAR LYMPHOMA

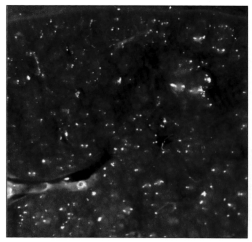

Follicular lymphoma involving the spleen. The lymphoma has a diffuse micronodular pattern enhancing white pulp. This is the most common pattern of follicular lymphoma involving the spleen.

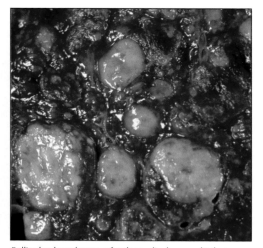

Follicular lymphoma of spleen displays multiple tumor masses effacing the splenic architecture. This is the 2nd most common pattern of follicular lymphoma involving spleen.

TERMINOLOGY

Abbreviations
- Follicular lymphoma (FL)

Synonyms
- Follicular center cell lymphoma, grades 1-3 (REAL classification)
- Follicular lymphoma, predominantly small cleaved cell, mixed small cleaved and large cell, or large cell (Working Formulation)
- Centroblastic/centrocytic lymphoma (Kiel classification)
- Nodular lymphoma, poorly differentiated, mixed, or histiocytic (Rappaport classification)

Definitions
- Mature B-cell neoplasm composed of germinal (follicle) lymphocytes (centrocytes and centroblasts) in variable mixture
- Histopathology usually shows follicular growth pattern; less frequently is purely diffuse

ETIOLOGY/PATHOGENESIS

Pathogenesis
- Bcl-2 overexpression as result of t(14;18)(q32;q21)/*IgH-BCL2* gene rearrangement
  - Bcl-2 inhibits programmed cell death, giving Bcl-2(+) lymphoma cells a survival advantage
  - Many other anti-apoptotic molecules (e.g., Bcl-x, Mcl-1, etc.)
- *IgH-BCL2* by itself is insufficient for lymphomagenesis
  - Other mechanisms are involved and needed for FL to develop

CLINICAL ISSUES

Epidemiology
- Incidence
  - FL is 2nd most common lymphoma in Western hemisphere
  - FL rarely arises in spleen
    - Splenic involvement is usually manifestation of systemic disease
- Age
  - Range: 30-83 years (median: 59 years)
- Gender
  - M:F = 1:1.4

Site
- Most cases of FL involving spleen are diagnosed by splenectomy
  - FL primarily affects lymph nodes, but also bone marrow, peripheral blood, and Waldeyer ring
  - FL involving extranodal sites usually reflects widespread nodal disease
- Primary FL of spleen is rare

Presentation
- Splenomegaly, abdominal pain, anemia, or thrombocytopenia
  - Usually associated with peripheral or abdominal lymphadenopathy with widespread disease
  - B-type symptoms in subset of patients

Laboratory Tests
- ~ 30% peripheral blood lymphocytosis

Natural History
- Splenectomy is not curative
  - May alleviate symptoms or cytopenias

Treatment
- Surgical approaches

FOLLICULAR LYMPHOMA

Key Facts

Terminology
- Follicular lymphoma (FL)

Etiology/Pathogenesis
- Bcl-2 overexpression is present in most cases of FL
  - Results from t(14;18)(q32;q21)/*IgH-BCL2*
  - Other factors are involved in pathogenesis

Clinical Issues
- Most cases of FL involving spleen are manifestation of systemic disease
- FL in spleen is commonly diagnosed by splenectomy
  - Performed for cytopenias or abdominal pain/discomfort
  - Splenectomy is rarely performed for diagnostic purposes
- FL is mostly clinically indolent disease

Microscopic Pathology
- Common patterns of involvement
  - Miliary pattern growing along preexisting follicles
  - Nodular effacement of architecture
- Neoplastic follicles are composed of centrocytes and centroblasts

Ancillary Tests
- Immunophenotype
  - Monotypic Ig(+), CD19(+), CD20(+)
  - CD10(+) and Bcl-6(+) in most cases
- Cytogenetics/molecular
  - t(14;18)(q32;q21)/*BCL2-IgH* in ~ 80-90% of cases

Top Differential Diagnoses
- Splenic marginal zone lymphoma (SMZL)
- Mantle cell lymphoma (MCL)

- Splenectomy performed usually for cytopenias, pain, or less usually, for diagnostic purposes
- Adjuvant therapy
  - Rituximab plus CHOP (cyclophosphamide, doxorubicin, vincristine, and prednisone)
  - Watchful waiting or rituximab alone are also alternatives depending on staging

Prognosis
- Usually considered an indolent lymphoma, but with frequent relapses
- International Prognostic Index for Follicular Lymphoma (FLIPI) is predictor of outcome
- 5-year overall survival is 55-70%
- Transformation to large B-cell lymphoma occurs
  - ~ 20% of patients with prolonged clinical follow-up

MACROSCOPIC FEATURES

General Features
- Variable gross appearance
  - Diffuse/miliary growth pattern, predominantly involving preexisting white pulp
  - Single or multiple tumor masses of variable size also can be observed
- Median weight: 1.1 kg (range: 0.5-2.7 kg)

MICROSCOPIC PATHOLOGY

Histologic Features
- Miliary pattern growing along preexisting follicles is most common pattern
  - Usually associated with marginal zone pattern and less red pulp involvement
  - Some researchers have suggested that this pattern is a form of in situ follicular lymphoma
    - Associated with or without disseminated disease
- Effacement of architecture is 2nd most common pattern
  - Follicles are packed and coalescent

- Correlates with grossly visible tumor mass
  - Can display diffuse areas
- Neoplastic follicles are composed of centrocytes and centroblasts
  - Variable cytologic predominance according to grade of tumor
    - Low grade (grades 1 and 2): Up to 15 centroblasts per high-power field on average
    - Grade 3: More than 15 centroblasts or immunoblasts per high-power field on average
    - Some high-grade cases have sparse centrocytes
- Marginal zone pattern in ~ 50% of cases
  - Lymphocytes acquire abundant, pale (monocytoid) cytoplasm
    - Typically present at periphery of neoplastic follicles
  - Splenic hilar lymph nodes also may show marginal zone pattern
- Red pulp infiltration as satellite aggregates
  - ~ 30% with diffuse red pulp involvement; mainly small FL lymphocytes
  - FL cells often appear smaller and less irregular than those in white pulp
- Bone marrow biopsy specimen is involved by paratrabecular aggregates
  - Other patterns are often present, but rare without paratrabecular pattern

Cytologic Features
- Fine needle aspiration performed uncommonly on spleen
  - Centrocytes and centroblasts are present in smears

Lymph Nodes
- Hilar or peripheral lymph nodes usually show features similar to those in spleen
  - Usually follicular pattern is present
  - Marginal zone pattern in ~ 10% cases

FOLLICULAR LYMPHOMA

ANCILLARY TESTS

Immunohistochemistry
- Positive for B-cell markers: CD19(+), CD20(+), CD79a(+), pax-5(+)
- CD10(+) and Bcl-6(+) in most cases
  - Stronger in white pulp; weaker in red pulp or in interfollicular areas
- Bcl-2 (variable [+]) in white and red pulp
  - Bcl-2 more frequently (+) in low-grade FL (65-90%) than in high-grade FL (50-80%)
- Follicular dendritic meshworks usually present
  - CD21(+), CD23(+), CD35(+), &/or CNA.42(+)
- T-cell antigens(-), Cyclin-D1(-)
- Variable proliferation rate as determined with Ki-67
  - Low-grade FL usually has low proliferation rate (< 20%)

Flow Cytometry
- Monotypic surface immunoglobulin(+)
- Heavy chains: IgM(+) or IgG(+), and IgD(-)
  - IgD(+) in rim of occasional residual mantle zone lymphocytes
- CD19(+), CD20(+), CD22(+), and CD79a(+)
- Usually CD10(+)
  - Occasional downregulation of CD10 in peripheral blood and bone marrow
- T-cell antigens(-)

Cytogenetics
- t(14;18)(q32;q21) in ~ 80-90%
- Other cytogenetic abnormalities are found in ~ 90% of FL and include
  - Losses of 1p, 6q, 10q, &/or 17p
  - Gains of 1, 6p, 7, 8, 12q, X, &/or 18q

In Situ Hybridization
- BCL2-IgH gene rearrangements can be demonstrated in almost all cases using fusion probes and FISH
  - Probes used are quite large and cover relevant regions of chromosomes 14 and 18
- BCL6 translocations in ~ 10% of cases

Molecular Genetics
- Monoclonal IgH gene rearrangements in 60-70% of cases
  - False-negative results are common
    - Result from presence of somatic hypermutation in IgH variable region genes
- BCL2-IgH gene rearrangements can be demonstrated in ~ 80% of cases
  - Most breakpoints in BCL2 on chromosome 18 occur on MBR (major breakpoint region)
    - Other minor breakpoints: Mcr (minor cluster region), icr (intermediate cluster region), etc.
    - PCR assays can sensitively detect most of these breakpoints
    - FISH assays, unlike PCR, can assess all breakpoints but are less sensitive
- It is important to remember that
  - PCR can detect BCL2-IgH fusions sequences in people without evidence of FL

- Frequency of (+) result correlates with increasing age
- This finding suggests that other molecular mechanisms are required for lymphomagenesis
- P53 gene mutations associated with transformation to high-grade lymphoma

DIFFERENTIAL DIAGNOSIS

Splenic Marginal Zone Lymphoma (SMZL)
- Micronodular infiltrate of white pulp centered on preexisting follicles
- Low-power magnification shows darker inner zone surrounded by paler marginal zone (biphasic pattern)
  - Residual germinal centers or mantle zones (-/+); usually not present
- Red pulp involvement usually as small aggregates
- Neoplastic cells are predominantly small with abundant pale cytoplasm, round nuclei, and small nucleoli
  - Scattered large cells always present
  - Plasmacytic differentiation is common; can be marked
    - Subset of cases associated with serum paraprotein; can be high level
- Proposed variant of SMZL diffusely involves red pulp of spleen
- Splenic hilar lymph nodes often show
  - Incomplete effacement with preservation of some sinuses
  - Marginal zone pattern that can colonize follicles and mimic FL
- Peripheral blood lymphocytes characterized by unipolar cytoplasmic projections (villous lymphocytes)
  - Subset of patients can present with marked lymphocytosis (~ 100 K)
- Bone marrow shows intertrabecular and sometimes paratrabecular lymphoid aggregates
  - Sinusoidal pattern of involvement in ~ 33-50% of patients
- Immunophenotype
  - IgM(+), IgD(+/-), CD19(+), CD20(bright [+]), CD22(bright [+])
  - CD11c(+), FMC7(+), CD5(-/+), CD10(-), Bcl-6(-)

Mantle Cell Lymphoma (MCL)
- Micronodular infiltrate of white pulp
- Small nodules or aggregates throughout red pulp
- Lymphocytes are uniform, intermediate in size, usually with irregular nuclear contours
- Immunophenotype
  - IgM(+), IgD(+), CD5(+), CD19(+), CD20(+), Cyclin-D1(+)
  - CD10(-), CD23([-/+] dim), CD43([+/-], dim), Bcl-6(-)
- Detection of t(11;14)(q13;q32)/CCND1-IgH is very helpful
  - FISH, conventional cytogenetics, or PCR assays can be performed

FOLLICULAR LYMPHOMA

Differential Diagnosis of Follicular Lymphoma in Spleen

	FL	SMZL	MCL	CLL/SLL
Clinical Features				
Age range (median)	40-78 y (59 y)	32-71 y (60 y)	34-78 y (68 y)	43-82 y (69 y)
Histopathologic Features				
Pattern	Nodular white and red pulp	Nodular white and red pulp	Nodular and diffuse	Nodular and diffuse
Marginal zone pattern	Frequent	Always	Occasionally	Unusual
Cytologic features	Centrocytes and centroblasts	Small cells ± monocytoid &/or plasmacytoid differentiation; scattered large cells	Uniform round to irregular cells; no large cells	Small lymphocytes, prolymphocytes, and paraimmunoblasts
Immunophenotype				
	CD10(+), Bcl-2(+), Bcl-6(+)	CD5(-/+), CD10(-), CD27(+)	CD5(+), CD43(+), Cyclin-D1(+)	CD5(+), CD23(+), CD43(+)
Heavy chain expression	IgM(+)/IgD(-/+)	IgM(+)/IgD(+/-)	IgM(+)/IgD(+)	IgM(+)
Lymphocyte stage of maturation	Follicle center stage	Recirculating memory B lymphocyte, post-follicular	Mantle cell, prefollicular	Virgin, prefollicular or antigen experienced cell
Cytogenetics				
	t(14;18)(q32;q21)	del(7q31-32)	t(11;14)(q13;q32)	+12, del(17p13), del(13q14.3), del(11q22-23), and del(6q21)
Molecular Genetics				
	IgH-BCL2	N/A	CCND1-IgH	N/A

FL = follicular lymphoma; SMZL = splenic marginal zone lymphoma; MCL = mantle cell lymphoma; CLL/SLL = chronic lymphocytic leukemia/small lymphocytic lymphoma; N/A = not available.

Chronic Lymphocytic Leukemia/Small Lymphocytic Lymphoma (CLL/SLL)
- Micronodular infiltrate of white pulp
- Expansion of white pulp forming uniform nodules with extensive involvement of red pulp
- Lymphocytes are round to oval with clumped chromatin and scant cytoplasm
  - Scattered admixed prolymphocytes and paraimmunoblasts
- Immunophenotype
  - Surface IgM([+] dim), IgD(+), CD5(+), CD19(+), CD20([+] dim), CD22([-/+] dim)
  - CD23(+), CD43(+/-), CD10(-), Bcl-6(-)

Diffuse Large B-cell Lymphoma (DLBCL)
- Can arise in spleen or be manifestation of systemic disease
- Large confluent nodules diffusely replacing white and red pulp, with frequent necrosis
- Large cells with variable composition: Centroblastic, immunoblastic, pleomorphic, lymphocyte/histiocyte-rich
- B-cell lineage: CD19(+), CD20(+), CD5(-), CD10(+/-), Bcl-6(+/-)

Lymphoplasmacytic Lymphoma (LPL)
- White pulp expansion and nodular aggregates in red pulp
- Periarteriolar aggregates of plasmacytoid cells, small lymphocytes, and immunoblasts
- Immunophenotype
  - Surface &/or cytoplasmic IgM(+), CD19(+), CD20(+/-), CD5(-), CD10(-)
- Often associated with Waldenström macroglobulinemia
  - Bone marrow involvement and serum IgM paraprotein

Follicular Hyperplasia or Marginal Zone Hyperplasia in Spleen
- Usually associated with autoimmune processes or idiopathic thrombocytopenic purpura
- Spleen often normal size but can be up to 1,000 g
- Well-demarcated white pulp and red pulp
- White pulp displays distinct germinal centers, mantle zones, and marginal zones (triphasic pattern)
- Red pulp is well preserved with only rare lymphocytes in sinuses or in splenic cords
- Immunophenotype shows polytypic B cells

SELECTED REFERENCES

1. Howard MT et al: Follicular lymphoma of the spleen: multiparameter analysis of 16 cases. Am J Clin Pathol. 131(5):656-62, 2009
2. Mollejo M et al: Splenic follicular lymphoma: clinicopathologic characteristics of a series of 32 cases. Am J Surg Pathol. 33(5):730-8, 2009
3. Swerdlow SH: Small B-cell lymphomas of the lymph nodes and spleen: practical insights to diagnosis and pathogenesis. Mod Pathol. 12(2):125-40, 1999
4. Falk S et al: Primary malignant lymphomas of the spleen. A morphologic and immunohistochemical analysis of 17 cases. Cancer. 66(12):2612-9, 1990
5. van Krieken JH et al: The distribution of non-Hodgkin's lymphoma in the lymphoid compartments of the human spleen. Am J Surg Pathol. 13(9):757-65, 1989

14

FOLLICULAR LYMPHOMA

Imaging and Microscopic Features

(Left) CT scan of the abdomen shows a 19 cm, diffusely enlarged spleen ⇗, without discrete masses, corresponding to follicular lymphoma with a micronodular pattern. Enlarged lymph nodes are also noted ➤ in this case of follicular lymphoma of the spleen. *(Right)* Follicular lymphoma with micronodular distribution. A neoplastic follicle replaces preexisting white pulp ➤. Small lymphoid aggregates ➔ are distributed throughout the red pulp.

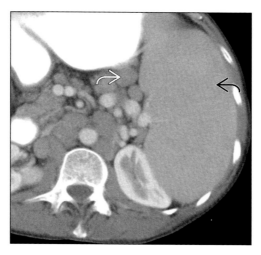
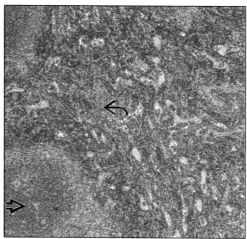

(Left) Follicular lymphoma (FL) of the spleen displays destruction of the architecture due to large confluent neoplastic follicles ➔. This pattern reflects the presence of large nodules or a tumor mass identified grossly. *(Right)* FL, grade 1, replacing white pulp of spleen. This field shows a predominance of small centrocytes (small cleaved lymphocytes) ➔ with only rare centroblasts (large noncleaved cells) ➤.

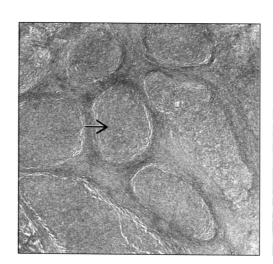
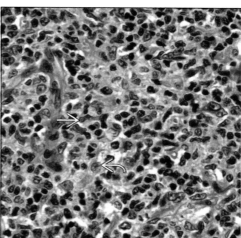

(Left) Follicular lymphoma, grade 3, involving spleen. The image shows the center of a neoplastic follicle with numerous large centroblasts ➤. Centrocytes are also present in the background. *(Right)* Follicular lymphoma involving splenic white pulp with a micronodular pattern. The follicle has a dark germinal center ➤ surrounded by lymphocytes with pale cytoplasm that impart a marginal zone pattern ➤, similar to the biphasic pattern of SMZL.

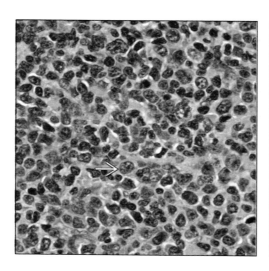
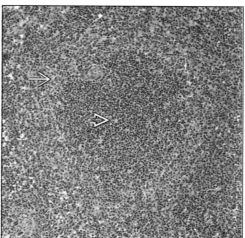

FOLLICULAR LYMPHOMA

Microscopic Features

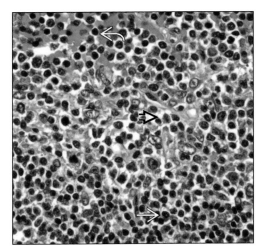
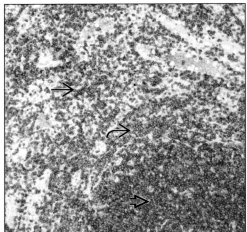

(Left) Higher magnification of the marginal zone of a neoplastic follicle of FL of the spleen shows that lymphocytes have more abundant cytoplasm ⇒ than lymphocytes in the center of the follicle ⇒ or in the red pulp ⇒. *(Right)* Immunohistochemistry for CD20 in FL of spleen demonstrates the distribution of neoplastic lymphocytes in the white pulp ⇒ as well as multiple aggregates in the red pulp ⇒. A marginal zone pattern is also apparent ⇒.

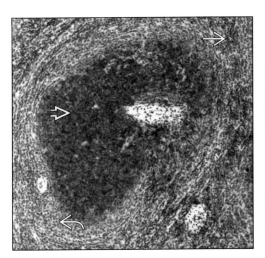
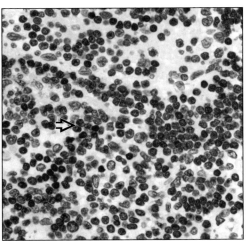

(Left) Immunohistochemistry for CD10 in follicular lymphoma of the spleen demonstrates that most cells in white pulp ⇒ are positive, while the reactivity is decreased in the red pulp ⇒ or in the marginal zone ⇒. *(Right)* Assessment for CD10 in FL of the spleen demonstrates that neoplastic lymphocytes in the red pulp ⇒ are negative, despite the fact that they are CD10(+) in the white pulp, suggesting an effect of the splenic microenvironment.

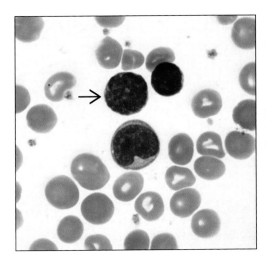
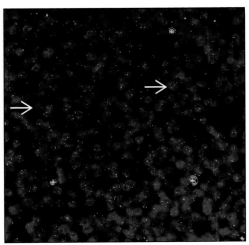

(Left) Peripheral blood smear of a patient with FL involving the spleen. This image shows 3 neoplastic lymphocytes in the blood, including a lymphocyte with markedly irregular nuclear contours ⇒. *(Right)* Follicular lymphoma of spleen assessed by fluorescence in situ hybridization (FISH) using Bcl-2 and IgH probes demonstrates that most nuclei have 3 signals ⇒, proof of BCL2-IgH fusion signals, consistent with the t(14;18)(q32;q21).

FOLLICULAR LYMPHOMA

Differential Diagnosis

(Left) Splenic marginal zone lymphoma (SMZL) with a micronodular distribution shows expansion of the white pulp ⇒ with a biphasic pattern and secondary red pulp involvement ➡. Follicular lymphoma involving the spleen may show a similar low-power appearance. *(Right)* SMZL replacing white pulp displays a biphasic pattern with central darker cells ⇒ and a relatively pale, peripheral marginal zone ➡. There is also secondary red pulp involvement ➡.

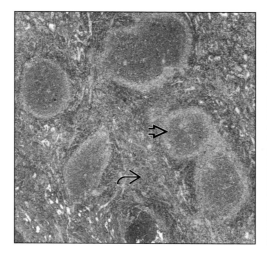
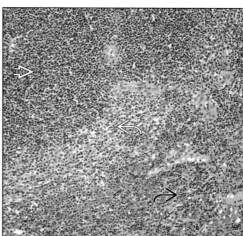

(Left) High magnification of SMZL in the middle of a tumor nodule displays a population of small lymphocytes with round to slightly irregular nuclear contours and variably abundant cytoplasm. Few cells in this field show monocytoid differentiation. *(Right)* Mantle cell lymphoma (MCL) involving the spleen displays expansion of the white pulp ⇒ in a micronodular pattern. There are also multiple lymphoid aggregates throughout the red pulp ➡ in this field.

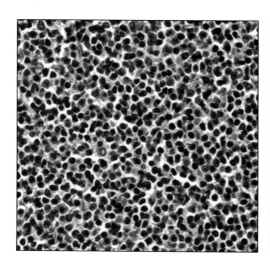
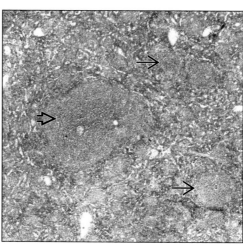

(Left) MCL displays expansion of the white pulp ⇒. Lymphocytes are uniform with irregular nuclear outlines. Adjacent red pulp shows sinusoidal infiltration ➡ as well as a small lymphoid aggregate ➡. Neoplastic cells at the interface between white and red pulp occasionally acquire abundant clear cytoplasm and impart a marginal zone pattern. *(Right)* MCL involving spleen. Cyclin-D1 immunostain highlights tumor expansion of white pulp ⇒ and smaller red pulp aggregates ➡.

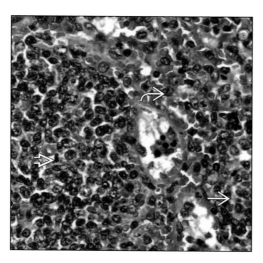
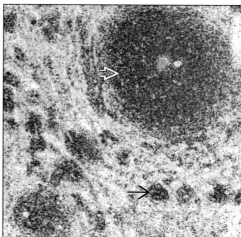

FOLLICULAR LYMPHOMA

Differential Diagnosis

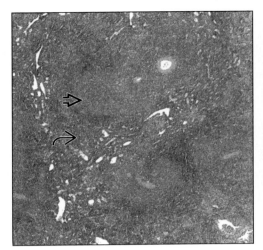
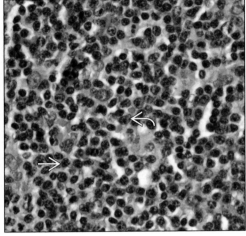

(Left) Chronic lymphocytic leukemia/small lymphocytic lymphoma (CLL/SLL) involving spleen displays prominent involvement of white pulp appearing as nodules in this field ⊳ as well as lesser red pulp involvement ⇨. *(Right)* CLL/SLL involving spleen. High magnification in the white pulp shows a predominance of small, round lymphocytes with clumped chromatin ➡, admixed with occasional prolymphocytes ➡.

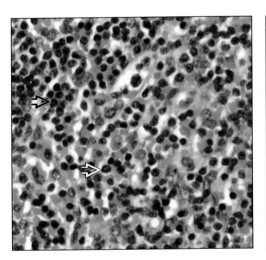
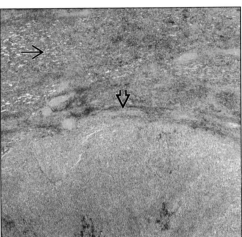

(Left) CLL/SLL involving spleen. High magnification of the red pulp shows small, round lymphocytes in the cords ⊳ as well as within sinuses ➡. *(Right)* Diffuse large B-cell lymphoma arising in the spleen (primary) demonstrates a well-circumscribed tumor mass ⊳ that diffusely replaces white and red pulp. In this field, uninvolved splenic parenchyma is also present ➡.

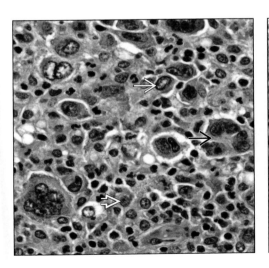
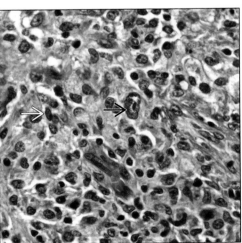

(Left) Diffuse large B-cell lymphoma arising in the spleen illustrates the spectrum of cells that can be detected in this type of tumor, ranging from intermediate ⊳ to large ➡ and multinucleated pleomorphic cells ➡. *(Right)* T-cell/histiocyte-rich large B-cell lymphoma arising in the spleen. Most of the cells are small benign lymphocytes ➡ &/or histiocytes with relatively few large neoplastic B cells ➡.

MANTLE CELL LYMPHOMA

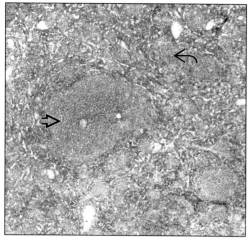

Mantle cell lymphoma involving splenic white pulp ⊃ with secondary red pulp involvement present as small aggregates ⇗.

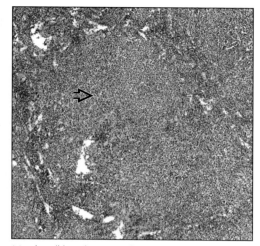

Mantle cell lymphoma involving splenic white pulp as a large nodule ⊃. A uniform cell population is noted.

TERMINOLOGY

Abbreviations
- Mantle cell lymphoma (MCL)

Synonyms
- Centrocytic lymphoma
- Intermediately differentiated lymphocytic lymphoma
- Intermediate lymphocytic lymphoma

Definitions
- B-cell lymphoma characterized by *CCND1-IGH*/ t(11;14)(q13;q32)
  - Most cases are composed of monomorphic small to medium-sized lymphocytes with irregular nuclear contours

ETIOLOGY/PATHOGENESIS

Pathogenesis
- *CCND1-IGH*/t(11;14)(q13;q32) with Cyclin-D1 overexpression occurs on most cases
  - Dysregulated Cyclin-D1 overexpression accelerates transition from G1 to S phase of cell cycle
    - Overcomes suppressive effects of retinoblastoma (RB1) and p27kip1
  - Other mechanisms are required for lymphomagenesis
- MCL is thought to arise from an antigen-naive, CD5(+) B cell (pregerminal center) in
  - Peripheral blood
  - Inner zone of mantle zone follicle

CLINICAL ISSUES

Epidemiology
- Age
  - Median: 7th decade (range: 34-78 years)

- Gender
  - M:F ratio = 2-3:1

Site
- Most cases of MCL involve lymph nodes, but extranodal sites are often involved
  - Common extranodal sites
    - Peripheral blood, bone marrow, gastrointestinal tract
    - Liver, spleen, Waldeyer ring
    - ~ 40% of patients with MCL have splenomegaly
- In some patients with MCL, splenic involvement is predominant
  - So-called splenomegalic form of MCL

Presentation
- Splenic involvement by MCL is usually associated with splenomegaly
  - Can be massive

Laboratory Tests
- Peripheral blood lymphocytosis in ~ 25% of cases; occasionally > 200 x 10⁹/L

Treatment
- Surgical approaches
  - Splenectomy performed usually for cytopenias or local symptoms (e.g., pain)
    - Rarely performed to establish diagnosis
- Adjuvant therapy
  - Rituximab (R) plus CHOP (cyclophosphamide, doxorubicin, vincristine, and prednisone)
  - R-plus-hyper-CVAD (fractionated cyclophosphamide, vincristine, doxorubicin, and dexamethasone)
  - Other aggressive chemotherapy regimens

Prognosis
- MCL is currently incurable and usually carries a poor prognosis
  - 27% overall survival at 5 years with R-CHOP

MANTLE CELL LYMPHOMA

Key Facts

Etiology/Pathogenesis
- *CCND1-IGH*/t(11;14)(q13;q32) resulting in Cyclin-D1 overexpression in most cases

Clinical Issues
- MCL is nodal-based disease but extranodal sites of involvement are common
  - Spleen is common site
- Splenectomy performed usually for cytopenias, pain, or less commonly, for diagnostic purposes
- Small subset of MCL patients present with massive splenomegaly and minimal lymphadenopathy
- Smaller subset of MCL patients have clinical picture that mimics B-PLL
  - Aggressive course and prominent splenomegaly
  - Marked peripheral blood lymphocytosis with many prolymphocytes

Microscopic Pathology
- Enlarged white pulp nodules with coalescence
- Red pulp involvement correlates with extent of MCL
- Typical: MCL cell population is uniform, small to intermediate size, with irregular nuclear contours
- Other morphologic variants of MCL can involve spleen
  - Pleomorphic, blastoid, prolymphocytoid

Ancillary Tests
- Surface Ig(+), CD19(+), CD20(+)
- CD22(+), FMC7(+), Bcl-2(+)
- CD5(+), Cyclin-D1(+), CD23(-)
- *CCND1-IgH*/t(11;14)(q13;q32)
- Additional chromosomal aberrations are very common

- 82% overall survival at 3 years with R-hyper-CVAD
- Blastoid and pleomorphic variants are associated with adverse prognosis
- Pure (> 90%) mantle zone pattern correlates with better prognosis

IMAGE FINDINGS

Radiographic Findings
- Splenomegaly can be detected by various imaging modalities
- MCL is usually fluorodeoxyglucose (FDG) PET negative/low
  - ± blastoid/pleomorphic variants

MACROSCOPIC FEATURES

General Features
- Median weight: 1.6 kg (range: 0.7-3.8 kg)
- Usually diffuse/miliary growth pattern
  - Occasionally large fleshy nodules

MICROSCOPIC PATHOLOGY

Histologic Features
- Enlarged white pulp nodules with frequent coalescence
  - Massive white pulp expansion in some cases
  - ± small residual germinal centers or marginal zone pattern
- Red pulp involvement correlates with extent of disease
  - Lesser disease: Small aggregates of MCL cells in cords and sinuses
  - Extensive disease: Diffuse infiltration of red pulp
- Scattered or clusters of histiocytes are common
- Tumor cell population is uniform and typically of small to intermediate size
  - Round to irregular nuclear contours
  - Clumped chromatin and occasionally distinct nucleoli

- Mitotic rate is variable
  - High in blastoid/pleomorphic variants
- Morphologic variants of MCL
  - Small round: Round nuclear contours and low mitotic rate
    - Mimics chronic lymphocytic leukemia/small lymphocytic lymphoma
  - Pleomorphic: Large cells with pale cytoplasm, more prominent nucleoli, and increased mitoses
    - Mimics diffuse large B-cell lymphoma
  - Blastoid: Medium-sized cells with immature chromatin
    - Mimics lymphoblastic lymphoma
  - Prolymphocytoid: Intermediate to large cells with prominent nucleoli
    - More easily recognized in touch imprints than in histologic sections
    - Mimics prolymphocytic leukemia
  - Monocytoid: Small cells with abundant pale cytoplasm
    - Mimics marginal zone B-cell lymphoma
- Examination of splenic hilar lymph nodes is helpful for diagnosis
  - Can assess pattern more reliably than in spleen
    - Diffuse, nodular, or mantle zone
    - Pure (> 90%) mantle zone pattern correlates with better prognosis
  - Cytologic features of MCL can be assessed more reliably
    - Environment of spleen or other extranodal sites alters cytologic features

ANCILLARY TESTS

Immunohistochemistry
- Pan-B-cell antigens(+), CD5(+)
- Bcl-2(+), CD43(+/-)
- CD3(-), CD23(-)
- CD10(-), Bcl-6(-)
- Cyclin-D1(+) with nuclear pattern

MANTLE CELL LYMPHOMA

- Proliferation index as determined by Ki-67 is variable and has prognostic significance
  - o > 40% correlates with poorer survival in R-CHOP-treated patients

Flow Cytometry
- Monotypic surface Ig(+), intermediate to strong
- IgM(+), IgD(+)
- CD19(+), CD20(+), CD22(+), CD79a(+)
- CD79b(+), FMC7(+)
- CD5(+), CD10(-), Bcl-6(-)
  - o Occasional cases are CD5(-), CD10(+), or Bcl-6(+)
    - ▪ More often pleomorphic/blastoid variants
- CD23 usually negative but dimly positive in ~ 10% of MCL cases
- Cyclin-D1 is technically difficult to assess by flow cytometry

Cytogenetics
- t(11;14)(q13;q32) is present in ~ 70-80% of cases
  - o Possible explanations for cases (-) by conventional cytogenetics
    - ▪ Poor growth of tumor cells in culture
    - ▪ Sampling error: e.g., only (-) BM assessed by conventional cytogenetics
    - ▪ Rare cases of of so-called Cyclin-D1(-) MCL
- Additional nonrandom chromosomal aberrations are very common in MCL
  - o Detected by conventional cytogenetics or comparative genomic hybridization
  - o Gains of 3q26, 7p21, 8q24, or trisomy 12
  - o Losses of 1p13-q31, 6q23-q27, 9p21, 11q22-q23, 13q11-q13, and 17p13-pter
- Blastoid/pleomorphic variants of MCL
  - o High frequency of additional chromosomal abnormalities
  - o Tetraploid clones are more frequent
  - o Higher frequency of abnormalities of 17p/*P53*, 9q/*P16*, and 8q24/*MYC*
- Prolymphocytoid variant of MCL
  - o High frequency of chromosome 17p/*P53* abnormalities

In Situ Hybridization
- FISH demonstrates the *CCND1/IgH* gene rearrangement in ~ 95% of cases

Molecular Genetics
- *CCND1-IgH* fusion gene can be shown by PCR in 30-40% of cases
  - o Commonly used primers detect only major translocation cluster (MTC)
- Southern blotting shows *BCL1* locus rearrangements in 60-70% of cases
  - o Multiple probes required for this detection rate
- Additional genetic changes in MCL
  - o Inactivating mutations of *ATM* gene at 11q22-23 in ~ 50% of cases
  - o *P53* mutations, *P15/16* deletions, *P18* deletion
  - o Loss of p16 and p21 expression
  - o *MYC* rearrangements or amplification
- Monoclonal *IgH* and *Ig* light chain gene rearrangements

- No evidence of monoclonal T-cell receptor gene rearrangements
- Somatic hypermutation of *Ig* variable region genes uncommon (~ 20%)

Gene Expression Profiling
- Expression of ~ 40 genes can reliably identify MCL cases
- Rare cases are Cyclin-D1(-), but show gene expression profile of MCL
  - o Can be Cyclin-D2(+) &/or Cyclin-D3(+)
  - o Other Cyclins may function as does Cyclin-D1 in nonphysiologic state

DIFFERENTIAL DIAGNOSIS

Chronic Lymphocytic Leukemia/Small Lymphocytic Lymphoma (CLL/SLL)
- Expansion of white pulp forming uniform nodules with extensive red pulp involvement
- Lymphocytes are round to oval with clumped chromatin and scant cytoplasm
  - o Variable admixture of prolymphocytes and occasional proliferation center formation
  - o ± proliferation centers/pseudofollicles
    - ▪ More common in spleens with extensive disease
- Immunophenotype is very helpful to distinguish CLL/SLL from MCL
  - o Surface Ig (dim, [+]), CD19(+), CD20(dim, [+])
  - o CD5(+), CD23(+), CD43(+/-)
  - o Cyclin-D1(-), FMC7(-/+)
- No evidence of *CCND1-IgH*/t(11;14)(q13;q32)

B-cell Prolymphocytic Leukemia (B-PLL)
- Usually massive splenomegaly and marked lymphocytosis
- Red pulp expansion with indistinct white pulp
- Intermediate to large cells with central, prominent nucleoli
  - o Perinuclear condensation of chromatin
- Immunophenotype
  - o Surface Ig (bright, [+]), CD19(+), CD20(bright, [+])
  - o FMC7(+), CD5(+/-), CD23(+/-), CD43(+/-)
  - o Proliferation index (Ki-67) high, Cyclin-D1(-)
- No evidence of *CCND1-IgH*/t(11;14)(q13;q32)
- Prolymphocytoid variant of MCL can closely mimic B-PLL morphologically
  - o Recognize as MCL by results of immunophenotypic and molecular studies

Hairy Cell Leukemia (HCL)
- Patients present with splenomegaly and pancytopenia
- Red pulp involvement with effacement of white pulp
- Red cell "lakes" and "pseudosinuses" represent areas of architectural disruption by tumor
- HCL cells have central indented nuclei without nucleoli and abundant pale cytoplasm
- HCL cytoplasmic "hairs" cannot be appreciated in histologic sections
  - o Touch imprints of spleen are useful to recognize
- HCL cells are tartrate-resistant acid phosphatase (TRAP)(+) by cytochemistry

MANTLE CELL LYMPHOMA

- Immunophenotype
  - Surface Ig(bright, [+]), CD19(+), CD20(+), CD22(+)
  - CD11c(+), CD25(+), CD103(+), annexin-A1(+)
  - CD5(-), CD23(-)
  - Cyclin-D1(+/-) with dim intensity in ~ 50% of cases

Follicular Lymphoma (FL)
- Most patients with FL involving spleen have systemic disease
  - Widespread lymphadenopathy, hepatomegaly, &/or bone marrow involvement
- FL in spleen exhibits miliary pattern growing along preexisting follicles
  - Most common pattern
- Follicles can enlarge and coalesce to form large, grossly visible masses
  - 2nd most common pattern
- Neoplastic follicles can exhibit marginal zone appearance at their periphery
- Immunophenotype
  - Surface Ig (bright, [+]), CD19(+), CD20(bright, [+])
  - CD10(+), Bcl-6(+), CD5(-)
  - Bcl-2 (+) in most cases
- BCL-2-IgH/t(14;18)(q32;q21) is present in most cases of FL

Splenic Marginal Zone Lymphoma (SMZL)
- Miliary pattern growing along preexisting follicles
  - Secondary red pulp involvement
- "Biphasic pattern" due to darker appearance of center of white pulp and lighter marginal zones
  - Center of white pulp composed of uniform, round, hyperchromatic lymphocytes
  - Marginal zone composed of small lymphocytes and intermediate to large cells with clear cytoplasm
    - Large cells are usually nucleolated
- Touch imprints of spleen helpful to show villous lymphocytes that are common in SMZL
- Bone marrow often shows sinusoidal pattern of involvement
- Immunophenotype
  - Surface Ig (bright, [+]), CD19(+), CD20(+)
  - CD5([-/+], ~ 20%), CD10(-), CD23(-/+), Bcl-6(-)

Splenic Diffuse Red Pulp Small B-cell Lymphoma
- Spleen cut surface is homogeneously brown-red without miliary-like nodularity
- Predominant red pulp involvement with effacement of white pulp (absence of nodularity)
- Peripheral blood shows villous lymphocytes
- Bone marrow may show sinusoidal involvement
- Immunophenotype is similar to SMZL

DIAGNOSTIC CHECKLIST

Clinically Relevant Pathologic Features
- Most patients with MCL have nodal-based systemic disease
  - Extranodal involvement is common in MCL patients

  - Blood, bone marrow, gastrointestinal tract, liver, and spleen
- Small subset of MCL patients can present with or develop clinical picture that mimics B-PLL
  - Aggressive clinical course
  - Prominent splenomegaly
  - Marked peripheral blood lymphocytosis with many prolymphocytes

Pathologic Interpretation Pearls
- Typical MCL is composed of uniform population of small to intermediate cells with irregular nuclear contours
  - Be aware of blastoid/pleomorphic variants
- Immunophenotype: B-cell(+), Cyclin-D1(+), CD5(+), CD10(-), and CD23(-)
- CCND1-IgH/t(11;14)(q13;q32) is present

SELECTED REFERENCES

1. Garcia M et al: Proliferation predicts failure-free survival in mantle cell lymphoma patients treated with rituximab plus hyperfractionated cyclophosphamide, vincristine, doxorubicin, and dexamethasone alternating with rituximab plus high-dose methotrexate and cytarabine. Cancer. 115(5):1041-8, 2009
2. Romaguera JE et al: High rate of durable remissions after treatment of newly diagnosed aggressive mantle-cell lymphoma with rituximab plus hyper-CVAD alternating with rituximab plus high-dose methotrexate and cytarabine. J Clin Oncol. 2005 Oct 1;23(28):7013-23. Epub 2005 Sep 6. Erratum in: J Clin Oncol. 24(4):724, 2006
3. Fu K et al: Cyclin D1-negative mantle cell lymphoma: a clinicopathologic study based on gene expression profiling. Blood. 106(13):4315-21, 2005
4. Ruchlemer R et al: B-prolymphocytic leukaemia with t(11;14) revisited: a splenomegalic form of mantle cell lymphoma evolving with leukaemia. Br J Haematol. 125(3):330-6, 2004
5. Thieblemont C et al: Small lymphocytic lymphoma, marginal zone B-cell lymphoma, and mantle cell lymphoma exhibit distinct gene-expression profiles allowing molecular diagnosis. Blood. 103(7):2727-37, 2004
6. Kansal R et al: Histopathologic features of splenic small B-cell lymphomas. A study of 42 cases with a definitive diagnosis by the World Health Organization classification. Am J Clin Pathol. 120(3):335-47, 2003
7. Angelopoulou MK et al: The splenic form of mantle cell lymphoma. Eur J Haematol. 68(1):12-21, 2002
8. Ruchlemer R et al: Splenectomy in mantle cell lymphoma with leukaemia: a comparison with chronic lymphocytic leukaemia. Br J Haematol. 118(4):952-8, 2002
9. Lai R et al: Pathologic diagnosis of mantle cell lymphoma. Clin Lymphoma. 1(3):197-206; discussion 207-8, 2000
10. Weisenburger DD et al: Mantle cell lymphoma. A clinicopathologic study of 68 cases from the Nebraska Lymphoma Study Group. Am J Hematol. 64(3):190-6, 2000
11. Wlodarska I et al: Secondary chromosome changes in mantle cell lymphoma. Haematologica. 84(7):594-9, 1999
12. Swerdlow SH et al: The morphologic spectrum of non-Hodgkin's lymphomas with BCL1/cyclin D1 gene rearrangements. Am J Surg Pathol. 20(5):627-40, 1996
13. Kraemer BB et al: Primary splenic presentation of malignant lymphoma and related disorders. A study of 49 cases. Cancer. 54(8):1606-19, 1984

MANTLE CELL LYMPHOMA

Microscopic Features

(Left) Mantle cell lymphoma involving splenic white pulp ➡ and secondarily involving red pulp as small aggregates or individual cells ➡. A dilated perifollicular sinus ➡ divides white from red pulp. *(Right)* Mantle cell lymphoma involving splenic red pulp as an aggregate in the cord ➡ shows a dilated sinus containing a mixture of cells ➡.

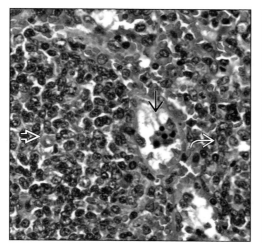
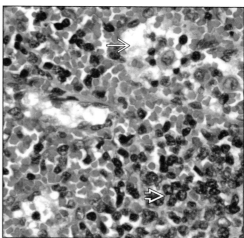

(Left) Immunohistochemistry for CD20 in mantle cell lymphoma of spleen shows marked expansion of white pulp ➡ and multiple tumor cell aggregates in the red pulp ➡. *(Right)* Immunohistochemistry for Cyclin-D1 in mantle cell lymphoma of spleen shows marked expansion of white pulp ➡ and multiple tumor cell aggregates in the red pulp ➡.

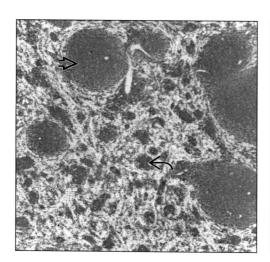
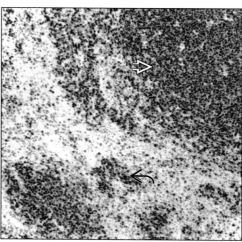

(Left) Mantle cell lymphoma involving a splenic hilar lymph node. This case shows a prominent mantle zone pattern. In general, tumor pattern is more readily appreciated in lymph nodes than in the spleen. *(Right)* Mantle cell lymphoma (MCL), prolymphocytoid variant, in peripheral blood. A small subset of MCL patients can have an aggressive clinical course, splenomegaly, and morphologic features suggestive of B-cell prolymphocytic leukemia.

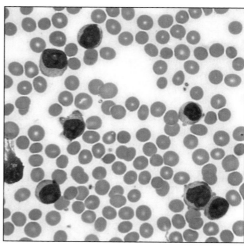

Variant Microscopic Features

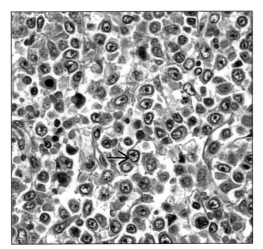

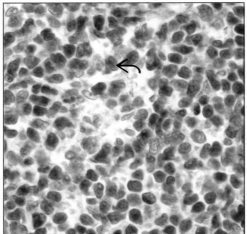

(Left) Pleomorphic variant of mantle cell lymphoma of the spleen shows that lymphocytes are large with vesicular nuclei and prominent nucleoli ⮕. *(Right)* Cyclin-D1 immunohistochemistry of pleomorphic variant of mantle cell lymphoma of the spleen shows strong reactivity in most neoplastic cells. Note the intermediate size and irregular nuclear outlines ⮕ of neoplastic lymphocytes.

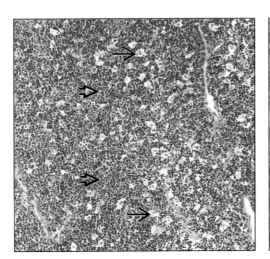

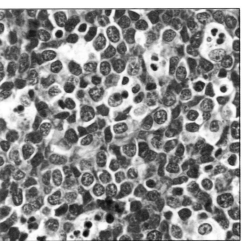

(Left) MCL, blastoid variant, shows a prominent starry sky pattern. The "stars" (highlighting 2 representative macrophages ⮕) are tingible body macrophages that appear pale in a "sky" of darker tumor cells ⮕. *(Right)* MCL, blastoid variant, with prominent "starry sky" pattern. The tumor cells are of intermediate size with immature chromatin resembling, in part, B-lymphoblastic lymphoma. This case had a chromosome 17p deletion (probably involving P53 gene).

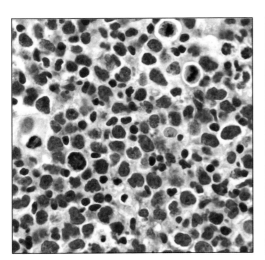

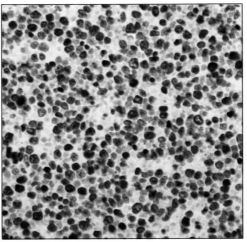

(Left) A case of mantle cell lymphoma, pleomorphic variant, associated with a t(2;8)(p12;q24) involving the Igκ and MYC genes. Note the varying size of the tumor cells, nuclei with prominent nucleoli, and high mitotic rate. *(Right)* Ki-67 stain of mantle cell lymphoma, pleomorphic variant, associated with a t(2;8)(p12;q24). Note the very high proliferation rate.

MANTLE CELL LYMPHOMA

Differential Diagnosis: CLL/SLL, B-PLL, and HCL

(Left) Chronic lymphocytic leukemia/small lymphocytic lymphoma (CLL/SLL) involving spleen shows expanded white pulp ⮂ with secondary red pulp ➔ involvement that is similar to MCL. *(Right)* CLL/SLL involving white pulp of spleen shows a predominance of small mature lymphocytes ➔ admixed with scattered prolymphocytes ➔, which are intermediate in size with distinct nucleoli. Proliferation centers are not common in spleen involved by CLL/SLL.

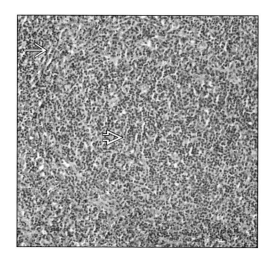
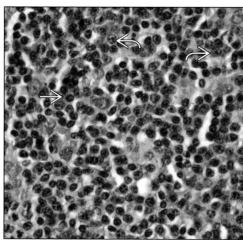

(Left) B-cell prolymphocytic leukemia of spleen shows extensive red pulp ⮂ infiltration leaving only remnants of white pulp ➔ around an arteriole. *(Right)* B-cell prolymphocytic leukemia of spleen shows red pulp infiltration. Neoplastic lymphocytes expand cords ➔ and sinuses ➔. Neoplastic lymphocytes are intermediate in size, many with distinct nucleoli ➔.

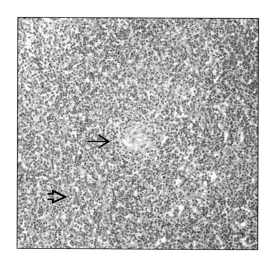
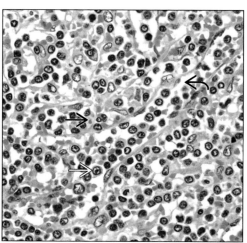

(Left) Hairy cell leukemia (HCL) involving spleen shows a diffuse infiltrate of red pulp. The HCL cells have a "fried egg" appearance with abundant pale cytoplasm and distinct cell membranes. *(Right)* HCL cells express Cyclin-D1 but only in a fraction of neoplastic cells, and the reactivity is faint.

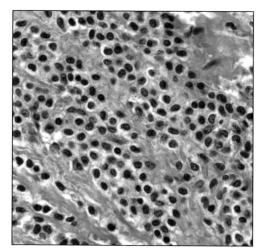
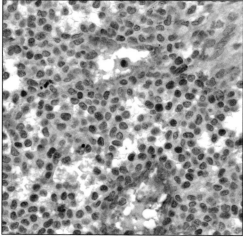

Differential Diagnosis: FL and SMZL

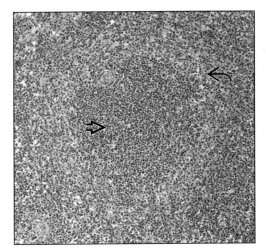
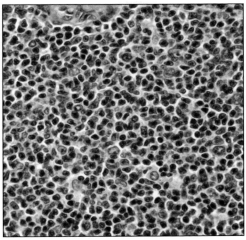

(Left) Follicular lymphoma (FL) involving the spleen shows a micronodular pattern characterized by a large neoplastic follicle ⇨ surrounded by marginal zone ➔. This appearance is that of "biphasic" pattern. (Right) Central area of germinal center in FL of spleen displays irregular centrocytes (small cleaved lymphocytes) admixed with larger centroblasts (noncleaved lymphocytes).

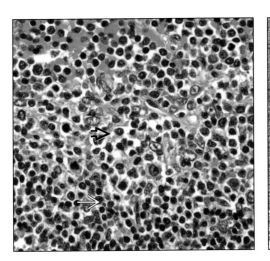
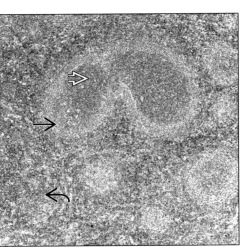

(Left) Marginal zone of follicular lymphoma involving spleen shows that lymphocytes have more abundant cytoplasm ⇨ when compared to lymphocytes in the central areas of the germinal center ➔. (Right) Splenic marginal zone lymphoma displays a "biphasic" pattern with a dark center of white pulp ⇨ surrounded by lighter marginal zone ➔. There is secondary red pulp involvement noted as nodular aggregates ➔.

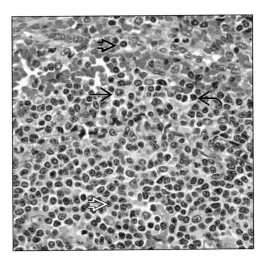
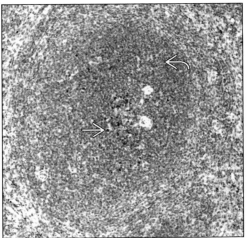

(Left) Splenic marginal zone lymphoma (SMZL) shows a mixture of small lymphocytes ➔ and intermediate to large cells with more abundant cytoplasm, some with a nucleolus ➔ compared with small uniform lymphocytes in the center of white pulp ⇨ or in the red pulp ➔. (Right) Bcl-6 immunohistochemistry of white pulp in SMZL shows scattered residual positive germinal center cells ➔, while most neoplastic cells are negative ➔.

CLASSICAL HODGKIN LYMPHOMA

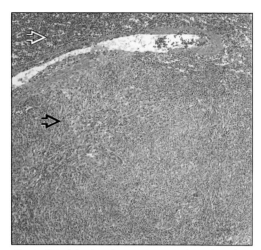

Classical Hodgkin lymphoma (CHL) involving the spleen characterized by an infiltrate ⊡ of large tumor cells in a background of inflammatory cells and fibrosis. Uninvolved spleen is also seen ⊡.

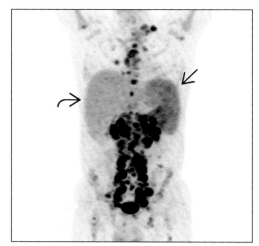

PET scan shows widespread CHL throughout the abdomen and pelvis. There is also enlargement of the spleen ⊡ and liver ⊡ due to lymphoma involvement.

TERMINOLOGY

Abbreviations
- Classical Hodgkin lymphoma (CHL)

Synonyms
- Hodgkin disease

Definitions
- Splenic involvement by CHL

CLINICAL ISSUES

Presentation
- > 80% of patients with CHL present with lymphadenopathy above diaphragm
  - Most common: Cervical, supraclavicular, and axillary lymph nodes
- 1/3 of patients present with B symptoms: Fever, night sweats, weight loss
- CHL can involve extranodal tissues
  - Common: Spleen, lungs, liver, and bone marrow
  - Primary splenic CHL is extremely rare
- Splenic involvement
  - 37% of patients have splenic involvement (mean from 17 published case series)
  - Splenic involvement is associated with bone marrow and liver involvement
- Staging laparotomy in CHL patients was performed in past
- Nowadays, staging laparotomy is no longer performed, mainly because
  - Routine use of chemotherapy is independent of stage (replacing wide-field radiotherapy)
  - Improvement of imaging studies
    - Positron emission tomography (PET) with fluorodeoxyglucose 18F (standard staging tool)

Treatment
- Drugs
  - Chemotherapy
    - Adriamycin, bleomycin, vinblastine, and dacarbazine (ABVD) is standard regimen

Prognosis
- CHL staging
  - According to Ann Arbor criteria modified at Cotswolds meeting
- Extranodal disease is adverse prognostic factor for localized CHL according German Hodgkin Lymphoma Study Group (GHLSG)

MACROSCOPIC FEATURES

Size
- Spleen may be large or normal size
- Variable patterns of splenic involvement
  - Multiple nodules, isolated or confluent (most common)
  - Solitary nodule
  - Miliary small nodules

MICROSCOPIC PATHOLOGY

Histologic Features
- All types of CHL can involve spleen
  - More frequent in mixed cellularity or lymphocyte-depleted types (up to 60%)
  - Less frequent in nodular sclerosis type
- Periarterial lymphoid sheath and marginal zones are initial sites of involvement
- Irrespective of type, fibrosis or sclerosis may surround tumoral nodules
- Determining type of CHL based on splenic morphology can be difficult and is usually unnecessary

CLASSICAL HODGKIN LYMPHOMA

Key Facts

Clinical Issues
- CHL can involve extranodal tissues
  - Most common: Spleen, lungs, liver, and bone marrow

Macroscopic Features
- Variable patterns of splenic involvement
  - Multiple nodules, isolated or confluent (most common)
  - Solitary nodule
  - Miliary small nodules

Microscopic Pathology
- All types of CHL may involve spleen
- More frequent in mixed cellularity or lymphocyte-depleted types (up to 60%)

- Periarterial lymphoid sheath and marginal zones are initial sites of involvement
- Irrespective of type, fibrosis or sclerosis can be seen
- Hodgkin/Reed Sternberg (HRS) cells &/or lacunar cells in inflammatory background

Ancillary Tests
- CD30(+), CD15(+), CD45/LCA(-) in most cases
- pax-5(+) with characteristic weaker expression than reactive B cells
- CD20(-/+), CD79a(-/+)
- Monoclonal *IgH* gene rearrangements usually detected by single cell PCR

Top Differential Diagnoses
- Splenic marginal zone lymphoma
- Diffuse large B-cell lymphoma

- Tumor cells
  - Hodgkin/Reed-Sternberg (HRS) cells and lacunar cells
- Background of mixed inflammatory cells
  - Granulocytes, histiocytes, eosinophils, neutrophils, plasma cells
- If cohesive sheets of lacunar or HRS cells: Syncytial variant of nodular sclerosis

ANCILLARY TESTS

Immunohistochemistry
- CD30(+), CD15(+), CD45/LCA(-) in most cases
- pax-5(+) with characteristic weaker expression than reactive B cells
- CD20(-/+), CD79a(-/+)
  - Weakly &/or variably (+) in ~ 20% of cases
- Small subset (~ 5-10%) of CHL express T-cell antigens
  - These cases also express pax-5

Molecular Genetics
- Monoclonal *IgH* gene rearrangements usually detected by single cell PCR
- Usually no evidence of monoclonal *IgH* or *TCR* gene rearrangements by routine PCR analysis

DIFFERENTIAL DIAGNOSIS

Splenic Marginal Zone Lymphoma
- Infiltration of white and red pulp by small cells with abundant pale cytoplasm
- Villous lymphocytes in peripheral blood smear
- pax-5(+), CD19(+), CD20(+), CD22(+), and CD3(-)
- Allelic loss of chromosome 7q11-36 (40%)

Diffuse Large B-cell Lymphoma (DLBCL)
- Most DLBCL of spleen represent systemic or secondary involvement
- Large nodule or mass
- pax-5(+), CD19(+), CD20(+), Bcl-6(+), and CD3(-)

Hairy Cell Leukemia
- Diffuse red pulp infiltrate by monomorphic small to intermediate lymphoid cells
- Atrophy of white pulp; red blood cell lakes
- "Hairy" cells in peripheral blood smear
- pax-5(+), CD19(+), CD20(+), annexin-A1(+), & CD3(-)
- CD11c(+), CD25(+), CD103(+)

T-cell/Histiocyte-rich Large B-cell Lymphoma
- Diffuse pattern of growth
- Few (< 10%) large lymphoma cells
- Numerous reactive small lymphocytes often associated with histiocytes
- Large neoplastic cells
  - CD45/LCA(+), CD20(+), CD79a(+)
  - CD30 is usually negative; CD15(-)

Hepatosplenic T-cell Lymphoma
- Red pulp infiltrate with atrophy of white pulp
  - Neoplastic cells are present within cords & sinuses (small to intermediate in size)
- CD3(+), CD4(-), CD8(-/+), CD16(+/-), CD56(+/-)
- TIA-1(+), GZM-B(-), perforin(-)

T-cell Large Granular Lymphocyte Leukemia
- Peripheral blood smear shows large granular lymphocytes (LGL)
- Spleen: Expansion of red pulp & sinusoids (tumor cells are small to intermediate in size)
- CD8(+/-), CD57(+/-), βF1(+/-) and CD56(-)
- GZM-B(+/-), perforin(+/-)

SELECTED REFERENCES

1. Paes FM et al: FDG PET/CT of extranodal involvement in non-Hodgkin lymphoma and Hodgkin disease. Radiographics. 30(1):269-91, 2010
2. Eberle FC et al: Histopathology of Hodgkin's lymphoma. Cancer J. 15(2):129-37, 2009
3. Butler JJ: Pathology of the spleen in benign and malignant conditions. Histopathology. 7(4):453-74, 1983

14

CLASSICAL HODGKIN LYMPHOMA

Microscopic and Immunophenotypic Features

(Left) Classical Hodgkin lymphoma (CHL) involving the spleen characterized by multiple neoplastic nodules ⮕, some confluent. Note the presence of uninvolved splenic parenchyma in the upper 1/2 of the field ⮕. *(Right)* CHL involving the spleen. The neoplastic nodules were composed of large Hodgkin-Reed-Sternberg (HRS) cells ⮕ in an inflammatory background with small lymphocytes and histiocytes. The inflammatory background can vary and may include a granulomatous reaction.

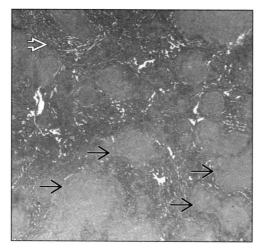
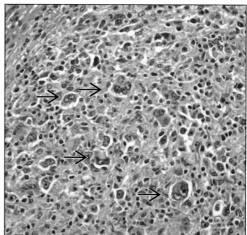

(Left) HRS cells ⮕ in CHL involving spleen. HRS cells are large with vesicular nuclei and prominent nucleoli (classically with owl-eye inclusion-like appearance). Nucleoli can have the same diameter as the background lymphocytes. *(Right)* HRS cells ⮕ are highlighted using an immunostain for CD30, which is an activation marker characteristically positive with a membranous and Golgi pattern in the HRS cells of CHL.

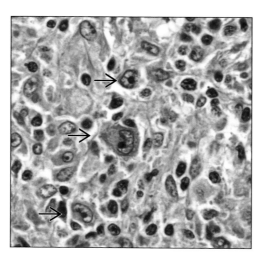
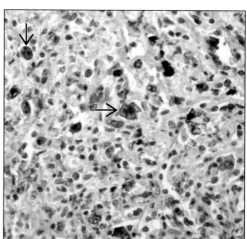

(Left) In CHL, Epstein-Barr virus (EBV) can be often detected by using immunostains for LMP1, as shown in the image, and by in situ hybridization analysis using an EBV small encoded RNA (EBER) probe. *(Right)* In CHL, the HRS cells ⮕ are characteristically negative for CD45 (LCA). In this image, the HRS cells are CD45(-) and are surrounded by many small reactive lymphocytes that are CD45(+).

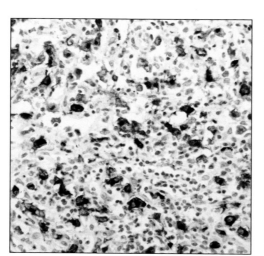
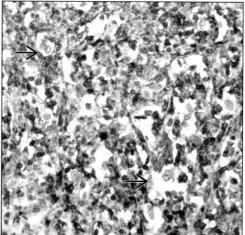

CLASSICAL HODGKIN LYMPHOMA

Differential Diagnosis

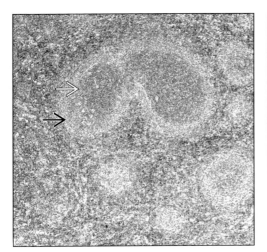
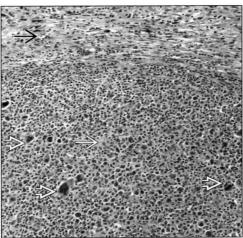

(Left) Hematoxylin and eosin shows splenic marginal zone lymphoma with nodular expansion of white pulp with a biphasic pattern: Dark center ⮞ and pale marginal zone ⮞. Both zones contain neoplastic lymphocytes. *(Right)* Diffuse large B-cell lymphoma involving spleen characterized by a well-circumscribed mass ⮞ surrounded by fibrous stroma ⮞. Note the pleomorphic tumor cells present ⮞.

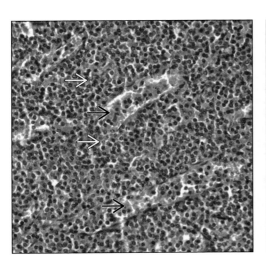
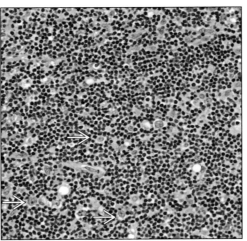

(Left) Hairy cell leukemia involving spleen shows many tumor cells diffusely infiltrating the red pulp ⮞, with occasional tumor cells also seen inside of the sinusoids ⮞. *(Right)* T-cell/histiocyte-rich large B-cell lymphoma composed of scattered large atypical cells, histiocytes, and numerous small lymphocytes. Note that the large lymphoma cells ⮞ are difficult to recognize at low magnification. CD20 or CD79a are very helpful to identify the neoplastic B-cells.

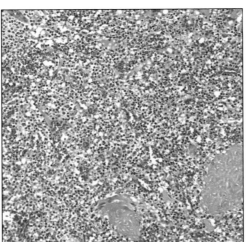

(Left) Hepatosplenic T-cell lymphoma infiltrating the red pulp of the spleen in a diffuse pattern. Residual, atrophic white pulp is noted ⮞ in this field. *(Right)* T-cell large granular lymphocyte leukemia expands the splenic red pulp cords and sinusoids by a relatively monomorphic population of small to intermediate large granular lymphocytes (LGL). The LGL morphology is easily recognized in peripheral blood smears.

HEPATOSPLENIC T-CELL LYMPHOMA

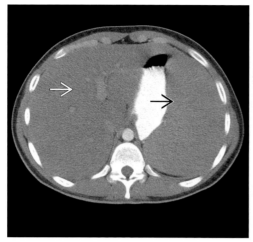

Abdominal CT of a 18-year-old patient with HSTCL shows the liver ➡ is enlarged, spanning at least 23 cm, & the spleen ➡ is also enlarged (15 x 9.5 x 23 cm). No focal lesions are detected.

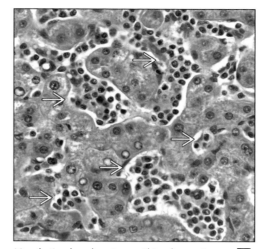

Neoplastic lymphocytes within liver sinuses ➡, characteristic of HSTCL. Immunohistochemical studies showed that cells were positive for CD2, CD3, and CD56, and negative for CD4 and CD8.

TERMINOLOGY

Abbreviations
• Hepatosplenic T-cell lymphoma (HSTCL)

Synonyms
• Erythrophagocytic T-gamma lymphoma

Definitions
• Aggressive extranodal, systemic T-cell lymphoma; usually TCR-γδ(+)
  ○ Hepatosplenomegaly and bone marrow involvement
  ○ Non-activated cytotoxic immunophenotype

ETIOLOGY/PATHOGENESIS

Associated with Chronic Immunosuppression
• Associated with 20% of cases
• Solid organ transplant recipients
• Long-term therapy for patients with inflammatory bowel disease (tumor necrosis factor α antagonists or thiopurines)

Etiology Unknown
• 80% of patients
• No association with infection by viruses, including HTLV-1, HHV8, or EBV

CLINICAL ISSUES

Epidemiology
• Incidence
  ○ < 1% of all non-Hodgkin lymphomas
• Age
  ○ Young adults; median age: 35 years
• Gender
  ○ Male predominance

Presentation
• Cytopenias are common
  ○ Thrombocytopenia is almost constant and severity correlates with progression
• Splenomegaly
• Hepatomegaly is very common
• Minimal or absent lymphadenopathy
• Systemic (B-type) symptoms
• High serum lactate dehydrogenase level
• Leukemic presentation is rare at initial diagnosis; can occur during course of disease

Treatment
• Standard anthracycline-containing chemotherapy regimens are not effective
• Platinum-cytarabine regimens and 2'-deoxycoformycin (pentostatin) have activity

Prognosis
• Poor
  ○ Median survival ~ 12 months
• No clinical features or biomarkers predict prognosis

MACROSCOPIC FEATURES

General Features
• Spleen
  ○ Diffuse enlargement
  ○ Homogeneous red-purple parenchyma; no gross lesions
• Liver
  ○ Diffuse enlargement; no gross lesions
• Lymph nodes
  ○ Usually not enlarged

HEPATOSPLENIC T-CELL LYMPHOMA

Key Facts

Terminology
- Clinically aggressive extranodal and systemic T-cell lymphoma
- Hepatosplenomegaly and bone marrow involvement

Clinical Issues
- Rare; < 1% of all non-Hodgkin lymphomas
- Young adults; median age: 35 years
- Hepatosplenomegaly
- Minimal or absent lymphadenopathy
- Poor prognosis

Microscopic Pathology
- Spleen: Red pulp infiltrate with white pulp atrophy
- Liver: Sinusoidal infiltration
- Cytologic features often change during disease course

- Early stage: Tumor cells are predominantly small to intermediate in size with irregular nuclear contours
- Late disease: Larger blastic cells

Ancillary Tests
- Typical immunophenotype
  - CD2(+), CD3(+), CD4(-), CD5(-), CD7(+/-), CD8(-), CD16(+/-), CD56(+), TCR-γδ(+)
  - TIA-1(+), GZM-M(+), GZM-B(-), perforin(-) (non-activated cytotoxic)
- Subset of cases express TCR-αβ
  - Similar clinicopathologic and cytogenetic features to TCR-γδ(+) cases
- Isochromosome 7q is consistent cytogenetic abnormality
- Trisomy 8 in subset of cases

MICROSCOPIC PATHOLOGY

Histologic Features
- Spleen
  - Red pulp infiltrate with atrophy of white pulp
    - Neoplastic cells present within cords & sinuses
  - Hemophagocytosis can be seen
  - Splenic hilar lymph nodes can show involvement (usually confined to sinuses)
- Liver
  - Sinusoidal pattern of infiltration
  - Mild portal and periportal infiltrate can be seen (usually is not prominent)
- Bone marrow
  - Subtle infiltration, difficult to recognize in H&E-stained sections
  - Pattern of infiltration and cytologic features often change during disease course
    - Early stage: Intrasinusoidal
    - Late stage: Interstitial or diffuse

Cytologic Features
- Early stage disease
  - Relatively monotonous tumor cells, predominantly small to intermediate in size with irregular nuclear contours
    - Nuclear chromatin loosely condensed with small nucleoli
    - Rare large blastic cells
- Late stage disease
  - Predominantly large blastic tumor cells

ANCILLARY TESTS

Immunohistochemistry
- CD2(+), CD3(+), CD4(-), CD5(-), CD7(+/-), CD8(-/+), CD16(+/-), CD56(+/-), and CD57(-)
- TIA-1(+), GZM-M(+), GZM-B(-), and perforin(-) (nonactivated cytotoxic)
- Most cases are TCR-γδ(+) (negative for βF1 antibody)

  - Loss of TCR-γδ expression can occur during disease progression
  - βF1 antibody reacts with epitope of framework of α/β TCR receptor
- Few cases express TCR-αβ(+) (positive for βF1 antibody)
  - Clinicopathologic and cytogenetic features similar to TCR-γδ(+) cases
- CD25(-), CD30(-), B-cell antigens(-)

Cytogenetics
- Isochromosome 7q is consistent abnormality (but not specific)
  - Detected in other lymphoma types: Nasal-type extranodal NK/T-cell lymphoma and ALK(-) anaplastic large cell lymphoma
- Trisomy 8 or loss of sex chromosome in subset of cases

Molecular Genetics
- Monoclonal gene rearrangements of *TCRγ* chain gene are frequently detected by PCR

DIFFERENTIAL DIAGNOSIS

Splenic Marginal Zone Lymphoma
- Spleen: Infiltration of white and red pulp
- Small neoplastic cells with abundant pale cytoplasm
- Villous lymphocytes in peripheral blood smear
- pax-5(+), CD19(+), CD20(+), CD22(+), and CD3(-)
- Allelic loss of chromosome 7q22-36 (40%)

Hairy Cell Leukemia (HCL)
- Older patients and indolent clinical course
- Red pulp infiltrate with atrophy of white pulp; red blood cell lakes
- "Hairy" cells in peripheral blood smear
- Interstitial pattern of bone marrow infiltration
- pax-5(+), CD19(+), CD20(+), CD25(+), CD103(+), annexin-A1(+), and CD3(-)

Intravascular Large B-cell Lymphoma
- Neurologic and dermatologic manifestations

HEPATOSPLENIC T-CELL LYMPHOMA

Differential Diagnosis with T-LGL and Aggressive NK-Cell Leukemia

Antibody	HSTCL	T-LGL	Aggressive NK-Cell Leukemia
CD3	+	+	- (surface)
CD4	-	-	-
CD5	-/+	+/-	+
CD7	+/-	+/-	-
CD8	-/+	+	-
CD16	+	+	+
CD56	+	-	+
CD57	-	+	-
βF1	-/+	+	-
TIA	+	+	+
GZM-M	+	+	+
GZM-B	-	+	+
Perforin	-	+	+
EBV	-	-	+

- Large cells filling splenic sinusoids and systemic small vessels (capillaries)
- pax-5(+), CD19(+), CD20(+), and CD3(-)

B-cell Prolymphocytic Leukemia
- Extremely high white blood cell count
- Spleen: Infiltration of white and red pulp
- Intermediate to large cells with prominent central nucleoli
- pax-5(+), CD19(+), CD20(+), CD3(-)

Peripheral T- or NK-cell Lymphomas with Intravascular Pattern
- Rare cases of T-cell lymphoma or NK-cell lymphoma can be intravascular
- Most cases not evaluated for TCR expression
- Some intravascular T-cell lymphomas reported may be HSTCL

T-cell Large Granular Lymphocytic Leukemia (T-LGL)
- Older patients
- Indolent clinical course often associated with infections
- Peripheral blood: Increased large granular lymphocytes (LGL)
- Spleen: Expansion of red pulp cords and sinusoids
- Bone marrow, usually interstitial pattern, but sinusoidal pattern can also seen
- Usually positive for CD8 (60%), GZM-B, perforin, βF1, CD5 (dim), CD16, and CD57, and negative for CD56
- Distinction between HSTCL and T-LGL can be difficult in some cases
  - Rare cases of T-LGL express TCR-γδ and lack cytoplasmic granules

Aggressive NK-cell Leukemia/Lymphoma
- Tumor cells have cytoplasmic azurophilic granules
- NK-cell markers(+), GZM-B(+), perforin(+), surface CD3(-), and EBV(+/-)

- No TCR gene rearrangements

T-cell Prolymphocytic Leukemia
- Extremely high white blood cell count
- Hepatosplenomegaly; generalized lymphadenopathy in subset
- Spleen: Red pulp infiltrate with atrophy of white pulp
- T-cell markers (+), CD52(bright, [+]), TCL1(+/-)
- Inv14q or t(14;14)(q11;q32)

T-Lymphoblastic Leukemia/Lymphoma
- Shares some clinicopathologic features of HSTCL
- Older children and adolescents
- Blasts are T-cells and TdT(+), CD1a(+), and CD99(+)

Myelodysplastic Syndrome (MDS)
- Cytopenias and blastic cells can resemble late stage HSTCL
- Blasts in MDS are usually myeloperoxidase(+), nonspecific esterase (+), myeloid antigens (+)

SELECTED REFERENCES

1. Falchook GS et al: Hepatosplenic gamma-delta T-cell lymphoma: clinicopathological features and treatment. Ann Oncol. 20(6):1080-5, 2009
2. Vega F et al: Hepatosplenic and other gammadelta T-cell lymphomas. Am J Clin Pathol. 127(6):869-80, 2007
3. Macon WR et al: Hepatosplenic alphabeta T-cell lymphomas: a report of 14 cases and comparison with hepatosplenic gammadelta T-cell lymphomas. Am J Surg Pathol. 25(3):285-96, 2001
4. Vega F et al: Hepatosplenic gamma/delta T-cell lymphoma in bone marrow. A sinusoidal neoplasm with blastic cytologic features. Am J Clin Pathol. 116(3):410-9, 2001
5. Alonsozana EL et al: Isochromosome 7q: the primary cytogenetic abnormality in hepatosplenic gammadelta T cell lymphoma. Leukemia. 11(8):1367-72, 1997
6. Kadin ME et al: Erythrophagocytic T gamma lymphoma: a clinicopathologic entity resembling malignant histiocytosis. N Engl J Med. 304(11):648-53, 1981

HEPATOSPLENIC T-CELL LYMPHOMA

Microscopic Features: Spleen and Liver

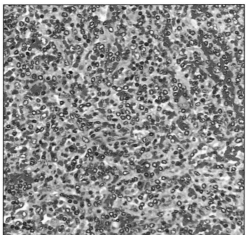

(Left) Hepatosplenic T-cell lymphoma (HSTCL). The neoplasm infiltrates the red pulp of the spleen in a diffuse pattern. Residual, atrophic white pulp is noted ➡️ in this field. *(Right)* HSTCL. The red pulp is infiltrated by cytologically atypical large lymphoid cells, some with a blastic appearance.

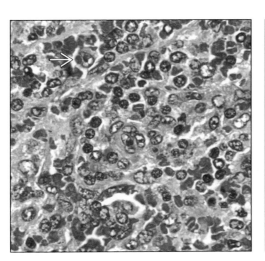

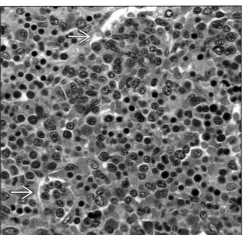

(Left) HSTCL involving the spleen. The tumor cells are large and exhibit a blastic appearance (vesicular nuclear chromatin). Hemophagocytosis is noted ➡️. These cytologic features are seen in late stage disease. *(Right)* HSTCL. The spleen revealed marked infiltration of the red pulp by atypical large lymphocytes, some with a blastic appearance. Some tumor cells are identified within the sinuses ➡️. This case of HSTCL expressed TCR-αβ.

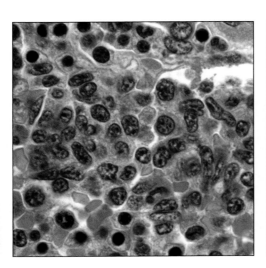

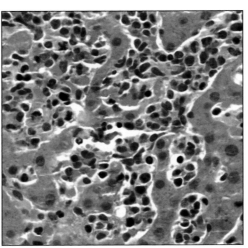

(Left) HSTCL. The tumor cells are variable in size, intermediate to large, with vesicular nuclear chromatin, irregular nuclear contours, and prominent nucleoli. This HSTCL has a TCR-αβ phenotype. *(Right)* Characteristic intrasinusoidal pattern of infiltration of liver by HSTCL. Note the distended sinusoids and the thinning of the plates of hepatocytes (usually 2 cells thick). The tumor cells are small to intermediate in size with condensed chromatin.

Immunophenotypic Features

(Left) HSTCL involving the spleen. The tumor cells are positive for CD3 and diffusely infiltrate the red pulp. Residual white pulp (B cells; CD3[-]) is seen in the lower right corner ➡. Note that CD3 expression is dim in the tumor cells in comparison with clusters of reactive T cells ➡. *(Right)* HSTCL involving the spleen. The tumor cells are negative for CD4. In this case, the tumor cells were also negative for CD8. Rarely HSTCL cases can be CD4(-) and CD8(+).

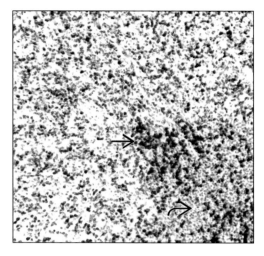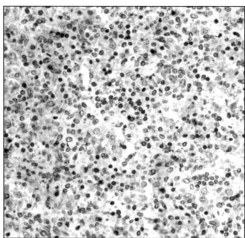

(Left) HSTCL involving the spleen. The tumor cells are negative for CD8 (some cases can be CD8[+]). In this field, CD8 highlights scattered reactive T cells within the sinuses and cords of the red pulp. Note that endothelial cells lining the sinuses are CD8 positive. *(Right)* The tumor cells are highlighted using an immunostain for T-cell intracellular antigen 1 (TIA-1), which is a cytotoxic enzyme characteristically positive in the cells of HSTCL.

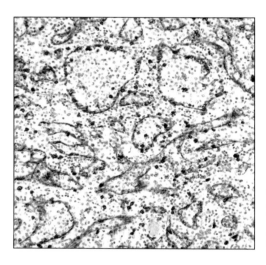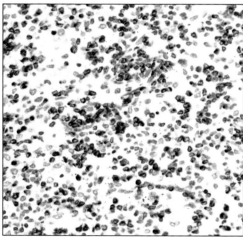

(Left) The tumor cells in HSTCL are characteristically positive for CD56 and negative for CD57. By contrast, T-LGL are usually negative for CD56 and positive for CD57. *(Right)* Most cases of HSTCL have a TCR-γδ immunophenotype and therefore are negative for the βF1 antibody. Currently, there are no known clinicopathologic differences between cases of HSTCL positive for either TCR-γδ or -αβ. The TCR-αβ HSTCL is considered a variant of HSTCL.

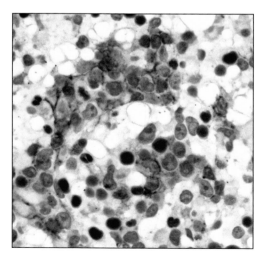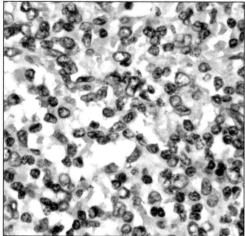

HEPATOSPLENIC T-CELL LYMPHOMA

Microscopic Features: Bone Marrow

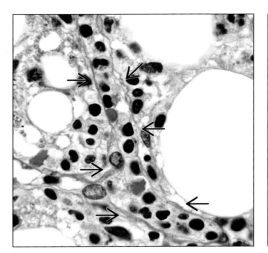

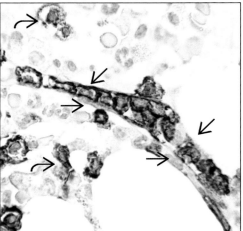

(Left) HSTCL involving bone marrow. The neoplastic cells are small and located predominantly in the sinusoids ➡. However, the intrasinusoidal infiltrate can be difficult to recognize in the H&E-stained slides, and it is useful to highlight the cells using immunostains specific for CD3. *(Right)* HSTCL involving bone marrow. The intrasinusoidal neoplastic cells ➡ are highlighted by the anti-CD3 antibody. Note the presence of scattered small, reactive T cells ➡.

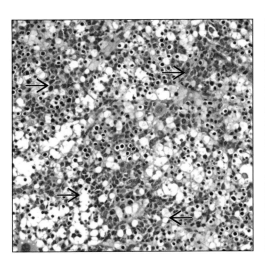

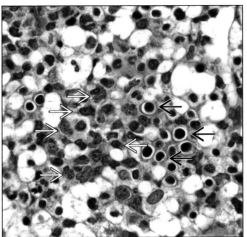

(Left) Hypercellular bone marrow in a patient with HSTCL. Note the presence of interstitial clusters of atypical lymphoid cells ➡. An intrasinusoidal pattern is not evident in this case. *(Right)* This case of HSTCL has an interstitial pattern of involvement. The tumor cells are variable in size, small to intermediate, with markedly irregular nuclear contours ➡. Note the round cell morphology of the erythroid precursors ➡.

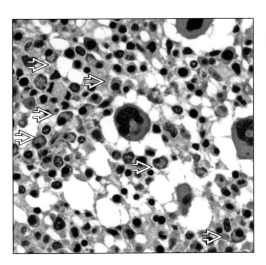

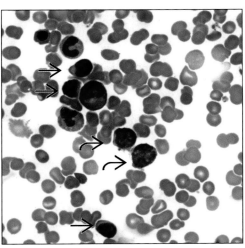

(Left) The uninvolved hematopoietic bone marrow in HSTCL is frequently hypercellular with trilineage hyperplasia. Moderate plasmacytosis ➡ and mild dysplasia can be seen. If the tumor cells are misinterpreted as blasts, the overall picture may be confused with a myelodysplastic syndrome. *(Right)* HSTCL. The neoplastic cells are intermediately sized with condensed nuclear chromatin ➡. Small reactive lymphocytes are seen ➡. Note the thrombocytopenia.

HEPATOSPLENIC T-CELL LYMPHOMA

Peripheral Blood, Bone Marrow, and Ancillary Features

(Left) In HSTCL, an overt leukemic picture is rare at initial examination and lymphocytosis is uncommon. However, a minor population of atypical lymphocytes can be identified in the peripheral blood smears. Note the presence of erythrophagocytosis ⊡. Historically, this lymphoma was initially termed as erythrophagocytic T-γ lymphoma. *(Right)* HSTCL lymphoma involving bone marrow. The bone marrow is hypercellular with numerous interstitial lymphocytes.

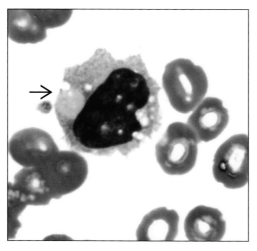
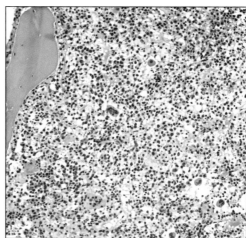

(Left) HSTCL. The tumor cells are large with a moderate amount of agranular basophilic cytoplasm, vesicular nuclear chromatin, and prominent nucleoli ⊡. A small lymphocyte ⊡ and a metamyelocyte ⊡ are also seen. *(Right)* HSTCL involving bone marrow. The tumor cells are positive for CD3 and are forming clusters inside the sinusoids ⊡. Note that CD3 expression is dim in the tumor cells in comparison with scattered reactive T cells ⊡.

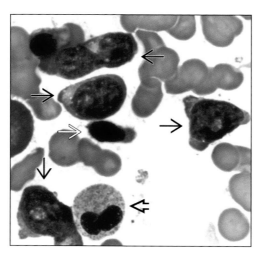
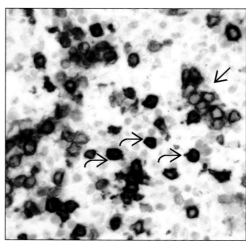

(Left) Monoclonal TCRγ gene rearrangements are frequently detected in HSTCL. The red peaks ⊡ represent a biallelic clonal rearrangement using V γ I genes. The other smaller peaks in red, blue, black, and green represent the polyclonal background of T cells. *(Right)* Positive FISH for presence of isochromosome 7q. This image shows an interphase cell with 3 red signals (3 7q31 regions) and 2 green signals indicating the presence of 2 centromeres for chromosome 7.

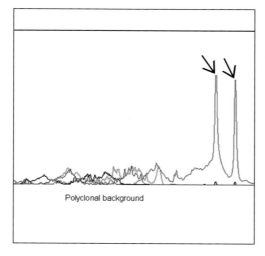

Polyclonal background

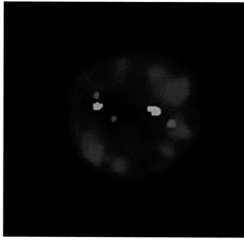

HEPATOSPLENIC T-CELL LYMPHOMA

Differential Diagnosis

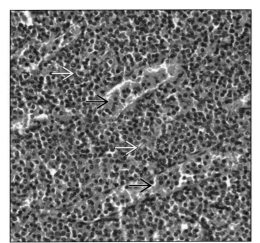 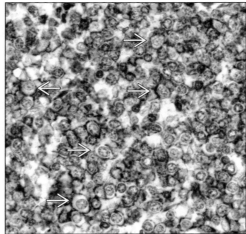

(Left) Hairy cell leukemia involving spleen. The tumor cells diffusely infiltrate the red pulp ➡, with occasional tumor cells also seen inside the sinusoids ➡. *(Right)* Tumor cells in hairy cell leukemia are positive for CD20. The membranous CD20 staining accentuates the presence of abundant cytoplasm ➡, a feature of "hairy" cells.

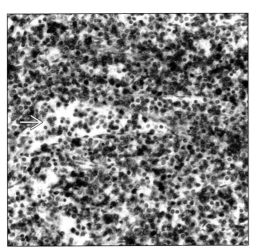 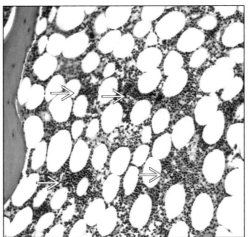

(Left) The diagnosis of hairy cell leukemia involving the spleen can be confirmed by annexin-A1 (ANXA1) stain, as the tumor cells are positive for ANXA1. Note the presence of occasional tumor cells within sinusoids ➡. *(Right)* Hairy cell leukemia involving bone marrow. The infiltrate is usually subtle, patchy, & interstitial ➡, but sometimes can be difficult to recognize in H&E-stained sections as the neoplastic lymphocytes can be confused with erythroid cells.

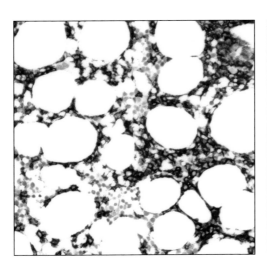 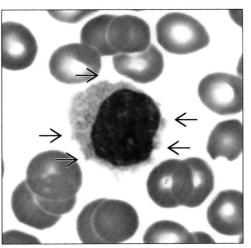

(Left) Interstitial bone marrow infiltrate characteristic of hairy cell leukemia. CD20, or other B-cell markers, are essential for the identification of "hairy" cells in bone marrow. *(Right)* Hairy cells are lymphoid cells, intermediate in size, with oval or indented (bean-shaped) nuclei and abundant and pale blue cytoplasm with circumferential "hairy" projections ➡.

Differential Diagnosis

(Left) Spleen involved by splenic marginal zone lymphoma (SMZL). Note the infiltration of the white pulp ➡ that, in this case, exhibits a biphasic appearance, with a central dark zone surrounded by paler marginal zones. Both zones contain neoplastic lymphocytes. **(Right)** Spleen involved by SMZL. In addition to the infiltration of the white pulp ➡, there is also infiltration of the red pulp, with small nodules of neoplastic cells ➡ and tumor cells in the cords.

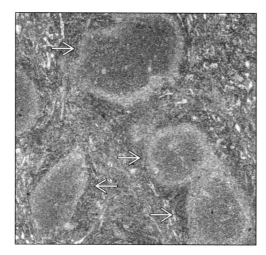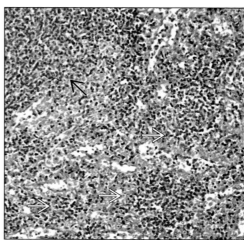

(Left) Some B-cell lymphomas involving bone marrow may have an intrasinusoidal pattern. This bone marrow specimen is involved by SMZL. The tumor cells are located within a sinusoid. The sinusoid is delineated by black arrows ➡. **(Right)** SMZL involving bone marrow. pax-5 confirms the B-cell lineage of the intrasinusoidal infiltrate ➡. The tumor cells were positive for CD20 and negative for CD5 and CD43.

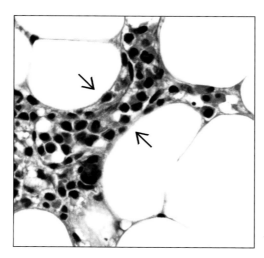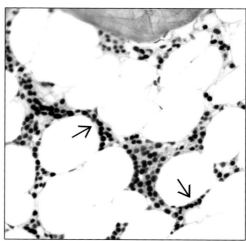

(Left) Brain biopsy shows T-cell lymphoma with clusters of large atypical lymphoid cells inside a small capillary. The neoplastic cells were negative for B-cell markers and were positive for CD3, CD8, CD56, TIA-1, and GZM-B. βF1 was negative. **(Right)** T-cell lymphoma diagnosed in a brain biopsy specimen. The neoplastic cells were positive for CD3 (shown), CD8, TIA-1, GZM-B, and CD56, and negative for βF1 and B-cell markers.

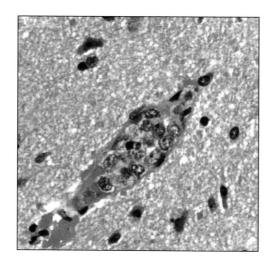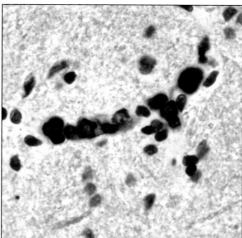

HEPATOSPLENIC T-CELL LYMPHOMA

Differential Diagnosis

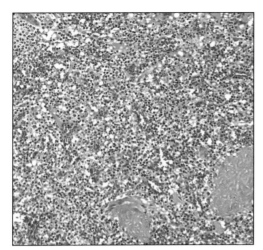 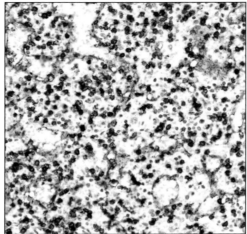

(Left) Splenic involvement by T-cell large granular lymphocyte leukemia (T-LGL) is characterized by expansion of the red pulp cords and sinusoids with sparing of white pulp. *(Right)* CD8(+) neoplastic T-LGL cells involving splenic red pulp cords. In addition, the neoplastic cells were also positive for CD3, TIA-1, and GZM-B. Note that the endothelial cells lining the splenic sinusoids are also CD8 positive.

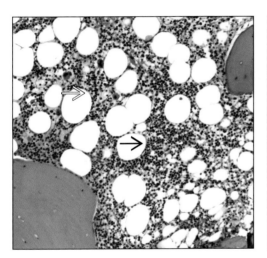 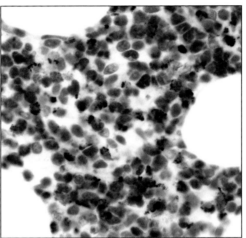

(Left) T-LGL involving bone marrow. Note the predominant interstitial ➡ and focally intrasinusoidal lymphocytic infiltrate ➡. *(Right)* T-LGL positive for the cytotoxic protein TIA-1. This stain highlights the interstitial lymphoid infiltrate. In addition, the tumor cells were positive for βF1, CD8, CD57, and GZM-B, and negative for CD56.

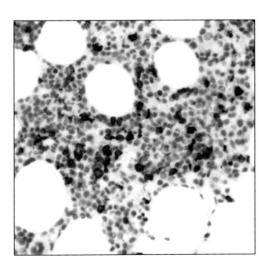 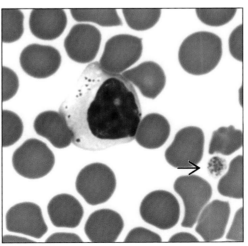

(Left) T-LGL positive for CD57. In addition, the tumor cells were also positive for TIA-1, βF1, CD8, CD57, and GZM-B, and negative for CD4 and CD56. This immunophenotype excludes the diagnosis of HSTCL. *(Right)* In T-LGL, the predominant lymphocytes in peripheral blood are LGL. They have moderate to abundant cytoplasm with fine to coarse azurophilic granules. The granules contain perforin and GZM-B (cytolytic enzymes). An unremarkable platelet is also seen ➡.

Antibody Index

ANTIBODY INDEX

Antibodies Discussed

Antibody Symbol/Name	Antibody Description	Clones/Alternative Names
β-2-microglobulin	component of MHC class I molecules	B2-MICROGLB
κ light chain	kappa light chain	KAPPA
λ light chain	lambda light chain	LAMBDA
Actin-HHF-35	actin, muscle (HHF35)	MSA, HHF-35
Actin-sm	actin, smooth muscle	SMA, ASM-1, CGA7, IA4, HUC-1
AE1/AE3	AE1/AE3; mixture of 2 anticytokeratin clones that detect a variety of both high and low molecular weight cytokeratins	
ALK1	anaplastic lymphoma kinase-1	5A4, ALK, ALKC
Androgen receptor	dihydrotestosterone receptor, nuclear subfamily 3, group C, member 4	AR441, F39.4.1, AR-N20, AR27
Annexin-A1	mediator of anti-inflammatory response and upregulated in hairy cell leukemia	ANXA1, LPC1, lipocortin
BAD	bcl-2-associated agonist of cell death	
Bartonella henselae	*B. henselae*	B-henselae, cat scratch fever agent
BAX	bcl-2-associated X protein	PU-347-P, B-9, BAX-P, P19, BAX-M
Bcl-2	B-cell CLL lymphoma 2; suppresses apoptosis in a variety of cell systems	ONCL2, BCL2/100/D5, 124, 124.3
Bcl-6	B-Cell CLL lymphoma 6	LN22, GI191E/A8, N-3, PG-B6P, P1F6, 3FR-1
BDCA-2	Monoclonal antibody directed toward immature plasmacytoid dendritic cells	CD303
BF1	T-cell antigen receptor	TCR
BOB1	B-cell OCT-binding protein 1	SC955, BOB.1
Caldesmon	actin interacting and calmodulin binding protein found in smooth muscle and other cell types	CAD, CALD1, caldesmon 1 isoform [1-5], CDM, HCAD, LCAD, MGC21352, NAG22
CD1a	T-cell surface glycoprotein	JPM30, CD1A, O10, NA1/34
CD2	T-cell surface antigen, LFA2	271, MT910, AB75, LFA-2
CD2AP	CD2 associated protein	
CD3	T-cell receptor	F7238, A0452, CD3-P, CD3-M, SP7, PS1
CD3-ε	T cell surface antigen T3/Leu-4 epsilon chain	CD3E, CD03e
CD4	T-cell surface glycoprotein L3T4	IF6, 1290, 4B12
CD5	T-cell surface glycoprotein Leu 1, T1	NCL-CD5, 4C7, 54/B4, 54/F6
CD7	T-cell antigen precursor Leu 9	272, CD7-272
CD8	T-cell coreceptor antigen, Leu 2, T-cytotoxic cells	M7103, C8/144, C8/144B
CD10	neutral endopeptidase	CALLA, neprilysin, NEP
CD11c	integrin alpha X chain protein	LEU-M5
CD12		CDw12
CD13	plays role in growth of DC/macrophage progenitors and precursors	
CD15	reacts with Reed-Sternberg cells of Hodgkin disease and with granulocytes	VIM-2,3C4, LEU-M1, TU9, VIM-D5, MY1, CBD1, MMA, 3CD1, C3D1, Lewis x, SSEA-1
CD16	Fc receptor of IgG	
CD19	B-cell antigen	
CD20	membrane spanning 4 domains of B-lymphocytes	FB1, B1, L26, MS4A1
CD21	CR2, complement component receptor 2, Epstein-Barr virus receptor	IF8
CD22	B-cell receptor	FPC1, LEU 14
CD23	Fc ε RII, low-affinity IgE receptor, IGEBF	1B12, MHM6BU38
CD25	If-2 receptor alpha	2A3, 4C9
CD26	ADA adenosine deaminase complexing protein 2, DPP4	44-4
CD27	TNF receptor	
CD29	fibronectin receptor, integrin beta 1 ITGB1	29C03, 7F10, HT29_12938
CD30	tumor necrosis factor SF8	BER-H2, KI-1, TNFRSF8
CD31	platelet endothelial cell adhesion molecule	JC/70, JC/70A, PECAM-1
CD33	SIGLEC lectin 3	PWS44

CD34	hematopoietic progenitor cell antigen	MY10, IOM34, QBEND10, 8G12, 1309, HPCA-1, NU-4A1, TUK4, clone 581, BI-3c5
CD35	erythrocyte complement receptor 1, immune adherence receptor, C3b/C4b receptor	CR1, BER-MAC-DRC, TO5C, E11
CD38	acute lymphoblastic T-cell antigen, T10	SPC32, VS38, T10
CD43	Major sialoglycoprotein on surface of human T lymphocytes, monocytes, granulocytes, and some B lymphocytes	LEU-22, DF-T1, L60, MT1, sialophorin, leukosialin, SPN
CD44	cell adhesion receptor for hyaluronic acid HCAM	9B5, HCAM, CD44H, B-F24, A3D8, 2C5, CD44S, F10-44.2, 156-3C11, DF1485, BBA10, VFF-14, CD44V10, CD44V3, 3G5, CD44V3-10-P, CD44V3-10, 3D2, CD44V4_5, CD44V5, VFF-8, VFF-7, 2F10, VFF-18, CD44V6, CD44V7, VFF-9, CD44V7_8, VFF-17
CD45	leukocyte common antigen	LCA, PD7/26, 1.22/4.14, T29/33, RP2/18, PD7, 2D1, 2B11+PD7/26
CD45RA	isoform of CD45 expressed by naive T cells	4Kb5, MT2, MB1
CD45RO	isoform of CD45 located on memory T cells	ICH1-L, low molecular weight isoform LCA
CD54	ICAM-1 (intracellular adhesion molecule 1)	23G12, CD54-P, ICAM
CD56	NCAM (neutral cellular adhesion molecule)	MAB735, ERIC-1, 25-KD11, 123C3, 24-MB2, BC56C04, 1B6, 14-MAB735, NCC-LU-243, MOC-1, NCAM
CD57	B-1,3-glucuronyltransferase 1 (glucuronosyltransferase P)	LEU-7, NK1, HNK-1, TB01, B3GAT1
CD68	cytoplasmic granule protein of monocytes, macrophages	PG-M1, KP-1, LN5
CD72	B-cell differentiation antigen	DBA.44
CD79-α	immunoglobulin-associated alpha, MB1	MB-1, 11D10, 11E3, CD79A, HM47/A9, HM57, JCB117
CD103		
CD117	C-kit; tyrosine protein kinase activity	C-19 (C-KIT), 104D2, 2E4, C-KIT, A4502, H300, CMA-767
CD123	receptor for IL-3 (IL-3R)	
CD138	syndecan; a useful marker for plasma cells	B-B4, AM411-10M, MI15
CD163	macrophage hemoglobin scavenging system	10D6
CD303	monoclonal antibody directed toward immature plasmacytoid dendritic cells	BDCA-2
CEA-M	carcinoembryonic antigen, monoclonal	CEA-B18, CEA-D14, CEA-GOLD 1, T84.6, CEA-GOLD 2, CEA 11, CEA-GOLD 3, CEA 27, CEA-GOLD 4, CEA 41, CEA-GOLD 5, T84.1, CEA-M, A5B7, CEJ065, IL-7, T84.66, TF3H8-1, 0062, D14, alpha-7, PARLAM 1, ZC23, CEM010, A115, COL-1, AF4, 12.140.10, 11-7, M773, CEA-M431_31, CEJO65, mCEA
Centerin	Serine proteinase inhibitor A11 antibody. May play an important role in GC-B cell physiology; expression in lymphomas can be important in differential diagnosis	GCET1, seprin A9, Serpina 11b, Serpina9
CK-PAN	cytokeratin-pan (AE1/AE3/LP34); cocktail of high and low molecular weight cytokeratins	keratin pan, MAK-6, K576, LU-5, KL-1, KC-8, MNF 116, pankeratin, pancytokeratin
CK20	Cytokeratin 20, low molecular weight cytokeratin with expression most commonly restricted to GI tract	KS20.8
CLA	cutaneous lymphocyte antigen	CLA-HECA452
Clusterin	clusterin, alpha chain specific	41D, E5
CMV	cytomegalovirus	
CRP	c-reactive protein	
CTLA-4	cytotoxic T-lymphocyte antigen 4	BN13
CXCL13	chemokine CXC ligand 13	53610, B lymphocyte chemoattractant (BLC)
CXCR3	chemokine CXC receptor R3	1C6

ANTIBODY INDEX

Cyclin-D1	Protein with important cell cycle regulatory functions; proto-oncogene; regulator of cell cycle progression (G1 to S-phase)	A-12, PRAD1, AM29, DCS-6, SP4, 5D4, D1GM, P2D11F11
Cyclin E	key regulator of G/S transition in cell cycle; overexpression observed in several malignancies associated with high proliferation	13A3, HE12
D11	homeobox D11	HOXD11
DBA.44	CD72, B-cell differentiation antigen	CD72
Desmin	class III intermediate filaments found in muscle cells	M760, DE-R-11, D33, DE5, DE-U-10, ZC18
E2A	immunoglobulin enhancer-binder factor E12/E47	
EBER	Epstein-Barr virus encoded RNA	
EBNA2	Epstein-Barr virus-associated nuclear antigen 2	
EBV-LMP	Epstein-Barr virus latent membrane protein	LMP1, CS 1-4
EBV-LMP1	viral protein produced during latent cycle of EBV infection	
EGFR	v-erb b1 erythroblastic leukemia viral gene, epidermal growth factor receptor	2-18C9, EGFR1, EGFR PHRMDX, NCL-R1, H11, C-ERBB-1, E30, EGFR.113, 31G73C6, 2-18C9
EMA	epithelial membrane antigen	GP1.4, 214D4, MC5, E29, MUC1, EMA/MUC1
Factor XIIIa	factor-XIIIA (fibrin stabilizing factor)	FXIIIA
FAS	CD 95 (Fas receptor (FasR)	CD95, fatty acid synthase, APO-1, UB2, B10
Fascin	singed-like protein	55K2, FAN1, Fascin 1, FSCN1, p55, SNL, singed like protein antibody
FOXP1	forkhead box transcription factor P3	JC12
GZM-B	Granzyme B; neutral serine protease	11F1, GR-B7, Granzyme B
H-caldesmon	high molecular weight caldesmon	HCAD, H-CD
Helicobacter pylori	*H. pylori*	H-pylori
HGAL	human germinal center-associated lymphoma	
HHV8	human herpesvirus-8 latent nuclear antigen-1	13B10, LNA-1, Kaposi sarcoma associated herpes virus, KSHV
HLA-DR	human leukocyte antigen DR	DK22, LN3, TAL.1B5, LK8D3
HMB-45	antigen present in melanocytic tumors such as melanomas	LB39 AA, CMM1, CMM, DNS, FAMMM, Mart1, Melan-A, MLM, tyrosinase
HPV	human papillomavirus	
HSV1/2	herpes simplex virus 1/2	HSV1/HSV2
ID2	DNA binding protein inhibitor	
IgA	immunoglobulin A	IGA
IgD	immunoglobulin D	IGD
IgM	immunoglobulin M	IGM
IL-13	interleukin 13	
IRF-4	interferon regulatory factor 4	MUM1P, clone MUM1, MUM1-IRF.4, MUM1, M17
J chain	immunoglobulin joining segment	NFGD11
Ki-67	Ki-67 (MIB-1); marker of cell proliferation	MMI, KI88, IVAK-2, MIB1
L1	neural adhesion molecule	UJ127, CD171
LANA1	latency associated nuclear antigen of HHV8	Human herpes 8 latent nuclear antigen, LN53
Langerin	CD207 molecule	CD207
LCA	leukocyte common antigen	PD7/26, 1.22/4.14, T29/33, CD45RB, RP2/18, CD45, PD7, 2D1, 2B11+PD7/26
LMP1	Epstein Barr virus- latent membrane protein	EBV-LMP, CS 1-4
Lysozyme	1,4-beta N-acetylmuramidase C	Lyz, Lzm, Ec3.2.1.17
M1	gastric superficial/foveolar cells	
M2	Cyclin dependent kinase 2	CDK2
Melan-A	melanoma antigen recognized by T cells 1 (MART-1); protein found on melanocytes; melanocyte differentiation antigen	M2-7C10, CK-MM
Melan-A103	clone of Melan-A	A103

ANTIBODY INDEX

met	met protooncogene	8F11, C-28, C-MET
MK	neurite growth promoting factor 2	Midkine, G2a,
MPO	myeloperoxidase	
MT	metallothionein	Clone E9
Mucosal homing receptor	role in lymphocyte homing to mucosal lymphoid tissues	Integrin-α4β7
MUM1	Interferon regulatory factor 4	IRF-4, MUM1P, clone MUM1, MUM1-IRF.4, M17
MxA	Protein induced by alpha interferon protein	
Myosin	motor protein responsible for actin-based motility	
N3	calponin	calponin, calp
NOTCH1	translocation-associated notch protein	
p16	cyclin-dependent kinase 4 inhibitor 2A	P16_INK4A, E6H4, sc1661, JC8, JZ11, P16, G175-405, F-12, DCS-50, 6H12, 16P07, 16P04
p21	cyclin-dependent kinase inhibitor 1A	WAF1, DCS-60.2, EA10, 6B6, 4D10, SX118, P21, P21_WAF1, WAFT
p53	p53 tumor suppressor gene protein	DO7, 21N, BP53-12-1, AB6, CM1, PAB1801, DO1, BP53-11, PAB240, RSP53, MU195, P53
p63	tumor protein p63	H-137, 7JUL
pax-5	paired box gene 2	Z-RX2, PAX-2
PD-1	programmed cell death protein 1	EH12, NAT105, Programmed death 1
Perforin		P1-8, PE-41-PU, 5B10
PR	progesterone receptor	10A9, PGR-1A6, KD68, PGR-ICA, PRP-P, PRP, PRI, 1A6, 1AR, HPRA3, PGR-636, 636, PR88, NCL-PGR
PU.1	transcription factor PU.1	G148-74
S100	Low molecular weight protein normally present in cells derived from neural crest (Schwann cells, melanocytes, and glial cells), chondrocytes, adipocytes, myoepithelial cells, macrophages, Langerhans cells, dendritic cells, and keratinocytes	S-100, A6, 15E2E2, Z311, 4C4.9, S100 protein
TCL1	trophoblast membrane protein 1	NDOG1
TCR	T-cell receptor antigen	T_Cell_AG_R, Beta-F1, 8A3, BF1
TCR-αβ	T-cell receptor heterodimer composed of an alpha and a beta chain	
TCR-β	Antibody directed toward the beta chain of the TCR-αβ heterodimer	
TCR-γ	T-cell receptor gamma chain	TCR-gamma
TCR-γδ	T cell receptor heterodimer composed of a gamma and a delta chain	
TdT	terminal deoxynucleotidyl transferase	SEN28
TF	Thomasen-Friedenreich blood group antigen	HB-T1
Thyroglobulin	dimeric protein specific to thyroid gland	DAK-TG6
TIA	T-cell intracellular antigen 1	NS/1-AG4, 2G9, TIA-1
TNF-α	Antibody directed toward the alpha chain of the TCR-αβ heterodimer	
TRAF1	tumor necrosis factor receptor 1	
TRAP	tartrate-resistant acid phosphatase	26E5, 9C5
Tryptase	serine proteinase contained in mast cells	AA1
Tyrosinase	catalyzes production of melanin	NCL-TYROS, T311
VEGF	vascular endothelial growth factor	JH121, 26503.11, VPF, VPF/VEGF, VEGF-A, VEGF-C, RP 077, VEGFR-1, RP 076, VEGFR-2, 9D9, VEGFR-3, FLT-4
Vimentin	major subunit protein of intermediate filaments of mesenchymal cells	43BE8, 3B4, V10, V9, VIM-B34, VIM
VS38	type II transmembrane glycoprotein expressed on many types of immune cells (i.e., activated T-cells, precursor and activated B-cells, plasma cells, monocytes, peripheral NK -cells, and early bone marrow precursor cells)	CD38, SPC32, VS38, T10
WT1	Wilms tumor gene 1	6F-H2, C-19
ZAP70	SYK-ZAP-70 protein	2F3.2, ZAP-70, ZAP-70-LR

INDEX

INDEX

INDEX

INDEX

INDEX

INDEX

INDEX

INDEX

INDEX

Index

INDEX

INDEX

INDEX

INDEX

W

Waldenstrom macroglobulinemia. *See* Lymphoplasmacytic lymphoma and Waldenstrom macroglobulinemia.

Wegener granulomatosis
    extranodal nasal type NK-/T-cell lymphoma vs., 10:12
    lymphomatoid granulomatosis vs., 7:88, 93

Whipple disease, 2:50–53
    chronic granulomatous lymphadenitis vs., 2:4
    clinical issues, 2:50–51
    differential diagnosis, 2:52
    lipid-associated lymphadenopathy vs., 3:107, 109
    lymphadenopathy associated with joint prostheses vs., 3:102, 105
    microscopic features, 2:53
    microscopic pathology, 2:51–52

Wiscott-Aldrich syndrome, autoimmune lymphoproliferative syndrome vs., 11:11–12

X

Xanthomatous pseudotumor. *See* Post-chemotherapy histiocyte rich pseudotumor.

X-linked lymphoproliferative syndrome, autoimmune lymphoproliferative syndrome vs., 11:11

Y

Yersinia infections, chronic granulomatous lymphadenitis vs., 2:5